EXPEDITION AND WILDERNESS MEDICINE

With an increase in visits to remote and dangerous locations around the world, the number of serious and fatal injuries and illnesses associated with these expeditions has markedly increased. Medical personnel working in or near such locations are not always explicitly trained in the management of unique environmental injuries, such as high-altitude illness, the bends, lightning strikes, frostbite, acute dehydration, venomous stings and bites, and tropical diseases. Many health care professionals seek training in the specialties of expedition or wilderness medicine to cope with the health risks faced when far removed from professional care resources, and the American College of Emergency Physicians has recently mandated that a minimum level of proficiency needs to be exhibited by all emergency medicine physicians in these disciplines. This book covers everything a prospective field physician or medical consultant needs to prepare for when beginning an expedition and explains how to treat a variety of conditions in a concise, clinically oriented format.

Dr. Gregory H. Bledsoe is a board certified Emergency Medicine physician and the founder and CEO of ExpedMed, LLC. After completing medical school and residency at the University of Arkansas for Medical Sciences, Dr. Bledsoe spent five years on faculty within the Johns Hopkins Department of Emergency Medicine, completing a fellowship in international emergency medicine and a master's degree in public health. He has worked as a field physician and medical consultant all over the world, served as an instructor and medical consultant for the U.S. Secret Service, and provided medical support during the African tours of both presidents Bill Clinton and George W. Bush. Each year Dr. Bledsoe directs the Expedition Medicine National Conference in Washington, DC.

Dr. Michael J. Manyak is vice president for medical affairs for Cytogen Corporation and a professor of Urology, Engineering Microbiology, and Tropical Medicine at The George Washington University. Dr. Manyak is a medical adviser to several field exploration organizations, was selected as a Fellow National of The Explorers Club in 1992, and received The Explorers Club's Sweeney Medal in 2004. His column on expedition medicine currently appears in *The Explorers Journal*.

Dr. David A. Townes is an associate professor at the University of Washington School of Medicine and Medical Director of AdventureMed in Seattle. He received his medical degree from the University of Massachusetts and completed his residency in emergency medicine and a fellowship in international emergency medicine and earned a master's degree in public health from the University of Illinois at Chicago. He earned a diploma in tropical medicine and hygiene from the London School of Hygiene and Tropical Medicine. Dr. Townes has worked as an on-site physician and medical consultant in remote and dangerous locations around the world, from Costa Rica to Antarctica.

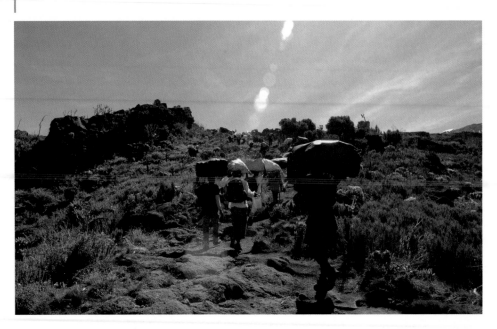

Photo courtesy of James A. Colderwood, Jr.

EXPEDITION AND WILDERNESS MEDICINE

Edited by

Gregory H. Bledsoe

Michael J. Manyak

David A. Townes

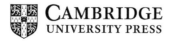

CAMBRIDGE
UNIVERSITY PRESS

CAMBRIDGE UNIVERSITY PRESS
Cambridge, New York, Melbourne, Madrid, Cape Town, Singapore, São Paulo, Delhi

Cambridge University Press
32 Avenue of the Americas, New York, NY 10013-2473, USA

www.cambridge.org
Information on this title: www.cambridge.org/9780521868730

First published 2009

Printed in the United States of America

A catalog record for this publication is available from the British Library.

Library of Congress Cataloging in Publication Data

Expedition and wilderness medicine / edited by Gregory H. Bledsoe, Michael J. Manyak, David
A. Townes.
  p. ; cm.
 Includes bibliographical references and index.
 ISBN 978-0-521-86873-0 (hardback)
 1. Outdoor medical emergencies. 2. First aid in illness and injury. I. Bledsoe, Gregory H.,
1973– II. Manyak, Michael J. III. Townes, David A. IV. Title.
 [DNLM: 1. Emergency Treatment – methods. 2. Expeditions. 3. Emergency Medical
Services. 4. Environment. WB 105 E96 2008]

 RC88.9.O95E96 2008
 616.02'52–dc22   2008006282

ISBN 978-0-521-86873-0 (hardback)

*For those who explore and those who
assist them, may their expeditions be
safer because of this knowledge.*

Contents

PART II. EXPEDITIONS IN UNIQUE ENVIRONMENTS

PART III. ILLNESS AND INJURIES ON EXPEDITIONS

Contributors

E. Wayne Askew, PhD
Professor and Director
Division of Nutrition
University of Utah
Salt Lake City, Utah, USA

Jeff Ayton, MBBS, MPHTM, FRACGP, FACRRM,
    FACTM, AFFTM
Chief Medical Officer
Polar Medicine Unit
Australian Antarctic Division
Australia

Howard D. Backer, MD, MPH
Past President, Wilderness Medical Society
Chief, Immunization Branch
Medical Consultant for Emergency Preparedness
California Department of Public Health
Medical Consultant, Mountain Travel-Sobek
Emergency Department, Kaiser Permanente,
Hayward, California, USA

Gregory H. Bledsoe, MD, MPH
CEO, ExpedMed, LLC
Director, Expedition Medicine National Conference
Emergency Medicine Physician
Saint Simons Island, Georgia, USA

Michael V. Callahan, MD, DTM&H (UK), MSPH
Director, Rescue Medicine Asia
Division of Infectious Diseases
Massachusetts General Hospital
Harvard Medical School
Boston, Massachusetts, USA

Richard Carmona, MD, MPH, FACS
17th Surgeon General of the United States
Distinguished Professor of Public Health
Mel and Enid Zuckerman College of Public Health
University of Arizona
Tucson, Arizona, USA

Craig Cook, MD
Medical Editor, *Sport Diver* magazine
Undersea Medical Consultants
Severna Park, Maryland, USA

Eugene F. Delaune III, MD
Medical Director, Europe Assistance USA
Assistant Clinical Professor
Department of Emergency Medicine
The George Washington University
Washington, DC, USA

Howard J. Donner, MD
Expedition Physician
Co-author, *Field Guide to Wilderness Medicine*
Family and Emergency Medicine
San Francisco, California, USA

M. Nicole Draghic
Vice President of Communications, BioSTAR Inc.
Germantown, Maryland, USA

Blair Dillard Erb, Sr., MD, FACP, FACC
Past President, Wilderness Medical Society
The Study Center
Townsend, Tennessee, USA

Timothy B. Erickson, MD, FACEP, FACMT, FAACT
Professor
Department of Emergency Medicine and Division
    of Clinical Toxicology
University of Illinois at Chicago, College
    of Medicine
Chicago, Illinois, USA

William W. Forgey, MD
Past President, Wilderness Medical Society
Associate Clinical Professor
Department of Family Medicine
Indiana University School of Medicine
Northwest Center for Medical Education
Gary, Indiana, USA

Luanne Freer, MD, FACEP, FAWM
Past President, Wilderness Medical Society
Founder and Director, Everest Base Camp Medical
    Clinic, Nepal
Medical Director, Yellowstone National Park
Bozeman, Montana, USA

Kevin B. Gerold, DO, JD
Program Medical Director
Tactical Medical Unit
Maryland State Police Special Operations Command
Assistant Professor
Department of Anesthesia and Critical Care Medicine
The Johns Hopkins University School of Medicine
Baltimore, Maryland, USA

Alan Gianotti, MD
Clinical Assistant Professor
Department of Surgery, Division of Emergency
    Medicine
Stanford University School of Medicine
Palo Alto, California, USA

Rajan Gupta, MD, FACS, FCCP
Associate Professor
Director, Trauma Program
Department of Surgery
Dartmouth Medical School
Dartmouth Hitchcock Medical Center
Lebanon, New Hampshire, USA

Peter H. Hackett, MD
Director, Institute for Altitude Medicine
Telluride, Colorado, USA
Clinical Director, Altitude Research Center
University of Colorado at Denver School of Medicine
Telluride, Colorado, USA

R. W. Bill Hamilton, PhD
Hamilton Research, Ltd.
Tarrytown, New York, USA

Jenny R. Hargrove, MD
Emergency Medicine Physician
Telluride Medical Center
Research Associate
Institute for Altitude Medicine
Telluride, Colorado, USA

Elliott R. Haut, MD, FACS
Assistant Professor of Surgery and Anesthesiology
    and Critical Care Medicine
Division of Acute Care Surgery: Trauma, Critical Care,
    Emergency and General Surgery
Department of Surgery
The Johns Hopkins University School of Medicine
Director, Trauma/Acute Care Surgery Fellowship
The Johns Hopkins Hospital
Baltimore, Maryland, USA

Peter J. Hotez, MD, PhD
President, Sabin Vaccine Institute
Editor-in-Chief, *PLoS Neglected Tropical Diseases*
Walter G. Ross Professor and Chair
Department of Microbiology, Immunology, & Tropical
    Medicine

The George Washington University
Washington, DC, USA

Edbert B. Hsu, MD, MPH
Associate Professor
Department of Emergency Medicine
Director of Training, Office of Critical Event
    Preparedness and Response
The Johns Hopkins University School of Medicine
Baltimore, Maryland, USA

Randall N. Hyer, MD, PhD, MPH
Former Winter-Over Medical Officer
Operation DEEP FREEZE, McMurdo and South Pole
    Stations
Antarctica

J. Lee Jenkins, MD, MSc
Assistant Professor
Disaster Control Physician
Department of Emergency Medicine
The Johns Hopkins University School of Medicine
Baltimore, Maryland, USA

Joyce M. Johnson, DO, MA
Rear Admiral, USPHS (ret)
Vice President, Health Sciences
Health and Life Sciences Global Business
Battelle
Arlington, Virginia, USA

Kenneth Kamler, MD
Vice President, The Explorers Club
Expedition Physician
Author, *Doctor on Everest*
Author, *Surviving the Extremes*
New York, New York, USA

Tracey Knutson, Esq.
Knutson & Associates
Girdwood, Alaska, USA

Kristin Larson, Esq.
Former Winter and Summer Research Manager,
    McMurdo Station, Antarctica
Board of Directors and Legal Committee, The
    Explorers Club
Attorney, Skadden, Arps, Slate, Meagher
    & Flom LLP
Washington, DC, USA

James Li, MD
Miles Memorial Hospital
Damariscotta, Maine, USA

Janet Y. Lin, MD, MPH
Assistant Professor
Director, International Emergency Medicine and
    Health Fellowship Program
Department of Emergency Medicine

University of Illinois at Chicago, College
    of Medicine
Chicago, Illinois, USA

**Desmond Lugg, AM, MD, FACOM, FAFOEM, FACRRM,
    Dip.Polar St.**
Former Head Polar Medicine, Australian Antarctic
    Division
Former Chief Medicine Extreme Environments
National Aeronautics and Space Administration
Washington, DC, USA

Christian Macedonia, MD, LTC, MC
United States Army
Chief of Research Operations
Telemedicine and Advanced Technology Research
    Center (TATRC)
Fort Detrick, Maryland, USA

Swaminatha V. Mahadevan, MD, FACEP, FAAEM
Associate Professor of Surgery/Emergency Medicine
Associate Chief, Division of Emergency Medicine
Medical Director, Stanford University Emergency
    Department
Editor, *An Introduction to Clinical Emergency Medicine*
Director, Stanford Emergency Medicine International
Department of Surgery, Division of Emergency
    Medicine
Stanford University School of Medicine
Palo Alto, California, USA

Michael J. Manyak, MD, FACS
Senior Medical Advisor, Global Rescue, Inc.
Vice President of Medical Affairs, EUSA Pharma
Professor of Urology, Engineering, Microbiology,
    and Tropical Medicine
The George Washington University
Washington, DC, USA

James M. Marinucci
Director, Wound Management Programs
Director, Continuing Medical Education
    and Training Programs
Adjunct Assistant Professor
Department of Emergency Medicine
The George Washington University
Washington, DC, USA

LTC John G. McManus, MD, MCR, FACEP, FAAEM
Assistant Chief, Academic Affairs
EMS Fellowship Director
Department of Emergency Medicine
Brooke Army Medical Center, Ft. Sam Houston, Texas
Medical Director, Fort Sam Houston and Camp
    Bullis Fire Department
Clinical Associate Professor
Department of Emergency Medicine
University of Texas Health Science Center
San Antonio, Texas, USA

Russell McMullen, MD
Co-director, Travel and Tropical Medicine Service
Associate Professor
Department of Medicine, Division of Emergency
    Medicine
University of Washington School of Medicine
Seattle, Washington, USA

Edward R. Melnick, MD
Department of Emergency Medicine
North Shore University Hospital
Manhasset, New York, USA

Kisha M. Moore, BA, MBBS, MRCS (Ed)
Specialist Registrar in Emergency Medicine
Northwest Thames – London Deanery
London, England

Bret P. Nelson, MD, RDMS, FACEP
Director of Emergency Ultrasound
Department of Emergency Medicine
Mount Sinai School of Medicine
New York, New York, USA

Martin T. Nweeia, DDS, DMD
Research Associate, Marine Mammal Program,
    Smithsonian Institution
Instructor, Advanced Dental Rotation
Harvard School of Dental Medicine
Boston, Massachusetts, USA

Christian F. Ockenhouse, MD, PhD
Deputy Director of the Division of Malaria Vaccine
    Development
Chief of the Department of Vivax Malaria Vaccine
    Discovery and Functional Genomics
Walter Reed Army Institute of Research
Silver Spring, Maryland, USA

David M. Parenti, MD, MScCTM
Professor
Department of Medicine, Microbiology, Immunology
    and Tropical Medicine
Division of Infectious Diseases
The George Washington University
    Medical Center
Washington, DC, USA

L. Alex Pranger
Vice President, BioSTAR Inc.
Germantown, Maryland, USA

R. Bradley Sack, MS, MD, ScD
Professor
Department of International Health
The Johns Hopkins Bloomberg School of
    Public Health
Baltimore, Maryland, USA

Marc A. Shepanek, PhD
Lead, Aerospace Medicine
Deputy Chief of Medicine of Extreme Environments
National Aeronautics and Space Administration
Washington, DC, USA

Noel E. Sloan, MD
Former Medical Officer, National Cave Rescue
    Commission
Team Physician, United States Deep Caving Team
Department of Anesthesiology
Methodist Hospital and Regional Trauma Center
Indianapolis, Indiana, USA

Stanley L. Spielman, MD
Chairman Emeritus, Southern Florida Chapter, The
    Explorers Club
Ophthalmology Consultant for South Florida
    Utilization Review
Former Adjunct Clinical Professor
Department of Ophthalmology
University of Miami Bascom Palmer Eye Institute
Miami, Florida, USA

Italo Subbarao, DO, MBA
Deputy Editor, *Disaster Medicine and Public Health
    Preparedness*
Director of the Public Health Readiness Office
Center of Public Health Preparedness and Disaster
    Response
American Medical Association
Chicago, Illinois, USA

Nelson Tang, MD, FACEP
Chief Medical Officer, Center for Law Enforcement
    Medicine
Assistant Professor
Director of Special Operations
Department of Emergency Medicine
The Johns Hopkins University School of Medicine
Baltimore, Maryland, USA

Marie Thomas
Deputy Director, Center for Advanced Research in
    Science and Technology
System Planning Corporation
Technical Advisor, Defense Advanced Research
    Projects Agency (DARPA)
Arlington, Virginia, USA

David A. Townes, MD, MPH, DTM&H
Medical Director, AdventureMed, LLC
Associate Professor
Associate Residency Program Director
Department of Medicine, Division of Emergency
    Medicine
University of Washington School of Medicine
Associate Medical Director for
    Utilization Management

University of Washington Medical Center
Seattle, Washington, USA

Michael J. VanRooyen, MD, MPH, FACEP
Co-director, Harvard Humanitarian Initiative
Associate Professor
Harvard Medical School and the Harvard School
    of Public Health
Chief, Division of International Health and
    Humanitarian Programs
Department of Emergency Medicine
Brigham and Women's Hospital
Boston, Massachusetts, USA

John Vonhof, EMT-P, OT
Paramedic, Orthopedic Technician
Author, *Fixing Your Feet: Prevention and Treatments
    for Athletes*
Manteca, California, USA

Alexander Vu, DO, MPH
Assistant Professor
Director, International Emergency Medicine Fellowship
Department of Emergency Medicine
The Johns Hopkins University School of Medicine
Center for Refugee and Disaster Response
The Johns Hopkins Bloomberg School of
    Public Health
Baltimore, Maryland, USA

COL Ian S. Wedmore, MD, FACEP, FAWM
United States Army Emergency Medicine Consultant
    to the Surgeon General
Adjunct Assistant Professor, Uniformed Services
    University of the Health Sciences
Clinical Instructor, University of Washington School
    of Medicine
Department of Emergency Medicine
Madigan Army Medical Center
Tacoma, Washington, USA

Zak H. Weis, DPM, MS
Department of Surgery
Amarillo Veterans Affairs Medical Center
Amarillo, Texas, USA
Team Podiatrist, Amarillo Gorillas Hockey
Weis Podiatry, Boulder, Colorado, and Amarillo, Texas
Amarillo, Texas, USA

William P. Wiesmann MD (COL, Ret.)
President and CEO BioSTAR Inc.
Germantown, Maryland, USA

Urs Wiget, MD
Expedition Physician
Medical Director, Reavita AG
Past President, Commission for Mountain Emergency
    Medicine (ICAR MedCom)
Zürich, Switzerland

Richard S. Williams, MD, FACS
Chief Health and Medical Officer
National Aeronautics and Space Administration
Washington, DC, USA

Bradford D. Winters, PhD, MD
Assistant Professor
Department of Anesthesiology and Critical
    Care Medicine
The Johns Hopkins University School of Medicine
Baltimore, Maryland, USA

Ken Zafren, MD, FACEP, FAAEM, FAWM
Medical Director, Alaska Mountain Rescue Group

Chairman, Medical Committee of the Mountain
    Rescue Association
Associate Medical Director, Himalayan
    Rescue Association
Vice President, International Commission for
    Mountain Emergency Medicine (ICAR MedCom)
Staff Emergency Physician, Alaska Native Medical
    Center, Anchorage, Alaska
Clinical Assistant Professor
Department of Surgery, Division of Emergency
    Medicine
Stanford University School of Medicine
Palo Alto, California, USA

Foreword

Jim Fowler

Honorary President, The Explorers Club

As we travel along life's sometimes convoluted and perilous path, we've always had one thing in common with our ancient ancestors: a desire to explore new territories. Whether to exploit natural resources, conduct research, or enjoy recreation, many of us still need to travel, explore, or seek outdoor adventure.

Natural survival of the fittest ensured an average life span much shorter in earlier days, and losing a few Vikings on trips was probably tolerated. Sailors were unaware of why they suffered from scurvy. If General Nobile had access to this textbook, his men may have survived their Arctic balloon crash depicted in *The Red Tent*. Today, we require permits and insurance to travel remotely, and everyone expects to come back alive!

However, life expectancy has increased and field medical care has improved considerably with better access to medicines, vaccines, and rapid transport. Before I first went to Africa in 1957 to produce a wildlife documentary that included an unwounded lion charging directly into camera, I was advised to consider having my appendix removed or learning to operate on myself in case it became inflamed. My choice was to have a former veterinarian turned missionary 200 miles away do the job if necessary. Today, I could consult this book on expedition medicine to prepare for such problems and potential evacuation.

My personal concerns in Africa were minimized when the expedition leader was bitten on the thumb by an Egyptian cobra and then, a few weeks later, temporarily blinded by a spitting cobra. The thumb bite was lucky because the fangs passed completely through before venom injection. The spitting cobra incident was more serious, but luckily a container of milk – handy as an ulcer remedy – was poured immediately into his eyes to dilute the venom. Otherwise, he faced the local treatment of a villager urinating into his eyes to wash out the poison. I made a note to always have milk available with spitting cobras in the neighborhood. The reader must determine whether this remains a good option.

This book should be read by everyone who enjoys nature, camps or conducts field research in distant areas, goes on safari, or just wants protection in remote places. Much information in *Expedition and Wilderness Medicine* has been learned the best way – the hard way – in the field by experienced explorers. If I had this book in the early 1960s, when I was deep in the Amazon forests on the first wild studies of the monkey-eating Harpy eagle, the world's largest, I may have avoided both the malaria and leishmaniasis that I contracted. Back in my hometown of Albany, Georgia, doctors did not diagnose the malaria for a week and never did figure out the leishmaniasis that was eating my ear for 6 months. Fortunately, a week of sun and saltwater on the Gulf of Mexico finally cured the infection.

Some things I have learned on my own to avoid:

- The brown jumping leach in Sumatra, which lives on land along trails and will latch on to you in a second, but a little tobacco juice or insect spray will keep it away.
- Amazonian red bugs or chiggers called Beta Rouge, big cousins to our North American variety.

- Green mambas in Africa. If you get bitten, you have time for one phone call – but you don't know who to call!

Though I have been charged by many animals, including 200 elephants led by an angry female, had my arm swallowed by a 22-foot-long anaconda, been bitten by piranhas in Peru, and been operated on by an Angolan witchdoctor, I have learned that the wilderness is not to be feared. Many undisturbed wilderness areas in the world are safe, healthy, beautiful, and full of life of all kinds. The dangerous places are usually where people are with their big cities, cars, electrical appliances, lawn mowers that cut people's legs off, and dangerous people themselves.

A great challenge facing our civilization is to keep people connected with the natural world since its existence is important to our lives. If we are uncomfortable or afraid of nature and its diverse life forms, big or small, then we may not save it. Human quality of life, even the very future of life on earth, would then be seriously threatened. This book provides a framework for health and safety in the field so that we can all enjoy nature, give it value, and try to preserve it for posterity.

Preface

Gregory H. Bledsoe, MD, MPH

Michael J. Manyak, MD, FACS

David A. Townes, MD, MPH, DTM&H, FACEP

As long as there have been expeditions, there has been expedition medicine. Whether it was Dr. David Livingstone treating his exploration party with quinine as they traveled up the Zambezi, Meriwether Lewis receiving medical training from Dr. Benjamin Rush, James McIlroy amputating frostbitten toes during Ernest Shackleton's Imperial Trans-Antarctic Expedition, or Dr. Jose Antonio Cajazeira treating Theodore Roosevelt on their Brazilian River of Doubt journey, expeditions and medicine have demonstrated a natural tendency to intersect.

In spite of this long and colorful history of medicine on expeditions, defining "expedition medicine" is no easy task. A medical professional providing medical care on an expedition might need to be a high-altitude expert one day and a tropical medicine expert the next. Exposure to envenomations, animal attacks, parasitic disease, and environmental extremes all may occur while traveling through remote areas on expeditions. It is this diversity of practice, and this intersection of medicine and nature, that initially draws many individuals to expedition medicine, and yet, when attempting to assimilate these varied topics into a single functional text, it is just this diversity that creates difficulty.

The editorial team has selected topics for this text that represent both the depth and the breadth of this expansive medical discipline. We recognize that even as individuals are drawn to different geographic environments, readers will use this text for different purposes. Depending on whether you plunge into the ocean depths, climb the highest peaks, or explore the deepest rainforest or jungle, certain chapters will apply to your journey more than others. Our goal was not to be completely comprehensive on every topic – as there are already excellent detailed texts dedicated to the various subtopics within expedition medicine – but rather to provide enough practical information to support a medical officer in a variety of field environments.

We strongly believed that for our text to truly help those in the field it needed to be written and edited by those in the field. Each of our authors was selected for their combination of both impeccable academic credentials and vast field experience. On any given day our authors could be climbing Everest, diving in the oceans, resuscitating patients on the battlefield, treating snakebites in the tropics, navigating hostile geopolitical environments, or rescuing stranded victims off mountains. These talented individuals do a lot because they know a lot; consequently, they also know a lot because they do a lot. Their perspective of medical care in these extreme environments is shaped by their field experience and translates into practical educational points for the reader. These chapters are not filled with tips for what one *might* do if he or she is ever in a particular situation, but what the author has done, and does, when faced with a specific decision point.

In the end, the book you now hold in your hands is the product of many thousands of hours of labor over the course of three years. It is not perfect – no text is, of course – but the editorial team hopes it will be a tool for those individuals who choose to venture into the many remote, extreme, and wilderness environments of our amazingly diverse world. We hope you find it helpful. We hope you find it interesting. We hope you find it inspiring. Most of all, we hope this text opens up a new level of understanding concerning medical care on expeditions and offers a resource to the expedition community that would make even a Livingstone, Lewis, Shackleton, or Roosevelt proud.

Acknowledgments

A special thanks to the following individuals who helped review chapters for this textbook:

- Christian Tomaszewski, MD
- Kimball Maull, MD
- Craig Cook, MD

Gregory H. Bledsoe expresses gratitude

- To my amazing wife, Sara, whose beauty is only surpassed by her kind, generous, and genuine spirit, who took my hand and leapt with me into this crazy world of international medicine. I love you, Honey; you are my best friend and the perfect partner for me in this adventure we are on together. Thanks for all your patience while I worked on this project.
- To my daughter, Taylor, the light of my life, whose smile melts hearts and lights up rooms, who has her mother's amazing energy and infectious enthusiasm, and who brings indescribable joy and purpose to my life. You are a gift from God, and your daddy loves you so very much. May He illuminate your path as He has mine and give you the opportunity to dream big dreams and live them. I am so proud of you.
- To my mother, Cecile Herndon Bledsoe, the quintessential "Southern Belle," whose grace and class are the stuff of legends, who poured her life into her family, whose voice I constantly hear inside my head, who taught her children the value of proper priorities and then lived a life of vision and sacrifice before us, and whose legacy will live beyond her through her children. Mom, you are amazing. Thank you for all your sacrifices in raising us. I am glad you have lived to hear your children rise up and call you "blessed." I love you.
- To my father, James H. Bledsoe, MD, FACS, the dedicated surgeon who took me to Haiti on a medical mission trip when I was in high school and consequently set the trajectory for my life. Thanks, Dad, for being such a man of integrity and for providing such an amazing example of discipline and hard work for us to follow. Thanks for being such a loving father and for being such a vocal encouragement to me during this project and throughout my medical training. I would rather have your approval than the applause of thousands. This book is as much yours as it is mine. I love you.
- To my siblings, Samuel E. Bledsoe, MD, and Patricia Bledsoe Freije, Esq., who are the iron that sharpens me. I am amazed by your talents and achievements. You are incredible. I love you both and am so proud of the people you have become.
- To the various in-laws in my life, Peter Freije, Kelly King Bledsoe, Jonathan Zebulske, David Zebulske, and my father- and mother-in-law, Dr. Terry and Faith Zebulske, thanks for the fun, the patience, the energy, and the support you have brought into my life. I love you all.
- To my extended family, all the Bledsoes, Zebulskes, Wards, Waters, Schiebers, and Braddys. You all are our "home base" as Sara, Taylor, and I live as medical vagabonds around

the world. Thanks for being such a great cheering section and safe haven. Home for us is where you are.

- To my mentors, Stephen M. Schexnayder, MD, and Guohua Li, MD, DrPH, who have spent countless hours prodding, directing, and encouraging me. Thanks for believing in me and for keeping me pointed in the right direction. You are the giants upon whose shoulders I have stood.
- To my friend and mentor Michael J. VanRooyen, MD, MPH, thanks for introducing me to the world of international emergency medicine. Your career is an inspiration to many.
- To my friends at the University of Arkansas for Medical Sciences and The Johns Hopkins University School of Medicine, thanks for the opportunity to expand my horizons and work alongside you.
- To all my friends in northwest Arkansas, too numerous to mention by name, thanks for investing in and helping raise me. No matter how long I am gone or how far I travel, I am still the boy from Rogers. You are ever present in my mannerisms, accent, and memories, and I always look forward to my visits with you. I miss you all greatly and leave you with two words: Go Hogs!

Michael J. Manyak offers his appreciation.

- So many to thank, so little time. First and foremost for dedication are the ones who keep the home fires burning. I am sincerely indebted to my most tolerant wife, Rebecca, who listens to my rantings and encourages me to dive the *Titanic*, hunt with pygmies in the African rainforest, seek artifacts on the *Atocha* treasure galleon, and break ice in Antarctica . . . and who is there waiting when I return. She is absolute proof that behind every successful man stands a surprised woman.
- Thanks to my children, Rachel, Susanna, and Tim, always companions on my expeditions . . . whether in my heart or by my side. Please try to remember some of my stories so you can tell them back to me when I forget them in later life.
- A sincere thanks to my many colleagues and friends in The Explorers Club who vividly inspire me on to the next challenge . . . many of you are authors in this text, and it does not happen without your invaluable contributions and camaraderie.
- Lastly, a special dedication to the memory of Dr. Roy Chapman Andrews, former director of the American Museum of Natural History, president of The Explorers Club, and inspiration for the Indiana Jones character . . . he was my first hero whose books ignited my scientific curiosity at age 5.

David A. Townes

I would like to thank my family, friends, and colleagues for all of their support and understanding during the creation of this text. Additional thanks go to those who have taught me along the way including my students from whom I have learned so much. Finally, thank you to all those individuals on the trail and in the field who serve as inspiration to continue to acquire knowledge.

PART 1. EXPEDITION PLANNING

1 | The Expedition Physician

Howard J. Donner

SIX LITERS

In 1988, I was asked to serve as expedition doctor on the first American ascent of Kangchenjunga, the world's third highest peak. I had provided medical support for numerous smaller expeditions of one to two weeks, but this trip was going to be different. Kangchenjunga was proposed as a three-month expedition into a then relatively little traveled region of Nepal. The Kangchenjunga region in 1988 was still closed to trekkers and required a climbing permit to access. Base camp was approximately 15 days by foot from the nearest road head, and in those days there were no satellite phones for security. This was to be my first significant expedition and as the launch date grew closer, I became increasingly apprehensive.

I was responsible for providing medical care and support to a 30-person expedition made up of climbers, Nepali porters, and Western support trekkers. A couple of mountain medicine handbooks existed in the late 1980s, but these references said little about operational issues of expedition medicine. How much intravenous fluid should an expedition like this carry? I had no clue. I realized that big expeditions carried intravenous fluids, but how much? That was another question. I quickly realized that the wilderness medical textbooks were completely inadequate for answering many practical questions. With mild consternation, I called my friend and mentor Dr. Peter Hackett. "Peter, I'm going to Kangchenjunga for three months, how much intravenous fluid should I take?" Peter responded calmly, "I don't know, just bring whatever you think you'll need." "Thanks, Peter." I then called my good friend, Howard Backer, and he suggested that I "ask Hackett." I went on to another mentor, Dr. Gil Roberts. Gil was living in Berkley in the late 1980s and had been one of my early mountain medical heroes. He was the physician on the first successful American Everest expedition in 1963, along with Whittaker, Hornbein, Bishop, Jerstad, and Unsoeld. Gil was known for being a bit of a nihilist, but he was clearly the reference I needed. I phoned him and queried, "Gil, how much intravenous fluid should I bring to Kangchenjunga?" "Well, Howard, it doesn't

really matter. Anybody that's going to live is going to live, and anyone that's going to die is going to die." I politely thanked Gil for his advice and dejectedly hung up the phone. Finally in complete desperation, I went to the appendices of Chris Bonington's books. The Brits, being very compulsive, typically included appendices, which carefully indexed the contents of the expedition medical kits. Unfortunately, these early British expeditions were much larger than ours and carried vast quantities of intravenous fluids (50 liters plus). Well, ultimately I empirically decided on 6 liters. This seemed like an adequate quantity for fluid resuscitation of one, moderate, nonsurgical trauma patient, or some form of moderately severe medical illness resulting in fluid loss or dehydration. On Kangchenjunga, we ended up using none of it. (See Figure 1.1.)

Coincidentally, shortly after my return, I was hired as a medical operations consultant for NASA. NASA was working then on Space Station Freedom, which was the conceptual forerunner for the international space station (ISS). At that time, Space Station Freedom was developing the capability for producing intravenous fluids via "ultra-filtration." They developed a process for converting drinking water into sterile water. Electrolyte salts were added to individually produce a variety of crystalloid solutions as needed. I was invited to speak at a large consultants' meeting in Houston. NASA was interested in my experience as a wilderness medicine doctor.

In due course, I was called to the podium and questioned in front of a very impressive group of international scientists and physicians. "Dr. Donner, on board Space Station Freedom we can produce intravenous fluids via ultra-filtration. As you know, ultra-filtration technique requires some time to produce these fluids. Our question for you is how much intravenous fluid should we have on hand, available to use immediately?"

Intimidated as I was by the caliber of scientist waiting for my reply, I managed to softly stammer, "uh, six liters." This somewhat arbitrary answer has personified my philosophy ever since; that is, expedition medicine is often an inexact discipline.

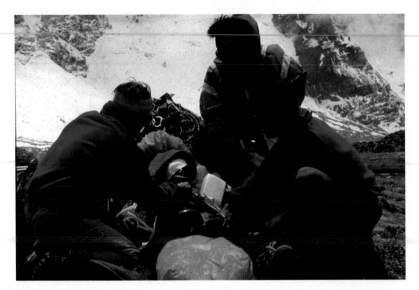

Figure 1.1. Medical training on Kanchenjunga. Photo courtesy of Howard Donner.

EXPEDITION MEDICAL MINDSET

Common Sense

The most important single attribute that an expedition doctor can possess is common sense, everything else can be learned. In Chapter 2, Dr. Forgey provides a well-thought-out and comprehensive chapter on the subject of preparing the expedition medical kit. You might keep in mind that ultimately no reference can provide a cookbook formula for successful medical preparation. Some textbooks provide algorithms for calculating drug types and quantities. "Let's see, I have 14 folks on a 9 day trip, I will therefore need 114 ibuprofen tablets." The arithmetic approach ignores the infinite nuances and intangibles of real-world expedition environments. A well-known, and well-respected, expedition physician came to one of my lectures years ago, at the start of her career. I was giving a talk on high-altitude illness. I described the ubiquitous nature of high-altitude cough, and the multiple etiologies, including dusty trails, smoke-filled guest houses, irritation to the respiratory mucosa secondary to cold dry air, and generally increased ventilation at altitude. Because of the high incidence of cough, I recommend bringing an adequate amount of cough drops on any high-altitude sojourn. She did some math . . . 30 members in her expedition, three months out, about 8 cough drops per person per day. The math resulted in a total of $30 \times 90 \times 8$ or 21,600 cough drops! This resulted in a number of dedicated porter loads entirely for cough drops, as well as a persistent legend of cough drops from that Everest expedition continuing to materialize around the Khumbu for years thereafter. Integrate a meticulous analytic assessment with a more generalized gestalt, based on knowledge, clinical experience, and, always, a bit of guesswork.

Complex Variables

The variables on any expedition are complex, making generic advice on "what to take" moot without an operational context. Major considerations should include

- The environmental extremes of the trip (e.g., arctic, high altitude, tropical, desert)
- Time of year (i.e., climatic conditions and disease conditions)
- Specific endemic diseases
- Your medical expertise (i.e., specialty and expertise of the expedition medical officer)
- The medical expertise of the other expedition members (i.e., neophyte tourists, a group of guides, other doctors)
- The total number of expedition members, including ancillary staff (i.e., porters, local guides, expedition staff)
- Duration of trip
- Team demographics (i.e., age and gender)
- Known preexisting medical problems of individuals within the group
- Distance from definitive medical care (e.g., are you traveling in the Alps or the Karakoram?)
- Availability of communications (i.e., cell phones, radios, satellite phones, tele-medicine capability)
- Availability and timeframe of rescue (i.e., organized rescue groups, proximity of airfields, availability and capability of helicopters and fixed-wing aircraft)
- Medical kit weight and volume limitations (i.e., will the kit be carried on your back, on others' backs, or on pack animals, sleds, rafts, or boats?)
- Who assumes the responsibility for providing local health care (i.e., on the trek in and out)

HEROIC FANTASY

Dr. Gil Roberts (see earlier reference) once stated that it was "heroic fantasy" to assume that an expedition doctor has the ability to manage any possible medical event occurring on a large expedition. Gil's hardened pragmatism runs counter to the idealized belief system with which many of us enter medicine. Get used to the idea that, at times, the medical needs of your patients may exceed your ability to do anything. This can be disconcerting for Western doctors who have been indoctrinated with the idea that something can always be done. Despite his slightly jaded view, Gil often pointed out that the single thing an expedition doctor should unfailingly be prepared for, and capable of, is providing pain relief. Remember that even when you can't fix it, you can generally help patients feel better. (See Figure 1.2.) Pay special attention to the discussion of analgesics in Chapter 3.

You Can't Carry a Hospital Formulary on Your Back

The process of organizing and obtaining the medical equipment for an expedition requires an enormous amount of planning and forethought. No matter how much equipment is ultimately hauled in, you cannot possibly prepare for every conceivable illness or accident. Philosophical approaches vary from "carry a SAM® Splint and some duct tape" to a collection that would stagger the local porters or sink a raft. Surgical types inevitably anticipate trauma, while internists favor meds. I frequently speak at wilderness medicine conferences on the subject of expedition medical preparation. Often, when I finish my talk, a small group of mildly irate looking doctors collect beneath the podium, "Uh-oh, what did I do wrong," I muse. Some specialists become indignant that I would suggest certain medications and leave out others. The anesthesiologist might remark, "I can't believe you recommended bringing

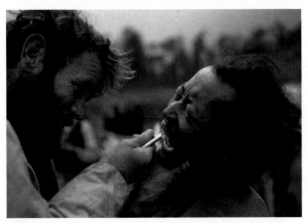

Figure 1.2. Gil Roberts and Sherpa on Everest 1963. Photo courtesy of Erica Stone.

morphine without mentioning fentanyl or ketamine." The psychiatrist might wonder why I only reference Haldol in my discussion of major sedatives. "Why don't you include newer agents such as Zyprexa or Symbyax?" The unhappy truth is that you can't carry an entire hospital formulary on your (or a porter's) back. Additionally, there is benefit in the concept of "tried and true" (i.e., using medications that you are familiar with from your daily practice). I continue to use ciprofloxacin (Cipro) in my medical kits. I am frequently asked why I don't use a third-generation quinolone such as levofloxacin (Levaquin). Clearly, newer third- and fourth-generation quinolones provide an increased spectrum against gram negative, and even some anaerobic, bacteria. These current generation quinolones could potentially be used as the ultimate expedition "super drug." Unfortunately, a few third- and fourth-generation quinolones were taken off the market following reports of serious adverse side effects. Side effects are problematic on expeditions, especially when the selection of backup drugs is limited, so I often choose to keep it simple. Ultimately, the choice of what to take will be individual, based largely on personal preferences and subjective "style." This element of "artistic license" is to some extent, what makes expedition medicine both challenging and fun. The recommendations in this, or any, book on expedition medicine should be viewed as guidelines, not gospel.

You're Definitely Forgetting Something

Years ago a friend of mine, Dr. Alan Gianotti, now an experienced expedition physician, called me late one evening. He explained that he was leaving the next morning for Pakistan on his first full-scale climbing expedition to the Karakoram. "Howard, I'm calling you because I'm really worried that I'm forgetting something."

After a short pause I responded, "Alan, I hope this will make you feel better, you're *definitely* forgetting something." My response to Alan, though flippant, was communicating a point. It is unrealistic to assume that you can travel to a remote region, on the other side of the planet, remain in isolation for three months, and manage to prepare for every conceivable illness or accident.

Another friend of mine, Brian Horner, served as medical officer on an extensive climbing expedition in the Antarctic. Unfortunately the large aircraft they were using for expedition support crashed on landing in poor visibility. Brian found himself confronted with the critical task of caring for multiple trauma patients with extensive injuries for many days. When Brian returned from that expedition, I asked him if there was anything, from a medical perspective, that he wished he had done differently. He replied, "Absolutely, I wish I had brought more morphine." He went on to say that he had included a typical quantity of narcotics, which were completely exhausted during the first few hours. For the next few days, Brian cared for these patients without any resources for providing analgesia. In retrospect, it is unlikely Brian could have anticipated a mass-casualty scenario extending for many days. Should we respond to Brian's experience by routinely including 50 ampules of morphine on every expedition? Ultimately, the expedition doctor must except that there are risks on expeditions that are not entirely predictable. These risks cannot always be planned for or entirely mitigated against.

Common Things Are Common

Remember, "Common things are common." It is natural to assume that patients in exotic locals will develop exotic disease entities. The reality is, patients in exotic places more typically develop fairly ordinary diseases. For example, before you make the diagnosis of schistosomiasis, consider more common causes of fever, cough, abdominal pain, or diarrhea. Include schistosomiasis in your differential, but initially, consider the common. Expedition populations are typically reasonably healthy, immune competent individuals. First-line treatment should reflect that.

General Guidelines for Expedition Drugs

- When possible, choose medications with low side-effect profiles (e.g., tinidazole over metronidazole).
- Choose medications with limited contraindications (e.g., Augmentin is contraindicated in penicillin-allergic patients). Do you want to carry additional drugs because a subset of your patients won't tolerate penicillin?
- When possible, choose medications that have multiple indications (e.g., drugs like Benadryl and prednisone have multiple uses on expeditions).
- Choose medications that have favorable dosing schedules (e.g., azithromycin over erythromycin). Compliance will markedly improve and you will greatly reduce the weight and volume of the medical kit.

If You Can't Steal Samples

Physicians with bulging sample cabinets may tend to favor anything they can get for free. Try to keep in mind what actual costs are if expedition members are paying the bill. Zymar (gatifloxacin) is an ideal drug for corneal ulcer, but should you provide a $60 antibiotic for routine pink eye? Consider bringing inexpensive drugs when possible and reserve the expensive "big guns" for serious indications. You may need to sequester them so that they remain available when really needed.

Often medicines are considerably more economical when purchased outside the United States. This is especially true in developing countries. You might look into the availability of commonly used drugs in the destination country. Quality control of foreign drugs can be an issue, and this should be investigated before arrival when possible.

What's Going On Up There?

Expedition and wilderness medicine is a constantly evolving field. Try not to let the conventions of those who have gone before you inhibit your creativity. I am often amused when teaching wilderness medicine courses that students feel uneasy about improving on a system or concept that I am teaching. Students should be encouraged to advance the field, and think independently. On my first expedition (see previous discussion) to Kangchenjunga, I went through each organ system systematically and reflected on how I could improve on the medical kits of my mentors. In the early 1980s urine beta-HCG test kits were becoming compact and user friendly. I wondered how I would manage a female support trekker on that expedition. For example, 15 days from the closest road head, a reproductive-aged female suddenly develops lower quadrant pain and/or vaginal bleeding. My first thought was "I need to know whether that patient is pregnant." The ability to rule out complications of first-trimester pregnancy (e.g., an ectopic pregnancy) would be key in any emergency department evaluation of those symptoms. Interestingly, I was not aware at that time of anyone carrying urine beta-HCG tests in their expedition kits. I threw one in and have continued to include it since. Ultimately I recommended that NASA include this capability for both space shuttle and space station. I was told recently that incredulous reporters still call Johnson Space Center from time to time and inquire, "We notice you're flying urine pregnancy kits on the space station and shuttle, what's going on up there?"

Why You Shouldn't Carry White Powder in Small Zip Lock Bags, and Other Customs Issues

One of the common expedition medical questions I receive is, "How do you get all of these medicines through customs?" The following suggestions will increase your odds of experiencing a relatively seamless customs experience:

- Don't carry white powder in zip lock bags. As obvious as this may sound, it is amazing how tablets of all sorts tend to break down with humidity and then slowly disintegrate in zip lock bags. A poorly identified zip lock bag, with pulverized white medicine inside, presents a rather suspect impression to a customs official. (See Figure 1.3.) Try to be meticulous with your drugs. Place your medicines in clearly labeled zip lock bags or medicine vials. If you choose

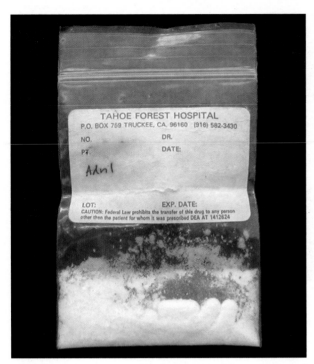

Figure 1.3. Pulverized ibuprofen in Patagonia. Photo courtesy of Howard Donner.

to use zip locks, protect them from physical damage inside of a sturdy kit or case. The more organized the kit looks, the less dubious the customs' officials seem to look.

- Carry a copy of your medical license. Showing a customs official a photocopy of your medical license carries a bit more credibility than stating, "But I'm a doctor, really."
- Present a letter of introduction. Customs officials seem to love embossed stationery or letters embellished with gold seals. These blank forms can be easily purchased through most office supply stores. Even if you're not traveling with the National Geographic Society, you can print up your own letter on embossed stationery. Introduce yourself as the expedition doctor for the "2008 blank blank expedition." As long as your name is on the letter, along with a signature from the sponsoring foundation (such as a friend of yours), custom officials seem to relax.

Despite all of your best efforts, remember that horror stories exist, and there are no absolute guarantees. Keep your fingers crossed.

ATTITUDES

Issues of Control

Most physicians revel in control. Most of us strive to avoid the unexpected and feel most comfortable when we can exert control over our surroundings. The inability to control outcomes in the expedition environment can catch the uninitiated physician off guard. In our customary practice, virtually everything possible is done for every patient, under every circumstance. I once cared for a young porter in the Himalayas who developed sudden onset of severe abdominal pain. He was carrying goods between villages in the Annapurna region and was not connected with any expedition. On physical exam, it was obvious that he had developed an acute abdomen. I explained to the patient that he needed immediate air evacuation to Kathmandu where he could be evaluated and treated by a surgeon. There was a small airfield, with evacuation capability, a few hours' walk down the trail. I wasn't quite ready for the patient's response. He said that he could simply not afford to fly to Kathmandu. He understood that he might die, but he also understood that when a person lived in the mountains, a surgical problem would probably result in death. That was simply the reality of living in a remote mountain region, and he seemed relatively comfortable with the notion. A group of us (Western trekkers) ultimately collected funds and financed his flight to Kathmandu. None of us were emotionally prepared for the alternative.

Differences in Fundamental Values

On another occasion, I treated a patient at the Himalayan Rescue Association clinic in Manang with a severe necrotizing fasciitis involving his forearm. I started the patient on a combination of emperic intravenous antibiotics. He also received extensive daily surgical debridement in our clinic. Despite our efforts, he developed fever and chills and began to deteriorate. (See Figure 1.4.) I asked our interpreter to inform his family that we needed them to collect enough money to fly the patient to Kathmandu. Although many Nepali families would not have had the means, this family did. Our interpreter discussed the options with the patient and his family. The family then asked, "If he goes to Kathmandu, is there still the possibility that he might die?"

I replied, "Yes, he could die even if he goes to Kathmandu." The family talked for a moment with the patient and then responded.

Our interpreter stated, "He doesn't want to go."

Incredulously I asked, "How can he not want to go?"

Our interpreter explained that the patient was worried that if he went to Kathmandu and died, his soul would remain lost and have difficulty returning to his family. The patient felt much more comfortable remaining at his home to die, even though evacuation would have most likely guaranteed survival. This episode reminded me that the most fundamental structure of human nature is often culturally based, and may offer surprises to Western physicians.

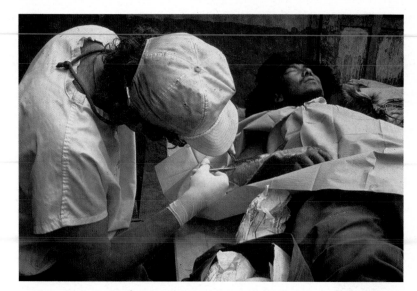

Figure 1.4. Debriding a necrotizing fasciitis in Manang, Nepal. Photo courtesy of Howard Donner.

Nonlinear

Linear-thinking Western expedition doctors may at times become frustrated working in developing countries with what could be perceived as a nonlinear approach to problem solving. In the world of expedition medicine, assume that frustration "comes with the territory." Many Westerners seek out adventure travel under one condition . . . that there is no adventure. On an expedition, be advised that adventure and chaos coexist, as do unforeseen trials and tribulations. There will be porter strikes, flat tires, landslides, and annoyances that can't even be imagined. On one trip in the Himalayas, I attempted to bring a large tank of medical oxygen up to a high-altitude clinic. The trek in was nine days. When the porter and his load of oxygen finally arrived at the clinic (nine days by foot later), alas, the oxygen cylinder was empty! It had not been filled at the supplier despite his assurance to the contrary. At times like this, it is often best to embrace the Nepali expression "Ke Garne," roughly, "Oh, well, what can you do?"

Lost in Translation

The complexities of language can be perplexing when providing medical care abroad, especially when the situation requires more than one interpreter. Once in Nepal, I needed to speak to an ill patient from Tibet. I went from English to Nepalese through our English/Nepali interpreter. From there we went through a Nepali interpreter who was fluent in the local dialect. We then had to go from the local dialect into Tibetan via a third interpreter. I remember inquiring "Does it hurt when he urinates?" The question passed through the three interpreters, eventually reaching the patient. Soon the three interpreters, the patient, and the patient's family were arguing and talking very excitedly in three dissimilar languages. After a minute of this, I stopped my interpreter and asked, "Please, what are they saying?" The interpreter paused, looked at me, and quietly replied "No." I was clearly losing something in the translation, but hey, "Ke Garne."

Feed It to the Yaks

When practicing medicine on international expeditions, you may feel overwhelmed by the plethora of medications that are completely unfamiliar to you. Even with the help of a physicians' desk reference (PDR) or similar work, you will find that many medications found in international settings simply don't exist in the North American database. My colleague Dr. Eric Weiss once told me, "If you are having trouble typifying unknown drugs, feed them to the yaks and categorize the medicine based on the yaks' reaction." Laughing in the face of frustration serves as a handy defense against despair. (See Figure 1.5.)

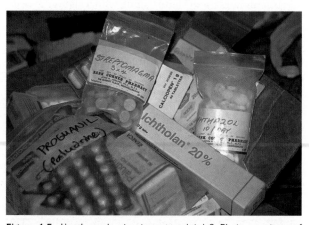

Figure 1.5. Used much streptomagma lately? Photo courtesy of Howard Donner.

Clinical Fundamentals

One of the most gratifying elements of expedition medicine is that the focus returns to clinical fundamentals. Clinical laboratory, imaging, and referral are not typically options in the expedition environment. You learn to rely on history and clinical findings. You may become so accustomed to treating routine illnesses without tests that it may seem odd when you return. Your hospital-based colleagues may order stool cultures for every case of "garden variety" diarrhea and you may find yourself longing for the commonsense and empirically based medicine that you practiced in the mountains.

Occam's Razor

In medical school, we are indoctrinated with the concept of "Occam's razor." Occam's razor suggests, "When given two equally valid explanations for a phenomenon, one should embrace the less complicated formulation." Or in simpler terms, "All things being equal, the simplest solution tends to be the best one." In my experience, this does not always hold true in the expedition environment. For example, it is quite common to see a patient with both altitude illness and a concomitant viral syndrome. It is the combination of infectious and environmental disease that puts the patient "over the edge," bringing them to your tent. Similarly, you may see a patient with high-altitude pulmonary edema and pneumonia in combination, yet our clinical conditioning suggests we should assume it's either one or the other. On an expedition, you may be treating a combination. On high mountains, the reality is that most patients have some combination of malnutrition, dehydration, insomnia, exhaustion, hypo- or hyperthermia, anxiety, and hypoxia in addition to their chief complaint.

East Meets West

We live in a culture where the relationship between those who practice allopathic medicine and those who practice alternative medicine is sometimes acrimonious. Fortunately, the chasm between these fundamental approaches to medicine seems to be narrowing. The first time I worked in Nepal, I was apprehensive about how I would interface medically with the local Lamas' practice of Eastern Tibetan medicine. I feared it would be "us against them." To my great surprise and relief the interplay between our Western clinic and the local Lamas' medicine was virtually seamless. When we had patients suffering from chronic conditions such as depression or intractable diseases such as cancer, I would often bring these patients to the Lamas. When the Lamas had patients with medical conditions that they felt uncomfortable with (e.g., trauma or infectious disease), they would often bring their patients to us. We adopted a philosophy and policy of "best tool for the job." It's a shame it can't be that painless in the States.

Intangibles

As stated earlier, there are times in the expedition environment when, apparently, nothing can be done. Some years back, I was called into a village where a young Tibetan mother was laboring unsuccessfully. The patient was tachycardic and weakening, and her labor was not progressing. I was traveling with a nurse practitioner who had worked as a midwife back in the States. I turned to her and said, "You're a midwife. Do something."

She then turned to me and replied, "You're the doctor. You do something."

I had the sudden realization, that despite my years of medical training, I was confronted with a situation where I had little to offer. No means for an emergency c-section, no availability of oxytocin, no vacuum extraction or forceps. I realized that I was unprepared to change the fate of this mother and her unborn child. Luckily for all, there was a Tibetan local in the crowd who came to me and politely said, "Doctor sahib, I have a powder that comes from a fish from a sacred lake in Tibet, sometimes we use it when the baby does not come."

I immediately replied, "Give it to her!" He disappeared and returned minutes later with a small satchel of some unknown dried substance and gave it to the patient. I realize that this scenario sounds improbable, but within 30 minutes the mother was laboring actively and within an hour she was delivering her baby. The infant was initially a bit limp, but following warming and towel stimulation, he "pinked up" and ultimately fared well.

To this day, I wonder what was in that "potion." Was it something tangible, such as an oxytocin analog, or perhaps something more enigmatic?

Remain open to new realms.

EXPEDITION MEDICINE 101

I'm often asked how one becomes competent as an expedition doctor. There is no single pathway, but this section will serve as an informal guide. There is no single specialty that prepares a person for expedition medicine. Generally, any primary care specialty such as family, internal, or emergency medicine will offer the broadest background. Historically, expedition doctors have come from essentially every discipline. Rescue doctors in the Alps, for example, are usually trained as anesthesiologists. No matter what your training, for most doctors, there is a general set of skills and knowledge that will enhance your competency in the expedition environment. If you're uncertain, review the following fundamentals before heading into the great unknown.

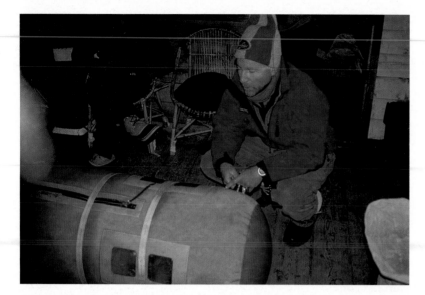

Figure 1.6. The Gamow bag saves lives at altitude. Photo courtesy of Howard Donner.

Tropical and Travel Medicine

Become familiar with the medical aspects of preparing for foreign travel. You will generally be considered the expert source for any questions regarding appropriate immunizations, malaria prophylaxis, and so on. These disorders can often be prevented if the team is instructed on specific precautions and prophylactic agents.

Familiarize yourself with the specific endemic diseases common in the area of your expedition, for example the local malaria risk, exotic diseases, local animal and arthropod hazards (e.g., dogs, snakes, scorpions, leeches). Depending on your destination, review common travel-acquired illnesses such as yellow fever, hepatitis, dengue, typhoid, paratyphoid fevers, meningococcal disease, and Japanese B encephalitis.

Learn all you can about intestinal protozoa and the all-pervasive diarrhea in travelers. Review preventative methods such as appropriate camp hygiene and other measures. Learn how to differentiate clinically between dysenteric and nondysenteric diarrheas, including when to treat conservatively and when to incorporate anti-infectives. Develop expertise in the principles of water disinfection methods, and be able to advise on which techniques provide efficacy for the specific pathogens in your part of the world.

See Chapter 17 for more information.

Environmental Concerns

Review the current management of cold injury, including prevention and treatment of hypothermia and frostbite for those heading toward cold environs. Consider learning more about heat illness, even if you're going to colder climes. Heat problems are common in overdressed climbers on sunny days, and, of course, in the tropics and desert. A comprehensive understanding of altitude problems, such as acute mountain sickness, high-altitude pulmonary edema, and high-altitude cerebral edema, is requisite for those "going higher." Review the latest drugs used for both prevention and treatment of altitude-related disorders. Become familiar with other high-altitude disorders such as periodic breathing, sleep disorders, retinal hemorrhage, and focal neurological deficits. Gain some experience in the use of the Gamow bag or other portable hyperbaric system. (See Chapter 19 on high-altitude medicine.) Consider other specific environmental concerns (e.g., marine envenomation and motion sickness on an ocean-based trip). (See Figures 1.6 and 1.7.)

Trauma

If it's been a while since you've managed emergencies and trauma, you should consider taking an advanced trauma life support (ATLS) course, which includes a thorough review of the initial evaluation and management of trauma. The course includes hands-on

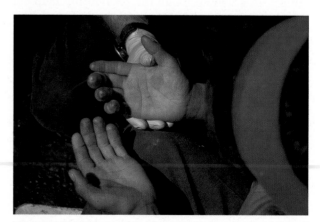

Figure 1.7. Frostbite on a Nepali porter. Photo courtesy of Howard Donner.

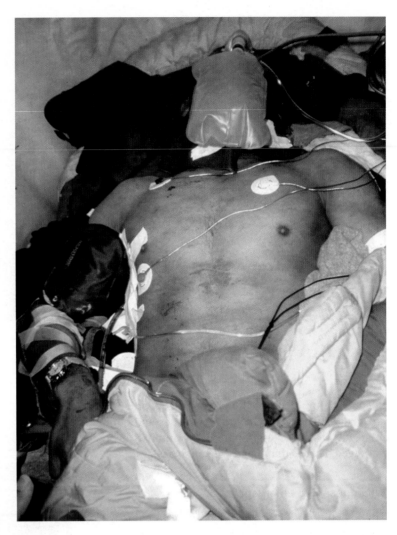

Figure **1.8**. Severe injuries on Denali including hemo-pneumothorax, midthoracic spine fracture with cord transection, suspected femur fracture, and hypothermia. Photo courtesy of Howard Donner.

training in important procedures such as endotracheal intubation, needle thoracostomy, and chest tube placement. These skills are key for providing a high level of trauma support on an expedition. If ATLS seems out of your scope, at least consider a course such as wilderness first responder (WFR) or its equivalent. Physicians sometimes wonder if a course like that would be too remedial. Remember that office-based doctors often get that "deer in the headlights" look when confronted with an emergency outside the confines of the office or hospital. These courses teach a systematic approach to evaluating trauma and help students become comfortable with handling and transporting injured patients in the outdoor environment. (See Figure 1.8.)

Orthopedics

You will need to be comfortable improvising splints for common orthopedic injuries and fractures, including the use of the SAM® Splint or other improvised splinting systems. The improvisation and application of femoral

traction should also be learned. Learn to recognize and treat common overuse syndromes that inevitably present as aches and pains on the trail (e.g., "sahib's knee" and tendonitis). You may also wish to review the use of adhesive tape for stabilizing the inevitable sprains and strains of expedition life (i.e., thumbs and ankles). Many dogmatic axioms such as "splint 'em as they lie" have become archaic and offer little merit when managing patients far from the road. If that statement surprises you, take a WFR course.

Wound Care

You will need to be adept at wound care management of basic lacerations and abrasions, including the use of suturing material (both skin and deep), surgical staplers, and tissue adhesives (e.g., glue). (See Figure 1.9.) Reexamine the optimal treatment for complicated blisters and burns, including new materials for treatment. Review the surgical management of ingrown toenails, subungual hematoma, and incision and drainage of abscesses.

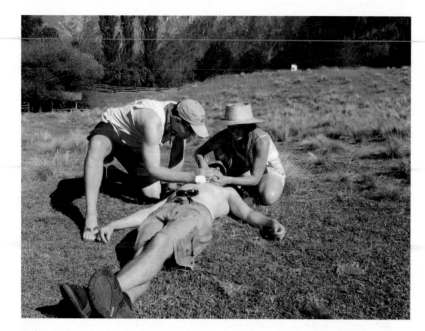

Figure 1.9. Simple wound repair with tissue adhesive in Patagonia. Photo courtesy of Howard Donner.

Epistaxis

Become familiar with the acute management of epistaxis. This should include techniques and equipment for nasal packing. There are a number of pre-packaged devices that make this much easier.

Wilderness Eye Emergencies

The expedition doctor should become familiar with the management of corneal foreign bodies, abrasions, and infections, including corneal ulcers. Familiarize yourself with the management and prevention of ultraviolet photokeratitis (snow blindness). (See Figure 1.10.)

Dental

My first extended medical experience in the Himalayas was with the Himalayan Rescue Association (HRA). I ran a small aid post in Manang, which is located in the Annapurna region of Nepal. I worked in Manang with an American nurse practitioner named Mariane Gilbert. On our first day of clinic operation, a visiting schoolteacher from the south presented with a severe toothache. He conveyed that he had recently had a molar extracted but felt that "they didn't get it all out." On exam there was an abscess surrounding residual roots remaining from the extraction. He was obviously suffering. My first reaction was to simply inform him that he needed to walk to the closest dental clinic, which was approximately three days down the trail by foot. Hearing my advice, Mariane asked me why we couldn't just do it for him.

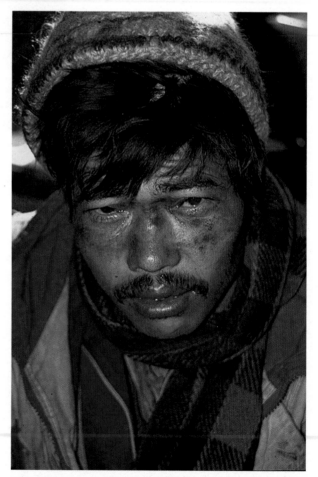

Figure 1.10. Severe ultraviolet photokeratitis in Pheriche, Nepal. Photo courtesy of Howard Donner.

I said, "I would love to oblige him; however, I don't have any dental equipment."

Mariane immediately pointed out that she had brought a small dental set from her personal dentist back in the States (including extractors, elevators, and dental syringes).

I said, "That's wonderful but I don't know how to perform any kind of dental procedures." In fact, like many medical students, I had received only a one-hour lecture on dentistry. Furthermore, I never really enjoyed working in patients' mouths.

Mariane gleefully announced that she had brought along a small handbook titled "Where There Is No Dentist" published by the Hesperian Foundation. At that point I was clearly defeated, and decided to attempt the procedure. The mandibular block went pretty well, and we proceeded to remove the remaining molar roots. To my surprise, the patient was satisfied. He thanked us, and left the clinic.

Following his departure I remarked, "I hope we don't see any more dental patients." The next day there was a small line in front of the clinic. The locals had heard that there was a "dentist" in town. For the rest of our time at Manang, we found ourselves intermittently attending to dental issues. We performed a lot of extractions that season. (See Figure 1.11.)

Develop some basic dental skills such as the use of temporary filling material (e.g., Cavit), and perhaps some more sophisticated skills such as the simple extraction of abscessed teeth. Your personal dentist can be a valuable resource.

Nursing Skills

Learn or relearn basic nursing skills. I can't emphasize this enough. This may frighten the overpampered physician, but you will need to administer all of the intramuscular and intravenous medications and fluids carried. Unless you're very fortunate, you won't be able

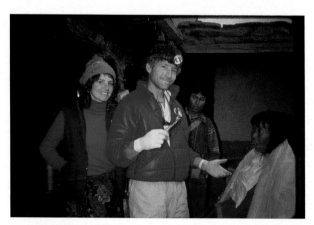

Figure 1.11. Tooth extraction in Manage, Nepal. Photo courtesy of Howard Donner.

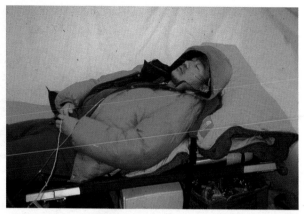

Figure 1.12. Severe HAPE on Denali. Photo courtesy of Howard Donner.

to "call a nurse." When is the last time you started an intravenous line?

Oxygen Delivery Systems

As with nursing skills, it may have been some time since you have needed to change regulators or fill and maintain oxygen bottles. Review the basics with an EMT or respiratory therapist. (See Figure 1.12.)

Basic Rescue Concepts and Skills

You won't be expected to rig for technical rescue, but you will be expected to know how to package a patient in a litter. Familiarize yourself with basic patient transportation and evacuation systems including improvised methods if necessary. Consider long-term care issues including bowel and bladder function during extended evacuation. (See Figures 1.13 and 1.14.)

Aeromedical Rescue Principles/Helicopter Operations

If you work in expedition medicine sooner or later you will be involved in a helicopter rescue. At the very least, you should learn how "not to be stupid" around a helicopter while loading a patient. Dangerous mistakes are easy to make around working helicopters. No matter how exciting helicopter rescue may seem, never get lulled into the idea that it's always the way to go. A helicopter mountain rescue operation is a high-risk endeavor for the pilot and crew as well as the patient. Always weigh the risk against the benefit. Often a ground-based evacuation makes more sense for noncritical patients. I have angered climbers on Denali for refusing to fly them out for frostbitten toes. "But that's how we do it in the Alps." Sorry, it's not how we do it on Denali. In the Alaska range, the risk of danger to pilot and crew does not justify the small

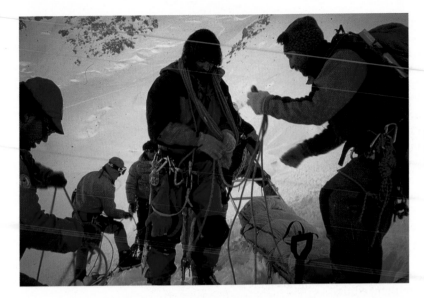

Figure 1.13. Climber rescue on Denali with volunteer guides and climbers. Photo courtesy of Howard Donner.

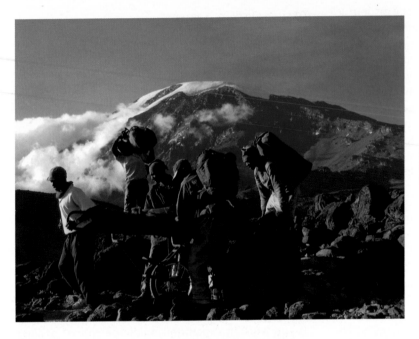

Figure 1.14. Transport of a HAPE patient off of Mount Kilimanjaro. Photo courtesy of Howard Donner.

advantage in tissue preservation of a toe. As always, use common sense. (See Figure 1.15.)

Environmental Specific Rescue Considerations

You should review avalanche rescue operations for ski- or snow-based mountaineering trips and crevasse rescue techniques for any glacial climbing trips. Additional skills may be required and will be dictated by the specific environment.

Expedition Communication Systems

Spend a little time familiarizing yourself with the proper use and etiquette of handheld radios. You won't want to sound like a "geek" when talking with guides and rescue personnel. As a rule of thumb, less is usually better. Satellite phones often provide an essential link in true expeditionary emergencies. Learn about the idiosyncrasies and nuances of your devices. One of the doctor's responsibilities should be to get to know the phone prior to departure. Don't wait until you need it to do this. Remember, you need to be "in sight" of the satellite for operation. Your location on the planet will change the relative position of the satellite, so read up. Learn the fundamentals of personal locator beacons (PLBs), or emergency position-indicating radio beacon (EPIRBs), if your expedition is using them. At the very least, learn how to activate them.

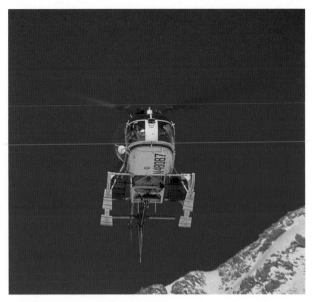

Figure 1.15. The "Denali Lama." Photo courtesy of Howard Donner.

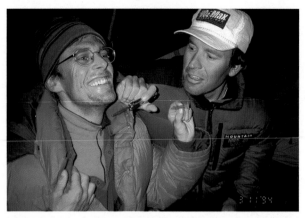

Figure 1.16. David Carter and Ed Viesters with improvised cricothy-rotomy tube and Leatherman. Photo courtesy of Howard Donner.

Wilderness Medical Improvisation

At the heart of expedition medicine is improvisation, using available gear and commonsense problem solving. Defined as "to fabricate out of what is conveniently at hand," improvisation encompasses many variations, is governed by few absolute rights and wrongs, and is limited more often by imagination than by personnel or equipment. When you work with an improvised system, you should test your creation on a noninjured person ("work out the bugs") before applying it to a victim. Include materials that lend themselves to improvisation in the expedition gear to enhance efficiency (e.g., duct tape). Creativity is needed when searching for improvisational materials.

One season I was working for the Himalayan Rescue Association (HRA) at the Pheriche clinic, located at 14,500 feet a couple of days below the Everest base camp. Normally the snow level during trekking season is about 17,000 feet. During that season, however, there was an enormous unseasonable snowfall, which blanketed the entire Khumbu region in deep snow down to 12,000 feet. Many trekking groups were caught off guard. The real casualties were the porters. We treated dozens of cases of severe frostbite of hands, knees, and feet. Many porters trek without sunglasses. With the unexpected snow and high UV reflectivity, we ended up treating dozens of cases of severe ultraviolet photokeratitis (snow blindness).

The standard treatment consists of topical therapy, pressure patching, and avoidance of further exposure. Unfortunately neither the local guesthouses nor our small clinic had the resources to house, much less treat, hundreds of porters. By now the sun was out and the bright snow and severe ocular symptoms made a

walkout by the porters impossible without sunglasses. Luckily, on a prior expedition, I had apparently had too much time on my hands. I had placed an emergency space blanket over my head, for reasons I can't remember, and realized that I could see through the aluminized Mylar. Remembering this, we quickly cut up an available space blanket, and duct taped strips over our patient's eyes. In this way we were able to fashion dozens of improvised Mylar sunglasses. The porters were able to make their way downhill, but for the next week we entertained a lot of trekker comments regarding the "disco porters."(See Figure 1.17)

Often you can harvest items from the victim (e.g., backpacks can be dismantled to obtain foam pads and straps). When possible, practice constructing improvised systems before they are required in an actual rescue. Courses that teach many of these techniques, such as WFR ("Woofer") or wilderness EMT, are invaluable (see earlier discussion). Consider taking a course like that; you'll be glad you did.

On the 1997 NOVA Everest expedition, climber David Carter came close to needing a cricothyrotomy. Dr. Eric Weiss had shown me how to create a "cric tube" out of a 3-mil syringe barrel cut off at 45 degrees. Fortunately, David did not require that intervention, but improvised tricks like that are good to know. (See Figure 1.16)

Proficiency in Expedition Specific Activities

The National Park System (NPS) maintains a medical rescue camp at 14,000 feet on the west buttress of Denali. No matter what the climbing resume of the doctor looks like, the NPS requires the rescue doctor to have climbed on Denali before working there. This is required because the extremes of the mountain could easily interfere with the medical mission. If the rescue doctor was inordinately distracted by the extreme arctic conditions, rescues and personnel could be compromised. Try to imagine your role

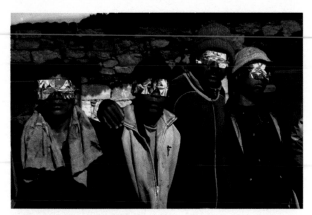

Figure 1.17. Improvised sunglasses from an emergency space blanket. Photo courtesy of Howard Donner.

as expedition doctor and do what you can to avoid becoming a liability. Get in shape, become proficient in that environment, and test your personal gear before you leave to "work out the bugs." Expedition life will force you out of your standard comfort envelope. (See Figure 1.18.)

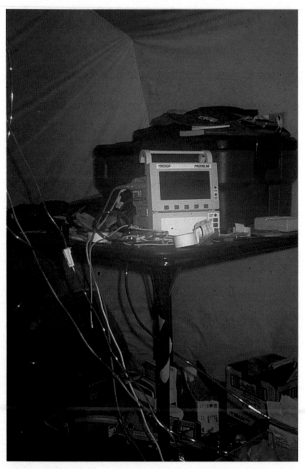

Figure 1.18. Austere working environment at 14,000 feet, Denali. Photo courtesy of Howard Donner.

Temperament

Most doctors learn to perform well under duress. This quality remains paramount in the expedition environment. As already noted, little in the expedition environment goes exactly as planned. Expedition doctors should cultivate their ability to remain cool under fire. In my experience, that ability is largely inherent in personality. Consider the following potentially stressful situations:

- How do you do in surgery when the intern drops the retractor?
- How do you respond in the emergency department when equipment malfunctions?
- How do you behave during a code?
- How do you respond to a flat tire?
- How do you react to an unexpected downpour on a day-hike?
- How well do you function without an interpreter?

These responses probably won't change when you go to work abroad.

Egos

Adventurers and expedition team members often have large egos associated with control issues. Part of the art of expedition medicine is learning diplomacy and control in the face of what may seem like tyrannical leadership. It helps to discuss the leadership hierarchy before you leave. Expedition doctors often assume that they will have the final word on medical decisions in the field. This is not always so. The expedition leader may feel that a medical decision will compromise the group dynamic or safety. In these cases, try to control your own ego and focus on your work as advocate for the patient. The ultimate game plan may not be yours.

It's Not Like the Textbooks

Just as in an office-based practice, it takes some time and experience to develop an expedition-oriented clinical acumen. Patients may not present as in the textbooks. For example, a patient with high-altitude pulmonary edema probably won't approach you and offer a history of increasing shortness of breath at rest. More likely their "presentation" will be coming into camp later than usual. Team members are often reluctant to offer an admission of early illness. Keep your radar going, go to the person's tent and ask, "What's up?"

PREEXPEDITION CONSIDERATIONS

Medical Fitness of Potential Team Members

Get involved early in the planning phases of the expedition. You can provide essential information relating to the physical abilities or medical fitness of potential team members. There may be a need for objective fitness testing, but keep in mind that certain intangible factors come into play on expeditions. I have seen some of the slowest and least probable members of expeditions slowly and steadily make their way to the summit (á la tortoise vs. hare). There are few absolutes and every team member will come to the expedition with his or her preexisting attitude toward risk. The sticky issue is addressing medical conditions that might compromise the quality or safety of the trip for other team members.

Preexpedition Medical History

A medical history should be obtained for all participants before heading out.

Rescue Preplan

Prearrange for formal rescue and become familiar with avenues to take should the need arise. This will include communication channels, insurance issues, local evacuation capabilities and resources, and medical facilities. These arrangements can usually be made through the embassy of the country sponsoring the expedition and augmented by local trekking or guiding agencies. The medical expertise within the team should be determined as well. That information will be key when managing a medical emergency or orchestrating a rescue. Prearrangements can greatly expedite the rescue process should the need arise.

Medical Oxygen Considerations

Although many high-altitude expeditions are getting away from the traditional use of climbing oxygen, it is certainly prudent to bring medical oxygen on most large-scale expeditions or treks. Remember that there are stringent regulations involving the shipping of medical oxygen via aircraft. Oxygen is considered a hazardous material. You have several alternatives:

- Ship your oxygen by surface at least three months in advance.
- Plan to purchase or rent your oxygen equipment in the country of your expedition. (*Note:* Oxygen is next to impossible to obtain in many developing countries.)
- Prearrange to have the oxygen shipped via airfreight utilizing the assistance of a hazardous materials shipper. Inquire well in advance!

Team Medical Training

Sometimes wilderness medical training for the team can be accomplished during the preexpedition planning meetings. These sessions can help to build team dynamics

as well. In reality, time and geography may make this difficult, and team members may be served by attending a WFR course prior to the expedition. (See earlier discussion.)

EXPEDITION CONSIDERATIONS

Camp Hygiene

Remain in control of camp hygiene, especially cooking practices. Expeditions that take camp hygiene seriously fare better in the battle against the ubiquitous gastrointestinal and respiratory illnesses that plague foreign travel in general and expeditions in particular. I have seen tyrannical (and successful) expedition leaders on Everest, ban other expeditions' climbers, with nothing more than a sniffle, from entering their base camp tents. Often team members will be naive to basic principles of hygiene. Use your clout as expedition doctor to promote wellness habits such as pre-meal handwashing.

Nutrition and Health Care Maintenance

The expedition environment is a notorious place for malnutrition and weight loss. On longer duration expeditions, especially at high altitude, nutritional consultation offered by the doctor can add to the medical well-being of the group and thereby the success of the expedition. Become familiar with the specter of high-altitude deterioration. Team members may lose a significant percentage of their body weight including lean muscle mass. Caloric and nutritional needs are discussed in Chapter 7; be ready to advise your group on optimizing diet in the expedition environment. Do not, however, insist on food that team members shun. Ultimately, expedition diets must taste good, or your team simply won't eat enough.

Medical Inventory

Continuously maintain the expedition medical kits. Strive to maintain an inventory of what has been used and remain mindful of specific drugs and equipment that may no longer be available. On some expeditions, restocking inventory from local towns or cities may be possible.

Medical Records

For many expedition doctors, the promise of escaping the world of medical bureaucracies and records is partly what beckons them to the wilds. Nonetheless, at least rudimentary records are important, especially for quality follow-up upon return. Attempt to maintain some form of medical record. A dedicated waterproof notebook will usually suffice as a patient log and ongoing medical record. You may choose to keep it simple, but always include the date, diagnosis, and treatment, including the specific drugs dispensed. Discuss potential signs and symptoms, which would prompt medical follow-up after leaving the expedition. Be prepared to notify the patient's primary care doctor upon returning home if necessary.

Medical Care of Individuals Not Part of the Expedition

As expedition physician, your primary responsibility is your expedition group. You will, however, invariably be called upon to help individuals who are not part of your expedition. On one of my first trips to Nepal, I was working as a doctor on a small expedition. It was early in the spring prior to the regular trekking season. Our team was carrying medical supplies for our trip, but I had no intention of making my medical presence known on our way in. As we approached each small village, dozens of villagers would surround our expedition and ask for medicine for various ailments.

After a few of these encounters, I approached our "sirdar" (head porter) and asked, "Why are you telling these villagers that there's a doctor coming through town, I'm not really prepared to provide medical care en route."

The sirdar replied, "I'm not telling anyone that you're a doctor, they just see an expedition coming through town and assume that we will have medicine and most likely a doctor."

Trekking groups and expeditions have historically provided extemporaneous medical care on the way in, but this routine practice has inherent shortcomings. Handing out wholesale medicines on the trail may seem innocuous, but there are potential drawbacks that should be considered. Doctors instinctively wish to help, but consider that in many developing countries, the government attempts to establish and maintain local health posts. It is common practice for nonmedical trekkers to hand out small handfuls of potentially inappropriate antibiotics. This may be in place of a specific antibiotic, in appropriate doses, for an appropriate duration. The patient may also require follow-up, which is typically nonexistent in this kind of interaction. Delivering wholesale medicine on the trail can undermine the confidence that locals have in their internal health care systems. Additionally, inappropriate or inadequate trailside treatment may destroy confidence in Western medicine, thus leading villagers away from appropriate care in the future.

Remember that many people in developing countries have little understanding of the basis of Western medical practice (e.g., the word for "germ" in Nepali is the same as that for "insect"). The use of pills is often misunderstood. More significance may be attributed to the shape or color of the pill than the medicine itself. Patients may attempt to collect medicines, which are then indiscriminately distributed to others at a later time. Consider teaching "self-care" methods (e.g., wound hygiene, hydration for diarrhea) rather than being eager to dispense medication. Be certain that if treatment is provided, full explanation and written instructions are given (using symbols or via interpreter). Perhaps more importantly, do not indulge in "heroic fantasy." The fact that you are trekking through does not imply that you must take on the responsibility for the village health care. Use common sense; clearly some trailside scenarios call for treatment.

Health Care for Local Staff

An often-neglected aspect of expeditionary medicine is the health care of the team's porters, local guides, and other staff. As obvious as this may seem, they should be treated with the same medical care as any other (Western) member of the expedition team. Historically, expeditions have not always abided by this ethic. A common misconception is that porters are natives and thus immune to the problems that affect Westerners. Unfortunately, serious illness and death continue to occur in porters because they simply were not observed for symptoms of hypothermia, frostbite, altitude illness, and the like. Remember, as expedition physician, your responsibilities extend to your ancillary staff as well as your Western expedition members. Remain proactive (i.e., if a porter is late coming into camp, find out why).

STANDARDS

This textbook includes a detailed chapter on medical legal considerations. There are however, a few points regarding standard of care that an expedition doctor should keep in mind. I'm not interested in making attorneys happy, but I am concerned about optimizing care. The standard of care is clearly a function of your environment. The standard of care on a dog sled expedition to the Antarctic is obviously going to differ from the standard of care in the emergency department of your local hospital. Standard of care issues, however, should not automatically be used as justification for suboptimal therapy. For example, in Nepal, I took care of a patient with a badly infected hand. The patient had been bitten on the hand by a dog while trekking through a remote village. Over time, the wounds became infected, and I was asked to see the patient. A doctor, along on the trek, had initially treated the patient. The treatment consisted of nothing more than the application of antibiotic ointment applied to the wounds. The doctor advised the patient that nothing more involved could be done in that environment. Clearly, even on a trek, standard of care would have been high pressure, syringe irrigation, with disinfected (or drinking quality) water. The attending physician should have realized that at best, the simple application of antibiotic ointment was less than the available standard of care.

Similarly, a physician who provides support for a high-altitude trek or expedition should become familiar with the probable medical entities that exist in that environment. Mistaking high-altitude pulmonary edema for pneumonia, and subsequently failing to descend that patient appropriately, would be a preventable mistake. It is assumed that any doctor agreeing to provide medical support for a high-altitude expedition would become somewhat versed in common high-altitude syndromes. If I have reason to believe that I'm providing a patient with less than the expected standard of care, I inform them. For example, if I'm treating a complicated wound infection in an expedition environment I might say to the patient, "at this point your treatment might include a wound culture, but that isn't possible here." "I'll choose the most appropriate antibiotic empirically, which should do the trick, but it's not optimal therapy." I inform the patient that it may not be the optimal antibiotic because we don't have cultures to guide our therapy. At that point, the patient has the information he or she needs to choose the best course of action. (Evacuate to obtain a higher level of care, and obtain a wound culture, or remain in the field and consciously accept some risk.) After discussing potential outcomes, I feel comfortable leaving it up to the patient. If the patient is someone I don't know very well, I might include the expedition leader or other responsible person in the discussion, as an informal witness. Reassure yourself with the following notion: In the rare case of potential malpractice, you will hopefully employ an expert witness that will present the standard of care from the wilderness medical perspective. More importantly, if you practice expedition medicine for prolonged periods, you'll never earn enough money to accrue enough equity, to worry about an adverse lawsuit. Moreover, you could pay attention to Chapter 5.

FINAL THOUGHTS – "PHYSICIAN, HEAL THYSELF"

The Doctor Is Not In

If you hope to survive an extended expedition in good form, when possible, be good to yourself. As an expedition doctor you are expected to be available "24-7" for any unexpected emergency. In my experience on larger expedition, there is a certain fatigue that comes with a never-ending 24-hour call. Although it may seem silly to arbitrarily designate "doctor's hours" on an expedition, it can be beneficial for your mental health. Set up specific hours during the day when expedition members can come to you with routine or chronic problems. On smaller trips or trips of shorter duration, this may not be necessary, but on large trips, it can prevent expedition doctor burnout. The first time I worked for the HRA, I made the mistake of bringing an old teaching

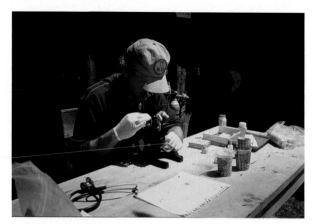

Figure 1.19. Stool samples and dining table may not be a good mix. Photo courtesy of Howard Donner.

microscope to the clinic. I figured it might be helpful for differentiating between bacterial and protozoan diarrheal etiologies. I realized that the system wasn't working because trekkers would walk in and set a steaming cup of stool next to my breakfast eggs. The clinic boundaries were weakening, so we discontinued evaluating stool samples. (See Figure 1.19.)

"I Felt Like a Band-Aid Dispenser"

Physicians returning from their first expedition often insinuate, "It wasn't as cool as in the slideshows." Those slideshows pack a lot of action into 50 minutes. It's usually not quite as exciting in "real time." Expedition life at times feels somewhat mundane. Expect to have "down" moments or days. Typically, just as things settle down, something unusual upsets the equilibrium. That's the normal ebb and flow of expedition life.

Returning doctors sometimes reflect on their experience, noting that instead of placing chest tubes they were handing out band-aids. One practical remedy for that is to advise your team prior to leaving that you expect them all to carry their own personal kits. You might offer them a list of items you expect them to carry. This technique also protects the neatly organized expedition medical kit from constant rummaging.

The personal kit includes commonly used items and might contain the following:

- Nonnarcotic analgesics (e.g., NSAIDs)
- Throat lozenges or cough drops
- Sunscreen and lip protection
- Basic blister care
- Minor wound care (e.g., band-aids)
- Insect repellant
- Vitamins
- Malaria prophylaxis (if indicated)
- Personal medications (for preexisting conditions)

Summation

Often we in the medical profession can begin to lose sight of the original motivations that attracted us to medicine. There is something extraordinarily fulfilling and rejuvenating about helping people in a natural realm, removed from technology, bureaucracies, and legal systems. Expedition medicine is all about common sense and creativity. Its challenges and freedoms can renew a sense of enthusiasm for medicine in its purest form.

In many ways, an old friend of mine, Redge Lake, summed it all up. He was a pioneer of kayaking first descents. He would tell friends that there were three things that were important when starting an expedition.

- "Don't be stupid." That essentially sums up what this book is about. Learn as much as you can and mitigate risks with proper preparation and judgment.
- "Stuff happens." This was his reminder that no matter how thorough your preparation, there will always be unanticipated events. It is the unexpected quality of expedition life that in fact, makes it compelling.
- "Bring beer." Redge was not advocating imbibing prior to steep river descents. He was using beer as a metaphor: to be in the moment, to have fun. No matter how dreadful the expedition, when you finally return, you'll be dreaming you were back in the wilds.

ACKNOWLEDGMENTS

As this chapter was based on my experience and not other written materials, I would like to use this space to acknowledge my career-long mentors and guiding lights.

Dr. Charles Houston, the visionary and prime inspiration for many of us in the field of expedition and wilderness medicine.

Dr. Peter Hackett, the quintessential expedition doctor, high-altitude scientist, and innovator. When will they build a Peter Hackett action figure?

Dr. Eric Weiss, my close friend and wilderness medicine partner in crime.

Dr. David Schlim, a brilliant doctor and source for practical information on myriad infectious diseases affecting the foreign traveler, trekker, and climber.

Mr. Lanny Johnson, a great friend with unparalleled wisdom in the arena of rescue medicine.

Dr. Joe Serra, my wilderness orthopedics guru, old friend, and original wilderness medicine coconspirator.

Dr. Paul Auerbach, my ongoing tor-mentor [sic].

Dr. Howard Backer, my close friend, mentor, and only friend who knows everything about water disinfection and disease.

Dr. Gene Allred, friend and wilderness medicine educator bar none.

Dr. Jim Wilkerson, his field guide, was innovative and far ahead of his time.

Dr. Cameron Bangs, the guy who taught me that teaching could be exciting if the teacher was electrified by the subject. Unfortunately, most medical school professors never met Cameron.

Evan Donner, Valeska Armisen, Martha Donner, Catherine Soutter.

2 | Assessing Expedition Medical Needs

William W. Forgey, MD

Having to evacuate a trip member for any reason, be it physical or psychological, disrupts, even can cancel, an expedition and places other trip members and rescuers at possible personal risk. The pretrip history and physical evaluation is the first defense in preventing the subsequent evacuation. Maintaining vigilance as to the trip members' medical and mental status during the trip is the second step toward prevention of this expensive and risky event.

A caveat that cannot be ignored, due to legal reasons, is that if you are going to request medical information of a participant, make certain that you do something appropriate with the information. Protect the access of this information from persons who do not have a need to know these personal medical details. Review the history and physical information and make decisions concerning the applicant's appropriateness for the trip or otherwise ensure that you will be able to manage any problems that are identified during the course of the expedition.

Legal actions taken against trip organizers always start with the material provided by the client before the trip making sure that the risk was appropriately described, that the participant understood it, and that health and other protective services were as indicated in the pretrip materials (see Chapter 5). One aspect that will be scrutinized is the information obtained by the medical history and physical. If the trip involves considerable physiological stressors, and the client was not informed of this and was not advised to have appropriate medical screening, you will be vulnerable to a tort action. If this was accomplished and you failed to note a condition that, in retrospect, would have disqualified the client from participating in the activity, you will also be at legal risk. If you take a person whose physical or mental ability does not seem reasonably able to manage the potential events of the expedition, you must provide an adequate safety net, or clearly describe to the client, in writing, your inability to do so. In this manner, you transfer some of the risk to the client. Remember that it is normally not the client, but a relative, who sues. The client's enthusiasm for participating may not be matched by a surviving family member. Their attorney will pick apart the management of any accident, basing the case not so much on how the accident was managed in the field (and you can believe this will be perused in detail also) but on that common medical concept of informed consent.

The way to protect your expedition from both legal and medical dilemmas is to develop a Risk Assessment and Management Plan (see Table 2.1). To accomplish this plan, you must be able to

1. Anticipate possible adverse events
2. Identify and eliminate causes of accidents
3. Determine what should be done if leadership becomes ill or killed
4. Develop an emergency response plan
5. Familiarize yourself with the medical history, general health, and stamina of each participant.

One of the most important tools is a medical history taken on every participant, even on your personal friends (see Table 2.2.) Eighty percent of a medical diagnosis is usually attributed to the medical history. Sometimes

---

Table 2.1. The risk assessment and management plan[a]

- Undertake pretrip medical evaluation and screening
  - Develop basis and indications for individual physiologic testing pretrip
  - Establish psychological predictors for success
  - Determine medical disqualifiers prior to initiating participant recruiting
- Analyze data
  - Identify special medical needs
  - Determine immunization status (see Chapter 4)
  - Establish appropriateness of participation approved
  - Augment group medical kit for individual needs (see Chapter 3)
- Develop a risk assessment and management plan
- Convey level of risk to participants
- Inform participants of medical capability and evacuation/ care plan

[a] This chapter will concentrate on the issues of the medical history and pretrip physical examination.

Table 2.2. Medical history form

Applicant Information
1. Name
2. Age
3. Date of birth
4. Gender
5. Home address
6. Daytime or cell phone
7. Home phone
8. E-mail address

Insurance Information
1. Insurance company
2. Policy number
3. Insurance company address
4. Insurance company telephone number – contact
5. Name of insured
6. Relationship

Health Questions
Indicate if you have had any of the following conditions in the past 2 years:
1. Respiratory/pulmonary disease (asthma, COPD, etc.)
2. Seizures
3. Heart condition or high blood pressure
4. Diabetes
5. Do you currently have an infectious condition?

Allergies
1. Please list all allergies to medications, food, or environment (insect stings, etc.)
2. List date of last reaction
3. Type of reaction
4. Treatment
5. Did you receive a prescription for epinephrine?

Medications
1. List all medications, both prescription and over-the-counter, which you are taking.
2. List dosage, specific times of day, and length of time which you have been on the medication.
3. Indicate the reason for taking each medication.

Do you have any medical condition that might interfere with your ability to fully participate on the proposed expedition?

When did you last see a physician or other medical professional and why?

Is there anything else you would like for the Expedition leadership to know?

the history is obvious, such as a witnessed accident. But usually, someone is suddenly ill, not feeling well, or having pain, and the major clues of the diagnosis have to be fished from the history. You might not be aware of critical details in even a close friend's history. His use of a beta-blocker to treat high blood pressure, for example, could result in a severe and unanticipated reaction to the use of epinephrine from your medical kit when treating anaphylaxis, which would otherwise have been an appropriate first-aid medication.

The proper medical history will have "qualifier" questions. An example is to request a list of current medications as well as to identify chronic medical conditions. A person might say that he does not have any chronic

condition, yet mention that he is taking an oral diabetic medication. To the client's way of thinking he does not have a chronic "medical condition." It is possible for an athlete to have knee surgery, be told that she is released, and not to consider that three months later she needs to report this recent surgery. An alerting qualifier question could be: "When was the last time you saw a doctor and for what purpose?" The answer "I have no medical problems" is thus clarified with the answer "I saw a doctor three months ago for release from my knee surgery."

The degree of isolation, possible environmental stress, and distance from medical care make the selection and medical knowledge concerning participants a critical part of the Risk Assessment and Management Plan.

HISTORY THRESHOLDS

History thresholds are clues in the medical history that alert the expedition medical planners or staff of levels of risk in the participant candidate.[1] Each component of the history that acts as a potential alert will be discussed with suggestions on how to further evaluate the possible concerns. Medical Alert thresholds can be divided into four classes of increasing concern.

Level One

A Level One threshold would not be a disqualification issue, but it would alert planners to the need for augmentation of the expedition medical kit, the need for the participant to bring appropriate personal medications, and the possibility for a problem with food or local allergens that might require adjustment of meal content or camping technique. A Level One threshold requires verification by directly questioning the participant candidate on the particulars. (See Table 2.3.)

The need for continued use of nonprescription medications is an indicator of a chronic problem that may have not been addressed by a physician or other appropriate medical professional. The reviewer should inquire about frequency and severity of symptoms. The response may indicate no further action or may suggest a medical evaluation by the participant's physician.

Birth control pills place users at a higher risk of phlebitis, especially if the woman also smokes. Their use may indicate a problem with frequency of menses or menorrhagia that requires hormonal control. It may indicate a person who is at risk of pregnancy and for whom a pregnancy test kit may be required in the medical kit for diagnostic purposes.

The use of one or two prescription medications should be noted. A reserve supply of the medications needs to be maintained in the expedition medical kit. The underlying problem being treated must be in stable condition and be a condition that the expedition medics will either

Table 2.3. Medical history alert level one Thresholds	
Category	**Concern**
Medication	Regular/frequent nonprescription use
Medication	Birth control pills
Medication	Fewer than 3 (nonpsychotropic)
Allergy	Ingestion – local reaction, not anaphylaxis
Allergy	Inhalation – local reaction, not anaphylaxis
Allergy	Injection/bite/sting – local, not anaphylaxis
Allergy	Physical contact – local, not anaphylaxis
Allergy	Eyes/nose – not anaphylaxis
Asthma	Use of rescue inhaler twice a month or less
Head injury	No impairment
Headaches/migraines	Fewer than two per month (average)
Heart condition	Functional murmur, age younger than 50
Hernia	No restriction on activity
Hospitalization	Over 1 year ago
Injuries (fractures, sprains)	Over 1 year ago
Scoliosis	No restriction on activity
Surgery	Over 1 year ago
Tobacco use	

not be expected to treat or that they would find manageable with their level of training.

Non-anaphylactic allergic reactions to ingestions of food, inhaled allergens, local irritations of eyes or allergic rhinitis, and contact dermatitis need to be addressed in the expedition planning phase to attempt to remove the known offending allergens from the person's environment. Changing diets so that the allergy can be avoided is frequently possible. An attempt can be made to avoid known causes of the participant's contact allergen. Avoiding inhaled allergens is more difficult and sometimes impossible to accomplish. The nature of the allergic reaction must be further questioned to ensure that the reaction is, indeed, nonsystemic in nature and only a less-serious local or delayed hypersensitivity reaction. The expedition candidate should be instructed to include the medication (frequently a nonprescription remedy) that he or she generally uses to treat or prevent the condition. An additional supply of this medication will also be added to the expedition medical kit to augment the person's supply of this medication.

Asthma episodes must be in good control or ceased being a significant medical problem. A threshold of requiring use of a rescue inhaler (albuterol) two times or fewer per month is an indication that the person's asthma is mild or under good medical management and control. The participant may be on multiple treatment medications.

A history of head injury with no impairment needs to be noted and further investigation conducted into the nature of the injury. If the person did not lose consciousness or only lost consciousness for 30 seconds or less, the injury can be considered minor, and no specific precautions are required.[2]

Headache is not a rare occurrence on wilderness expeditions as was indicated by Welch (see Chapter 3, Table 3.2) who demonstrated a rate of 10.1 incidents per 10,000 person days.[3] However, it was not a significant reason for terminating a trip in data provided by Boulware when looking at 280 long-distance Appalachian Trail hikers, representing 38,940 person-days of experience.[4] Headaches with a frequency of two per month on an average should suggest a medical review to determine the severity and diagnosis of the type of headache, whether or not the headache can be managed by the patient with nonprescription or prescription medications, and if the patient is incapacitated and for how long when the attacks occur. Provisions for personal and backup medications adequate to treat the patient's headaches must be available.

Generally a comment on the medical form that the expedition candidate has no restriction of activity even though he has an inguinal hernia needs clarification or confirmation from their personal physician. Strangulated hernias were a common cause of death amongst the voyageurs of the fur trade in Northern Canada and would certainly be a medical emergency on a modern expedition.

A history of hospitalization, fracture, sprain, or surgery over one year ago would generally not be of current medical concern. Briefly asking the candidate to ensure that there are no residual issues will suffice. Orthopedic issues, such as old injuries and scoliosis that carry no physical restrictions will be of no current concern if they are asymptomatic.

Tobacco use is a major risk factor for cardiovascular disease and may be a source of disagreement between smoking and nonsmoking members of the party. The medical reviewer should note the age of the participant and judge the number of pack-years of smoking history as a rough clue to potential personal health issues that the participant might have.

Level Two

Level Two thresholds are also generally not disqualification issues, but they do require further inquiry to complete the medical screen. Frequently, this can be through verification by directly questioning the participant candidate. At times permission to directly contact the participant's physician to confirm the participant's suitability will be appropriate. If this is necessary, the physician must have a clear understanding of the level of physical and mental stress to which the participant will be subjected in order to give informed advice.

A Level Two threshold issue might also require that the participant assume responsibility for a greater medical risk than he or she would otherwise have in civilization. The participant must be aware of the expedition medical staff's ability, or lack thereof, to deal with the medical issue which exists. (See Table 2.4.)

Persons on psychotropic medications who have not required a dosage change in three months can be considered stable. The medical reviewer should contact the participant and inquire if he or she plans to have a medication holiday during the expedition. This should be discouraged unless the underlying condition is mild or the person has experienced programmed lapses in medication without relapses or behavioral difficulties in the past.

Significant allergies to food items, bites, stings, injections, or contact must have a plan for avoidance and symptom management if avoidance fails. In the case of anaphylaxis, the affected expedition member must have a prescription for epinephrine from their physician, with an extra quantity for supply to the expedition medical kit. The person should have been desensitized by an allergist if possible. If there are multiple food allergens, it may be impossible to accommodate the individual as the basic food stocks for other trip members may require an adjustment that would not serve their best nutritional requirements or personal likes.

Anxiety that is mild enough not to require medication or that has been successfully treated with the same medication for the past three months should be a stable condition. A direct questioning of the client should confirm the status of this condition.

A youth participant's medical history may indicate autism or Asperger's syndrome. An inquiry to the client or his or her guardian or parent should indicate the social level of function the participant is capable of maintaining and the apparent suitability for the expedition.

A history of back pain needs further inquiry of the participant as to the need for medication for pain relief or muscle spasm treatment, the level of physical function that he or she is capable of performing, and if the person is occasionally restricted from physical activity. Has the participant had back surgery? In the case of frequent medication need, the use of routine pain medication, or a history of surgery, further inquiry is required. Ask when the last time medication was required, what medications were required, and how long the episode lasted. Judgment will have to be made as to the potential for capable performance on the expedition, and this might require sending an inquiry to the person's physician for a physical evaluation.

Like anxiety, depression that is mild enough not to require medication or that has been successfully treated with the same medication for the past three months should be a stable condition. A direct

Table 2.4. Medical history alert level two thresholds

Category	Concern
Medication	Psychotropic – stable for 3 months
ADD/ADHD	See medications for further thresholds.
Allergy	Ingestion – anaphylaxis
Allergy	Injection/bite/sting – anaphylaxis
Allergy	Physical contact – hypersensitive
Anxiety	On no medications
Anxiety	Stable on medication or medical plan for 3 months
Autistic/Asperger's syndrome	
Back pain	
Depression	No medications
Depression	Stable on medication for 3 months
Dizziness, syncope, malaise	Food/water intake related
Headache/migraines	More than two per month
Hernia	Restriction on duty
Hospitalizations	6 months to 1 year ago
Injuries (fracture/sprains)	3 months to 1 year ago
Physician restriction	Dietary restrictions
Physician restriction	Special considerations or restrictions
Scoliosis	Restriction on activity
Surgery	6 months or 1 year ago
Weight	Over 300 pounds or greater than threshold weights indicated in Table 2.5

questioning of the client should confirm the status of this condition.

Dizziness, syncope, or malaise that appears to be related to food or water intake are common complaints that, when made, need to be questioned. Generally, the applicant will state that either too little or too much water results in episodes of weakness, or that the symptom is either aggravated or made better by eating. Complaints of this nature will require inquiry of the participant's physician, and a clear diagnosis will need to be established. If the episode was a one-time occurrence, was trivial in nature, or can be controlled with appropriate diet and hydration, the complaint should not be significant.

Headaches that occur more than two per month would be acceptable if this is a stable pattern, diagnosis has been established, and the condition responds to treatment readily.

Untreated hernias that have a restriction on activity require inquiry to the treating physician as to the potential for strangulation or the exact limitations that need to be imposed. The answers to these questions would determine the appropriateness of the candidate's participation in the expedition.

Hospitalization from 6 months to 1 year ago, fractures or sprains that occurred 3 months to 1 year ago and a history of surgery from 6 months to 1 year ago need further inquiry to the participant. If insufficient detail or concern arises, the treating physician should be contacted. Physician inquiry should be made for all cases that have physician restrictions placed on them or special monitoring requirements or physical restrictions.

Obesity can be determined by height–weight measurements reported on the physical history form. Analysis of data from the National Health and Nutrition Examination Survey III 1988–1994 demonstrates that persons with a body mass index (BMI) equal to or greater than 27 kg/m^2 have high risk for other significant medical conditions: 70% have type 2 diabetes, 56% have hypertension, and 47% have high cholesterol.[5] The medical reviewer must be aware that these participant candidates are at a higher risk for cardiovascular events. It has also been shown that obese patients are significantly more likely than lean patients to experience complications and death after a traumatic injury.[6,7] (See Table 2.5.)

The recommended maximum weight equals a BMI of 31 kg/m^2, while the upper range of an acceptable weight for a person 35+ years is a body mass index of 27 kg/m^2. (See Table 2.6.)

The Boy Scouts of America National Sea Base has an absolute maximum weight of 300 pounds for a very practical reason: The ladders installed on their boats have a load limit rating for that amount.[8]

Table 2.5. Recommended weight for participation in strenuous activities

Recommended Weight (lb)			
Height	19–34 Years	35+ Years	Maximum[a]
5'0"	97–128	108–138	166
5'1"	101–132	111–143	172
5'2"	104–137	115–148	178
5'3"	107–141	119–152	183
5'4"	111–146	122–157	189
5'5"	114–150	126–162	195
5'6"	118–155	130–167	201
5'7"	121–160	134–179	207
5'8"	125–164	138–178	214
5'9"	129–169	142–183	220
5'10"	132–174	146–188	226
5'11"	136–179	151–194	233
6'	140–184	155–199	239
6'1"	144–189	159–205	246
6'2"	148–195	164–210	252
6'3"	152–200	168–216	260
6'4"	156–205	173–222	267
6'5"	160–211	177–228	274
6'6"	164–216	182–234	281

Note: This is the recommendation by the Boy Scouts of America for youth and adult participation in the sailing programs conducted through the Florida National Sea Base.
[a] Maximum weight equals a body mass index of approximately 31. Byrnes MC, McDaniel MD, Moore MB, Helmer SD, Smith RS. The effect of obesity on outcomes among injured patients. *J Trauma.* 2005;58(2):232–7.

Table 2.6. Weight standards

BMI (kg/m^2)	Weight Status
Below 18.5	Underweight
18.5–24.9	Normal
25.0–29.9	Overweight
30.0 and above	Obese

Evacuation of obese persons can be complicated by plane lift limitations for aeromedical rescue or place severe stress on persons attempting stretcher transport. These issues must be considered when identifying a potential participant who is obese.

The medical reviewer should also inquire into the candidate's general level of physical fitness, to ensure that his or her participation on a strenuous trip would be appropriate. Total weight is not always an indication of obesity or lack of aerobic fitness, but it should trigger a medical review that can usually consist of directly questioning the individual candidate.

Level Three

Level Three thresholds are usually not disqualification issues, but they might be depending upon the demands and resources of the expedition. These items do require further inquiry to complete the medical screen. This might be accomplished by simply directly questioning the candidate concerning the stability of the events that have been flagged as a Level Three threshold; however, usually verification of the fact will be necessary directly from the treating physician. As mentioned previously, the physician must have a clear understanding of the level of physical and mental stress to which the participant will be subjected in order to give informed advice. (See Table 2.7.)

A Level Three threshold issue requires that the participant assume responsibility for a greater medical risk than he or she would otherwise have in civilization. The participant must be aware of the expedition medical staff's ability, or lack thereof, to deal with the medical issue which exists.

If a candidate is taking three or more medications for any cause, there is increased responsibility for the expedition's medical team with regard to ensuring that the person is compliant with his or her medication schedule, that a "back-up" supply is obtained (usually from the individual) for the expedition medical kit, and that the medical condition(s) can be adequately managed in the field.

It is particularly important that certain conditions, such as asthma and the need for psychotropic medications, be stable. Generally this means that there has been no need to adjust the medications for the past 3 months. Chronic conditions that required a dosage or medication modification within the last 3 months may not be

Table 2.7. Medical history alert level three thresholds

Category	Concern
Medications	3 or more
Medications	Changed within previous 3 months when used to treat chronic condition
Medications	Medication usually taken but suspended for expedition
Allergy	Inhaled – anaphylaxis
Allergy	Physical contact – anaphylaxis
Allergy	Through eyes/nose – anaphylaxis
Anxiety	On medication less than 3 months
Asthma	Episodes more than twice a month
Asthma	Triggered by allergen likely to be encountered on expedition, regardless of attack frequency
Bipolar	
Blood pressure	High or low
Chest pains	
Depression	On medication less than 3 months
Diabetes	
Dizziness, fainting, syncope episodes	Not related to food or water intake
Ear infections	Frequent within the past 2 years
Eating disorder	
Head injury	Impairment
Heart condition	Other than functional murmur
Hospitalization	Within previous 3 months
Infection disease	Chronic
Injuries (fractures/ sprains)	Within previous 3 months
Respiratory disease	
Surgery	Within previous 6 months
Ulcer	Gastric or duodenal

optimally treated. Physician inquiry should be made when a recent medication alteration has been necessary.

Generally medications should not be suspended during the expedition. At times, such as with mild ADD/ADHD, this may be appropriate, and perhaps a "medication holiday" will be approved by the physician. Usually this should be discouraged. It must be particularly discouraged without prior experience with drug-free intervals or without the treating physician's approval.

Allergic reactions resulting in anaphylaxis, whether from inhaled, contact, or ingested allergens, are a great concern. It is possible that avoidance will not be possible on the expedition. Treating a life-threatening condition can be problematic and may be impossible in a wilderness area. The participant candidate must understand that epinephrine prescribed for his emergency use by his physician will only last 20 minutes and may not be effective at all when treating his/her reaction. The onset of the reaction may be too quick for the medical team to respond, and the patient will need to be capable of self-administering epinephrine. A back-up supply of epinephrine must be supplied by the participant for inclusion in the expedition medical kit, in addition to the supply carried in his or her personal medical kit. There may not

be an adequate local emergency rescue team available to evacuate the patient to definitive medical care. The expedition medical team must consider providing additional treatment capabilities such as intravenous solutions, steroids, airway management materials, and antihistamines. If the person has had to use epinephrine in the past, a person traveling with the potential patient must be capable of administering the epinephrine. At times the reaction may be so sudden that the victims cannot inject themselves. Not only will persons having anaphylactic reactions require emergency treatment with epinephrine, but they will also need to be evacuated. This may place a tremendous strain on the expedition, regarding both its function and its financial resources.

A history of bipolar depression or depression will require careful questioning of the participant to ensure that he or she plans to remain on medication during the expedition. A medication review is necessary. If the person is under current therapy, medications have not been altered during the past 3 months, and no drug holiday is planned, the condition can be considered stable. Ensure that duplicate medications are available for the expedition medical kit.

A medical history of high or low blood pressure requires inquiry as to the current treatment results. If normotensive with a regimen that has been well tolerated, with stable blood chemistries with regard to electrolytes, renal function, and liver function, the candidate would be acceptable. Adequate provision for replacement medication must be made within the expedition medical kit.

Diagnosis of the etiology of chest pain reported in the history must be established. The candidate's physician would need to be contacted if uncertainty is apparent or if the cause is cardiac or pulmonary. Musculoskeletal problems must be controlled adequately so as not be incapacitating. Cardiac conditions must be stable, and the suggested evaluations must be performed as indicated in the section in this chapter on Cardiology Clearance.

Persons with diabetes need to indicate that the condition can be self-managed, that fasting blood sugars are not fluctuating, that the HbA1C is below 8, and that no significant co-morbid conditions have complicated the clinical picture. It is particularly important to identify a person with peripheral neuropathy because foot blisters or infections can be devastating on a wilderness expedition. A peripheral neuropathy is a condition that will probably disqualify the participant, unless it is certain that blisters can be prevented or managed in the field. Additional insulin and needles must be available in the expedition medical kit, but all insulin-dependent diabetics must also carry an adequate supply in their personal kits. Non-insulin-dependent diabetic patients will require both a personal and a back-up supply of oral medications. All diabetics will need a glucometer and testing supplies (e.g., test strips, lancets, alcohol wipes). If more than one diabetic is on the expedition, a limited number of glucometers can be carried that could be shared. Expedition members must be able to recognize the symptoms of hypoglycemia and ketoacidosis and have the skill and medications to respond (i.e., glucagon, intravenous dextrose or glucose paste, regular insulin).

A history of repeated attacks or vertigo, near syncope, or the claim of dizzy spells must have a clear medical diagnosis as to etiology. The participant's physician will need to be contacted for appropriate documentation, and the condition must be either preventable, very limited in duration and not a risk to the patient, or treatable in the field.

Ear infections, either otitis media or externa, that have been frequent within the last 2 years will require appropriate medications in the expedition medical kit. The participant's treating physician needs to provide advice on treatment protocols for the patient's condition.

Eating disorders must be stable with no unusual weight for height at the time of application, and a stable weight for the previous 3 months. Medication use must be noted, and an additional supply must be obtained for the expedition medical kit. The person's treating physician should be contacted for confirmation of the condition's stability and the suitability for candidate's participation.

Head injuries resulting in impairment will need clarification and participation approval from the treating physician. It should be especially noted if there are requirements for specific monitoring, treatment capability for seizures, unusual intolerance of climate extremes, or behavioral abnormalities. These requirements must be within the capability of the group to manage; otherwise, participation is not appropriate.

If the history report identifies a heart condition, other than a functional murmur, follow the instructions in the Cardiology Clearance section in this chapter.

A hospitalization within the previous 3 months requires further inquiry as to cause and may result in requiring clearance from the treating physician. If the cause precipitates one of the history thresholds, follow the advice of that paragraph.

Chronic infectious disease must be suppressed, not significantly symptomatic, not contagious, and potential exacerbations must be within the capability of the members of the expedition to manage. Additional supplies of current medications must be available for the expedition medical kit as well as carried by the participant. A treatment protocol must be in place and acceptable to the expedition leadership as well as participant.

Orthopedic injuries that have occurred within the past 3 months will require an inquiry to the treating physician for clearance for participation on the expedition. As with all physician contacts, there must be a communication

Table 2.8. Limitations for moderate altitudes	
2,000 feet	CHF, myocardial infarction less than 8 weeks before
4,000 feet	Severe cardiac disease with recent decompensation
6,000 feet	Myocardial infarction 8 to 24 weeks before, angina, sickle cell disease, cyanosis, cor pulmonale, or respiratory acidosis
8,000 feet	Marked ventilatory restriction, more than mildly symptomatic heart/lung disease
10,000 feet	Symptomatic heart/lung disease or suspected disease

Forgey WW. *Traveler's Medical Resource*. Merrillville, Ind.: ICS Books; 1990:4–29.

to the physician that adequately describes the physical demands of the trip.

Chronic obstructive pulmonary disease must be stable, and the expedition member must be able to participate in the level of activity required for the trip. Disqualifiers would be inadequate PO_2 on room air or a $PO_2 < 50$ mm Hg projected for an altitude of 6,000 feet. Table 2.8 indicates several of the contraindications for participation at various altitudes. Chapter 21 in this book discusses high-altitude medicine in great detail.

If any surgery has taken place within the previous 6 months, clearance for participation must be obtained by the treating physician. Even though patients who have completed a surgery without complications may feel that the issue has been resolved, they may not be aware of restrictions or risks that may pose a hazard to them from participating on an expedition to a remote area.

A history of duodenal or gastric ulcer is not an excluding issue, but the condition must be well controlled or asymptomatic for the past 6 months. Expeditions into unknown or unfamiliar regions can be a cause for significant stress. The diet may not be ideal, regardless of the planning that has been performed. If the patient requires chronic medical management to control ulcer symptoms, additional medication must be available for the expedition medical kit and an adequate supply carried by the participant.

Level Four

Level Four thresholds are disqualification issues if the expedition is not medically capable of handling the attendant clinical situations that may or will develop on the trip. These conditions may result in greater risk to the candidate or to other members of the expedition. The treating physician must be consulted, and the physician must have a clear understanding of the risks, hardships, and medical capabilities of the expedition to treat the candidate.

Table 2.9. Medical history alert level four thresholds	
Category	Concern
Cancer	Symptomatic
HIV/HBV positive	Symptomatic
Life-threatening condition	Management, repatriation
Pregnancy	Delivery, management of infant
Refusal of medical treatment	Inability to manage medical issues

A Level Four threshold issue requires that the participant assume responsibility for the medical risk. The participant must be aware of the expedition medical staff's ability, or lack thereof, to deal with the medical issue which exists, if acceptance of the person on the expedition is approved. (See Table 2.9.)

The issues brought to light by a Level Four medical history threshold would require the expedition leadership to approve participation and the participant to assume risk. Because other members of the expedition might well be affected by the medical conditions which are potentially going to be encountered with regard to these individuals, the safety of other trip members and the impact upon the expedition mission must be considered in addition to the proposed participant's desires.

THE PHYSICAL EXAMINATION

The Mountain Travel Sobek Company uses what many consider to be an ideal approach to a preexpedition physical. The various components of the exam and history used by this company are described with a brief discussion.[9]

MOUNTAIN TRAVEL SOBEK: HISTORY AND PHYSICAL FORM

INSTRUCTIONS TO PARTICIPANT:

Please list on this Medical Certificate all abnormalities in your health and medical history. Most medical problems do not preclude participation in our trips. However, environmental factors and remote destinations with no medical facilities or means of rapid evacuation may create a risk that is beyond your expectations or that we find inadvisable. Most trips do not have designated trip doctors. Accurate disclosure will allow us to advise you of necessary preparations or alternatives and will allow your trip leader to be knowledgeable in the event of a problem.

Comments: This introductory material sets the tone of defusing enthusiastic client's fears that they may be precluded from a great adventure if they honestly fill out the medical history. It informs of the importance of the material, indicates an alternative and more appropriate trip may be suggested but also indicates an assumption of risk if the participant rejects the alternative. This would be more clearly spelled out in subsequent correspondence if management felt the risk was too high for the participant.

HISTORY SECTION FOR PARTICIPANTS:

This part should be completed by all trip members.

Do you have or have you been told by a doctor that you had:

- Epilepsy
- Diabetes
- Asthma or lung disease
- Heart disease: congestive failure, angina, prior heart attack or bypass surgery
- Significant foot, leg, or back problems
- Ulcers
- High blood pressure
- Colitis or recurrent intestinal trouble
- Arthritis
- Recurring thrombosis in legs or lungs

If yes, please explain in detail.

Do you have any other significant medical problems which have required the regular care of a doctor? Explain.

Have you been HOSPITALIZED in the last three years? Explain.

Do you have any ALLERGIES or have you had any bad reactions to any drugs? Which ones and what side effects?

Are you currently taking any regular medications? If so, please list.

Describe regular exercise habits and comparable outdoor activities or recent trips.

Special warning and qualifying section for participants.

If you are an applicant for a high altitude climbing expedition, please sign. "I have received and read Mountain Travel Sobek's letter on health problems at high altitude."

If you are age 65 or above, or the box is checked, your physician must complete the following. Please provide physician with trip itinerary, this form, attached note to physician and letter of health problems at high altitude.

The physical form is simply as listed below.

The applicant _____ Age____ has been examined and was found to be physically qualified to participate in a trip of the type checked below:

☐ "Easy"

☐ "Moderate"

☐ "Strenuous"

☐ "Mountaineering"

Mountain Travel Sobek would check the appropriate box indicating trip severity level

I have discussed the above matters with my patient.

(Physician's signature block with address and telephone number)

Comments: The form asks for no particulars concerning the physical examination, even vital signs. The entire matter of evaluating the physical qualification is left to the physician's discretion, yet it is clear that the physician is being provided with guidance as to the level of the trip's physical exertion requirements and remoteness.

The guidance provided the physician by Mountain Travel Sobek is well organized and easy to use. It is reproduced here as an indicator of the information a physician requires, and what should be expected of the physician's assessment.

Note to the Physician

In the Mountain Travel Sobek Catalog, each of our trips has a descriptive line indicating what conditions can be expected on the trip. Some examples are: "Easy to moderate walking, medium elevation, no camping," "Rugged road travel, optional walking, high altitude, no camping," or "Strenuous walking, high elevation, 15 nights camping."

"Easy" generally indicates short hikes of 2–4 hours or optional walks at low elevation. "Moderate" indicates hiking over varied terrain for 4–6 hours per day at elevations usually less than 15,000 feet. "Strenuous" signifies hiking over potentially steep terrain, longer hikes and/or high altitudes. "Mountaineering" incorporates "Strenuous" hiking conditions at altitudes that may reach 20,000 feet. Some trips have no hiking but are strenuous, particularly for persons over age 65, because of high altitude and long jarring vehicle travel by bus or jeep on remote mountain roads – or more unconventional means of travel such as camel or elephant.

For details of this trip, please read the Trip Itinerary which is provided to each trip member, paying special attention to the "Qualifications" paragraph.

Medical facilities may not be available on Mountain Travel Sobek trips; on mountaineering trips, local facilities are non-existent, and evacuation is prolonged and difficult. A trip physician may not accompany the trip.

High altitude mountaineering expeditions pose a special health risk to participants. Please read the letter prepared by Mountain Travel Sobek on health problems at high altitudes that is intended for both client and physician. It will help you counsel your patient as to whether or not he or she should participate in such an expedition.

We do not have a standard physical form but do expect a thorough medical examination with emphasis on cardiovascular and respiratory status, peripheral circulation, blood pressure and any potentially debilitating problems – e.g., gall bladder disease, kidney stones, asthma, active ulcer, colitis, hernia, back problems, etc. Lab data should include a CBC, urinalysis, blood sugar, BUN or creatinine, and resting cardiogram. Testing of pulmonary function, a recent chest x-ray and an exercise EKG are appropriate, if history indicates. A published protocol that you may find helpful for cardiac evaluation of travelers to altitude is included with this form.

If you have any questions concerning the difficulty and environmental factors on any trip or the specific risks to your patient, please call Mountain Travel Sobek at 1-800-227-2384.

Comments: The Mountain Travel Sobek material provides the consumer with incentive to correctly answer questions, provides information to both the consumer and the physician to encourage a focused and educated examination, and provides alerts to the company concerning chronic and acute medication conditions. This allows the company to provide consultation to the consumer concerning alternate trips if it detects inappropriate results in the history and physical.

CARDIOLOGY CLEARANCE

Four separate criteria require various levels of cardiac pretrip evaluation: participant's age, presence of symptoms, history of coronary-related diagnosis, and severity of the trip.

Because coronary artery disease increases with age, one of the determinants for a cardiology clearance is age related.[10] This fact coupled with the anticipated physical work required by the expedition suggests the extent of the clinical evaluation must increase by both age and the anticipated severity of the physical demands of the expedition.

Herbert Hultgren published an evaluation of travelers to high altitude in the *Journal of Wilderness Medicine* that has become the current standard for cardiac evaluation.[11] He stratified individuals into two diagnostic groups: low risk and high risk. The low risk group was considered to be a minimal risk for a coronary event (angina, infarct, sudden death) over 5 years of 2–4%, whereas the high risk group would have a substantial risk for a coronary event in 5 years of 10–20%. To place persons in these grouping the following history and diagnostic criteria were applied:

1. Asymptomatic without evidence of coronary disease, no risk factors for coronary disease. Risk category: Low. Treadmill test optional.
2. Asymptomatic, with one or more risk factors for coronary disease. Treadmill test indicated.

   Treadmill test negative or minimally positive. Risk category: Low.

   Treadmill test strongly positive; thallium scan indicated.

   Thallium scan normal. Risk category: Low.

   Thallium scan strongly positive. Risk category: High. Coronary arteriography indicated.

3. Known coronary artery disease, such as history of prior infarct, ECG evidence of prior infarct, history of

unstable angina, presence of unstable angina, prior bypass surgery, or angioplasty. Treadmill indicated.

Treadmill test strongly positive. Risk category: High.

Treadmill negative or minimally positive. Risk category: Low.

4. Age under 50 years.

One or more risk factors for coronary artery disease. Treadmill test optional.

No risk factors for coronary disease. Treadmill test not indicated.

Hultgren identified to following as risk factors for coronary disease:

1. Family history (sudden death, infarct, angina before 55 years in family members)
2. History or presence of hypertension
3. ST segment depression of any magnitude in the resting electrocardiogram; and
4. Prior episode of chest pain

With regard to the treadmill test, it was regarded as negative or minimally positive if the patient could walk 9 minutes or more (through Stage 3 Bruce protocol) without chest pain and with equal to or less than 1 mm ST segment depression. It was considered strongly positive if the patient walked 6 minutes or less (Bruce protocol) and had either chest pain and/or equal to or greater than 2 mm ST segment depression.

Expedition leaders must identify medical and psychological conditions that are disqualifiers from participation. Mountain Travel Sobek does not list any disqualifiers in its initial participant information, but other organizations do. An example is the Boy Scout of America Florida Sea Base. The program, specifically excludes persons who:

• Weigh more than 300 pounds
• Have significant heart disease, asthma, or hypertension
• Have incompletely controlled psychiatric problems
• Are subject to anaphylaxis
• Do not meet age requirements (minimum 14 years of age)

Persons who have any of the following conditions must have an isotope cardiac stress test as a condition of participation:

• Angina
• Myocardial infarction
• Surgery or angioplasty; surgery to treat congenital heart disease, or other heart surgery
• Stroke or transient ischemic attacks (TIAs)
• Claudication
• Family history of heart disease or a family member who died unexpectedly before age 50
• Diabetes
• Smoking
• Excessive weight (see Table 2.5)

Possible additions to this list would include persons with an abnormal resting electrocardiogram or those with a serum cholesterol >240 mg/dL.

The physical form indicates to the participant that "even if the stress test is normal, the results of testing done without the exertions of a high adventure program do not guarantee safety."

Persons are excluded from participating in the scuba program if they have diabetes that requires insulin for control, epilepsy, asthma, heart trouble, current cold, or a severe medical problem or if they are under the influence of alcohol or drugs. There are some exceptions. They state, "Any asthma history regardless of control, unless documented by a methacholine challenge test and found to be resolved, disqualifies an individual from participation in the scuba program."

AGE-RELATED RISK

In physically fit persons younger than 40 years of age, sudden death, while rare, is usually not caused by coronary artery disease and would not be reliably discovered by echocardiography or exercise stress testing.[12] Persons older than 40 years, who have exertionally related symptoms, generally have coronary atherosclerosis which can be detected by cardiac stress testing.[13]

Persons older than 40 who plan to participate in an expedition with strenuous activity (60–80% VO_2 maximum, 70–90% maximum heart rate) should have exercise testing. There is general agreement that persons without risk factors undertaking moderate intensity exercise (40–60% VO_2 maximum, 50–70% maximum heart rate) do not need an exercise test prior to participating.[14]

CONTINUED MONITORING DURING THE TRIP

During the course of the expedition, various members of the group will tolerate environmental and physical and mental stress differently. The trip leader and physician must monitor the basic condition of all members. Establishing open lines of confidential communication can best do this. Make certain that you encourage participants to tell you of problems with constipation, foot problems, headache, or other signs or symptoms of medical problems during the earliest stages.

The most apparent nonverbalized sign that something is going wrong is for a person to have a change in personality or for them to begin to complain or show evidence of loss of coordination. National Outdoor Leadership School calls these signs "grumble, mumble, and stumble." Loss of appetite and inability to sleep are subtle signs that something is wrong. Other symptoms are not so subtle, such as dyspnea, diarrhea, and vomiting. Regardless, it will be up to the trip leadership to identify problems as they initially develop and provide a change in environment or work activity level that allows the participant to have a safe and enjoyable (if possible) conclusion to the trip. This is where compassion and the art and science of medicine come together.

It is critical to have the knowledge base that was obtained as part of the pretrip history and physical examination available to appropriate persons on the expedition medical team for utilization during the trip. This requires control of the information as well as access issues (see Chapter 5). The expedition medical kit must be adjusted to the problems identified as unique to various trip participants as well as general requirements for adequate care and evacuation plans for the expedition in general. In case of serious injury, death, or other local catastrophe, the ability to inform expedition headquarters, appropriate next of kin, and even local and international media must also be managed.

The basis of success in these many areas is an adequate pretrip history on all participants and an appropriate physical evaluation as indicated by the strenuous level of exertion required by the expedition members, taking into account their unique individual issues. With this as the basis of the medical decision making, the appropriate management of medical emergencies should be accomplished in a professional and successful manner.

REFERENCES

1. The Student Conservation Association (SCA) recruits both youth and adults for six-week backcountry trail conservation programs. These projects involve construction work in remote areas, some of which require hiking for several days to reach. Founded in 1957, the SCA places 3,000 volunteers into conservation projects yearly. Due to the remoteness and difficulty of medical evacuation, proper medical screening and safety are driving principles behind the SCA success story. This is accomplished by establishing medical history review thresholds to alert staff members of various degrees of medical risk that candidates might posses. The medical threshold principles were developed by the SCA Chief Medical Reviewer Kris Wright with senior staff input from Kurt Merrill, Jay Satz, and physician adviser William Forgey, MD.

2. Forgey, WW, ed. Traumatic brain injury. In *Wilderness Medical Society Practice Guidelines for Wilderness Emergency Care*. Butte, Mont.: Falcon Press, 2006.

3. Welch TP. Data-based selection of medical supplies for wilderness travel. *Wilderness Environ Med.* 1997;8(3):148–51

4. Boulware, DR, Forgey WW, Martin WJ, II. Medical risks of wilderness hiking. *Am J Med.* 2003;114:288–93.

5. Data on file: Reference 038–014, Hoffman-La Roche, Nutley, N.J.

6. Byrnes MC, McDaniel MD, Moore MB, Helmer SD, Smith RS. The effect of obesity on outcomes among injured patients. *J Trauma.* 2005;58(2):232–7.

7. Neville AL, Brown CV, Weng J, Demetriades D, Velmahos GC. Obesity is an independent risk factor for mortality in severely injured blunt trauma patients. *Arch Surg.* 2004; 139(9):983–7.

8. Recommended weight for participation, BSA Florida Sea Base, 2006.

9. Mountain Travel Sobek Company, General Health Form. 1–888-MTSOBEK (687–6235) or 1–510-594–6000. *http://www. mtsobek.com.*

10. Diamond GA, Forrester JS. Analysis of probability as an aid in the clinical diagnosis of coronary artery disease. *N Engl J Med.* 1979;300:1350–8.

11. Hultgren, HN. Coronary artery disease and trekking. *J Wilderness Med.* 1990;1:154–61

12. Thompson, PD. Athletes, athletics, and sudden cardiac death. *Med Sci Sports Exerc.* 1992;24:981–4.

13. Herbert, WG, Froelicher, VF. Exercise tests for coronary and asymptomatic patients. *Physician and Sportsmedicine.* 1991;19:55–62.

14. Backer, H. Medical limitations to wilderness travel. *Emergency Medicine Clinics of North America.* 1997;15:17–41.

3 | Expedition Medical Kit

William W. Forgey, MD

Medical kits serve two basic functions: to provide transportable medical provisions and convenience in case of emergencies. From early history, evidence of medical kits can be found in archeology sites.[1] Trajan's Column in Rome depicts scenes of wounded soldiers being treated by their fellow soldiers, an event that would require access to transported accessible supplies. Over the past 50 years, journal articles have discussed emergency medical kits for physicians or other health care professionals to use in their offices[2,3,4,5,6] or during travel.[7,8] Kits for professional or lay use have been advocated for emergency medical treatment in special circumstances such as foreign travel,[9,10,11,12,13] in-flight emergencies,[14,15,16,17,18] and wilderness expeditions.[19,20,21,22,30,31]

Multiple factors impacting upon the design of a medical kit for remote area expedition use are indicated in Table 3.1.[23] These basic factors have been described in the *Wilderness Medical Society Practice Guidelines for Wilderness Emergency Care.*

PURPOSE OF THE TRIP

Focusing upon the expedition goals and understanding the mission of the trip is the most basic requirement that needs to be clarified when designing a medical kit (Figure 3.1). If the group intends on only managing injuries and illness that will be encountered by expedition participants, then an analysis of those potential disorders will influence the kit content and quantity of materials. As quoted in the *Practice Guidelines*: "Because a search and rescue (SAR) team must be equipped to handle the medical emergencies that they expect to encounter, they can justify carrying specialized medical gear. On recreational trips, however, the medical kit displaces other equipment that might be needed. Hikers, white water enthusiasts, and climbers all need different medical kits to meet their specialized needs."[23]

A study published by Timothy Welch in 1997 examined incident data for injury and medical kit component use for a high adventure Boy Scout adventure travel program that canoed and hiked into remote areas of the

Adirondack State Park, New York.[20] There were 565 participants between 14 and 18 years of age on programs of one week in duration, thus the data represented 3,955 person-days of wilderness travel. Table 3.2 represents the injury rates in the program in total incidents and incidents per 10,000 person days. Table 3.3 shows the actual supply use the programs experienced. This evidence-based information produced a recommended kit content for similar programs, as shown in Table 3.4.

Similar incidence data have been published by several of the large outdoor training schools, National Outdoor Leadership School (NOLS), Colorado Outward Bound, and the Student Conservation Association.[24] These groups take slightly older students for longer trips (up to 6 weeks) into remote areas, generally in national parks or wilderness areas within the United States. NOLS data reporting experience from 630,937 program days from 1998 through 2002 show that 46% of the injuries occurred while hiking with a pack, while other activities including mountaineering, river boating, sea kayaking, and skiing each accounted for less than 5%. Seventeen percent of the NOLS injuries occurred within the campsite.[24]

Table 3.1. Medical kit architecture: factors that determine medical kit design
A. Purpose of the Trip
B. Level of Medical Training
C. Destination
D. Participant Medical Conditions and Age
E. Length of Trip
F. Time for Evacuation or Medical Rescue
G. Size of the Party
H. Bulk, Weight, and Cost
I. Accessibility
J. Risk of Loss or Diversion
K. Replenishment
L. Preservation
M. Expectations
N. Diagnostics
O. Improvisation

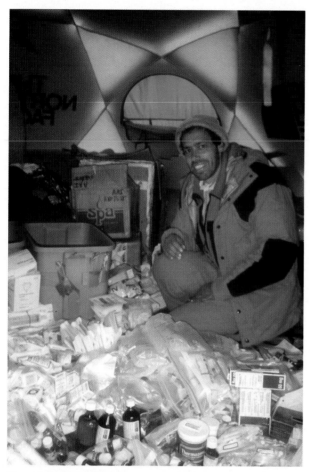

Figure 3.1. The medical kit and gear to be taken on an expedition should be designed with the destination in mind. Here an expedition physician sits with his expedition medical gear on Mount Everest. Photo courtesy of Kenneth Kamler.

An organization dedicated to reducing wilderness travel risk and gathering incident data is the Wilderness Risk Managers' Committee. Information about their yearly conference and contact information can be found at their Web page published through the NOLS Web site at *http://www.nols.edu/wrc*. [25]

An evaluation of the medical risks of wilderness hiking performed by Boulware, Forgey, and Martin on Appalachian Trail through hikers and section hikers is summarized in Table 3.5.[26] Foot blisters (64%), skin chafing (51%), and diarrhea (56%) were the most frequently encountered medical problems by this group of 280 long-distance hikers.

Others have published estimates of medical kit content based upon the multiple parameters of anticipated degree of risk, length of expedition, and numbers of participants to produce tables or diagrams of how to pick out the amount and type of supplies to be packed for an expedition.[9–12,19] The difficulty with other than basic equipment and supplies being included in these estimates is that none of them can accommodate all the variation of factors described in Table 3.1.

Table 3.2. Association of Adirondack scout camp wilderness trip incident rates[a]

Injury	Total Incidents	Incidents/10,000 Person-days
Leech wound	1	2.5
Dehydration	1	2.5
Contact dermatitis	2	5.1
Sunburn	3	7.6
Headache	4	10.1
Nosebleed	1	2.5
Abdominal pain	2	5.1
Ankle sprain	1	2.5
Open wound	14	35.4
Abrasion	3	7.6
Blister	19	48.0
Superficial foreign body	1	2.5
Bruise	1	2.5
Conjunctiva foreign body	3	7.6
Burn	5	12.6
Hypothermia	1	2.5

[a]Data are reported for 3,955 person-days of exposure of adolescents taking 1-week hikes and canoe trips in the Adirondack Park. Welch TP. Data-based selection of medical supplies for wilderness travel. *Wilderness Environ Med.* 1997;8(3):148–51.

Table 3.3. Association of Adirondack scout camp wilderness trip incident supplies used in program[a]

Item	Units Used	Units Used Per 10,000 Person-days
Adhesive bandages	9	22.8
Adhesive tape	17	43.0
Antacid (tablet)	1	2.5
Antibiotic ointment	15	37.9
Antihistamine (tablet)	1	2.5
Bismuth subsalicylate (tablet)	2	5.1
Conforming gauze bandage	10	25.3
Elastic bandage	2	5.1
Hydrocortisone cream 1%	1	2.5
Ibuprofen (tablet)	7	17.7
Moleskin	19	48.0
Povidone-iodine (solution)	15	37.9
Scissors		
Sterile gauze pads	11	27.8
Steristrips	2	5.1
Thermometer		
Tincture of benzoin	9	22.8
Tweezers		

[a]Data are reported for 3,955 person-days of exposure of adolescents taking 1-week hikes and canoe trips in the Adirondack Park. Welch TP. Data-based selection of medical supplies for wilderness travel. *Wilderness Environ Med.* 1997;8(3):148–51.

Table 3.4. Medical kit recommended content based upon association of Adirondack scout camp wilderness trip incident data[a]

Item	Quantity
Dressings and Wound Care	
Adhesive bandage (Band-Aid®)	12
Adhesive tape (2-inch roll)	2
Conforming gauze roll bandage 3-inch	2
Elastic bandage 3-inch	1
Moleskin (15.5-square-inch sheets)	2
Spenco Second Skin® (4-inch squares)	4
Sterile gauze compresses (4-inch squares)	6
Equipment	
Scissors	1
Thermometer	1
Tweezers	1
Oral OTC Preparations	
Antacid (chewable tablets)	6
Antihistamine (diphenhydramine 50 mg)	6
Bismuth subsalicylate chewable	6
Ibuprofen 200-mg tablets	6
Topical OTC Preparations	
Alcohol swabs (for cleaning equipment)	10
Triple antibiotic ointment (0.9-g packets)	6
Hydrocortisone 1% cream (30-g tube)	1
Povidone/iodine swabs	8
Tincture of benzoin (30-ml bottle)	1

[a]Evidence-based recommendation for a medical kit designed for a group of 12 individuals on a 2-week wilderness trip.

Welch TP. Data-based selection of medical supplies for wilderness travel. *Wilderness Environ Med.* 1997;8(3):148–51.

Table 3.5. Heat and cold stable medications frequently included in expedition medical kits

Substance	Effective after Heat Stress	Effective after Cold Stress
Adrenaline (epinephrine)	Yes	Yes
Atropine	Yes	Yes
Ringer lactate	Yes	Yes
Lidocaine	Yes	Yes
Metaprolol	Yes	Yes
Nifedipine	Yes	Yes
Nitroglycerine	Yes	Yes

Kupper TEAH, et al. Drugs and drug administration in extreme environments. *J Travel Med.* 2006;13:35–47.

Clearly defining the expedition mission can help designers exclude, as well as include, expedition medical kit contents. Evidence-based medicine has demonstrated the low risk of contracting infectious blood-borne pathogens from other healthy companions, thus challenging the need for barrier protective gloves, even though most authorities suggest, and all large commercial medical kits include, these items.[27] Search and rescue crews will very likely be encountering traumatized nonparticipant victims and will need to have protection using universal precautions against blood-borne pathogens. Expeditions that plan to care for indigenous populations or other groups of persons with whom they may have contact would also require blood-borne pathogen protective barriers.

Evidence-based incident usage or kit design can be expected to be applicable only to identically repeated programs (with regard to length, leadership, terrain, weather, and level of individual experience). In forming an expedition, the medical kit will have to be built from the ground up relying upon the architecture of Table 3.1 for guidance. The foundation of the kit design will be the purpose (mission) of the trip. Taking a group of dedicated explorers into uncharted territory will result in a different level of risk than leading weekly hikes through an established trail system in a national park, a group of adventurous college students for 6 weeks through a wilderness area, or individuals hiking for 1 to 3 months on low-altitude, yet steep trails. Other than the portions of the expedition that repeat access routes commonly used by trekkers, once the group starts burrowing into the unknown, experiential published risk factor tables will be of minimal use. Personal experience from participation in similar explorations will provide the most reasonable basis for forming a content list that will anticipate the severity of trauma and illness expedition members are likely to encounter. Without that experience, an expedition heading into the remote unknown can design an appropriate kit adhering to the Table 3.1 principles and studying the contents of the first two sections of this book. Purpose of trips includes degree of risk from the exploration activity as well as the approach march or transportation, uncooperative or hostile local population, and the willingness of the party to "back down" when the level of risk appears to be very high. If the accomplishment of the mission takes precedence over individual safety, then one might expect massive trauma or death as a real possibility that would have to be managed. Conquering a military objective brings to mind a level of risk of this magnitude. Many times in the past "conquering" an unknown area, climbing a difficult peak, or descending a raging torrent, have similarly resulted in significant morbidity and mortality.

LEVEL OF MEDICAL TRAINING

The *Wilderness Medical Society Practice Guidelines* states that, "It is inappropriate to include medications and equipment that no trip member has the requisite knowledge or experience to use safely. Trip members responsible for medical care of the group should have direct input into the contents of the medical kit. Levels of training and experience can differ widely among groups of physicians, nurses, and EMS personnel. A degree or license may not guarantee knowledge in any specific area. Pre-trip training to supplement the knowledge base of the providers is advisable." [23]

The inclusion of specialized medical equipment is not a function of awarded degrees, but of training and necessity. Non-physician-staffed air medical crews, trained to diagnose conditions requiring chest tubes and proper placement techniques, have shown a similar complication rate comparing their field chest tube thoracostomy outcomes to those of a physician trauma service.[28] Physicians not trained or without sufficient experience in performing chest tube thoracostomies should not carry or expect to use chest tubes in the field. It makes sense to include chest tubes, or items that could be used in lieu of a chest tube, only if the level of risk of potential need and the ability of the expedition team members to properly use the equipment exists simultaneously. This caveat holds true for every item in the medical kit.

DESTINATION

"Consider the terrain, altitude, weather, propensity for endemic diseases, and other inherent dangers. Groups heading into remote areas where local inhabitants may request medical help must consider this potential demand on their supplies, and must consider whether they intend to respond."[23]

Obtaining information on disease risk can be accomplished by accessing the foreign travel databases available on various international Web sites. The primary U.S. source is the Centers for Disease Control and Prevention at *http://www.cdc.gov/travel/*. The World Health site is: *http://www.who.int/ith/*. Many private travel medicine sites reproduce material from these two sites. An informative pharmaceutical industry portal site is *http://www.surf-for-safe-travel.com*, which is financed by GlaxoSmithKline (GSK). It in turn will link you to *http://www.fitfortravel.com/en/*, the Web site of the University of Munich Tropical Institute; and *http://www.travelmedicineweb.org/*, which is also funded by GSK containing articles especially written for this site and links to many outside sites such as commercial CME offerings. Another portal site is *http://www.us.aventispasteur.com* recently renamed *http://www.sanofipasteur.us* with multiple resource areas for both professional and public access.

The International Association for Medical Assistance to Medical Travelers (IAMAT) is a nonprofit membership that maintains a network of physicians – general practitioners and specialists, hospitals and clinics around the world – who have agreed to treat IAMAT members in need of medical care during their journey. Their aim is also to advise travelers about health risks, the geographical distribution of diseases, immunization requirements, sanitary conditions of water, milk and food, and environmental and climatic conditions around the world. Its Web site, *http://www.iamat.org*,

contains unique, non-government-filtered disease risk information and specific recommendations for international immunization compiled by its international scientific advisory board. Membership in IAMAT is free, and access to the Web site is immediate even without membership.

The International Society for Travel Medicine (ISTM) Web site at *http://www.istm.org* has a particularly useful link to non-ISTM information resources, which is hosted at *http://info.dom.uab.edu/gorgas/geomed/links2.html*.

Special risks associated with high altitude, diving, and aeronautics are discussed in detail in other chapters of this book. It will be necessary to incorporate suggestions made in these chapters for special medication and appropriate devices specific to your expedition.

PARTICIPANT MEDICAL CONDITIONS AND AGE

Evaluation of trip participants is discussed in this book in Chapter 2. Suffice it to say that if trip members who have underlying medical conditions requiring specialized equipment and/or medications are accepted for participation, these items must be included in the trip medical kit. Generally the best technique is to allow the participant to carry their own medications, with an adequate back-up supply in the group medical kit to allow continuing treatment if the principle supply is lost or damaged.

Pediatric populations, older participants, and special needs expedition members will necessitate an adjustment to the formulary. Individual medical problems need to be identified during the pretrip assessment. Consideration for acceptance on an expedition will, in part, be made based on the ability to manage any unique morbid conditions that the individual has. Part of the management issue is the ability to properly carry, maintain, and administer an individual's unique medications or treatments.

LENGTH OF TRIP/RESUPPLY

Some nomograms use length of trip to determine quantities and varieties of medical supplies to use in an expedition medical kit;[19] however, the quantities of materials and length of duration of the trip is not a linear relationship. You do not necessarily need three times the number of blister pads for a 3-week trip as you do a 1-week trip. Additionally, some conditions, such as blisters, are much more likely to occur earlier in a trip, while others, such as parasitic infectious diseases, occur later in a trip.

Length of trip could affect the requirement for definitive care items. Even though a 1-week trip may not require the provisioning of wound closure material (closure strips, sutures, staples, bonding glue), a trip in a remote area lasting months may well wish to consider these items.

Long trips may pass through inhabited areas that would allow restocking of basic materials, or even obtaining medications not available in the country of origin. Many useful medications can be obtained in Europe or Asia that are not available in the United States, for example. Even though relying on resupply while en route or on the expedition is a risky technique, it makes for a very convenient and sometimes a less costly acquisition. The principle concern would be to not devastate a local resource for your expedition's needs. Restocking en route should only be anticipated if the expedition planner has personal familiarity with the locale.

TIME FOR EVACUATION OR MEDICAL RESCUE

The *Wilderness Medical Society Practice Guidelines* state: "Some trips progressively distance themselves from medical care. On other trips, time required to obtain help may be deceptive. A river raft trip into a canyon, for instance, may last only hours, but evacuation in the event of an accident may take many days of dangerous and laborious effort."[23]

A number of factors increase time to rescue and may place additional demands upon a medical kit:

1. A delay in the decision to request rescue by the party
2. A breakdown in communications to the outside for help
3. Long distance for rescuers to travel
4. Being uncertain in location
5. Local natural disasters or political instability
6. Prohibitive rescue cost
7. Expecting rendezvous with rescuers or another party, if delayed

The medical kit plan must consider the possibility of unusual delay and the extended requirement for the medical kit to be used beyond the normally expected expedition length or evacuation time.

SIZE OF THE PARTY

Medical kits have been classically designed with the size of the group as a primary characteristic. An increase in participant numbers will influence the quantity of some medications and bandaging supplies, but the increased requirement is not linear. As seen from the injury rates of a typical adolescent wilderness program noted in Tables 3.2, 3.3, and 3.5, with the use of a personal medical kit, an increase in numbers of participants would not greatly affect total quantities of supplies consumed.[20] Equipping each member of the expedition with a personal kit containing antibiotic ointment, a few bandages, blister supplies, an antiinflammatory and personal medications can reduce the size of the main medical kit for a large party and will accommodate treatment of blisters, chafing, and muscle or joint pain, which are predominate medical incidents on 1- to 6-week trips.

Major expeditions would augment these supplies in the main kit, but in general the expedition kit would have antibiotics, diagnostic equipment, and major wound management items, if appropriate.

Table 3.6 provides guidance for evidence-based medical kit contents for a group of 12 adolescents traveling for 1 week in remote wilderness canoeing and hiking areas at low altitude. Appendix A contains recommended allowances for a party of six adults traveling into very remote areas for up to two months. Please see specific chapters to find recommendations of items suggested by the authors of the specialized chapters in this book.

Appropriate quantities of supplies for large expedition medical kits are best calculated using experience from similar expeditions in the past. After action reports,

Table 3.6. Incidence of injuries and illness encountered by Appalachian Trail section or through hikers[a]

Complaint	Incidents (n = 280)	Percentage
Musculoskeletal		
Acute joint pain	102	36
Numbness	78	28
Back pain	64	23
Chronic joint pain	62	22
Muscle cramps	55	20
Achilles heel pain	55	20
Shin splints	39	14
Tendonitis	38	14
Muscle strain	36	13
Ankle sprain	32	11
Fracture	11	2
Cutaneous		
Feet blisters	180	64
Skin chafing	143	51
Lost toenails	83	30
Sunburn	72	26
Tick bites	68	24
Poison ivy	57	20
Skin rash	44	16
Skin infection	15	5
Infectious		
Respiratory infection	40	14
Flu-like symptoms	20	7
Lyme disease	9	3
Urinary tract infection	2	1
Diarrhea	156	56
Miscellaneous		
Dehydration	55	20
Allergies	22	8
Constipation	15	5
Heat exhaustion	13	5
Hypothermia	13	5

[a]Data compiled from 280 long-distance hikers, representing a combined 38,940 days of wilderness exposure.
Boulware DR, Forgey WW, Martin WJ, II. Medical risks of wilderness hiking. *Am J Med.* 2003;114:288–93.

journals, or direct contact with previous expedition members are viable methods of obtaining this information. The Explorers Club in New York City has a library that is available for research of this nature. Researchers interested in gaining access to the James B. Ford Library, Sir Edmund Hillary Map Room, or The Explorers Club archives must make an appointment with the curator. The Research Collections are open by appointment Monday through Thursday, 12 noon to 4 P.M.[29]

BULK, WEIGHT, AND COST

Even if cost is not a consideration, the weight and bulk of a kit are potential limiting factors (Figure 3.2). Because bandaging and splints are bulky and possibly awkward to carry, the use of improvised materials, such as clothing for bandaging and local fabrication of splints, might need to be incorporated into plans for the medical kit.

Using multifunctional components and cross-therapeutic components may also reduce medical supplies and equipment.[30,31] If one piece of equipment or a drug can be used for many different purposes, weight can be significantly reduced. Knowledgeable medical team members are needed to optimize this tactic.

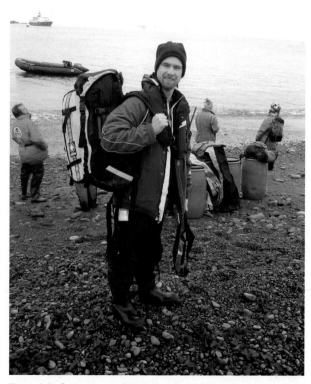

Figure 3.2. On most expeditions, the size of the medical kit is a consideration. Here the medical officer carries a portable medical kit for landings in Antarctica while the majority of medical gear remains on the ship. Photo courtesy of Gregory H. Bledsoe.

An example of a multifunctional item is Benadryl (diphenhydramine), which can be used to treat allergies and congestion, to suppress cough, as a topical anesthetic to oral mucosa, as a sleep aid, as an antianxiety medication, to treat muscle cramps, to treat nausea, and to prevent motion sickness.

An example of cross-therapeutic components would be to include Percogesic in the same medical kit, as this compound can be used to treat pain and fever, but it also can be used to help treat muscle cramps and congestion, as an antianxiety agent, and as a sleeping aid. While diphenhydramine and Percogesic do serve different primary therapeutic purposes with FDA approval, they are both multifunctional (allowing other items with similar therapeutic effects to be omitted), they also are cross-therapeutic allowing many of their therapeutic effects to be achieved by the other compound.

Table 3.7 illustrates examples of cross-therapeutic compounds. The Appendix describes modular medical kits with an explanation of component choices that reflects these concepts.

ACCESSIBILITY

Medical kits have to be packed in such a way that appropriate members of the team can easily obtain and utilize them. This requires obvious marking (unless security precautions dictate otherwise). Generally red is the color of choice for medical kits, but regardless of color, it should be clearly distinguished from other packages, and it should also stand out from local environmental markings. This helps prevent it from being left behind on portage trails or misplaced in equipment dumps on larger expeditions.

Placement of the medical kit, or at least its most likely required components, needs to be considered within the expedition planogram so that emergency items can be accessed during the different phases of the expedition movement from point to point in civilization and during different phases of the expedition in the wilderness.

This placement, or staging, of portions of the kit is most easily accomplished when the kit has been divided into functional modules. Cardiac module for treatment of acute coronary syndrome, orthopedic modules with specialized splints, and wound care modules with irrigation and closure supplies are examples of functional modules.

Specific components of the medical kit that have urgent priority must be marked and positioned for their ready accessibility. Cardiac medications require immediate access, while a delay of hours would be acceptable for acquiring the splinting materials. Urgently needed medical supplies will be of no help when packed in a cargo hold under tons of food, or stuffed mysteriously within unmarked bags.

Table 3.7. Examples of over-the-counter (OTC) and prescription (Rx) multifunctional medications with cross-therapeutic capabilities[a]

Medication	Pain	Muscle Cramps	Cough	Itch	Fever	Nausea	Inflammation	Diarrhea	Anxiety	Allergy	Gastritis	Sleep Aid	Menstrual Cramps
Percogesic (OTC)	xxx	xxx	x	X	xxx				xx	xx	x	xx	xxx
Ibuprofen (OTC)	xxx	xx		X	xxx		xxx						xxx
Diphenhydramine (OTC)		xxx	xxx	Xxx		xx			xxx	xxx	x	xxx	x
Cimetadine (OTC)		x		X		x				x	xxx		x
Loperamide (OTC)								xxx			x		x
Acetaminophen-hydrocodone (Rx)	xxx	xxx	xxx	X	xxx			xxx	x		x	xx	xx
Hydroxyzine (Rx)	x	xx	x	Xxx		xxx			xxx	xxx	X	xxx	x

[a]Choosing medications with multiple therapeutic functions allow greater therapeutic coverage using fewer items. This also gives greater depth to the medical kit as there are alternate medications to use for treatment if there is loss or consumption of primary items.
Forgey W. *Basic Essential of Wilderness First Aid*. Butte, Mont: Falcon Books; 2007. Forgey, W. *Wilderness Medicine*. Globe, Conn: Globe Pequot Press; 2003.

RISK OF LOSS OR DIVERSION

Some components of the medical kit may require specific security and limited access, such as narcotic medications or items that are considered valuable and that might be subject to pilferage. Even though this may restrict general accessibility, the location of these items should be well known to appropriate expedition members.

Respect of the kit use needs to be instilled into expedition members. Needless consumption of materials for trivial reasons might lead to shortages at critical times later. Conversely, medical kits can also make great barter items or gifts for local inhabitants. This tends to happen for a variety of reasons. Among the most important is their perceived importance among local people. A kit contains items that are simply not available in the indigenous economy. The expedition may find itself short of a food item or other perceived necessity and bartering away a medical kit component may make good sense at the time. In fact, if things are going well the kit will have been of no use, and there you are – out of coffee.

Local emergencies, natural disasters, and political upheaval, all can place the local population at great medical risk. If it is anticipated that the expedition will play a role in providing local medical aid, this usage factor must be considered when designing stock levels and even components of the expedition medical kit.

If the purpose of the expedition is to provide local medical relief, then a difference must be made between the materials being brought into the country for relief efforts and the items that have been deigned for the expedition's succor and survival. Certainly the decision to divert assets from the expedition medical kit to local use must be made with great care and approved by the expedition leadership.

REPLENISHMENT

The opposite of loss or diversion is the planned replenishment of items during the trip from local resources. As mentioned earlier, some items might not be available in the country of departure (such as medications not released in the United States).

Personal familiarity with a geographic area will be the best guide as to whether or not it is feasible or appropriate to plan on replenishing medical kit materials from local sources. Under some circumstances, indigenous materials may make ideal additions to the expedition kit, but at other times local supplies may be strained and consuming items that are in short supply would be unethical.

Large expeditions can be an economic boon to local economies. Medical supplies are seldom the object of local vendors, whereas foodstuffs, clothing, and equipment may provide local vendors with profit and local porters with wages. While seldom a viable option, the planned replenishment or acquisition of medical supplies while in inhabited areas is a seldom used but potential possibility.

Arranging reshipment of supplies from a home base is a common technique used on long solo hikes. Food, replacements for clothing items, and augmentation of medical supplies can be drop shipped to way points on the trail thus allowing the management of load weight. The technique of arranging resupply shipments to be delivered en route is a commonly used military and expedition tactic. If the reshipment technique is dependable, it could cut the initial weight and bulk of the expedition medical kit significantly. Excess supplies shipped to the expedition's requirements usually can be disposed of locally quite easily.

PRESERVATION

While some medications can withstand an enormous temperature storage range, such as atropine and lidocaine, others can be expected to be temperature-sensitive.[32,33] Table 3.5 contains a list of frequently used emergency medications with indications of cold and heat stability.[34]

Storage can be affected by the type of container and placement of these containers within the expedition equipment stores. Even though dark red may make a container more visible, such a container would absorb heat better than a reflective white color.

Placement of medical supplies deep within other containers restricts their accessibility, but it can also provide some temperature modulation, preventing fluctuations of hot and cold during modest diurnal variations. Very heat-sensitive materials will require special handling in refrigerated or insulated containers. Items suggested for the modular medical kit in this chapter do not require sensitive temperature control. Some items advised for inclusion in the specialty chapters of this book in Parts 2 and 3 do require careful, heat-stable storage.

EXPECTATIONS

Although it is more of a legal consideration than a purely medical one (see Chapter 5), expedition members need to understand what medical care will be offered them on the trip from internal resources and what other resource will be available from outside agencies. Certainly, the onus of bringing personal medications should be on each member. The group expedition medical kit needs to be supplied with a reserve supply of these medications in case the personal supply is lost.

More importantly, expedition members need to have a clear idea of what level of medical care the group can expect from its medical officers. This includes not only the care provided from expedition internal resources but also the level of evacuation and medical assistance that is expected of local nationals.

There are obvious implications for the medical kit for such expectations. Will blood transfusion equipment be included? What about cardiac defibrillation capability and oxygen availability? Sometimes these additions are appropriate and necessary. Other times, they are impractical and probably unnecessary. But if capabilities have been promised or are expected by expedition members, the inclusion of these capabilities must be clarified.

DIAGNOSTICS

Even though a thorough history and clinical examination can diagnose most medical conditions, having the ability to diagnose and record physiological parameters can be of great importance to the clinician. Often wilderness expeditions have a medical research component, where very sophisticated diagnostic equipment is utilized. For nonresearch exploration, the weight, bulk, cost, and medical training required for appropriate use limits the diagnostic items that will be carried.

The pulse can be felt by palpation, and the heart, lungs, and abdomen can be auscultated by the ear against bare skin. But for aesthetic purposes, and to amplify the findings, a stethoscope might be worth the weight, cost, and bulk. A field expedient of measuring minimal blood pressure by palpation is listed in Table 3.8; otherwise, a sphygmomanometer and stethoscope must be included.

Abdominal pain differential might require the use of pregnancy test kits and urine test strips that indicate leukocyte and nitrite presence. High-altitude illness diagnosis can be augmented with oxygen saturation readings from a portable pulse oxymeter. Special populations may require additional diagnostic items such as blood glucose monitors or urine-testing supplies for diabetics. Hypothermia signs and symptoms are notoriously difficult to use to determine core temperature, thus a rectal thermometer may be a useful addition to the medical kit. A headlamp will help conduct oral and superficial ear examinations, but an otoscope will enable a more thorough examination of the auditory canal.

Some diagnostic equipment can also be used for therapeutic care, such as automatic external

Table 3.8. Estimation of blood pressure by palpation[a]

Blood pressure estimate	Pulse detected by palpation
90	Carotid
80	Femoral
80	Radial – standing
70	Radial – sitting

[a]Wilderness medicine frequently relies on clinical evaluation and treatment improvisation without the benefit of equipment and medical supplies. This table provides an estimate of blood pressure without the use of a sphygmomanometer and stethoscope by palpation of various arterial pulses.

defibrillators. The use of diagnostic equipment requires a level of training, investment, and capability of managing the extra weight, which pose limiting factors for many expeditions.

IMPROVISATION

Improvisation is a fundamental skill in wilderness medicine. Virtually all general courses in wilderness medicine teach techniques of designing splints from backpack stays, ski poles, or other appropriated equipment or from natural products. Appendix A describes a modular medical kit. Realizing that the medical kit may be destroyed or inaccessible, alternative techniques or improvisational therapies are described for many of the items.

Many practical programs on exploration technique, which often include tips on improvisation, are offered through the Explorers Club in New York City. Updates of program listings can be found on the club's Web site at *http://www.explorers.org/calendar/month.php*. A list of current wilderness medicine courses sponsored by the Wilderness Medical Society is on their Web site at *http://wms.org/conf/calendar.asp*.

MODULAR KITS

Dividing the expedition kit into modular units has many advantages. It aids with kit dispersal, allowing allocations of the kit to be placed at multiple locations thus preserving segments of the kit in the case of major disasters, such as the loss of portions of the transported goods.

As mentioned in *Wilderness Medical Society Practice Guidelines*,[23] some organizations and search and rescue teams use a modular approach to medical kits for control purposes. Separate kits, with increasing sophistication and for various purposes, are available for individuals and situations requiring more advanced equipment. The basic kit is designed for use by lay personnel, but only specially trained individuals can use the more advanced kits, and they carry them into the field only when required.

Modular kits also increase accessibility as specific kits can be marked or color coded to increase visibility.

Some authorities categorize medical kits by portability. An example of this system is the one advocated by Goodman et al. with kits identified as (1) items to carry on person; (2) items to carry in individual packs; (3) items to distribute among personal packs or carry in central supply packs; and (4) items to store in vehicles.[19] This technique identifies survival and first-need items in the individual packs and accomplishes disbursement of supplies among individuals and various levels of expedition kit storage areas.

Medications and specialty supplies recommended in other specialized chapters would form the basis of additional modules for the expedition medical kit.

REFERENCES

1. Jackson R. An ancient British medical kit from Stanway, Essex. *Lancet.* 1997;350(9089):1471–3.
2. Scarez A. Contents of the emergency kit of the practicing physician. *Strasbourg Med.* 1961;12:320–6.
3. Roberts MW, Morrill GS. Medical emergencies and a standardized emergency kit for the dental office. *J Acad Gen Dent.* 1972;20(5):36–9.
4. Bradley BE, Dworin AM, Gobetti, JP. Medical emergencies in dental practice. Part II: Emergency kit and equipment. *J Mich Dent Assoc.* 1979;61(3):199–203.
5. Fourn P. Medical kit. *S Afr Med J.* 1977;52(4):158–9.
6. McCarthy FM. A minimum medical emergency kit. *Compendium.* 1994;214, 216, 218–20.
7. Rehder K, Shampo MA, Kyle RA. Physician's personal in-flight medical kit. *JAMA.* 1982;247(7):1011
8. Margulies RA, Cowan ML. A personal medical emergency kit. *Aviat Space Environ Med.* 1984;55(4):319–20.
9. Marsden PD. Tropical medical kit. *Practioner.* 1966;196 (174):555–6.
10. Marsden PD. Medical kit for tropical voyage. *Practioner.* 1968;200(197):418–21.
11. Dardick KR. Travel medicine. General advice and medical kit. *Med Clin North America.* 1992;76(6):1261–76.
12. Lewin M, Kuhn M. The Gobi Desert medical kit. *Lancet.* 2003;362 Suppl.:S4–5.
13. Sakmar TP. The traveler's medical kit. *Infect Dis Clin North Am.* 1992;6(2):355–70.
14. Mohler BR. Idealized inflight airline medical kit: A committee report. *Aviat Space Environ Med.* 1976;47(10):1094–5.
15. Cottrell JJ, Callaghan JT, Kohn GM, et al. In-flight medial emergencies. One year of experience with the enhanced medical kit. *JAMA.* 1989;262(12):1653–6.
16. Emergency Medical Kit Ad Hoc Task Force. Aerospace Medical Association. Report of the inflight emergency medical kit task force. *Aviat Space Environ Med.* 1998;69(4):427–8.
17. DeJohn CA, Veronneau SJ, Wolbrink AM, et al. An evaluation of the U.S. in-flight medical kit. *Aviat Space Environ Med.* 2002;73(5):496–500.
18. Thibeault, C. Emergency medical kit for commercial airlines: An update. *Aviat Space Environ Med.* 2002;73(6):612–3.
19. Goodman PH, Kurtz KJ, Carmichael J. Medical recommendations for wilderness travel. 3. Medical supplies and drug regimens. *Postgrad Med.* 1985;78(2):107–15.
20. Welch TP. Data-based selection of medical supplies for wilderness travel. *Wilderness Environ Med.* 1997;8(3):148–51.
21. Townes DA. Wilderness medicine. *Prim Care.* 2002;29(4): 1027–48.
22. Schimelpfenig T. *NOLS Wilderness Medicine.* Mechanicsburg, Penn: Stackpole Books; 2006.
23. Forgey W, ed. Wilderness medical kits. In: *Wilderness medical society practice guidelines for wilderness emergency care.* Butte, Mont.: Falcon Press: 2006.
24. Leemon D, Schimelpfenig T. Wilderness injury and evacuation: National Outdoor Leadership School's incident profile, 1999–2000. *Wilderness Environ Med.* 2003;14:174–82.
25. *http://www.nols.edu/wrc,* last accessed September 15, 2006.

26 Boulware DR, Forgey WW, Martin WJ II. Medical risks of wilderness hiking. *Am J Med.* 2003;114:288–93.

27 Henderson DK, Fahey BJ, et al. Risk for occupational transmission of human immunodeficiency virus type 1 (HIV-1) associated with clinical exposures: A prospective evaluation. *Ann Intern Med.* 1990;113:740–6.

28 York D, Dudek L, Larson R., Marshall W, Dries D. A comparison study of chest tube thoracostomy: Air medical crew and in-hospital trauma service. *Air Med J.* 1993;12(7):227–9.

29 *http://www.explorers.org/res_col/res_col.php,* last accessed October 8, 2006.

30 Forgey W. *Basic Essential of Wilderness First Aid.* Butte, Mont: Falcon Books; 2007.

31 Forgey W. *Wilderness Medicine.* Guilford, Conn: Globe Pequot Press; 2000.

32 Johansen, RB, Schafer, NC, Brown, PI. Effect of extreme temperatures on drugs for prehospital ACLS. *Am J Emrg Med.* 1993:11:450–2.

33 Hogerzeil, HV, Battersby A, et al. Stability of essential drugs during shipment to the tropics. *BMJ.* 1992;304:210–12

34 Kupper TEAH, Schraut B, et al. Drugs and drug administration in extreme environments. *J Travel Med.* 2006;13:35–47.

4 | Immunizations

David A. Townes MD, MPH, DTM&H, and Russell McMullen, MD

INTRODUCTION

Becoming ill far from home is a risk shared by all participants in expeditions. Even though it is impossible to completely eliminate the occurrence of illness, the risk can be reduced through a combination of behavior modification, immunization against vaccine-preventable diseases, and pharmacologic disease prophylaxis. Immunizations are a safe, reliable, and cost-effective component of this three-part approach. With proper preexpedition evaluation and planning, appropriate immunization is often easier and more reliable than behavior modification or pharmacologic disease prophylaxis. Immunizations fall into three categories: routine, required, and recommended.

Routine immunizations are those administered in childhood and/or at regular intervals during adulthood. Measles vaccine and tetanus vaccine are common examples. There is some variation in routine immunizations among countries: as an example, while Bacille Calmette-Guerin (BCG) may be included in the routine immunization schedule in certain areas of the world, it is not in the United States. Similarly, varicella immunization has become part of the routine immunization schedule in the United States but not in other areas of the world. Routine immunizations are listed in Table 4.1.

Required immunizations are those that are necessary for entry into certain countries. Yellow fever vaccine is required for entry into many countries. Meningococcal vaccine is required for entry into Saudi Arabia during the annual Hajj and Umrah pilgrimages. Prior to any expedition, it is important to check updated information about required immunizations for the country or countries of the expedition and those entered in transit. Required immunizations are listed in Table 4.2.

Recommended immunizations will depend on the specific expedition. Participants should be inoculated when there is a risk of contracting the disease and the potential morbidity and mortality from the disease on the well-being of the participants, and its impact on the expedition, outweigh any potential risk of the vaccine

itself. This will vary from expedition to expedition and may vary among individuals on the same expedition. For each potential vaccine, it is also important to consider the availability, cost, recommended schedule for administration, route of administration, and side-effect profile. Recommended immunizations are listed in Table 4.3.

This chapter includes general guidelines for routine, required, and recommended immunization of adult expedition participants. For each vaccine, the type, formulation, route, and schedule of administration reflect current recommendations for the United States. In some instances, additional vaccines, different formulations, and alternative or accelerated dosing schedules are discussed. These vaccines may only be available in other countries and thus not approved by the Federal Drug Administration (FDA); also, the FDA may not endorse alternative schedules used for vaccines within the United States. Complete information about immunization of children, pregnant women, and immunocompromised individuals is not included in the text, but references for further information are provided.

When possible, the general geographic distribution of each disease is listed by region, continent, or country. It is essential to remember, however, that there may be significant variability within a region, continent, or individual country. There may also be significant seasonal variability within a specific area. For example, only part of Ethiopia lies within the sub-Saharan "meningitis belt" of Africa. The risk of meningococcal meningitis may be significantly higher in this area than in other areas of Ethiopia. There is also seasonal variation with the risk substantially increased during the dry season from December to July.

As with other aspects of expedition planning, appropriate immunization begins with a careful evaluation of the expedition including the type, location, time of year, and duration of the expedition; the activities and conditions the participants will encounter; and the general health status and immunization history of the participants. This is a dynamic process due to constant changes in the incidence, prevalence, and distribution of

Table 4.1. Routine immunizations

Diphtheria	Pertussis
Haemophilus influenza type b	Poliomyelitis
Hepatitis A	Rubella
Hepatitis B	*Streptococcus pneumoniae*
Influenza	Tetanus
Measles	Varicella
Mumps	

Table 4.2. Required immunizations

Meningococcal disease	Yellow fever

Table 4.3. Recommended immunizations

Cholera	Smallpox
Japanese encephalitis	Tick-borne encephalitis
Lyme	Tuberculosis
Plague	Typhoid
Rabies	

diseases, government regulations and requirements, and scientific developments.

In the end, it is important that expedition participants obtain up-to-date information about the specific areas they intend to visit. There is a variety of excellent print and World Wide Web resources; many of the latter can be accessed for free, including the particularly useful Web sites of the Centers for Disease Control and Prevention (CDC; *http://www.cdc.gov*) and the World Health Organization (WHO; *http://www.who.int*).

BACKGROUND

Common to all vaccines is the induction of antibody production to a given antigen. The antibody then prevents or reduces the severity of illness if the individual is exposed to the disease at a later time. There are four major types of vaccines.

1. *Live attenuated vaccines* contain bacteria or viruses that have been altered so they do not cause disease. Examples include the measles, mumps, rubella vaccine (MMR), and oral polio vaccine (OPV). In general, live attenuated vaccines are contraindicated in pregnancy and immunocompromised individuals.
2. As the name implies, *inactivated or killed vaccines* contain inactivated or killed viruses. Inactivated polio vaccine (IPV) is an example.
3. *Toxoid vaccines* contain toxins produced by bacteria that have been altered to render them harmless. Antibodies against these toxoids can then prevent clinical disease due to the toxin. Common examples include the single antigen vaccine for tetanus and combination vaccines containing tetanus and diphtheria toxoids.

4. Finally, *component* or *conjugate vaccines* contain part of the bacteria or virus. *Haemophilus influenza* type b vaccine (Hib) is one example.

Adverse reactions may occur to any vaccine. The majority are mild local or systemic reactions; however, severe reactions do occur rarely. Reaction may be to any of the components of the vaccine including the animal proteins, antibiotics found in trace amounts in the vaccine, preservatives, stabilizers, or the vaccine antigen.

In general, all commonly used vaccines may be administered on the same day without significantly impairing the immune response or the production of antibody or increasing the risk or severity of side effects beyond the cumulative local effects of receiving injections at several sites on a given day.

Inactivated or killed vaccines usually do not interfere with the immune response to other inactivated or killed vaccines, nor do they interfere with the response to live attenuated vaccines. Therefore, inactivated or killed vaccines may be given with, before, or after other inactivated or killed vaccines, plus they can be given at any time with regard to live attenuated vaccines.

In contrast, the response to the latter of multiple live attenuated virus vaccines may be reduced if they are not administered on the same day or else with an acceptable interval of 28 days between them. If two live attenuated virus vaccines are not given the same day but fewer than 28 days apart, the second vaccine should eventually be readministered at least 4 weeks later. Live attenuated virus vaccines may also interfere with tuberculosis skin testing, which should be repeated 4–6 weeks after administration of the vaccine.

Individuals with severe or moderate acute illness should not have vaccines administered. Postponement is not necessary in those with mild illness. With the exception of the oral typhoid vaccine, it is safe and acceptable to administer vaccines to individuals on antibiotics.

Specific contraindications for the administration of vaccines are included with the description of individual vaccines.

ROUTINE IMMUNIZATIONS

Diphtheria, Tetanus, Pertussis

Diphtheria causes an illness that may affect the respiratory tract, skin, or other sites including eyes, nose, and vagina. It is caused by toxin-producing strains of the gram-positive bacteria *Corynebacterium diphtheriae* and *Corynebacterium ulcerans*. Disease is spread through respiratory droplets or personal contact. Diphtheria is found worldwide including in parts of the Americas, Africa, Asia, the South Pacific, the Middle East, Europe, and all countries of the former Soviet Union.

Clostridium tetani is the toxin-producing gram-positive anaerobic bacterial causative agent of tetanus. It is found in soil worldwide; disease is particularly common in the Philippines, Vietnam, the Asian subcontinent, Indonesia, and Brazil. Toxin generated during infection may result in muscle contraction and rigidity resulting in laryngeal spasm, autonomic dysfunction, and respiratory failure.

Infection with the gram-negative bacterium *Bordetella pertussis* may result in pertussis, a respiratory infection characterized by coughing paroxysms. Similar to diphtheria and tetanus, pertussis has a worldwide distribution.

As part of their routine immunization, children under 7 years of age are given a combination vaccine for diphtheria, tetanus, and pertussis containing diphtheria and tetanus toxoids and acellular pertussis antigens (DTaP). The vaccine containing whole cell pertussis antigen (DTwP) is no longer available in the United States. The vaccine is administered before the child's seventh birthday with five doses of DTaP at 2, 4, and 6 months and then between 15 and 18 months and 4 to 6 years. The fifth dose may not be necessary if the fourth was given after age 4 but before age 7.

Adults should receive the adult formulation containing tetanus and diphtheria toxoids (Td). Until recently, there was no adult formulation that included a pertussis vaccine (see discussion below). In adults who did not receive a primary series as a child or if there is uncertainty, one dose of Tdap and two doses of Td should be administered intramuscularly (IM), the first two doses 4–8 weeks apart and the third 6–12 months later. If this schedule is not possible, then the third dose should be given 4–8 weeks after the second. Two doses provide some protection, but one dose is of little benefit. Adults who did receive the full series require a booster every 10 years.

Because adults are susceptible to pertussis once childhood immunity wanes, an adult booster for tetanus and diphtheria vaccine that also contains acellular pertussis antigen has recently been introduced (Tdap). This is a one-time substitute for a dose of Td vaccine and can be administered at anytime starting at 11–12 years of age. If there is a particular concern about exposure to pertussis in adults, Tdap can be administered as close as 2 years after the last dose of Td. This may be a consideration for members of an expedition traveling to areas where preventive health care for the local population is poor.

Haemophilus Influenza Type B

Haemophilus influenza type b may be the causative agent in bacterial meningitis, pneumonia, bacteremia, septic arthritis, and epiglottitis. There are three conjugate Hib vaccines licensed for use in infants and children in the United States. The administration schedule varies depending on the specific vaccine used, but regardless, the series is completed with a booster administered at 12–15 months. There is no adult formulation of the vaccine.

Hepatitis A

Hepatitis A is a viral infection spread through ingestion of the hepatitis A virus (HAV) via fecal–oral transmission, either through person-to-person contact or contaminated food or water. It is perhaps the most common vaccine-preventable disease for travelers. Illness in young children tends to be mild, often without causing jaundice, and results in natural immunity. In the developing world, most of the population will have been infected when they were quite young. In adults, signs and symptoms of the illness include fever, nausea, abdominal pain, malaise, jaundice, and dark urine. The distribution is worldwide, although the risk to travelers is much higher in the developing world where water resources and sanitation may be poor.

In the United States, there are two currently licensed monovalent vaccines. Both are made from inactivated hepatitis A virus. The vaccine is administered in a single IM dose in the deltoid resulting in a protective concentration of antibodies in 94–100% of individuals in 4 weeks. A booster is recommended in 6–12 months to promote protection for at least 10 years, possibly lifelong.

Purified serum immune globulin was used for prevention of hepatitis A prior to the introduction of hepatitis A vaccine. It may still play a role in prevention of hepatitis A for a very small number of people at particular risk. If the expedition begins in significantly less than 4 weeks, and there will likely be almost immediate exposure to a large native population and primitive sanitation conditions, and the person has never received a dose of hepatitis A vaccine, administration of purified human immune globulin along with the first dose of vaccine may provide temporary immunity until antibody production from the vaccine begins. The antibody titer generated by the vaccine may be lower in these individuals than if one receives just the vaccine. These individuals should receive their booster dose of hepatitis A vaccine at 6–12 months to generate a long-term protective response similar to that expected in individuals who did not receive immune globulin.

Immune globulin can interfere with the response to some live virus vaccines. Measles, mumps, rubella vaccines, and varicella vaccine should be administered at least 2 weeks before IM immune globulin or else 3 months afterward. Yellow fever vaccine does not appear to be significantly affected.

Hepatitis B

Hepatitis B is a viral infection spread through contact with blood or other body fluids infected with the hepatitis B virus (HBV). High-risk behaviors include engaging in sexual activity, sharing needles, receiving blood transfusions, having medical or dental procedures, and getting a tattoo. Participants in expeditions involving delivery of health care to the local population may be at risk as well. HBV has a worldwide distribution, but high-risk areas where the incidence of chronic carriage in the native population is high include Africa, Southeast Asia, the Middle East, the South and Western Pacific Islands, the Amazon River basin, and parts of the Caribbean.

Two monovalent hepatitis B vaccines are currently available. They are made using recombinant DNA technology in yeast cells to replicate hepatitis B surface antigen (HBsAg); this is then purified. Standard administration is IM at 0, 1, and 6 months. An accelerated administration at 0, 1, and 2 months with a booster in 12 months has been approved for one of the vaccines.

Some individuals may not develop sufficient levels of antibodies. Individuals at risk include smokers, obese individuals, those with chronic medical conditions, and those who received the vaccine in the buttocks, where it was administered when first introduced in the 1980s. If a person will be providing health care or will be at continued significant risk or exposure, it may be advisable to measure the hepatitis B surface antibody (HSsAb) level 4 weeks or more after completion of the series. If insufficient antibodies are measured after the standard course, then one additional dose should be administered and the titer repeated in 4–12 weeks. If the antibody titer is still insufficient, the full course should be completed and the titer measured again.

As of 2001, there is a combination vaccine for hepatitis A and hepatitis B that is administered at 0, 1, and 6 months. For individuals traveling in less than a month, there is also an accelerated schedule administered at 0, 7, and 21 days that has recently been approved by the FDA. This accelerated administration results in virtually 100% seroconversion rate to hepatitis A; the seroconversion rate for hepatitis B is lower, but better than that achieved with a single dose of hepatitis B vaccine. A booster is recommended at 12 months if the accelerated schedule is used.

Influenza

Influenza is a viral illness characterized in adults by the abrupt onset of constitutional and respiratory signs and symptoms. The etiological agents are the influenza A and B viruses. Influenza tends to occur seasonally in the United States but may occur year round in the tropics. While the disease affects all age groups, morbidity and mortality are highest in certain groups including those whose members are older than 50 years of age; those with pulmonary disease, asthma, renal disease, ischemic heart disease, and other chronic medical conditions; transplant recipients; immunocompromised individuals; persons on chronic aspirin therapy (who

are at risk of Reye syndrome); and women who may become pregnant. Immunization should be considered routine in these high-risk groups.

There are currently two types of vaccines available. Both contain three strains of influenza virus and are administered annually. One vaccine contains inactivated or killed virus and is administered IM. The other contains live attenuated influenza virus (LAIV) administered as a nasal spray. The LAIV is intended only for healthy persons between 5 and 49 years of age.

Measles

Measles is a viral illness with a worldwide distribution most common in the developing countries of Europe and Asia. The clinical syndrome includes fever, cough, coryza, Koplik spots, and a characteristic rash. Less severe complications include middle ear infections and diarrhea. More severe complications include pneumonia and encephalitis, often leading to death.

The measles vaccine contains a live attenuated measles virus either alone or in combination with the mumps vaccine or the rubella vaccine, or both (MMR). A single dose is administered IM at 12–15 months resulting in immunity in 95% of individuals. A second dose may be given as soon as 28 days later, but it is routinely given in the United States between 4 and 6 years of age. If an adult has not had a second dose of measles or MMR vaccine, it should be given before travel to the developing world.

Mumps

Mumps is a viral illness characterized by fever, headache, myalgia, malaise, anorexia, and parotitis.

The mumps vaccine contains a live attenuated mumps virus administered alone or in combination with measles and rubella (MMR). The recommended dosing schedule for MMR is a first dose at 12–15 months and a second dose at 4–6 years of age.

Rubella

Rubella is a mild viral illness that is characterized by fever and rash. Rubella is most concerning if it is contracted during pregnancy because it may lead to serious birth defects or fetal loss.

The vaccine contains a live attenuated rubella virus administered alone or in combination with measles and mumps (MMR) with the first given at 12–15 months and the second given at 4–6 months of age. It is important that women avoid getting pregnant for at least 1 month after receiving the vaccine.

MMR may be given with any other live attenuated or inactivated vaccine. Inactivated vaccines and the live attenuated typhoid vaccine may be given at any time before or after the live attenuated measles vaccine; however, if MMR and the current live attenuated yellow fever vaccine are not given simultaneously, they should be separated by at least 28 days.

Poliomyelitis

Poliomyelitis is a potentially serious acute viral infection spread by the fecal–oral route. Infections may be asymptomatic or may feature gastrointestinal symptoms, but of most concern is the central nervous system disease resulting in flaccid paralysis, respiratory failure, and, rarely, death. The program for global elimination of poliomyelitis has been largely successful and today there are four countries in which it is endemic (Afghanistan, India, Nigeria, Pakistan). Outbreaks do still occur both in these and other countries.

There are two vaccines currently available: an inactivated (IPV) formulation and a live attenuated oral formulation (OPV). Adequate primary immunization results from administration of at least three doses of OPV or four doses of IPV or a combination of both.

Due to the risk, albeit very low, of developing polio when a person receives primary vaccination with OPV, in the United States children now routinely receive only IPV given at 2, 4, 6–18 months, and 4–6 years. Adults who did not receive primary vaccination in childhood should receive two doses of IPV, 4–8 weeks apart and a third dose 6–12 months after the second. Several accelerated dosing schedules are utilized. If protection is required in less than 4 weeks, one dose of IPV should be administered. If 4–8 weeks is available for dosing, two doses of IPV should be administered 4 weeks apart. If more than 8 weeks are available, three doses of IPV should be administered at least 4 weeks apart. In each case, the remaining doses may be given later at the normal schedule intervals. Adults who received their primary series as a child but are planning to travel to countries where poliomyelitis is endemic or regions that have not been declared polio-free by the World Health Organization should receive a "one time" dose of IPV prior to travel.

Streptococcus pneumoniae

Pneumococcal disease caused by the bacterium *Streptococcus pneumoniae* ranges from mild illness to life-threatening infections including pneumonia, bacteremia, and meningitis. Even though the distribution of the disease is worldwide and may affect all age groups, high-risk groups are very similar to those at risk for influenza. Concurrent immunization for both diseases should be considered in these individuals. Those at particular risk for pneumococcal disease include individuals older than 65 and individuals between 2 and 64 years of age who have chronic cardiovascular, pulmonary, or liver disease; diabetes mellitus; alcoholism; or who are immunocompromised.

There are two vaccines, both designed to induce antibodies against the pneumococcal capsule. The conjugate vaccine is part of the routine infant immunization schedule, with extension into childhood for certain groups; the polysaccharide vaccine is part of the routine adolescent and adult vaccination schedule for at risk individuals.

Varicella

Varicella-zoster virus (VZV) is the cause of chickenpox (varicella) in primary infection and herpes zoster as a reactivation of a latent infection. Varicella is a generally mild infection in children characterized by fever, malaise, and a characteristic rash. Serious complications, although rare, are more common in infants, adults, and immunocompromised individuals. These include secondary bacterial infection of the skin lesions, pneumonia, and encephalitis.

The varicella vaccine contains live attenuated VZV. It is now routinely administered to children starting at 12–18 months of age, but should be given to at-risk older children and adults. Children getting the first dose at 12–18 months should receive a second dose at least 3 months later, although it is routinely given at 4–6 years. Children over 13 years of age and adults should receive two doses given 4–8 weeks apart. Individuals with a reliable history of chickenpox do not need to be immunized. If there is uncertainty, prior disease is not a risk for immunization.

The live attenuated varicella vaccine may be given simultaneously with any other live attenuated or inactivated vaccine. It should not be given at the same time as immune globulin (see preceding discussion). The live attenuated oral typhoid vaccine may be administered at any time before or after the varicella vaccine. If the live attenuated varicella vaccine, the live attenuated MMR vaccine, and the live attenuated yellow fever vaccines are not given simultaneously, they should be separated by at least 28 days.

REQUIRED VACCINATIONS

Yellow Fever

Yellow fever is a viral illness transmitted to humans by the bite of various infected mosquitoes, including *Aedes aegypti*, in equatorial South America, southern Panama, and sub-Saharan Africa. Clinically, yellow fever may range from an influenza-like syndrome, to hepatitis, and in the most severe cases, hemorrhagic fever.

Yellow fever vaccine is required for entry into several countries listed in Table 4.4. In addition, certain countries require proof of vaccination or booster within 10 years when traveling to or from a yellow fever endemic country. A complete list of these countries and specific requirements are available through the CDC. Yellow fever endemic zones are shown in Figures 4.1 and 4.2.

Table 4.4. Countries that require vaccination against yellow fever for entry

Benin	Bolivia	Burundi
Burkina Faso	Cameroon	Central African Republic
Congo	Cote d'Ivoire	Democratic Republic of Congo
French Guiana	Gabon	Ghana
Liberia	Mali	Niger
Mauritania	Rwanda	Sao Tome and Principe
Sierra Leone	Togo	

Source: Centers for Disease Control and Prevention. *Health Information for International Travel* 2008. Atlanta: U.S. Department of Health and Human Services, Public Health Service; 2005.

The World Health Organization regulates yellow fever vaccine production, administration, and documentation. The vaccine is a live attenuated vaccine administered as a single subcutaneous (SQ) injection. This single administration leads to seroconversion in approximately 95% of recipients and provides at least 10 years immunity.

Immunization against yellow fever is recorded on the "International Certificate of Vaccination" commonly known as the Yellow Card, which is approved by the WHO. If the vaccine is contraindicated and the person is traveling to a country requiring proof of vaccination, there is a place on the Yellow Card where a physician can certify that the person should not receive a particular vaccine. However, it is recommended that a statement signed by a physician on letterhead stating that yellow fever vaccine could not be administered should also be obtained and carried by the individual.

The yellow fever vaccine may be given with all other available vaccines. If other live attenuated viral vaccines are not given concurrently with the yellow fever vaccine, 28 days should be allowed to elapse between sequential vaccinations. Chloroquine, a drug commonly used for malaria prophylaxis, inhibits replication of the yellow fever virus in vitro but does not adversely affect antibody response to yellow fever vaccine. Likewise, IM immune globulin dose not inhibit the effectiveness of yellow fever vaccine, unlike other live virus vaccines.

There have been cases of vaccine-associated neurological disease (4–6 cases per 1,000,000 given) and vaccine-associated viscerotropic disease, clinically and pathophysiologically similar to naturally occurring yellow fever (3–5 cases per 1,000,000). The data suggest the latter complication is more common in persons older than 60 years of age receiving their primary immunization. Careful examination of the true risk of yellow fever should be done and immunization reserved for those who are at genuine risk of acquiring yellow fever. This is especially important for individuals older than 60 who require a primary vaccination. In these individuals, consideration should be given to altering travel plans to reduce the risk of yellow fever and eliminate the need for the vaccine. Additionally, individuals with a history of thymus disease, thymoma, and myasthenia gravis should not get the vaccine due to increased risk of complications.

Meningococcal Disease

Meningococcal disease is an acute bacterial illness characterized by fever, headache, nausea, vomiting, an ecchymotic rash, and meningitis. Occurrence is worldwide but is increased in certain areas including the "meningitis belt" across sub-Saharan Africa during the dry season of December through July as shown in Figure 4.3. Epidemics also occur throughout the world, with recent examples being Saudi Arabia in 2000 and in Burkina Faso in 2004.

Proof of vaccination is *required* for entrance into Saudi Arabia for travelers to Mecca during the annual Hajj and Umrah pilgrimages during late spring. Vaccination is *recommended* for those going to affected countries in sub-Saharan Africa. The vaccine is a polysaccharide quadrivalent vaccine against serogroups A, C, Y, W-135 administered as a single dose providing 3–5 years immunity. There is also a bivalent vaccine against serogroups A and C but not Y and W-135; this is not available in the United States. Monovalent vaccines are available outside the United States including in Canada and Europe.

A recent advance in the United States is the release of the quadrivalent vaccine conjugated with diphtheria toxoid (MCV4). This formulation appears to stimulate a stronger immune response and induce protection for a longer period. It is now the recommended vaccine for individuals between 11 and 55 years of age.

RECOMMENDED VACCINATIONS

Cholera

Cholera is an acute intestinal infection caused by the toxigenic bacteria *Vibrio cholerae* group O1 (classical or El Tor) or group O139; it is transmitted by contaminated food and water and rarely from person to person. It may occur anywhere but especially where sanitation and living conditions are poor. Refugees and other displaced persons are particularly at risk. Outbreaks have occurred in Indonesia, Asia, Eastern Europe, Africa, the Iberian Peninsula, Peru, and the city of New Orleans. Cholera vaccination is not generally recommended because of the low risk to the majority of travelers and the relatively low efficacy of the vaccine. It may be considered for individuals who will be traveling or working in refugee settings.

Despite not being required by the WHO, in certain areas local authorities may request evidence of a

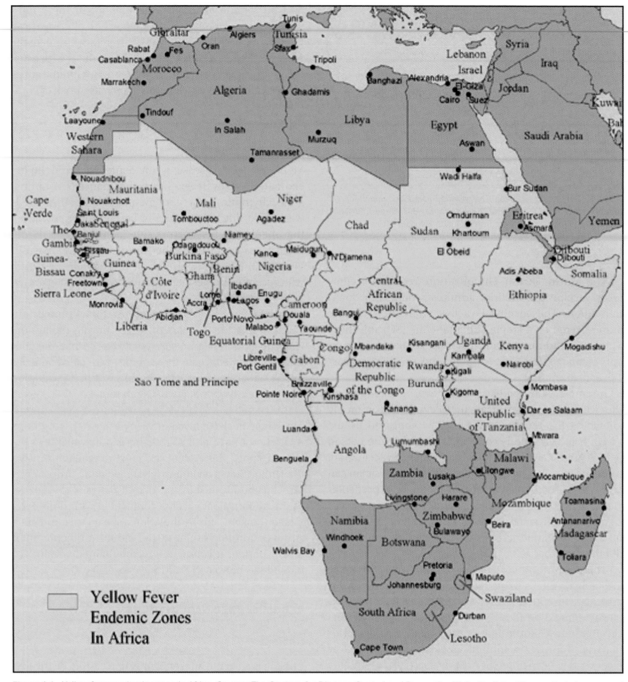

Figure 4.1. Yellow fever endemic zones in Africa. Source: The Centers for Disease Control and Prevention Web site *(http://www.cdc.gov)*, accessed June 15, 2007.

cholera vaccine from individuals arriving from or going to an endemic area. In these cases, one recent dose of the current cholera vaccine recorded on the Yellow Card may meet the criterion. Others may be required to pay a "fee" for a "waiver."

There are two oral cholera vaccines, but neither is available in the United States. They are live attenuated vaccines given as a single dose resulting in protection for 6 months, perhaps longer. Cholera is better avoided through careful food and water precautions. Cholera is

very sensitive to gastric acid; therefore, individuals on medications that reduce gastric acid may be at additional risk.

Japanese Encephalitis

Japanese encephalitis (JE) is a flavivirus infection transmitted by *Culex* mosquitoes in East, Southeast, and South Asia where it is the leading cause of childhood encephalitis. It occurs seasonally, primarily in rural

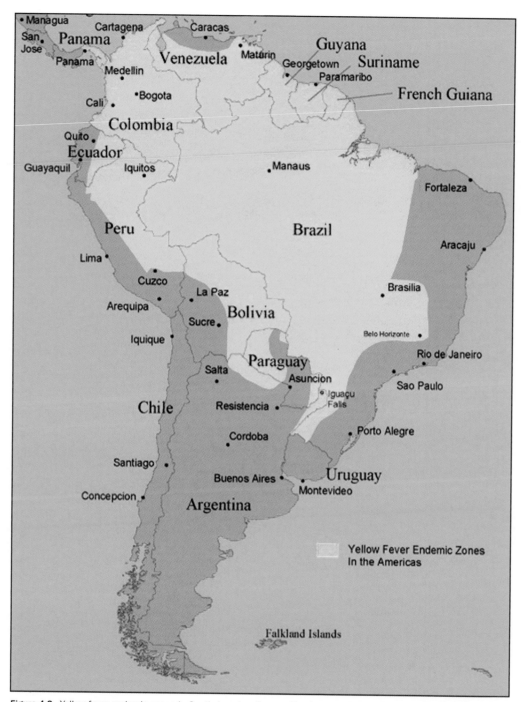

Figure 4.2. Yellow fever endemic zones in South America. Source: The Centers for Disease Control and Prevention Web site *(http://www.cdc.gov)*, accessed June 15, 2007.

agricultural areas where flooding irrigation is utilized. In many parts of Asia, these areas border urban centers. The vaccine should be considered for people with even short-term overnight outdoor rural exposure during the high transmission season. The endemic zones for JE are shown in Figure 4.4.

The vaccine is an inactivated viral vaccine, given SQ at 0, 7, and 30 days. It may also be administered at 0, 7, and 14 days, although the seroconversion rate may

be less. Two doses given 7 days apart provide short-term immunity to about 80% of recipients. Because of the potential for delayed side effects, the series should be completed at least 10 days before travel. There is an additional risk of reaction to the vaccine in those allergic to hymenoptera envenomation. A booster is recommended after 2 years or more in the event of return to the endemic area. A vero-cell derived vaccine, requiring only two doses and with a better side-effect

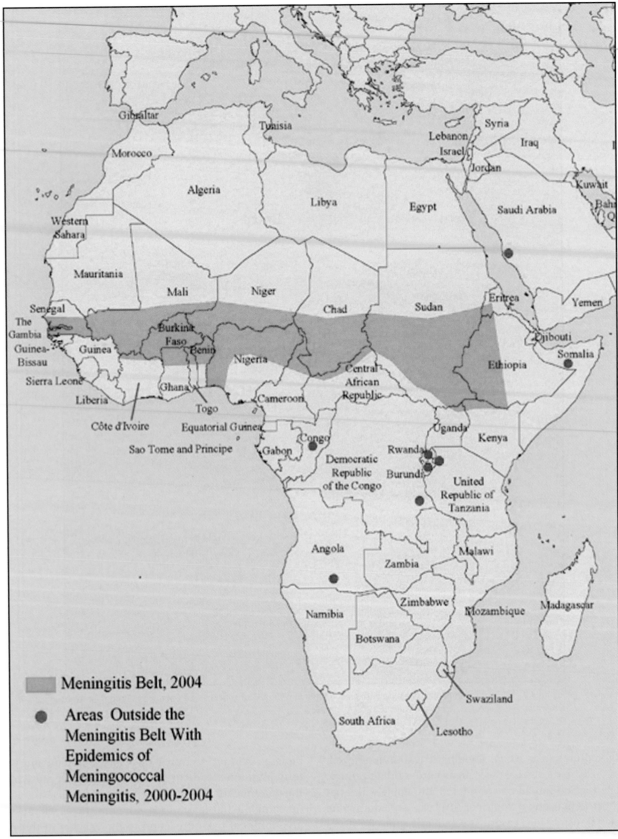

Figure 4.3. Meningitis belt in Africa, 2004. Source: The Centers for Disease Control and Prevention Web site *(http://www.cdc.gov)*, accessed June 15, 2007.

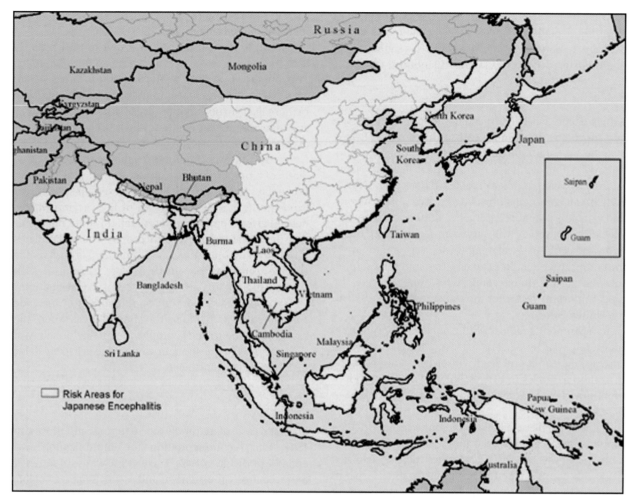

Figure 4.4. Risk areas for Japanese encephalitis. Source: The Centers for Disease Control and Prevention Web site (*http://www.cdc.gov*), accessed June 15, 2007.

profile, should soon be available to replace the current vaccine.

Lyme

Lyme disease is caused primarily by infection with the spirochete *Borrelia burgdorferi.* It occurs in Asia, Europe, and North America. Clinical presentation includes the characteristic rash called erythema chronicum migrans (Figure 4.5), as well as fever, arthritis, and neurological manifestations.

The vaccine was removed from the market in 2002 and is no longer commercially available.

Plague

Plague is caused by the bacteria *Yersinia pestis,* which is endemic in wild rodents. It is transmitted to humans either by fleas, through direct contact with infected animals, or via person-to-person respiratory secretions. The vaccine is an inactivated or killed bacteria vaccine. Its efficacy and thus utility have not been fully documented, and it is no longer commercially available in the United States. It is not recommended for general travel

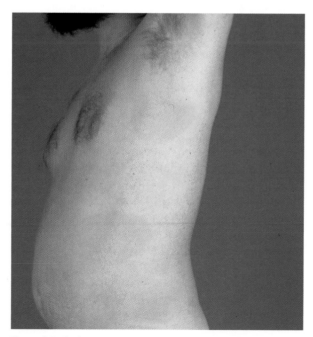

Figure 4.5. Erythema chronicum migrans. Photo courtesy of J. Dick MacLean, McGill University Centre for Tropical Diseases.

but may be prudent in certain high-risk groups such as scientific expeditions involving field biologists where exposure to potentially infected animals is significant. It is administered as 3 doses IM over 10 months.

Rabies

Rabies occurs when an infected animal bites a person and inoculates the wound with a rhabdovirus. It may also be transmitted via a lick to an open wound. Although some countries, particularly isolated or island nations, appear to be free of rabies, it does occur worldwide on all continents except Antarctica. All carnivores and bats are potential reservoirs; the importance of a species as a reservoir will vary from region to region. In many areas of the developing world, dogs are the most important reservoir. Bats can also transmit rabies, often through almost undetectable bites, and they are the most important vector for the transmission of rabies in the United States.

Rabies presents clinically with a nonspecific prodromal phase followed by paresis, spasms, paralysis, delirium, convulsions, coma, and death. Onset of symptoms can be in as short as a week to 10 days, but incubation periods of months and perhaps years following exposure have been noted.

Rabies vaccines available in the United States include human diploid cell rabies vaccine (HDCV), purified chick embryo cell vaccine (PCEC), or rabies vaccine adsorbed (RVA). All contain inactivated or killed rabies virus. In addition, rabies immune globulin (RIG) is an important part of postexposure prophylaxis in most individuals.

All individuals who have had a significant exposure to potentially infected animals require postexposure treatment and vaccination against rabies. For postexposure treatment, if no preexposure vaccination was administered, the individual should receive one dose of RIG and a series of five doses of IM vaccine initiated as soon as possible after the exposure. The vaccine is given on day 0 and subsequently on days 3, 7, 14, and 28. The dose of RIG is 20 IU/kg. It should be administered with as much as possible infiltrated around the wound and the rest administered at a remote site, preferably the glutei to avoid any chance of the subsequent vaccine doses being given at the site where RIG was administered. If not immediately available, RIG may be given up to 7 days after the first dose of rabies vaccine.

It is important to consider that both RIG and rabies vaccine may be difficult to locate in remote settings and developing countries. Due to cost, even if RIG is available, it may be horse-derived (equine RIG, or ERIG) rather than human-derived. These preparations have been associated with an increase risk of serum sickness. Similarly, locally produced vaccine may be derived from infected brain tissue of lab animals. These vaccines may be less effective than tissue-culture-derived vaccines used in the developing world and also appear to have a more serious side-effect profile.

Bearing in mind all of the above, preexposure prophylaxis may make sense for certain expedition members. This applies especially to those going to areas where even pet animals are not immunized against rabies and to those likely to be in remote areas where it may be difficult to readily access adequate and safe care in the event of an exposure.

Preexposure vaccination for rabies consists of three doses of a modern tissue-culture-derived vaccine given IM on days 0, 7, and 21 or 28. In the event of subsequent exposure, two additional doses of the vaccine will be needed given 3 days apart. Although this does not eliminate the need for postexposure prophylaxis, it eliminates the need for RIG and decreases the number of doses of the vaccine needed in the event of exposure. It may also lessen the time urgency in receiving postexposure vaccination.

Preexposure vaccination should therefore also be considered for individuals traveling to areas where the vaccine may be in short supply, the quality or safety of the vaccine is in question, or when there is a likely delay in obtaining the vaccine.

Smallpox

The last case of naturally occurring smallpox was in 1977, and recommendation for immunization was ended worldwide in 1982. The vaccine was subsequently removed from the market and is no longer available commercially.

The vaccine is a live virus vaccine containing vaccinia virus, an orthopoxvirus related to smallpox that provides cross-protection. It is available through the CDC on a case-by-case basis and is generally reserved for individuals working with the virus, certain military personnel, and potential outbreak investigators and first responders.

Tick-Borne Encephalitis

Tick-borne encephalitis (TBE) is caused by infection of the central nervous system with a flavivirus. The two main serotypes are the Central European encephalitis virus and the Russian spring-summer encephalitis virus; they are both transmitted to humans through the bite of the *Ixodes ricinus* tick in Europe, *Ixodes persulcatus* in Northeast Asia, or more rarely through ingestion of unpasteurized dairy products. The distribution of TBE is shown in Figure 4.6.

A vaccine is not currently available in the United States. In some countries in Central Europe (e.g., Austria), a majority of the population has been vaccinated. One formulation of the vaccine used in Europe is administered as three IM injections over the course of 1 year. This vaccine is not commercially available in Canada

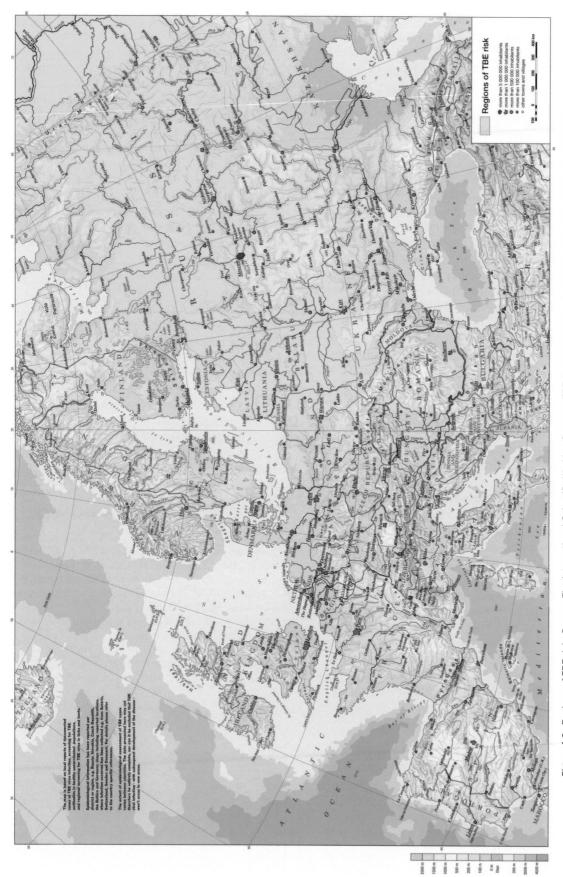

Figure 4.6. Regions of TBE risk. Source: The International Scientific Working Group on TBE (*http://www.tbe-info.com/tbe.aspx*), accessed June 15, 2007.

but may be obtained through Canadian providers on a special access basis. The second formulation available in Europe has a similar schedule but may also be administered as an accelerated schedule on days 0, 7, and 21 with a booster in 12–18 months and at 3–5 years.

Tuberculosis

The bacterium *Mycobacterium tuberculosis* is the cause of tuberculosis. Once thought to be a disease of the past, it has reemerged and is now one of the largest health problems worldwide, especially in the developing world. The clinical manifestations are diverse but can be generally categorized as pulmonary and extrapulmonary.

There is no general consensus for the use of Bacille Calmette-Guerin in adults. Investigations have not consistently demonstrated efficacy in adults, and it is not routinely recommended in the United States. In infants and children, however, the use of BCG has been demonstrated to reduce the incidence of severe disease including meningitis and disseminated disease. It is routinely administered to infants and children in the developing world. BCG is a live attenuated vaccine and is thus contraindicated during pregnancy and in immunocompromised individuals.

Typhoid

Typhoid, or enteric fever, is caused by the gram-negative bacterium *Salmonella typhi*. Enteric fever can also be caused by *Salmonella paratyphi* A and B, although the symptoms are typically less severe. Available vaccines offer protection against typhoid but are less or not effective against the paratyphi strains. Typhoid is acquired by consumption of contaminated food and drink. The potentially life-threatening clinical syndrome consists of high fever, malaise, headache, anorexia, splenomegaly, and relative bradycardia.

There are two vaccines available in the United States. One formulation containing a live attenuated form of the bacterium is administered orally as four capsules given every other day for a week. Revaccination is recommended in 5 years. The protection provided may be overcome by ingestion of large amounts of the bacteria, so food and

water precautions are still necessary. Because it is a live attenuated bacterial vaccine, it should not be given to immunocompromised individuals or in pregnancy.

There may be concern with oral typhoid vaccine in those planning on using Malarone for malaria prophylaxis. Proguanil, a component of Malarone, has been shown at 200 mg/day to decrease the immune response to the oral typhoid vaccine, but standard Malarone dosing contains only 100 mg/day. Ideally one would want to wait for 10 days after the oral typhoid vaccine to start Malarone.

There is also an IM typhoid vaccine that utilizes the polysaccharide Vi capsular antigen as its immune stimulus. Considered safe in both pregnant and immunocompromised individuals, it is administered as a single dose with ongoing booster doses given after 2 years as needed.

CONCLUSION

A key component of expedition planning is determination of the necessary immunizations for each participant. This includes a careful evaluation of both the expedition and its participants. It is essential to begin the process early enough to allow for appropriate administration of all vaccinations. In combination with pharmacologic disease prophylaxis and behavior modification, immunization against vaccine-preventable disease is a safe, reliable, and cost-effective way to protect the health and safety of expedition participants and thus help ensure the success of the expedition itself.

SUGGESTED READINGS

Centers for Disease Control and Prevention. *Health Information for International Travel 2008*. Atlanta: U.S. Department of Health and Human Services, Public Health Service; 2008.

Gill GV, Beeching NJ. *Lecture Notes on Tropical Medicine*. 5th ed. Malden, Mass.: Blackwell Science; 2004.

Jong EC, McMullen R. *The Travel and Tropical Medicine Manual*. 3rd ed. New York: Elsevier Science; 2003.

Peters W, Pasvol G. *Tropical Medicine and Parasitology*. 5th ed. St. Louis: Mosby International Limited; 2002.

Plotkin SA, Orenstein WA. *Vaccines*. 4th ed. New York: Elsevier; 2004.

5 Legal Considerations during Expedition Planning

Kristin Larson, Esq., and Tracey Knutson, Esq.

No matter your personal view of risk, trips away from home can involve certain unknown and unforeseen risks and unplanned surprises. Such contingencies can be as innocuous as a flight delay or as serious as a week-long white-out at high altitude. And even though advanced planning will not eliminate such surprises, it will mitigate the impact of such events on the goals and enjoyment of the endeavor, as well as on the legal liabilities stemming from unexpected incidents.

Expeditions are inherently risky, and it is this risk quotient that differentiates garden variety trips from expeditions. Most risk exposure on expeditions is derived from the potential for bodily harm, and for this reason books such as this one, providing specialized information on medical care in expedition contexts, are important references. Knowing what types of medical risks will be present and methods for preventing and/or treating them in the field are vital pretrip evaluations, but simply knowing the medical risks is not enough. Often overlooked in the expedition planning phase are steps and methods for reducing the entire range of risks and the legal liabilities that may be present. For instance, after the medical triage is complete, considerations inevitably turn to the rights and obligations of those involved, and if the proper framework is in place prior to the trip, such matters can be resolved in an orderly fashion with minimal dispute. Moreover, the risk of liability does not always end with the expedition itself but may arise long after the crampons have been hung up. For example, disputes concerning intellectual property generated in relation to the expedition may arise, but with proper advanced consideration and planning such aggravations can be minimized.

The purpose for this chapter then is to provide expedition leaders and planners with an overview of legal considerations – a checklist of sorts – to assist in evaluating legal risks and developing mitigation measures at the early planning stages rather than waiting until the accident/conflict/incident occurs to consider legal implications. Such planning includes developing documentation memorializing agreements and relationships; understanding how legal liabilities occur and are judged; establishing a robust and context-appropriate organizational structure; conducting adequate due diligence on the destination and participants; and considering potential postexpedition products. Because this is but a single chapter in a comprehensive medical text, the scope and detail is necessarily limited. Thus, for instance, it does not include a discussion on country-specific permits and licenses that may be required for a particular type of activity in a particular location, nor does it cover legal regimes of different countries. Rather, this chapter should serve as a starting point for planning and further consultation with legal specialists.

RISK MANAGEMENT PLANNING

Due to the types of activities involved and the huge growth in participation within the adventure and recreation sports industry (including, by analogy, expeditionary undertakings), it is vital that the leaders of such entities undertake methodical and responsible assessments of the risks associated with the planned activities, and then employ risk and safety management practices.[1] Generally, an adventure- or expedition-styled entity needs to consider two types of risk management: first, minimizing the risks or hazards of the actual activity that it is conducting and, second, minimizing the risks of loss or damage to the expeditionary entity (and/or its members). Because of the high costs of litigation, insurance, and legal liabilities in general, it is clear that, to attain the second goal of minimizing risks of loss and damage to expedition entities, it is worthwhile investing significant time considering the issue of minimizing the risks associated with planned activities. For this reason, critical consideration should be given to each element of the expedition. This analysis or risk management planning should be done with expedition leaders and members and should, at a minimum, involve the following four elements:

1. **Risk identification:** This element relates to the range of activities and their potential for exposing the

expedition to safety and negligence liabilities, property loss, contract disputes or personnel issues (e.g., fidelity).

2. **Risk evaluation:** This element relates to a determination of the potential severity and frequency of risk incidents.

3. **Risk treatment:** Is the expedition and/or its members willing to retain the risk? Will the planners need to reduce it, treat it, or avoid it?

4. **Implementation:** This element relates to the development and execution of policies and procedures, warnings, brochures, and training.[2]

Risk is subjective, and each member of an expedition will view it differently based on his or her level of confidence, experience, personal wealth, and physical capabilities. Depending on the diversity of the expeditionary group, one approach for determining a preliminary range of risks is for the expedition leaders to canvas the members directly. This will allow the group leader(s) to get an initial read on the range of risk-adversity among the members, as well as assist in zeroing in on the level and the types of risks the members anticipate and/or will tolerate.[3] For a successful endeavor, the level of risk management must correlate well with the risk tolerance of the participants. If risk is mitigated to a point consistent with a particular level of group or member tolerance, participant experience and satisfaction will be positively affected.[4] And, although undoubtedly obvious, it bears repeating that more planning effort toward minimizing and mitigating should be spent on risks that produce or present severe or frequent consequences. Remember, it is not that an expedition entity has a duty to ensure that participants/members are kept away from *all* risk; rather the goal of risk management is to ensure that participants are not exposed to risks that would be considered unreasonable given the circumstances under which the expedition is forming. See, generally, the section entitled "Tort Liability or Negligence, Generally" in this chapter.

The remainder of this chapter is broken into specific areas that will allow expedition planners to focus on and understand the risks of liability that may be associated with the expedition, as well as approaches for minimizing such risks. A threshold consideration is deciding the form of organization that the expedition will take. Will it be a loose-knit group of individuals? A hierarchy of leaders and members? A team of professionals? As explained in the next section, this decision can substantially impact the degree of liability exposure the group as a whole may be shielded from.

STRUCTURING THE EXPEDITION TO OPTIMIZE ITS GOALS AND MINIMIZE LIABILITY

History is littered with the launchings of people to unknown territories. However, until relatively recently, governmental sponsorship and patronage played a significant role in such campaigns, providing not only the incentives, funds, and other resources but also the goals and deliverables of such trips. Risks for loss and damage were borne primarily by the sponsor. In modern times, trips to uncharted territories have all but disappeared, and two primary expedition formats have taken their place: (1) remote field activities focused on gaining scientific or cultural knowledge; and (2) forays undertaken principally to fulfill personal goals such as endurance and inspiration. Government funding continues to play a primary role in supporting field research, as well as extraterrestrial exploration. Other types of expeditions are now almost exclusively private endeavors and have therefore assumed all the risks attendant to such endeavors.

For this reason, expedition groups now expend increasingly longer periods of "lead-up" time to their trips, raising the necessary capital and/or finding sponsors and developing plans that will guard against failure or loss.[5] Depending on a number of factors (e.g., financial needs, scope of activities, number and roles of expedition personnel, planning lead-time, and postexpedition products such as documentaries, books, and/or product endorsements), formation of a formal organizational structure for such private expeditions may facilitate reaching these goals. During the planning phase, consideration should be given to any one of a number of different recognized organizational forms, and a lawyer should be consulted to determine which structure best fits the needs of a specific expedition.

The organization of choice for most large-scale modern-day expeditions is the nonprofit corporation. This is largely due to its advantages for attracting donors and the liability protection afforded by its corporate structure. Formation of such a structure can also help define the legal relationships within the group, as well as the group's relationships with outside parties. This section of the chapter summarizes the process and potential benefits of setting up a nonprofit corporation. Small expedition groups may determine that formation of such a legal entity is too cumbersome and represents too much of a trade-off against the need for nimbleness. In such instances, the execution of liability releases and other agreements among the members, as discussed in "Avoiding and Defending against Tort Liability in Adventure or Expeditionary Contexts" section of this chapter may provide sufficient definition of legal relationships and liability mitigation measures. However, for larger expeditions involving multiple forms of legal relationships and potential liabilities, formation of a corporate entity may prove to be the best solution.

The Expedition as a Nonprofit Organization

Most expeditions want to get and to give. They want to get support and financial sponsors, and to give time educating or publicizing their experiences or endeavors. For this reason, expeditions are uniquely positioned to take advantage of the two primary benefits offered by nonprofit laws: facilitated access to benefactors/ sponsors and credit for community service. Modern nonprofit law has its roots in many cultures as an outgrowth of religious traditions and through the encouragement of private pursuit of "good works" by governmental entities. Philanthropy likewise is not new, with evidence of its existence dating back more than 4,000 years to both ancient Greek and Egyptian cultures. However, as observed by Alexis de Tocqueville more than 150 years ago, only in America has the caliber of charitable activities and nonprofit associations risen to such high levels of sophistication and importance.

Threshold Considerations in Forming a Nonprofit Corporation

As summarized earlier, there are significant payoffs associated with forming a nonprofit corporation, but going this route also involves a fair amount of work, both in the initial setup and as ongoing obligations. A summary of factors to consider when addressing the pros and cons of the nonprofit incorporation question follows:

Lawful Purpose

While for-profit corporations can be formed for any lawful purpose, nonprofit corporations can only be established if their goal is to accomplish one or more specific purposes, as delineated in the tax code, which will

---

Nonprofits may earn money!

The value that Americans place on nonprofit organizations is reflected in the tax code as exclusions from certain tax obligations of the organization and as deductions for donors. Thus, one of the most basic reasons for forming a nonprofit organization is to qualify for the significant cost offsets such as tax exemptions that are available to the nonprofit sector. Other benefits include eligibility for grants earmarked for or restricted to qualified nonprofit organizations, as well as incentives for donors in the form of individual tax deductions for contributions. Also, by incorporating the nonprofit organization, its directors, officers, and members are afforded a valuable form of legal protection from personal liability for claims brought against the nonprofit corporation, a feature that provides an especially salient benefit for organizations undertaking potentially risky activities. Even though incorporation is not a necessary prerequisite for becoming a qualified nonprofit organization, by taking the extra step of incorporating, additional valuable organizational benefits may be realized. For purposes of this chapter, it is assumed that a decision to form a nonprofit organization will also include incorporation and thus the term "nonprofit corporation" is used throughout this chapter.

---

benefit a segment of the community or society as a whole. There are many different recognized types of nonprofit associations ranging from labor organizations to social clubs and fraternal lodges, each governed by specific provisions of the tax code; however, our discussion is limited to the most common nonprofit form employed by large-scale expeditions. Such nonprofit organizations are governed by Section 501(c)(3) of the tax code and can only be formed for religious, charitable, scientific, literary, and/ or educational purposes. These categories are broadly defined, and if an expedition includes elements of data-collection, public educational outreach, or humanitarian objectives, it will likely qualify.

Official Paperwork

Record-keeping is an essential part of administering and maintaining a nonprofit corporation and is dictated in large part by the state laws governing both corporations and nonprofit organizations. Once the corporation is set up, there will be annual tax and reporting requirements, as well as bookkeeping requirements for tracking income and expenses. After a 501(c)(3) designation has been received, the corporation will be required to incorporate Generally Accepted Accounting Principles (GAAP) into their practices and comply with applicable state and federal laws and regulations. Bookkeeping becomes more complex if a payroll is provided to any members of the organization. Thus, an essential threshold consideration is whether the expedition members are willing to put in the extra time and effort (or to pay the costs) associated with maintaining the necessary infrastructure of a nonprofit corporation.

Restrictions on Activities

Restrictions imposed on 501(c)(3) organizations may limit the organization's freedoms by prohibiting it from distributing profits or other private benefits to members and by controlling the means by which assets of the organization are disposed of upon its dissolution. Additionally, even though a nonprofit may realize many benefits from its tax-exempt status, the income that qualifies for the exemption must be earned while furthering the goals of the organization. Income earned in ways unrelated to the organization's nonprofit status is usually taxed as unrelated business income under both state and federal corporate income tax rules. However, a nonprofit corporation may form a for-profit subsidiary if it finds that a large percentage of its activities are generating unrelated business income. Seeking the advice of competent professionals (legal and tax) from the very beginning is essential for maximizing the benefits of these statutes and for avoiding costly mistakes.

Donations

Many public and private granting organizations are required by their own operating rules and tax regulations to donate their funds only to 501(c)(3) organizations; therefore by forming a nonprofit corporation, the expedition may be eligible for a broader range of funding. Whether or not the expedition is soliciting donations, funds, grants, and sponsorship from organizations that restrict such support only to 501(c)(3) entities, the provision of any financial support will usually be accompanied by formal agreements and understandings. Such legal arrangements will generally be facilitated when an organizational entity represents the expedition as opposed to one or more individual members of the group entering into such legal arrangements.

Liability Protection

Protecting members from personal liability is one of the primary drivers for forming corporations (both nonprofit and for-profit). Once incorporated, the directors, trustees, officers, employees, and members of the corporation will generally be shielded from personal liability for the debts, judgments, and other liabilities of the corporation. Recourse by creditors will be limited to the corporate assets to satisfy debts and liabilities incurred. To maintain this liability shield, members are held to certain conduct standards (e.g., they cannot act recklessly with respect to corporate duties or co-mingle funds), and it is essential to maintain the separate existence of the corporate identity. The importance of maintaining such formalities cannot be overemphasized, especially as nonprofit adherence to such norms is of increasing interest to states' attorney general offices.

Formal Organizational Structure

Some of the less obvious benefits flowing from the formation of a nonprofit corporation are derived from the fact of its own "legal personality." Thus, a corporation's own separate identity will continue to exist, independent of the people who formed it and who work for it, thereby ensuring that the corporation will continue to exist despite changes in personnel. Additionally, as a legal entity, the corporation may also serve as an employer of its principals, providing them with employee fringe benefits not available within unincorporated forms, and the corporate entity may also enter into contracts, make purchases, and procure its own insurance policies. Such benefits may be particularly attractive for organizations supporting risky expeditions and/or entering into book or film deals or hiring third-party contractors such as guides and subject matter specialists. The formality of a corporate structure also facilitates delegation of authority and favors orderly decision making. Within such organizations, specific operating rules are delineated in the articles of incorporation and bylaws, thereby reducing the potential for divisive or counterproductive interactions. Sponsors, donors, and granting organizations will also be more likely to support and enter into agreements with an organization that presents a business-like structure for its interactions.

The Process of Forming a Nonprofit Corporation

There are many resources available both in texts and online to aid a group in setting up a nonprofit organization (see References). However, once the group has reviewed the basic parameters and completed the preliminary work of defining goals and scope of the expedition enterprise, it should consult a lawyer specialized in the applicable nonprofit and corporate laws. Consultation with a tax specialist is also advisable. The preliminary steps for setting up a nonprofit corporation are as follows:

- Determine if the expedition and/or organization will be pursuing a valid purpose recognized by Section 501(c)(3) of the federal tax code.
- Determine if the goals of the expedition organization can be met or enhanced within the operating confines imposed by nonprofit and corporate statutes and regulations.
- File your articles of incorporation (the basis for which can be obtained through the applicable state secretary of state).
- Prepare the organizational bylaws, which include the organization's objectives and purposes, number of directors, and related organizational protocols.
- Apply for federal 501(c)(3) tax exemption.
- File related state tax exempt forms.
- Set up bookkeeping, hold the first board of directors meeting, and review and take steps necessary to ensure compliance with other state laws related to both corporations and nonprofit organizations.

Summary

There are many potential benefits in forming a nonprofit corporation, but there are a number of formalities that must be met and maintained in order to reap these benefits. Strategic questions such as the importance of a liability shield for individual expedition members and the need for providing donors with charity deductions must be examined by the organization's principals and weighed against the paperwork burdens and restrictions attendant with any decision to move forward with such an undertaking.

Assuming your organization meets the legal criteria but is still uncertain whether to take on the extra layer of administration, you should consider the less tangible benefits accorded by the organizational structures outlined in this section. Specifically, it is the authors' view that clear-cut legal relationships and delineation of authority and responsibility, as well as limitations on legal liability, weigh strongly in favor of nonprofit corporation formation. At the outset of an expedition, complications imposed by forming contracts, allocating intellectual property rights, and sorting out liabilities may not be obvious. However, once they do arise, they can be dealt with more cleanly within a formal organizational structure. But there are many caveats to this preference. Primary among them is whether the expedition organization is sufficiently large and possesses a long enough planning horizon (or intends to undertake or support multiple expeditions) to justify the added layers of administrative hassle related to setting up a formal, government-regulated structure. Additionally, as outlined in the next sections of this chapter, it is possible to delineate the rights, responsibilities, and liabilities of the organization's members through agreements, releases, and formal contracts outside the confines of a nonprofit corporation, however residual risk of personal liability for actions and debts of the group may remain and should be carefully considered.[6]

UNDERSTANDING AND MINIMIZING OR MITIGATING LIABILITIES

In the expedition context, legal liabilities are most likely to arise in the form of a tort claim. As demonstrated by a recent study conducted by the Society for the Study of Legal Aspects of Sports and Physical Activity, 55% of the cases studied involved claims of negligence (tort liability).[7] Such liabilities may arise among expedition members or third parties or may be brought against the expedition as a whole. As discussed more fully later, the basis for tort liability is harm caused to persons and property as a result of intentional or negligent acts of others, and generally involves a violation of a duty imposed by law upon persons having a legal relation to each other. There is no action in tort if there is no resulting economic loss.

There are many avenues by which tort liability may be visited on an expedition and such liability risks increase with the complexity of the undertaking. Although an expedition may have disputes concerning contracts, when litigation arises it is usually as a result of an injury or fatality that has occurred. Where emergency response is remote, unavailable, or improperly delivered, and medical or emergency extrication costs are high, the chances that a lawsuit will arise to recover those costs increase dramatically. These lawsuits are most commonly prosecuted by the injured, his or her family, or his or her insurance company. In addition to participant-based claims, there is an increasing trend of litigation by third parties who do not understand the risks inherent in most expeditions. For instance, parents or spouses of deceased expedition members may seek redress for perceived negligence on the part of other expedition members, even where the expired expedition member accepted those risks. Additionally, nonrelated third parties may be exposed to the expedition's risks involuntarily through their role in search and rescue activities, evacuation, or unintentional fire and other natural resource damage caused by the expedition. Compromise of such third-party interests may

result in collateral costs and legal disputes implicating expedition members.

Fortunately, numerous layers of protection that will shield against or fix liability at a pre-agreed level can be put in place. Such protections include a reasonable understanding of how tort liabilities arise, specialized insurance policies, well-written liability releases, and, as already discussed, structuring the expedition entity as a nonprofit corporation. This section of the chapter provides an overview of tort liability and the types of liability claims most commonly brought in the adventure activity or expedition context. This section also provides expedition planners with information on liability releases, insurance coverage and products, and other approaches for addressing these risks in advance of field deployment.

Tort Liability and Negligence, Generally

Because the vast majority of legal liability claims likely to arise in an expedition or adventure-oriented context will involve allegations of negligence, proactive risk management involves a fundamental understanding of negligence, how it arises, and how it will be alleged. Negligence is in the field of legal liability known as "torts" and involves unintentional injury to a person or property. Negligence under the law is generally defined as the failure to use ordinary care (i.e., failing to do what a person of ordinary prudence would have done under the same or similar circumstances). Essentially, a court or other trier of fact will look to determine whether an expedition operator, member, guide, or perhaps some other entity hired or recruited to provide some service to the expedition could or should have recognized an unreasonable risk and then did nothing to warn the expedition or its members or did nothing to reduce or eliminate the unreasonable risk. To examine negligence in behavior or conduct, the basic inquiry will look to see whether the risk encountered was foreseeable and whether the risk encountered was unreasonable under the circumstances.[8] Negligence may be simple, ordinary, or gross, *and* it may apply to expedition entities as well as their individual members.

Simple Negligence

In order to achieve a finding of negligence, the entity bringing the claim must prove each of four elements necessary to sustain the cause of action: duty, standard of care, causation, and damages.

Duty. Duty refers to one party's responsibility to take reasonable care for the protection of another party. Duty is societal, thus courts and legislatures will determine which members of society have a duty to each other. As societal relationships change or are formalized by contract so will the duties owed between parties. Duty usually stems from three sources: (1) from a relation-ship inherent in the situation such as the special rela-tionship that will exist between expedition leaders or organizers and the expedition members; (2) from a voluntary assumption such as when off-duty mountain rescue personnel voluntarily become involved in a res-cue situation (the would-be rescuer will then have the duty to perform the rescue with care); or (3) from a duty mandated by a statute or regulation of some sort such as the regulatory requirements associated with pro-viding medical care.[9]

Standard of Care and Breach of That Standard of Care or That Duty. Standards of care, which vary according to activity and context, can be thought of as the act or omission – the thing that was done or not done to protect the expedition or its members, which was not consistent with what a reasonably prudent expedition should do under those particular circumstances. Gener-ally, determining what a reasonable person[10] would have done under the circumstances *is* establishing the stan-dard of care. Standards may be set by statute, ordinance, or regulation, or by the profession. A standard of care will take into account who is delivering the service and what their level of knowledge should be. In other words, the standard of care will be what would be expected of a reasonable and careful person carrying out the same activity (e.g., a reasonable guide, instructor, medical provider, experienced expedition leader, etc.). The stan-dard of care then for a professional person such as an expedition guide or leader or medical care provider, is that degree of care that is shown by a reasonably pru-dent expedition leader or physician operating in like or similar circumstances.[11] In order to minimize liability risks, it is crucial to understand established professional customs and practices in the field or style of your expe-dition.

Causation. In order to be found legally liable for a mem-ber's injuries or death, the expedition or its members (or any other third party for that matter) must have caused the injury. This is the foundation of the American fault-based tort liability system. The idea is that there must be a plausible connection between the defendant's miscon-duct and the plaintiff's injury. Another way of expressing this is that the injury must not be too remote from the actions of the person alleged to have caused it. It can be difficult sometimes to determine and establish an actual cause.

Damages. The last element required for a finding of negligence is that the injured or deceased person must suffer some type of compensable harm. There are four types of damage or harm generally recognized under the law: (1) economic loss (lost wages, medical care costs, custodial care); (2) physical pain and suffering; (3) emo-

---

Explanatory case law on simple negligence

A few explanatory cases illustrate how simple negligence may occur and how it is adjudicated. In *Licato v. Eastgate*,[12] a gentleman named Licato was injured on property imme-diately adjacent to defendant's motorcycle track when Licato lost control of the new motorcycle he was testing and struck an invisible or hidden excavation ditch on the adjoining property. Evidence showed that there were no boundaries or barriers between the two properties, and that Licato had not been warned, even though the track owners knew of the ditch, and also knew that the track was frequently used for testing. The court found that it was foreseeable that motorcyclists would lose control in testing situations and that the adjacent ditch was an unreasonable danger given these circumstances. In *Saffro v. Elite Racing Inc.*,[13] Saffro experienced a grand mal epi-leptic seizure while returning home on an airplane, several hours after completing a marathon running race in San Diego. Saffro sued the race organizer saying it was neg-ligent in organizing and supervising the race. Specifically, Saffro stated that the organizer negligently failed to provide adequate water and fluids to the runners during the race. Elite Racing defended saying that Saffro's injuries resulted from an inherent risk of the sport – dehydration in distance running. The evidence showed that prerace written materi-als assured racers of 23 water stations, 11 of which would have electrolyte fluids; on the day of the race, however, the first few stations were not prepared to distribute any fluids, and there was no electrolyte fluid available at all during the race. An appeals court overturned a lower court ruling and held that a race organizer has a duty to organize and conduct a reasonably safe event; this duty requires the organizer to take reasonable steps to minimize the risks without altering the nature of the sport. In this case, it meant the race organizer's duty included minimizing the risks of dehydration by providing adequate fluids along the course.

---

tional distress (fright, anxiety, loss of peace of mind and happiness, humiliation, and embarrassment); and (4) physical impairment (permanent or temporary, total or partial).

Contributory Negligence

Beyond the responsibility of the expedition as an entity to act reasonably on behalf of its members or participants, the actual expedition members have a corresponding legal duty to take reasonable care to prevent injury to themselves. When an expedition member engages in conduct that is unreasonable and contributes to his or her own harm, that member is contributorily negligent for any "damages" he or she may suffer. If a member par-ticipates or engages in the expedition's risky activities in an unreasonable manner, depending on the state law involved, any award ultimately made in litigation either is reduced by the percentage of the member's own fault (contributory negligence), or may be a complete defense to the claims (comparative fault). Where an injured or deceased expedition member's own conduct fell below the standard of what a reasonably prudent participant would have done in similar circumstances, any resulting claim made will likely be reduced or eliminated on the basis that he or she was proximately responsible for that harm.

Gross Negligence

Grossly negligent conduct involves acts or omissions that are considered more egregious than those of simple or ordinarily negligent conduct because those acts demonstrate willful or reckless misconduct. An important aspect of a gross negligence claim is that the liability release agreement between the expedition and its members (see section "General Liability Release and Waiver Documents") will not act as a shield from claims of gross negligence. Four things are usually considered in cases where gross negligence is alleged, although not all four elements must be alleged:[17] (1) an intentional act or intentional failure to perform a duty but not a conscious intent to harm; (2) an awareness that the conduct will create a risk of harm to another, even though the extent might not be appreciated; (3) knowledge of acts that could have been undertaken to assist the operator in appreciating the risk of harm; and (4) creation of a risk that is extreme and outrageous – this will be measured by the probability of risk of harm and the severity of the harm that might result.

Types of Claims Brought against Recreation or Adventure Entities

The foregoing summary is meant to provide expedition planners with a working knowledge of negligence. This

Explanatory case law on contributory negligence

A few explanatory cases serve to illustrate how contributory negligence may occur and how it is adjudicated. In the famous Canadian heli-ski case of *Scurfield v. Cariboo Heli-Skiing Ltd.*,[14] a client/participant was found to be contributorily negligent for his own death when he failed to follow the guides' instructions not to enter an avalanche area before another client had finished traversing it and for ignoring verbal avalanche warnings. In *Voight v. Colorado Mountain Club*,[15] Voight was injured and suffered a frostbite amputation when she became separated from her commercial hiking group. In her lawsuit, Voight alleged that the designated trip leader failed to monitor and/or otherwise supervise the hiking group thereby allowing or causing her to become separated. Experts testified it was the designated leader's duty to keep the group together, though a jury later found that Voight had a concomitant duty to pay attention and stay with her hiking group; the club was found to be 70% negligent, and the hiker was found to be 30% negligent.

Explanatory case law on gross negligence

A few explanatory cases serve to illustrate how simple negligence may occur and how it is adjudicated. In *Martinez v. Swartzbaugh*,[16] Martinez won an opportunity to ride in a charity McLaren race car. During the ride, he was not provided with a helmet, seat belt, or other safety devices, and he was seriously injured when the driver suddenly accelerated to 140 mph, lost control, and crashed the car. The court agreed with the allegation of gross negligence. In *Hatch v. V.P. Fair Foundation*, a bungee jump operator arrived late to his business on a day when clients were booked and in his rush then violated written policies in the company safety manual by failing to inspect the equipment as required, failing to conduct a preclient test jump, failing to attach the bungee cord to the crane, operating the jump with five rather than six people, and using an 18-year-old controller even though the manual specified a person 25 years of age older. A participant was seriously injured, and the court found that this cumulative conduct was grossly negligent.

next section provides a brief description of negligence claims commonly brought in the adventure and recreation sport context. With knowledge of these types of liability-producing situations, a well-conceived expedition can evaluate and manage the risks associated with the endeavor both before and during its execution.

Coparticipant Liability

It is generally thought that coparticipants engaged in active sports or adventures are not liable to one another except where reckless or intentional conduct is involved. See, for example, *Mankoski v. Mieras*,[18] a case in which Mankoski and Mieras went to an indoor rock climbing gym and signed a liability release in favor of the gym before commencing their climbing activities. During a climb, while Mieras was on belay, Mankoski fell from the climbing wall and then later sued his buddy, alleging that Mieras had too much slack in the rope and couldn't effectively operate the brake device. Mieras argued that Mankoski was hurt by an inherent risk of climbing – falling – so that Mieras had no duty to protect him from these risks and/or injuries. The court dismissed Mankoski's case, finding that he was indeed hurt by an inherent risk of climbing. In *Dare v. Freefall Adventures, Inc.*,[19] a skydiver sued a coparticipant for injuries sustained while attempting to avoid an in-air midjump collision; the court found that the suing skydiver had the burden of proving the coparticipant was reckless or grossly negligent.

Premises Liability

Premises liability refers to the doctrine that landowners or other possessors of property being used for recreational or adventure-oriented endeavors can be held liable for injuries sustained by folks who are using their land or facilities. Generally, landowners or possessors will have the duty to inspect their property/facilities to discover defects, to remove or repair dangers, to warn users of hazards, and to make their land/facilities reasonably safe.[20] See *Estate of Adam Harshman v. Jackson Hole Mountain Resort and USA*,[21] a case where 16-year-old Adam Harshman was killed after landing on his head and neck after snowboarding off of a 20-foot tabletop jump in a fenced off man-made terrain park. Allegations in the lawsuit brought by Harshman's family included premises liability, negligent management, negligent maintenance, and negligent operation of the terrain park. The Court reviewing the case found that Jackson Hole owed no duty to protect Harshman from those dangers or conditions that are characteristic of or intrinsic to or such an integral part of snowboard jumping because providers of these types of opportunities are not required to eliminate, alter, or control these inherent risks. In finding that the risks Harshman encountered were inherent to snowboard or terrain park jumping, the court found that the subject terrain park contained posted warnings and had been inspected the day of the accident and that Harshman himself was known to have been an experienced snowboarder who had used the jump many times before.

Negligent Rescue, Response, or Medical Care

Expedition and adventure providers should be concerned about providing adequate response in the event of a foreseeable incident.[22] When improper or inadequate rescue or response occurs, or when the provider has no procedure in place, the member/participant will argue that an accident of some sort was certainly foreseeable and having a poor or nonexistent response plan exposed the participant to an unreasonable risk of harm. See *Jaffee et al. v. Pallota Teamworks*, where Jaffee died after participating in a charity bike ride sponsored by Pallota to raise money for AIDS research. During the subject four-day bike ride, one afternoon Jaffee approached a medical aid station and complained of dizziness and nausea. Volunteers gave her IV fluids and when her condition failed to improve and she began vomiting they gave her more IV fluids. When Jaffee's blood pressure dropped and she collapsed, only then was she transported to a hospital where she died the next day of a brain hemorrhage. Jaffee's parent and estate sued the race organizer claiming that it had negligently trained and equipped the aid stations, and then negligently failed to diagnose, monitor, treat, and care for Jaffee. It is unknown what liability would have been ascribed to the race event had Jaffee not signed a liability release and waiver document which expressly acknowledged the risk of injury or death, stated that she was physically capable of participating, stated that her medical care provider had approved her participation, *and*

included the medical care providers in the list of individuals to be released.

Negligent Supervision or Instruction

Expedition and adventure entities need to be aware that they may have a duty to supervise participants. Supervising generally includes overseeing, managing, regulating, and teaching.[23] For instance, in *Dunn v. So. Calif. 7th Day Adventists*,[24] a 14-year-old boy fell while rock climbing on a church-sponsored camping trip and suffered severe brain injury. His parents claimed that the church provided negligent supervision and undertook a high-risk activity without sufficient experience. (The case was settled out of court.) This case illustrates not only the types of claims made but also that nonprofit entities like religious organizations are routinely sued these days.

Negligent Hiring or Use of Inexperienced Guides, Instructors, and Others

Hiring professionals in support of your expedition involves careful evaluation and judgment, especially where such professionals will be responsible for a key element of success or the safety of the participants. Lack of due diligence in the hiring and management of third parties or failing to ensure that service contracts adequately allocate any resulting liability can open the expedition entity or its leaders to liability. For additional details on employment, see the section "Employment-Related Issues."[25] An expedition entity should have written documentation of the experience and certification levels of all third-party entities and/or employees (including, as appropriate, that of the group's leaders and medical professionals). An expedition can be successfully sued and held legally liable if there is an accident and the entity failed to properly screen its personnel. Motor vehicle (i.e., automobiles, aircraft, boats, etc.) use is another particularly big area to look into with respect to authorizing expedition personnel.[26] Expedition entities should establish in their risk management reviews and any resulting policies and procedures, which personnel will operate motor vehicles or be responsible for leasing vehicles and under what circumstances.

Failure to Warn

One of the most common allegations in lawsuits against adventure-oriented operations is that they failed to warn and inform participants of the risks involved and/or that the leader failed to give adequate instructions. Expedition leaders and organizers must inform members of the known risks that they are likely to encounter on the expedition and, where appropriate, that there may be unknown risks associated with the activity or area of travel. The legal duty to warn can usually be satisfied by setting good policies or rules, posting warnings on equipment or facilities, oral warnings and safety briefings, thorough documentation (e.g., in the liability release and waiver agreements), encouraging safe participation, and ensuring that all participants are aware of the inherent risks of the expedition. An effective warning is thought to be specific, obvious and direct, unambiguous, easy to understand, simple, and complete.

Depending on the type of expedition organization, it is also worth considering whether to base the participant's understanding of the risks on a traditional model of authoritative leading where the guide or leader makes all decisions, or alternatively to use the expedition leaders to educate participants about the options and include them in the decision-making process so that members are actively accepting and assuming the risks.[27] See section "Other Defenses to Claims of Negligence."

Equipment Issues

The field of "products liability" has generated volumes of text dedicated solely to its consideration, and as such is beyond the scope of this chapter. However, it is important for all expedition members to be aware that product manufacturers, distributors, retailers, and *others who provide equipment* can be sued on the basis of negligent or faulty equipment design or manufacture that results in injury or harm to a participant.[28] Operators or other providers can also be sued for improper fitting, lack of maintenance, or noncompliance with standards or manufacturer's instructions. If an expedition entity or a participant alters equipment or uses it in a manner that is inconsistent with the manufacturer's suggestions, the warranties on the product can be voided, thereby exposing the trip organizers or participants to liabilities. Equipment modifications should be done only by trained and authorized personnel. As appropriate, and especially where the expedition entity is providing equipment to its participants, inventories of equipment should be maintained, along with individual piece identification numbers. Additionally, inspections of equipment should be done routinely and should be documented; damaged or overused equipment should be repaired by qualified persons or replaced. Maintain all manufacturer warranties and make sure the warranties are registered.

Avoiding and Defending against Tort Liability in Adventure or Expeditionary Contexts

Beyond the ordinary tort defenses (i.e., lack of evidence or failure of proof, statute of limitations, etc.), three types of defenses are commonly employed for defending against expedition or adventure-styled liability claims. These are (1) existence of well-drafted liability release and waiver documents, (2) evidence that the risk encountered was an "inherent risk," and/or (3) evidence that the participant "assumed" the risks of the injury-producing activity.[29] Understanding these defenses will assist the developing expedition in its risk management processes, both before embarking on the expedition and while in the field.

General Liability Release and Waiver Documents

Liability releases are the basic tool used by travel organizations and in the outdoor recreation industry to shift legal liabilities and prevent litigation. These documents are contractual in nature and are meant to effectuate an agreement from the participant to relinquish the right to sue the entity (e.g., the provider, organizer, or operator) in the event that either the negligence of the entity or an inherent risk results in injury to the participant.[30] For a contract to be valid, there must be a "meeting of the minds" between the signatories (e.g., there must be indicia that all parties understood the meaning, intent, and desired outcome of the agreement). To prove this element, there must be not only evidence of an understanding of the primary rights and obligations being memorialized in the contract, but also some form of "consideration" flowing between the parties. In most cases, consideration is money flowing in one direction and goods or services flowing to the other. In the expedition context, consideration in support of a liability release usually takes the form of expedition support services to be furnished to the person signing the release.

Courts routinely strike down releases that are not clearly identified as such or that are hidden in another document. For this reason, it is important for the liability release to be a separate, stand-alone document that is clearly identified (e.g., entitled in bold at the top: PARTICIPANT AGREEMENT, RELEASE, WAIVER, AND ACKNOWLEDGMENT OF RISK FOR ABC EXPEDITION). There should be no attempt to downplay or otherwise minimize the importance of the liability release or it will fail entirely in its purpose. Additionally, if the persons being asked to sign the liability release do not speak English as their native language or are not well educated, it is incumbent on the expedition leaders or organizers to ensure such participants receive proper counseling before signing it (and it may be worthwhile memorializing such counseling in the liability release). A crucial point in understanding the exculpatory effect of a well-drafted release and waiver document is that it can deflect claims deriving from the inherent risks of the activity (See section "Inherent Risk"), and in some states will also shield from claims of simple negligence. However, note that no release and waiver document, no matter how competently drafted, will protect an entity from its grossly negligent conduct.

Releases must be in writing and, as will become clear upon reading this section of the chapter, should be developed with the assistance of an attorney with knowledge of the governing laws covering releases, as well as the goals and concerns of the expedition parties. Remember also that the manner in which a liability release is

Proper administration of a release and waiver contract

Proper administration of a liability release includes the following elements:[31]

- Allow the participants time to read the document
- Nonreaders should have the document read to them, and you should be able to account for language barriers.[32]
- Educate your staff so that, through their words and actions, they don't render your release meaningless.
- Don't let people cross out words on their release – they either sign it or don't participate.
- Have a witness present (e.g., a staff member or spouse) during the signing.
- Don't allow intoxicated individuals to sign the release because they lack the capacity to understand and therefore bind themselves.
- Retain the agreements!! They should be kept at least as long as the applicable statute of limitations period, and the expedition entity should consult an attorney for information on the applicable statute of limitations. Retain all waivers because they also give you lists of other witnesses who were participating in the activity on that day or at that time.
- Organize the executed release agreements and store them in secure fireproof places. Lost or destroyed waivers will generally not be upheld.
- Send a copy of the release document you are using to your insurance company.

administered will have a direct impact on its effectiveness. For instance, courts have decided not to uphold a release when the person administering the release made certain oral representations about the release (e.g., representations such as "it is only for check in," "it is only for our records," or "it is only for insurance purposes"), or if there is some allegation that the signature was obtained by false representations of the administrator or where material facts are withheld from the signer, or where the important exculpatory language is not obvious.[33]

Now that you are aware of how to administer a liability release, we turn to the question of what should be included in the actual release, waiver, and acknowledgment of risk contract (referred to hereinafter as the "liability release" or "release"). Again, you need to have competent legal counsel review whatever you are using. That said, there are several good sources available for help in both understanding written liability releases and in drafting them. Many of these sources are listed in the bibliography to this chapter.[34] What follows is a basic description of the primary elements of a liability release as well as rationale for including them:

- Use clear typeface that is not too small. It must be easy to read, no flowery or crazy typefaces. Don't put in anything untrue or that could be construed as a guarantee ("our guides *all* have *extensive* back country experience"; "you *will* have a safe trip"). Have a bolded title to the document. Do not bury your release/waiver in another document – it should be separate. Use the phrase "including but not limited to" throughout the agreement.
- Name all persons and entities to be released.
- Name all parties in addition to the signer who are relinquishing their rights to sue by virtue of the document.
- Include language of consideration – this is what makes it a contract under the law.
- Address liability for inherent risks by including a lengthy description of the inherent risks, or what you consider to be the range of inherent risks, and make reference to coparticipant behaviors.
- Address ordinary negligence separately from the inherent risks. These are two separate issues and courts confuse them regularly. When something shows up as two separate issues, judges are more likely (based on the rules of legal construction) to perceive these as two separate issues.
- Use a separate paragraph for the assumption of the risk language. This paragraph should also affirm that the member's participation is voluntary and should also include language that the signatory agrees to abide by the rules/regulations/safety warnings of the entity and/or the guides and others with responsibility.
- The document should clearly state that the signatory is releasing the operator/entity from responsibility for injury or death or property damage caused by the ordinary negligence of the operator or its employees or contractors or agents.
- Include a paragraph concerning health issues: (1) acknowledgment that they have no health problems, physical disabilities, or mental impairments that would preclude their participation; (2) acknowledgment that they have sufficient skill and fitness to participate in the expedition; (3) acknowledgment that they are not under the influence of drugs or alcohol and there is no reason why they lack capacity to sign the liability release document; (4) acknowledgment that they have insurance that will cover the costs of emergency medical treatment and/or transportation related to the activity or that they are willing to bear these costs themselves; (5) acknowledgment that they authorize the operator to administer emergency first aid, CPR, or AED (defibrillator) when deemed necessary; (6) acknowledgment that they authorize the operator/provider to secure emergency transport and or medical care when deemed necessary; and (7) authorization for the operator to release or share participant medical information with medical care providers.[35]
- Include a forum selection clause (which will determine the state court system any disputes stemming from the liability release will be litigated in).

- Include an indemnity agreement that the signatory agrees to bear all costs and fees incurred by the operator or institution in defending themselves against the claims of the participant or his family, estate, and the like.
- As appropriate include a photographic or intellectual property rights assignment for promotional and/or commercial use of the signatory's likeness (see section "Intellectual Property Rights" for a discussion of intellectual property considerations).
- Include a statement that if any part of the document is found to be void or illegal by a court the other parts will remain in full force and effect and will be given the broadest construction possible by the courts in the state that you have referred to in your forum selection clause.
- Include an affirmation toward the bottom of the document that the signatory has read and fully understands the information and agrees to be bound by its terms. This should be in bold.
- Include a signature area, which should include spaces for name, address, and phone number. If you serve minors, it should have a place for both the parent's and minor's signatures. (Note: If you serve minors, you need to understand what the applicable courts are saying about minors and releases, and make sure the entire language of the release is consistent with this.)
- If you can't get the release information on one page (small type should be avoided), include acknowledgments (e.g., initial block) at the bottom of each page. If possible, include a third party witness who will initial the liability releases when they are signed by the participant.
- Do not cut-and-paste, employ boilerplate language, or adopt some other liability release you find at a conference or online. Liability releases are contracts and will be construed carefully by the courts. They must be very context-specific and never overly inclusive or vague. If written and administered correctly, liability releases will be the cornerstone of your risk mitigation and liability defense plan.
- Most importantly, get your liability release reviewed by competent legal counsel.

Medical Release and Permission to Treat

The medical liability release and permission to treat form is an agreement that is often separate and apart from the general liability release discussed in the last section. One of the primary differences is that the medical agreement is solely between each individual member of the expedition and the expedition's medical professional(s). It is not a document that broadly releases the potential liability of a group of persons. For this reason, it is recommended that the medical release document be presented as a separate agreement, though there are many instances where the medical release is tagged on to the bottom of a participant liability release form.

At a minimum the medical release form should include the following elements:

- Acknowledgment by the signatory of potential injuries and illnesses (and death) that may occur on the expedition
- Acknowledgment by the signatory of the potentially primitive or nonexistent medical treatment facilities and limited emergency response capabilities likely to be encountered during the expedition
- Authorization for transportation and treatment deemed necessary either by the expedition medical personnel or by other medical or dental professionals appropriated by the expedition medical professional(s)
- An agreement to hold harmless the expedition medical professional(s), as well as any other expedition personnel for medical treatment undertaken pursuant to and consistent with the terms of the medical release
- A disclosure statement by the participant of any medical, physical, and psychological conditions that may be relevant for medical treatment and/or emergency evaluation by the expedition medical professional(s) (in most cases, this statement should not replace the requirement for a documented medical evaluation by the participant's physician)
- Permission for the expedition medical professional(s) to provide confidential medical information to other parties as reasonably necessary for addressing medical emergencies

When developing the medical liability release and permission to treat form, the expedition's medical professional should consider some additional points. First, not all expeditions will have a physician as part of the expedition; instead, if any medical personnel are brought along at all, the expedition may instead opt to employ nurses, physician assistants, paramedics, emergency medical technicians, or simple first-aid providers for this role. Even if a physician is on the expedition, the initial treatment may be made by someone other than the physician. Each of these different professions possesses different abilities to treat, as well as limitations, and the scope of medical capability within the expedition team should be disclosed in the medical liability release. Second, permission to treat should also cover any transportation after the illness or injury has occurred. Injured expedition members have been transported out of the wilderness on the backs of sherpas, on mules and donkeys, or on litters carried by fellow expedition members. Such primitive transportation modes can increase the injury or cause additional injuries and may be the only way to get an injured participant to more advanced medical facilities. As such, the medical release needs to address evacuation and transportation in its coverage. Third, confidentiality of medical information may be an issue. Porters, locals, or other members of the expedition are most likely going to be involved in any extraction, rescue, and first-aid provided to an injured participant, and medical conditions are likely to be communicated via nonprivate modes or observed by a broad cross section of persons. After the rescue is complete and the patient is transferred to local hospitals, there may not be any confidentiality as we know and expect in the United States. Information about a patient's medical condition may be posted on the wall of the hospital or broadcast to any person asking questions (including the press). For this reason, expedition participants should be warned of this potential lack of confidentiality, acknowledge it, and waive any claims they might otherwise have.

It is vital for all participants to be fully informed as to the level of sophistication of the medical care that is likely to be available throughout the expedition. Inexperienced Western travelers may expect that the same or similar medical care that is available by calling 911 will exist wherever they may travel. Stories are told of such travelers refusing field care believing that an ambulance or flight for life is coming shortly in a country where a donkey may be the only transportation available. This expectation may be fostered by the availability of satellite telephones and computer connectivity during the expedition.

In addition to the medial release form, participants should be reminded during safety briefings (see the next section, "Other Defenses to Claims of Negligence"), about the availability and quality of medical care that can be expected on each leg of the expedition. All participants must understand that the only medical personnel that will be available, at least part of the time, are the other people on the expedition. This discussion should also include expectations regarding the level of assistance that may be required from every other member of the expedition, along with the potential curtailment of the expedition.

Other Defenses to Claims of Negligence

The liability releases described previously (both general and medical) will form the backbone of your legal defense and liability mitigation strategy; however, expedition personnel and entities may also employ other defenses against claims of liability that frequently arise in the adventure context. The two most common defenses involve arguments that the risks causing claimant's harm were "inherent" to the activity and could not reasonably be controlled or mitigated by the expedition entity and/

or that the claimant voluntarily "assumed" the risks of harm (which can be evidenced by the liability release form and through statements and conduct of the claimant. A brief description of these defenses is provided next.

Inherent Risk. As discussed earlier in the section entitled "Simple Negligence," expedition-styled entities bear some legal liability for exposing participants to risks that are both foreseeable *and unreasonable* under the circumstances. It is also true, however, that adventure entities have no duty to protect participants from the "inherent risks" associated with an activity and there will be no corresponding liability for injury or loss resulting from such inherent risks. An inherent risk may be foreseeable, but it is not considered *unreasonable* because it is the type of risk that, if removed from the activity, would alter the essential nature of the activity, and therefore the activity would lose its integrity. For instance, if a person wants to go white-water rafting in Class V rapids, an inherent risk of the activity is falling in the water and possibly drowning. If a person wants to go rafting without encountering the risk of falling overboard and drowning, they will have to alter the essential nature of the activity (i.e., they will need to raft on calmer waters). Courts vary in their interpretation of this as a common law doctrine. Some hold that a participant doesn't need to know and understand, in advance, the particular inherent risks. Others hold that participants have to possess some subjective understanding of the specific inherent risk that caused the injury before the doctrine applies. Additionally, many states have promulgated inherent risk statutes covering specific sports, in which attempts are made to define the inherent risks of those individual sports such as horseback riding or white-water rafting. An expeditionary entity should work with competent counsel who is conversant in the law on this issue.[36]

Assumption of Risk. At one time, it was reasonable to assume that participants voluntarily undertaking a risky expedition understood and assumed the risks of the endeavor, while the expedition's wealthy patrons participated vicariously. However the current trend is toward participation by patrons as actual expedition members. Such "expeditioneers" are increasingly populating the wildest rivers, highest peaks, and most remote quarters in the world in exchange for their role as financial underwriters. Many of this ilk are physically trained and may have experience in off-grid locations; however, such participants may not fully appreciate the implications of a field appendectomy or the perils of a sprained ankle when out of helicopter range until they are stricken patients with unrealistic expectations as to the standard of care available to them. This is particularly true if the expedition equipment includes sophisticated communication capability such as satellite phones and EPIRBs,[37] which often impart a false sense of security and safety. Thus, the importance of informed risk assumption by all participants is significant and should be approached thoughtfully and thoroughly, especially with respect to the standard of care likely to be available in the event of a medical emergency.

Assumption of the risk can serve as a complete defense to a plaintiff's claims. The theory is that a participant may not sue or prevail in a suit for injuries when the person voluntarily exposed themselves to a risk or danger that they were aware of or that is obvious or commonly understood.[38] Usually assumption of risk is either express or implied. Express assumption is usually when a liability release document covering the risk has been signed. Implied assumption is where the participant agrees to participate and thereby impliedly agrees to the inherent risks of the sport. The risks of an activity most properly belong to both the participants and the expedition; in other words, risks are generally "shared" between the entity and the participants, and risks can be effectively "assumed" by participants when the participants are warned or understand the risks. (See section "Contributory Negligence"). To pretend that the guide or expedition leader is solely or fully accountable or to

pretend that the member/participant is fully responsible is wrongheaded. If an expedition member has been adequately informed and warned, the expedition entity can make the argument in a time of conflict that the member legally assumed the risks.

Postaccident Behavior. In closing out this section on defenses to negligence-oriented legal liabilities, it is worth mentioning an important but often overlooked element that can be very effectively employed to reduce or eliminate the probability of lawsuits: postaccident conduct. This category includes both the creation and maintenance of goodwill during the postaccident time frame and the avoidance of admissions that could be construed as accepting responsibility for the incident. First of all, expedition members should never assume that an injured member is getting appropriate medical care; the expedition members should follow up, visit, call, and, as appropriate, interact with family members. The expedition entity should also notify its insurance company right away to get advice on the proper course of conduct for the expedition entity and/or its members to follow and to determine what the insurance company may be willing to pay for.

Essentially, when considering expedition risk management, remember that the more serious the incident, the more elevated the expedition's response should be in both rescue efforts and preparation for or anticipation of litigation. In terms of communicating with an injured person or their families, do say that the expedition is sorry that so-and-so is hurt; but don't say the expedition is sorry for the accident or takes responsibility for it. A single designated person should act as the spokesperson. Finally, be mindful of materials to include in the "Incident File."[40]

- Witness statements, complete lists of participants and addresses
- Staff/guide statements
- Law enforcement files/contacts (do you need to notify your public land administrator?)
- Photographs/videotapes – Did your members or others shoot photos? Can you get them?
- Participant agreements
- Releases/exculpatory agreements
- Radio logs or trip manifests
- Media reports

Shifting the Risk of Liability or Damage with Insurance Products/Coverages[41]

Insurance coverage[42] is one of the most effective means of protecting against extraordinary costs arising from accidents, damages, and in some cases costs associated with litigation. The topic of insurance coverage is examined in detail in another chapter, thus this section serves only to supplement that chapter by providing an

---

Elements of a good (verbal) safety briefing

In order to ensure that an expedition member has been adequately informed so as to preserve the assumption-of-risk defense, it is important not only to include the range of risks likely to be encountered as part of the liability release agreement but also to provide frequent safety briefings or discussions as the expedition moves along.

The basic elements of a good safety briefing include:[39]

- **Specifics of the activity:** Area, weather, what can be expected on the trip and/or for that day, inherent dangers/risks, proper equipment use, proper techniques demonstration, emergency preparedness and procedures, the requirement to follow the leaders' directions at all times.
- **Participant responsibility:** The level of physical demands, acknowledgment that no one has a medical or physical condition that would prevent their participation or ability to help in the event of an emergency, explanation that no drugs or alcohol are to be consumed during the activity, the requirement that members notify guides/leaders of any problems with equipment or other members.
- **Closing:** Confirm that all participants signed the liability release and other forms required for participation in the expedition, actively solicit questions members might have, arrive at consensus that the group understands and accepts what is required of them in the activity and that they accept the risks of the activity, and provide an "out" for members who do not want to participate in any given "optional" activity so that participation is deemed to be voluntary.

overview of additional legal-based factors to consider when evaluating insurance options.

There are numerous reasons to insure: to comply with permitting agencies, to protect the assets of the expedition and its members, to be financially responsible to the expedition and its benefactors, and to be professionally or morally responsible to the members and any third parties who may be affected by the expedition and its risks. However, as emphasized at several points throughout this chapter, liability mitigation measures should be tailored to address the range of risks expected to be encountered, as well as the structure and makeup of the expedition members. Purchase of insurance is no exception to this rule. The destination and types of activities planned will have significant bearing on the type of mitigation measures to be employed, but the size and funding of the expedition are also realistic considerations.

Obviously, the more dangerous the expedition, the more desirable it is to have broad and robust protection. However such protection comes at a cost, which may be beyond the means of expedition members, and even then, full protection is never guaranteed. Thus, it is possible that payment of even the biggest insurance premium will not ensure a safe return, especially from uncharted territories. In such cases, the right liability mitigation mix may involve minimal or moderate insurance coverage, mutual liability releases, and decent cash reserves to serve as self-insurance.

Unless costs have no bearing whatsoever, it is essential to perform a risk assessment of the entire expedition plan (including the capabilities of the participants) in order to determine the range of possible risks and, in so doing, develop reasonable case and reasonable worst case scenarios. (See section "Risk Management Planning" at the beginning of this chapter.) Only then is it possible to perform a cost–benefit analysis to determine the scope of appropriate mitigation measures, including insurance products that are best suited to address the risks of the expedition at a level that is affordable to the participants. In reaching this decision, consensus among the participants is recommended.

Types of Insurance Products, Generally

Health Insurance. Almost all people hold some form of health insurance coverage, but typical policies may not cover accidents resulting from unusual and/or risky activities such as alpine or rock climbing, extreme diving (e.g., deep diving, wreck diving, or cave diving), or other high-risk activities or the so-called "adrenaline sports" (e.g., sky diving and Class V kayaking), especially when such activities are pursued outside the United States. Additionally, standard medical insurance coverage usually excludes coverage for a preexisting health condition, which could have major implications in the expedition

context if it is possible to conclude that the rigors of the expedition triggered a relapse or complicated the existing condition (e.g., heart failure).

Because medical insurance is one of the best means of protecting against unusual emergency costs and for ensuring that such costs are at least partially covered, it is also therefore one of the best measures that expedition members can take not just to protect their own bank account from personal injuries but also to protect against litigation, reducing the likelihood of claims against the expedition. For instance, by setting a requirement for all members of the expedition to hold certain types of insurance policies, each with prescribed coverages and minimum coverage limits, the expedition participants are afforded a substantial risk mitigation benefit because doing so reduces the likelihood that the injured member or his family will be personally responsible for the potentially significant expenses stemming from an expedition accident. Specialized medical insurance policies can be obtained through companies offering a wide range of travel insurance options as discussed in greater detail in Chapter 11 but is summarized here. Additionally, by joining certain organizations such as the American Alpine Club or Divers Alert Network (DAN), participants are afforded access to specialized insurance policies that may cover evacuation and activity-specific emergency care such as recompression chamber treatments. However, always carefully review the policy to determine limits of coverage, especially with respect to evacuation. For instance, the DAN insurance policy includes transportation to a hyperbaric chamber but no evacuation from there.

Supplements to Homeowners or Renters Insurance Policy. Homeowner's (or renter's) insurance will often cover losses experienced while traveling but using it for this purpose could raise your premium well above the cost of the individual premium you might otherwise pay to obtain trip-specific travel insurance. Additionally, most home insurance policies only cover losses of items in your possession, and not for medical issues or trip cancellation. Thus, it is advisable to purchase insurance designed specifically for travelers, and further tailored to cover the types of risks inherent in the expedition.

Travel Insurance. Insurance policy coverage for travelers can be as simple as lost or stolen baggage coverage, but it can also provide coverage for trip cancellation due to personal injury or illness in the family and for certain high-risk activities, damage to rental cars, and medical evacuation in foreign places. Within the ambit of travel insurance, there is a panoply of options both in terms of scope of coverage and claim thresholds. For starters, there are two basic policy types: primary and secondary. Primary insurance covers you from the first penny, and secondary insurance kicks in after your own private (pre-existing) insurance has paid out. With secondary coverage a claimant may be waiting months for the preexisting homeowner's or medical insurance to pay before the insured is able to apply to get reimbursement from the secondary policy, and in the case of medical expenses, the claimant may be sending receipts back and forth for months before seeing a dime of the insurance purchased for the trip. With a primary policy, you are paid for the event or loss outright, but with a secondary policy, you are paid the difference between your out-of-pocket costs and what has already been paid. For obvious reasons, the primary insurance route is preferable, not only in terms of the hassle factor but also for ensuring that your homeowners policy is not increased as a result of your travel predilections. In the expedition context, the primary policy is also preferable because it will reduce or eliminate the potential for financial disputes among expedition participants.

Medical Malpractice Insurance. Standard medical malpractice insurance is limited in its geographic coverage and generally covers the medical professional for specific practice venues and a prescribed list of medical care activities. For this reason, it is essential for the medical professional(s) affiliated with the expedition to contact their own medical malpractice insurance carriers to ensure that adequate coverage exists for the anticipated duties and requirements potentially imposed on the medical personnel for the trip.

Insurance Coverage for the Nonprofit Corporation. Even though individual members of a nonprofit corporation are generally shielded from personal liability, it is a myth that nonprofit organizations possess "charitable immunity" from liability. As with individual insurance policies, several levels of insurance coverage are available, and nonprofit corporations – depending on the structure of the organization (e.g., existence of employees) and the types of activities it will be engaging in – should consider this type of coverage. At a minimum, the nonprofit organization should carry a policy that covers general liability and a standard directors and officers (D&O) policy. D&O policies are purchased in order to protect both the organization and its directors and officers, and the D&O also supplements indemnification protection appearing in the nonprofit's articles of incorporation. General liability policies for nonprofit corporations provide basic liability protection and coverage for bodily injury and property damage losses arising from the premises, operations, and products. Based on the organization's risk assessment, it may be desirable to include additional insurance endorsements as modifications to the existing insurance contract or policy.

In addition to insurance coverage, the nonprofit organization may be in a position to provide liability protection beyond what is covered in its insurance policies. For instance as summarized in "Structuring the Expedition to Optimize Its Goals and Minimize Liability" of this chapter, by selecting the corporate form, individual members and their personal assets are generally protected from liability of the organization. Additionally, where permitted by state law and the organization bylaws, an organization can promise to reimburse board members for legal costs they incur, but paltry financial resources frequently necessitate the purchase of supplemental insurance protection to make such indemnification provisions meaningful.

Participant's Proof of Insurance Coverage

As a means of reducing the risk of unexpected personal costs due to losses, cancellations, and accidents, the expedition planners and/or medical professional should set out specific guidelines delineating precisely the types of insurance coverage each member must have for the period of the expedition. Additionally, it is highly advisable for the expedition leaders to require a signed statement by each participant showing proof of the coverages they deem necessary, which may include

- Trip cancellation and interruption
- Emergency medical evacuation and assistance
- Accidental death and sickness
- Loss of baggage and personal effects

These signed statements should also include participant disclosures concerning any preexisting health condition that could limit the coverage under applicable medical insurance programs. Additionally, such a statement should include an acknowledgment that the expedition entity and/or leadership has advised the participant to obtain and carry in full force the prescribed insurance policies and a pledge to hold the expedition entity, its employees or members or any related parties harmless for the participant's failure to purchase adequate insurance coverage or sufficient coverage limits. Obviously, when evaluating the need and efficacy of requiring particular types of insurance coverage for the expedition participants, the leaders must determine if insurance will do any good. For instance, if the expedition is going into an area where an organized evacuation is not possible, then it will be more important to amass a pile of crisp $100 bills than to pay for pricey insurance. This question and others should be addressed with your insurance brokers as described in the next section.

Questions and Issues to Discuss with the Insurance Broker

Seek out an insurance company that specializes in outdoor or adventure-type risks so they understand the range of potential losses that the expedition is likely to encounter. Also such professionals can be of service to the expedition in their risk management and loss control analyses. Be proactive in the expedition's own risk management and demonstrate this to the insurance company. Insurance companies are more comfortable with an entity that appears as a reasonable risk. Where outdoor adventure programs are unique risks already, expeditionary entities will need to work a bit harder selling themselves. Do a good professional job on the application, call the broker, invite the broker to meet with the expedition organizers, use a good waiver and release form, and emphasize all the things this expedition will do to run a tight ship and use experienced personnel. If applicable, show the broker the expedition's procedures, staff or guide training and certifications, staff (criminal) background certifications, safety reviews, equipment checks and templates/tickle sheets, and awareness and enforcement of industry standards. If the expedition has one, show the broker your Web site (have it reviewed by counsel first!) and any other marketing or promotional materials that have been created by the expedition. Here are some examples of questions for your broker:

- Ask whether any of the following should be considered: comprehensive general liability (CGL), commercial auto (CA), worker's compensation, umbrella policies for extra coverage over and above the CGL and CA, errors and omissions (E&O), directors and officers (D&O), Kidnap & Ransom, Evacuation, and any other specialized coverage.
- Discuss whether any or all of the coverages you are seeking are available for groups (e.g., if the expedition forms a nonprofit corporation) as well as for individuals? Determine if there are any savings to be had by purchasing policies for a group and holding the policy through a nonprofit corporation?
- Ask how to ensure that the expedition medical professionals are covered.
- Determine whether standard health insurance will cover accidents during dangerous and/or foreign activities planned for the expedition (e.g., diving, rafting, and climbing).
- Can other expedition members and/or the expedition organization be added as named insureds on individual policies?
- Can insurance companies sue or claim against other expedition members as individuals or against a nonprofit organization for the insured losses if there is a liability release in place?

ADDITIONAL LEGAL CONSIDERATIONS FOR THE EXPEDITION'S MEDICAL PROFESSIONAL

In addition to the medical liability release and permission to treat form and medical malpractice insurance issues discussed in the previous section, some other issues are unique to expeditionary medical professionals and may possess liability implications and/or relate to compliance with law. The following are the most salient of those considerations.

Physical Evaluation of Participants

When planning the expedition, the medical professional must make threshold determinations concerning the minimum physical (and sometimes psychological) requirements necessary for each potential member's participation in the expedition. In the past, persons interested in participating in the expedition would fill out a medical questionnaire and someone from the expedition would evaluate it based on their training and experience to determine if the applicant "passed muster." However, performing the participant's medical evaluation by such means can generate legal liability for both the evaluator and the expedition organization as a whole. By deeming someone to be appropriately fit, the expedition itself is assuming some of the risk that would otherwise have remained solely with the applicant participant. Additionally, most states do not allow anyone but a licensed physician to diagnose a patient based on a questionnaire.

For these reasons, the person in the best position to assess the medical, physical, and other conditions of the applicant is that person's personal doctor. The most "bullet-proof" means of assuring that the applicant meets the physical requirements is to provide two documents to the evaluating physician: (1) a simple statement to be signed by that doctor indicating his or her impressions: "I find no medical conditions that I consider to be incompatible with XYZ activities"; and (2) a description of the planned undertaking and conditions that the applicant/participant is likely to be exposed to during the expedition. Both the Boy Scouts of America and the Professional Association of Diving Instructors (PADI) are good resources for such medical evaluation forms and related releases.

Prescription Drugs

Participants' Prescription Drugs

Like the medical evaluation, the participant's personal prescription drugs are best acquired by the participant in the participant's own name and carried by the participant. However, the participant should disclose all drugs he or she is taking either on a regular basis or may take to address certain conditions during the expedition so that the medical professionals can make informed assessments of the participant should emergency treatment become necessary. A good safety precaution is to require each participant to obtain double the quantity of prescription drugs needed. Key prescriptions should not be transported in checked baggage unless unavoidable and the extra quantities may be transported by the physician as a safety precaution against loss.

The Physician's Medical Kit

Drugs and other prescription materials that the expedition physician includes in the expedition kit should be carried by the physician, and they should remain in their original containers. For all controlled drugs, including narcotics, records pertaining to use and disposal should be maintained throughout the expedition, including the date of receipt, the name and address of the person from whom they were received, and the kind and quantity received. The records should also reflect the date and time of administration, dispensing, or disposal; the name of the person to whom they were administered, dispensed, or disposed; and the kind and quantity of drug. The U.S. Drug Enforcement Administration (DEA), and possibly their foreign counterparts, will likely request this information both when leaving and returning to the United States. Even though it is often considered a humanitarian action to leave supplies and medications with appropriate responsible parties upon return to the United States, the DEA requires detailed accounting for any Class I narcotics (opiates and other regulated medications) that you had in your possession when you departed from the United States. Thus, it is fine to leave bandages and other medical equipment and nonrestricted medications, but strong pain medications such as morphine, Demerol, oxycodone, and similar medications must be accounted for.

Good Samaritan Laws

Good Samaritan laws in the United States protect those who come to the aid of others who are injured or ill from blame or liability for any circumstances arising from the voluntary assistance provided.[43] These laws are intended to reduce bystanders' hesitation to assist, for fear of being prosecuted for unintentional injury or wrongful death. The existence of some type of relationship (e.g., relationships that impose a legally recognized duty on the actor) may render the Good Samaritan laws inapplicable. For instance, from the medical professional's perspective, it is important to note that if there is an agreement in place to provide medical services whether or not the medical professional is receiving any form of compensation for his or her services, such a person will generally be precluded from employing the Good Samaritan defense.[44] Thus, if a physician is on an expedition wholly or in part to provide medical care to members of the expedition, then a relationship has been created, and as a result the physician may not rely on the Good Samaritan Laws to defend against a claim. However, if that same physician provided assistance to a member of an unrelated expedition, for instance, in the next tent over, he or she would

likely fall within the immunity protections of the Good Samaritan provisions.

It is well to note that the Good Samaritan laws differ from state to state, and that several countries impose widely varying versions of such laws. For instance Italy, Japan, France, Belgium, and Spain actually impose a duty to render care. In such countries, Good Samaritan laws describe a legal requirement for citizens to assist people in distress, unless doing so would put them in harm's way.[45] In Germany, a citizen is obliged to provide first aid when necessary and is immune from prosecution if assistance given in good faith turns out to be harmful. The authors could find no case law that would impose these countries' duties on noncitizens.

Because the Good Samaritan laws are applied in widely varying fashion, both within and outside of the United States, it is not really possible to delineate when exactly a medical professional will be able to seek immunity under such laws. For this reason (and many others), physicians and other medical professionals should always confirm that his or her malpractice carrier will provide coverage for the scope of professional activities to be encountered while on an expedition.

OTHER LEGAL CONSIDERATIONS FOR THE EXPEDITION

This section is the chapter's "catch-all" and covers three widely divergent topics that nonetheless may be of assistance to expedition planners when examining liability risks and entering into contracts.

Intellectual Property Rights

Expeditions are increasingly making use of global communications technology and combining it with digital imagery and high definition motion pictures. Using this infrastructure, expeditions are creating intellectual property that may be as simple as a real-time daily log of activities or as complex as feature-length documentaries. Preparations for such activities form an integral part of expedition planning, and such planning should include more than equipment evaluations and acquisitions. Thorough consideration should also be given to who will "own" the resulting media products, who will have rights to use the resulting intellectual property, and in what manner it may be used. For instance, if there is a copyright, will it belong to individual members or to the group as a whole?[46] If royalties are generated by the resulting books/photos/films or speaking engagements, who will they go to and in what proportion? Additionally, contracts governing production/publication rights (and possibly cash advances) may need to be negotiated with educational organizations, television content providers, and/or book publishers. Who will conduct those negotiations and on whose behalf?

Depending on the nature and makeup of the expedition group, it is advisable in advance to have a full discussion among members concerning the development and use of expedition-derived intellectual property as well as any resulting proceeds flowing from it. It may be that the expedition members adopt an "eat what you kill" approach and allow individual members to go after their own story-dissemination activities, be it a tell-all adventure travel book, photo exhibit, the Rotarians' lecture circuit and/or a lived-to-tell-about-it film (any of which could trigger privacy rights issues if the likeness, etc., of another expedition member is included). However, it may be advisable to take a more organized approach to the development of such postexpedition products and the allocation of any resulting fame, profits, and copyrights. Additionally, assuming that a nonprofit corporation has been formed in relation to the expedition, the development and enforcement of intellectual property agreements may be facilitated if made in the context of such an entity. In any case, a discussion among expedition members on this subject should not be postponed until after the trip, as doing so invites, at a minimum, bad feelings and could result in litigation and delays in bringing the products into the public sphere.

The following list includes some of the considerations related to expedition intellectual property that should be addressed prior to finalizing expedition plans:

- Who will own the copyrights in produced materials and who will have related or delegated rights in them? If the expedition members as a group will retain rights, it may be advisable to form an organization (e.g., nonprofit corporation) as discussed previously in this chapter.[47] Under such an arrangement, agreements with agents and publishers and/or production companies may be with the nonprofit corporation rather than with individual members. Royalties, if any, could also flow to the corporation, although different arrangements can be made through agreements and licenses. A legal professional familiar with copyright law should be consulted to optimize, protect, and help determine how and when to delegate these rights.
- If a nonprofit corporation is formed, will the marketing of the publications align with the stated purpose of the organization (e.g., educational/scientific)? If no, it may be advisable to form a separate for-profit subsidiary of the nonprofit to handle commercial activities. However, taking this step may not be necessary, depending on the degree of work and income such endeavors represent relative to the nonprofit. A knowledgeable attorney should be consulted first.
- If more than one of the expedition members intends to independently market "the story," it is advisable to understand the scope of each member's plans and to obtain agreements among the members not to compete with one another, at least for a set amount of time

after the conclusion of the expedition. Additionally, it will be important to discuss privacy issues and rights of publicity. Such a discussion may include whether other expedition members have a right of pre-approval for use of their name and/or likeness in any resulting films, books, stories, slide shows, and so on.

- Before reproducing, distributing, and/or making commercial use of the name, likeness, or voice of any person, "model releases" should be obtained for each such person.
- If the leadership of the expedition intends to own all resulting publications, findings, publicity, imagery, and the like (as well as any product endorsements) stemming from the expedition, and if they are requesting other members to assist them, but not share in the production and any resulting proceeds, such plans and intentions should be clearly communicated and agreed to in writing in advance by all affected members.

Employment-Related Issues

A critical issue that expeditionary entities need to assess in their risk management planning is the fact that both the expedition and its employees or guides/leaders can be held liable in the event of an incident or accident that injures or kills a participant. In the absence of some type of immunity, if the guide or leader breaches a duty to a participant, and that breach is shown to be the proximate cause of the injury, then the guide/leader is negligent and can be held legally liable for damages.[48] The expedition entity (e.g., the nonprofit corporation) may be generally liable under the doctrine of *respondeat superior* or vicarious liability. This doctrine holds that, if the person is an employee and is acting within the scope of his or her employment responsibility and authority and if the act was not grossly negligent, the negligence of the employee will be imputed to the entity as well. If the employee was acting outside his or her scope of authority the act is *ultra vires* (without authority) and the employing entity is generally relieved of liability.[49] Volunteers/trainees/interns to an organization are generally responsible for their own negligence. However, if they are acting under the control of the entity, then the corporate entity is generally liable under a *respondeat superior* theory. Volunteers of public or nonprofit organizations are immune from liability from their own negligence if they qualify under the Federal Volunteer Protection Act or a state volunteer immunity statute.[50]

Because of the various exposures employers face, it is more and more common for entities to attempt to classify employees as independent contractors in their businesses. The main reasons to claim that someone is an independent contractor are to avoid having to pay certain insurances and contributions for state and federal taxes and to try to reduce the amount of liability faced by the operator. The general rule is that if an injury results from the negligence of an independent contractor, liability for negligence is shifted from the operator (in this case an expeditionary entity) to the independent contractor. However, there are substantial risks in trying to establish that a third-party working for an expedition is an independent contractor as opposed to an employee. For instance, if the agent (guide, etc.) is misclassified with respect to paying wages, the entity could be liable for back taxes and interest and penalties (up to 100 percent in some cases). This is federal law. Also if someone employed by the expedition is hurt on the job and the expedition entity did not properly apply the test as to whether that person was genuinely an independent contractor, the penalties for failing to provide worker's compensation insurance can be staggering. Individual state laws govern here. Usually the appropriate state agency dealing with worker's compensation (generally the Department of Labor) will have information available to employers by phone on how the state, through its regulations, classifies employees versus independent contractors.

There is also the matter of unemployment benefits. If the entity has misclassified and not paid appropriate withholding to account for its employee's state unemployment benefit calculations, it could be liable for back payments and penalties. Classifying someone as an independent contractor also doesn't mean the expedition entity won't be sued for negligent hiring or supervision or retention of your independent contractor. See previous section on negligent hiring.

As with practically all issues discussed in this chapter, this is an area in which the expedition entity will want to seek competent advice from professionals knowledgeable in its state, region, and type of business (tax advisers and lawyers).

Body Repatriation

We all expect to come home . . . ALIVE. As such, body bags and the abandonment of mortal remains are topics that rarely receive enthusiastic discussion. The potential death of expedition members should be planned for, at least among the expedition leaders and its medical professionals, and should be discussed among all expedition members. Additionally, as emphasized throughout this chapter, one of the most important components for defending against claims is evidence that full and complete warnings and risk disclosures were made to all participants. For this reason, it is necessary that the expedition members clearly understand any potential obstacles to body repatriation and the potential costs to their estate and/or families that may be incurred. Trip organizers should make inquiries with local public land administrators (assuming such exist) as to the

> **Tests to help determine whether a person really is an independent contractor:[51]**
>
> - Employee = hired, paid a set wage or salary, trained by the employer, works on an ongoing basis, performs work as directed by the employer, paid by the hour, week, or month, uses the employer's tools.
> - Independent contractor = engaged only for a specific project usually for a set sum and is usually paid at the end of the project, can do the job his or her own way and usually furnishes own equipment, has minimal restrictions, and is only responsible for satisfactory completion of the project, may have his or her own business license, should be reporting income as self-employed and not as an employee.

availability of search and rescue groups and also to determine the level of support that may be expected from local officials. Doing so will allow members to assess local conditions, human resources, and potential costs.

The extent that any real advanced planning can occur for this contingency, like other considerations in this chapter, is context driven. For instance, if the expedition involves high-altitude climbing or other "transport-challenged" destinations, or if body retrieval would present a danger to surviving expedition members, it is likely that the body will need to remain in situ. The various scenarios need to be discussed with all expedition members so that they can acknowledge these risks and fully assume them. Written agreements among the expedition members should be made memorializing the discussion as well as the arrangements agreed upon by the group (e.g., that the expedition will not be responsible for costs or actions involved in extracting and repatriating bodies from remote or high-altitude locations). Such statements should be part of the liability waiver (discussed previously) and may also be more particularly covered in a separate stand-alone agreement. It is also important to include an acknowledgment in the section of the liability waiver on possession of required insurance policies, that the participant either possesses insurance for, or otherwise agrees to bear costs associated with body repatriation.[52] Putting such agreements in place is vital for ensuring that the expedition will not become liable for costs of recovery that family members may undertake to bring the body home.

In the event of a death in a remote location, and to the extent possible, one or more written statements should be obtained from witnesses and/or the examining medical professional verifying the time and location of the death as well as the cause (if ascertainable). Photographs are also advisable.

While familiarizing the expedition with the capabilities of the local authorities concerning the availability of emergency response (including moving bodies) is crucial to pretrip planning, once a foreign-based death has occurred, the U.S. Consulate can provide a broad range of services to assist with getting an American citizen's body back to the United States.[53] For example, the U.S. consular officer in the foreign country will assist the family in making arrangements with local authorities for preparation and disposition of the remains. Options available to a family depend upon local law and practice in the foreign country and certain documents are required before remains can be sent from one country to another. In most instances, a U.S. consular mortuary certificate is required to ensure orderly shipment of remains and to facilitate U.S. Customs clearance. The U.S. consular officer will prepare the certificate and ensure that the foreign death certificate (if available), affidavit of the foreign funeral director, and transit permit, together with the consular mortuary certificate accompany the remains to the United States. Expedition leaders, members, and their families should be aware that arrangements for local burial or return of the remains to the United States is affected by local laws, customs, and facilities, which are often vastly different from those in the United States. Additional considerations or delays may result to the extent circumstances of death require investigation or involve a "quarantinable" disease.

The U.S. State Department's website provides detailed information (including contact telephone numbers) on this subject and should be consulted as part of the expedition planning process.

CONCLUSION/SUMMARY

Lawyers are often accused of being killjoys for their tendencies to anticipate worst case scenarios. In reality, nothing could be further from the truth! The typical lawyerly approach is to draft protective agreements with clauses ensuring that the allocation of culpability, costs, and benefits has been accomplished in advance of an incident or conflict. Far from being pessimistic spoilsports, it is our goal, in providing the foregoing materials on risk management and legal liability assessment, that you (and we) will spend more time enjoying expeditionary pursuits and less time haggling over disputes about "he said – she said."

In conclusion we provide a big-picture checklist of the considerations that we covered in this chapter and believe expedition leaders and medical professionals should consider when developing and executing their expedition plan:

- Determine as early as possible whether your organization would benefit from the twin advantages offered by forming a nonprofit corporation: liability protection of its members and employees and fund-raising tax offsets.
- Conduct a thorough risk assessment both at the outset of your expedition and on a rolling basis:

brainstorm with the expedition participants and consult professional risk managers (e.g., specialized insurance brokers), and others with experience in the types of activities planned for your expedition as you elaborate your risk management plans. To the extent possible, gather information from local authorities on conditions, capabilities, and services (e.g., search and rescue) that may be available should the expedition require them.

- Find the balance between the level of risk tolerance you will expect or need from your expedition coparticipants and the types of activities and risk exposures you as the leader and/or medical professional want to incorporate into the expedition plan. Then take affirmative steps to mitigate risk levels accordingly (e.g., ensure that proper screening procedures are in place and that insurance and waivers are robust enough to cover the plan).
- Make sure that all participants are fully apprised of risks that they will be exposed to throughout the expedition. To the extent possible, try to forecast as many of these risks in advance so they can be included in the liability waiver and screened for in the medical evaluation. However, as plans and conditions change (as they inevitably will) during the expedition, take time to hold safety briefings and discussions to ensure that all members continue to fully understand and are *voluntarily assuming* the risks on a rolling basis.
- To understand the types of possible litigation exposure the expedition may face, try putting yourself in the shoes of the expedition members' family or loved ones. What level of professionalism and emergency preparedness would they expect of the guides/leaders/expedition entity under the circumstances being contemplated?[54]
- Think of managing risks as being not so much minimizing them but optimizing your resources and the situation – of making the most effective use of a given situation. Optimizing is caring for the expedition, its staff and guides, participants, benefactors, and the adventure industry as a whole, and that is good risk management.
- Consider the range of postexpedition "products" that may be developed including photo exhibits, lecture circuits, books, and documentaries. To the extent possible, discuss these opportunities in advance of the expedition to ensure that there is no competition after the expedition, and take steps to develop, protect, and allocate resulting copyrights and trademarks.

Even though we have tried to discuss the current state of the law on various issues that may affect the legal liabilities of an expedition, nothing in the law is black and white. Work with good competent counsel. Stay abreast of what's happening with the activities/sports planned for your expedition, as well as with what others in similar expeditions are doing with respect to risk mitigation. Look at risk management with a positive, goal-oriented view. It is about creating a good, competent, and smoothly run expedition. Moreover, it is about *getting out there*, whether it's on the knife edge of a high-altitude ridge or the deepest white-water chasm extant: Have fun, be safe, and especially avoid liability!

REFERENCES

1. See Moran S, Glenn L. Trends in risk management: A look at the risks involved in outdoor adventure programming. *The Outdoor Network*. 2002;13(1).

2. See Hronek BB, Spengler JO. Overview of trends, risk and legal liability. *Legal Liability in Recreation and Sports*, 2nd ed. Champaign, Ill.: Sagamore Publishing; 2002:22–3. See also Cloutier R with Garvey D, Leverette W, Moss J, Vadade G. Preparing risk management documents. *Legal Liability and Risk Management in Adventure Tourism*. Kamloops, British Columbia: Bhudak Consultants; 2000: Chapter 9; Cotton DJ, Wolohan JT. Risk management. *Law for Recreation and Sports Mangers*. 3rd ed. Dubuque, Iowa: Kendall/Hunt Publishing Comp.; 2000; Garvey D, et al. Risk management. *Manual of Accreditation Standards for Adventure Programs*. Boulder, Colo.: Association for Experiential Education; 1999.

3. See Hronek BB, Spengler JO. Overview of trends, risk and legal liability. *Legal Liability in Recreation and Sports*. 2nd ed. Champaign, Ill.: Sagamore Publishing; 2002: Chapter 1, 22–3.

4. See Cloutier R with Garvey D, Leverette W, Moss J, Vadade G. Risk management. *Legal Liability and Risk Management in Adventure Tourism*. Kamloops, British Columbia: Bhudak Consultants; 2000: Chapter 8, 96.

5. The correlation between fund-raising and risk mitigation is not coincidental. As an expedition seeks and brings in sponsors, benefactors, and grants, they will also need to demonstrate that the expedition has a sound plan and a high probability of success. Risk assessment and management are key elements of this plan.

6. These forms and agreements should also be executed within the context of an expedition nonprofit corporation.

7. This study was based on a review of several hundred published adventure or recreational cases tried in court, and after tort liability, the next highest percentage (11%) of claims were based on employment issues (wrongful termination, breach of employment contracts, wrongful demotion). See Fried, G. Why do we need risk management? *Safe at First, A Guide to Help Sports Administrators Reduce Their Liability*. Durham, N.C.: Carolina Academic Press; 1999: 10.

8. See Cloutier R with Garvey D, Leverette W, Moss J, Vadade G. Tort law. *Legal Liability and Risk Management in Adventure Tourism*, Kamloops, British Columbia: Bhudak Consultants; 2000: Chapter 2. See also Cotten DJ, Wolohan JT. Negligence law. *Law for Recreation and Sports Managers*, 3rd ed. Dubuque, Iowa: Kendall/Hunt Publishing Company; 2000: Chapter 2; Hronek BB, Spengler JO, The negligence cause of action, *Legal Liability in Recreation and Sports*, 2nd ed. Champaign, Ill.: Sagamore Publishing; 2002: Chapter 5; Fried G. Applicable legal terms and principles. *Safe at First, A Guide to Help Sports Administrators Reduce Their Liability*. Durham, N.C.: Carolina Academic Press; 1999, Chapter 3; Hicks E. A defense lawyer's perspective on risk management and crisis response. In: Ajango D. ed., *Lessons Learned, A Guide to Accident Prevention and Crisis Response*. Anchorage: University of Alaska Press; 2000.

9. See Cotten DJ. Wolohan JT. Elements of negligence, *Law For Recreation and Sports Managers*, 3rd ed. Dubuque, Iowa: Kendall/Hunt Publishing Company; 2000: Chapter 2.11, 57.

10. See The elusive reasonable person. *The Outdoor Education and Recreation Law Quarterly*. 2001;1(Spring).

11. See Cloutier R with Garvey D, Leverette W, Moss J, Vadade G. Tort law. *Legal Liability and Risk Management in Adventure Tourism*. Kamloops, British Columbia: Bhudak Consultants; 2000: 16–17.

12. See *Licato v. Eastgate*, 499 N.Y.S. 2d 472 (A.D. 3 Dept. 1986).

13. See *Saffro v. Elite Racing Inc.*, 98 Cal. App. 4th 173 (Ct. App. California, May 7, 2002) (rev. denied, 2002 Cal. Lexis 5268 (July 2002)).

14. See *Scurfield v. Cariboo Heli-Skiing Ltd.*, 74 B.C.L.R. (2d) (1993).

15. See *Voight v. Colorado Mountain Club*, 819 P. 2d 1088 (Colo. App. 1991).

16. See *Martinez v. Swartzbaugh*, 2002 Cal. App. Unpub. LEXIS 12192.

17. See Cotten DJ, Wolohan JT. Elements of negligence. *Law For Recreation and Sports Managers*, 3rd ed. Dubuque, Iowa: Kendall/Hunt Publishing Company; 2000: Chapter 2.11, 59.

18. See *Mankoski v. Mieras*, 1999 WL 33453871 (Mich. App.).

19. See *Dare v. Freefall Adventures, Inc.*, 2002 WL 432370 (N.J. Super A.D.).

20. See Cotten DJ, Wolohan JT. Premises liability, *Law For Recreation and Sports Managers*, 3rd ed. Dubuque, Iowa: Kendall/Hunt Publishing Company; 2000: Chapter 2.30, 209.

21. See *Estate of Adam Harshman v. Jackson Hole Mountain Resort and USA*, 379 F. 3d 1161 (2004).

22. See, generally, Cotten DJ, Wolohan JT. Emergency care. *Law for Recreation and Sports Managers*, 3rd ed., Dubuque, Iowa: Kendall/Hunt Publishing Company; 2000: Chapter 2.31.

23. Ibid. at Chapter 2.32.

24. See *Dunn v. So. Calif. 7th Day Adventists*, San Bernadino Sup. Ct. (1998).

25. See Pearson JV. Staffing issues in the adventure and recreation industry. Presented at: Recreation and Adventure Program Law & Liability Conference; April 2004; Denver, Colo. CLE International.

26. See Fried G. Transportation. *Safe at First: A Guide to Help Sports Administrators Reduce Their Liability*. Durham, N.C.: Carolina Academic Press; 1999: Chapter 27, 296. See also Cotten DJ, Wolohan JT. Transportation. *Law for Recreation and Sports Managers*, 3rd ed. Dubuque, Iowa: Kendall/Hunt Publishing Company; Chapter 2.34; Anglin B, Chatfield R. A crash-bang ride around transportation safety. Presented at: Outward Bound 2002 Wilderness Risk Management Conference Proceedings; October 2002; Reno, Nev.

27. See Cloutier R with Garvey D, Leverette W, Moss J, Vadade G. Tort law. *Legal Liability and Risk Management in Adventure Tourism*. Kamloops, British Columbia: Bhudak Consultants; 2000: 19.

28. See Horton LL. Sports and recreational liability. Presented at Recreation and Adventure Program Law and Liability Conference; April 2004; Denver, Colo.

29. See Hronek BB, Spengler JO. Defenses to negligence. *Legal Liability in Recreation and Sports*, 2nd ed. Champaign, Ill.: Sagamore Publishing; 2002: 65, 68–9.

30. Ibid. at Chapter 7. See also Cotton DJ, Wolohan JT. Waivers and releases. *Law for Recreation and Sports Mangers*, 3rd ed.

Dubuque, Iowa: Kendall/Hunt Publishing Company; 2000: Chapter 2.23; Hansen-Stamp C, Gregg CR. Is it really worth the paper it is written on? *The Outdoor Education and Recreation Law Quarterly.* 2003;3(3) and 2004;3(4).

[31] See Cloutier R with Garvey D, Leverette W, Moss J, Vadade G. Use of waivers. *Legal Liability and Risk Management in Adventure Tourism.* Kamloops, British Columbia: Bhudak Consultants; 2000: Chapter 6, 57–8.

[32] Ibid. at page 65.

[33] See, *Sexton v. Southwestern Auto Racing Assoc.*, 394 N.E. 2d 49 (Ill., 1979); *Talbert v. Lincoln Speedway*, 33 D&C. 3d 111 (Pa., 1984); *Johnson v. Robert Dunlap and Racing, Inc.*, 280 S.E. 2nd 759 (N.C. 1981); *Hobby v. Gilpin*, 1984 Tenn. App. LEXIS 26906.

[34] See Cotton DJ, Cotton MB. *Waivers and Releases of Liability,* 4th ed. Statesboro, Ga.: Sport Risk Consulting; 2004. See also Cloutier R. with Garvey D, Leverette W, Moss J, Vadade G. *Legal Liability and Risk Management in Adventure Tourism,* Kamloops, British Columbia; 2000: Chapter 6, 57–8; Van Gorder C. Parents' signatures on release forms: Is one enough?, *The Outdoor Education and Recreation Law Quarterly.* 2002;2(3).

[35] Note: Some of the health issues covered in the general liability release and waiver agreement will overlap with and be redundant with the medical release document discussed in the next section; however, for a number of reasons, it is important to maintain these as separate agreements, among them is the fact that the parties will not be the same in both agreements, and the circumstances triggering their applicability may also differ.

[36] See, generally, *Allan v. Snow Summit*, 51 Cal. App. 4th 1358 (1996); *Cooperman v. Wyoming Rivers & Trails,* 214 P. 3d 1162 (10th Cir. June 2000); *Distefano v. Forester*, 85 Cal. App. 4th 1249 (Jan. 2001); *Loney v. Adirondack River Outfitters, Inc.*, 30 A.D. 2d 747 (N.Y. Supp. App. Ct. July 2003); *Madsen v. Wyo. River Trips*, 31 F. Supp. 2d 1321 (Wyo. D.C. 1999).

[37] Emergency position-indicating radio beacons (EPIRBs) are designed to facilitate search and rescue operations by alerting rescue authorities and indicating the party's location. The signal from most EPIRBs is detectable by aircraft and satellite.

[38] See Cotton DJ, Wolohan JT. Defenses against liability. *Law for Recreation and Sports Managers*, 3rd ed. Dubuque, Iowa: Kendall/Hunt Publishing Company; 2000: Chapter 2,21, 79–83. See also Hansen-Stamp C, Gregg CR, eds. Assumption of risks. *The Outdoor Education and Recreation Law Quarterly.* 2003;3(1).

[39] Ibid. at Chapter 9, pages 126–7, quoting Will Leverette on safety talks.

[40] See Knutson T. Litigation issues: Lessons learned in the courtroom. Presented at: Recreation and Adventure Program Law and Liability Conference; April 2004; Denver, Colo., CLE International. See also Clouotier R with Garvey D, Leverette W, Moss J, Vadade G. Accident guidelines. *Legal Liability and Risk Management in Adventure Tourism* Kamloops, British Columbia: Bhudak Consultants; 2000: Chapter 10.

[41] See Freeman F. Insurance issues in the industry. Presented at: Recreation and Adventure Program Law and Liability Conference; April 2003; Denver Colo., CLE International. See also Freeman F. Insurance issues. Presented at: Recreation and Adventure Program Law and Liability Conference; April 2004; Denver Colo., CLE International; Clouotier R with Garvey D, Leverette W, Moss J, Vadade G. insurance. *Legal Liability and Risk Management in Adventure Tourism*, Kamloops, British Columbia: Bhudak Consultants; 2000: Chapter 13.

[42] See Freeman F. Insurance issues in the industry. Presented at: Recreation and Adventure Program Law and Liability Conference; April 2003; Denver Colo., CLE International. See also Freeman F. Insurance issues. Presented at: Recreation and Adventure Program Law and Liability Conference; April 2004; Denver Colo., CLE International; Clouotier R with Garvey D, Leverette W, Moss J, Vadade G. Insurance. *Legal Liability and Risk Management in Adventure Tourism.* Kamloops, British Columbia: Bhudak Consultants; 2000: Chapter 13.

[43] See *Van Horn v. Torti*, 148 Cal. App. 4th 1013 (2007), where a friend in a following car stopped to assist a friend get free from a crashed car, and the helping friend (defendant) was later alleged to have aggravated injuries sustained in the crash and caused plaintiff's permanent paraplegia. The court reversed defendant's grant of summary judgment holding (1) that the defendant's actions were not in response to a medical emergency (even though she thought the crashed car was about to catch fire), and she therefore was not entitled to immunity under California's Good Samaritan law, and (2) that there were sufficient questions of fact that it was proper to remand the claim for further proceedings, particularly as to whether defendant's actions constituted negligence. This case seems to indicate that a Good Sam (at least in California) should confine their emergency responses to actions that are strictly medical in nature. Perhaps the defendant should have waited for the car to catch fire before assisting?

[44] See *Boccasile et al. v. Cajun Music Ltd*, 694 A.2d 686 (1997) (Sup. Ct. R.I.), where two medical professionals were volunteering in the first-aid tent at a music festival, when a man succumbed, and later died due to anaphylactic shock (from consumption of seafood gumbo). The court held that the physician and nurse attending to the man were not liable for the man's wrongful death because the widow failed to establish an applicable standard of care against which the defendant's conduct could be measured. The medical professionals sought and received summary judgment on the basis that they were volunteers and therefore protected by Rhode Island's Good Samaritan laws. However, the court stated that the decision was based on standard of care criteria and did not rule on whether care rendered at a first-aid tent would be gratuitous. This case demonstrates that even where Good Sam defenses are not availing, it is possible for medical professionals to defend their actions on the basis of the context in which the medical care was rendered.

[45] One well-known application of this duty was in relation to the photographers at the scene of Princess Diana's fatal car accident. They were investigated for violation of the French Good Samaritan law.

[46] Even where copyrights are owned by individuals or corporations, their use may be delegated through a collaboration agreement and/or through licensing agreements (exclusive or nonexclusive), which may delineate in detail the rights and responsibilities of the licensee/user, and include, for instance, whether each use will be subject to the copyright owner's approval and whether the use right extends to commercial, creative, and/or business matter usage. Such agreements should also be used to delineate how revenues will be collected and disbursed. In the expedition context, it is also worth deciding whether an expedition member's rights to any intellectual property created will stay with other expedition members or will flow to that participant's heirs should the member die or become incapacitated.

[47] If the understanding is that the corporation owns the intellectual property rights, the corporation will also retain rights

to any copyrightable materials generated by any employee of the corporation.

[48] See Cotton DJ, Wolohan JT. Which parties are liable? *Law for Recreation and Sports Managers*, 3rd ed., Dubuque, Iowa: Kendall/Hunt Publishing Company; 2000: Chapter 2.12, 66.

[49] Ibid. at page 68. See also Pearson JV. Staffing issues in the adventure and recreation industry. Presented at: Recreation and Adventure Program Law and Liability Conference; April 2004; Denver, Colo. CLE International.

[50] Cotton DJ, Wolohan JT. Which parties are liable? *Law for Recreation and Sports Managers*, 3rd ed. Dubuque, Iowa: Kendall/Hunt Publishing Company; 2000: Chapter 2.12, 69.

[51] Ibid. at pages 70–1. See also Van Gorder C. Employee or independent contractor: Guidelines for classifying your workers. *The Outdoor Network*. 2002;13(2).

[52] Medical evacuation insurance often has a clause for repatriation of remains, and it is prudent to review your policy. This subject is covered in more detail in other chapters.

[53] The authority and responsibilities of a U.S. consular officer concerning return of remains of a deceased U.S. citizen abroad are based on U.S. laws (22 U.S.C. 4196; 22 CFR 72.1), treaties, and international practice.

[54] See Cloutier R with Garvey D, Leverette W, Moss J, Vadade G. Risk management. *Legal Liability and Risk Management in Adventure Tourism*. Kamloops, British Columbia: Bhudak Consultants; 2000: Chapter 8, 99, quoting Will Leverette.

SUGGESTED READINGS

For additional information, the authors suggest consulting the following resources.

Cloutier R, with Garvey D, Leverette W, Moss J, Vadade G. Preparing risk management documents. *Legal Liability and Risk Management in Adventure Tourism*. Kamloops, British Columbia: Bhudak Consultants; 2000.

Hicks E. A defense lawyer's perspective on risk management and crisis response. In: Ajango D, ed. *Lessons Learned, A Guide to Accident Prevention and Crisis Response*. Anchorage: University of Alaska Press; 2000.

Hopkins BR. *Nonprofit Law Made Easy*. New York: John Wiley & Sons; 2005.

Hopkins BR. *Starting and Managing a Nonprofit Organization: A Legal Guide*. 4th ed. New York: John Wiley & Sons; 2005.

Manuso A. *How to Form a Nonprofit Corporation*, 7th ed. Berkeley, Calif: Nolo; 2005.

Moran S, Glenn L. Trends in risk management: A look at the risks involved in outdoor adventure programming. *The Outdoor Network* 2002;13(Winter).

Paulsson J. *Denial of Justice in International Law*. New York: Cambridge University Press; 2005 (reprinted in 2006).

Pelton RY. *The World's Most Dangerous Place*s. 4th ed. New York: Harper Resource; 2000.

Vartorella WF, Keel DS. *Funding Exploration: The Challenge and Opportunity for Funding Science and Discovery in the 21st Century*. Marco Polo Monographs; 2004.

State of Risk - Risk Management in the Outdoor Industry, A Training DVD produced by Knutson & Associates for Commercial Guides, Adventure Sports Operators, Public Land Administrators and Adventure Insurers; see *www.traceyknutson.com*.

Michael J. VanRooyen, MD, MPH, FACEP

Many travelers are seeking exotic, remote, and potentially dangerous venues. These may include extremes of altitude, temperature, isolation, and potential political instability.

Most expeditions are planned by professionals with experience in handling local climates, cultures, and conditions. Whether you are traveling with a scientific expedition or a remote tourist adventure, most serious expeditions take planning down to the last detail. Despite preparations, many expeditions are subject to severe conditions and both natural and man-made calamities. It is essential, therefore, that regardless of the degree of leadership or external preparation, the adventure traveler must take ownership of his or her own safety.

The objectives of this chapter are to provide practical insights pertaining to travel safety as it relates to man-made hazards, such as transportation safety, theft, assault, and imprisonment, with a particular emphasis on avoiding problems while traveling. The chapter is intended to provide useful suggestions that may, to some, seem very basic and obvious but that, for many reasons, are important to ensure safe and unobstructed travel, especially to remote or unfamiliar destinations. For additional information about conflict areas or regions of political instability, see Chapter 14.

NEW TRENDS IN TRAVEL: GROWTH IN THE NONTRADITIONAL TRAVEL INDUSTRY

The rapidly expanding market of adventure and remote travel, as well as the massive international tourist industry, has increased travelers' exposure to all sorts of travel-related hazards, both natural and man-made. Travelers now have access to a greater number of adventure tours, remote explorations, and exotic cultures. These individuals include

- Wilderness and remote travelers
- Adventure and "high-impact" travelers
- Travelers on expeditions to extreme locations, including mountaineering and caving

- Travelers who take on eco-challenges and outdoor adventure sports
- Long-term remote travelers
- Travelers to conflict areas and politically unstable regions

And with these adventures come exposure to areas with high crime rates, insecure political climates, and areas with complex local political insecurity, where assault, theft, and even kidnapping have become far more common. Whether you are leading an expedition to a remote area of the Amazon or are part of a tour of the Vatican, you need to make certain preparations and take a few precautions prior to traveling.

HEALTH RISKS: REAL VERSUS PERCEIVED RISKS

One of the great anxieties associated with travel to foreign countries and exotic lands is fear of the unknown. A surprising number of travelers have a disproportionately intense fear of death by certain spectacular means and ignore the far more likely causes of injury and death posed by everyday occurrences like car accidents. To dispel a few myths for those not inclined to follow the population-based evidence, here is a list of the most feared but least likely causes of death to travelers:[1]

Airplane crashes: Over 30 million Americans have significant anxiety due to fear of dying in a plane crash. The statistics, of course, point out the amazing safety of air travel. The risk of death for an American, for example, is one death for every 7.4 million flights. This means that you can fly everyday for 19,000 years before being killed in an airplane crash.

Shark attacks: Americans, in particular, have a visceral fear of being attacked and killed by a shark. The International Shark Attack File (ISAF) lists all shark attacks and deaths. Only 1,909 confirmed shark attacks have occurred around the world in the last 350 years, 737 of which occurred in the United States, resulting in 38 fatalities. The odds of being attacked by a shark are therefore about one in 11.5 million, and your chances of being killed are about one in 264.1 million.

Murders: Murder scares people because of its unpredictability, yet the vast majority of the 520,000 people murdered around the world (WHO statistic) are a result of political unrest or hostile intent, not random murders of civilians. The true risk of being randomly murdered is incredibly low.

Terrorist attacks: Terrorism has been on the minds of travelers for the last decade, and recent surveys indicated that many Americans fear travel to foreign countries for fear of a terrorist attack. While the odds are certainly higher in Iraq and Afghanistan, the overall risk of being killed in a terrorist attack are spectacularly low, about one in 9.3 million.

Natural disasters: Tsunamis, earthquakes, hurricanes, floods, and other natural disasters all create significant fear. The odds of being killed by a natural calamity is about one in 3,357, although the vulnerable are by far more likely to die in a natural disaster, so travelers and tourists are much less likely to be killed.

MOST COMMON RISKS TO TRAVELERS

Although expedition and adventure-type travel has its own inherent risks, the epidemiology of travel-related illness and death is fairly predictable. Prior studies have noted that 64% of foreign travelers get some sort of illness, with each day of travel increasing the chances of getting ill by 3–4%. Of all those traveling abroad, the likelihood of becoming ill is noted in Table 6.1.

Causes of death while traveling abroad are most commonly due to underlying cardiovascular illnesses and injuries. Given that many foreign travelers are elderly, the risk of cardiovascular illness is disproportionately high. Of all those traveling abroad, the likelihood of dying is noted in Table 6.2.

In preparing to travel abroad, many travelers pay close attention to issues like proper immunizations and precautions for eating and drinking safely. Even though this is indeed important, it is also important to consider ways to ensure your safety from accidental and intentional injuries as well.

Table 6.1. Foreign travelers' illnesses

Diarrheal illness	46%
Respiratory infection	26%
Skin disorder	8%
Acute mountain sickness	6%
Motion sickness	5%
Accidents and injuries	5%

Freedman DO, et al. Spectrum of disease and relation to place of exposure among ill returned travellers. *N Eng J Med.* 2006;354: 119–30.

Table 6.2. Causes of death while traveling abroad (all ages)

Cardiovascular illness	49.0%
Unintentional injury	22.0%
Other medical (noninfectious)	13.7%
Suicide/homicide	2.9%
Infectious diseases	1.0%

MacPherson DW, Guérillot F, Streiner D, Ahmed K, et al. Death and dying abroad: the Canadian experience. *J Travel Med.* 2000;7: 227–33.

PERSONAL SAFETY: START WITH PROPER PACKING

As you prepare for travel, it is important to adapt your packing so that you reduce your risk and possible problems in foreign venues. Plain, conservative dress is almost always a good bet, with attention to local customs. It typically helps to blend in, which means dark, conservative clothing in Eastern Europe, head coverings for women in Muslim states, and no shorts and sleeveless shirts in many conservative countries.

Leave valuables or flashy looking jewelry at home. It almost always draws the wrong type of attention. Limit the amount of valuables you take with you. Consider getting an inexpensive watch for your trip, and leave rings and necklaces behind. The hotel safe is usually a good place to temporarily store cash and valuables. Plan to conceal your cash, credit cards, and identification. Avoid fanny packs and around-the-neck pocket carriers, and handbags as these are an easy target for theft. Do not put your valuables in a day pack, but keep them close and concealed.[2]

Seasoned travelers always keep a copy of their passport back at home, and also have a copy with their luggage, apart from the original. An extra copy of your passport can save you a lot of trouble at customs or when attempting to get a replacement. Also, keep several extra passport-sized photos, especially if you are traveling to areas that may require additional travel authorization. If you are traveling in Chad, for example, the government requires an additional travel permit after you arrive. As a rule, leave the rest of your wallet at home, including extra credit cards and other forms of ID.

TRAVEL INTELLIGENCE AND INFORMATION GATHERING PRIOR TO TRAVEL

The U.S. State Department issues travel warnings about countries they deem a risk. Even though depending on this list may severely restrict your travel options, it is a good idea to read the advisories and be familiar with the perceived threats. One of the best methods for collecting region- or country-specific information is by contacting people who live there, if you have access. Ground intelligence is usually more fine-grained and more contextual than general warnings and news bulletins. The Internet is a good source of information, but requires some degree of context and screening to sort out the major threats or problems with a particular location.

LOCAL CUSTOMS, LAWS, AND CONDUCT

Your travel safety and security can be enhanced by some basic understanding of your destination. It is amazing how many tourists go to a location without knowing the customs, currency, basic geography, and general political landscape. Learn as much as you can about local customs, habits, styles of dress, currency, major cities. Also, know where you are staying in relationship to other large hotels, as they are often a safer alternative because they have better security arrangements and controlled access. Even if you are not staying at a major hotel, the hotel staff can be a good source of information when in-county.[3]

TRAVEL INSURANCE

Numerous travel insurance companies offer travel insurance, as well as evacuation insurance. Check with your current insurance provider first to determine the extent of your coverage, international coverage, provisions for evacuation, and whether medical services abroad are covered. Many policies will not cover injuries suffered as a direct result of an altercation in a conflict area. Policies may be obtained for your specific scenario, such as employment in a politically insecure environment, war and terrorism insurance, and political evacuation insurance.[4] War and terrorism insurance is often extremely expensive, but evacuation services can be acquire reasonably for short-term travelers.

The U.S. Department of State Web site (*http://travel. state.gov/travel/index.html*) provides a list of travel insurance and medical evacuation companies. The Centers for Disease Control and Prevention (CDC) lists these companies in a noninclusive list of providers:

> **International SOS** (*http://www.internationalsos. com*): International SOS offers 24-hour physician-supported medical assistance. Members have access to online services, safety tips, travel advisories, and travel recommendations. Policies include medical evacuation and repatriation coverage and access to international clinics and emergency services.

> **MEDEX** (*http://www.medexassist.com*): MEDEX travel assistance services include 24-hour access to case managers who can help locate medical care providers and help with payment of medical expenses. Insurance policies include medical evacuation and repatriation services, emergency dental coverage, and assistance with replacement of medications.

International Association for Medical Assistance to Travelers (*http://www.iamat.org*): IAMAT is a nonprofit organization that maintains an international network of physicians, hospitals, and clinics who have agreed to treat IAMAT members in need of medical care while abroad. Membership is free, although a donation to support IAMAT efforts is appreciated.

PLANES, TRAINS, AND AUTOMOBILES

Remember that, despite the impressive threats of exotic infectious diseases or political instability, the most likely cause of death and disability in travelers younger than age 55 is motor vehicle accidents. With the exception of cram-packed minibuses in less industrialized settings, mass transit is far safer than driving in an individual car. U.S. health statistics compare the death rate per billion passenger miles of airplanes (0.01), trains (0.02), and transit buses (0.03) to passenger cars (0.89). The International Road Traffic and Accident Database (Organisation for Economic Co-operation and Development [OECD]) notes that death rates per 100 million kilometers driven are 43 times higher in Egypt, 36 times higher in Kenya, and 12–20 times higher in Northern Africa.[5]

An astounding number of people (the author included) maintain vigilant seat-belt use in their home country, where there are also airbags, safety devices, and reasonably compliant drivers and then ride unrestrained in a taxi heading though downtown Cairo. This is especially true of travelers to remote areas who often use precarious means of transportation to get to more remote locations, including buses, local adapted pickups, and flatbed trucks. It is because of this tendency that we offer a few basic vehicle safety tips.

VEHICLE SAFETY TIPS

Consider a few practical tips for traveling via automobile when traveling abroad. This includes avoiding the temptation to get behind the wheel and drive. If you can hire a local driver, you might get a better sense of the region in which you are traveling, and if there is a traffic mishap, you are not held directly (and financially) accountable. If you have to drive, take your time, know where you are going, and seek major routes. It is also wise to avoid driving at night. Navigating the poorly lit roads in Nairobi in an unfamiliar vehicle, with many pedestrians walking along the road (as there are very few sidewalks), is a recipe for disaster, both for the person or persons you may hit and for you.

Here are some helpful hints for driving abroad:[6]

- Become familiar with your vehicle in less-crowded conditions.
- Don't drive at night.
- Drive slowly and in control.

- Avoid large gatherings or busy markets.
- Wear a seat belt, always.
- Avoid driving when you are suffering from jet lag.

If you need to rent a car, look for a common type vehicle from a reputable dealer, and make sure the car is in good working order, making note of any preexisting body damage. Consider getting a car with air-conditioning so that you can have the windows rolled up and the car locked when you are in it. If you encounter what appears to be an informal roadblock or rocks across the road creating a makeshift barrier, there is a good likelihood that these are ploys to get you to stop. Turn around and drive away. Carjackers and thieves work in very organized groups around service stations, parking lots, markets, and along major highways. Be suspicious of anyone who flags you down, points to your car to indicate a flat or an oil leak, hails you or tries to get your attention when you are in or near your car.

Also, it is generally unwise to rent a motorcycle or motor scooter. Even though locals may be whirring conveniently around, nimbly navigating through traffic, as an outsider you have a reasonable chance of becoming a hood ornament and being forced to be content with the local health care system. Many organizations that deploy field staff, the U.S. Peace Corps included, have long since discouraged the use of motorcycles or scooters for their staff.

WALKING AND USING LOCAL TRANSPORT

When traveling in a foreign county, use the same common sense that you would at home. Know your route, have a good sense of where you are going, and pay attention to your surroundings. Avoid using short cuts, side streets, narrow alleys or poorly lit streets. If you need to ask directions, ask someone who appears to be an official or in a position of authority, or stop in a local store.

Be especially alert in areas that have high tourist traffic. Although it may be unavoidable, try to avoid large public demonstrations, civil disturbances, roadblocks, and large festivals. In these settings, as well as in markets, on trains, or in any crowded public area, keep your belongings close to you and beware of pickpockets or thieves. If you are confronted and requested to relinquish your cash or valuables, give them up. They can be replaced, and you can avoid an encounter with the aforementioned local health care system.

The more common scenario is general harassment by eager porters or taxi drivers at airports or tourist destinations. The aggressive nature of people selling goods, offering taxis and tours, or volunteering to carry your bags can complicate your arrival in a new country. Here are a few helpful tips:

- Study the map of the region where you are going before arrival.

- Know your plan and how you will get out of the airport or bus/train station.
- Carry your own luggage, hold it firmly, and wave off any would-be porters.
- Walk purposefully away from the crowd, to a place that is not crowded.
- Be polite but very firm with people who jostle you and attempt to carry your bags.

If you are taking a taxi, ask a local person while still on the train or plane about the range of fares. Then proceed to a registered taxi and tell him where you need to go and ask how much, and compare to the price you've been quoted. Come to an agreement before departing. Also, be sure to ask where the taxi is, as many will have you walk quite a distance to load the taxi.

TRAINS AND RAIL STATIONS

Because of the rapid flow of tourists and travelers through major rail stations, they are a frequent setting for thieves, scams, and hustlers. Pay close attention to your baggage. It's generally a good idea not to carry valuable items in the first place. Keep your bag attached to you at all times, taking care not to put it down, even for a moment. Lock the strap around your shoulder or wrist, and consider wearing backpacks backward in every crowded setting. Simple distractions such as two teenagers fighting nearby or someone tapping you on the shoulder are enough to divert your attention and allow your bag to be lifted. Traveling in a group is almost always a good idea, especially on trains or buses.

HOTELS AND LODGING SAFETY

The most common place to be subject to a theft is a hotel room. Hotel rooms are often not secure, and theft typically occurs when you are out of the room, or occasionally as you sleep. When you book a hotel, ask for a room on the second or third floor. Check the room for functioning locks, and be sure they work. Check for problem areas such as access to common patios or externally accessible windows. If the room is not easily secured, go back to the desk and request another room. It is also helpful to put the "do not disturb" sign on your door and leave the television and light on to give the impression that the room is occupied. When you leave the room, carry the room key with you instead of leaving it at front desk.[6]

SEXUAL HARASSMENT

Sexual harassment of women is a common occurrence in both industrialized and less industrialized settings. Harassment can take the form of jeering and whistling, unwanted advances, physical contact, and outright attack. This is a particular issue for women traveling to places where women have restricted freedom and, to one degree or another, suffer the daily oppression of fewer rights and less social, economic, or personal freedom. The presence of a Western woman who dresses entirely appropriately by Western standards can be viewed as inappropriate and provocative in some cultures.

Avoiding sexual harassment, especially when traveling to settings where women enjoy a lesser standard of freedom, can be accomplished by planning ahead. Do a little background checking on the local customs and habits, and try to dress appropriately for the setting. Even though you may not agree with cultural standards or condone a style of dress, you should accept that other cultures have very different customs and acceptable standards of dress. It is best to conform as much as possible to avoid confrontation. This includes choosing loose, conservative, and nonrevealing clothing and observing local customs to determine how much exposure of arms and legs is appropriate, or if scarves for head covering may be necessary. The more female travelers dress like the local women, the fewer difficulties they will experience from local men.

It is also very helpful to keep the company of other travelers. Sexual advances and true harassment rarely occur when people travel with a group, and there is certainly safety in numbers. Many women in other cultures literally walk arm in arm with each other, and collectively ignore unwanted advancements. Be cautious of public displays of affection with men, as this is often seen as inappropriate in many cultures.

Travelers who are in a public setting and subjected to jeering and comments should make all attempts to ignore them and avoid engaging the provocateurs with comments and retorts. Women should avoid being alone in groups of foreign men or getting into crowded vehicles with unknown local men. Also avoid casual touching, as this can be interpreted in many countries as provocative behavior, and never give out personal information in the course of a conversation, including your full name, hotel, or where you are going next.

Violent sexual attacks are rare, but they can occur in some settings. Be aware of the possibility that sexual predators may follow travelers to an isolated area or to their hotel. Travelers should check to see if they are being followed and should be wary if they encounter a stranger coincidentally in more than one venue. Travelers who are staying alone should be absolutely sure that their hotel room is secure and that they are not followed. It is probably not necessary to be paranoid, but taking the proper precautions can help travelers avoid unwanted advances and sexual assault.

AVOIDING LEGAL PROBLEMS

When you are traveling outside your home country, you are subject to the laws and regulations of the country where you are traveling, not your home country. The rights and assurances you have as a U.S. citizen, for

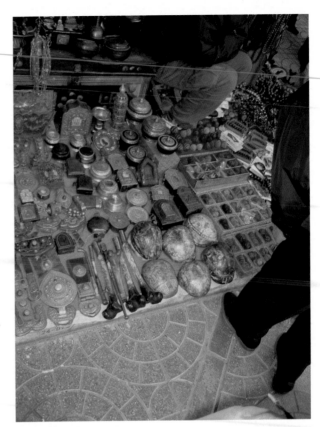

Figure 6.1. Be careful what you buy in local markets. Items that turn out to be illegal to own or transport such as national artifacts or, in the case of this photo, human bones will cause problems in customs. Photo courtesy of Gregory H. Bledsoe.

example, no longer apply abroad. What may have been a minor infraction in the United States can be a major problem abroad, resulting in large fines, detention, and even incarceration. Some of the most common reasons for detention of American and European travelers abroad are listed below.

Theft: Stealing antiquities or walking off with souvenirs from temples or monuments can land you in a foreign prison. Even purchasing souvenirs that turn out to be national artifacts can be a major offense (Figure 6.1). In the 1990s, this was a major issue in the former Soviet states, and it remains a significant problem in Mexico, Central America, Egypt, Turkey, and around the Middle East. If you buy something on the market that can be construed as an antique, obtain documentation from the vendor.

Drug possession: Possessing a controlled substance accounts for one-third to one-half of all long-term incarcerations abroad. Possession of even small amounts of cocaine, narcotics, or marijuana can land unwary travelers in jail for years. Many countries do not distinguish between personal use and drug trafficking, and some have mandatory sentences. Although there have been reports of arrests for possession of prescription medication, this is very unusual. Simple precautions, like keeping medications in original prescription containers, will prevent misunderstandings at the border.

Photography: In most situations, it's acceptable to photograph people and the scenery. This does not apply, however, to foreign military installations or anything that the local or national military deem to be of strategic importance. Photographing local militia, roadblocks, or even groups of people gathered in a city setting can prompt the local guards and military (legitimate or not) to question, harass, and sometimes confiscate your photographic equipment. The more conspicuous the equipment and your behavior, the more likely you will be to have it confiscated. The best policy is to apologize profusely, show them that you are putting the camera away, agree to go back to your hotel if needed, but avoid surrendering the equipment if possible.

If you do have legal problems, you have the right under international law to locate and talk to a U.S. Consulate Officer. The consulate can send someone to you who not only speaks English but knows local officials, customs, and the major issues that you will be facing if you are detained for some reason. Consular officers will also notify your family members if you wish and can ensure that you are being held in humane conditions.

TRAVEL TO HIGH-RISK AREAS

In traveling to many expedition and wilderness destinations, you can pass through or near areas that are experiencing significant social or political unrest. It is important to get information ahead of time so that you can make proper arrangements and get detailed information about the ground situation. If you must travel in an area where there has been a history of terrorist attacks or kidnapping, be sure to have contact with a well-connected local resource and be in touch with them about the threats to foreigners. It can be helpful to register with the U.S. embassy upon your arrival, as they can track your whereabouts and inform you of sudden political changes, security alerts, or evacuation orders. Before departing, thoroughly review the political and security threats in the country where you will be traveling, including a review of major hotels, corporations, relief agencies, and other organizations working on the ground.

TRAVEL HEALTH

Although travel health issues are covered in greater detail elsewhere in the text, there are a few common-sense tips to take into consideration as you plan your trip. If you are traveling to an exotic region or into a region that requires immunizations and malaria prophylaxis, be sure to visit a travel health clinic. Travel agents are not typically the best source of information. To accomplish your complete immunization schedule, you may need to visit the travel clinic 6 to 8 weeks ahead of time, although many immunizations can be accelerated. The best online resource for travel health is the Centers for Disease Control and Prevention in Atlanta (*http://www.cdc.gov*). The Web site is easily navigated and has the information that most travel health clinics use to give advice.

MANAGE YOUR MONEY

Take special care to handle your money appropriately. It is not a good idea to carry large amounts of cash, and traveler's checks are an excellent choice if you have to carry large amounts of money for extended travels. Every seasoned traveler has his or her preferences for holding cash and/or credit cards. One common approach is to have a flat pouch that carries your credit cards, money, passport and a few passport photos next to your skin, either around your neck or around your waist, tucked into your pants. The money belt is probably the safest because it's hardest to take from you by a thief, and, more importantly, you are less inclined to take it off and leave it somewhere.

Fanny packs and wallets in backpacks are common targets for thieves, as is a pouch hanging from your neck, even if it is under your shirt. If you must carry large amounts of cash, you can wrap the bills in a small plastic sandwich bag and slide it into your shoe. Keep local currency, singles and some of your cash in your pocket and available so you don't have to take your shoe off every time you buy something at the market, and if you get approached by a would be assailant, you can give up the money in your pocket with out losing everything.

IF YOU ARE VICTIM OF A CRIME

If you become a victim of a crime such as theft or assault or encounter legal problems, and you are a U.S. citizen, contact the nearest U.S. embassy as well as the local police. Consular personnel can assist with replacing travel documents and providing contact with family members, as well as obtaining medical care, and, in the case of severe illness or injury, assisting with evacuation. They can also assist by helping through the legal process (see the earlier discussion of avoiding legal problems) and obtaining an attorney who can assist you.

TAKE HOME POINTS

Here are a few major points to keep in mind when planning a trip or expedition:

Know what to expect on your trip: Be diligent about getting information about your trip, including information about itinerary, accommodations, food, and water. Know the size and makeup of your travel group. Find out about endemic illnesses and local security risks, including personal safety issues like local transportation. Know local weather conditions so you can pack properly.

Assess the skills as well as the physical and mental stamina that will be required of you for the trip: Carefully evaluate your level of preparedness, and respect your personal capabilities and limitations. For strenuous or technical expeditions, take the time to get in condition and upgrade your skills. If that is not possible, don't go. If you are older than 40, and going on a strenuous expedition, consult your physician to get some objective advice.

Choose experienced guides and regional experts when planning an expedition or remote travel and research their track records: Such companies should provide a system for rating the risk and employ good risk management practices. They should have a reasonable cancellation policy. They should also use appropriately certified guides and instructors, who speak the local language and are first-aid trained.

Find out if your destination is dangerous in either physical or political terms: In many countries, there is political instability, police and judicial corruption, an ongoing war, insurgencies, or sporadic unrest. Be sure that you know, and your group knows, the political and social landscape prior to traveling. Also, address issues of personal security, including evaluation of accommodations, local crime, and local transportation. Remember that you are a lucrative target.

Take a medical kit that suits the needs of your expedition: Resist the temptation to bring a huge amount of medication and supplies. A simple first-aid kit with appropriate medications for diarrhea, malaria, and commonly encountered illnesses is usually sufficient.

Have an evacuation plan and health insurance: Buy comprehensive health, travel, and life insurance. Many insurance policies do not cover activities that involve risk such as scuba diving or skydiving, and most will not cover events related to war or terrorism. Check with the restrictions of your health insurance policy, and consider supplemental coverage for medical evacuation.

Observe basic practices of personal security: As discussed in this chapter, you can do a number of things to minimize your risk of injury or assault. Personal security starts with awareness of your surroundings and the potential for problems.

Take the time to make contingency plans: Planning for emergencies includes establishing communication links with home or local resources and for communication in an emergency. Keep copies of essential documents with you and be prepared for theft or lost items.

SUMMARY

Expedition and wilderness travel carries with it unique risks of injury and exposure. Many travel-related injuries, mishaps, and altercations can be avoided by knowing well the region where you will be traveling and taking the appropriate preparatory steps to account for local conditions, endemic illnesses, political issues, and logistical issues. Ultimately, regardless of planning and proper packing, travel to foreign settings requires some degree of situational awareness while traveling. Being aware of your situation requires preparation and knowledge of local customs, anticipation of problem scenarios, and experience. If you lack the latter, it will be important to know more about the culture, customs, threats, and potential problems than if you were traveling someplace more familiar. Remember, travel safety is largely in the hands of the traveler.

REFERENCES

[1] http://www.sixwise.com/newsletters/05/07/13/the_six_most_feared_but_least_likely_causes_of_death.htm.

[2] Safe Trip Abroad. Department of State Publication 11285, Bureau of Consular Affairs, November 2005. http://travel.state.gov.

[3] Pelton RY. The World's Most Dangerous Places, 5th ed. New York: HarperResource; 2003.

[4] http://www.travelinsurancecenter.com. Accessed November 20, 2006.

[5] International road traffic and accident database (OECD). http://www.irfnet.org/.

[6] http://danger.mongabay.com/hotel_crime.htm.

7 | Nutritional Support for Expeditions

E. Wayne Askew, PhD

INTRODUCTION

Food and Its Role in the History of Exploration

Food has played a prominent role in "expeditions" from the days of early sailing voyages and turn of the century arctic explorations up to the present-day conquest of outer space. Almost every account of exploration expeditions contains descriptions of food (or the lack thereof). In his book *Polar Journeys*, food scientist Robert Feeney observes that "An adequate supply of food and water has always been the primary need of any group of explorers" (1998). The technology of food packaging, fortification, and preservation has changed dramatically over the past century along with our *understanding* of nutritional requirements. Man's nutritional requirements, however, are still basically the same as they were years ago, only our understanding of nutrient requirements has changed. Man still requires basically the same amount of protein, vitamins, minerals, and water as did the sailors aboard Christopher Columbus's voyage to the new world in 1492, Robert Peary's conquest of the North Pole in 1909, and Will Steeger's first confirmed dogsled journey to the North Pole (without resupply) in 1986, as well as Tom Avery's retracing of Peary's route to the North Pole in 2005. Nutrition, in particular energy requirements, may be somewhat altered in modern expeditions due to better equipment, more efficient clothing, and, in some cases, motorized conveyances; however, this often simply permits an expedition to push harder and cover more miles in a day. The net result is a similar total daily caloric macronutrient (carbohydrate, fat, and protein) and micronutrient (vitamin and mineral) requirement, regardless of the time period in history the expedition was conducted. The most noticeable difference between classic expeditions of the past and modern ventures is the rapidity with which expedition members can be inserted into the wilderness settings and the rapidity with which they can be extracted. The change in the amount of time explorers must subsist upon their expedition food stores is a definite advantage to modern expeditions; for example, it is

probable that Shackleton's and Scott's men were not in tip-top nutritional shape to begin their expedition after weeks at sea on marginally adequate shipboard rations traveling from England to Antarctica (Feeney 1998). They had to subsist upon marginal nutrient intakes at best for the duration of their expeditions, which only worsened during the long arduous return route. Contrast this with Ranulph Fiennes and Michael Stroud's 1993 trek across the South Pole; they started the expedition well fed and in good condition, they became nutritionally depleted by the strenuous journey but were extracted by an airplane within 24 hours of accomplishing their objective and back in England within 10 days (Stroud 1994). Despite high-tech gear and rapid deployment and extraction prior to and at the end of their trans-Antarctica sledge journey, Stroud and Fiennes experienced nutritional challenges (Stroud 1994):

Breakfast...was meager by any standards...for men working as hard as we were. We consumed it before it had time to thicken; our hunger overwhelming our patience....From time to time our hands strayed without thinking, popping squares of chocolate into our mouths. We...chewed and consumed them with urgency...we were starving and had lost all self-control. Our ration of two bars (per day) was gone before we knew it and nothing was left to fuel the long day. It was incredibly stupid but very human.

Expedition planners should not be lulled into a "technology-induced" false sense of security when it comes to planning the nutritional support of an expedition. High-technology equipment and commercial sources of conveniently packaged and preserved food items abound; yet the paramount importance of achieving the right amount of food and the right mix of nutrients to support the physical activity anticipated, the duration of the expedition, and the climatic conditions into which the expedition will venture remains as important now as it was to an earlier Antarctic expedition planner, Robert Scott. Scott's five-man polar exploration party succumbed to starvation and hypothermia following an attempted conquest of the South Pole in 1912 (King 1999). Although a seasoned veteran and careful planner,

Scott encountered exceptionally harsh weather conditions, which slowed his team's progress and strained his limited food supplies. The addition of an additional man to the originally planned team without a proportional adjustment in food also contributed to the food shortage. Although the lack of vitamin C in Scott's food provisions may have contributed to the scurvy-like symptoms that beset team members toward the end of their ill-fated journey, it was ultimately the cold and the lack of calories that stopped the expedition short of the next life-saving food cache (Solomon 2001).

Importance of Food and Morale

Food plays an important role in staying healthy and building and repairing body tissue and energy reserves. It is the fuel that powers expedition members carrying heavy packs over difficult terrain. It also helps keep us mentally alert and helps keep the attitude of expedition members positive. Without good nutrition, the disposition and attitude of team members can deteriorate rapidly.

Bradford Washburn, explorer, mountaineer, photographer, cartographer, and past director of the Boston Museum of Science knew the value of food to an expedition and was an advocate for good nutrition planning: "It is almost unnecessary to emphasize the importance of an adequate diet for the production of body heat. There is no better investment in the well being, safety and efficacy of a party (expedition) than food-plenty of it, well prepared" (1962).

This wisdom notwithstanding, in some instances, a somewhat "Spartan" approach can be adopted toward nutrition without total disaster, depending upon the "stoicism" and experience of the individual(s) involved. No one has been more successful at conquering extreme environmental challenges than Reinhold Messner whose focus is always upon achieving the objective of his personal expedition to the exclusion of food when it was not convenient to eat or carry many supplies. Messner, by his own accounts, trained himself to go for extended periods of time without food during critical points in his ascent of high elevations (Alexander 2006). Messner is an experienced mountaineer and is well aware of his own personal reserves and limitations. However, not all expedition members can be expected to be this focused and disciplined when it comes to food and their understanding of their own personal need for sustenance. Nor need they be when it is possible to plan good nutritional support that can serve the dual purpose of renewing psychological "stores" such as spirit and morale as well as physiological energy "stores" (Marriott 1995). The success of expeditions composed of several team members depends in large part upon teamwork. Group dynamics and morale can be affected by many factors, especially when faced with unexpected environmental challenges. It is important to use food as a positive morale factor, or at the very least, not a negative morale factor. A hot,

filling meal at the end of a hard day can go a long way toward the preparation for the next challenging day to come.

The Lack of Food – Starvation and Its Consequences

Adequate energy (calories) appears to be the biggest nutritional problem facing early explorers, notwithstanding descriptions of debilitating but seldom fatal vitamin and mineral deficiencies (Feeney 1998). The inability to include enough calories for the team members because of space and weight considerations often became catastrophic when unexpected delays were encountered en route due to bad weather (e.g., Scott's ill-fated conquest of the South Pole, Solomon 2001), when food spoilage or contamination occurred (e.g., possible lead poisoning of canned provisions of the Franklin expedition to find the Northwest Passage, Beatty and Geiger 1988), when catastrophic loss of food supplies occurred (e.g., Mawson's polar expedition's loss of a sledge containing most of their food supplies into a crevasse, Bicknell 2000) or when local food resupply proved unreliable (e.g., Lewis and Clark's expedition to map the Northwest Territory, Devoto 1953; Duncan and Burns 1997). Depending upon animal and plant foods found along the expedition route can be "chancy" and in some instances detrimental to the health of the expedition members (Mawson's encounter with vitamin A toxicity, Bickel 2000; Camas root identification uncertainty and illness of members of the Lewis and Clark expedition, Duncan and Burns 1997; Gunderson 2003).

The physical environment into which the expedition must venture can have a strong influence upon food and water requirements (Askew 1989; 1995; 1997; 2002b). The interaction of extreme wilderness environments and food, water, and physical performance is depicted in Figure 7.1. Paradoxically, it is at the time when food and water are at their shortest availability that man's physiological needs for these items peaks. An increased need for energy or water coupled with a dwindling supply of either or both can spell disaster. One of the best examples of an unanticipated consequence of an increasingly harsh environment and depleted food supplies can be found in that of the Donner Party of 1846. While crossing the Sierras bound for California, it became snowbound by an early winter storm. Marooned by deep snow and cold, the party bivouacked until help could arrive but in the intervening 2 months of bitter cold, 47 out of 90 party members died from starvation (McCurdy 1994). The demise of many of the male members of the party was probably a consequence of expending unreplenished energy unsuccessfully hunting for food.

Nutrition–Environment Interaction and Expedition Performance

Nutrition for work in environmental extremes is often modeled after principles of performance nutrition

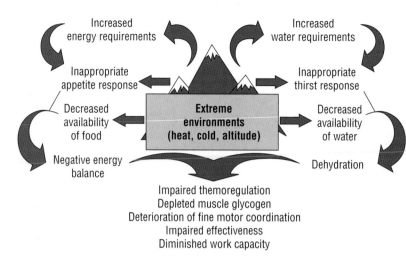

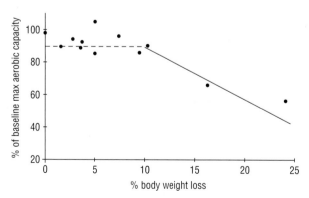

Figure 7.1. The interaction of extreme wilderness environments on food and fluid intake and physical and mental performance. With permission from Askew EW. Nutrition, malnutrition and starvation. In: Auerbach PS. *Wilderness Medicine*, 4th ed. St. Louis: Mosby; 2001:271–84.

gained from sports nutrition applications. Many of the work physiology principles are the same, but an important distinction exists. The success of a sporting event often hinges upon even the smallest component of the performance equation (genetics, training, motivation, and nutrition); however, the success of an expedition may be a bit more flexible or "forgiving." Expeditions can be, but most often are not, competitive endurance events. The speed with which an expedition progresses is important, but usually time delays for one reason or another are expected. Long periods of food deprivation can be disastrous to expeditions, but short periods of food deprivation (less than 5–7 days and less than 10% body weight loss) usually do not have a great influence upon physical performance capacity (Taylor et al. 1957; Consolazio 1967; Askew et al. 1987; Friedl 1995), although the lack of food may considerably "dampen" morale. Friedl (1995) has assimilated data from several studies of food restriction and performance. The results depicted in Figure 7.2 illustrate the relationship between the capacity for aerobic work and weight loss in non-obese subjects. It can be seen that weight losses of less than 10% have only a small influence upon the capacity for aerobic work; however, actions that require strength or power may respond differently (Friedl 1995). Strength response to weight loss due to caloric restriction depends to some degree upon the measurement utilized to evaluate strength and the time period over which the weight loss occurs, but most studies show only small declines (< 8%) in muscle strength with body weight losses of less than 5% over time periods of less than 30 days (Askew et al. 1987). Longer periods of energy deficiency resulting in more weight loss, however, can result in significant strength reductions (Friedl 1995). Taken together, and applied to expedition work, it would appear that some food deprivation can be accommodated for time periods of less than 10 days without the expedition grinding to a halt. The overall speed or the progress of the expedition along the trail and the ability to carry heavy packs without frequent rest periods may be somewhat reduced and fine motor coordination may be impaired, mainly due

to glycogen depletion. In real terms, this may mean that a gradual trek to the summit objective might be accommodated with less than adequate caloric intake during good weather, but with impending bad weather, which normally requires an all out push to the summit, power output may be compromised. Good expedition food planning can help remove this limitation from the team's performance objectives.

Energy shortfalls resulting in depleted glycogen stores are an immediate concern when food restriction occurs, but vitamin and mineral deficiencies are of lesser urgency because they usually take weeks, not days, to develop and do not greatly influence physical performance until after 3–4 weeks of suboptimal intakes (van der Beek et al. 1988; 1994). Hard physical work involving increased oxidative energy metabolism can increase the dietary requirement for certain B vitamins (Woolf and Manore 2006) and significant tissue depletion of water-soluble vitamins can occur on a calorie-adequate, but vitamin-restricted diet. Van der Beek (1988; 1994) found that 8 weeks of a calorie-adequate diet with reduced water-soluble vitamin intake (10–30% of requirement) resulted in approximately a 20% decrease in work

Figure 7.2. Changes in maximal oxygen uptake compared to corresponding loss of body weight in young healthy soldiers. By permission from Friedl KE. When does energy deficit affect soldier physical performance? In: Marriot BM. *Not Eating Enough*. Washington, DC: National Academy Press; 1995:253–83.

capacity with no significant performance decrements evident at the 4-week point in his study. This can be extrapolated to suggest that expeditions lasting less than a month will fare relatively well with energy intakes adequate to prevent excessive weight loss (<5% body weight), even with a marginally adequate vitamin content. While the situation of a vitamin-reduced dietary intake is not recommended, the ability to perform the physical tasks at hand may be less than desired, but adequate to proceed. However, if food deprivation is accompanied by temperature extremes such as extreme cold or extreme heat, physical performance will be seriously challenged (Askew 2002b). Food, and particularly carbohydrate, is important for shivering thermogenesis in the cold. In hot weather accompanied by heavy sweating, sodium intake may be critical. Usually the sodium content of the ration is adequate to replace sweat sodium losses, but reduced food intake coupled with heavy sweat loss can compromise this important electrolyte. It is always a good idea to include a separate supply of salt in each backpacker's pack in case of emergency. Salt is light, not bulky, and airline or restaurant packets of 3–5 g NaCl are easy to include in group and private provisions. Usually 6–12 g of NaCl per day from food will be adequate to replace sodium sweat losses in most cases (Askew 1997). An average mixed meal contains approximately 3–8 g NaCl. Liberal salting of food can supply additional sodium replacement if needed.

Factors Influencing Nutrition Requirements

A multitude of factors can influence the nutritional requirements of expedition members. These principally include the sex, body size, and activity level of the individuals involved as well as the physical environment into which the expedition will proceed. These factors will play a major role in determining the level of exertion and hence the amount of food energy required. The duration of the expedition is a key factor in determining the total energy requirements that need to be planned to support the expedition. The guidance in this chapter for planning nutritional support of expeditions is not meant to be prescriptive for individuals who may be at either end of the normal distribution, but it should be viewed as a target from which adjustments may need to be made depending upon the individual, the environment, the day's activities, and the duration of the expedition.

PLANNING NUTRITION SUPPORT

First Step: Choose the Food Planner Carefully

Some experienced planners have learned through trial and error to fairly accurately predict and plan their own individual nutrition provisions. This may work well enough for the individual on solo treks, but it often does not "multiply up" or translate well into group provision plans. For example, one anecdote known to the author involved a peanut butter "fanatic" who provisioned a 4-day backpacking trip for a group of himself and two friends by glomming onto a "target" daily calorie requirement of 3,500 kcal/day, multiplying that by 3 people times 4 days to arrive at a total of 42,000 kcal and dividing that by the number of kcal in a jar of peanut butter (in this case 3,300 kcal/jar) and provisioned the party with 13 jars of peanut butter and as many crackers as could be packed in around the provisions in the packs as "bonus" carbohydrate calories. The first day all agreed that these provisions were novel but okay: Appetites were keen and peanut butter was plentiful. The diet seemed rather repetitious on the second day and downright monotonous by the third day. By the fourth day, peanut butter revulsion had set in, and the other two campers were earnestly trying to catch fish and scrounge for berries while referring to the food planner as the "squirrel." Thereafter, upon return to civilization, even the peanut butter fanatic could not bring himself to eat peanut butter without a shudder of revulsion.

It is best to designate one reasonably well-balanced individual to be in charge of food planning (not a person who has strong dietary preferences he or she wishes to impose upon the group). Some of the most pathetic stories I have heard regarding food have come from members of my Wilderness Nutrition Class recounting food-related experiences such as vegetarians forced to endure Spam[TM] (the canned edible kind sold by Hormel) and conversely, meat-loving campers forced to subsist upon a menu of granola, couscous, and lentils. Food preferences are real and can be problematic if the party members have not been consulted and some staples that all can agree to eat are provisioned. Although it is axiomatic that hunger will compromise human dietary principles – for example, refer to accounts of cannibalism among members of the marooned Donner party (Stewart 1960) and the Columbian soccer team whose airplane crashed in the Andes (Read 1974) – expedition members should be consulted for dietary preferences and especially food allergies before the provisions are assembled. It is best to permit individuals with "food issues" (e.g., participants with gluten or nut allergies, lactase deficiencies, or hypoglycemia) to be in charge of packing some specific food items in their own packs if they do not think they can eat all the food items planned for the expedition. These individuals will usually be well versed on how to handle their own unique dietary challenges and can generally manage their issues quite well. Vegetarians can be accommodated by cooking meat items separately and permitting campers to mix the food items on their plate as they see fit. For example, a pot of vegetable soup can become a meat stew by cooking the vegetable soup and the diced meat separately, browning the meat with flour and then mixing the flour-coated meat with the hot vegetable soup after the vegetarian diners have taken their portions of the soup.

Second Step: Establishing Energy Requirements

The overriding concern for most nutritional planners is to ensure that enough energy (kcal) is contained in the day's ration of food to sustain the level of performance desired. Sustaining moderate physical performance capability usually means at least enough food energy to prevent excessive weight loss. On an expedition, a weight loss of more than 2 lb per week should be viewed as undesirable. Insufficient food energy intake is almost always accompanied by a suboptimal intake of other important nutrients such as vitamins and minerals; therefore, an important first step is important to plan for caloric adequacy. There are several commonly used methods of predicting nutritional requirements for an expedition, ranging from the approximate to the more precise:

1. Experience gained by trial and error
2. Rules of thumb
3. Tables based upon anticipated workload
4. Equations for calculating resting energy requirements and multiples of resting energy expenditure
5. Bulk rationing planning methods such as that used by the National Outdoor Leadership School (NOLS)

Most planners will use one or sometimes a combination of these procedures to develop a plan for nutrition support of the expedition. It goes without saying that the larger the expedition party will be, the more remote the destination will be, and the more days the expedition will encompass, the more precise should be the planning.

Estimating Energy Requirements

The first step to establishing requirements is to choose a "system" for estimating energy requirements. The choice of a planning system will depend upon both the purpose of the expedition and the length of time it will encompass as well as weather conditions. These considerations will determine if a "caloric" rule of thumb can be used or if more exact tables based upon workload or energy-predicting equations based upon gender, body size, and environment should be employed. These techniques can be applied to individuals, but for the purposes of this chapter, it will be used to plan for groups of individuals who have similar characteristics but upon whom measurements have not been individually made.

Rule-of-Thumb Approach

As an example, a recreational excursion into the backcountry during temperate weather for less than one week could probably adequately be provisioned by using what can be referred to as "the military rule of thumb" because it is based upon what active individuals (soldiers) are projected to require for field operations. This guidance for U.S. soldiers can be found in AR 40–25: Nutrition Standards and Education: Nutritional Standards

for Operational and Restricted Rations (NSOR) (2001). This document can be accessed at *http://www.army. mil/usapa/epubs/pdf/r40_25.pdf*. The military generally assumes that the average soldier (which in our case can reasonably be considered comparable to an active backpacker) will require an average day's ration of food of 3,600 kcal/day in support of moderate physical activity. A table of military ration nutrient recommendations from AR 40-21 is given in Table 7.1 and is useful as a planning guide for ration assembly. It is not intended to be a table of recommended dietary allowances for individuals but rather a guide for assembling an adequate day's supply of food. If heavy physical activity is anticipated, this amount of calories will not be optimal, but the vitamin and mineral content should be reasonably adequate.

Estimates Based upon Tables of Energy Requirements

If a bit more information is available about the general intensity of the predicted activities, AR 40-25 also permits an estimate of caloric requirements with respect to gender and activity level (Table 7.2) that will be more accurate than the more general 3,600 kcal/day NSOR energy standard given in Table 7.1. Caloric estimates based upon such a general classification of a day's activity and duration can sometimes suffice for general planning purposes for a mixed group of expedition members. Other planners such as Consolazio (1966) have published convenient energy requirement tables based upon climate, body weight, and physical activity levels (Table 7.3). The requirements in Table 7.3 are not gender specific but should be adequate for both sexes.

WHO/FAO Tables for Resting and Physical Activity Level Energy Estimates

More precise estimates of total daily energy expenditure utilize resting energy expenditure for the basis of their calculation of total energy expenditure. Resting energy expenditure can be calculated from equations derived from nomograms or found in tables. The World Health Organization/Food and Agriculture Organization (WHO/FAO) have simplified the use of resting energy prediction equations by providing a table based upon age, sex, and body weight that can be found in their publication, "Human energy requirements" (FAO report, 2001). Alpers et al. (1995) lists a convenient version of this table, which is shown in Table 7.4. Physical activity levels (PALs) applied as multipliers to the underlying resting energy can provide an estimate of total daily energy requirement. PAL coefficients have been derived from measurements of average 24-hr energy expenditures (TEE) and resting energy expenditures (REE) by the following relationship: PAL = TEE/REE. WHO/FAO PAL coefficients derived for daily activities that can be characterized or categorized

Table 7.1. Ration nutrient composition targets: Nutritional standards for military operational and restricted rations (NSOR)[a] useful as a guide for planning expedition rations

Nutrient	Unit	Operational rations	Restricted rations
Energy	Kcal	3600	1500
Protein	G	91	50
Carbohydrate	G	494	200
Fat[b]	G	(see footnote b)	(see footnote b)
Vitamin A[c]	g RE	1000	500
Vitamin D[d]	G	5	3
Vitamin E[e]	Mg	15	8
Vitamin K	G	80	40
Vitamin C	Mg	90	45
Thiamin (B1)	Mg	1.2	0.6
Riboflavin (B2)	Mg	1.3	0.7
Niacin[f]	mg NE	16	8
Vitamin B6	Mg	1.3	0.7
Folic Acid[g]	g DFE	400	200
Vitamin B12	G	2.4	1.2
Calcium	Mg	1000	500
Phosphorus	Mg	700	350
Magnesium	Mg	420	210
Iron	Mg	15	8
Zinc	Mg	15	8
Sodium[h]	Mg	5,000–7,000	2,500–3,500
Iodine	G	150	75
Selenium	G	55	28
Fluoride	Mg	4.0	2.0
Potassium	Mg	3,200	2,000

[a] Based upon Table 2-2 in Army Regulation 40–25 (2001). Values are minimum standards for ration nutrient content, except for fat (which does not have an absolute standard value) and sodium (which presents minimum and maximum content levels). Nutritional standards for rations are based on the MDRIs established for healthy, active military personnel. Energy (kcal) is generally adequate for moderate physical activity but may need to be adjusted higher or lower depending upon body size, activity level, and environment.

[b] Total energy from fat should not exceed 35% of total kcal.

[c] The unit of measure is microgram retinol equivalent (μg RE). 1 μg RE = 1 μg retinol or 6 μg β-carotene. 1 μg RE = 10 International Units (IU) vitamin A if from β-carotene. 1 μg RE = 3.33 IU vitamin A if from retinol.

[d] As cholecalciferol. 1 μg cholecalciferol = 40 IU vitamin D.

[e] The unit of measure is milligram α-tocopherol that includes RRR-α-tocopherol, the only form of α-tocopherol that is found in food and the 2R-stereoisomeric forms that are found in fortified foods and dietary supplements. This does not include the 2S-stereo-isomeric forms that are also found in fortified foods and dietary supplements.

[f] The unit of measure is niacin equivalent (NE). 1 mg NE = 1 mg niacin or 60 mg dietary tryptophan.

[g] The unit of measure is dietary folate equivalent (DFE). 1 μg DFE = 1 μg food folate, 0.5 μg synthetic folic acid taken on an empty stomach, or 0.6 μg synthetic folic acid taken with meals.

[h] These values do not include sodium from salt packets. The sodium content of restricted rations may not be adequate for military personnel operating in hot environments, especially if they are not acclimatized. In these situations, an electrolyte beverage may be indicated to provide additional electrolytes.

Table 7.2. Rule-of-thumb estimates of total energy requirements based upon activity level[a]

Activity level	Male (kcal/day)	Female
Light (relaxing around camp)	3,000	2,200
Moderate (short day hike, no pack)	3,250	2,300
Heavy (half day on the trail with pack)	3,950	2,700
Very Heavy (full day on the trail with pack)	4,600	3,150

[a] Based upon Table 2–1 of Army Regulation 40–25, Military Dietory Reference Intakes (2001).

Table 7.3. Total daily energy requirements for physical activity in temperate, hot, or cold climates

Physical activity level	Temperate	Environment[a]	
		Cold (kcal/kg body weight)	Hot (kcal/kg body weight)
Light	32–34	35–46	40–54
Moderate	45–52	47–55	55–61
Heavy	53–63	56–68	62–75

[a] Altitude not shown, similar to the high range of Temperate. From Consolazio (1966).

Table 7.4. WHO/FAO tables of estimates of resting energy expenditure based upon age, sex, and body weight

Age (yr)	Male	Female
3–10	22.7 (wt in kg) − 495	22.5 (wt in kg) + 499
10–18	17.5 (wt in kg) + 651	12.2 (wt in kg) + 746
18–30	15.3 (wt in kg) + 679	14.7 (wt in kg) + 996
30–60	11.6 (wt in kg) + 879	8.7 (wt in kg) + 829
>60	13.5 (wt in kg) + 987	10.5 (wt in kg) + 596

From Alpers et al. (1995), p. 78.

considering the day's collective efforts are shown in Table 7.5. With enough diligence, PAL coefficients can be applied to specified blocks of the day's activities, but for our purposes we will use an overall 24-hr PAL and apply it to the REE for predicting energy expenditure (TEE = PAL × REE). Note that broad categorization of a day's activities may not adequately represent the overall 24-hr energy expenditure and may need to be modified depending upon the individual's activities, physical condition, climate, and the like. A PAL of 1.4 would be the lower level for short-term survival with little activity, whereas PALs as high as 4.5–4.7 have been recorded for hauling sleds across the arctic. PALs at this higher range are usually not sustainable for longer periods of time. PALs are similar in concept to the method of multiples of resting energy expenditure utilizing the Harris Benedict equation to calculate resting energy expenditure, which will be described next.

Table 7.5. Classification of the day's activities into an intensity of habitual activity, the physical activity level (PAL)

Activity category	PAL coefficient
Sedentary or light	1.4–1.69
Activities that do not demand much physical effort	
Active to moderately active	1.70–1.99
Moderate to vigorous physical activities such as walking long distances as part of daily routine	
Vigorously active	2.00–2.40
Regular engagement in strenuous work such as walking long distances over rugged terrain carrying heavy load	
Extremely active	2.50–4.50[a]
Strenuous physical activity for prolonged periods such as man hauling sledges across frozen terrain	

[a] PALs in this range are usually not sustainable by most people for time periods longer than 2–3 weeks.
PAL values from WHO/FAO report (2001).

Harris Benedict Equation Estimate of Resting Energy Expenditure and Multiples of Resting Energy Expenditure

More exact methods to predict caloric requirements based upon energy equations derived from or modified after the Harris Benedict equation can be found in numerous clinical nutrition references (Alpers et al. 1995). The Harris Benedict equation is given in Table 7.6 for both males and females and requires knowledge or estimate of body height and weight and sex (male or female). Although this equation was developed for calculating the energy needs of an individual person, it can be used for group projections provided an "average" or "typical" group member can be described. This equation is useful for predicting resting energy expenditure but requires activity or workload multipliers called activity coefficients (ACs) to add on energy for specific activities or "work" occurring throughout the day. This procedure is called "multiples of resting energy expenditure" (Pellet 1990). The utility of the calculation of resting energy expenditure for an individual or a representative

Table 7.6. Harris Benedict equation for estimating resting energy expenditure: formula for predicting basal (resting) energy expenditure from individual sex, age, height, and weight measurements

Men:
Energy expenditure (kcal) = 66 + 13.7 (wt in kg) + 5.0 × (ht in cm) – 6.8 (age in years)

Women:
Energy expenditure (kcal) = 655.1 + 9.6 (wt in kg) + 1.8 × (ht in cm) – 4.7 (age in years)

Alpers et al. (1995).

member of the group is in its use as the basis for applying multiples of REE coefficients (ACs) appropriate to the day's categorized activities and their duration in order to predict TEE. An example of prediction for planning purposes of a typical daily energy requirement arrived at by three methods – tables of total daily energy expenditure, WHO/FAO table/PALs, and the Harris Benedict equation/multiples of REE (AC) – is given in Table 7.7.

Table 7.7. Sample calculation of estimates of total daily energy expenditure by three methods

Expedition member information: Geology field expedition consisting of men between the ages of 30–60, average weight of 75 kg. Typical 24-hr day projected to consist of 8 hr sleeping, 3 hr very light camp chores (pitching tent, cooking, toilet, etc.), 1 hr light work collecting and cutting wood, 5 hr hard work carrying 55-lb packs along unimproved trail, 3 hr of rest and lunch breaks along the trail and in camp, 4 hr moderate work collecting rock specimens.

Activity coefficients (AC) based upon those of Pellet (1990)
Resting	1.0
Very light work	1.5
Light work	2.5
Moderate work	5.0
Heavy work	7.0

Method #1 Tables of activity and energy requirements

Based upon description of activities, this looks like a heavy to very heavy day's workload, therefore something between the "heavy" and the "very heavy" male classification from Table 7.2 of 3,950–4,600 kcal/day would be chosen (take the higher estimate if uncertain). Using Table 7.3 and choosing the high level of activity for temperate environment, one would predict 63 kcal/kg × 75 kg = 4,725 kcal/day.

Method #2 WHO/FAO table of REE and PALs

REE based upon male age group from Table 7.4 = 11.6 × 75 kg + 879 = 1750 kcal/day.

Calculate TEE by first classifying the activity projections for the day into one of the overall PAL categories for the day given in Table 7.5 and multiplying the PAL value chosen x the REE. Based upon the description of the activities, I would estimate that this is a "Vigorous" activity day. TEE = REE x PAL = kcal to support that day's activities:

Total energy expenditure, kcal/24 hr = 2.4 × 1750 = 4,200

Method #3 Harris Benedict equation and multiples of resting energy expenditure (AC)

Calculate REE based upon Harris Benedict equation:
REE = 66.5 + (13.8 × 75 kg) + (5 × 155) – (6.8 × 40) = 1,600 kcal/24 hr

Calculate TEE by first classifying hours of the day's activity projections into resting, very light, light, moderate or heavy activity, and then apply this equation:

TEE = AC × fraction of day engaged in that activity × REE = kcal to support that activity, sum all activities to get 24-hr energy expenditure estimates:
Resting:	1.0 × 11/24 × 1,600 =	733
Very light work	1.5 × 3/24 × 1,600 =	300
Light work	2.5 × 1/24 × 1,600 =	166
Moderate work	5.0 × 4/24 × 1,600 =	1333
Heavy work	7.0 × 5/24 × 1,600 =	2333
Total energy expenditure, kcal/24 hr 4,865		4,865

Using the rule-of-thumb projection from Table 7.7, we would estimate the daily energy requirements for a typical expedition member described in Table 7.6 to be approximately 4,600 kcal/day. Alternatively, using the climate and activity level categories from Table 7.3 to establish energy expenditure at 63 kcal/kg, we would predict approximately 4,700 kcal/day. Using the more involved calculations of the Harris Benedict equation for REE and multiples of REE or the WHO/FAO table for REE and applying a PAL to account for the day's activities, we would estimate an energy requirement of between 4,200 and 4,800 kcal/day. Which of these estimates is correct? The answer to that is probably none of them due to the vagaries of climate and unpredictable physical activity variations and the choice of the size, sex, and activity of a "typical" expedition member to permit us to accomplish these calculations. However, one can rest assured that the energy demands for most of the expedition team members will be somewhere in the ballpark of these estimates (4,500 kcal per person per day would be a reasonable choice); missing the mark on an occasional day by 500 kcal one way or the other is not going to inflict great hardship upon the expedition members. For example, a 500 kcal/day deficit for 14 days would create feelings of hunger and some discontent but would most likely result in an average weight loss of only 2–3 lb.

After energy (caloric) requirements have been projected, determining the rest of the nutrient content (macronutrients, vitamins, and minerals) is easier. Because of the large number of kcal expedition members will consume to meet energy demands, it is likely that protein and most of the vitamin and mineral requirements will be met along the way to caloric sufficiency, quite by accident if not by "intelligent" design. It is always best to check, however, because it is easy to remedy potential nutrient deficiencies with some sound food item choices in the planning stages. For example, hard physical work in all environments, but in particular at higher elevations, will require plentiful antioxidant nutrients to counter elevated levels of oxidative stress (Askew 2002a). Foods particularly high in vitamin C (dried fruit, dehydrated juices), vitamin E (nuts, whole grains, wheat germ, canola oil), and beta carotene (dried sweet potato, mango, apricots) can be included on a daily basis. Calcium is particularly a concern for female expedition members during long expeditions. A plentiful supply of powdered milk is one of the best ways to help meet calcium requirements in the trekker's meals. Powdered milk (~70 mg calcium/tbsp) can be reconstituted with water or better yet, mixed into soups, stews, instant mashed potatoes, coffee, tea, and hot chocolate. That failing, a supply of a calcium-based antacid such as Tums™ (~200 mg calcium/tablet) or an over-the-counter calcium supplement, can help female members increase their calcium intakes. Typical expedition food intakes at 3,600 kcal/day will most likely supply 800–1,000 mg of calcium per day, whereas the Reference Dietary Intake (RDI) for calcium for females is 1,200 mg/day. Supplemental iron may be needed for female expedition members; this may best be met with a multivitamin supplement that contains ferrous iron. Males will usually not need more iron that what is supplied in the food.

A guide to what macronutrients (carbohydrate, fat, and protein) and micronutrients (vitamins and minerals) humans need to meet their daily requirements can be found by consulting the current dietary reference intakes (DRIs) published by the National Academy of Sciences (Otten et al. 2006). A simple approach to ration planning can be achieved by comparing what the day's food *should contain* to reasonably meet dietary reference intake recommendations to what the food selected *actually contains* based upon known nutrient content of the selected foods. The nutrient composition of a day's planned food ration can be conveniently checked for overall nutrient adequacy by comparing the analyzed nutrient content of the projected day's food to a standard such as the Nutritional Standards for Operational Rations (NSOR) shown in Table 7.1, or, assuming the entire ration is eaten, the nutrient content can be compared to the DRI (Otten et al. 2006). For example, if one wishes to check the adequacy of the vitamin C content of the planned day's food, the DRI as well as the NSOR lists 90 mg as the adequate target and the NSOR gives 45 mg as a minimum for short periods of time (restricted rations, usually for fewer than 10 days). One can then total up the vitamin C content of the day's food items by checking the nutrition facts label on each food, looking up the food in a standard reference such as *Food Values of Portions Commonly Used* (Pennington and Douglass 2005), or utilizing a computer software program designed for nutrient analysis of food such as the Food Processor™ (ESHA Research, Salem Oregon). Serious expedition food planners should utilize a nutrient analysis software package to evaluate the nutrient profile the foods contain to make sure their final food selections are meeting energy projections. Although it is not essential to achieve 100% of the DRI every day for every nutrient, the content of other nutrients should be at least 75% of the current DRI, especially if the expedition is expected to last longer than 14 days. Even for relatively short expeditions, one might as well make the nutrient profile as close to optimal as possible even though there may not be any short-range consequences anticipated from nutrients that fall a bit short of what is recommended in the DRIs.

Macronutrient Requirements

Energy in terms of kcal is the overriding macronutrient requirement and is met by the collective sum of the calories supplied by carbohydrate, fat, and protein. There is no specific requirement for fat, per se, except for its contribution to calories and a small amount of essential fatty acids. Likewise, there is no specific requirement for carbohydrate except for its contribution to calories and replenishment of glycogen stores. Some recommendations for the fat and carbohydrate content of the ration may influence satiety and endurance and perhaps the logistics of food planning; however, these two nutrients are not as prescribed as the protein content of the ration. Protein, to be efficiently utilized for the replacement of tissue turnover, needs to have an adequate essential amino acid profile. Adequate protein intake, like vitamins and minerals, is usually not much of a problem in expedition rations due to the relative large daily intake of food required to meet caloric demands. Even a relative low total protein content of 10% of the ration kcal will provide approximately 90 g of protein with a 3,600 kcal/day energy intake. The RDI for protein for an unstressed 70-kg individual at low to moderate everyday energy expenditure levels is 56 g/day (0.8 g/kg body weight). A more generous goal of 1.0 g/kg is a better target because it provides some insurance that enough protein will be available to maintain the lean body mass of expedition members, considering that some protein may be deaminated and converted to glucose for energy utilization during days of heavy energy expenditure. Foods such as dried jerky, lentils, beans, and peas have high-quality protein. Soy protein approaches the essential amino acid profile of casein, which is considered close to ideal. When a mixture of high-quality vegetable source protein is included with food prepared with casein-containing protein such as powdered milk or an albumin-containing protein such as dried eggs, a healthy and adequate protein intake is virtually assured. If high-protein quality food items such as cheese, jerky, or fish are offered at least one meal per day, protein and amino acid profiles should be excellent. Other nonmeat protein sources from grains particularly worth considering are quinoa and amaranth. Quinoa and amaranth are two ancient, high-protein plants that hail from South America. The quality of the nutrients and the amino acid profile they offer surpasses that of more common grains such as corn, wheat, or rice (Table 7.8). The protein content of these two foods has a good essential amino acid balance approaching that of soybeans and casein. They are high in the amino acid lysine, which is limited in most cereal grains such as wheat, sorghum, corn, and barley. Quinoa and amaranth both contain about 16% protein, B and E vitamins, calcium, iron, and phosphorous. Their simple distinctive taste gives them great versatility for cooking purposes. They can be substituted for other grains in many recipes. Because they are not true cereal grains, they can be eaten by people who suffer from cereal grain allergies. Amaranth is gluten-free and is appropriate for consumers who have wheat and gluten allergies. Amaranth is high in lysine, well balanced

Table 7.8. Nutritional profiles of some common grains (100 g dry uncooked)

Grain	kcal	Protein(g)	CHO(g)	Fat(g)	Fiber(g)
Quinoa	374	13	69	6	6
Amaranth	374	14	66	7	15
Rice (white)	379	8	84	0	2
Rice (wild)	357	15	75	1	6
Oats (oatmeal)	375	10	78	4	7
Corn (grits)	347	9	79	1	5
Wheat (couscous)	376	13	77	1	5

Note: Values from *http://www.elook.org/nutrition*. 100g = 3.5 oz = approximately ½ cup.

in other amino acids, has a protein content of around 14–16%, and is high in fiber. When including food items from grains in the expedition food packs, be sure to seek out the presteamed or precooked dried grain products (quick or instant) that require less boiling and hence less fuel for preparation. Adequate carbohydrate intake (400–600 g/day) is necessary daily to replace muscle glycogen. When glycogen stores decline, perceived exertion increases (Wilmore and Costill 1999). This means that carrying heavy packs along steep trails will seem particularly exhausting if muscle glycogen stores are not replenished each day. A daily reference dietary value for carbohydrate (CHO) is 300 g, although this level does not permit work with high power outputs and should be considered a minimum. Trail days encompassing hard work (heavy packs, steep and difficult terrain) will be better supported with up to twice this amount of carbohydrate. The danger of glycogen depletion without dietary repletion is that body protein (lean muscle) will be lost as the body attempts to supply glucose derived from gluconeogenesis from amino acids and both strength and endurance will suffer. Sixty percent of a day's kcal or 7–10 g CHO/kg body weight (BW) would be an ideal carbohydrate target but sometimes difficult to achieve with expedition foods. A reasonable check to make during ration planning would be to ensure that the day's food will supply at least 6 g CHO/kg BW (e.g., for a 75-kg individual: $6 \times 75 = 450$ grams CHO).

Carbohydrate is necessary for work requiring intermittent high power outputs but is less important when work is at a low to moderate sustained level. Some expeditions (Steger 1987) have taken advantage of the concentrated energy of fat and utilized rations relatively high in fat to save weight and space to good logistical advantage. The use of high-fat rations, although feasible, should be implemented with care because a period of "adaptation" to higher than normal levels of fat in the diet is required to permit tissue-level enzymic adaptation to oxidizing fat as an energy source (Phinney et al. 1983; Steger 1987). A classic example of what might be expected when a high-fat diet is abruptly thrust upon an expedition not accustomed to low-carbohydrate intakes can be found in the 1943 Army evaluation of pemmican for hard physical work in the cold (Kark et al. 1946). Soldiers abruptly subjected to a high-fat pemmican diet soon became glycogen depleted, ketotic, and exhausted and were not capable of performing their daily work schedule. Whenever possible, it is usually a better plan to ensure a reasonable level of carbohydrate intake (350–500 g/day) compatible with higher power outputs. Although this discussion puts fat in a rather "unflattering" light, it should also be remembered that if the pace of the expedition is relatively slow and not interspersed with intermittent arduous trail challenges or if extreme cold is to be encountered, fat may be a useful energy source in the diet. Cold challenge studies conducted during World War II by Mitchell et al. (1961) indicated that meals high in fat may help improve cold tolerance. Although follow-up research to Mitchell's findings are lacking in the literature, other investigators have shown that a small mixed meal prior to a period of cold exposure (e.g., sleeping in a sleeping bag at subzero temperatures) may help the body maintain extremity temperatures (fingers and toes) at higher levels that permit a more restful sleep (Kreider and Buskirk 1957; Kreider 1961). A synthesis of the sports medicine and cold physiology literature suggests that frequent small meals or snacks while on trail will help replenish muscle glycogen levels and may improve cold tolerance (Askew 1989). During physically challenging stretches of the trail, ingestion of 30–60 g CHO per hour (a typical sports energy bar contains 30–50 g CHO per bar) will help prevent excessive glycogen depletion.

No discussion of macronutrients would be complete without considering the staple of most arctic explorers, pemmican. Most turn-of-the-century accounts of arctic exploration mention the use of pemmican. There was probably good reason to incorporate this staple of the diet of indigenous peoples into the explorer's food supplies; pemmican was nutritious (an excellent source of high-quality protein, and even vitamin C depending on whether berries were added to the meat and tallow mix). It was very energy dense and filling, typically 60–70% of the kcal in pemmican was from fat. The melted fat acted both as an energy source and as a barrier to oxygen, thus helping to keep the pemmican preserved without refrigeration. Pemmican served equally well as a food supply for man and dogs, thus simplifying logistics of arctic explorers even further. Modern advances in food preservation, preparation, and packaging have long since eclipsed the need for pemmican on most expeditions; indeed, it is difficult now even to find a commercial source of true traditional pemmican. Those so inclined can find numerous recipes for pemmican on internet postings (e.g., *http://www.natureskills.com/pemmican_recipe.html*). Those put off by the taste of lard or the idea of saturated fat may wish to substitute peanut butter in

place of the melted tallow. This substitution improves the palatability of the mixture but decreases the caloric density a bit. A stock of pemmican as an "emergency" provision to accompany expedition food supplies or as a meal for an unanticipated "cold" camp is not a bad idea, but the author would not recommend it day in and day out as the expedition staple.

Micronutrient Requirements

Deficiencies of micronutrients take weeks to develop, so day-to-day angst over whether the DRIs of expedition members have been met is somewhat academic with respect to everyday health and expedition food planning. As mentioned earlier, there is a good chance a reasonably adequate intake of vitamins and minerals will be achieved quite by accident if the traveler eats a mixed expedition diet that meets their energy requirement. Expeditions projected to last longer than 2–3 weeks should give more consideration to the content of B vitamins, vitamin C, sodium, potassium, calcium, iron, and zinc because the body does not store these water-soluble nutrients to an appreciable extent. Fresh food resupply often can be arranged after several weeks in the field. When this is not possible, a good expedition plan will include a multivitamin/multimineral tablet per day for expedition members. A supplement supplying 100% of the RDI for vitamins and minerals is low in cost, doesn't take up much space in the pack and makes adherence to the RDIs in food nutrient planning less of an issue.

Water Requirements

Water is just as important as energy in planning food for an expedition (Askew 1997). The planner must have a good plan for providing potable water to expedition members. It is likely that natural water flows or snow will be encountered, and these should be considered nonpotable until treated or disinfected by chemicals, filtering, or boiling. Please refer to Chapter 8 for water purification methods. It is important to consider a guide to determine the quantity of water needed. As a rule of thumb, 4–6 liters of canteen water will be needed per day for food and drinking in temperate climates. A good hydration plan would consist of a liter of fluid upon rising in the morning with breakfast, a liter on the trail before lunch, a liter with lunch, a liter in the afternoon before dinner, and a liter with dinner in the evening. A canteen less or a canteen more may be needed in cold or hot climates, respectively. There is no DRI for water, not because it is not an essential nutrient, but because water requirements are influenced by so many variables including temperature, humidity, workload, solar load, and even salt and protein in the diet. When water is plentiful it is a relatively simple task to encourage everyone to drink to avoid dehydration. Sometimes thirst is overridden by the activities of the day, and expedition members can become involuntarily dehydrated. Food plans that include lots of fluid and encourage fluid intake such a soups, stews, rehydrated cereals, powdered beverage bases, and even tea and coffee can help team members stay hydrated. Heating water during breakfast and putting the hot water in thermos bottles prior to hitting the trail can encourage fluid intake in cold weather conditions and provides a convenient way to hydrate soup packets during a quick stop on the trail.

Translating Energy Requirements into Food Projections

The basic structure for the expedition food plan is framed by energy and water requirements. As soon as the daily energy target is established and multiplied up to encompass the size and duration of the expedition, the food planner can begin to choose food to meet the energy needs. This can be done several ways. A menu that repeats itself every 3 days provides some variety and is a reasonable approach to meal planning. Small variations in menu items can be included, if desired, to relieve food "boredom." A one-day sample menu for one person supplying approximately 3,600 kcal (enough for a day's moderate work) is given in Table 7.9. This simple menu consists of easy-to-prepare heat-and-eat or snack items and provides for an almost continuous intake of calories and nutrients throughout the day to continually replenish muscle glycogen stores. The carbohydrate content (478 g) is good but might need to be increased by 100 g (400 kcal) if hard physical work is anticipated. The protein, fiber, and vitamin and mineral content generally meet requirements with the exception of a few of the vitamins. This is where a simple multivitamin tablet can fill in the shortfalls in the DRIs or, with a bit of menu "tweaking," food items can be selected that are good sources of the "low" vitamin. For example, another serving of a powdered fortified fruit beverage would bring the vitamin C content up from the current 60 mg in the sample ration to the 90 mg DRI value. Once the menu cycle meeting predicted daily energy demands is decided upon, the individual food items can be multiplied up to encompass the duration of the trip (e.g., 5 times the 3-day quantities would be needed for a 15-day expedition).

If large groups will make up the expedition, menus for the entire group can be planned and scaled up or down to meet the size (energy demands) of the group. Usually food preparation for larger groups will involve a good deal of food item assembly from individual ingredients at each day's campsite and should be well thought out in advance. Clear written food preparation instructions with quantities and preparation steps are advised, even if the food planner is also the cook. Sometimes memory

Table 7.9. One day sample individual menu for one person, minimal preparation[a]

Menu Item	kcal
Breakfast	
2 servings instant oatmeal	594
1 cup Instant juice (Tang)	90
Snack	
1 energy bar	140
3 slices jerky	243
Lunch	
1 soup packet (instant ramen)	290
1 serving wheat crackers	53
Snack	
1 serving granola	383
3 slices jerky	243
Dinner	
2 servings instant macaroni & cheese	820
1 soup packet (instant ramen)	290
1 serving wheat crackers	53
1 chocolate bar	225
Bedtime snack	
½ serving granola	191
Total kcal/day	3,615

[a]This sample menu provides (of the kcal) approximately 13% protein, 51% CHO, and 36% fat; in terms of grams, the menu provides 126 g protein, 478 g CHO, 152 g fat, and 36 g fiber, it meets over 100% of the RDI for Vitamins A, E, thiamine, riboflavin, niacin, B6, but meets about 36–67% of the Vitamin C, D, K, B12, and pantothentic acid RDIs.

Most all mineral requirements are well met with this menu, supplying 1,568 mg calcium, 18 mg zinc, 68 mg iron, and 8,000 mg sodium.

fails and even the cook needs a day off once in a while; clear concise written preparation instructions will permit any expedition member to prepare the meal. A day's sample menu with preparation instructions for a group of 10 people is given in Table 7.10.

NOLS Bulk Ration Planning

Another good way to plan food, especially for a longer expedition where a good deal of food preparation will be done by cooking from ingredients at the campsites, is the National Outdoor Leadership School ration planning system (Pearson 2004). Pearson suggests the following steps for bulk ration planning (note that an energy estimate is included within this planning system in step #1). The information in steps 1–5 is reproduced from *NOLS Cookery* (Pearson 2004) with permission; further details can be gained by referring to pages 3–11 of that publication.

Steps in Food Planning Using the NOLS ppppd System

Step #1: Estimate the total amount of "generic" food that will be needed during the trip by determining the

Table 7.10. One sample day group menu for 10 people, moderate preparation required[a]

Breakfast
Hydrate hash browns. Drain off excess water and set aside
In fry pan heat oil and sauté onions.
Add the hash browns until they cover the bottom of the pan.
Fry until crispy. Dice or grate cheese and add to hash browns.
Fry until cheese melts. Top with salsa (optional).
Serve with coffee and Tang breakfast drink.

Cheesy Hash Browns and Tang
2 lb dry hash browns
2 cups cheddar cheese
1 cup dried onions
10 packets Tang juice mix
salsa

Lunch
Boil two pots of water (10 cups/pot).
Provide each person with a packet of dried soup mix,
   one packet of crackers, and a packet of hot chocolate mix
   and a packet of instant coffee mix.
The coffee and hot chocolate can be mixed for a "mocha."
Beverage or consumed alone.

Soup, Crackers, and Mocha
10 packets dried soup mix
10 packets of wheat crackers

10 packets hot chocolate mix
10 packets instant coffee

Dinner
Reconstitute dehydrated food items separately
   according to instructions. In pot one add milk,
   margarine, salt and pepper, then add potatoes
   slowly, stir until thick and fluffy.
Rehydrate onions. Grate or cube cheese.
Open corn, drain and set aside.
In second pot, add rehydrated chili mix,
   stir, then add onions and corn. Mix well.
   Continue to cook until chili is done.
   Layer ingredients in dutch ovens,
   placing chili mixture on bottom, then
   potatoes. Sprinkle cheese on top.
   If desired place some cheese in
   the chili mixture. Place lid on top
   of dutch oven and put over a very
   low heat on the stove. Remove from
   heat once cheese has melted.
   Be careful that the bottom doesn't burn!

Chili Pie
4 cups dry chili mix
6 cups instant potatoes
10 tbsp margarine

1 cup powdered milk
1 cup dried onion
4 cups drained corn
4 cups cheddar cheese

[a]This sample 10-person menu provides approximately 2,200–2,300 kcal/day/person. Snacks must be added morning, afternoon, and evening or adjust serving sizes to bring the total daily calorie intake up to meet predicted energy expenditure. Alternatively, central expedition meal planning can provide the basic three meals per day and individual expedition members can supplement with their own snacks as they see fit. Each day's menu items, quantities, and preparation instructions should be listed for each day of the trip that a particular menu is planned.

pounds of food per person per day (ppppd). Pearson offers these guidelines in choosing an estimate for ppppd:

1.5 ppppd for leisure camping of short (3–5 days) duration provides 2,500–3,000 kcal/day
1.75–2.0 ppppd for temperate weather hiking with full packs, 7–10 days, 3,000–3,500 kcal/day
2.0–2.25 ppppd for hiking or skiing with full packs, cool weather, 7–10 days, 3,500–4,500 kcal/day
2.5 ppppd for very strenuous hiking or skiing with packs or pulling sleds in very cold mountainous environments, 4,000–5,000 kcal/day

Step #2: Calculate the total amount of food needed for the entire trip

Number of people × Number of days × ppppd =
   Total poundage of food needed

Step #3: Partition the total poundage of food into food "categories" according to the following chart:

	Category multipliers (ppppd)				
Food category	1.5	1.75	2	2.25	2.5
Breakfast	0.24	0.28	0.33	0.35	0.38
Dinner	0.27	0.32	0.35	0.37	0.40
Cheese	0.19	0.22	0.24	0.26	0.28
Trail foods	0.32	0.35	0.37	0.45	0.49
Flour and baking[a]	0.11	0.13	0.16	0.09	0.10
Sugar and fruit drinks	0.10	0.12	0.14	0.15	0.18
Soups, bases, desserts	0.06	0.09	0.13	0.15	0.19
Milk, eggs, margarine, cocoa	0.21	0.24	0.28	0.31	0.33
Meats and substitutes[b]	0	0	0	0.12	0.15

[a]The need for baking ingredients is lower in winter conditions, when only quick pan baking is feasible.
[b]High-fat and high-preservative meats are added in winter to meet higher fuel needs.

Step #4: Calculate the total pounds of each food category based upon the category multipliers from step #3 and the number of people and the number of days. An example is shown in the following chart for four people on an 8-day trip at 1.75 ppppd:

Food category	Calculation	Rounded (lb)
Trail foods	0.35 × 4 × 8 = 11.5	
Dinner	0.32 × 4 × 8 = 10.5	
Breakfast	0.28 × 4 × 8 = 9.0	
Milk, eggs, margarine, cocoa	0.24 × 4 × 8 = 7.5	
Cheese	0.22 × 4 × 8 = 7.0	
Flour and baking	0.13 × 4 × 8 = 4.0	
Sugar and fruit drinks	0.12 × 4 × 8 = 4.0	
Soups, bases, desserts	0.09 × 4 × 8 = 3.0	
Meats and substitutes	(none in this instance)	
Total pounds		~56.5 lb

Step #5: Choose and add specific foods under each category until the total weight for each category is approximately equal to the amount calculated in Step #4. For example, for the milk, eggs, margarine, cocoa category, 3 lb dried milk, 2 lb dried eggs, 1 lb margarine, 1.5 lb cocoa = 7.5 lb. NOLS offers the option that if you do not plan using the foods in a particular category such as baking, take the poundage allotted to "Flour and baking" (in this example shown here, 4 lb), and add the pounds to another category such as breakfast or dinner. Don't just omit it or you will ultimately come up short on energy and other nutrients contained in that food category. Refer to pages 3–11 of *NOLS Cookery* for greater detail and pages 19–28 of *NOLS Cookery* for some specific food selection suggestions.

LOGISTICS: WEIGHT/VOLUME CONSIDERATIONS

Expeditions utilizing some means of conveyance such as sleds, horses, pack mules, or ATVs will be less concerned with the weight and physical space the food supplies will occupy than will the expedition where each member or designated members carry the food in packs. It is usually easier to distribute the food items among two or three "food bearers" for the trip depending upon the weight of the food because this tactic permits a more organized approach to food item packing and ultimately being able to readily locate the item after you reach camp. Food items should either be packaged by the day, if possible, or at least by like components (e.g., spices in one container, staples such as flour and margarine in another, and soups in another). Packaging all food items in as few packs as possible facilitates hanging food from tree branches in bear country, but may lend a feeling of "insecurity" to members with just trail snacks in their packs. Expeditions in hazardous terrain such as frozen snow with crevasses or precipitous cliffs might consider parceling out the food supplies to several expedition team members so that if disaster befalls one member with food not all the food is lost. One need only consider Antarctic explorer Gregory Mawson's expedition's unexpected encounter with a crevasse that swallowed up the entire sledge containing most of their provisions leading to life-threatening starvation (Bickel 2001).

If you have made your calculations and food selections and the weight or bulk is too prohibitive, several options are available: (1) reduce the duration of the expedition, (2) reduce the number of people in the expedition, (3) arrange resupply, or (4) remove bulky heavy food items and replace them with more concentrated energy food selections. Assuming the first three options are not available, the food supply list can be examined for items such as canned soups and vegetables that can be substituted and supplied in dehydrated form. Be aware that this will increase water requirements for food preparation. Food items containing large amounts of carbohydrates such as pasta, crackers, biscuits, or bread tend to be cherished by campers, but their calorie-per-gram figure of merit is low. Some of these items can be replaced with high-fat food items such as peanut butter, salami sticks, cheese, and nuts to reduce volume. Be aware that some substitutions cannot be made on a calorie-for-calorie basis. For example, substituting peanut butter for pasta calorie for calorie greatly reduces the carbohydrate content of the ration and may lead to less "vigor" on the trail because of less muscle glycogen repletion.

The guiding thoughts to keep in mind during food planning are: "Can I carry it"? and "Will I eat it"? Remember, food is "food" whether eaten or not, but it only becomes "nutrition" after it is consumed. Do not provision food only starving expedition members would be willing to eat if you want to be asked to plan the food for the next expedition!

PRACTICAL GUIDANCE AND SUGGESTIONS

Sanitation

Sanitation is as important in the field as it is at home, but it is harder to achieve. Designated cooks who understand the importance of washing hands before food preparation and food serving as well as cleaning pots and pans and utensils after use are the first line of defense between food-borne illness and expedition members. Bacteria do not thrive in extremely cold weather so sanitation and food preservation may not be as critical in arctic expeditions as they are in hot or temperate climates. Serving food dry or hot will help reduce food-borne pathogens. Food leftovers should be considered not safe and discarded (burned, buried, or packed out) if means of refrigeration are not available.

A chlorine solution used to disinfect water is useful to disinfect surfaces used to prepare food such as a thin rollup plastic cutting board. A simple sanitizing rinse consists of 1/3 cup chlorine bleach per 5 gallons of *filtered/potable* water or ½ oz (1 cap full) per 1 gallon of *filtered/potable* water. Air drying of washed and rinsed eating and cooking utensils is preferable to drying them with a dirty camp towel. If water and fuel is plentiful, dipping washed utensils into a pot of boiling water as a final step will help destroy bacteria. Hand-washing stations can be set up with a collapsible plastic water jug and a bar of antibacterial soap between the tents and the eating area to encourage handwashing. That failing, a squeeze bottle or tube of commercial handwashing disinfectant "dry wash" should be made available to all expedition members, and they should be encouraged to use it prior to consuming food.

Practical Advice

You can't control the weather on an expedition, but you can control the food to help counter the weather. Plan on some "bail out" foods to fall back upon when the weather is bad or everyone is worn out: Instant soups, bouillon cubes, hot chocolate, energy bars, and jerky can be very useful in these instances. Another great suggestion modified from a recipe in Dorcas Miller's *Backpacker: More Backcountry Cooking* (2002) is an emergency breakfast for those who just can't start their day without coffee but don't have time to prepare a pot of hot coffee before hitting the trail due to rain or time contingencies (Table 7.11). A recipe modified from Pearson (2004) is given in Table 7.12 for a "power peanut butter" for the trail, which keeps well if kept in sealed containers (such as prepackaging the mixture in rollup tubes available at outdoor specialty stores). This mix is quite palatable, useful for trailside lunch breaks or in "cold" camps and contains more nutrients

---

Table 7.11. Quick-start cold trail breakfast[a]

½ cup cashews or walnuts
½ cup raisins
½ cup chocolate-covered coffee beans

[a]This mixture can be prepackaged in zip lock bags and is equivalent to approximately 1,000 kcal, 14 g protein, 110 g CHO, 63 g fat, and 11 g fiber, and the caffeine equivalent of about one cup of coffee. Granola can be substituted for raisins.

Table 7.12. "Trail power" peanut butter[a]

2 cup peanut butter
1 cup honey
1 cup margarine (soft safflower based)
1 cup powdered milk

[a]This recipe makes forty 2 tbsp servings containing 157 kcal, 11 g CHO, 4 g protein, 12 g fat, 36 mg calcium, and 1 g fiber/2 tbsp serving.

(in particular carbohydrate and calcium) than peanut butter alone. Energy bars are convenient, a quick source of calories, and, if chosen wisely, a multivitamin in a bar. A handy listing of the nutrient content of many popular energy bars can be found in the pocket-sized book *Sports Nutrition Guide* (Stephenson and Bader 2005).

The *NOLS Nutrition Field Guide* (Howley 2002) is an excellent guide to nutrition planning to accompany the *NOLS Cookery* (Pearson 2004). Carole Latimer provides some good practical advice to consider in her excellent book *Wilderness Cuisine* (1991). I have expanded upon some of her suggestions here:

1. **Eat frequently.** This helps replenish glycogen stores as they are depleted throughout the day, lessening fatigue and increased perceived exertion. This becomes more important as appetite increases after the first couple of days on the trail or after adjustment to altitude.

2. **Avoid constipation.** Eat fiber, and drink lots of water. Include some bran cereal, dried prunes, or packets of Metamucil™ (a natural fiber laxative) in your pack. Including beans in the daily food will also help. You should try to achieve a minimum of 20 g fiber/day and more is usually desirable. The author is reminded of an associate who was the physician on a cold weather trek in Pakistan who had to digitally remove impacted feces from the distal colon of a particularly miserable and constipated expedition member 10 days into the trek.

3. **Good food makes for good spirits.** Provide "comfort" foods such as coffee, tea, cocoa, chocolate, bacon, and chicken soup. Morale is important; always eat something even at the end of an exhausting day when all you want to do is crawl into your sleeping bag. You will sleep better and warmer (Askew 1989), and you will arise in better spirits with your glycogen restored ready for the next day's challenge. A good expedition leader will encourage group meals and check to make sure that team members are eating and drinking as they should.

4. **Prevent hypothermia.** This important aspect of expedition safety is a function of clothing management, shelter, and food. Dress warmly, stay dry, avoid exhaustion and overexposure, snack frequently, don't skip meals, don't become dehydrated, drink hot liquids at every opportunity (a thermos for each expedition member is indispensable in colder weather). Frequent small meals throughout the day during cold weather expeditions will improve cold tolerance by helping to maintain core temperature at a more constant level. A 600-kcal snack before climbing into the sleeping bag in cold weather will help keep the skin temperature of the toes and fingers warmer leading to more restful sleep (Askew 1989).

One final reminder, gear is good, but you can't eat it – your expedition food plan is as important as your gear, plan wisely!

SUGGESTED READINGS

Alexander C. Murdering the impossible. *National Geographic*. 2006;210(6):42–67.

Alpers DH, Stenson WF, Bier DM. *Manual of Nutritional Therapeutics,* 3rd ed. New York: Little, Brown and Company; 1995: 73–114.

Askew EW. Nutrition for a cold environment. *Physician and Sportsmedicine*. 1989;17:77–89.

Askew EW. Environmental and physical stress and nutrient requirements. *Am J Clin Nutr*. 1995;61:631S–637S.

Askew EW. Nutrition and performance in hot, cold and high altitude environments, In: Wolinsky I, ed. *Nutrition in Exercise and Sport*, 3rd ed. Boca Raton, Fla.: CRC Press; 1997: 597–619.

Askew EW. Work at high altitude and oxidative stress: antioxidant nutrients. *Toxicology*. 2002a;180:107–19.

Askew EW. Nutrition, malnutrition and starvation. In: Auerbach PS, ed. *Textbook of Wilderness Medicine*, 4th ed. St. Louis: Mosby; 2002b:1271–84.

Askew EW, Munro I, Sharp MA, Siegel S, Popper C, Rose MS, Hoyt RW, Martin JW, Reynolds K, Lieberman H, Engell D, Shaw CP. *Nutritional Status and Physical and Mental Performance of Special Operation Soldiers Consuming the Ration, Lightweight or the Meal, Ready-to-Eat Ration.* U.S. Army Research Institute of Environmental Medicine Technical Report No. T7–87. Natick, Mass.: U.S. Army Research Institute of Environmental Medicine; 1987.

Beatty O, Geiger J. *Frozen in Time: Unlocking the Secrets of the Franklin Expedition.* Saskatoon: Western Producer Prairie Books; 1988.

Bickel L. *Mawson's Will: The Greatest Polar Survival Story Ever Written.* South Royalton, Vt.: Steerforth Press; 2000.

Consolazio CF. Nutrient requirements of troops in extreme environments. *Army Research and Development Magazine*. 1966;7:24–7.

Consolazio CF, Nelson RA, Johnson HL. Metabolic aspects of acute starvation in normal humans: performance and cardiovascular evaluation. *Am J Clin Nutr*. 1967;20:684–93.

Devoto B. *The Journals of Lewis and Clark.* New York: Houghton Mifflin; 1953: 240.

Duncan D, Burns K. *Lewis & Clark: The Journey of the Corps of Discovery.* AUDIOBOOK; 1997.

Feeney RE. *Polar Journeys: The Role of Food and Nutrition in Early Exploration.* Washington, DC: American Chemical Society; 1998: 5–13.

Friedl KL. When does energy deficit affect soldier physical performance? In: Marriott BM, ed. *Not Eating Enough.* Washington, DC: National Academy Press; 1995: 253–83.

Gunderson M. *The Food Journal of Lewis and Clark: Recipes for an Expedition.* Yankton, SD: History Cooks; 2003: 109, 129.

Howley M. *NOLS Nutrition Field Guide.* Lander, Wyo.: National Outdoor Leadership School; 2002.

Human Energy Requirements. Report of a Joint FAO/WHO/UNU Expert Consultation. Rome, 17–24 October 2001 (+CD-ROM). A copy in PDF format is available at: *ftp://ftp.fao.org/docrep/fao/007/y5686e/y5686e00.pdf*. A summary of this report was subsequently published in *Food and Nutrition Bulletin*. 2005;26(1):166.

Kark RR, Johnston R, Lewis J. Defects in pemmican as an emergency ration for infantry troops. *War Med*. 1946;8:345–352.

King, P. *Scott's Last Journey.* New York: Harper Collins; 1999: 169–80.

Kreider MB. Effect of diet on body temperature during sleep in the cold. *J Appl Physiol*. 1961;16:239–42.

Kreider MB, Buskirk ER. Supplemental feeding and thermal comfort during sleep in the cold. *J Appl Physiol*. 1957;11:337–43.

Latimer C. *Wilderness Cuisine: How to Prepare and Enjoy Fine Food on the Trail and in Camp.* Berkeley, Calif.: Wilderness Press; 1991: 17–26.

Marriott BM. *Not Eating Enough.* Washington, DC: National Academy Press; 1995: 3–40.

McCurdy SA. Epidemiology of disaster – the Donner party. *Western J Med*. 1994;160:338–42.

Miller DS. *Backpacker: More Backcountry Cooking.* Seattle, Wash.: The Mountaineers; 2002: 11.

Mitchell HH, Glickman N, Lambert EH, Keeton RW, Fahnstock MK. The tolerance of man to cold as affected by dietary modification: carbohydrate vs fat and the effects of frequency of meals. *Am J Physiol*. 1961;16:239–42.

_____. *Nutrition Standards and Education.* Army Regulation 40–25. Washington, DC: Headquarters, Department of the Army, Navy and Air Force; June 2001.

Otten JJ, Hellwig JP, Meyers LD, eds. *Dietary DRI Reference Intakes: The Essential Guide to Nutrient Requirements.* Washington, DC: The National Academies Press; 2006: 529–41.

Pearson C. *NOLS Cookery,* 5th ed. Mechanicsburg, Pa.: Stackpole Books, 2004: 3–11.

Pellett PL. Food energy requirements in humans. *Am J Clin Nutr*. 1990;51:711–22.

Pennington JA, Douglass JS. *Food Values of Portions Commonly Used,* 18th ed. New York: Lippincott Williams & Wilkins; 2005.

Phinney SD, Bistrian BR, Evans WJ, Blackburn GL. The human metabolic response to chronic ketosis without caloric restriction: preservation of submaximal exercise capacity with reduced carbohydrate oxidation. *Metabolism*. 1983;37:758–65.

Read PP. *Alive: The Story of the Andes Survivors.* New York: Avon, Harper and Collins; 1974.

Solomon S. *The Coldest March: Scott's Fatal Antarctic Expedition.* New Haven, Conn.: Yale University Press; 2001: 232–46.

Steger W with Shurke P. *North to the Pole.* New York: Times Books; 1987.

Stephenson J, Bader D. *Sports Nutrition Guide.* Mankato, Minn.: Appletree Press; 2005: 136–45.

Stewart GR. *Ordeal by Hunger: The Story of the Donner Party.* Lincoln: University of Nebraska Press; 1960.

Stroud M. *Shadows on the Wasteland: Crossing Antarctica with Ranulph Fiennes.* Woodstock, NY: Overlook Press; 1994.

Taylor HL, Buskirk ER, Brozek J, Anderson JT, Grande F. Performance capacity and effects of caloric restriction with hard physical work on young men. *J Appl Physiol*. 1957;10:421–9.

van der Beek EJ, van Dokkum W, Schrijver J, Wedel M, Gaillard AWK, Wesstra A, van de Weerd H, Hermus RJJ. Thiamin, riboflavin, and vitamins B-6 and C: impact of combined restricted intake on physical performance in man. *Am J Clin Nutr*. 1988;48:1451–62.

van der Beek EJ, van Dokkum W, Wedel M, Schrijver J, van den Berg H. Thiamin, riboflavin and vitamin B-6: impact of restricted intake on physical performance in man. *J Am Coll Nutr*. 1994;13:629–40.

Washburn, B. Frostbite: what it is – how to prevent it – emergency treatment. *N Engl J Med*. 1962;266:974–89.

Woolf K, Manore MM. B-vitamins and exercise; does exercise alter requirements? *Int J Sports Nutr Exer Metab*. 2006; 16:453–84.

Wilmore JH, Costill DL. *Physiology of Sport and Exercise.* Champaign, Ill.: Human Kinetics; 1999: 146.

Howard D. Backer, MD, MPH

The views and opinions expressed in this chapter are those of the author and do not necessary represent those of the California Department of Public Health.

FIELD WATER DISINFECTION

Waterborne disease is a risk for international travelers who visit countries that have poor hygiene and inadequate sanitation and for wilderness users relying on surface water in any country, including the United States. The main reason for treating drinking water is to prevent gastrointestinal illness from fecal pollution with enteric pathogens.[1] Appearance, odor, and taste are not reliable means to estimate water safety (Figure 8.1).

Of the 1.7 billion square miles of water on earth, less than 0.5% is potable. Almost none of the surface water in the United States is drinkable without treatment.[2] Few areas are now without human or animal activity, the major risk for contaminating water. Expeditions may go to very remote areas but still encounter risk on arrival in developing countries and on the approach to their destination. Even common high-altitude climbing routes are littered with human feces that contaminate streams below during snowmelt or rains. Prevention of enteric infections during an expedition involves three main areas: (1) water disinfection; (2) personal and camp hygiene; and (3) food safety.

Treatment of drinking water provides enormous benefits with minimal risk. Without disinfection and filtration, waterborne disease would spread rapidly in most public water systems served by surface water.[3] Where treatment is in place, disasters, such as floods and hurricanes, often overwhelm treatment facilities and contaminate groundwater, requiring point-of-use disinfection.

The combined roles of safe water, hygiene, and adequate sanitation in reducing diarrhea and other diseases are clear and well documented. Sanitation, including water treatment, is considered one of the ten great public health achievements that helped conquer infectious disease as a main cause of mortality in the United States.[4,5] Recent studies of simple water interventions in households of developing countries clearly document improved microbiological quality of water as well as reduced incidence of diarrhea illness independent of other measures to improve sanitation.[6,7] There are little data to demonstrate benefits of water disinfection in the U.S. wilderness, and some argue that it is not necessary.[8,9] Boulware et al. demonstrated that drinking untreated water correlated with higher rates of diarrhea among Appalachian Trail hikers.[92]

RISK AND ETIOLOGY

Infectious agents in contaminated drinking water with the potential for waterborne transmission include bacteria, viruses, protozoa, and parasites.[1,14] The long list of pathogenic microorganisms capable of waterborne transmission is similar to that of potential etiologic agents of travelers' diarrhea; almost all enteric pathogens and opportunistic pathogens that are transmissible by the fecal–oral route can be transmitted through water (Table 8.1). Separating the contribution of waterborne transmission of these pathogens from food-borne and person-to-person transmission is impossible; in fact, the latter two are probably more common. However, in developing countries, 15–20% of diarrhea is estimated to be waterborne. In developed countries, as much as 15–30% is attributed to municipal drinking water.

Risk of waterborne illness depends on the number of organisms consumed, which is determined by the volume of water, concentration of organisms, and treatment system efficiency[10] (Table 8.2). The excretion and loading of microbial contaminants in water are dynamic and change over time. Additional factors include virulence of the organism and defenses of the host. Infection and illness are not synonymous; the overall likelihood of illness from multiple studies for all three categories of microorganisms (bacterial, viral, protozoan) is 50–60%. Total immunity does not develop for most enteric pathogens, and reinfection may occur.[10]

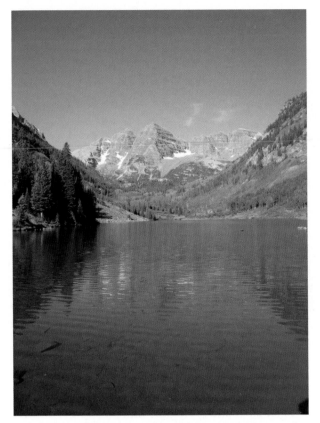

Figure 8.1. Though water may look clean, it can still contain contaminants. Photo courtesy of Howard Backer.

Table 8.1. Waterborne enteric pathogens

BACTERIAL
Escherichia coli
Shigella
Campylobacter
Vibrio cholerae
Salmonella
Yersinia enterocolitica
Aeromonas

VIRAL
Hepatitis A
Hepatitis E
Norovirus
Poliovirus
Miscellaneous enterics (more than 100 types: adenovirus, enterovirus, calcivirus, ECHO, astrovirus, coronavirus, etc.)

PROTOZOAL
Giardia lamblia
Entamoeba histolytica
Cryptosporidium
Blastocystis hominis
Isospora belli
Balantidium coli
Acanthamoeba
Cyclospora

PARASITIC
Ascaris lumbricoides
Ancylostoma duodenale (hookworm)
Taenia spp. (tapeworm)
Fasciola hepatica (sheep liver fluke)
Dracunculus medinensis
Strongyloides stercoralis (pinworm)
Trichuris trichiura (whipworm)
Clonorchis sinensis (Oriental liver fluke)
Paragonimus westermani (lung fluke)
Diphyllobothrium latum (fish tapeworm)
Echinococcus granulosus (hydatid disease)

Data from References 5, 14, 32, 33.

Some bacterial pathogens (*Shigella, Salmonella typhosa*) occur exclusively in human feces, whereas others (*Yersinia, Campylobacter,* non-typhoidal *Salmonella*) may be present in wild or domestic animals. The pathogenic enteric viruses seem to occur exclusively in human feces.

Recreational water contact may result in risk of enteric infection due to inadvertent ingestion during swimming and white-water boating, mainly from microorganisms that require only small infectious dose. Recreational water activities have resulted in giardiasis, cryptosporidiosis,[11] typhoid fever, salmonellosis, shigellosis, *E. coli* O157 infection,[12] viral gastroenteritis, and hepatitis A, as well as in wound infections, septicemia, and aspiration pneumonia due to *Legionella*.[3]

Developing Countries

The World Health Organization (WHO) estimates that worldwide, 25% of the population (1.5 billion rural and 200 million urban people) lack safe drinking water and 50% lack adequate sanitation. In Africa and Asia, nearly 20% of rural water supplies (Figure 8.2) are not functioning at any one time. Only 35% of wastewater is treated in Asia and 14% in Latin America.[13] In urban areas, the quality of water has deteriorated because of the lack of

Table 8.2. Estimated infectious dose of enteric organisms

Organism	Infectious Dose
Salmonellae	10^5
Shigella	10^2
Vibrio	10^3
Enteric viruses	1–10
Giardia	10–100
Cryptosporidium	10–100

Data from Reference 10.

water treatment chemicals, laboratories for monitoring, and operators to control the processes.

An estimated 80% of the world's diseases are linked to inadequate water supply and sanitation.[10] Between 10 million and 25 million people die each year (28,000 to 68,000 persons each day) from diseases caused by contaminated water and unsanitary conditions.

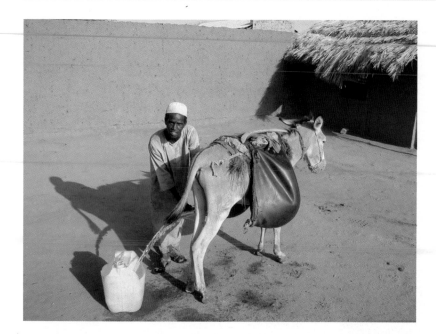

Figure 8.2. In developing countries, potable water may be difficult to come by. Here a local worker brings well water into a campsite by donkey. Photo courtesy of Gregory H. Bledsoe.

In developing countries, these illnesses account for 1 billion cases of diarrhea every year and 95% of deaths in children younger than 5 years of age.[14,15]

In certain tropical countries, the influence of high-density population, rampant pollution, and absence of sanitation systems means that available raw water is virtually wastewater.[16] Contamination of tap water must be assumed because of antiquated and inadequately monitored disposal, disinfection, and distribution systems. Water from springs and wells and even commercial bottled water may be contaminated with pathogenic microorganisms.

United States

Waterborne pathogens regularly cause outbreaks of infectious diarrhea acquired in U.S. parks, campgrounds, and recreation and wilderness areas.[3] Between 1970 and 1990, gastroenteritis of undefined etiology accounted for most cases overall, while *Giardia* caused the most cases of defined etiology.[3] Enteric bacteria are still associated with 12% of waterborne outbreaks in the United States.[17] The general pattern and etiology of waterborne outbreaks in the United States was little changed in 1999–2000 compared to the prior decades.[18]

Few data are available on microbiologic content of remote water sources. The source of fecal contamination in water may be either human or animal. High coliform levels were found in backcountry lakes and streams in the Sierra Nevada, associated with high-impact human use or cattle grazing, whereas most remote sampling sites without this activity were free of coliform or pathogenic organisms.[19,20]

More than 100 different virus types are known to be excreted in human feces.[21] All surface water supplies in the United States and Canada contain human enteroviruses.[22] Even remote surface lakes and streams tested in California showed disturbing levels of viral contamination.[21] In 2002, a series of outbreaks was reported on 17 different Colorado River raft trips involving more than 130 individuals. Lab evaluation of effluent from portable toilets found Norovirus, which was also isolated from river water at Lee's Ferry on the south branch of the river.

Protozoa

Six protozoa cause enteric disease and may be passed via waterborne transmission: *Giardia lamblia, Cryptosporidium parvum, Entamoeba histolytica, Cyclospora cayetanensis, Isospora belli,* and the microsporidia.[14,23] The first two are the most important for wilderness travelers. *Cryptosporidium* is an emerging enteric pathogen that has overtaken *Giardia* as the most common waterborne protozoa.[14] Waterborne transmission of *E. histolytica* is common in developing countries. *Giardia* cysts are widespread in surface water, found as frequently in pristine water and protected sources as in unprotected waters, with a direct correlation between numbers of cysts and levels of human use or beaver habitation.[17,24–26]

A zoonosis with *Giardia* is known, but the extent of cross-species infection is not clear.[27] Many of the species apparently capable of passing *Giardia* cysts to humans, including dogs, cattle, ungulates (deer), and beaver, are present in wilderness areas.[24] *Cryptosporidium* is now found more frequently than *Giardia* in surface water, but in smaller numbers, and also has a large zoonosis.[28,29]

The low numbers of cysts recovered from the environment indicate that the risk of ingesting an infectious dose of *Giardia* cysts is small.[30] However, the likely model that poses a risk to campers is pulse contamination; a brief period of high cyst concentration from fecal contamination, similar to a recreational outbreak among lap swimmers in a swimming pool contaminated with fecal material.[31] Surface water is subject to frequent, dramatic changes in microbial quality as a result of activities on a watershed.[32]

Parasitic organisms other than protozoa are seldom considered in discussions of disinfection. The frequency of infection by waterborne transmission is unknown because food and environmental contamination or skin penetration is more prevalent. The most obvious risk is from nematodes, with no intermediate hosts, that are infectious immediately or soon after eggs are passed in stool. *Fasciola hepatica*, a liver fluke of herbivores and humans, is normally acquired by ingestion of encysted metacercariae on water plants or free organisms in water. The Guinea tapeworm, *Dracunculus medinensis*, is a tissue nematode of humans and causes the only such disease transmitted exclusively through drinking water. Worldwide eradication of *Dracunculosis* has nearly been accomplished.

Bacterial spores can cause serious wound and gut infections but are not likely to be waterborne enteric pathogens. *Clostridium* is ubiquitous in soil, lake sediment, tropical water sources, and the stool of animals and humans.

Chemical hazards are also becoming an alarming source of pollution in surface water. The greatest risks to wilderness travelers are pesticides from agricultural runoff and heavy metals from old mine tailings.

Persistence of Enteric Pathogens in the Environment and Natural Purification

After environmental contamination has occurred, a natural inactivation or die-off begins. However, enteric pathogens can retain viability for long periods.[33] Cold temperatures prolong survival in water, which explains the risk of transmission in mountain regions. In temperate and warm water, survival is measured in days. However, tropical water creates a microbiologically rich environment where coliform bacteria, including *E. coli* and *Vibrio cholerae*, can survive several months and may even proliferate.

Most enteric organisms, including *Shigella*, resist freezing.[34] Other organisms, including *Cryptosporidium*, may also survive weeks to months in freezing temperatures.[35]

It is widely believed that streams purify themselves and that certain water sources are reliably safe for drinking. These concepts have some truth but do not preclude the need for disinfection to ensure water quality. Self-purification is a complex process that involves settling of microorganisms after clumping or adherence to particles, sunlight providing ultraviolet destruction, natural die-off, predators eating bacteria, and dilution. The process is time dependent and less active during wet periods and winter conditions. Hours needed in flow time downstream to achieve a 90% bacterial kill by natural self-purification vary with pollution inflow and rate of water flow.[32]

Storage in reservoirs or lakes also improves microbiologic quality, with sedimentation as the primary process. Generally, 80–90% of bacteria and viruses are removed by storage, depending on inflow and outflow, temperature, and no further contamination. Cysts, with a larger size and greater weight should settle even faster than bacteria and viruses. Spring water is generally of higher quality than surface water, provided that the true source is not surface water channeling underground from a short distance above the spring. Wells and aquifers can be polluted from surface runoff.

Drawing conclusions from the preceding factors is difficult:

- In wilderness water, most sediment is inorganic, and clarity is not an indication of microbiologic purity.
- The major factor in determining the amount of microbe pollution in surface water is human and animal activity in the watershed.
- Streams do not adequately purify themselves.
- The settling effect of lakes may make them safer than streams, but care should be taken not to disturb bottom sediments when obtaining water.
- Groundwater is generally cleaner than surface water because of the filtration action of overlying sediments.
- Remove the top 4–5 cm of snow to obtain snow for melting. Avoid discolored snow.

Drinking water treatment standards acknowledge the impracticality of trying to eliminate all microorganisms from drinking water, allowing a small risk of enteric infection. Likewise, field treatment may not eliminate all risk from drinking water.

Standards for Portable Disinfection Products: EPA Registration

The Environmental Protection Agency (EPA) does not endorse, test, or approve mechanical filters; it merely assigns registration numbers. Current registration of mechanical filters requires only that the product make reasonable claims and that the location of the manufacturer be listed; no disinfection studies are required. However, many companies now use the standards as their testing guidelines. For mechanical filters, the standards should be applied only for those microorganisms against which claims are made, such as protozoa and bacteria, excluding viruses.

EPA standards require that challenge water at various temperatures and seeded with specific amounts of different microorganisms and contaminants be pumped through the filters at given intervals during the claimed volume capacity of the filter. A 3-log reduction (99.9%) is required for cysts, 4-log reduction (99.99%) for viruses,

Table 8.3. Definition of terms

Clarification	Techniques that reduce turbidity of water.
Coagulation–flocculation	Removes smaller suspended particles and chemical complexes too small to settle by gravity (colloids).
Contact time	The length of time that the halogen is in contact with microorganisms in the water.
Disinfection	A process that kills or destroys nearly all disease-producing microorganisms, with the exception of bacterial spores. As applied here, refers to pathogenic waterborne microbes and is the desired result of water treatment.
Enteric pathogen	Microorganisms capable of causing intestinal infection after ingestion; may be transmitted through food, water, or direct fecal–oral contamination.
Halogen	Oxidant chemical that can be used for disinfection of water.
Halogen demand	The amount of halogen reacting with impurities in the water.
Potable	Implies "drinkable" water, but technically means that a water source, on average, over a period of time, contains a "minimal microbial hazard," so that the statistical likelihood of illness is acceptable.
Purification	Frequently confused with "disinfection," but is more accurately used to indicate the removal of organic or inorganic chemicals and particulate matter to improve offensive color, taste, and odor.
Residual halogen concentration	The amount of active halogen remaining after halogen demand of the water is met.
Reverse osmosis	A process of filtration that uses high pressure to force water through a semi-permeable membrane that filters out dissolved ions, molecules, and solids.
Sterilization	A process by which all forms of microbial life, including bacteria, viruses, protozoa and spores are destroyed.

and 5- to 6-log reduction for bacteria. Testing is done or contracted by the manufacturer; the EPA neither tests nor specifies laboratories.

To be labeled a "microbiologic water purifier," the unit must remove, kill, or inactivate all types of disease-causing microorganisms from the water, including bacteria, viruses, and protozoan cysts so as to render the processed water safe for drinking. An exception for limited claims may be allowed for units removing specific organisms to serve a definable environmental need, for example, removal of protozoan cysts.

Chemical products that are used for treating municipal or private water supplies for drinking are considered pesticides and must be registered by the EPA Pesticide Branch. Registration signifies that the composition is such as to warrant the proposed claims without unreasonable adverse effects on the environment.

DISINFECTION METHODS

Definitions

Multiple techniques that can achieve potable water from source water of poor quality can be used in the field. Disinfection, the desired result of field water treatment, means the removal or destruction of harmful microorganisms. The goal of disinfection is to achieve potable water, indicating only that a water source, on average over a period of time, contains a "minimal microbial hazard," so that the statistical likelihood of illness is acceptable. Water sterilization is not necessary because not all organisms are enteric human pathogens.[36] Purification is frequently used interchangeably with disinfection, but

it more accurately refers to the removal of contaminants and particulate matter as well as the removal of offensive color, taste, and odor. Purification may not remove or kill enough microorganisms to ensure microbiologic safety (Table 8.3).

Heat

Heat is the oldest means of water disinfection. It is used worldwide by residents, travelers, and campers to provide safe drinking water. In countries with normally safe drinking water, it is often recommended as backup in emergencies or when water systems have become con-

Table 8.4. Heat

Advantages	Disadvantages
Does not impart additional taste or color to water	Does not improve the taste, smell, or appearance of poor quality water
Single-step process that inactivates all enteric pathogens	Fuel sources may be scarce, expensive, or unavailable
Efficacy is *not* compromised by contaminants or particles in the water, as FOR halogenation and filtration	Does not prevent recontamination during storage
Can pasteurize water without sustained boiling	
Relative susceptibility of microorganisms to heat	Protozoa > Bacteria > Viruses

Table 8.5. Heat inactivation of microorganisms	
Organism	Lethal temperature/time
Giardia	70°C (158°F) for 10 min
Cryptosporidium	72°C (161°F) heated up over 1 min
Salmonella, Shigella, and Campylobacter	75°C (167°F) or 3 min
V. cholerae	60°C (140°F) for 10 min 100°C (212°F) for 10 s
E. coli	60°C (140°F) for 5 min 70°C (158°F) for 1 min
Enteric viruses	56 (133°F) –60°C (140°F) in 20–40 minutes < 1 minute above 70°C (158°F)
Hepatitis A	85°C (185°F) for 1 min

Table 8.6. Boiling temperatures at various altitudes	
Altitude (m/ft)	Boiling point (°C/°F)
1,524/5,000	95/203
3,049/10,000	90/194
4,268/14,000	86/187
5,793/19,000	81/178

taminated by floods or a lapse in water treatment plant efficacy. Fuel availability is the most important limitation to using heat (Table 8.4).

Heat inactivation of microorganisms is time and temperature dependent; the thermal death point is reached in shorter time at higher temperatures, whereas lower temperatures are effective with a longer contact time.[37] Pasteurization uses this principle to kill enteric food pathogens and spoiling organisms at temperatures between 60 and 70°C (140 and 158°F).[38] Therefore, the minimum critical temperature is well below the boiling point at any terrestrial elevation.

Microorganisms have varying sensitivity to heat; however, all common enteric pathogens are readily inactivated by heat (Table 8.5). Bacterial spores (e.g., Clostridium spp.) are the most resistant; some can survive 100°C (212°F) for long periods, but are not likely to be waterborne enteric pathogens. Boiling is not dependent on water quality like filtration or chemical disinfection. Heat kills or inactivates all enteric waterborne pathogens, regardless of whether they are freely suspended or present in particles.[5] Protozoal cysts, including Giardia and Entamoeba histolytica, are the most susceptible to heat. Cryptosporidium and parasitic eggs and larvae are also inactivated at these lower pasteurization levels.

Common bacterial enteric pathogens (E. coli, Salmonella, Shigella, V. cholerae) as well as viruses are killed by standard pasteurization temperatures;[38–40] death occurs in less than 1 minute above 70°C (158°F).

Boiling Time

The boiling time required is important when fuel is limited. The old recommendation for treating water was to boil for 10 minutes and add 1 minute for every 1,000 feet (305 m) in elevation. However, available data suggest this is not necessary for disinfection. In the wilderness, the time required to heat water from 55°C (131°F) to boiling temperature counts toward disinfection.

Therefore, any water brought to a boil should be adequately disinfected.[41] An extra margin of safety can be added by boiling for 1 minute or by keeping the water covered for several more minutes, which will maintain high temperature without using fuel, or by allowing it to cool slowly. Although the boiling point decreases with increasing altitude, this is not significant compared with the time required for thermal death at these temperatures (Table 8.6). Although attaining boiling temperature is not necessary, it is the only easily recognizable end point without using a thermometer. Many other sources, including the World Health Organization, now agree with the recommendation to simply bring water to a boil. Because of scant data for hepatitis A, the Centers for Disease Control and Prevention (CDC) and EPA still recommend boiling for 1 minute to add a margin of safety.[42] Other sources still suggest 3 minutes of boiling time at high altitude to give a wide margin of safety.[28,42]

When no other means are available, the use of hot tap water may pasteurize water in developing countries, if water has been sitting in a tank near 55–60°C (131–140°F) for a prolonged period.[43] Tolerance to touch is too variable to be a reliable gauge of pasteurization temperatures.[39]

Solar Heat

Pasteurization has been successfully achieved using solar heating. A solar cooker constructed from a foil-lined cardboard box with a glass window in the lid can be used for disinfecting large amounts of water by pasteurization. Bottom temperatures of 65°C (149°F) have been obtained for at least 1 hour in up to three 3.7-L containers. Exposure to full sunshine in Kenya destroyed E. coli in 2-L clear plastic bottles within 7 hours, if the maximum temperature reached 55°C (131°F). Inactivation in this situation was a combination of thermal and ultraviolet irradiation[44,45] No thermal inactivation occurs below 40°C (104°F). This could be a low-cost method for improving water quality, especially in refugee camps and disaster areas.

Physical Removal

Turbidity and Clarification

River, lake, or pond water is often cloudy (turbid) and unappealing due to suspended organic and inorganic

Table 8.7. Summary of clarification techniques

Technique	Process	Uses, advantages
Sedimentation	Settling by gravity of large particulates	Requires only time; Greatly improves water esthetics
Coagulation–flocculation	Removes suspended particles, most microorganisms, some dissolved substances	Simple process, easily applied in field; Greatly improves water quality; Improves efficacy of filtration and chemical disinfection
Activated charcoal	Removes organic and some inorganic chemicals	Removes toxins such as pesticides and will remove chemical disinfectants; Improves taste esthetics of water
Filtration	Physical and chemical process	Removes microorganisms; If charcoal stage, may improve taste and remove chemicals

matter, such as clay, silt, plankton, and other microscopic organisms, and often associated with unpleasant odors and tastes. Removing particulate matter can greatly improve the taste of water, as well as decrease the number of microorganisms. Bacteria and viruses may be attached to particulate matter or be embedded in it, affording some protection from disinfectants. Clarification to remove turbidity is an important first initial step that greatly improves the efficacy of filtration or chemical disinfection.[46] Sedimentation and coagulation–flocculation are clarification techniques that can be easily applied in the wilderness for pretreatment of cloudy water, followed by disinfection with microfiltration or halogenation (Table 8.7).

Sedimentation

Sedimentation is the separation of particles large enough to settle rapidly by gravity, such as sand and silt. This is particularly effective for glacial streams and rivers after rain has mixed large amounts of sediment into the water. Water is allowed to sit without agitation. After sediment has formed on the bottom of the container, the clear water is decanted or filtered from the top. The time required depends on the size of the particle. Generally, 30 minutes to a few hours are adequate for large particles such as inorganic sands and silts. Microorganisms, especially protozoal cysts, eventually settle (as discussed with reservoirs); reductions up to 90% may be achieved overnight or in 1–2 days.[16] How-

ever, the organisms are easily disturbed during pouring or filtering.

Coagulation–Flocculation

Smaller suspended particles and chemical complexes too small to settle by gravity are called colloids. Most of these can be removed by chemical precipitation, known as coagulation–flocculation. This technique is used routinely in large municipal disinfection plants but is simple enough to be used at the household level and in the outdoors[41] (Table 8.8).

Coagulation is achieved with addition of an appropriate chemical, causing particles to stick together on contact because of electrostatic and ionic forces.[33] Aluminum salts (alum), iron salts, and lime are commonly used, readily available coagulants. The second stage, flocculation, is a purely physical process obtained by prolonged gentle mixing to promote the formation of larger particles. Coagulation–flocculation removes most coliform bacteria (60–98%), viruses (65–99%),[47] *Giardia* (60–99%), helminth ova (95%), heavy metals, dissolved phosphates, and minerals.[48] Despite removal of most microorganisms, a subsequent disinfection step is advised.

To clarify water by coagulation–flocculation in the field, add 10–30 mg of alum per liter of water. The exact amount is not important, so it can be done with a pinch of alum, lime (calcium oxide), or both for each gallon of water, using more if the water is very cloudy. Next, stir or shake briskly for 1 minute to mix the coagulant and then agitate gently and frequently for at least 5 minutes to assist flocculation. Settling requires at least 30 minutes, after which the water is carefully decanted or poured through a cloth or paper filter. The process can be repeated, if necessary. Finally, microfiltration or halogenation should be used to ensure disinfection.

Alum is a common chemical used by the food industry in baking powder and for pickling. It can be found

Table 8.8. Coagulation–flocculation

Advantages	Disadvantages
Highly effective to clarify water and remove many microorganisms	Unfamiliar technique and substances
Improves efficacy of filtration and chemical disinfection	Adds extra step unless combined flocculent-disinfectant tablet
Inexpensive and widely available	
Simple process with no toxicity	
Relative susceptibility of microorganisms to coagulation–flocculation	Protozoa > Bacteria = Viruses

in some food stores or at chemical supply stores. In an emergency, baking powder or even the fine white ash from a campfire can be used.[49] Various crushed beans and seeds have been used traditionally by native peoples as coagulation–flocculation agents.[16]

Adsorption

Adsorbents such as charcoal, clay, and other types of organic matter (e.g., burnt rice hulls or coconut shell) have been used for water treatment for millenia.[50] These processes are often combined with filtration or coagulation because these substances can also serve as the filter media and even can act as coagulants.[41]

Granular Activated Carbon

When activated, charcoal becomes highly reactive and adsorbs dissolved chemicals (thus its role for medical detoxification). Granular activated carbon (GAC) is the best means to remove toxic organic and inorganic chemicals from water (including disinfection by-products) and to improve odor and taste.[33,51] GAC is a common component of field filters. Compressed into block form, it can act as both a depth filter and an adsorbent.

GAC does not kill microorganisms; in fact, bacteria colonize charcoal beds and are resistant to chlorination because the chlorine is adsorbed by the GAC.[33,50] Therefore, an alternative means of disinfection should always be used in conjunction with GAC.

GAC can be used before or after disinfection. Before disinfection, GAC removes many organic impurities that result in bad odor and taste. GAC is best used after chemical disinfection to make water more palatable by completely removing the halogen[22] and other chemical impurities.

Eventually, the binding sites on the carbon particles become saturated and no longer adsorb; some molecules are released as others preferentially bind.[51]

Filtration

Portable water treatment products are the third highest intended purchase of outdoor equipment after backpacks and tents. Filters are appealing because they are simple to use and require no holding time (Table 8.9).

Filtration is both a physical and chemical process, so many variables influence filter efficiency. The characteristics of the filter media and the water, as well as flow rate, determine the interactions. Filtration can reduce turbidity, bacteria, algae, viruses, color, oxidized iron, manganese, and radioactive particles.

The size of a microorganism is the primary determinant of its susceptibility to filtration (Table 8.10). Waterborne pathogens often adhere to larger particles or clump together, making them easier to remove by physical processes. Therefore, observed reductions are often greater than expected based on their individual sizes.[41] Portable filters can readily remove protozoan cysts

Table 8.9. Filtration

Advantages	Disadvantages
Simple to operate	Adds bulk and weight to baggage
Mechanical filters require no holding time for treatment (water is treated as it comes out of filter)	Most filters not reliable for removal of viruses
Large choice of commercial products	Expensive relative to chemical treatment
Adds no unpleasant taste and often improves taste and appearance of water	Channeling of water or high pressure can force microorganisms through the filter
Rationally combined with halogens for removal or destruction of all pathogenic waterborne microbes	Eventually clogs from suspended particulate matter; may require some maintenance or repair in field
Susceptibility of microorganisms to filtration	Protozoa > Bacteria > Viruses

and bacteria, but they may not remove viruses, which are another order of magnitude smaller than bacteria. However, adsorption and aggregation during passage through mechanical filters reduce viruses. Virus particles may adhere to the walls of diatomite (ceramic) or charcoal filters by electrostatic chemical attraction, which can be enhanced by a coating on the filter or a positive charge.[52]

Many filters constructed with various designs and materials are marketed for field use (Table 8.11). Surface, membrane, and mesh filters are very thin with a single layer of fairly precise pores, whose size should be equal

Table 8.10. Microorganism susceptibility to filtration

Organism	Average size (μm)	Maximum recommended filter rating (μm)
Viruses	0.03	N/S
Escherichia coli	0.5 × 3–8	0.2–0.4
Campylobacter	0.2–0.4 × X 1.5–3.5	0.2–0.4
Microsporidia	1–2	N/S
Cryptosporidium oocyst	2–6	1
Giardia cyst	6–10 × 8–15	3–5
Entamoeba histolytica cyst	5–30 (average 10)	3–5
Cyclospora	8–10	3–5
Nematode eggs	30–40 × 50–80	20
Schistosome cercariae	50 × 100	Coffee filter or fine cloth
Dracunculus larvae	20 × 500	Coffee filter or fine cloth

N/S = Not specified.

Table 8.11. Portable field water filters and purification device

Manufacturer, product / Manufacturer's web site[a]	Microbial claims[b]	Operation	Primary filter, additional elements, stages, comments[c]	Capacity	Retail price[d]
Aquamira *http://www.mcnett.com*	P	Sport bottle	Carbon filter, 2 µm, in squeeze bottle. May be used in conjunction with Aquamira water treatment – chlorine dioxide stabilized solution.	1–2 person	$19
AquaRain *http://www.aquarain. com*					
AquaRain 200	P, B	Gravity drip	Stacked bucket filter with 2 ceramic elements. Carbon core, stainless steel housing.	Small group	$189
AquaRain 400	P, B	Gravity drip	Bucket filter, 4 ceramic elements. Carbon core, stainless steel housing.	Large group	$199
British Berkfeld *http://www.jamesfilter. com*					
Big Berkey	P, B	Gravity drip	Bucket filter, 4 ceramic elements with carbon matrix. Available in stainless steel or lexan housing.	Large group	$249
LP-2	P, B	Gravity drip	Bucket filter, 2 ceramic elements. Plastic housing.	Small group	$145
General Ecology *http://www. generalecology.com*			Claims for viral removal are based on electrostatic attraction in Structured Matrix compressed carbon block filter. Variety of sizes and configurations also available for in-line use and electric powered units.		
Microlite	P	Hand pump	Intake strainer, GAV, Biocide tablets for suspected bacterial and viral contamination.	1–2 person	$30
First-Need Deluxe	P, B, V	Hand pump	Compressed charcoal.	Small group	$90
Base Camp	P, B, V	Hand pump or electric	Compressed charcoal element similar to First Need. High flow, high capacity. Stainless steel housing. Prefilter. Electric models also available.	Large group	$500
Trav-L-Pure	P, B	Hand pump	Same compressed charcoal filter element as First Need in plastic housing.	Small group	$150
Hydro-Photon *http://www.hydro-photon.com* Steri-Pen Classic	P, B, V	Handheld purifier	Ultraviolet purifier uses 4 AA batteries with timer. Active end of unit is held in bottle or other small container of water.	1–2 person	$150
Steri-pen traveler	P, B, V		Smaller and lighter than classic, uses 2 CR123 lithium batteries; optional solar charging case	1–2 person	$130 $49 (solar charger)
Katadyn *http://www.katadyn.com*			Unless otherwise specified, filter elements are 0.2 µm ceramic depth filter.		
Exstream Exstream XR	P, B, V	Sport bottle	Iodine resin with filter for protozoan cysts, and granular activated charcoal.	1–2 person	$45 $50
Hiker Guide	P	Hand pump	Pleated glass-fiber 0.3 µm filter with granular activated charcoal core and prefilter. For high-quality source water, removes "most" bacteria.	1–2 person	$60 $85

Basecamp	P, B	Gravity drip	Pleated glass fiber 0.3 μm with activated carbon. Reservoir bag with in-line filter.	Small group	$60
Mini	P, B	Hand pump	Ceramic filter with prefilter	1–2 person	$90
Pocket	P, B	Hand pump	Ceramic filter with prefilter	Small group	$190
Ceradyn Gravidyn	P, B	Gravity drip	Bucket filter, 3 ceramic candles; optional activated carbon core filters with Gravidyn.	Small–large group	$160 $190
Combi	P, B	Hand pump	Ceramic filter and activated carbon cartridge; can be converted for in-line faucet use.	Small group	$160
Expedition	P, B	Hand pump	Ceramic filter with intake prefilter. Stainless steel housing.	Large group	$890
Survivor 06 Survivor 35	P, B, V	Hand pump	Reverse osmosis filter. Desalinates as well as disinfects, for ocean survival. Very low flow rate. Power units available.	1–2 person	$750 $1900
MSR *http://www.msrcorp. com/filters*					
Sweetwater MicroFilter	P, B	Hand pump	0.2 μm depth filter with granular activated carbon and prefilter. Purifier solution (chlorine) as pretreatment to kill viruses.	Small group	$60
Miniworks EX	P, B	Hand pump	Ceramic filter with activated carbon core and prefilter.	Small group	$80
Waterworks EX	P, B	Hand pump	Ceramic filter with activated carbon core, prefilter, and third-stage membrane filter.	Small group	$160
Miox Purifier	P, B	Chemical purifier	Battery operated 1 × 6 inch device produces disinfectant through electrolysis of water and salt.	Small group	$130
Sawyer *http://www. sawyerproducts.com*					
Water filter	P, B	Sport bottle or in-line gravity drip	Hollow fiber filter, 0.1 μm. Drink-through water bottle, in-line gravity drip from reservoir bag, or faucet attachment.	1–2 person or small group	$50
Water purifier	P, B, V	Sport bottle or in-line gravity drip	Hollow fiber filter 0.02 μm membrane. Drink-through water bottle or in-line gravity drip from reservoir bag, or faucet attach.	1–2 person or small group	$120–150
Stern's Outdoor Products *http://www.stearnsinc. com/*					
Outdoors Filter Pump	P	Hand pump	Ceramic 0.5 μm filter and prefilter	1–2 person	$26
Outdoors High Flow	P	Gravity drip	Ceramic 0.5 μm filter with activated carbon core. Plastic collection bag.	Small group	$70
Timberline *http://www. timberlinefilters.com*					
Eagle	P, B	Hand pump	1 μm filter; ultralight and unbreakable.	1–2 person	$26
Basecamp	P	Gravity drip	2 μm filter; coated nylon reservoir bag.	Small group	$66

[a] This is not a comprehensive list. Models change frequently. Manufacturer site provided if it contains product information; otherwise, search manufacturer and brand with any major search engine to find large retail sites that provide detailed product information.
[b] P = protozoa, B = bacteria, V = viruses
[c] Consider additional features, such as flow rate, filter capacity, size, and filter weight.
[d] Prices vary.

to or less than the smallest dimension of the organism. These filters provide little volume for holding contaminants and thus clog rapidly, but they can be cleaned easily by washing and brushing without destroying the filter. Maze or depth filters depend on a long, irregular labyrinth to trap the organism, so they may have a larger pore or passage size. Contaminants adhere to the walls of the passageway or are trapped in the numerous dead-end tunnels. Granular media, such as sand or charcoal, diatomaceous earth, or ceramic filters, function as maze filters. A depth filter has a large holding capacity for particles and lasts longer before clogging but may be difficult to clean effectively because many particles are trapped deep in the filter. Flow can be partially restored to a clogged filter by back flushing or surface cleaning, which removes the larger particles trapped near the surface. Surface cleaning is highly effective for ceramic filters.

Little objective comparable data are available on different filters.[46,53] The ceramic filters have been tested most extensively and generally consistently perform well.[54–56] Some ceramic filters now remove 99–99.9% of viruses, but the fourth log required by water treatment units remains a challenge. First Need charcoal block filter (General Ecology, Exton, Pa.) and Sawyer Water Purifier microtubule filter (Sawyer, Safety Harbor, Fla.), have been able to meet the EPA standards for water purifiers, including 4-log removal of viruses.[52] Most of the filters containing iodine resins have been withdrawn from the market.

The semipermeable membranes in reverse-osmosis filters are inherently capable of removing viruses. A reverse-osmosis filter uses high pressure (100 to 800 psi) to force water through a semipermeable membrane that filters out dissolved ions, molecules, and solids.[33] This process can desalinate water as well as remove microbiologic contamination. If pressure or degradation causes breakdown of the membrane, treatment effectiveness is lost.

Small hand-pump reverse-osmosis units have been developed. Their high price and slow output currently prohibit use by land-based wilderness travelers, but they are important survival items for ocean travelers. Battery- or power-operated units are standard equipment on large ships. The U.S. Department of Defense uses large-scale mobile reverse-osmosis units for water treatment.[49]

For domestic use and in pristine protected watersheds where pollution is minimal and the main concerns are bacteria and cysts, filtration can be used as the only means of disinfection. However, for foreign travel and for surface water with high levels of human use or sewage contamination, most filters should not be used as the sole means of disinfection.[54] Additional treatment with heat or halogens before or after filtration guarantees effective virus removal. Filters are also useful as a first step to remove parasitic and *Cryptosporidium* organisms that have high resistance to halogens.

Table 8.12. Halogenation

Advantages	Disadvantages
Inexpensive	Potential toxicity (especially iodine)
Iodine and chlorine are widely available	Corrosive, stains clothing
Very effective for bacteria, viruses and most protozoa	Ineffective for *Cryptosporidium*
Taste can be removed	Imparts taste and odor
Flexible dosing	Flexibility requires understanding of disinfection principles
As easily applied to large quantities as small quantities	
Relative susceptibility of microorganisms to halogens	Bacteria > Viruses > Protozoa

Many different types of filter media, from sand to vegetable products to fabric, have been used throughout history in various parts of the world. Filtration using simple, available products is of interest for use in developing countries and in emergency situations.[41] Sand filtration, capable of removing turbidity and greater than 99% of organisms, can be improvised with stacked buckets or barrels. Rice hull ash, crushed charcoal, sponges, and various fabrics have all been used in filtration. Fine woven cotton fabric is effective at removing larger parasites, such as schistosoma cercariae, *Fasciola* species, and guinea worm larvae. Fine woven fabrics, such as sari material can filter out 99% of *Vibrio cholerae*, since the organism often adheres to algae.[57]

Halogens

Worldwide, chemical disinfection is the most widely used method for improving and maintaining microbiologic quality of drinking water and is well suited for use in the field. (Table 8.12) Chemical disinfectants used for water disinfection are strong oxidants. Halogens, chiefly chlorine and iodine, are the most common chemical disinfectants used in the field. In addition, chlorine dioxide is now available in small use applications. Extensive data support the efficacy of halogens. Studies of field technique that find failure of specific methods or products can usually be attributed to inadequate contact time in cold water or failure to clarify turbid water.[46,55,58]

Variables with Halogenation

Understanding the principal factors of halogen disinfection allows intelligent and flexible use[36,51,59] (Table 8.13).

Sensitivity to halogen is determined by the cell wall or capsule and the relative susceptibility of proteins to denaturation and oxidation.[51] Organisms, in order of

Table 8.13. Factors affecting halogen disinfection

	Effect	Compensation
Primary factors		
Concentration	Measured in milligrams per liter (mg/L) or the equivalent, parts per million (ppm); higher concentration increases rate and proportion of microorganisms killed.	Higher concentration allows shorter contact time for equivalent results. Lower concentration requires increased contact time.
Contact time	Usually measured in minutes; longer contact time ensures higher proportion of organisms killed.	Contact time is inversely related to concentration; longer time allows lower concentration.
Secondary Factors		
Temperature	Cold slows reaction time. Each 10°C increase in temperature increases inactivation rate at least twofold.	Some treatment protocols recommend doubling the dose (concentration) of halogen in cold water, but if time allows, exposure time can be increased instead, or the temperature of the water can be increased.[69]
Water contaminants, cloudy water (turbidity)	Halogen reacts with organic nitrogen compounds from decomposition of organisms and their wastes to form compounds with little or no disinfecting ability, effectively decreasing the concentration of available halogen. In general, turbidity increases halogen demand.	Doubling the dose of halogen for cloudy water is a crude means of compensation that often results in a strong halogen taste on top of the taste of the contaminants. A more rational approach is to first clarify water to reduce halogen demand.
Halogen demand	The amount of halogen reacting with these impurities.	In general, chlorine demand rises with increased turbidity. Clear water is assumed to have minimal demand (1 mg/L) and cloudy water high demand (3–5 mg/L).
Residual halogen concentration	The amount of active halogen remaining after halogen demand of the water is met. To achieve microbial inactivation in aqueous solution with a chemical agent, a residual concentration must be present for a specified contact time.	Testing chlorine residual in the wilderness with simple swimming pool test kits may be reasonable for large groups, but it is not practical for most. Smell of chlorine usually indicates some free residual. Color and taste of iodine can be used as indicators.
pH	The optimal pH for halogen disinfection is 6.5–7.5. As water becomes more alkaline, approaching pH 8.0, much higher doses of halogens are required.	Most surface water is neutral to slightly acidic, so compensating for pH is not necessary. Tablet formulations of halogen have the advantage of some buffering capacity.

increasing resistance to halogen disinfection, are enteric (vegetative) bacteria, viruses, protozoan cysts, bacterial spores, and parasitic ova. Review literature frequently attributes exaggerated resistance of *Giardia* to halogens. There are adequate data that demonstrate susceptibility of *Giardia* to halogens, given sufficient concentration and contact time.[24,58,60–62] *Cryptosporidium* oocysts differ greatly from other protozoan cysts and are highly resistant to halogens, 14 times more resistant that *Giardia* cysts.[63,64] Although halogens can achieve disinfection of *Cryptosporidium* in the field, this is not practical. Both *Cryptosporidium* and *Giardia* are susceptible to chlorine dioxide.[63,65] The relative potency of common disinfectants to inactivate waterborne microbes is ozone > chlorine dioxide > electrochemically generated mixed species oxidant > free chlorine or iodine > chloramine.

Chlorine

Chlorine is currently the preferred means of municipal water disinfection worldwide and the preference of CDC and WHO for individual household disinfection of drinking water. Extensive data support its use.[22]

The major disinfectant is hypochlorous acid (HOCl). Both calcium hypochlorite ($Ca[OCl]_2$) and sodium hypochlorite (NaOCl) readily dissociate in water to release HOCl.[22,36] Chloride ion (Cl^-, NaCl, or $CaCl_2$) is germicidally inactive. Chlorine reacts with ammonia (organic waste) to form chloramines that have weak disinfecting power. Chlorine has no known toxicity when used for water disinfection.

Free chlorine is the most widely available and affordable means of chemical water disinfectants.[6] For household or field water treatment, free chlorine can be obtained in liquid, granular, or tablet forms, or generated from electrolysis of salt (Tables 8.14 and 8.15).

Superchlorination–Dechlorination

The process of superchlorination–dechlorination uses high doses of chlorine (generally in the form of calcium hypochlorite) to achieve concentrations of 30–200 ppm of free chlorine. These extremely high levels are above

Table 8.14. Iodine and chlorine formulations and doses

Iodination techniques (added to 1 liter or quart of water)	Amount for 4 ppm	Amount for 8 ppm
Iodine tabs	1/2 tab	1 tab
Tetraglycine hydroperiodide		
EDWGT (emergency drinking water germicidal tablet)		
Potable Aqua		
Globaline 2% iodine solution (tincture)	0.2 ml 5 gtts	0.4 ml 10 gtts
10% povidone-iodine solution[a]	0.35 ml 8 gtts	0.70 ml 16 gtts
Saturated solution: iodine crystals in water	13 ml	26 ml
Saturated solution: iodine crystals in alcohol	0.1 ml	0.2 ml
Chlorination techniques	**Amount for 5 ppm**	**Amount for 10 ppm**
Sodium hypochlorite	0.1 ml	0.2 ml
Household bleach 5%	2 gtts	4 gtts
Calcium hypochlorite		
Redi Chlor (1/10 gm tab)		¼ tab/ 2 quarts
Sodium dichloroisocyanurate		
AquaClear		1 tab (8.5 mg NaDCC)
Chlorine plus flocculating agent		1 tab
Chlor-floc		

Measure with dropper (1 drop = 0.05 ml) or tuberculin syringe.
[a] Povidone-iodine solutions release free iodine in levels adequate for disinfection, but scant data are available.

Table 8.15. Recommendations for contact time with halogenations in the field

Concentration of halogen	Contact time in minutes at various water temperatures		
	5°C	15°C	30°C
2 ppm	240	180	60
4 ppm	180	60	45
8 ppm	60	30	15

Note: Data indicate that very cold water requires prolonged contact time with iodine or chlorine to kill *Giardia* cysts. These contact times have been extended from the usual recommendations in cold water to account for this and for the uncertainty of residual concentration.

the margin of safety for field conditions and rapidly kill all bacteria, viruses, and protozoa and could kill *Cryptosporidium* with overnight contact times. After contact time of at least 10–15 minutes, several drops of 30% hydrogen peroxide solution are added that reduces hypochlorite to chloride, forming calcium chloride (a common food additive), which has no taste or smell. Excess hydrogen peroxide reacts with water to form oxygen and water.

This is a good technique for highly polluted or cloudy water and for disinfecting large quantities. It is the best technique for storing water on boats or for emergency use. A high level of chlorine prevents growth of algae or bacteria during storage; water is then "dechlorinated" in needed quantities when ready to use.

The ingredients can be easily obtained and packaged in small Nalgene bottles. The two reagents must be kept tightly sealed to maintain their potency. Properly stored, calcium hypochlorite loses only 3–5% of available chlorine per year. Thirty percent hydrogen peroxide is corrosive and burns skin, so it should be used cautiously.

Sodium Hypochlorite

Household Bleach: Liquid household bleach is a hypochlorite solution that comes in various concentrations, usually 5.25%. This has the convenience of easy availability, low cost, high stability, and administration with a dropper. Sodium hypochlorite solutions are vulnerable to significant loss of available chlorine over time; stability is greatly affected by heat and light. If bleach containers break or leak in a pack, the liquid is corrosive and stains clothing.

Drinkwell from Katadyn (Katadyn Produkte AG, Switzerland; Katadyn North America, Minneapolis, Minn): 10 ml bottle can treat 100 liters using 3 drops/liter. It is stable for 3 years if stored at temperatures lower than 25°C (77°F).

SweetWater Viral Stop (Cascade Designs, Seattle, Wash): 2-oz squeeze dropper bottle.

Calcium Hypochlorite (Dry Chlorine)

Calcium hypochlorite is a stable, concentrated, dry source of hypochlorite that is commonly used for chlorination of swimming pools. It is widely available in tablets or tubs of granules through chemical supply or swimming pool supply stores.

Redi-Chlor (Continental Technologies, Little River, Kan): Tablets come in different sizes and can be broken in half or fourths to treat different quantities of water. Recommended dose results in 2–5 mg/L residual chlorine. Add more for very cold water or if a faint chlorine smell is not detected after contact time. Available in blister packs with fifty 0.1-g tablets to treat 1 gallon per tablet, or blister packs of fifty 0.25-g tablets to treat 5 gallons per tablet. This is a convenient source of hypochlorite, which can also be used for superchlorination.

Chlorination–Flocculation Tablets

Tablets contain alum and 1.4% available chlorine in the form of dichloroisocyanurate (sodium dichloro-s-triazinetrione) with proprietary flocculating agents. Bicarbonate in the tablets promotes rapid dissolution and acts as a buffer. One 600-mg tablet yields 8 mg/L of free chlorine.

Testing by the U.S. military demonstrated biocidal effectiveness similar to iodine tablets under most conditions.[66–68] Extended contact time was necessary for complete viral removal in some of the tests. Because of the ability to flocculate turbid water, the action was superior to iodine in some poor-quality water.

Chlor-floc (Deatrick & Associates, Alexandria, Va): Thirty tablets individually sealed in foil packets; weight 1.6 oz.; capacity: 30 L (8 gal). Chlor-Floc is widely available through military surplus and survival Web sites.

One tablet is utilized for the clarification and disinfection of 1 liter of water from polluted sources at temperatures of 25°C (77°F). At 5°C (41°F), use two 600-mg tablets to provide 2.8% available chlorine. To strain the sediment, pour the water through the cloth provided. The tablets are stable for 3 years if stored in their packaging out of the heat.

This is one of the individual field methods for U.S. military troops and suggested for potential use in developing countries by the WHO. It is an excellent one-step technique for cloudy and highly polluted water. Alum is a widely used flocculent that causes suspended sediment, colloids, and many microorganisms to clump, settle to the bottom and readily be filtered or strained. Most *Cryptosporidium* oocysts would be removed by the flocculation. Some chlorine reacts with contaminants and is inactivated. It is important to confirm some chlorine taste and smell at the end of the contact time. For added safety, prolong the contact times up to 1 hour contact time in cold polluted and dirty water.

In clear water without enough impurities to flocculate, the alum causes some cloudiness and the chlorine residual is strong. After treatment, water should be poured through a special cloth to remove floc and decrease turbidity.

Tablets lose effectiveness with exposure to heat, air, or moisture. To extend shelf life, many tablets are individually wrapped in foil.

PUR Purifier of Water (Proctor and Gamble, Cincinnati, Ohio): This new product is a packet with chlorination and flocculation powder now available to large relief organizations for use outside the United States in disaster and conflict situations. The company plans to begin distribution for individual users in the developing countries.

Sodium Dichloroisocyanurate

Sodium dichloroisocyanurate (NaDCC) is a stable, non-toxic chlorine compound that releases free active chlorine and forms a mildly acidic solution, which is optimal for hypochlorous acid, the most active disinfectant of the free chlorine compounds. Free chlorine is in equilibrium with the available chlorine that remains in compound, providing greater biocidal capacity. NaDCC is more stable and provides more free active chlorine than other available chlorine products for water disinfection.

Aquatabs (Global Hydration Water Treatment Systems, Kakabeka Falls, Ontario, Canada): Similar product may be available under the brand Aquaclear and Puritabs. Each tablet contains NaDCC in a paper–foil laminate. When dissolved in one liter of water, each effervescent tablet releases 10 mg of free chlorine, with 50% of the available chlorine remaining in compound and released as free chlorine is used up by halogen demand. Tablets are available in multiple strengths and can be broken to treat smaller quantities of water. Larger quantities are available in tubs. Aquatab also makes slow-dissolving tablets for larger quantities of water that contain trichloroisocynauric acid (TCCA), which acts similarly to NaDCC. The tablets have a 3-year shelf life; cost depends on size and quantity of tablets.

Surface water disinfection of clear water is accomplished at 10 mg/L in 10 minutes, 1 mg/L for tap water, and 2–5 mg/L for well water. NaDCC can also be used to wash fruits and vegetables in concentrations of 20 mg/L. This good source of chlorine is available in multiple dosage forms, including individually wrapped tablets. Larger concentration tablets allow for disinfection of large quantities of water and for shock chlorination of tanks and other storage systems.

Iodine

Iodine is effective in low concentrations for killing bacteria, viruses, and cysts, and in higher concentration against fungi and even bacterial spores, but it is a poor algicide.[51,69] Despite several advantages over chlorine disinfection, its use has been limited by concerns of its physiologic activity.

Only elemental (diatomic) iodine (I_2) and hypoiodous acid (HOI) play major roles as germicides. Their relative concentrations are determined by pH and concentration of iodine in solution; under field conditions, I_2 is the major disinfectant. Iodide (I^-) is important because it readily forms when reducing substances are added to iodine solution. This can be used to remove the taste of iodine as is discussed later. Iodide ion is without any effect for water disinfection and also has no taste or color, but is still physiologically active.

Iodine Toxicity

There is concern with iodine because of its physiologic activity, potential toxicity, and allergenicity. Iodine is an essential element for normal thyroid function and health in small amounts of 100–300 µg/day, but excess amounts can result in thyroid dysfunction. Although most persons can tolerate high doses of iodine without development of thyroid abnormalities,[70] iodine-induced hyperthyroidism can result from iodine ingestion by persons with underlying thyroid disease or when iodine is given to persons with prior iodine deficiency.[70,71] Iodine-induced hypothyroidism or goiter is much more common from excessive iodine intake, but the mechanism through which iodide goiter is produced is not well understood. Changes in thyroid function tests are common with excess iodine intake, but they usually remain within the range of normal values. Even when they are outside the normal range, changes in thyroid function remain subclinical, and values revert to normal within weeks to months without persistent thyroid disease.

Goiters were discovered among a group of Peace Corps volunteers in Africa and were linked epidemiologically to the use of iodine resin water filters. Forty-four (46%) of the volunteers had enlarged thyroids, but 30 of these had normal thyroid function tests.[72,73] Several studies have investigated prolonged ingestion of iodine in low concentrations and found minimal thyroid changes and no clinical problems.[74]

The EPA and the WHO, supported by the American Water Works Association (AWWA), have recommended iodine use for water disinfection only as an emergency measure for short periods of about 3 weeks. However, this period of short use appears arbitrary.

Data recently reviewed suggest the following guidelines as appropriate:[75]

- High levels of iodine (16–32 mg/day) such as those produced by the higher recommended doses of iodine tablets should be limited to short periods of 1 month or less.
- Iodine treatments that produce a low residual ≤1–2 mg/L appear safe, even for long periods of time in people with normal thyroid glands.
- Anyone planning to use iodine for prolonged periods should have their thyroid examined and thyroid function tests done to ensure that they are initially euthyroid. Optimally, repeat thyroid function test and examine for iodine goiter after 3–6 months of continuous iodine ingestion and monitor occasionally for iodine-induced goiter thereafter. If this is not feasible, assure low-level iodine consumption (see previous discussion) or use a different technique.

Certain groups should not use iodine for water treatment:

- Pregnant women (due to concerns of neonatal goiter)
- Individuals with known hypersensitivity to iodine
- Persons with a history of thyroid disease, even if controlled on medication
- Persons with a strong family history of thyroid disease (thyroiditis)
- Persons from countries with chronic iodine deficiency

Products and Techniques for Iodination

Iodine is available in solution, tablet, and crystals for field use (Table 8.14).

Iodine Solutions. Iodine solutions commercially sold as topical disinfectants are inexpensive and can be measured accurately with a dropper but are staining and corrosive if spilled. These solutions contain iodine, potassium, or sodium iodide in water, and ethyl alcohol or glycerol. Iodide improves stability and solubility but has no germicidal activity and adds to the total amount of iodine ingested and absorbed into the body. "Decolorized" iodine solution contains iodide and should not be used for water disinfection.

In aqueous solution, povidone-iodine provides a sustained-release reservoir of halogen; free iodine is released in water solution depending on the concentration (normally, 2–10 ppm is present in solution).[69]

Iodine Crystals (Saturated Solution). Because of limited solubility in water, iodine crystals may be used for disinfection. In one technique for field use, 4–8 g of crystalline iodine is put in a 1- to 2-oz bottle, which is then filled with water. A small amount of elemental iodine goes into solution (no significant iodide is present); the saturated solution is used to disinfect drinking water. Water can be added to the crystals hundreds of times before they are completely dissolved.

An alternative technique is to add 8 g of iodine crystals to 100 ml of 95% ethanol. Increased solubility of iodine in alcohol makes the solution less temperature dependent and allows much smaller volumes to be used (8 mg/0.1 ml), which can be measured with a 1 ml syringe or dropper (2 drops).

The stability and simplicity of iodine crystals have led to their testing for in-line systems that provide continuous water disinfection for remote households and small communities. In these designs, residual iodine is removed with GAC.

Polar Pure (Polar Equipment, Saratoga, Calif): 8 gm of iodine crystals in a 3-oz glass bottle filled with water; 30- to 50-μm fabric prefilter provided; capacity: 2,000 quarts; weight: 5 oz. The bottle cap (approximately 6.5 cc) is used to measure iodine solution. Directions and color dot thermometer are printed on the bottle. Recommended dose (2 capfuls if iodine solution is 20°C [68° F]) yields 4 ppm iodine when added to 1 quart of clean water. Contact time depends on temperature of the water to be consumed; warm water to 20°C (68° F) before adding iodine to shorten contact time.

Saturated aqueous solution of crystalline iodine is an excellent and stable source of iodine. Recommendations are adequate for clear, warm water; but because it is not feasible to warm all water, extend contact time 1–2 hours for very cold water. Temperature of the bottle affects the concentration of iodine in the saturated solution (200 ppm at 10°C [50°F], 300 ppm at 20°C [86°F], 400 ppm at 30°C [86°C]), which is the reason for the color-dot thermometer on the bottle. In the field, it may be easier to warm the bottle in an inner pocket than to estimate temperature and adjust the dose. The supernatant should be carefully decanted or filtered to avoid ingestion of the crystals; this is aided by the weight of the crystals, which causes them to sink and by a lip in the bottle to catch crystals when pouring off water. Many people prefer crystalline iodine because of its large disinfectant capacity, small size, and light weight; however, the glass bottle can break.

Iodine Tablets. The tablets used by the U.S. military and sold in the United States for water disinfection contain tetraglycine hydroperiodide, which is 40% I_2 and 20% iodide. Tetraglycine hydroperiodide was originally developed and chosen as a preferred technique by the military for individual field use because of its broad-spectrum disinfection effect, ease of handling, rapid dissolution, stability, and acceptable taste.[76,77]

Each tablet releases 8 mg/L of elemental iodine into water. An acidic buffer provides a pH of 6.5, which supports better cysticidal than virucidal capacity, but it should be adequate for both. Tablets have the advantages of easy handling and no danger of staining or corroding if spilled. They are stable for 4–5 years under sealed storage conditions and for 2 weeks with frequent opening under field conditions, but they lose 30% of the active iodine if bottles are left open for 4 days in high heat or humidity.

Potable Aqua (Wisconsin Pharmacal Co, Jackson, Wis.): 50 tablets; with P.A. Plus Neutralizing tablets, weight 2 oz; also sold as Globaline and EDWGT (emergency drinking water germicidal tablets): One tablet is added to 1 quart of water. In cloudy or cold water, add two tablets. Contact time is only 10–15 minutes in clear, warm water, much more in cold, cloudy water. "Neutralizing" tablets are made of ascorbic acid, which converts iodine to iodide, removing the taste and color.

This method was developed by the military for troops in the field. Advantages are unit dose and short contact time, but these concentrations create strong taste that is not acceptable to many wilderness users. The military requirements dictated a short contact time (10 minutes in clear, warm water), thus the relatively high concentration of iodine (8–16 ppm). With adequate contact time and moderate temperatures, one tablet can be added to 2 quarts of water to yield 4 ppm of free iodine. Rather than use two tablets in cloudy water, clarify the water first.

Iodine Resins

Iodine resins are considered demand disinfectants. The resin has low solubility, so that as water passes through, little iodine is released into aqueous solutions. On the other hand, when microorganisms contact the resin, iodine is transferred and binds to the microorganisms, apparently aided by electrostatic forces.[78,79] Bacteria and cysts are effectively exposed to high iodine concentrations, which allow reduced contact time compared with dilute iodine solutions. However, some contact time is necessary, especially for cysts. Resins have demonstrated effectiveness against bacteria, viruses, and cysts, but not against *Cryptosporidium parvum* oocysts or bacterial spores.[80]

Iodine resins are effective disinfectants that can be engineered into attractive field products, including large-scale units for international disasters. The effectiveness of the resin is highly dependent on the product design and function. A microfilter, generally 1 μm, effectively removes *Cryptosporidium*, *Giardia*, and other halogen-resistant parasitic eggs or larva to avoid prolonged contact time. Because iodine resins kill bacteria and viruses rapidly, no significant contact time is required for most water. Cloudy or sediment-laden water may clog the resin, as it would any filter, or coat the resin, inhibiting iodine transfer.

Several companies recently have abandoned iodine resin-containing portable hand-pump filters due to testing that demonstrated viral breakthrough, despite initial premarketing testing that passed the EPA protocol. It was not clear whether failure was related to inadequate contact with the resin or insufficient contact time with the iodine residual. Only one drink-through bottle remains on the U.S. market, but other products are still available via the Internet from outside the United States. Iodine resins may prove useful for small communities in undeveloped and rural areas where chlorine disinfection is technically and economically unfeasible.

Chlorine versus Iodine

A large body of data proves that both iodine and chlorine are effective disinfectants with adequate concentrations and contact times (cold temperatures equate with slow disinfection time for both). Chlorine and iodine tablets have been directly compared and found to be similar in their biocidal activity in most conditions using recommended dose and contact time.[66]

Iodine has several advantages over chlorine. Of the halogens, iodine has the lowest oxidation potential, reacts least readily with organic compounds, is least soluble, is least hydrolyzed by water, and is less affected by pH, all of which indicate that low iodine residuals should be more stable and persistent than corresponding concentrations of chlorine.[51,69] Taste tolerance or preference for iodine over chlorine is individual. Opposite preferences have been documented when direct comparisons are done.[67,81]

Improving Halogen Taste

Objectionable taste and smell limit the acceptance of halogens, but taste can be improved by several means. One method is to use the minimum necessary dose with a longer contact time. Several chemical means are available to reduce free iodine to iodide or chlorine to chloride, both of which have no color, smell, or taste. These chemical species also have no disinfection action, so these techniques should be used only after the required contact time. The best and most readily available agent is ascorbic acid (vitamin C), which is available in crystalline or powder form. A common ingredient of flavored drink mix, ascorbic acid accounts for their effectiveness in covering up the taste of halogens. Other safe and effective means of chemical reduction are sodium thiosulfate and hydrogen peroxide, which act as catalysts to reduce free iodine and chlorine through an electrochemical reaction. GAC will remove the taste of iodine and chlorine partially by adsorption and partially by chemical reduction. The relationship between halogen concentration and time allows use of the minimum necessary dose, with a longer contact time. Finally, alternative techniques such as filtration or heat that do not affect taste can be used in many situations.

MISCELLANEOUS DISINFECTANTS

Mixed Species Disinfection (Electrolysis)

Passing a current through a simple brine salt solution generates free available chlorine, as well as other "mixed species" disinfectants that have been demonstrated effective against bacteria, viruses, and bacterial spores.[82] The process can be used on both a large and a small scale. The resulting solution has greater disinfectant ability than a simple solution of sodium hypochlorite and has even been demonstrated to inactivate *Cryptosporidium*, suggesting that chlorine dioxide is among the chemicals generated.[83]

Miox Purifier (MSR, Seattle, Wash.): New technology created by the military uses salt, water, and electrical current generated from camera batteries to produce a mixed species disinfectant solution that is added to water. The kit comes with instrument, batteries, salt packet, indicator strips, instructions, and storage sack. Refills of salt cartridge are available. Weight of pen 3.5 oz, kit 8 oz. Add water, shake, and press a button. Solution generated is then added to drinking water. Inactivates all bacteria, viruses, and protozoa. Viruses and bacteria require dwell time of 15 min; *Giardia,* 30 min; *Cryptosporidium,* 4 hours. Can be used for individuals or groups. LED lights

indicate if there is a low battery or inadequate reagents (salt and water). Test strips are used to test water for adequate chemical residual.

The science has been known for some time and is used in large commercial processes, but it was not available previously in portable design. According to the instructions, the extended dwell time indicates low concentrations of the active disinfectant and the need to plan for prolonged contact time if *Cryptosporidium* is a strong concern. The high-technology approach will appeal to some, but it may be intimidating to others. The indicator lights and test strips add reassurance that the process is proceeding effectively. Although this technique can be used for large volumes, this instrument generates enough for only 1 liter at a time and may be cumbersome to use for larger volume containers.

Chlorine Dioxide

Chlorine dioxide (ClO_2), a potent biocide, has been used for many years to disinfect municipal water and for numerous other large-scale applications. Recently, it has gained wider use for disinfection of both community and point-of-use drinking water supplies in developed countries. Chlorine dioxide is capable of inactivating most waterborne pathogens, including Cryptosporidium parvum oocysts, at practical doses and contact times. [63,65] It is at least as effective a bactericide as chlorine; in many cases, it is superior. It is far superior as a virucide.[22] Chlorine dioxide does not produce a lasting residual.

Until recently, chlorine dioxide could be used only in large-scale water treatment applications, because it is a volatile gas that must be generated onsite by sophisticated equipment. Several new chemical methods for generating chlorine dioxide onsite can now be applied in the field for small quantity water treatment. Advantages of chlorine dioxide are greater effectiveness than chlorine at equivalent doses and the ability to inactivate *Cryptosporidium* oocysts with reasonable doses and contact times (Table 8.16).

Katadyn MicroPur MP-1 tablets (Katadyn Produkte AG, Switzerland; Katadyn North America, Minneapolis, Minn.): Chlorine dioxide release agent in various strength tablets, and powders that are EPA registered for a wide range of disinfection tasks.

These tablets generate chlorine dioxide in contact with water through a well-known acid chlorite reaction. Shortly after a tablet is immersed into water, a saturated solution of the soluble solid constituents forms within the matrix of the tablet. ClO_2 is rapidly formed within the pores and then carried into the bulk solution by CO_2 effervescence, which ensures that the resultant solution is well mixed without the user having to agitate the container. After the chlorine dioxide gas is released, the material reduces into common salts.

Table 8.16. Chlorine dioxide	
Advantages	**Disadvantages**
Effective against all microorganisms, including *Cryptosporidium*	Volatile, so do not expose tablets to air and use generated solutions rapidly
Low doses have no taste or color	No persistent residual, so does not prevent recontamination during storage
Portable device now available for individual and small group field use and simple to use	Sensitive to sunlight, so keep bottle shaded or in pack during treatment
More potent than equivalent doses of chlorine	
Less affected by nitrogenous wastes	
Relative susceptibility of microorganisms to chlorine dioxide	Bacteria > Viruses > Protozoa

Company testing shows killing of bacteria and viruses within 15 minutes in any water conditions, and inactivation of *Giardia* and *Cryptosporidium* within 30 minutes in clear warm water and 4 hours in cold and dirty water. One tablet is used for treating 1 quart of water. Instructions are to insert rapidly into water after removing from package and avoid exposure to sunlight during disinfection contact time.

The product is EPA registered as an antimicrobial water purifier. The extended contact time in cold, dirty water ensures that sufficient chlorine dioxide is generated and adequate residual remains for sufficient time to treat water in all conditions. It is more reasonable and provides a margin of safety to clarify the water to improve taste and esthetics and warm the water to reduce contact time. Company testing is well designed with multiple controls. They also have documentation that residual concentrations of chlorine dioxide were well maintained during the recommended contact times. Chlorine dioxide does not have extended persistence in water, so it should not be used to maintain microbiologic purity of stored water. Sunlight breaks down chlorine dioxide, so for optimal effect, keep the water bottle in a dark location, such as inside a pack or bag, during disinfection time.

AquaMira (McNett Corp, Bellingham, Wash.), **Pristine** (Pristine Water Treatment Systems, Port Coquitlam, BC, Canada): A stabilized solution of chlorine dioxide is mixed with phosphoric acid, which activates the chemical and is then mixed with water for disinfection. Contact times for inactivation of *Cryptosporidium* by Pristine range from 15 minutes in warm water using a triple dose to 7 hours using a single dose in very cold water. The two solutions are mixed together in a mixing cap and added to the water for treatment. Advantages include effectiveness across a broad range of water, temperature, and pH; no aftertaste or odor; unaffected by freezing. AquaMira is now also available in tablet form.

The chemistry of generating chlorine dioxide through a similar method is well described. The product is still pending EPA approval as a purifier in the United States. It does have limited approval now for bacteria. The Canadian product makes full claims, including *Cryptosporidium*. Testing data will be available from the company when EPA approval is obtained. Given the volatility of chlorine dioxide and slow reaction times, concentrations may be variable due to mixing process and time delay. The EPA delay is likely related to performance in cold and dirty "worst case" test water, which may be an issue in disaster situations, but it is not often encountered by wilderness users.

AquaMira has recently marketed tablets that are EPA registered as a purifier, making the pills preferred over the liquid.

Silver

Silver ion has bactericidal effects in low doses, but the literature on antimicrobial effects of silver is confusing and contradictory.[22,51,84] Water disinfection systems using silver have been devised for spacecraft, swimming pools, and other settings.[22]

The advantage is absence of taste, odor, and color. Short-term field use is limited by its marked tendency to adsorb onto the surface of any container (resulting in unreliable concentrations) and interference by several common substances. Because silver is physiologically active and permanent discoloration of the skin and mucous membranes may result from prolonged use, a maximum limit of 50 ppb of silver ion in potable water is recommended. At this concentration, disinfection requires several hours. Persistence of residual silver concentration allows reliable storage of disinfected water. Silver impregnation of filters neither prevents microbial contamination of the filter nor sustains its action as a bactericide in the effluent water.[85]

The use of silver as a drinking water disinfectant has been much more popular in Europe where silver tablets are sold widely for field water disinfection. They have not been approved by the EPA for this purpose in the United States, but they were approved as a water preservative to prevent bacterial growth in previously treated and stored water.

MicroPur Forte tablets from Katadyn: Widely available in Europe, but not marketed in United States, these tablets contain silver and sodium hypochlorite. The chlorine kills viruses, bacteria, and *Giardia*. The silver adds to the disinfection capacity, as well as preventing recontamination if water is stored for up to 6 months. Contact time is 20–120 minutes, depending on the temperature of the water. Shelf life is 2 years, stored in cool dry conditions. It is available as tablets or liquid. This is a rational combination for water that will be stored for some period of time.

MicroPur from Katadyn: This product releases silver ions. It is available in two sizes of tablets (for 1 quart or 5 quarts), liquid (10 drops/gal), or crystals for treating larger quantities of water. In addition to poorly documented effects on all many different types of microorganisms, there is some difficulty controlling the residual concentration and concern over chronic effects. This product makes no claims for viruses and protozoa because concentrations may not be adequate to kill these organisms. It has been approved by the EPA to be marketed in the United States as a "water preservative" to maintain bacteria-free water for up to 6 months.

Potassium Permanganate

Potassium permanganate is a strong oxidizing agent with some disinfectant properties. It was used extensively before hypochlorites as a drinking water disinfectant. It is still used for this purpose and also for washing fruits and vegetables in parts of the world. It is usually employed in a 1–5% solution for disinfection.

Bacterial inactivation can be achieved with moderate concentrations and contact times, but it cannot be recommended for field use because quantitative data are not available for viruses or protozoan cysts, despite the chemical's frequent use in some parts of the world. Packets of 1 g to be added to 1 L of water are sold in some countries. A French military guide from 1940 instructed users: "To sterilize water, use a solution of 1 gram of $KMnO_4$ for 100 grams of water. Add this solution drop by drop to the water to sterilize until the water becomes pink. The operation is considered sufficient if the water remains pink for half an hour." The solutions are deep pink to purple and stain surfaces.

Hydrogen Peroxide

Hydrogen peroxide is a strong oxidizing agent but a weak disinfectant.[86] Small doses (1 ml of 3% H_2O_2 in 1 L water) are effective for inactivating bacteria within minutes to hours, depending on the level of contamination. Viruses require high doses and longer contact times. Although information is lacking on the effect of hydrogen peroxide on protozoa, it is a promising sporicidal agent in very high (10–25%) concentrations.

Hydrogen peroxide is popular as a wound cleanser; for odor control in sewage, sludges, and landfill leachates; and for many other applications. It is considered safe enough for use in foods, yielding the innocuous end products oxygen and water; it is considered nature's disinfectant because it is naturally present in milk and honey, helping to prevent spoilage.

Lack of data for protozoal cysts and quantitative data for dilute solutions prevents it from being useful by itself as a field water disinfectant.

Ultraviolet Light

Ultraviolet (UV) lamp disinfection systems are widely used to disinfect drinking water at the community and household level. In sufficient doses, all waterborne enteric pathogens are inactivated by UV radiation. Bacteria and protozoan parasites require lower doses than enteric viruses and bacterial spores. *Giardia* and *Cryptosporidium* are susceptible to practical doses of UV and may be more sensitive because of their relatively large size.[87] The germicidal effect of UV light depends on light intensity and exposure time. UV treatment does not require chemicals and does not affect the taste of the water. It works rapidly, and extra dosing to the water presents no danger; in fact, it is a safety factor. UV irradiation with lamps requires a power source and is costly. UV light has no residual disinfection power; water may become recontaminated, or regrowth of bacteria may occur.[54] Particulate matter can shield microorganisms from UV rays (Table 8.17).

Steri-Pen (Hydro-Photon Inc, Blue Hill, Me.): Portable, battery-operated ultraviolet water disinfection system disinfects up to 16 oz of clear water in less than one minute and 32 oz in 90 seconds by stirring the UV element in water. Uses 4 AA batteries (disposable or rechargeable: alkaline batteries provide 20–40 treatments; lithium batteries, 130–140 treatments); weight 8 oz, with batteries; length 7.6 inches; width 1.5 inches; lamp lasts 5,000 treatments (625 gallons). It comes with a nylon carrying case, and a prefilter is available for removing particulate matter. It has a dosage selector for 16- or 32-oz water treatment. A new product design (SteriPEN Adventurer) is smaller and lighter, uses two CR123 batteries, and has

Table 8.17. Ultraviolet irradiation

Advantages	Disadvantages
Effective against all microorganisms	Requires clear water
Imparts no taste	Does not improve water esthetics
	Does not prevent recontamination during storage
Portable device now available for individual and small group field use and simple to use	Expensive
	Requires power source
Available from sunlight	Requires direct sunlight, prolonged exposure; dose low and uncontrolled
Relative susceptibility of microorganisms to ultraviolet	Protozoa > Bacteria > Viruses

an optional solar recharging panel on the case for use with rechargeable batteries.

Microbiological testing conducted at the University of Arizona, the University of Maine, the Oregon Health Sciences University, and Hydro-Photon against multiple types of bacteria, viruses, *Giardia,* and *Cryptosporidium* shows that SteriPEN meets the standard as set forth in the U.S. EPA Guide Standard and Protocol for Testing Microbiological Water Purifiers, destroying in excess of 99.9999% of bacteria, 99.99% of viruses, and 99.9% of protozoa and *Cryptosporidium* oocysts.

In general, UV light for water disinfection is well established and widely used for water treatment in many large and varied applications. Until now, these have required a larger, fixed power and light source. The use of this portable technology is currently limited to small volumes of clear water; however, the potential is great for further advances that will increase its uses in the field and make it less expensive. The testing for this device can be found on their Web site. Testing was only successful in clear water, not in EPA "worst case scenario" water unless prefiltered with microfiltration. The simplicity and rapidity of this technique is appealing.

Solar Irradiation

UV irradiation by sunlight in UV-A range can substantially improve microbiologic quality of water and reduce diarrheal illness in developing countries. Recent work has confirmed efficacy and optimal procedures of the solar disinfection (SODIS) technique.[41,88,89] Transparent bottles (e.g., clear plastic beverage bottles), preferably lying on a dark surface, are exposed to sunlight for a minimum of 4 hours, but some investigations demonstrate improved benefit from several sequential days. Oxygenation induces greater reductions of bacteria, so agitation is recommended before solar treatment in bottles.

UV and thermal inactivation are synergistic for solar disinfection of drinking water in transparent plastic bottles. Above 55°C (131°F), thermal inactivation is of primary importance. Use of a simple reflector or solar cooker can achieve temperatures of 65°C (149°F), which will pasteurize the water (see previous discussion of heat disinfection).

Where strong sunshine is available, solar disinfection of drinking water is an effective, low-cost method for improving water quality and may be of particular use in refugee camps and disaster areas.

Citrus

Citrus juice has biocidal properties. Lemon or lime juice has been shown to destroy *V. cholerae* at a concentration of 2% (equivalent of 2 tablespoons per liter of water) with a contact time of 30 minutes. A pH less than 3.9 is essential, which depends on the concentration of lemon juice and the initial pH of the water. Lime juice also killed 99.9% of cholerae on cabbage and lettuce and inhibited growth of *V. cholera* in rice foods, suggesting that adding sufficient lime juice to water, beverages, and other foods can reduce disease risks.[41] More research is needed before this can be recommended as more than an ancillary or emergency measure. Commercial products using citrus cannot yet be recommended as primary means of water disinfection.

PREFERRED TECHNIQUE

The optimal technique for an individual or group depends on the number of persons to be served, space and weight available, quality of source water, personal taste preferences, and availability of fuel (Tables 8.18, 8.19, and 8.20). The most effective technique may not always be available, but all methods will greatly reduce the load of microorganisms and reduce the risk of illness. The preferred method of treatment for the military, when large-scale equipment can be brought to the site, is reverse osmosis water purification unit because it can produce high-quality water from a low-quality source. For smaller groups, the military relies mainly on monitored chlorine. Individual means include iodine tablets, chlor-floc tabs, and chlorine liquid bleach.[49]

The only limitation for halogens is *Cryptosporidium* cysts, but in high-quality pristine surface water, the cysts are generally found in insufficient numbers to pose significant risk. Chlorine dioxide is currently the only one-step chemical processes available. Any surface water in undeveloped countries where there is human and animal activity should be considered contaminated with enteric

Table 8.18. Summary of effectiveness of field water disinfection techniques

	Bacteria	Viruses	Giardia/ Ameba	Cryptosporidium	Nematodes/ Cercarea
Heat	+	+	+	+	+
Filtration	+	+/−[a]	+	+	+
Halogens	+	+	+	-	+/−[b]
Chlorine dioxide	+	+	+	+	+/−[b]

[a] Most filters make no claims for viruses. Reverse osmosis is effective. General Ecology and Sawyer Purifier have test data to support virus removal.

[b] Eggs are not very susceptible to halogens but have very low risk of waterborne transmission.

Table 8.19. Choice of method for various source water

Source Water	"Prisitine" wilderness water with little human or domestic animal activity	Tap water in developing country	Developed or developing country	
			Clear surface water near human and animal activity [a]	Cloudy water
Primary concern	Giardia, enteric bacteria	Bacteria, Giardia, small numbers of viruses	All enteric pathogens, including Cryptosporidium	All enteric pathogens
Effective methods	Any single-step method[b]	Any single-step method[b]	1. Heat 2. Filtration plus halogen (can be done in either order); iodine resin filters (see text) 3. Chlorine dioxide 4. Ultraviolet (commercial product, not sunlight)	CF followed by second step (heat, filtration, or halogen)

CF = Coagulation–flocculation
[a] Includes agricultural runoff with cattle grazing, or sewage treatment effluent from upstream villages or towns.
[b] Includes heat, filtration, halogens, chlorine dioxide, or ultraviolet.

pathogens. Optimal protection requires either heat or a two-stage process of filtration and halogens. Currently First Need, the Exstream iodine resin-containing water bottle, and Sawyer Viral Purifier are the only filters with test-supported claims to meet requirements for viral removal.

Water from cloudy low-elevation rivers, ponds, and lakes in developed or undeveloped countries that does not clear with sedimentation should be pretreated with coagulation–flocculation, and then disinfected with heat or halogens. Filters can be used but will clog rapidly with silted or cloudy water. Even in the United States, water with agricultural runoff or sewage plant discharge from upstream towns or cities must be treated to remove *Cryptosporidium* and viruses. In addition, water receiving agricultural, industrial, or mining runoff may contain chemical contamination from pesticides, other chemicals, and heavy metals. A filter containing a charcoal element is the best method to remove most chemicals.

Halogens need to be used when water will be stored, such as on a boat, in a large camp, or for disaster relief. When only heat or filtration is used before storage, recontamination and bacterial growth can occur. Hypochlorite has advantages, including cost, ease of handling, and minimal volatilization in tightly covered containers.[90] A minimum residual of 3–5 mg/L should be maintained in the water. Superchlorination–dechlorination is especially useful in this situation because high levels of chlorination can be maintained for long periods, and when ready for use, the water can be poured into a smaller container and dechlorinated.

For prolonged storage, a tightly sealed container is best. Narrow-mouth jars or containers with water spigots prevent contamination from repeated contact with hands or utensils.[6,91]

On oceangoing vessels where water must be desalinated during the voyage, only reverse-osmosis membrane filters are adequate. Halogens or silver should then be added to the water in the storage tanks.

PREVENTION AND SANITATION

Studies in developing countries have demonstrated a clear benefit in the reduction of diarrheal illness and other infections from safe drinking water, hygiene, and adequate sanitation.[6,7] Wilderness travelers essentially live in conditions similar to the developing world, without running water or sanitation. Unfortunately, many wilderness travelers confuse the importance of hygiene with the need to relax their concern about living on the ground.

A study of Appalachian Trail hikers showed that water disinfection, routine handwashing, and proper cookware cleaning were all associated with decreased diarrhea.[92] A *Shigella* outbreak among river rafters on the Colorado River was finally traced to infected guides who were shedding organisms in the stool and contaminating food through poor hygiene.[93] Personal hygiene, mainly handwashing, prevents spread of infection from food contamination during preparation of meals.[93] A widely publicized study in the United States demonstrated that only 67% of Americans wash hands after using a public toilet. Simple handwashing with soap and water purified

Table 8.20. Summary of advantages and disadvantages of disinfection techniques

	Heat	Filtration	Halogens	Chlorine dioxide	Two-step process	UV
Availability	Wood can be scarce	Many commercial choices	Many common and specific products	Several new products generate ClO$_2$	Filtration plus halogen or clarification plus second stage	New portable commercial device; sunlight
Cost	Fuel and stove costs	Moderate expense	Cheap	Depends on method, generally inexpensive	Depends on choice of stages	Commercial device relatively expensive
Effectiveness	Can sterilize or pasteurize	Most filters not reliable for viruses	*Cryptosporidium* and some parasitic eggs are resistant	All organisms	Highly effective, should cover all organisms	All organisms
Optimal application	Clear water	Clear or slightly cloudy; turbid water clogs filters rapidly	Clear; need increased dose if cloudy	Clear water, but ClO$_2$ less affected by nitrogenous compounds	May be adapted to any source water	Requires clear water, small volumes
Taste	Does not change taste	Can improve taste, especially if charcoal stage	Tastes worse unless remove or "neutralize" halogen	Unchanged, may leave some chlorine taste	Depends on sequence and choice of stages: generally improves	Unchanged
Time	Boiling time (minutes)	Filtration time (minutes)	Contact time (minutes to hours)	Prolonged hours, if need to ensure *Cryptosporidium* disinfection	Combination of time for each stage	Minutes
Other considerations	Fuel is heavy and bulky	Adds weight and space; requires maintenance to keep adequate flow	Works well for large quantities and for water storage; some understanding of principles is optimal; damaging if spills or container breaks	More experience and testing would be reassuring. Likely to replace iodine for field use.	More rational to use halogens first if filter has charcoal stage; C-F is best means of cleaning very turbid water followed by halogen, filtration, or heat	Sunlight for emergency situations with no other method available; commercial product for high-quality source water and small groups

with hypochlorite (bleach) significantly reduced fecal contamination of market-vended beverages in Guatemala.[94] No one with a diarrheal illness should prepare food.

Sanitation should extend to the kitchen or food preparation area. In addition to handwashing, dishes and utensils should be disinfected by rinsing in chlorinated water, prepared by adding enough household bleach to achieve a distinct chlorine odor.[95]

Prevention of food-borne contamination is also important in preventing enteric illness. Washing fruits and vegetables in purified water is a common practice, but little data support its effectiveness. Washing has a mechanical action of removing dirt and microorganisms while the disinfectant kills microorganisms on the surface. However, neither reaches the organisms that are embedded in surface crevices or protected by other particulate matter.[96] Chlorine, iodine, or potassium permanganate are often used for this purpose. Higher concentrations can be used than would normally be palatable for drinking water.

The ultimate responsibility is proper sanitation to prevent contamination of water supplies from human waste. Leaving feces in the open for UV disinfection is not reliable, and feces may wash into the watershed with rain runoff. Moreover, it will be repulsive to other campers. In the Sierras, feces left on the ground generally disappeared within 1 month, but it was not known whether disinfection occurred before decomposition or whether the feces washed away, dried, or were blown in the wind.[97] Despite more rapid decomposition in sunlight rather than underground, burying feces is still preferable in areas that receive regular use.

In the soil, microorganisms can survive for months. A Sierra Club study found more prolonged survival in alpine environments.[97] Microorganisms may percolate through the soil. Most bacteria are retained within 20 inches of the surface, but in sandy soil this increases to 75–100 feet;[49] viruses can move laterally 75–302 feet.[98] When organisms reach groundwater, their survival is prolonged, and they often appear in surface water or wells.

The U.S. military and U.S. Forest Service recommend burial of human waste 8–12 inches deep and a minimum of 100 feet from any water. Decomposition is hastened by mixing in some dirt before burial. Shallow burying is not recommended because animals are more likely to find and overturn the feces. Judgment should be used to determine a location that is not likely to allow water runoff to wash organisms into nearby water sources. Groups larger than three persons should dig a common latrine to avoid numerous individual potholes and inadequate disposal. To minimize latrine odor and improve its function, it should not be used for disposal of wastewater.

In some areas the number of individual and group latrines is so great that the entire area becomes contaminated. Therefore sanitary facilities (outhouses) are becoming common in high-use wilderness areas. Popular river canyons require camp toilets, and all waste must be carried out in sealed containers.

REFERENCES

1 Theron J, Cloete TE. Emerging waterborne infections: contributing factors, agents, and detection tools. *Crit Rev Microbiol.* 2002;28(1):1–26.
2 EPA. *National Water Quality Inventory Report.* Environmental Protection Agency; 2000.
3 Craun G. *Waterborne Disease in the United States.* Boca Raton, Fla.: CRC Press,1986.
4 CDC. Ten great public health achievements – United States 1900–1999. *MMWR.* April 2, 1999;48(12):241–3.
5 Schoenen D. Role of disinfection in suppressing the spread of pathogens with drinking water: possibilities and limitations. *Water Res.* 2002;36:3874–88.
6 Sobsey M, Handzel T, Venczel L. Chlorination and safe storage of household drinking water in developing countries to reduce waterborne disease. *Water Sci Technol.* 2003;47(3):221–8.
7 Quick RE, Kimura A, Thevos A, et al. Diarrhea prevention through household-level water disinfection and safe storage in Zambia. *Am J Trop Med Hyg.* 2002;66(5):584–9.
8 Rockwell RL. *Giardia lamblia* and Giardiasis with particular attention to the Sierra Nevada. *Sierra Nature Notes (Yosemite Association).* 2002;2.
9 Welsh T. Evidence-based medicine in the wilderness: the safety of backcountry water. *Wilderness Environmental Med.* 2005;15:235–7.
10 Hurst C, Clark R, Regli S. Estimating the risk of acquiring infectious disease from ingestion of water. In: Hurst C, ed. *Modeling Disease Transmission and Its Prevention by Disinfection.* Melbourne: Cambridge University Press; 1996: 99–139.
11 CDC. Protracted outbreaks of Cryptosporidiosis associated with swimming pool use – Ohio and Nebraska, 2000. *MMRW.* 2001;50(May 25):406–10.
12 Feldman K, Mohle-Boetani J, Ward J, et al. A cluster of *Escherichia coli* O157: non-motile infections associated with recreational exposure to lake water. *Public Health Reports.* July–August 2002;117: 380–5.
13 World Health Organization. *The Global Water Supply and Sanitation Assessment 2000.* Geneva: WHO and UNICEF; 2000.
14 Ford TE. Microbiological safety of drinking water: United States and global perspectives. *Environmental Health Perspectives.* 1999;107(Suppl 1):191–206.
15 Pruss A, Kay D, Fewtrell L, Bartram J. Estimating the burden of disease from water, sanitation, and hygiene at a global level. *Environ Health Perspect.* May 2002;110(5):537–42.
16 Chaudhuri M, Sattar S. Domestic water treatment for developing countries. In: McFeters G, ed. *Drinking Water Microbiology.* New York: Springer-Verlag; 1990.
17 Rose J, Gerba C, Jakubowski W. Survey of potable water supplies for *Cryptosporidium* and *Giardia. Environ Sci Technol.* 1991;25:1393–1400.

18 CDC. Surveillance for waterborne-disease outbreaks – United States, 1999–2000. *MMWR*. November 22, 2002;51(SS-8): 1–48.

19 Derlet RW, Carlson JR. An analysis of wilderness water in Kings Canyon, Sequoia, and Yosemite national parks for coliform and pathologic bacteria. *Wilderness Environ Med*. Winter 2004;15(4):238–44.

20 Derlet RW, Carlson JR, Noponen MN. Coliform and pathologic bacteria in Sierra Nevada national forest wilderness area lakes and streams. *Wilderness Environ Med*. Winter 2004;15(4):245–249.

21 Gerba C, Rose J. Viruses in source and drinking water. In: McFeters G, ed. *Drinking Water Microbiology*. New York: Springer-Verlag; 1990: 380–99.

22 White G. *Handbook of Chlorination*. 3rd. ed. New York: Van Nostrand Reinhold; 1992.

23 Marshall M, Naumovitz D, Ortega Y, Sterling C. Waterborne protozoan pathogens. *Clin Microbiol Rev*. 1997;10:67–85.

24 Hibler C, Hancock C. Waterborne giardiasis. In: McFeters G, ed. *Drinking Water Microbiology*. New York: Springer-Verlag; 1990: 380–99.

25 Monzingo D, Stevens D. *Giardia* contamination of surface waters: a survey of three selected backcountry streams in Rocky Mountain National Park. Fort Collins, CO: National Park Service; 1986.

26 Suk T, Sorenson S, Dileanis P. The relation between human presence and occurrence of *Giardia* cysts in streams in the Sierra Nevada, California. *J Freshwater Ecol*. 1988:4.

27 Bemrick W. Some perspectives on the transmission of giardiasis. In: Erlandsen S, Meyer E, eds. *Giardia and Giardiasis: Biology, Pathogenesis and Epidemiology*. New York: Plenum Press; 1984.

28 Rose J. Occurrence and control of *Cryptosporidium* in drinking water. In: McFeters G, ed. *Drinking Water Microbiology*. New York: Springer-Verlag; 1990:294–322.

29 LeChevallier MW, Norton WD, Lee RG. Occurrence of *Giardia* and *Cryptosporidium* spp. in surface water supplies. *Appl Environ Microbiol*. 1991;57(9):2610–16.

30 Zell S. Epidemiology of wilderness-acquired diarrhea: implications for prevention and treatment. *J Wilderness Med*. 1992;3:241–49.

31 Porter J, et al. *Giardia* transmission in a swimming pool. *AJPH*. 1988;78:659.

32 Geldreich E. Microbiological quality of source waters for water supply. In: McFeters G, ed. *Drinking Water Microbiology*. New York: Springer-Verlag; 1990:3–32.

33 U.S. Environmental Protection Agency Drinking Water Health Effects Task Force. *Health Effects of Drinking Water Treatment Technologies*. Chelsea: Lewis Publisher; 1989.

34 Dickens D, Dupont HL, Johnson P. Survival of bacterial enteropathogens in the ice of popular drinks. *JAMA*. 1985; 253:3141–3.

35 Steiner T, Thielman N, Guerrant R. Protozoal agents: what are the dangers for the public water supply? *Annu Rev Med*. 1997;48:329–40.

36 Laubusch E. Chlorination and other disinfection processes. *Water Quality and Treatment: A Handbook of Public Water Supplies*. New York: McGraw Hill; 1971.

37 Joslyn L. Sterilization by heat. In: Block S, ed. *Disinfection, Sterilization, and Preservation*. 4th ed. Philadelphia: Lea and Febiger; 1991:495–527.

38 Frazier W, Westhoff D. *Preservation by use of high temperatures*. New York: McGraw-Hill; 1978.

39 Groh C, MacPherson D, Groves D. Effect of heat on the sterilization of artificially contaminated water. *J Travel Med*. 1996;3:11–13.

40 Alder V, Simpson R. Sterilization and disinfection by heat methods. In: Russel A, Hugo W, Ayliffe G, eds. *Principles and Practice of Disinfection, Preservation, and Sterilization*. 2nd ed. Oxford: Blackwell Scientific; 1992:483.

41 Sobsey M. Managing water in the home: accelerated health gains from improved water supply. Geneva: World Health Organization; 2003. WHO/SDE/WSH/02.07.

42 CDC. *Health Information for International Travel 2005–2006*. Atlanta: U.S. Department of Health and Human Services, Public Health Service; 2005.

43 Bandres J, Mathewson J, DuPont H. Heat susceptibility of bacterial enteropathogens. *Arch Intern Med*. 1988;148: 2261–3.

44 Joyce T, McGuigan K, Elmore-Meegan M, Conroy R. Inactivation of fecal bacteria in drinking water by solar heating. *Appl Environ Microbiol*. 1996;62:399–402.

45 McGuigan KG. Solar disinfection: use of sunlight to decontaminate drinking water in developing countries. *J Med Microbiol*. 1999;48:785–7.

46 Schlosser O, Robert C, Bourderioux C, Rey M, de Roubin MR. Bacterial removal from inexpensive portable water treatment systems for travelers. *J Travel Med*. 2001;8:12–18.

47 Rao V, et al. Removal of hepatitis A virus and rotavirus by drinking water treatment. *J Am Water Works Assoc*. 1988; 82:59–67.

48 Binnie C, Kimber M, Smethurst G. *Basic Water Treatment*. 3rd ed. London: IWA; 2002.

49 U.S. Army. *Sanitary Control and Surveillance of Field Water Supplies*. Washington, DC: Departments of the Army, Navy, and Air Force; 1999. Dept. of Army Technical Bulletin (TB Med 577).

50 Le Chevallier M, McFeters G. Microbiology of activated carbon. In: McFeters G, ed. *Drinking Water Microbiology*. New York: Springer-Verlag; 1990:104–20.

51 National Academy of Sciences Safe Drinking Water Committee. The disinfection of drinking water. *Drinking Water and Health*. 1980;2:5–139.

52 Gerba C, Naranjo J. Microbiological water purification without the use of chemical disinfection. *Wilderness Environ Med*. 2000;11:12–16.

53 U.S. Army. *Preventive Medicine Concerns of Hand Held Water Treatment Devices*. Aberdeen Proving Ground, Md.: U.S. Army Center for Health Promotion and Preventive Medicine; March 10, 2003. Water Quality Information Paper No 31–032.

54 Environmental Health Directorate Health Protection Branch. Assessing the effectiveness of small filtration systems for point-of-use disinfection of drinking water supplies. Ottawa: Department of National Health and Welfare; 1980. 80-EHD-54.

55 Ongerth J, Johnson R, MacDonald S, Frost F, Stibbs H. Backcountry water treatment to prevent giardiasis. *AJPH*. 1989;79:1633–7.

56 Tobin R. Testing and evaluating point-of-use treatment devices in Canada. *J Am Water Works Assoc*. 1987;79:42–45.

57 Huo A, Xu B, Chowdhury MA, Islam MS, Montilla R, Colwell RR. A simple filtration method to remove plankton-associated *Vibrio cholerae* in raw water supplies in developing countries. *Appl Environ Microbiol*. 1996;62(7): 2508–12.

58 Jarroll E, Hoff J, Meyer E. Resistance of cysts to disinfection agents. In: Erlandsen S, Meyer E, eds. *Giardia and Giardiasis: Biology, Pathogenesis and Epidemiology*. New York: Plenum Press; 1984:311.

59 Dychdala G. Chlorine and chlorine compounds. In: Block S, ed. *Disinfection, Sterilization, and Preservation*. 4th ed. Philadelphia: Lea & Febiger; 1991:131–52.

60 Sobsey M, Fuji T, Hall R. Inactivation of cell-associated and dispersed hepatitis A virus in water. *J Am Water Works Assoc*. 1991;83:64–7.

61 Jarroll E, Bingham A, Meyer E. *Giardia* cyst destruction: effectiveness of six small water disinfection methods. *Am J Trop Med Hyg*. 1980; 29:8–11.

62 Gerba C, Johnson D, Hasan M. Efficacy of iodine water purification tablets against *Cryptosporidium* oocysts and *Giardia* cysts. *Wilderness Environ Med*. 1997;8:96–100.

63 Korich DG, Mead JR, Madore MS, Sinclair NA, Sterling CR. Effects of ozone, chlorine dioxide, chlorine, and monochloramine on *Cryptosporidium parvum* oocyst viability. *Appl Environ Microbiol*. May 1990;56(5):1423–1428.

64 Carpenter C, Fayer R, Trout J, Beach MJ. Chlorine disinfection of recreational water for *Cryptosporidium parvum*. *Emerg Infect Dis*. 1999;5(4):579–84.

65 Clark RM, Sivagnesan M, Rice EW, Chen J. Development of a Ct equation for the inactivation of *Cryptosporidium* oocysts with chlorine dioxide. *Water Res*. 2003;37:2773–83.

66 Powers E. Efficacy of flocculating and other emergency water purification tablets. Natick, Mass: U.S. Army Natick Research, Development and Engineering Center; 1993. Report Natick/TR-93/033.

67 Powers E, Hernandez C. Efficacy of Aquapure emergency water purification tablets. Natick, Mass: U.S. Army Natick Research, Development and Engineering Center; 1992. Technical Report Natick/TR-92/027.

68 Powers E, Boutros C, Harper B. Biocidal efficacy of a flocculating emergency water purification tablet. *Appl Environ Microbiol*. 1994;60:2316–23.

69 Gottardi W. Iodine and iodine compounds. In: Block S, ed. *Disinfection, Sterilization, and Preservation*. 4th. ed. Philadelphia: Lea & Febiger; 1991:152–67.

70 Braverman L. Iodine and the thyroid: 33 years of study. *Thyroid*. 1994;4:351–5.

71 Roti E, Vagenakis A. Effect of excess iodide: clinical aspects. In: Braverman L, Utiger R, eds. *Werner and Ingbar's The Thyroid*. Philadelphia: Lippincott-Raven; 1996.

72 Kettel-Khan L, Li R, Gootnick D, et al. Thyroid abnormalities related to iodine excess from water purification units. *Lancet*. 1998;352:1519.

73 Goodyer L, Behrens RH. Safety of iodine based water sterilization for travelers. *J Travel Med*. January 2000;7(1):38.

74 Freund G. Effect of iodinated water supplies on thyroid function. *J Clin Endocrinol Metab*. 1966;26:619–24.

75 Backer H, Hollowell J. Use of iodine for water disinfection: iodine toxicity and maximum recommended dose. *Environ Health Perspectives*. 2000;108(8):679–84.

76 Powers E. *Inactivation of Giardia Cysts by Iodine with Special Reference to Globaline: A Review*. Natick, Mass.: U.S. Army Natick Research, Development and Engineering Center; 1993. Technical Report Natick/TR-91/022.

77 Rogers M, Vitaliano J. Military and small group water disinfecting systems: an assessment. *Milit Med*. 1979;7:267–77.

78 Marchin G, Fina L. Contact and demand-release disinfectants. *Crit Rev Environ Control*. 1989;19:227–90.

79 Fina R, et al. Virucidal capability of resin I3 disinfectant. *Appl Environ Microbiol*. 1982;44:1370–3.

80 Upton S, Tilley M, Marchin G, Fina L. Efficacy of a pentaiodide resin disinfectant on *Cryptosporidium parvum* oocysts In vitro. *J Parasitol*. 1988;74:719–21.

81 O'Connor J, Kapoor S. Small quantity field disinfection. *J Am Water Works Assoc*. 1970;62:80–84.

82 Rutala WA, Weber DJ. New disinfection and sterilization methods. *Emerg Infect Dis*. 2001;7(2):348–53.

83 Venczel L, Arrowood M, Hurd M, Sobsey M. Inactivation of *Cryptosporidium parvum* oocysts and *Clostridium perfringens* spores by a mixed-oxidant disinfectant and by free chlorine. *Appl Environ Microbiol*. 1997;63:1598–1601.

84 Hurst C. Disinfection of drinking water, swimming pool water and treated sewage effluents. In: Block S, ed. *Disinfection, Sterilization, and Preservation*. 5th ed. New York: Lippincott Williams and Wilkins; 2001:713–30.

85 Bell F. Review of effects of silver-impregnated carbon filters on microbial water quality. *J Am Water Works Assoc*. 1991;83:74–6.

86 Block S. Peroxygen compounds. In: Block S, ed. *Disinfection, Sterilization, and Preservation*. 5th ed. New York: Lippincott, Williams & Wilkins; 2001:182.

87 Linden KG, Shin GA, Faubert G, Cairns W, Sobsey M. UV disinfection of *Giardia lamblia* cysts in water. *Environ Sci Technol*. 2002;36(11):2519–22.

88 Oates PM, Shanahan P, Polz MF. Solar disinfection (SODIS): simulation of solar radiation for global assessment and application for point-of-use water treatment in Haiti. *Water Res*. Jan 2003;37(1):47–54.

89 Conroy RM, Meegan ME, Joyce T, McGuigan K, Barnes J. Solar disinfection of drinking water protects against cholera in children under 6 years of age. *Arch Dis Child*. 2001;85(4):293–5.

90 Mintz E, Reiff M, Tauxe R. Safe water treatment and storage in the home. a practical new strategy to prevent waterborne disease. *JAMA*. 1995;273:948–53.

91 Wright J, Gundry S, Conroy R. Household drinking water in developing countries: a systematic review of microbiological contamination between source and point-of-use. *Trop Med Internat Health*. 2004;9(1):106–17.

92 Boulware DR. Influence of hygiene on gastrointestinal illness among wilderness backpackers. *J Travel Med*. 2004;11(1):27–33.

93 Merson R, et al. An outbreak of *Shigella sonnei* gastroenteritis on Colorado river raft trips. *Am J Epidemiol*. 1974;100:186–96.

94 Sobel J, Mahon B, Mendoza C, Passaro D, Cano F, et al. Reduction of fecal contamination of street-vended beverages in Guatemala by a simple system for water purification and storage, handwashing, and beverage storage. *Am J Trop Med Hyg*. 1998;59:380–7.

95 Hargreaves JS. Laboratory evaluation of the 3-bowl system used for washing-up eating utensils in the field. *Wilderness Environ Med*. 2006;17(2):94–102.

96 Ortega YR, Roxas CR, Gilman RH, et al. Isolation of *Cryptosporidium parvum* and *Cyclospora cayetanensis* from vegetables collected in markets of an endemic region in Peru. *Am J Trop Med Hyg*. 1997;57(6):683–6.

97 Reeves H. Human waste disposal in the Sierran wilderness. In: Stanley J, Harvey H, Hartesveldt R, eds. *A Report on the Wilderness Impact Study: The Effects of Human Recreational Activities on Wilderness Ecosystems with Special Emphasis on Sierra Club Wilderness Outings in the Sierra Nevada*. San Francisco: Sierra Club; 1979:129.

98 Sattar S. *Viruses, Water and Health*. Ottawa, Canada: University of Ottawa Press; 1978.

9 Special Considerations

Elders, Women, Pregnant Women, Children, and the Immunocompromised

Blair Dillard Erb, Sr., MD

The spirit of adventure is alluring. For some the attraction comes from an irresistible personal need to explore; for others the song of the mountains, deserts, rivers, seas, ice caps, and even skies beckons. The gentle touch of a breeze on the cheek, the crunch of scree underfoot, and the scent of trees and flowers tickle the senses and, once experienced, leave a memory that calls for revisiting in the future.

Many who have experienced such wilderness activities share their reactions with others who may respond to the call and join them. The exploring community is no longer made up predominantly of scientists but of individuals of varying physical abilities, skills, experiences, and health. Some may require special consideration if they are to participate in the activity. This chapter will deal with special considerations for populations with possibilities for limited physical and environmental tolerance: elders, women, pregnant women, children, and the immunocompromised. These individuals add to the rapidly growing number of participants in a wide assortment of adventures led by organized groups.

Many ventures are quite demanding in a physical, mental, emotional, and environmental sense. Some may even be unsafe and hazardous. As a result, the degree of attention placed on planning, organizing, and undertaking the venture may warrant the term "expedition" to define the activity. Defined as "a journey, voyage, excursion or venture undertaken for a specific purpose," an expedition may vary considerably in its characteristics, demands, and hazards.[1]

In an expedition, three components must be meshed in the planning stages: type of expedition, the features of the venture, and the characteristics of the participants. This chapter will first review the features to which all participants will be exposed followed by those that require special consideration.

CLASSIFICATIONS OF EXPEDITIONS, VENTURE ACTIVITIES, AND PARTICIPANTS

Classification of Expeditions

Expeditions can be differentiated according to the primary activity, which has implications for participant preparation. Goal-oriented professional expeditions, such as conservation studies, specific scientific projects, or adventures represent a classical type. Commercial travel or quality expeditions led by experienced travel guides, such as those found on an eco-travel trip, are a specific subset of expeditions. A third type consists of recreational expeditions, exemplified by midrange mountaineering, treks, and hiking. Educational and training expeditions are a fourth, and quite common, classification of expedition, which consists of school programs. Last, a distinct set of expeditions occur for medical skill training and experience, which may involve research or teaching.[2]

A classification such as this helps identify and describe the project and its goals. It introduces some of the characteristics needed for planning for costs, travel, gear, supplies, academic or scientific requirements, life experience expectations, and administrative and training demands.

Classification of Wilderness Ventures

As planners address the selection of participants, it is critical to understand the physical challenges presented by the terrain, the environment, and the hazards. The classification of venture demands then can be matched with the physical abilities and needs for healthy participation in the venture.

Wilderness ventures should be evaluated and classified according to the degree of physical exertion required.

Extreme performance ventures comprise a separate class reserved for individuals with extensive skill sets and physical conditioning; high-altitude technical mountaineering such as a Mount Everest ascent is a good example of this category. High-performance ventures (e.g., remote hunting activities or jungle trekking) are significantly demanding but are generally more forgiving. Recreational activities (e.g., Alpine hiking, National Park trail walking) constitute the largest and most familiar category of ventures. A fourth category is reserved for therapeutic activities whose participants are usually those with manifest illness or disability where rehabilitation is a goal.[3]

Classification of Participants

Participants should be classified in order to address their physical characteristics, functional capacity, and experience. The members of an expedition presented to the physician may fit the Bell distribution curve for the five classifications of participants. This rather intricate classification system is a tool that can be useful for assessment of medical suitability of an individual candidate or group for the proposed venture.

The five categories in which participants in wilderness ventures may be classified are as follows:

Group A: Demonstrated high-performance individual. Some who approach wilderness ventures have already been through a form of natural selection. For example, nearly every person interested in participating in an extreme high-altitude mountain expedition such as to Mount Everest will have trained or participated in other high-altitude activities and will have proven their capacity to function at altitude.

Group B: Healthy vigorous individual. They usually participate in regular exercise and are in good, though not necessarily competitive, physical condition but still enjoy periodic wilderness ventures.

Group C: Healthy deconditioned individual. The examiner must be alert to the apparently healthy businessman or professional person who does not participate in regular exercise and is "deconditioned" but still ambitious to participate in vigorous activities. These individuals may have occult medical problems, hidden risk factors, and may even be in health jeopardy.

Group D: Individual with risk factors. Some prospective participants may seem healthy but have risk factors that may warrant a complete medical assessment.

Group E: Individual who is manifestly ill. Therapeutic outdoor exercise programs may be prescribed as a form of physical therapy for persons who are in cardiac rehabilitation programs, have metabolic illnesses such as diabetes, need stroke rehabilitation, or have other disorders in which structured or limited physical activity is desired. Individuals in this group often have special requirements that will not be offered in a larger group situation, and their inclusion may be detrimental to the overall group objective. These people should be advised to participate in a personalized program.[4]

The idealized distribution curve in participants reflects a rather small number of high-performance participants with peaks in the normal healthy and healthy-appearing but deconditioned groups with the curve tapering to a rather small number of persons with an overt illness. Some may have known risk factors, while others possess unrecognized risk factors. All participants may be vulnerable to some challenges unique to the venture that call for universal consideration. Others may require special consideration because of limitations or conditions that may put them or others in jeopardy. Prospective participants with functional limitations are often burdensome to the entire expedition and may compromise the mission. It is also clear that some seemingly healthy individuals may provide a hint, a clue, or body language observed during the interview that calls for personalized and possibly more extensive medical assessment.[3] It is a well-known fact that prospective members in a venture will hide or trivialize medical information in order to avoid being denied participation.

UNIVERSAL CONSIDERATIONS

Universal Medical Considerations apply to all participants in any venture and call for awareness and detailed planning by the leaders because of their impact on the physical performance of the individual or group. These considerations include the medical history, physical demands that cause fatigue, and environmental factors such as heat, cold, and altitude. Other areas of concern such as trauma, nutrition, water quality and supply, infections, and animal and insect bites are covered in detail in other chapters. The classification of activities helps participants and leaders review the hazards attendant with the activities and, in turn, initiate a response to health demands and medical needs. These considerations are potentially present for any expedition and for all populations.

Medical History

Experienced teachers of the art and science of medicine have observed that if you talk to the patient, and, more importantly, listen, the patient will tell you the diagnosis. Perhaps the patient will not use the technical terms, but the description is so lucid that the physician can interpret clearly. So it is with the medical selection of suitability for wilderness ventures and expeditions.

A study on predictors of success (or failure) in wilderness ventures published by the Austrian Society of Alpine and High Altitude Medicine evaluated a medical examination that included personal data, past and family medical history, psychological status, physical examination, and physiological assessment.[3] Of the five components of the exam, only physical examination and physiologic assessment were of a technical nature while the other three components could all be derived from an interview. Weighted scoring of participating medical/leader experts indicated that the most dependable (over 50%) predictor of success was a history of a successful previous similar venture. The most reliable predictor of failure was a history of failure in a similar venture or of psychological or interpersonal problems (also over 50%).

These predictors could easily be determined by interview. Technical medical and physiological components were recognized as support data. This validates empiric observations by experienced and senior medical/wilderness leaders who, confident in their selection of successful participants, insist on being able to interview applicants prior to higher level ventures for personal observation of the candidates' prospects for safe and successful outcomes. This study gave rise to the expression that an experienced old "Salty Dog" medical/wilderness leader can recognize an experienced and stable "Salty Dog" participant with a degree of confidence.

Physical Demands

The common denominator among outdoor ventures is physical activity. Attendant with physical activity is the prospect for fatigue. Fatigue can interrupt an expedition and increase the risk of injury. The experience of both the participant and leaders in estimating the physical condition of the individual and matching that with the estimated physical demands is of major value in predicting success or failure of the entire venture.

An estimate of physical demands can be obtained by measuring the oxygen consumption of the individual and comparing it to the energy cost of the task. Energy requirements for a particular task can be estimated by measuring oxygen consumption using a Douglas bag, Max Planck respirometer, oxylog, or other device. The energy consumption is defined in ml/kg/min body weight oxygen uptake, which can be translated into calories (expressed in kcal) or METs. One MET represents the energy cost of sitting quietly (3.5 ml O_2/kg/min) and is a useful term for reporting both the energy cost of the task in multiples of the resting rate and the tolerance of the participant.

The tolerance an individual exhibits for exercise can be determined by measuring maximal oxygen

Table 9.1. Some human energy costs in METs often expended on expeditions

Walking 2mph, level	2 METs
Walking 3 mph, level	3 METs
Walking 4 mph, level	4 1/2 METs
Walking 3 mph, 5% grade	5 METs
Jogging, level	6 METs
Running (mouth breathing)	10 METs

Notes: One [1] MET is the energy cost of sitting quietly and is normalized to 1 kg body weight. Technically the MET is accepted as 3.5 ml/min/kg body weight, It a *rate* of energy expenditure and can be converted to Calories by the formula:
Cal.= METs × kg body wt × 0.0167 × Time$_{min}$.
Altitude, temperature, terrain characteristics, snow, and other variables can influence metabolic costs.

consumption (PWC_{max}) while performing on a treadmill, cycle, or step ergometer and is reported as maximal oxygen uptake (VO_2) in ml/kg/min of oxygen consumption or as calories or METs.[5] Since the maximal physical work capacity, PWC_{max}, of the average 40-year-old male in the United States is 10 METs, the range from resting (1 MET) to 10 METs results in a useful scale of 1–10, which is convenient for comparing the workload of an activity with the PWC_{max} (Table 9.1). From this comparison, the duration of exercise tolerance for the activity in question can be estimated. Some highly trained athletes can be measured above 20 METs, but the 1–10 range is useful for the average person.

Most activities of daily living require less than 3 METs. Fatigue occurs when the rate of energy expenditure exceeds tolerance of the participant. Most people can expend energy costs of activities representing about 30% of their PWC_{max} during an 8-hour task. Greater physical requirements with higher energy expenditure may be sustained only for shorter periods of time (Table 9.2). Short bursts of high-energy expenditure are required in many outdoor ventures and for certain tasks but cannot be sustained as long as lower rates of energy expenditure. Consequently, it is of value for participants to learn to pace themselves.

Table 9.2. Percentage of maximal work capacity that can be maintained for given periods of time

Work duration (hours)	Maximal work capacity (percentage)
1	64
2	54
3	48
4	44
5	41
6	39
7	37
8	35
9	33

Based on Bink and Bonjer equations (21, 22).

An experienced leader can often recognize prospects for success or failure of a candidate simply by spending time with the candidate interviewing, watching body language, and taking some physical and physiological measurements. Experience provides the best parameter to judge physical functional capacity, but technical measurements make an excellent research and educational tool and can help answer some clinical questions.

A physical training program featuring aerobic, anaerobic, and skill techniques can be an invaluable aid to prepare the candidate for the venture. Three components make up the exercise prescription: frequency, intensity, and duration. Most aerobic programs suggest participation at least 3 days per week, 20 minutes to 1 hour of activity and at least 40–50% of personal functional capacity. For those in ill health or beyond 35–40 years of age, an individualized and supervised training program may be prudent. Tolerance for the physical demands of expeditions is essential because fatigue not only can interrupt the venture but also can increase the risk of injury or illness.

Environmental Concerns: Heat

When the stress of ambient environmental heat is added to the physical demands of an expedition, risk of illness, injury, and even death may result. [6,7] Regulation of body heat is influenced by functional changes in the cerebral thermoregulatory center located in the anterior preoptic hypothalamic nuclei and by altered skin sensors. Weight, body mass, cardiovascular, renal, or pulmonary status can influence the individual response to heat. Tolerance to heat is affected by medication (such as beta-blockers, anticholinergics, antidepressants, tranquilizers), frequency and duration of exposure, acclimatization, and intensity and duration of physical activity. Tolerance to future heat exposure can be improved by a physical conditioning program employing 60–100 minutes of low-intensity exercise daily at less than 50% of the individuals' maximal work capacity (PWC_{max}) at tolerable ambient temperatures for 7–14 days before the planned expedition. Other factors aiding prevention of heat injury include adequate hydration, nutritional status with adequate electrolyte intake, and weight control.

Extensive discussion about thermal extremes is found in other chapters in this text. However, briefly, there are two types of serious heat illness: heat exhaustion and heatstroke. Heat exhaustion may be slower in onset and more subtle and is associated with hypovolemia from dehydration. Manifestations include thirst, weakness, confusion, paleness, and sweaty appearance, along with those characteristics associated with hypovolemic shock. Heatstroke, on the other hand, may be more abrupt and is characterized by hot flushed skin, tachycardia, and high oral temperature [45°C (105°F)], agitation, stupor, or coma, along with the signs and symptoms of shock. Heatstroke is a true emergency.

Less serious heat illnesses include heat cramps and heat syncope usually associated with exercise or prolonged exposure to sun or intense hot weather.

Environmental Concerns: Cold

Cold-induced injuries include systemic hypothermia or localized frostbite. Hypothermia is potentially lethal and refers to a body core temperature below 35°C (95°F). There are three levels of hypothermia: mild where the core temperature decreases to as low as 33°C (90°F), moderate with core temperature between 32°C and 27°C (90°F and 80°F), and severe where core temperature is below 80°F (27°C).

During expeditions in cold and demanding environments, physical exhaustion associated with dehydration and hypoglycemia may set the stage for potentially fatal loss of body heat. [8] Other physical environmental influences such as wind, humidity, altitude, ultraviolet and infrared radiation may contribute to the hazard. The wind chill index is a useful measurable parameter in the urban environment but impractical in a remote setting; the experienced outdoorsman is aware that a breeze felt blowing across the cheek indicates that wind velocity is over 5 knots/hr. Wet clothing contributes to heat loss. [9] Adequate food intake is essential to maintain adequate core body temperature.

The combination of cold, dampness, wind, and physical exhaustion may prove fatal especially to those vulnerable from decreased physical reserves. Medical conditions with impaired peripheral circulation can exacerbate hypothermia and contribute to frostbite.

Environmental Concerns: Altitude

Demographic data regarding the effect of altitude illness have been gathered from recreational skiing sites or have been anecdotal and associated with mountaineering, at times with commercial tours and guides. Honigman reported that 25% of visitors to moderate altitude develop altitude illness and report some protective effect from living at moderate elevations of 1,500–2,000 m (4,921–6,562 feet). The most frequent predictors of acute mountain sickness are altitude of residence less than 1,000 m, history of previous episode of altitude illness, and age younger than 60 years. [10] Prevention and management of acute mountain sickness will be addressed in other chapters.

Nutrition and Water

Although covered extensively in other chapters, a few words about nutrition and water are appropriate in this context. Proper nutritional planning is essential to preparation for expeditions, not only because it serves as the fuel supply for physical activity, but because it is required for mental clarity and tolerance to environmental stress.

Principal food components consist of carbohydrate, protein, and fat, minerals, vitamins, and water (the most important). Nutritional dietary content is critical during environmental temperature stresses especially during physical activity in temperature extremes.[11–15] Average nutritional needs for an expedition consist of about 4,000 kcal/day for men and 3,500 kcal/day for women. Marked environmental stresses require 4,000–6,000 kcal/day.

Individuals can tolerate deprivation of food much longer than inadequate water intake and subsequent dehydration. Total water deprivation can be tolerated for only about 6–14 days.[11] In addition to usual fluid loss of between 1,000 and 1,500 ml/day, physical activity and environmental influences such as extreme heat and altitude can increase the rate of fluid loss making maintenance and replacement of adequate fluid essential.

SPECIAL CONSIDERATIONS

Among those who warrant special consideration when they seek participation in expeditions are elders, women, pregnant women, children, and those who are immunocompromised. These groups require extra planning beyond review of universal considerations, inclusion of supplies not usually taken on an expedition, and special attention with close observation by expedition leaders and medical personnel. Determining medical suitability of prospective participants is best accomplished by competent medical personnel experienced in providing medical services in environments that include the features, illnesses, and hazards peculiar to the proposed expedition. Consultation should be sought from medical specialists about management issues for the disorders or special physical conditions of participants in anticipation of an adverse medical event.

Elders on Expeditions

Many elders have reached their advanced age in good physical and financial health. As a result, more than ever before, seniors in our society remain vigorously active and often participate in demanding goal-oriented activities. Longevity, economics, worldwide transportation, and communication services combined with available time from their retirement make it possible for their participation in previously unreachable activities. Simultaneously, the past few decades have seen an increase in the numbers of both nonprofit and commercial organizations that have made such ventures more easily available, organized, and administered.

Health risk associated with physically demanding ventures increases with age because of altered physical and physiologic function, unrecognized medical problems, or consequences of previous illnesses or injuries. Caution through planning and open assessment will help provide a venture appropriate for the individual.

How do you define an elder? Aging is a natural consequence of living and every organ system is affected by the aging process. Age-related changes may occur slowly, but they eventually result in anatomic and functional changes. Furthermore, degenerative disorders and diseases may result in anatomic, biochemical, and physiologic changes. An elder is generally recognized as someone older in age with the implication that some of the aging process is occurring or has occurred.

The simplest classification is by chronologic age. Smith suggested the following definition: athletic old (younger than 55 years of age), young old (55–75 years of age), and old old (older than 75 years old).[16] Barry and Eathorne emphasized function by simply dividing elders into the "hale" and the "frail".[17] Preferred by this author is a comprehensive classification that includes three factors: the chronologic age in years, a pathologic description of morphologic changes, and a functional description of features affecting participation in venture activities.

Loss of function in the various organ systems can be estimated by using the "1% Rule," which claims that most organ systems lose function at roughly 1% per year after age 30.[18] Both specific and diverse effects on the organ systems of elders affect their overall function during an expedition.[19] Physical and physiological alterations in function may occur so slowly in elders that they are not recognized until the person ventures into a demanding environment.

Physical Function

The average 40-year-old male has a maximal physical work capacity (PWC_{max}) of about 10 METs. Most males lose about one MET of their PWC_{max} per decade after age 40. Until the most recent generation, females have been viewed traditionally as having a PWC_{max} of about 2 METs less than males. Now, with a major increase in female participation in athletics and training activities and a better understanding of physiology, there has been an adjustment in estimation of between 1 and 2 METs in their PWC_{max}. As previously stated, most activities of daily living require about 3 METs and healthy individuals are estimated to tolerate about 30% of their PWC_{max} during sustained activity lasting 8 hours or more. Consequently, an average healthy 40-year-old male with a 10 MET PWC_{max} can sustain the usual levels of daily activity and still be able to get out of bed the next morning and repeat the workload. Expeditions, however, usually have a much higher energy cost, sometimes demanding up to 10 or more METs in short bursts. Time to develop tolerance to higher levels of activity has theoretically been estimated using the Bink and Bonjer equation.[20,21]

Rapid onset of fatigue may be a signal indicating the need for assessment and a physical conditioning program. In view of the advanced years of elders and the possibility of underlying cardiovascular disease, vigorous programs should be supervised. One can usually expect to enhance the PWC_{max} by greater than 15% in a sustained 3–6 month program. A conditioning program should include flexion and extension exercises during a warm-up, an active aerobic cardiovascular conditioning component, and a cool-down component. The aerobic component should last at least 20 minutes at a level of about 50% PWC_{max} at least 3 days a week. The participant is encouraged to learn to read "body signals," generated from the body during physical activity, that provide an indication of the activity effect on the body (Table 9.3).

This theoretical description of the physiologic requirements of physical activity serves as a quantifiable approximation but cannot replace the judgment of an experienced expedition leader. So, look at the trail, read the terrain, feel the temperature, and read your body signals.

Changes in Organ Systems in the Elderly

The aging process leads to some generally irrevocable changes for which expedition leaders and medical officers should have some appreciation. It has often been noted that elders often feel they are still teenagers in spirit and are only limited in activity by their decreased physical capacities. Awareness of this attitude promotes understanding the desire for an elder to participate in an activity that may appear beyond their capacity. Knowledge about the changes in organ systems will help the medical officer evaluate an elderly individual for the proposed venture.

Cardiovascular System

Cardiac output is usually decreased by 20–30% by age 70 and maximal heart rate is decreased 6–10 beats/min/decade. This loss of physiological capacity decreases cardiovascular tolerance to activity.[22] A feeling of pressure in the chest and dyspnea (shortness of breath) both alert the participant to seek rest and, if at altitude, move to a lower elevation for help. Rest periods of 5 min/hr or more may be needed to tolerate the exertion. It is important to pace the speed of walking for prolonged activity, and caloric intake should be included at the rest break. Fluid replacement is absolutely necessary in the elderly because their reserves may be less than a younger person and problems with dehydration can be exacerbated by medication use. Heat and altitude may cause a significant increase in fluid demands.

Respiratory System

Decreased elasticity of the lungs adds to a reduction in pulmonary vital capacity of roughly 30 ml/yr after age 30. Changes in pulmonary function are more noticeable in situations of increased exertion or more extreme climates or altitude. Certain pulmonary changes such as dyspnea, productive cough, and hemoptysis (blood in the expectorant), especially at altitude, may be the first harbinger of serious medical problems like pulmonary edema.

Renal System

Aging also leads to loss of kidney function over time and the usual laboratory screening determinant of renal function, serum creatinine, only provides a crude estimate that may underestimate renal physiologic capacity. Dehydration and cardiovascular deficits may induce renal deterioration in the elderly who already have a lower reserve. Renal clearance changes and fluid retention may result in swelling of the lower extremities known as edema.

Gastrointestinal Tract

Decreased number of taste buds, salivary flow, and decreased gastric acid production may modify appetite and food intake as one ages. Constipation may occur as a result of decreased dietary fiber and intestinal motility with dehydration contributing significantly to this condition. Therefore, constipation, especially in elders, is frequently seen on extended ventures. Other problems such as hemorrhoids, pain during defecation, and

Table 9.3. Body signals	
Primary body signals	**Secondary body signals**
Cardiovascular	**Musculoskeletal**
Heart rate: estimate physiologic effect of physical workload	Tremulousness, weakness, cramps, dehydration, low salt
Head pulsing; ? hypertension	Shivering: cooling < 35.5°C (96°F)
Chest awareness or pain	Shivering stops, confusion: $T < 33.9$°C (93°F)
Fluttering, arrhythmia	
Respiratory	Sweating > 7 METs
Mouth-breathing: > 60% of PWCmax	**Genitourinary**
Breathing too hard to talk > 85% PWCmax	Urinary frequency at altitude
Cough or Cheyne-Stokes respiration: altitude	"Hochdiurese" of climbers
Cyanosis of nailbeds, nose, earlobes: hypoxia	Sensory effects
	Tubular vision: altitude
	Loss of color/night vision: altitude
Neurologic	Wind on cheek: 5 mph breeze
Headache: altitude; with confusion:	
Cerebal edema	

Note: Energy expenditure of physical activity results in physiologic responses that can be recognized by the active person. Learn to read these "body signals" as an indication of intensity and reserve. Make your own list. *Always keep your reserve!*

bleeding may result from or contribute to gastrointestinal problems with evacuation.

Genitourinary System

There is an increased susceptibility for urinary tract infections in the elderly due to changes in natural resistance, changes in pelvic floor musculature in women, and the development of lower urinary tract obstruction from the prostate in men. Dehydration again can contribute to the development of a urinary tract infection in both sexes. On occasion, difficulty with hygiene and chafing from extended walking can contribute to female urinary tract infections though they are not causative. Another reason to avoid dehydration is because of its direct relationship to urinary stone formation, an excruciatingly painful occurrence that can be a medical emergency. Most common medications for colds and allergies should be avoided by men who experience lower urinary tract voiding symptoms because the obstructive symptoms can be exacerbated. Any medical kit should include a urinary catheter to relieve total obstruction if elders are involved.

Musculoskeletal System

Decreased height from loss of skeletal calcium, osteoporosis, sarcopenia with increased fat/muscle mass ratio, decreased synovial fluid in joints with changes in cartilaginous surfaces, and hypertrophic changes in joints often result in loss of as much as 20% muscle mass and strength by age 65 years.

Central Nervous System

Atrophic changes of the central nervous system occur as one ages, and elders may have one or more symptoms of this natural progression. Decreased brain size and weight and decreased cortical cell count may result in impaired cerebral function, loss of agility and balance, and sensory impairment. Subtle changes in altitude tolerance, early symptoms of Alzheimer's disease, mood swings, and memory loss may reflect impending symptomatic organic brain disease and any elder with these characteristics should be assessed for central nervous system function.[19] Unrecognized alcoholism may become full-blown withdrawal psychosis during altitude exposure especially under physical stress. Development of inappropriate behavior or confusion during extended hiking or other exertion may be mitigated by providing some source of glucose to the elderly participant to help restore a degree of rational behavior for return to the base camp. Heat intolerance from impaired heat sensors as well as decreased cardiovascular dissipation of heat may result in hyperthermia in elders. Likewise, intolerance to cold from decreased circulatory function is more prominent in the elder population and can lead to cold injury more readily.

Eyes

Decreased translucency of the lens with cataract formation, decreased pupil size and potential increase in intraocular pressure with glaucoma, decreased vision especially at night and with color, and impaired accommodation are some of the major ophthalmologic problems that occur in an elderly population. These issues cause major concern for walking on rough terrain or at night and must be taken into consideration with altitude changes.

Ears

Loss of hearing especially in the high tones results in a decrease in directional discrimination.

Skin

Decreased skin thickness and turgor result in decreased resistance to bruising and tearing. This is a common development in the elderly and may contribute to greater skin damage from trauma as well as a decrease in wound healing.

A group that has recognized the special circumstances of elderly participation in venture type of activities is the Gray Eagles. The Gray Eagle hiking group was founded by retired Memphis pathologist, Dr. John Duckworth and his hiking partner, Mr. John Johnson, retired Kraft food executive. Qualifying as "Salty Dogs" because of their wisdom and their experience, they have led their senior group through much of the Rocky Mountain West. Their experiences have led to the formulation of principles of preparation, which are invaluable for elders and form a useful prerequisite checklist:

1. Preselection based on interview, medical history, experiences of previous similar ventures, and medical assessment.
2. Stringent 6-month conditioning program including hiking in well-fitted boots with at least 100 miles use with the hiker's feet in them.
3. Carrying a backpack on the conditioning walk weighing one-third of the body weight.
4. Orientation and regular meetings prior to embarking featuring safety, risk, expectations, and discussion of current and future clinical problems including those associated with hypothermia, altitude, and dehydration. This also promotes dynamic social interaction among the venturers.
5. Counseling regarding clothing for the trip including the three-season principle to prepare for sudden weather change.
6. Meeting with officials at the trailhead departure site.

As a result of their rigorous approach, the Gray Eagles have experienced very few medical problems over the years, the most significant of which have resulted from subtle year-to-year central nervous system changes in participants, which manifest as cognitive or behavioral changes.[19] They have confirmed the observation that "Remember, the elderly still climb mountains. It's just that their definition of mountains has changed considerably!".[23]

Problems Particular to Females

With their welcome involvement, women make up the largest percentage increase in the growing number of expedition travelers to remote and hazardous areas. Their physical constitution, physiological stamina, and skill levels may be a major contribution to any venture, from mountaineering, to underwater expeditions, to space travel. Because of certain anatomical and physiological differences from men, there are some considerations, however, that should be recognized and accommodated.

Prior to a lengthy expedition, especially in a remote area, a personalized history should be obtained incorporating age of menarche, history of pregnancies, gynecologic abnormalities and/or surgery, menopause if it has occurred, abnormal uterine bleeding, sexually transmitted diseases, and medications currently prescribed. The use of contraceptives should be carefully detailed and emphasized if sexual relationships are considered by the person during the venture.[24]

Physical Activity

Experience during expeditions and wilderness ventures indicates that there is virtually no limitation to female participation in endurance activities when compared with the endurance of males. Except for weight lifting and carrying, there is virtually no distinction in physical activity of expeditions made because of gender. Just as with males, it is prudent for prospective participants in expeditions to undergo a regular training program using essentially the same principles as males.

Oxygen consumption studies are valid and identical principles are used for female evaluation as for males. Similarly, the energy cost of various activities is the same because the O_2 consumption is normalized for weight (1 MET = 3.5 ml O_2/min/kg).

Altitude

There appears to be virtually no gender-related difference in the incidence of acute mountain sickness between males and nonpregnant females.[25] In a recent consensus paper on medical recommendations for women going to altitude, no difference was found between men and women in the incidence of acute mountain sickness and the incidence is not significantly affected by the menstrual cycle.[26] The incidence of high-altitude pulmonary edema appeared to be lower in women than in men while peripheral edema is higher in women than in men.[26] A female in very early pregnancy or who becomes pregnant on an expedition to altitude may put the embryo at risk, and participation in such a venture is not recommended during pregnancy.

Thermal Extremes

Females have lower sweat rates and, consequently, less evaporation and cooling from the skin making heat dissipation more dependent on circulatory mechanisms. In hot dry climates, however, a greater amount of sweating is helpful for cooling, and a 2-week exercise program may help prepare the participant for a hot dry environment through acclimatization. As with males, increased fluid intake is important for replacement.[6,7]

Adaptation to hot dry heat may be influenced by the menstrual cycle. Women may tolerate hot environments better in the follicular phase of the menstrual cycle than in the luteal phase. Although it is unlikely to be necessary in most cases, the phase of the cycle may be estimated by determining the resting core body temperature, which is approximately 0.4°C (0.7°F) higher in the follicular phase.[27]

It has been postulated that the insulation effect of body fat distribution may benefit women in cold environments, but there have been no definitive studies. However, extreme cold may be less well tolerated in females than in males because of decreased heat production from less muscle mass. As with men, clothing protection of the extremities is critically important for prevention of cold injury.

Genitourinary Considerations

A history of gynecologic disorders, such as cystocele or rectocele, alerts the team health care leader to the prospects of genitourinary difficulty during the expedition. Urinary tract symptoms should be fully evaluated by a physician and an existing urinary tract infection needs to be treated.[24] Vulvovaginitis, a common condition, can develop into an extremely painful and disruptive disorder and should be addressed before departure on a venture. Appropriate antibiotics and antifungal medications should be part of the medical kit if females are involved in a remote venture.

Contraception

The health of the embryo and the effects of altitude or a demanding environment take precedence in the continued debate over exposure of pregnant women to such circumstances. Women are urged to consider contraception if still fertile and a sexual relationship will occur on the venture. It is advised that the method of contraception be selected in consultation with her physician and ideally tried for at least 3 months before embarkation to establish techniques and tolerance. Women planning high-altitude ventures should consider the lowest dose of oral contraceptives to reduce the attendant thromboembolic risk that is increased in this environment.[24]

Pregnancy and Remote Travel

There is universal agreement that the effect of vigorous wilderness ventures on pregnant women, especially those that involve altitude, is a primary concern when planning expeditions.[24] Potential risks to both mother and fetus make pregnancy a relative contraindication for participation in such activities in the view of many leaders. Pregnant women have increased risks for hypertension, diabetes, and cardiovascular problems due to significant changes in fluid and hormonal regulation. Alterations in blood flow, venous stasis, and pelvic pressure especially with prolonged seating increase the risk of deep venous thrombosis and pulmonary embolism in this population. Complications of pregnancy are higher among teenage girls and women in the later childbearing years, and the risk of complications rises with subsequent pregnancies.

The three stages of pregnancy have different potential problems caused by the physiological stresses of expeditions. The effect on the unborn child especially in the early first trimester can result in undesired serious consequences. Principal maternal problems in the first trimester are miscarriage and ectopic pregnancy. Miscarriage usually occurs before 15 weeks and can be caused by maternal/fetal stresses caused by physical demands. Complications may include pain, vaginal bleeding, and infection especially when there is incomplete evacuation of the uterine contents. A miscarriage should be considered an emergency if it occurs in the field and evacuation of the mother is advised. Ectopic pregnancy is one that develops outside the uterus, usually in the fallopian tube, and often occurs prior to 6 weeks after conception. Ectopic pregnancy is a surgical emergency because rupture of the tube and significant hemorrhage can ensue. Although ectopic pregnancy is a potentially serious occurrence in the first trimester, it is not caused or exacerbated by increased exertion or environmental rigors.

Although there are very few complications in the second 3 months of pregnancy, the most common complication of early labor can be associated with placental detachment and significant vaginal bleeding. Blood pressure problems, excessive weight gain, and diabetes may become evident during the second trimester. In remote areas, early labor and delivery is extremely difficult and women in this intermediate stage of pregnancy should be highly discouraged from participation in physically demanding ventures. As for advanced pregnancy, it is not advised for a woman in the third trimester to be on a wilderness expedition.

Special Considerations for Children

Educational travel tours and selected adventure activities have become more inclusive of children and young adults, and data collected from such activities give us insight into the spectrum of medical problems that can arise among young travelers. Youth groups now actively participate in organized tours. One source of information about medical problems encountered by youths during travel is provided by World Challenge Expeditions, Ltd., who accompanied 2,915 youths aged 15–18 on expeditions between June and September 2001. Data collected by adult team leaders on 2,402 people (82%) revealed medical problems occurred in 64% of participants with 6% defined as serious and 1% required hospitalization. Girls were affected 19% more frequently than boys, and illness and injury were more prevalent in South America than in Australasia. There was one fatality reported in this group, which demonstrated a relatively high overall incidence of health risks.[28] Other sources of information about medical problems in youths exist with the Boy Scouts of America who have records from many years of ventures at national scouting camps.

Behavior

Responsibility for children is vested in adult supervisory authority to provide leadership and direction. Children need to understand the mechanics of the venture, communicate, and comply with the rules to minimize risk from inherent hazards of the trip. Adult leadership must begin with teaching prior to the venture, and discipline is required from both children and adults. The appropriate ratio of adult leaders to youths varies with the activity, location, and environment of the venture.

Altitude

Symptoms of acute mountain sickness (AMS) in children may be difficult to recognize. Most symptoms are constitutional; may consist of fatigue, headache, nausea, and restless sleep; and may be difficult to differentiate from standard side effects of protracted travel. The incidence of acute mountain sickness in children seems to be essentially the same as adults, occurring in approximately 20% of children as young as 3 years ascending to an altitude of 3,500 meters and above.[29,30] There is also evidence that young children who travel to high altitude, especially with preexisting upper respiratory symptoms, may be more prone to develop high-altitude pulmonary edema (HAPE). Treatment for children with AMS or HAPE mirrors that of adults with rapid descent the hallmark of therapy. Prophylactic and therapeutic doses of acetazolamide have not been clearly established for children.[31,32]

Thermal Extremes

Thermoregulation is less efficient in children than in adults; consequently, children are more susceptible to heat- and cold-related illness than adults. Cardiovascular heat dissipation is reduced due to lower cardiac output in children making conductive, convective, and radiant cooling relatively ineffective. Decreased perspiration in children impairs cooling from evaporation. Likewise, children are more susceptible than adults to hypothermia. Lack of adequate fat insulation and physical inactivity with decreased heat production from metabolism increase vulnerability to cold, which may be poorly communicated by children. Maintenance of hydration is mandatory for children in both thermal extremes because of this decreased thermoregulation and lack of reserve.

Infections and Immunization

Children are especially vulnerable to infection on travel. Serious respiratory, gastrointestinal, or neurological infections such as tuberculosis or bacterial meningitis can result from exposure to the causative microorganisms harbored by indigenous people. Children are susceptible to parasitic diseases due to poor water or food quality, and malaria is particularly lethal for children. Once again, even more so than in adults, attention must be paid to rapid fluid replacement in children due to losses by vomiting or diarrhea. It is imperative that children have current inoculations to diseases we rarely consider in the developed world such as polio.[33]

Child Abductions and Custody

Both domestic and international child abductions are a continuing concern, and it is prudent to have a consent letter for children traveling with a nonparental adult. Travelers in Europe are advised to have photographic identification of adult and child and a letter of consent for travel purposes; other international border identification requirements may vary.[34] A letter of consent by proxy will help expedite medical treatment in instances of nonurgent pediatric care. To this end, the Committee on Medical Liability of the American Academy of Pediatrics has produced useful clinical guidelines with information about circumstances and delegation of informed consent and the limitations of such action.[35]

Medical Considerations for the Immunocompromised

Immunodeficiency can be classified as primary (genetic) or secondary (acquired) and derives from many causes. One estimate suggests that the birth prevalence of primary immunodeficiency is approximately 1/100,000.[36] However, secondary immunodeficiencies are much more prevalent and have a wider range of etiologies and clinical features. Secondary causes of immunosuppression include sequelae from chemotherapy, organ transplantation medication, surgical absence of the spleen, and infection with HIV/AIDS.

Populations lacking full immunocompetence include the very young or very old, pregnant women, and those with diabetes mellitus and end-stage renal or liver disease. Population-based data are not precise, but it

has been estimated that acquired immunodeficiency in the United States from all causes may range from more than 3% of the population up to as much as 20% (36). The most commonly encountered immunodeficient conditions on adventure travel are caused by HIV/AIDS; chemotherapeutic agents for treatment of malignancy with immunosuppressant drugs used for organ transplants and asplenia are less common causes.

One would think that immunodeficient high-risk candidates who pose a risk to both themselves and members on the trip would avoid such circumstances. Behavioralists suggest that persons facing potential end-of-life treatment may seek that one last venture, recognizing that they risk opportunistic infection and greater hazards from enteric and respiratory pathogens. No controlled studies are available to document this increased risk for immunocompromised patients on adventure trips. However, opportunistic infection with gastrointestinal or respiratory organisms is well known in the immunocompromised patient, and these risks increase in the less-controlled environment of travel. Furthermore, energy requirements differ for immunocompromised patients and must be considered for participation in a strenuous event.[37,38] The decision to travel for these individuals is complex, and it is essential that the participant be fully informed of the risk and make that decision in consultation with the health care providers and expedition leaders.

SUMMARY

Expedition leaders should take into consideration the special needs of expedition participants. While some activities may be better suited for various types of persons, most individuals can participate in potentially remote excursions with minimal risk. It is up to the expedition leader to properly inform potential expedition participants and to help assess their appropriateness in planned expedition activities.

EPILOGUE

What a joy it is to feel the soft, springy earth under my feet once more, to follow grassy roads that lead to ferny brooks, where I can bathe my fingers in a cataract of rippling notes, or to clamber over a stone wall into green fields that tumble and roll and climb in riotous gladness!

– Helen Keller

REFERENCES

1   *Webster's Third International Dictionary of the English Language Unabridged*, Gove PB, ed. Springfield, Mass: Merriam-Webster Inc.; 1961.
2   Leggat PA. *Preparing Medical Personnel for Expeditions*. Townsville, Australia: Anton Breinl Centre for Public Health and Tropical Medicine, James Cook University. Lecture presented March 2006.

3 Erb BD. Determining medical suitability for wilderness ventures. *Jahrbuch 2005.* Innsbruck, Austria: Austrian Society for Alpine and High Altitude Medicine. 2005; 11–30.

4 Bowman WD. *Outdoor Emergency Care, Comprehensive First Aid for Non-urban Settings.* The National Ski Patrol, National Ski Patrol System; 1988: 288–307.

5 McCauley RL, Smith DJ, Robson MC, Heggers JP. Frostbite. In: Auerbach PS, ed. *Wilderness Medicine.* St. Louis: C. V. Mosby; 2001: 178–206.

6 Honigman B, et al. Acute mountain sickness at moderate altitudes. *J Int Med.* 1993;118:587.

7 Zell SC, Goodman PH. Wilderness preparation, equipment, and medical supplies. In: Auerbach PS, ed. *Wilderness Medicine.* St. Louis: C. V. Mosby; 2001: 1680.

8 Strauss MB. *Familiar Medical Quotations.* Boston: Little Brown and Co.; 1968.

9 Askew EW. Water. In: Ziegler EE, Filer LJ, Jr, eds. *Present Knowledge in Nutrition.* Washington, DC: ILSI Press; 1996.

10 Murlin JR, Miller CW. Preliminary results of nutritional surveys of United States army camps. *Am J Public Health.* 1919; 9:401.

11 Askew EW. Nutrition, malnutrition and starvation. In: Auerbach, PS, ed. *Wilderness Medicine.* St. Louis: C. V. Mosby; 2001: 1271–84.

12 Armstrong LE, et al. Responses of soldiers to 4 gm and 8 gm NaCl diets. In: Marriott BM, ed. *Nutritional Needs in Hot Environments.* Washington, DC: National Academy Press; 1993.

13 Pike J. Water supply planning. *http://www.globalsecurity.org/military/library/policy/army/fm/10–52/ch3.htm,* last accessed May 13, 2008.

14 Adolph EE. *Physiology of Man in the Desert.* New York: Interscience; 1947.

15 Taubes G. A mosquito bites back. *NY Times Magazine.* August 24, 1997; 40–6. In: Auerbach PS, ed. *Wilderness Medicine.* St. Louis: C. V. Mosby; 2001: 754.

16 Jong EC. Travel medicine. In: Auerbach PS, ed. *Wilderness Medicine.* St. Louis: C. V. Mosby; 2001: 1554–1577.

17 Smith EL (reported by Howley EH). Speed considerations in developing exercise programs for the older adult. In: *Behavioral Handbook of Environmental Enhancement and Disease Prevention.* New York: John Wiley and Sons; 1984.

18 Barry HC, Eathorne SW. Exercise and aging. *Med. Clin of North America.* 1994;78:357.

19 Kane RL, Auslander JG, Abross IB. *Essentials of clinical geriatrics,* 3rd ed. New York: McGraw-Hill; 1994.

20 Erb BD. Elders in the wilderness. In: Auerbach PS, ed. *Wilderness Medicine.* St. Louis: Mosby; 2001:1795-1811.

21 Bink B. Physical working capacity in relation to working time and age. *Ergonomics.* 1962;5(1):25–31.

22 Bonjer, FH. Actual energy expenditure in relation to physical working capacity. *Ergonomics.* 5:29–31, 1962.

23 Erb BD. The elderly in the wilderness. *Wilderness Med Lett.* 1995;12:6.

24 Trofotter KF, Jr, Dahl B. Women in the wilderness. In: Auerbach PS, ed., *Wilderness Medicine.* St. Louis: C. V. Mosby; 2001: 1761–94.

25 Hackett P, Rennie D. The incidence, importance and prophylaxis of acute mountain sickness. *Lancet.* 1976;2: 1149.

26 Jean D, Leil C, Kriemler S, Meijer H, Moore LG. Medical recommendations for women going to altitude. *High Altitude Medicine Biol.* 2005;6(1):22–31.

27 Shapiro Y, et al. Physiological responses of men and women to humid and dry heat. *J Appl Physiol.* 1980;49:1.

28 Shapiro Y, et al. Heat balance and transfer in men and women in hot-dry and hot-wet conditions. *Ergonomics.* 1981;24:375.

29 Frascorolo P, Schutz Y, Jequier E. Decreased thermal conductance during the luteal phase of the menstrual cycle in women. *J Appl Physiol.* 1990;69:2029.

30 ISMM. Concensus statement on children at high altitude. *High Altitude Med Biol.* 2001:389.

31 CIWEC Clinic. Trekking with children. CIWEC Clinic Home Page. Available at: *http://www.ciwec-clinic.com.* Accessed August 16, 2006.

32 Luks A, Jean D, Zafren K. Any thoughts about acetazolamide in children on Kilimanjaro? ISSM Discussion Forum. Available at: *http://www.digest@list.ismmed.org.* Accessed August 29, 2006.

33 Pattinson K. Altitude sickness in youth groups. *Wilderness Environ Med.* 2003;14:153.

34 Sadnicka A, Walker R, Dallimore J. Morbidity and determinants of health on youth expeditions. *Wilderness Environ Med.* 2005;16(1):60.

35 Bacaner N, Stauffer B, Boulware D, Walker D, Keystone J. Travel medicine considerations for North American immigrants visiting friends and relatives. *JAMA.* 2004;291: 2856–62.

36 Sample Consent Letter. Consular Affairs, Foreign Affairs and International Trade. August 30, 2006. Canada

37 Berger J, Committee on Medical Liability. Consent by proxy for non-urgent pediatric care, guidance for the clinician in rendering pediatric care. *Amer Acad Pediatrics.* 2003;112:1186–95.

38 Buckley RH. Advances in the understanding and treatment of human severe combined immuno-deficiency. *Immuno Res.* 2000;22:237–51.

39 Gerba CP, Rose JB, Haas CV. Sensitive populations: who is at risk? *Int J Food Microbiol.* 1996;30:112–23.

40 Trevejo RT, Barr MC, Robinson RA. Important emerging bacterial zoonotic infections among the immuno-compromised. *Vet Res.* 2005;36:493–506.

41 Dupont HL, et al. Prevention of travelers diarrhea by the tablet formulation of bismuth subsalyciate. *JAMA.* 1987;257: 1347.

42 Ericsson CD, Dupont HL. Travelers diarrhea, approach to prevention and treatment. *Clin Inf Dis.* 1983;16:298.

43 Dupont HL, et al. Prevention of travelers diarrhea with trimethaprim and sulfa-methaxyzole. *Rev Infect Dis.* 4;1982:533.

44 Keller H. *The Story of My Life,* Macy JA, ed. New York, Toronto, London, Sydney, Auckland: Bantam Books; 1962: 94. (By special arrangement with Signet.)

10 | Communications Planning for the Expedition Medical Officer

Christian Macedonia, MD, LTC, MC

The planet earth is a sphere with a surface area of 509,600,000 square kilometers. With vast amounts of the earth's surface remote from population centers and city services, there is plenty of room for expeditions to roam. Exploring is all about discovering new things off the beaten track. When a medical emergency arises, however, the very remoteness that makes exploring so interesting can also make it dangerous or sometimes even deadly.

In days past, expedition organizers had few alternatives for mitigating medical risk. Expedition participants were chosen for their exceptional physical fitness, and usually an expedition doctor or medic with experience in expedition medicine was included, but in the end the team prayed for a little luck. There was an expectation and acceptance that exploring was an inherently dangerous undertaking that might result in serious disability or even death.[1]

Things have changed in the twenty-first century. With advancements in medicine and telecommunications have come elevated expectations among those who wish to explore. We read almost every month about someone with a serious disease or disability taking on a challenge that daunted even the most robust individuals in decades past – amputees are summiting Everest, the blind take trips into the Amazon, and septuagenarian retirees cruise to the Antarctic on icebreakers.[2] Extreme sports literally take athletes to new heights.[3] If one of these modern-day explorers is hurt or falls ill, there is an expectation that a communication system will be in place to enable the delivery of medical care to that patient. Expedition physicians need to be aware of this modern expectation and have appropriate knowledge about communications and telemedicine.

MODERN COMMUNICATIONS AND TELEMEDICINE

Satellite communications have flattened the earth and brought some of the greatest minds in medicine to some of the most remote corners of the planet. Digital cameras show the waxy hands of a recently frostbitten climber, a satellite phone call to a doctor in Washington, DC, helps an expedition medic select medication for a trekker in the Andes, and a solo transoceanic sailor is instructed in the steps for lancing of an abscess via satellite e-mail.[4] All of this is possible through modern communications systems (Figure 10.1).

Telemedicine is simply "medicine at a distance" using the combination of the Greek word for "far," τελε (tele), and the English "medicine" (see Chapter 22 for a more detailed discussion of telemedicine). Telemedicine involves the use of telecommunications technologies to support the diagnosis and/or treatment of medical or surgical disorders. The first telemedicine systems used simple telephone or cable video connections.[5] These technologies can be something as simple as a phone call or as sophisticated as a telerobotic surgery performed over broadband communications links (Figure 10.2).[6]

The early days of communication in expeditions were themselves explorations of new technological territories rather than just exploration of new physical territories.[7,8] As such, these expeditions hauled gear that was often larger and heavier than the actual expedition survival gear. In modern days, communication and telemedicine technologies have reached a level of maturity and price point where a typical expedition can expect to have sophisticated technologies that would have been unavailable even in the recent past.

The expedition physician must have an understanding of the role of communications systems and its application to providing medical care in remote locations. The depth and breadth of the equipment available for any particular expedition is daunting, and the medical officer must understand how to properly assess for communications needs depending on the type of expedition and the characteristics of the expedition participants (Figure 10.3). Choosing a proper communications system for an expedition is imperative not only for proper patient treatment in the field but also for triage and evacuation of a critically ill patient when necessary.

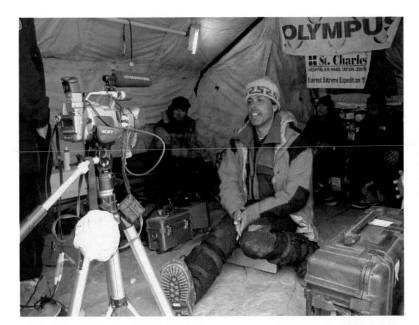

Figure 10.1. Dr. Kenneth M. Kamler, gives a class on cold weather injury prevention from a clinic at the base camp of Everest (situated at 5,500 m) to students and doctors at Yale University. Photo courtesy of Robert Hyman.

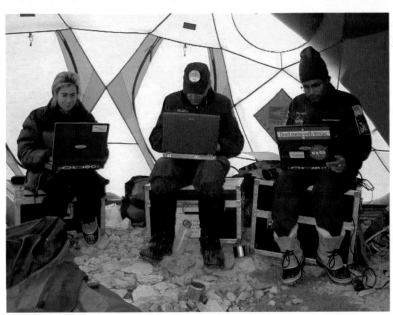

Figure 10.2. Despite the wide availability of video teleconferencing tools, e-mail remains the most widely used telemedicine application. Photo courtesy of Robert Hyman.

COMMUNICATIONS PLANNING

There is no substitute for good planning on expeditions, and this is particularly true for the expedition physician.[9] Once the organization of medical assets is established, it is best to draft a written plan. The plan does not have to be exhaustive, but it does need to be detailed well enough to be followed by another member of the team in case the medical team leader is incapacitated.

Planning also should demonstrate appropriate understanding of the telecommunications requirements versus the available resources. The scale of the telecommunications plan needs to fit within the scope, budget, and location of the expedition. There are no one-size-fits-all telecommunications systems in existence. Some telecommunications services offer massive amounts of voice and data capabilities but may come at an unacceptably high cost or be provided in limited geographical locations. It would be just as foolish to pack a 3-m satellite dish for a recreational journey to Machu Picchu as it would be to pack crampons for a Sahara expedition. Being overequipped can be as bad as being underequipped.

The medical officer should download any necessary manuals, texts, Centers for Disease Control and Prevention (CDC) or World Health Organization (WHO) health advisories and have these stored not only on a computer or personal digital assistant (PDA), but also on a flash drive as a backup. These should be linked as appendices to the telemedicine plan. The medical officer should also bookmark essential pages for easy linking, if

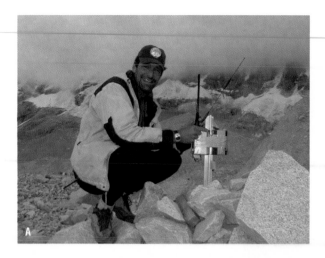
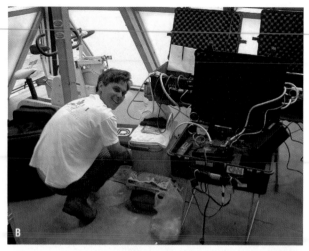
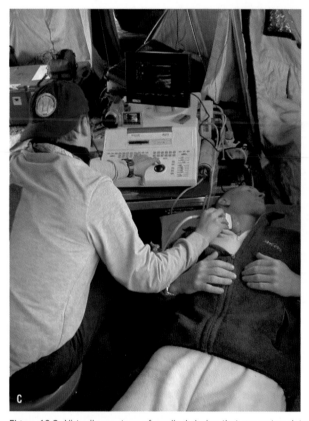
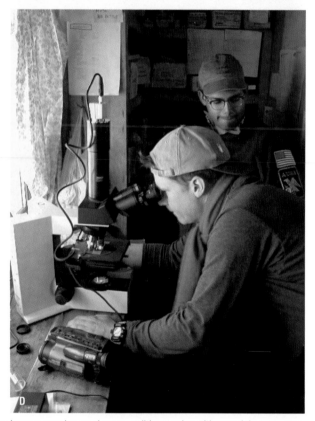

Figure 10.3. Virtually any type of medical device that generates data or images can be used on expeditions using either real-time or store-and-forward telemedicine techniques. Photo courtesy of Christian Macedonia.

communications bandwidth and equipment that support Web navigation are available. For instance, bookmarking weather services can be valuable in helping determine what kinds of environmental countermeasures the expedition needs to perform such as added layers of clothing or sunscreen.

EXPEDITION FOCUS

Expeditions are task-organized, based on the objectives (summit a mountain, search for a particular deep ocean species, document the trade routes of an ancient

civilization, measure radiation in the polar regions). When developing a communications plan, the expedition team needs to ask some basic questions:

- Is the expedition for entertainment, adventure, scientific research, commercial exploration for resources, or historical research?
- Will it be large or small?
- Will it be in a hostile environment?
- Will it take place among a culture with a language and social conventions far different from those of the expedition party?

These basic questions can help begin the discussion to determine what type of communications equipment the team will need on the expedition. Each of these factors, along with others, will help determine what gear would be most appropriate.

USING TELECOMMUNICATIONS EQUIPMENT

This is often an underappreciated part of the planning. Does the medical staff know how to use the telecommunications equipment? This is not a small point. Sometimes the communications package is managed by people other than the medical staff due to the high price of the equipment and airtime. The culture of medicine has become habituated to the availability of quick and easy access to e-mail and telephone.[10] Naturally, the expedition physician should ask some questions prior to the expedition's departure:

- What kind of access does the medical staff have to the communications gear?
- How quickly can an emergency communications link be set up?
- Does the medical team need its own dedicated means of communication independent of the expedition's own?

It is wise to perform drills and to make up "cheat sheets" similar to the way one prepares for cardiac arrest code situations. The medical team member should know how to turn their communications equipment on, how to enter access codes, and how to dial in contact numbers. This may seem trivial to anyone who has not had to do this on an expedition. Even something as simple, however, as dialing a phone number may be a complicated affair as satellite phone number prefixes may change based on which satellite you choose to use. Furthermore, there are no standard menus under which telecommunications terminals operate. Each manufacturer has its own proprietary interface or user menus despite the fact that it may use standard telecommunications protocols.

The medical team members need to be as qualified on their communications equipment as they are on their medical equipment. Just like any medical skill, this usually involves practice, practice, and more practice.

EXPEDITION ENVIRONMENT

To know what kind of medical support package is required, the expedition medical officer needs to have total awareness of the situations under which they will be practicing. This information should be used to adjust the plan accordingly. For instance, if a group is planning a diving expedition but has limited capabilities to handle hyperbaric emergencies, then the medical team should prepare its communications system with that in mind. Such a plan might include steps for contacting the nearest hyperbaric facility in case of emergency,

having links stored to Web-enabled information support sites, and/or having medical evacuation services speed-dial information preprogrammed into communications devices.

MEDICAL RECORDS

The expedition physician is responsible for informing the expedition team leader what requirements they have for the health and safety of the expedition *before* departing on the expedition, including any needed medical records and immunization records. Ideally, the expedition physician has at least access to abbreviated medical records on all the expedition team members, but an alternative may be to have all the expedition members carry scanned (Adobe PDF files) copies of their medical and immunization records on a rugged USB flash drive (Figure 10.4). This is a poor man's version of an electronic dog tag.

With the knowledge of the state of health within the expedition members, the expedition medical officer can develop a plan that optimizes the medical supplies and determine what kind of medical specialty support, if any, is required. The expedition medical officer can then produce a contact list either on a laminated card, stored on their flash drive, or on a PDA (the author recommends all three) that allows for consultation either by teleconferencing or e-mail. It is useful to make contact with any consulting facility prior to departure, if possible, not only to test the links but also to develop a rapport with any consulting specialists.

CHOOSING EQUIPMENT AND SERVICES

The equipment available to expedition medical teams is improving steadily, and the costs are decreasing

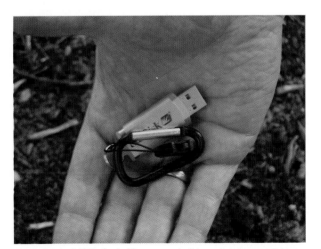

Figure 10.4. A USB flash drive connected to a simple snap-link can store valuable information such as a summarized medical record, emergency contact info, and even digital photos of the owner's passport and visas. Ruggedized and encrypting versions of these devices can be found through many retail sources. Photo courtesy of Christian Macedonia.

or remaining flat. The availability of services is also expanding so that territories only accessible by one modality are often supported by another. When developing the communications plan, the expedition physician (or expedition communications specialist) needs to contract for the appropriate equipment and realize that the communications needs might change during the course of the expedition. For example, an expedition may first travel from one country that uses one type of cell phone standard to a country with a different cell phone standard. Should one rely on satellite phones and bypass the problem, or might it be simpler to rent a local cell phone during the time the expedition will be in a foreign city? To make reasonable decisions regarding the choice of equipment, consider the three C's: Cost, Capabilities, and Customs.

Cost

Communications equipment is often the most expensive part of an expedition. Equipment costs, however, are only part of the equation because, as anyone who has ever gotten a "free" mobile phone can attest, airtime and service charges can be onerous. When choosing telecommunications equipment, one cannot divorce it from the service charges unless one is using purely point-to-point FM radio communications. All other forms have some service fee. Some providers break down the cost by straight airtime while others charge by the data bit. If voice communications are all that is required, then airtime it the key cost consideration. If the expedition is expected to use Internet services with varying degrees of bandwidth then data rate charges may apply. These issues should be explored with the communications retailer *before* the expedition starts.

Capabilities

Simple voice communications need minimal telecommunications bandwidth. High-speed data network services, particularly video links, require much more robust communications links (Figure 10.5). Wider capabilities also cost in terms of the overall power and equipment footprint. The latest technologies in telemedicine have improved dramatically in this regard but are still a consideration, particularly if the medical team must carry its own equipment.

Customs

Many countries have duties and tariffs placed on telecommunications gear and satellite systems. Some have legal prohibitions or actually block their usage. A little research can save huge headaches at border crossings. When in doubt, contact your embassy or consulate.

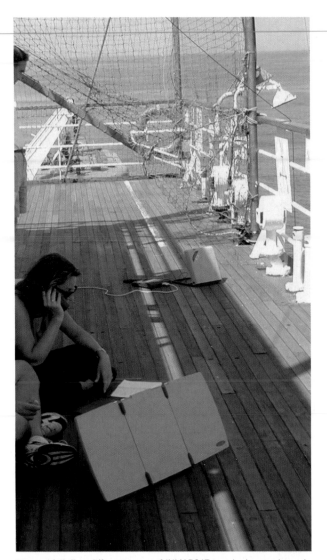

Figure 10.5. Two different types of INMARSAT terminals are shown in use during a marine archeology expedition to the RMS *Titanic*. The larger terminal in the foreground is used for voice and moderate speed data, while the smaller terminal is used primarily for voice but can be used to send data at very low data rates. Photo courtesy of Christian Macedonia.

COMMUNICATIONS PACKAGES FOR MEDICAL USE

Virtually any digital medical tool from microscopes to sphygmomanometers can be connected to a computer. (See Table 10.1.) If the expedition medical officer is contemplating using anything other than the basics, he or she should contact any number of retailers or manufacturers of medical devices. Unless the team is conducting purely a "telemedicine expedition," it is unlikely that one would need anything other than the following basic communications tools:

- Communications terminal (cell phone, satellite phone, broad satellite terminal)
- Rugged computer loaded with appropriate software (laptop, touchpad, or PDA)
- Flash drive or drives for secure data storage

Table 10.1. Matrix of available telecommunications services

Service	Location/ availability	Type	Terminal size	Mod/high	Typical user	Price voice	Price data	Terminal price and overhead cost
GSM/CDMA cellular	Variable, strongest near cities	Cellular	Very small; handheld	Low/mod	Everybody	*	**	*
Globalstar satellite phone	60% of the earth's surface	LEO	Small; handheld	Low	Travelers to remote locations	**	***	***
Iridium satellite phone	Worldwide	LEO	Small; handheld	Low	Travelers/military	**	***	***
Inmarsat terminal Voice/ BGAN	Worldwide	GSO	Moderate (briefcase)	Low/mod	Maritime, travelers, military, news channels	**	**	****
Thurya satellite phone	Middle East	GSO	Small; handheld	Low	Travelers in the Middle East	**	***	***
VSAT C-band terminal	Asia, Africa, Latin America	GSO	Large shipping container	Mod/high	Businesses, rural villages	*	*	*****
VSAT ku band terminal	Europe/North America	GSO	Large shipping container	Mod/high	Businesses processing credit card transactions, most gas stations, WalMart	*	*	*****

Note: Polar expeditions usually require specialized telecommunications plans because satellite service providers are focused on providing services to the 99% of the population that live between the Arctic and Antarctic zones.

- Reliable power source (solar or using on-site generation with lithium battery backup)
- Durable digital camera (with or without video capability)

The basic package does not have to be a burden to an expedition. It can take up a space as small as a daypack and cost as little as U.S. $2,000. Size and cost, however, should be a function of the expedition safety goals relate to the environment to be explored. These kits can be purchased à la carte or can be rented through a telecommunications retailer specializing in remote business telecommunications. These retailers usually support the maritime, petroleum, transportation industries as well as diplomatic and military missions.

SUMMARY

Communications systems are now common components of expedition medicine, but they can never eliminate the medical risks of expeditioneering. They can, however, elevate the level of safety to a level that affords more people the opportunity to enjoy the richness of this beautiful planet and even the heavens above. The wise expedition physician fully understands the strengths and limits of technology and prepares the team for their proper use.

REFERENCES

1 Fodstad H, Kondziolka D, Brophy BP, Roberts DW, Girvin JP. Arctic and Antarctic exploration including the contributions of physicians and effects of disease in the polar regions. *Neurosurgery.* 1999;44(5):925–39; discussion 939–40.

2 Prociv P. Health aspects of Antarctic tourism. *Travel Med.* 1998; 5(4):210–2.

3 Townes DA. Wilderness medicine: Strategies for provision of medical support for adventure racing. *Sports Med.* 2005;35(7):557–64.

4 BBC World Service. Sailor operates on own elbow. Thursday, November 19, 1998.

5 Moore GT, Willemain TR, Bonanno R, Clark WD, Martin AR, Mogielnicki RP. Comparison of television and telephone for remote medical consultation. *N Engl J Med.* 1975; 292(14):729–32.

6 Grigsby J, Sanders JH. Telemedicine: Where it is and where it's going. *Ann Intern Med.* 1998;129(2):123–7.

7 Satava R, Angood PB, Harnett B, Macedonia C, Merrell R. The physiologic cipher at altitude: telemedicine and real-time monitoring of climbers on Mount Everest. *Telemed J E Health.* 2000;6(3):303–13.

8 Otto C, Pipe A. Remote, mobile telemedicine: the satellite transmission of medical data from Mount Logan. *J Telemed Telecare.* 1997;3 (Suppl 1):84–5.

9 Tek D. Medical planning for expeditions. *Emerg Med Clin North Am.* 1992;10(2):449–66.

10 Coile RC, Jr. The digital transformation of health care. *Physician Exec.* 2000;26(1):8–15.

APPENDIX

Telemedicine Glossary

A

Analog signal: A continuous signal that carries information through modulation of a continuous carrier signal's amplitude or frequency (in contrast to a digital signal). Old cellular phone systems and many handheld and conventional FM radio systems operate using analog signals.

Airtime: The time spent transmitting over a mobile phone or satellite network.

Asynchronous communication: Two-way communication in which the data rates of the sender or uplink of the communications is different from that of the receiver or downlink.

B

Bandwidth: The carrying capacity of a particular data link, usually defined by uplink and downlink data rates listed in kilobits or megabits per second.

Bit: Binary encoded information is stored and transmitted in a series of ones (on) or zeros (off). The bit is a single binary digit. It is the fundamental unit of binary math.

Bluetooth: A very short-range wireless communications standard providing connectivity to electronic devices such as personal computers, wireless phones, some medical devices, printers, and PDAs. Operates in the 2.4-GHz range and is limited to 10 m.

Broadband: Communications (e.g., broadcast television, microwave, and satellite) capable of carrying a wide range of frequencies; refers to transmission of signals in a frequency-modulated fashion, over a segment of the total bandwidth available, thereby permitting simultaneous transmission of several messages.

Byte: Eight bits. Data storage is usually described in terms of bytes (kilo: 1,000, mega: 1,000,000, giga: 1,000,000,000, tera: 1,000,000,000,000)

C

Cellular: A wireless telephone network that is divided into regularly spaced interconnecting "cells" consisting of antennae and base stations.

Channel: Any communications path between two points using any medium.

Codec: Short for "code/decode" this is a piece of software or hardware that converts one type of signal or encoding to another for the purposes of transmission or ease of signal processing.

Code division multiple access (CDMA): An encoding processing algorithm for both speech and text developed by Qualcomm.

Compression (of files or signal; photos, video, voice): A mathematical simplification of a dataset in order to reduce the dataset to a smaller size. This is performed to either reduce storage or transmission bandwidth requirements.

D

Digital communications: Communications using binary (on-off) encoded signals. Compare to *analog signal.*

Digital imaging and communication in medicine (DICOM): An ACR/NEMA (American College of Radiology – National Electrical Manufacturers Association) standard for communication, classification, interoperability, and storage of medical image information. This is primarily a communications standard and not an imaging standard.

Digitiziation: The conversion of information into digital form. For example, a fax machine converts a scanned paper document into digital information for telephone transmission.

Direct digital capture: The capture of audio, video, or still image information directly into a digital form.

Downlink: The earthward received path of information from a transmitting station or satellite. Also called a reverse link.

DS1 (T1): A digital carrier capable of transmitting 1.544 Mbps of electronic information. The general term for a digital carrier available for high-value voice, data, or compressed video traffic.

DS3 (T3): A carrier of 45-Mbps bandwidth. One DS3 channel can carry 28 DS1 channels.

Duplex: See *full duplex.*

E

Encryption: The systematic scrambling (or coding) of an analog or digital signal to avoid unauthorized access to voice or data that is stored or transmitted. An encryption key or decryption device is required to decode the encrypted signal or file.

F

Federal Communications Commission (FCC): The agency of the U.S. government responsible for the regulation of telecommunications modalities, frequencies, commercial entities, and hardware within the United States.

Fiberoptic: Durable glass fibers used to transmit high-bandwidth digital communications utilizing pulses of laser light.

Film digitizer: A film-scanning device that converts sheet film into a digital image file for storage or transmission.

Firewall: A hardware device or specialized software program that blocks unauthorized users or network queries from access through a protected network.

Full duplex: A system capable of simultaneous bidirectional communications. Contrast to *half duplex*.

Full-motion video: A video stream with refresh rates approximating that of the flicker frequency of human eyesight. This translates to approximately 24 frames per second.

G

Geostationary earth orbiting satellites (GEOS): Satellite system that orbits at a distance 36,000 km above the earth, and remains in a stationary position relative to any fixed point on the earth.

Global positioning system (GPS): A system of satellites launched and maintained by the United States used for terrestrial navigation. The satellite system broadcasts time-encoded information to terrestrial systems enabled with GPS decoders to calculate extremely accurate position date utilizing triangulation.

Global system for mobile communications (GSM): A digital cellular phone technology introduced in 1991 and now used around the world. GSM operates in various countries under one of three different frequency bands: 900 MHz, 1800 MHz, and 1900 MHz. GSM utilizes TDMA.

H

Half-duplex: A communication channel over which both transmission and reception are possible, but only in one direction at a time.

Health Insurance Portability and Accountability Act (HIPAA): Although titled as an insurance act, it is primarily regarded as the definitive statute governing patient privacy in the United States. This includes information transmitted or stored over telemedicine links.

Health Level-7 Data Communications Protocol (HL-7): Defines industry standards for transmitting and storing billing, hospital census, order entries, and other health-related information between devices and data repositories.

I

International Telecommunication Union (ITU): An agency of the United Nations, headquartered in Geneva, Switzerland.

Image processing: Use of algorithms to modify images, usually to enhance important characteristics in them such as contrast or magnification.

Integrated services digital network (ISDN): A specific digital telecommunications technology that allows for the integrated transmission of voice, data, and video; a protocol for medium-bandwidth digital transmission.

International Mobile Satellite Organization (INMARSAT): An international satellite consortium now privatized as Inmarsat PLC.

Internet: A loosely affiliated international computer network linking computers and computer networks around the globe. Originally started by the U.S. Department of Defense in the late 1960s as ARPANET.

J

JPEG: Joint Photographic Experts Group. The most widely used and accepted digital compression standard used in telemedicine as well as in consumer digital camera imaging.

L

Land Earth Station Operator (LESO): Commercial or governmental enterprise that provides a link from a space satellite network to the terrestrial telecommunication grid.

Local area networks (LANs): Private networks that facilitate the sharing of information and computer resources by members of a specific group.

Low earth orbit satellites (LEOS): Satellite systems operating in low earth orbit (500–2,000 km above earth). The major commercial LEOS communications providers are Iridium LLC and Globalstar.

M

Mobile terminal: A portable data or voice communications tool used at the distal end of a digital communications network.

Modem: A modulator/demodulator. This device converts information into a transmissible form and can demodulate signals sent from another modem remotely.

Multiplexing: When multiple signals (cell phone, satellite) are carried in the same frequency band at the same time. The major wireless multiplexing methods include TDMA and CDMA.

N

Narrowband: A telecommunications medium that uses (relatively) low-frequency signals, exceeding 1.544 Mbps.

Network: An interconnected group of digital devices.

Non-geostationary satellites (NGSOs): System of satellites that orbit the earth in motion relative to the earth's surface. These can be singular or in an orbital constellation. They are divided into low earth orbit

(LEO; about 1000 km above the earth's surface) and medium earth orbit (MEO; about 10,000 km from the earth's surface; GPS is in MEO).

O

Optical character recognition (OCR): Automated scanning and computerized identification of printed characters used to convert written or printed documents into digitized text documents.

P

Picture archiving and communications system (PACS): A radiology image archiving system that acquires, transmits, stores, retrieves, and displays digital images along with HL-7 data from a variety of imaging sources.

Pixel: Picture element. The smallest fundamental display element of a digital image.

R

Repeater: A device that receives a radio signal and retransmits an amplified signal in a new direction.

S

Short message service (SMS): The transmission of short alphanumeric text messages to and from mobile devices or computers. Messages cannot be longer than 160 characters.

Store-and-forward: To capture and store medically relevant information for later forwarding of that information for interpretation, usually not in real time. This is the most common and the least expensive means of conducting telemedicine today.

T

Telecommunications: The use of wire, radio, optical, or other electromagnetic channels to transmit or receive signals for voice, data, and video communications.

Teleconsultation: The use of telecommunications to conduct medical consultation whereby the consultant is in a geographic location remote from the point of consultation.

Telemedicine: The use of audio, video, and other telecommunications and electronic information processing technologies to provide health services or assist health care personnel at distant sites.

Telementoring: The use of telecommunications technologies to provide guidance or instruction to another health care provider or sometimes even to the patient.

Telemonitoring: The use of audio, video, and other telecommunications and electronic information processing technologies to monitor patient status at a distance.

Telepresence: The use of robotic and other technologies to provide "presence" of an individual from a remote location enabled through a telecommunications link. Telepresence systems usually provide an essential element of presence required for a task. For instance, a surgical telepresence system provides robotic graspers as surrogates of a remote surgeon's hands.

Transmission control protocol/Internet protocol (TCP/IP): A communications protocol governing data exchanged over the Internet.

Third generation (3G): A new wireless standard for high-bandwidth applications utilizing wideband frequency carriers and a CDMA air interface.

Time division multiple access (TDMA): An older method of digital wireless communications transmission allowing multiple users to access over a single radiofrequency.

Transmission speed: The speed at which information passes over a channel specified in either bits per second (bps) or baud.

U

Uplink: The skyward transmit path of information to a receiving station or satellite. Also known as forward link.

V

Video teleconferencing: Real-time, usually two-way transmission of digitized video images between two or more locations.

Virtual reality: Complex computer-synthesized environment(s) that interact with humans utilizing artificial stimuli to one or more senses.

W

Wireless application protocol (WAP): An open standard for wireless communication between cellular phones and the Internet. WAP was specifically designed to deliver Web data to wireless devices with smaller screens.

World Wide Web (WWW): An ad hoc interconnected system of Internet nodes linking computers and servers around the globe utilizing hypertext markup language encoded software. This term is used synonymously with the Internet in popular culture, although not all Internet traffic is part of the World Wide Web.

The Phonetic Alphabet

A Alpha

B Bravo

C Charlie

D Delta

E Echo

F Foxtrot

G Golf

H Hotel

I India

J Juliet

K Kilo

L Lima

M Mike

N November

O Oscar

P Papa

Q Quebec

R Romeo

S Sierra

T Tango

U Uniform

V Victor

W Whiskey

X X-ray

Y Yankee

Z Zulu

0 Zero

1 One

2 Two

3 Tree

4 Four

5 Fife

6 Six

7 Sev-en

8 Ate

9 Nin-er

11 | Minimizing Risk on an Expedition

Medical Coverage and Evacuation Insurance in Remote Environments

Michael J. Manyak, MD, FACS

INTRODUCTION

You are making flight arrangements for that special trip: an exotic locale, an adventure tour, or a scientific expedition. The immediate excitement has been tempered by sobering thoughts of health and safety. You have searched the Internet for travel advisory information about your developing world destination. The travel agent may have been to the area but probably stayed in a nice hotel in the capital city, not in the tent or hammock you will call a temporary home. You have been advised to sign up for travel insurance. You are inundated with confusing choices about insurance, and there is very generic advice about the site – drink only bottled water, get immunization for hepatitis and meningitis, have a tetanus shot within the last 10 years, eat only well-cooked food. Your local physician has little experience with travel medicine. Information about local health resources is nonexistent or unreliable. Geopolitical information resources say the area is reasonably stable, but there has been sporadic violent insurgent activity in the northern regions for years, and travel is advised with caution. Bird flu has been reported in the adjacent country. What should you do to prepare for your travel safety?

RISK ASSESSMENT AND INSURANCE

International travel, once a daunting proposition reserved for those with significant financial means, has now become commonplace with approximately 50 million annual travelers from industrialized countries to the developing world.[1] Although business travel accounts for a significant segment of this population, there has been a tremendous increase in travel for educational, recreational, or adventure purposes. The past 20 years have witnessed a continuing upsurge in travel to places previously deemed inaccessible, exemplified in the extreme by those private citizens fortunate enough to experience space travel.

Standard health and safety issues, which have become mundane or taken for granted in an industrialized urban society, become more prominent in remote areas where risk is increased and quality health care is less accessible. Travelers face a different subset of potential problems than those remaining in their familiar environments. Health problems are self-reported in 22–64% of people traveling to the developing world.[2] Though most of these problems concern gastrointestinal, respiratory, and skin infections that tend to be self-limiting, about 8% (4 million) of the 50 million travelers become ill enough to seek medical care abroad or upon reaching home.[3]

Much of the data on travel had been collected approximately two decades ago, but recent data has been reported either from surveys or through use of the GeoSentinel program for disease surveillance.[3,4] The GeoSentinel database, coordinated by the International Society of Travel Medicine and the Centers for Disease Control and Prevention, consists of information gathered at 30 travel or tropical medicine clinics on six continents. The sites consist of academic as well as free-standing clinics and reflect a mixed population of patients requiring both outpatient and tertiary services. Between 1996 and 2004, this database recorded the characteristics of over 17,000 patients who had traveled to 230 countries. The data revealed that 67% of the travelers had medical problems concentrated in 4 of the 21 major syndrome categories. This concentrated group was comprised of, in decreasing order of incidence, systemic febrile illness (malaria, dengue, etc.), acute diarrhea, skin disorders, and chronic diarrhea; another 18% were affected by nondiarrheal gastrointestinal, respiratory, and genitourinary disorders (Table 11.1).[4] Eighty percent of the patients overall had exposure in one of six developing regions of the world, and more than 50% of them had received documented medical advice from a medical provider before travel.

Difficulty with access for health care is exacerbated for those involved in expeditions, exotic adventure travel, and scientific or corporate endeavors that take people to remote locations. The mining engineer in the central Indonesian highlands faces the same issues

Table 11.1. Most common sources of traveler medical problems[a]

Systemic febrile illness
Acute diarrhea
Dermatologic disorders
Chronic diarrhea
Nondiarrheal gastrointestinal disorders
Nonspecific symptoms or signs
Genitourinary disorders

[a]Reasons for travel included tourism (59%), family visits (15%), business (14%), volunteer activities (8%), and educational travel (4%). Adapted from 17,353 patients reporting to travel clinics in the GeoSentinel Program (Europe, United States, Canada, Israel, Australia, New Zealand) after travel to 230 countries.[4] The disorders account for 85% of complaints in decreasing order of occurrence.

of receiving quality health care for an adverse medical event as those presented to polar travelers. Although a catastrophic event is unlikely in the home environment for most people, these unexpected disastrous events pose serious threats and can be more likely in remote destinations. Events like the recent tsunami in Southeast Asia cannot be anticipated, but general preparation for a potential evacuation due to an adverse event should be considered. Increasing political unrest, violent crime, and terrorism make it prudent for travelers to take certain precautions in locations where there is potential for these types of disturbances. This chapter addresses considerations for expedition leaders and medical officers regarding risk assessment and management for travelers in the developing world.

EXPEDITION MEDICINE

The dramatic increase in travel to remote locations and the accompanying stories of medical misadventures have raised the awareness of the need for better preparation to avoid problems when possible and to deal with them judiciously when they arise. Equally important, and often overlooked, is the follow-up required after return to industrialized society; both legal and medical issues can arise in the aftermath of an expedition with an adverse event. This burgeoning need to address health and safety in the field has stimulated the rapid growth of a medical subspecialty concerned with management of medical problems for adventure travel and wilderness experiences. Expedition medicine is an evolving subset of this discipline with a narrower focus on remote environments.

Expedition medicine has been likened to military medicine for the civilian. Elements common to both include preventive medicine, field communication, transportation, experience with tropical and infectious disease, knowledge of medical problems peculiar to extreme environments, and emergency medicine.

Furthermore, expedition medicine requires awareness of public health and local environmental issues as well as knowledge about local health resources. In time of crisis, the expedition medical officer is often expected to be calm in the midst of chaos and to provide services that may exceed his or her specific medical training, increasing the already stressful circumstances.

Greater awareness of the need for information has spawned a plethora of literature on travel, with many articles addressing travel health. The sophisticated international traveler is likely to be more informed about travel health issues but also may be confused because of differing opinions on preparation and management. This confusion also exists in health care providers who seek advice for patients on travel-related health care.

Although travelers often profess to be concerned about health and safety on the road in remote environments, one just as often discovers that not all areas are adequately addressed before departure. Two such aspects that are underappreciated concern security and proper travel medical insurance. Neglect of proper preparation in these areas can be due to inattention but is often related to a lack of understanding of potential areas of concern and an inability to identify sources for assistance. One should not assume that tour operators or travel companies offer more than very basic services for security and medical care. They are certain to carry liability insurance to protect themselves against legal action for an adverse medical event on their activity, but services for the client often do not exceed minimal temporary medical care and emergency transportation to a regional medical facility, which may be inadequate for anything other than basic first aid. Inadequate medical care and evacuation often is a result of not knowing what you do not know about your coverage.

THE IMPACT OF TRAVEL AND THE NEED FOR INSURANCE

The evolution of travel medical insurance over the past several years mirrors the changing perception about the need for coverage. For example, prior to the terrorist attacks on the World Trade Center, less than 10% of Americans purchased travel medical insurance. However, post 9/11, no insurance sector has shown greater popularity than travel insurance: current estimates place travel insurance coverage at more than 30% of the travel population.[2] The greatest fear of 74% of American travelers is an adverse medical event. This same survey by a major insurer also revealed that 92% of the responders desired immediate access to U.S.-quality health care and the option to be transported home to receive treatment.[5]

Most illnesses reported by travelers are mild and self-limited but anywhere from 0.01 to 0.1% of the 50 million people who travel to developing countries will need evacuation for a medical reason.[6,7] Approximately 1 in 100,000 will die during travel. In a review of all American deaths overseas, as reported to the U.S. Passport Office by the Consular Representatives, the major cause of death was injury from motor vehicle accidents or drowning.[8] Causes of death vary with the age and gender of the traveler, with females less likely to die on the road. Infectious disease as a cause of death was surprisingly low, and deaths from circulatory (myocardial infarction, stroke) or cancer causes were lower than corresponding domestic death rates.

THE BASICS OF TRAVEL INSURANCE

The actual benefits of travel insurance are not obvious despite the promotional byline. Programs with titles like "Rapid Rescue" can be anything but, and "Travel Shield" can be quite porous, whereas "Gold Protection Preferred" may define exactly what you need to get out of a medical predicament – gold. In its fundamental form, travel insurance is designed to protect the traveler from the *economic* impact of unforeseen expenses incurred while traveling. Under this type of coverage, emergency hospital bills, lost luggage, and perhaps even a medical evacuation will be reimbursed if receipts are submitted. However, most travelers do not realize that travel insurance is *secondary* (subrogated, in insurance parlance) to other insurance policies under which the travelers are covered. This means that if you receive emergency medical treatment in a developing country and it is covered by your health insurance, your health insurer pays, not the travel insurance company. This is an important distinction because if your health insurance specifically excludes treatment outside the United States or you do not have health insurance, the purchase of travel insurance becomes imperative.

The traveler who seeks an insurance policy for a trip of any kind needs to differentiate among components of coverage (Table 11.2). Services may include a portion dedicated to the trip logistics itself. These are classified

Table 11.2. Key components of travel insurance policies[a]

Travel assistance
- Lost luggage
- Trip cancellation
- Visa services
- Inoculation advice

Medical coverage
- Medical expenses with limits

Evacuation
- Evacuation of injured
- Evacuation of spouse
- Return of mortal remains

[a]The traveler is advised to carefully read when the policy is activated and exclusions for coverage. Policies may not include all components.

as assistance services and consist of reimbursement for loss of luggage, trip interruption, trip cancellation, provision of visa and immunization information, and similar services peripheral to health care and safety. Many of us have been irritated when these circumstances arise, but these events are not critical for health and safety. The upside for this benefit is that the addition of this type of coverage to your package comes at a low cost.

The second component is medical coverage itself, which has various limits of reimbursement that may differ based on the policy premium. This premium can vary with the level of deductible amount selected if different levels are offered. Clients are usually required to pay for the medical services incurred at the location or in transit and seek reimbursement upon return from the trip. Although costs of medical services in other countries may be lower in comparison to the United States, the overall expenses for hospitalization and treatment can be quite high because of the perception of the traveler's personal wealth and the lack of recourse for the impaired traveler. An extended stay in a foreign hospital is not desirable for most travelers because of the questionable quality of care and the mounting expense, which quickly gobbles up the insurance amount, thus making an evacuation or medical transfer more urgent.

The third component is the actual evacuation in the event of an adverse medical event. Although they are frequently presented as bundled services in the same policy, each insurance product is different and may lack one of these characteristics. Each component can be purchased separately depending on the personal needs of the individual on travel. The products of insurance companies vary, and it is important to review the circumstances under which each part of the policy takes effect and the limits of what is actually covered.

THE NEED FOR EVACUATION

Despite growth in recognition of need and the emergence of many options for coverage, many forms of insurance or travel-related services fall short of the standards anticipated for adequate medical assistance by most travelers. One needs to avoid the American Express syndrome of presupposing full medical and evacuation coverage in domestic insurance policies or through ownership of a particular credit card. Most medical insurance policies associated with credit cards or organizational memberships have significant restrictions on international medical services and do not include appropriate evacuation. In addition, many adventurous activities are excluded from policy coverage even in supposedly inclusive policies (Table 11.3).

Travelers with broad private medical insurance coverage on domestic policies generally have similar coverage when on international travel. However, this is not true universally, and the wise traveler will verify coverage

Table 11.3. Common exclusions for medical and evacuation insurance

Travel to countries in armed conflict
Older than age 75
Hazardous adventure (e.g., skydiving, bungee jumping, helicopter skiing)
Adverse event due to alcohol or illicit drug use
Withdrawal from chronic alcohol or drug abuse
Exacerbation of known psychoses

limits before embarking on a trip. Medicare and most health maintenance organizations do not provide coverage for international travel. *It is imperative to understand that even comprehensive medical insurance policies do not cover evacuation.* Only a few major insurance companies provide evacuation coverage, emphasizing the need to acquire a separate policy. Without supplemental insurance coverage for medical problems and evacuation, the injured or ill patient generally has no recourse but to pay the local charges for transportation and treatment. These costs can be considerable with evacuation expenses alone frequently ranging over $100,000.[7] Specific details about evacuation should be determined as well since there have been several instances where the

quality of transportation and the final destination of the evacuation have been far below the clients' expectations. In these cases, the company has technically discharged its legal duties, but the patient may be only marginally better than at the limited facilities in the vicinity of the site of injury or illness. So, to avoid being transported by oxcart (interpreted by the insurance company as the most readily available means of transfer) to the outpatient clinic in the next village (designated regional medical facility), establish before departure what would happen in the case of a serious medical event. (See Figures 11.1 and 11.2.)

The inherent desire for Americans to return to the United States for health care is strongly supported by outcomes data comparing domestic care to that in other countries. Access to U.S.-quality health care is important because it places the odds in your favor for a positive outcome. For example, recent reports in the *European Heart Journal* and the *British Journal of Surgery* reveal that even in Western Europe, surgical mortality is almost 20% higher than it is in the United States. This figure rises to nearly 30% in Eastern Europe and to over 70% in Latin America.[9,10] No data are available for the rest of the world. If you want the best possible medical outcome, it remains true that no country compares to the

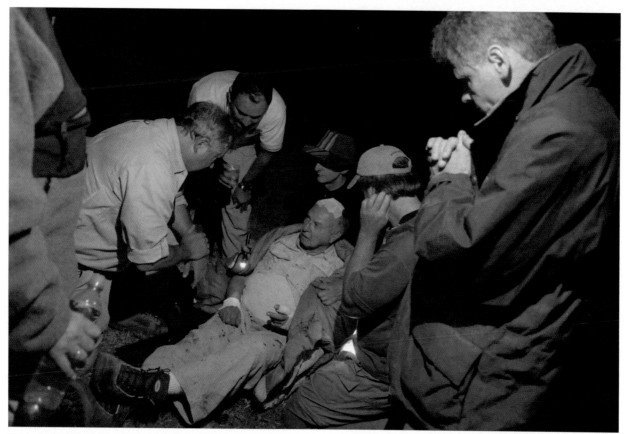

Figure 11.1. Patient assessment and determination of need for evacuation is dependent on accurate on-site information. This patient was determined to be stable enough to await safer daylight helicopter high-altitude evacuation after serious fall. Photo courtesy of Zbigniew Bzdek, *Chicago Tribune.*

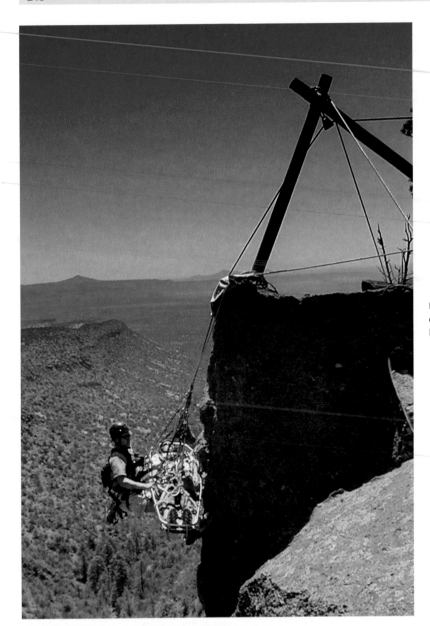

Figure 11.2. Roped high-altitude rescue procedure in New Mexico. Photo courtesy of Global Rescue, Inc., Boston.

United States. However, in nearly all cases, the insurer will determine whether evacuation is necessary and the destination for the evacuee, regardless of patient and family desires. A few companies like Global Rescue (Boston) do provide this service to the patient-desired medical facility, but, in most instances, the patient and family will not have a vote for the evacuation destination. This is another important point to consider when acquiring evacuation insurance.

The decision about evacuation is complex, and the traveler and his or her family usually do not understand it. The initiation of evacuation occurs when an attending physician at the site or one contacted by authorities determines that the patient's medical needs exceed the available resources. Evacuation then proceeds if the physician in charge determines that the patient is in need of better quality care and will survive the move.[7]

Immediate evacuation after stabilization is usually indicated for cardiac, neurological, orthopedic, surgically correctable, and obstetrical conditions.[11] Evacuation is usually delayed for patients with acute psychosis, alcohol or drug withdrawal, uncontrolled seizures, and other unstable disorders because there is little benefit for relocation, and management is difficult, especially in an airplane. Furthermore, conditions that would not ordinarily preclude ground transportation at standard atmospheric pressures may be contraindicated when changes in atmospheric pressure during flight could cause tragic consequences due to low oxygen content or gas expansion.[7]

Other reasons for rapid evacuation for a more stable patient include hospitalization in a facility that has inadequate hygiene or adherence to universal precautions (reusable syringes or intravenous tubing, lack of

Potential disaster averted but expensive

The Colca Canyon in southern Peru, purportedly the deepest in the world, is beautiful, but its descent is strenuous due to the altitude and frequently very narrow ledges. An adverse medical event would most likely require evacuation on foot because helicopters cannot fly to the high-altitude areas where hikers are stranded or cannot land due to the terrain (Figure 11.3). On a recent expedition to this canyon, a participant sustained serious injuries after a 50-foot fall stopped only by a large cactus patch. Evacuation was required, but the 5-hour ascent by mule would be very difficult and painful at best with potential for deterioration. The physician on site contacted the company whose "evacuation" policy the patient had purchased, a well-known organization that markets its services internationally. The company refused to evacuate the patient, stating that they were only required to transport him and that required him to be at a medical facility – which was inaccessible.

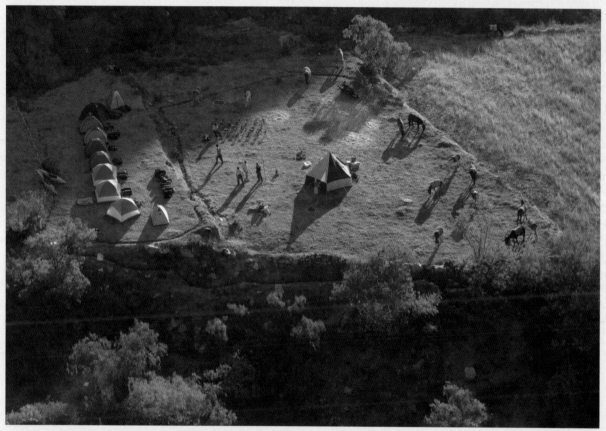

Figure 11.3. Medical evacuation in a remote location can be very challenging with limited means. Evacuation from this site in the Peruvian Andes would require transport by mule to an area suitable for a helicopter. High-altitude evacuation by helicopter is not always feasible due to air density and atmospheric conditions. Photo courtesy of Zbigniew Bzdek, *Chicago Tribune*.

A second company with a known track record of successful evacuations was contacted and provided an immediate response. Unfortunately, because the patient had not purchased the policy from the second company, he bore the full cost of the expensive evacuation. Predictably, several months later, the first company, which refused to evacuate the patient, now claims repeatedly that it did not refuse evacuation. Fortunately, the patient recovered without complication because he received timely care.

The moral of this story is to carefully read your insurance policy. Even though the first company technically fulfilled its legal obligation for transport, the language in the policy is deceptive because it does not specify evacuation and the interpretation of transportation is provided by the company. Therefore "evacuation" only occurs when convenient. Unfortunately, this is not an uncommon occurrence among travelers and is not the first instance associated with this company. With travel insurance coverage, the old Roman warning *Caveat Emptor* ("Buyer Beware") is very applicable.

disposable gloves, etc.), lack of surgical instruments or supplies required for the procedure required (such as orthopedic implants), unscreened blood products needed for hemorrhagic conditions, or unavailability or substandard critical drugs.[11] In these cases, risk of creating an unnecessary complication can be avoided by transporting the patient to an appropriate facility with such services.

An important consideration not often pondered by travelers is the return of a spouse or family members in case of a debilitating medical event. Even less contemplated in most cases is the return of mortal remains in the event of a death. Many evacuation policies will provide a return benefit for family as well as return of mortal remains subject to the limits of the policy; this benefit may be part of an assistance package that accompanies evacuation. If a death has occurred and return is a covered benefit, the insurance company will assist in the arrangements for return of the deceased. This becomes very important to deal with legal ramifications of transport across international boundaries, compounded by familial bereavement.

POLICY COVERAGE EXCLUSIONS

Another aspect of insurance often overlooked is the exclusion for coverage for problems that occur on travel in some developing countries (Table 11.3). Many of these countries have had a history of political instability but may now be stable and not considered by most travelers to be dangerous. Despite the perceived decreased risk, these countries may remain as a destination excluded from coverage.

Age is often an exclusion, with most insurance companies not providing coverage for a person older than age 75. Most companies will consider coverage for people between the ages of 75 and 85 on an individual basis after review of the medical history, but the premium may be more costly.

Other exclusions that are important to note involve sporting or adventurous activities. Bungee jumping and skydiving are obvious exclusions for coverage, but activities usually considered less dangerous like skiing and scuba diving may be excluded; in fact, some of these activities may be a major reason for travel to that locale. Some insurance companies provide a product that covers adventurous activities with an additional premium. Likewise, certain organizations do provide coverage for specific activities that are excluded in most insurance packages. For example, the Divers Alert Network (DAN) provides insurance coverage in case of a diving accident, but evacuation is not included. Once again, this points out the need to scrutinize your policy to determine whether evacuation is a provided service.

Problems that arise from some chronic disorders may not be covered by travel policies for treatment or evacuation. Exacerbation of known psychoses, sequelae from chronic drug or alcohol abuse, and appearance of withdrawal from chronic drug or alcohol abuse are commonly excluded. In fact, it is not well known that many policies will not cover anything stemming from an alcohol-related event. So, someone who sustains a serious injury from falling off a barstool after too much holiday cheer may have a very sobering experience upon discovery that coverage may not be provided in some circumstances.

SELECTION OF SERVICES

Clearly, the first issue to determine before selecting any insurance product is existing protection. (See Table 11.4.) If you have examined your domestic medical policy and confirmed appropriate coverage for overseas or travel to a remote area, you may have adequate coverage and not require the medical expense component of a policy. However, it is important to find out the algorithm for response in the case of an adverse medical event. You should find out if you can speak directly to a doctor from a remote site. Furthermore, you should also determine whether you have direct access to a specialist if you need that type of communication for a specific problem. The reason for queries about these processes that are standard for domestic medical problems is that insurance companies do not employ doctors. Despite brochures that suggest otherwise, insurers do not have doctors on staff, do not have relationships with health care facilities (other than for billing and reimbursement), and do not have the ability to send someone to assist you. Most companies outsource these services to other companies beyond their control, frequently located overseas beyond the reach of the U.S. legal system.

The second step is to determine if you need evacuation insurance. Once you have ascertained that fact, and in most instances travelers will need evacuation insurance, there are important points you need to understand regarding exercising this type of policy. Limits of reimbursement and conditions of exclusion are obviously key issues, but other serious aspects should be understood by the traveler. The first step of communication should be clear, and you should know the qualifications of the responder (i.e., will you have immediate access to an accredited physician?). You and your family also need to understand who makes the decision to evacuate and to where that evacuation will occur. Lastly, you should address the transport of mortal remains and traveling companions in case of a tragedy. If the company you have selected cannot answer these questions to your satisfaction, you should keep looking for an organization that can provide the protection you seek.

Table 11.4. Travel medical resources (partial list)

International Association for Medical Assistance to Travelers (IAMAT): *http://www.iamat.org*
International Society of Travel Medicine: *http://www.istm.org*
International SOS: *http://www.internationalsos.com*
U.S. Department of State: *http://www.travel.state.gov/travel/overseas*
Center for Disease Control: *http://www.cdc.gov*

SUMMARY

As you have seen, the issue of travel medical insurance and evacuation coverage can be complex and the subtleties of application of your policies to your situation may not be apparent until you are in the midst of a crisis. Essentially, three points matter when it comes to travel and evacuation insurance: the quality and capability of the organization you have contracted with to protect you from risk, the determination of the services covered, and the exclusions for coverage. If these questions are answered to your satisfaction, you will have minimized the risk to you on your proposed travel. Remembering an oft-repeated definition of an adventure as an expedition that went wrong, make sure you maximize your protection and comfort level while on the road.

REFERENCES

1 Ryan ET, Wilson ME, Kain KE. Illness after international travel. *N Engl J Med.* 2002;347: 505–16.

2 Steffen R, deBernardis C, Banos A: Travel epidemiology – a global perspective. *Int J Antimicrob Agents.* 2003; 21:89–95.

3 Hill DR. Health problems in a large cohort of Americans traveling to developing countries. *J Travel Med.* 2000;7:259–66.

4 Freedman DO, Weld LH, Kozarsky PE, et al. Spectrum of disease and relation to place of exposure among ill returned travelers. *N Engl J Med.* 2006;354:119–30.

5 Richards DL. What tour operators and adventure travelers need to know about travel "risk mitigation" insurance. *Adventure Travel Trade Association.* March 2006.

6 Steffen R, Rickenbach M, Wilhelm U, et al. Health problems after travel to developing countries. *J Infect Dis.* 1987;156:84–91.

7 Teichman PG, Donchin Y, Kot RJ. International aeromedical evacuation. *N Engl J Med.* 2007;356:262–70.

8 Baker TD, Hargarten SF, Guptill K. The uncounted dead – American civilians dying overseas. *Public Health Rep.* 1992;107:155–9.

9 Bennett-Guerrero E, Hyam JA, Shaefi S, et al. Comparison of P-POSSUM risk-adjusted mortality rates after surgery between patients in the USA and the UK. *Br J Surg.* 2003;90:1593–8.

10 Giugliano RP, Llevadot J, Wilcox RG, et al. Geographic variation in patient and hospital characteristics, management, and clinical outcomes in ST-elevation myocardial infarction treated with fibrinolysis. *Euro Heart J.* 2001;1702–15.

11 Thomson DP, Thomas SH. Guidelines for air medical dispatch. *Prehosp Emerg Care.* 2003;7:265–71.

12 | The Expedition Returns

Responsibilities and Reports

Randall N. Hyer, MD, PhD, MPH

INTRODUCTION

The Return Should Be Planned before the Expedition Leaves Home

In any expedition, the overriding goal is to ensure the safety and health of the expedition members. These duties extend to the communities where they reside and those they have visited. Carrying out these responsibilities and reports is a primary medical and public health obligation. Careful preexpedition planning will help ease the burden and ensure their prompt and satisfactory completion.

What are the expedition's responsibilities? What reports are needed upon return? When should these be considered and planned for? Who should be accountable? What are the full spectrum and most likely illnesses associated with the expedition's return? Who should follow through with these? What reports are needed when? To whom should they be made?

Travel is associated with medical risks. Generally, 15–50% of all travelers to developing countries will report some illness (Cossar et al., 1990; Yung and Ruff, 1994). The most likely event is diarrhea and the most likely fatal event is a motor-vehicle accident (Steffen et al., 2003). Figure 12.1 shows monthly incidence rates of health problems during stays in developing countries. In one study, 64% of those who traveled to developing countries became ill, of whom 8% sought medical care (Hill, 2000). In a general survey in the United Kingdom, 42% of respondents reporting travel had become ill while abroad and nearly half required further medical attention upon return (McIntosh et al., 1994). A 2-year study of 784 American travelers, being abroad a mean of 19 days and having visited some 123 countries, showed that upon return 26% of travelers were ill and of those 56% became ill after return (Hill, 2000).

Even with exhaustive pretravel planning and prevention, people still get sick. In a study of 150 primarily well-educated travelers who were given free vaccinations, medications, and travel medicine consultation, in which personal preventive measures were presented in numerous formats by a physician specializing in infectious diseases, 64% of travelers developed illness abroad, and 20% developed illness upon return. These travelers were very compliant with their prescriptions (98%) and antimalarial chemoprophylaxis (77%). The most frequent illnesses were diarrhea and upper respiratory illness, and 10% of travelers were forced to change their itinerary (Horvath et al., 2005).

Expeditions probably do not represent a standard cross section of travelers and are frequently associated with exotic travel either to places or to peoples that are infrequently visited. Particularly with sponsored expeditions, expeditioners are likely to represent a selected, motivated, and otherwise above-average healthy people. On the other hand, some commercially oriented expeditions may have economic interests that predispose them to take even those who are not medically and physically qualified. Some expeditions are certainly higher risk like mountaineering with one study showing a 15-fold increased likelihood of death (Pollard and Clarke, 1988). In addition, medical and health events that would have otherwise gone unnoticed or undetected may present themselves during the stress and extremes of an expedition.

Despite the apparent risk associated with expeditions, one retrospective questionnaire survey of 246 expeditions taking 2,381 participants to more than one hundred countries showed 65 expeditions (26%) reporting no medical incidents and the remaining 181 reporting 835 medical incidents in 130,000 person-days (6.4 per 1,000 person-days). Of the 835 medical incidents, 59% were preventable (one-third being gastrointestinal upsets), 78% were classified as minor, and only 5% as serious. No excess of serious incidents was reported in any particular organizational group or environment (Anderson and Johnson, 2000). In a more physically exhausting and aggressive expedition, a study of 671 adventure racers revealed 243 medical encounters and 302 distinct injuries. Skin and soft tissue injuries and illness were the most frequent (48%), with blisters on the

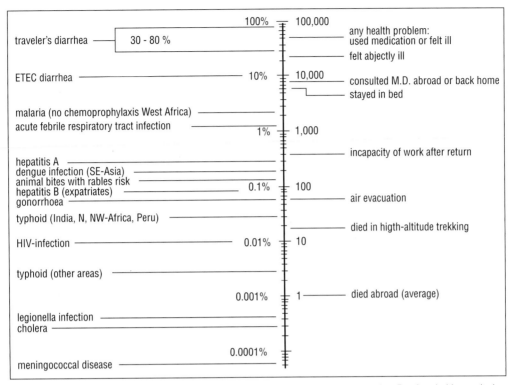

Figure 12.1. Monthly incidence rates of health problems during stays in developing countries. Reprinted with permission from Steffen et al. (2007).

feet being the most common (32.8%). Respiratory illness was second (18.2%) and the most likely medical reason for event withdrawal (Townes et al., 2004).

Clearly, no two expeditions are the same, whether the itineraries, conditions, seasons, or people change, and thus the actual risk of bringing illness home will vary. One must also be vigilant that some illnesses may be associated with travel itself, such as venous thrombo-embolism, and that some ill, returned expedition members may have contracted their illness before going or after returning. In any case, preexpedition medical planning will help, but should not be considered exhaustive nor final. Illnesses can present postexpedition, and the expedition medical officer has specific responsibilities and reports to follow up with upon return.

RESPONSIBILITIES

The expedition leadership, usually delegated to the expedition medical officer, is primarily responsible for the health and safety of the expedition. Broadly speaking, the expedition has a fiduciary responsibility to expedition personnel, their families and communities, the host country, and finally to medical science. This responsibility continues after the expedition has returned, and the medical officer must be sensitive to both internal and external medical events that occurred during the expedition. For medical events and particularly treatments rendered, the records should be obtained and made a permanent part of expedition records or individual medical records as appropriate.

There are also public health responsibilities to communities that the expedition has visited as well as to those where expedition members reside. To communities that have been visited, expeditions must be sensitive to the needs and circumstances of the local populations. In some cases, expeditions can bring local people in contact with an infectious organism to which they have no or weak natural immunity. One example might be bringing an influenza strain currently circulating in the developed world to a remote and isolated population.

Additionally, some expeditions may wish or be required to include a humanitarian health component for local populations encountered. These interventions must be carefully planned with attention paid to local resources and practices with plans and provisions for follow-up. Expedition members may often be exposed to local flora and fauna and may pick up and return home with diseases either wholly new or not native to the populations in which they live. This phenomenon could cause an outbreak of something common like malaria, exotic like viral hemorrhagic fever, or even a previously undescribed illness.

Many expeditions have medical and scientific research as their primary, secondary, or even tertiary purpose. When the expedition returns, it is imperative that all relevant data gathered either directly or indirectly are made available to sponsors of research or in reports to the appropriate authorities. Data and observations collected should always be considered for publication in appropriate peer-reviewed journals.

The Returned Expeditioner Who Is Ill

Expeditioners who either have returned or become ill after returning can have physical, psychological, and emotional ailments. Physical ailments can be acute or chronic as well as communicable or noncommunicable. One must also be attuned to potential acute and chronic psychological or emotional ailments.

A classic syndrome is the post-traumatic stress syndrome (PTSD), often observed following a uniquely dramatic, serious, or emotionally difficult experience (American Psychiatric Association, 1994). PTSD is sometimes referred to as post-traumatic stress reaction to emphasize that it is a routine result of traumatic experience rather than a manifestation of a preexisting psychological weakness.

Returned expeditioners can also suffer from survivor syndrome, where feelings of guilt and abandonment come from a seemingly random event, where one survives and others perish. Standard screening questionnaires for PTSD are available and can be used for initial evaluation and referral to appropriate specialist expertise.

Beyond the better-described PTSD, the emotional consequences of the loss of the expedition's community are another more routine syndrome to be aware of. After spending weeks, if not months, together in close company and potentially stressful or very impressionable circumstances, a community usually forms among the expedition members. New social hierarchies, support structures, and emotional bonds that support the expedition while in progress are formed. Upon return, these bonds abruptly break. Expedition members may also feel estranged from their lives, families, communities, and workplaces. As has been observed in wintering-over communities in Antarctica, the more simplified, goal-directed daily life of an expedition may cause members to question their preexpedition circumstances upon return (Oliver, 1991).

These possible adjustment difficulties can be addressed or ameliorated through follow-up expedition activities, meetings, and other social events to help ease the transition. In some cases, individuals may require specialist help.

Key Steps in the Approach to the Ill, Returned Expeditioner

Following the return, expedition members can be classified into three broad categories (Churchill et al., 1993). All three groups may express concern about passing diseases onto others or their ability to return to future expeditions. Individuals may seek care for:

- Specific symptoms
- Screening investigations that reveal latent infections
- Retrospective diagnosis of illnesses suffered abroad

The expedition medical officer must keep in mind that though common diseases are common, expeditions may go to uncommon places. Expedition members may easily come into contact with rare or unusual, or in some cases, undescribed illnesses. Though expedition members, in general, may be more attuned to their exotic travels and exposures, it may very well be that a primary care provider will be the first point of contact in the medical system. As such, both medical and nonmedical expedition members will need to be able to help educate and inform primary care providers regarding potential exposures, risks, and possible diagnoses. In some cases, they will require careful evaluation with specialists.

Expedition History

One of the principal risk factors for the ill, returned expedition member is travel to unusual locations and exposures to foreign flora and fauna. Thus, the expedition's travel features and history may be the single most important part of diagnostic work-up. Table 12.1 outlines some key considerations of the expedition's history and features. A recent study using data from 30 GeoSentinel sites (specialized travel or tropical medicine clinics on six continents) showed a strong association with travel destination and the diagnosis of certain diseases (Freedman et al., 2006). Additionally, these data may assist with the identification of travel-acquired illness and prevention of spread to others (Shaw et al., 2003).

Stressor-specific PTSD checklist

The PCL (PTSD Checklist) is a 17-item self-report measure of the 17 DSM-IV (Diagnostic and Statistical Manual of Mental Disorders) symptoms of PTSD. Respondents rate how much they were "bothered by that problem in the past month." Items are rated on a 5-point scale ranging from 1 ("not at all") to 5 ("extremely"). The version printed here is the PCL-S (specific), which asks about problems in relation to an identified "stressful experience" (Weathers, 1993).

The PCL can be scored in several different ways. A total score (range 17–85) can be obtained by summing the scores from each of the 17 items. Cutoff scores for a probable PTSD diagnosis have been validated for some populations but may not generalize to other populations. A second way to score the PCL is to follow the DSM-IV criteria. It has been suggested that a combination of these two approaches (i.e., the requisite number of symptoms are endorsed within each cluster AND the total score is above the specified cutoff point for a specific population) may be best (further details on evaluation are available at *http://www.ncptsd.va.gov/ncmain/ncdocs/assmnts/ptsd_checklist_pcl.html* (accessed 31 Jan 2007).

Table 12.1. Key considerations in the expedition's history and features in the approach to the ill returned expeditioner

Expedition History	Expedition features
Chronology and itinerary of expedition	Altitude
Situation reports/leader's notes	Climate
Exposure history	Cultural
• Infections	Environmental
• Environmental	Exertion
• Toxicological	Geographical
• Native fauna and flora	Physical
• Native populations	Seasonal
	Stress
	Urban versus rural

The health care provider must remain aware that illness may have been the result of travel or could have been contracted either before or after the expedition. Timing is perhaps one of the most useful tools. Different infections have characteristic incubation periods and these can help with diagnostics as shown in Table 12.2. Though 90% of infections acquired abroad will generally present themselves within 6 months, some infections acquired during the expedition, for example leprosy, filariasis, tuberculosis, onchocerciasis, and Chagas' disease, may not even present for months or even years after exposure (Yung and Ruff, 1994).

Another important part of the history is the activities of the expeditioners. Were they in a rural or agricultural area? Perhaps even unexplored or unknown terrain? Were they hunting, swimming in freshwater lakes, or providing health care to local populations? Where and what were they eating? Food from street vendors in developing countries, for example, is notoriously risky. Did expedition members engage in certain high-risk activities, either known or unknown to others? If multiple expedition members are ill, this would suggest a common

exposure, possibly infectious or perhaps toxicological. It is also possible that ill, returned expeditioners will harbor multiple infections.

Medical Workup

The medical workup for the ill, returned expeditioner will generally follow standard medical practice taking into account the expedition history and the patient's medical history, followed by a directed physical exam with appropriate laboratory testing to help establish a differential or even definitive diagnosis. There should be a low threshold for referral to specialist care, though the primary health care provider and/or expedition physician will need to ensure that the appropriate treatment and follow-up are carried out.

With the patient's medical history, attention should closely be paid to which immunizations were obtained and when they were received. Ideally, the complete vaccination record for all expedition members should be available, as different vaccines, different manufacturers, and different durations of efficacy exist. One should be careful, however, to not be misled. Just because someone has received a vaccination for a given disease does not imply immunity. For example, the influenza vaccine changes yearly for both the northern and southern hemispheres. In the tropics, influenza occurs year-round and as such, influenza illness has been reported as the most frequent vaccine-preventable infection among travelers to subtropical and tropical countries (Mutsch et al., 2005). Further confounding can come from antibiotics or chemoprophylaxis, especially indiscriminate, incomplete, or inappropriate use. Table 12.3 has some important questions for history taking, and Table 12.4 suggests some possible infectious etiologies based on the history.

Following a thorough review of the expedition and medical history, a careful physical examination and appropriate laboratory testing are indicated. Often, distinctive physical findings are not seen in returning travelers. Some findings on exam can suggest certain

Table 12.2. Relative incubation periods of selected infections potentially carried home

Fewer than 10 days	Up to 3 weeks	More than 3 weeks
Anthrax	African trypanosomiasis	American trypanosomiasis
Arboviral infections	Brucellosis	Amoebic liver abscess
Enteric bacterial infections (including paratyphoid)	Cutaneous myiasis/tungiasis/scabies	Enteric helminthic infections
Enteric viral infections	Enteric hepatitis	Enteric protozoal infections
Influenza	Enteric protozoal infections	Filariasis
Plague	Leptospirosis	HIV
Pneumonia	Lyme	Leishmaniasis
Rickettsioses: louse, flea-borne, typhus	Malaria (especially *P. falciparum*)	Malaria
Seafood poisoning	Rickettsioses: scrub typhus, spotted fever group, Q fever	Schistosomiasis
Viral hemorrhagic fevers	Strongyloides	Tuberculosis
	Typhoid fever	Viral hepatitis

Adapted from Spira (2003) and Yung and Ruff (1994).

Table 12.3. Some relevant medical history questions
Animal contact?
• Bites, licks
Other bites?
• Insect
• Arachnid
• Reptile
• Mammal
Contact with sick persons?
High-risk sexual activity?
Food sources, exposures?
Water, liquid sources?
Vaccination history?
Medications?
• Routine
• Travel-related?
Injuries and illnesses?
Treatment history?
Injections?
Transfusions?
Surgeries?

Table 12.4. Potential infections related to various exposures

Exposures	Possible Infections
Bites	
Mosquitoes	Malaria, dengue, yellow fever, encephalitis, filariasis
Ticks	Borreliosis (Lyme, tick bite fever, relapsing fever), rickettsioses (typhus, Rocky Mountain spotted fever), Congo-Crimean hemorrhagic fever, Q fever, tularemia, encephalitis, ehrlichiosis
Flies	African trypanosomiasis, onchocerciasis, leishmaniasis, bartonellosis, salmonella, myiasis
Fleas	Plague, tungiasis
Triatomids (reduviids)	American trypanosomiasis (Chagas' disease)
Mammals	Rabies, sodoku (rat-bite fever), tularemia, anthrax, Q fever, cellulitis
Ingestion	
Untreated water	Hepatitis A/E, cholera, Norwalk/caliciviruses, salmonella, shigella, giardia, poliomyelitis, cryptosporidium, cyclospora, dracunculiasis
Unpasteurized dairy	Brucella, tuberculosis, salmonella, shigella, Listeria
Raw or undercooked food	Enteric bacteria (*Salmonella*, Shigella, *E. coli*, *C. jejuni*, etc.); helminths [ascaris, trichinella, taenia – including cysticercosis, whipworm, capillaria, Angiostrongylus; protozoa (amoebiasis, toxoplasma)]
Freshwater skin contact	Leptospirosis, schistosomiasis, acanthamoeba, or naegleria
Sand/dirt/mud skin contact	Hookworm, cutaneous larva migrans, visceral larva migrans, leptospirosis
High-risk sexual contacts	HIV, hepatitis B/C, syphilis, gonorrhea, Chlamydia, herpes
Contact with ill persons	Pneumonia, tuberculosis, Epstein-Barr, meningitis, rheumatic fever, Lassa fever

Adapted from Spira (2003).

expedition-related diseases. Table 12.5 shows a differential diagnosis for some physical findings, and Table 12.6 provides a differential for some cutaneous findings. Though specialist referral is likely, Table 12.7 suggests some initial laboratory studies that can be considered with the initial presentation and may help guide specialist care. Several reports may help guide the clinician in establishing a differential and eventual definitive diagnosis (diagnoses) (Spira, 2003; Freedman et al., 2006; Ryan et al., 2002; Yung and Ruff, 1994; Hill et al., 2006).

Two Most Likely Presentations in the Ill, Returned Expeditioner

Diarrhea

With common things being common, diarrhea is likely to be the single most likely postexpedition complaint (Shaw et al., 2003). Persistent diarrhea must be carefully evaluated. Diarrhea can be confusing because it can be caused by multiple pathogens and can have multiple episodes each with different etiologies. Many diarrheal episodes do not have a determined cause. It should be noted that a recent study showed no impact of the use of alcohol hand gel sanitizers on the development of either diarrhea or respiratory illnesses (Horvath et al., 2005).

Diarrhea associated with expeditions can be broadly categorized as acute and chronic. Acute diarrhea is normally of short duration (typically 4 days) and can be categorized as either inflammatory or noninflammatory depending on whether fecal leukocytes are present. Though acute diarrhea is likely to have occurred and resolved during the expedition, it can certainly present in a returned traveler. Chronic diarrhea usually lasts 19 days or more. A common pathogen is *Giardia*, though an enteric infection can cause a persistent irritable bowel syndrome resulting in a chronic diarrhea presentation.

Table 12.8 shows different pathogens commonly associated with acute and chronic diarrhea.

Fever

Fever is perhaps the most common clinical sign in a returned expeditioner. Common causes include malaria, typhoid, hepatitis A, and possibly dengue fever, depending on where the expedition was. Fever requires a careful evaluation (Ryan et al., 2002).

Table 12.5. Physical findings and potential differential diagnoses for potential expedition-acquired diseases

Exposures	Possible infections
Abdominal tenderness	Yesinia enterocolitica, colonic ameboma, anisakiasis, hepatitis, Clonorchis or Opisthorchis, biliary obstruction
Ataxia/paresis/ paraesthesia	Rabies, toxic seafood ingestion, envenoming, neurocysticerocosis, neuroschistosomiasis
Hepatomegaly	Malaria, leishmaniasis, amoebic liver abscess, typhoid, hepatitis, leptospirosis
Jaundice	Hepatitis, malaria, leptospirosis, relapsing fever, cholelithiasis, pancreatitis
Lymphadenopathy	Plague, HIV, rickettsioses, brucellosis, leishmaniasis, lymphogranuloma venerum, Lassa fever
Nystagmus/diplopia	Rabies, botulinum poisoning, neurotoxic snakebite envenoming
Petechiae/ecchymosis	Meningococcemia, yellow fever, dengue, rickettsioses, viral hemorrhagic fevers, envenoming
Splenomegaly	Malaria, leishmaniasis, trypanosomiasis, typhoid, brucellosis, typhus, dengue
Wheezing	Loeffler's syndrome, Katayama fever, tropical pulmonary eosinophilia

Adapted from Spira (2003).

Malaria is the most common cause of febrile illness in travelers returning from endemic areas, and prompt evaluation is essential to initiating timely treatment (Antinori et al., 2004). A recent World Health Organization (WHO) report has found malaria to be grossly underreported and imported cases have seen an increase in the most serious variant, *Plasmodium falciparum* (Muentener et al., 1999). Malaria has no specific signs and symptoms and can often appear as other disorders. Additionally, most health care providers in developed countries, especially those in primary care, are unlikely to have ever seen a case. One axiom is that unexplained fever in a returned traveler is malaria until proven otherwise.

Malaria is treatable and if this diagnosis is included in the differential, serial blood samples should be taken every 6–12 hours for examination by an experienced technician. Malaria usually presents after travelers return home, often secondary to inadequate chemoprophylaxis. Figure 12.2 shows the approximate risk for mortality and morbidity from malaria for a 1-month exposure without chemoprophylaxis. Suspected malaria should be promptly referred to a specialist with experience in current treatments (Smithuis et al., 2004; White and Warrell, 1996; White, 1996).

In a 2-year study of 784 American travelers, being abroad a mean of 19 days and having visited some 123 countries, the incidence of documented malaria was 3.8 cases per 1,000 travelers. Complete compliance with antimalarials was 80%. Side effects were reported by 4% of those taking chloroquine, 11% of those tak-

Table 12.6. Selected cutaneous manifestations of potential expedition-acquired diseases

Exposures	Possible disease
Erythema migrans	Lyme
Eschar	Typhus, anthrax, African trypanosomiasis, Congo-Crimean hemorrhagic fever, tularemia, spider bites
Hypopigmentation	Tinea (pityriasis) versicolor, tinea corporis, leprosy, vitiligo
Linear	Photodermatitis, cutaneous larva migrans, gnathostomiasis, larva currens, flea bites, *M. marinarum*, sporotrichosis, nematocyst stings, lymphangitis
Maculopapular	Drug reaction, dengue, acute HIV, rickettsia, syphilis, leptospirosis, brucellosis, typhus, bartonellosis, typhoid, rubeola, rubella, scarlet fever, insect bites, cercarial dermatitis, seabather's eruption, eczema, tungiasis, myiasis, scabies, arthropod bites, miliaria rubra
Migrating	Cutaneous larva migrans, larva currens, gnathostomiasis, loiasis, myiasis, paragonimiasis sparganosis
Nodules	Onchocerciasis, bartonellosis, myiasis, paracoccidioidomycosis
Papulosquamous	Superficial mycoses or exacerbations of eczema or psoriasis
Petechial/ecchymoses	Rickettsia, meningococcemia, yellow fever, viral hemorrhagic fevers, dengue, leptospirosis
Swelling/edema	*Loa loa* calabar swellings, trichinosis (especially facial/periorbital)
Ulcers	Leishmaniasis, tropical ulcers, anthrax, tularemia, cutaneous diphtheria, ecthyma, syphilis, yaws, tuberculosis, granulomas inguinale, lymphogranuloma venereum, plague, arthropod bite (e.g., brown recluse spider)
Urticaria	Drug reactions, filariasis, onchocerciasis, cutaneous larva migrans, larva currens (strongyloidiasis), acute schistosomiasis, fascioliasis, hymenoptera stings, insect bites, enterobiasis, gnathostomiasis, scabies, cercarial dermatitis, seabather's eruption, nematocyst stings
Vegetation/verrucae	Bartonellosis, histoplasmosis, leishmaniasis, maduromycosis, paracoccidioidomycosis, pinta, syphilis, tuberculosis, yaws
Vesicular	Varicella, herpes simplex, drug reactions, sunburn, photodermatitis

Adapted from Spira (2003).

Table 12.7. Suggested initial laboratory studies

General
- Complete blood count to include platelets and microscopy
- Glucose-6-phosphate dehydrogenase level if primaquine therapy for malaria may be needed
- Blood films for malaria; repeat every 12 hr up to three if previous films negative; attempt to obtain blood samples during fever. Tests should include both thick and thin Giemsa-stained blood smears
- Liver function tests and electrolytes
- Urine analysis and culture as indicated; urine microscopy for S hematobium eggs
- Culture: blood, urine, sputum, stool, cerebrospinal fluid, lesions as indicated
- Serologies: amoebae, schistosomes, arboviruses, hepatitis (Be cautious about interpreting serologies not done at the appropriate time. In addition, helminthic serologies are not standardized, and there is cross-reactivity between helminths. Furthermore, one cannot distinguish between a current versus past infection in frequent travelers or expatriates.)
- Sputum microscopy as indicated
- Lumbar puncture as indicated
- Tuberculosis skin testing and follow-up radiograph as necessary
- Biopsies of lesions or of bone marrow, especially if suspected typhoid, leishmaniasis, or tuberculosis
- Radiographic tests such as radiograph, ultrasonography, computed radiography, or MRI. Radiographs useful with tuberculosis and other pulmonary infections including *Paragonimus* and trichinosis and cysticercosis whose calcified cysts can be visualized on soft-tissue films; ultrasonography is useful for abscesses, especially amoebic liver abscess and echinococcal cysts

For diarrhea
- Stool microscopy: fresh, with iodine, acid-fast and trichome or iron-hematoxylin stains
- Stool hemoccult
- Stool culture and sensitivity for enteric pathogens
- Stool serology for *Giardia* antigens as well as C difficile antigen (Blood tests should also include complete blood count with a differential, amoebic serology and chemistries. Urine can be tested for D-xylose.)
- In cases of chronic diarrhea, consider a lactose tolerance test or a Schilling test with intrinsic factor
- Endoscopy with biopsy and duodenal aspirate or colonoscopy with biopsies and cultures should follow if initial testing in nondiagnostic; also consider ultrasonography, computerized or magnetic imaging studies

Less common tests
- Day and night blood concentrations for filarial blood smears
- Skin snips for onchocerciasis
- Rectal snips for schistosomiasis
- Urine concentration for schistosomiasis
- Sputum for ova and parasites in suspect paragonimiasis and migrating larvae

Adapted from Spira (2003).

Table 12.8. Different pathogens commonly associated with acute and chronic diarrhea

Acute		Chronic
E. coli (various including enterotoxigenic, enteroaggregative, enteropathogenic, etc.)	20–75%	Bacterial – *Campylobacter, Clostridium difficile, Aeromonas hydrophila, Plesiomonas shigelloides, Yersinia enterocolitica*, small bowel bacterial overgrowth, *Mycobacterium tuberculosis*
Campylobacter	Common, especially in Southeast Asia	Protozoal – *Giardia lamblia, Entamoeba histolytica, Cryptosporidium, Cyclosporidium*
Rotavirus (in adults)	Rare	Helminthic – hookworm, *Strongyloides stercoralis, Schistosoma mansoni* and *S. japonicum, Trichuris tri*
Salmonella	1–3%	Tropical sprue
Vibrio parahaemolyticus	< 1%	Noninfective travel-related – disaccharidase (including lactase) deficiency, irritable bowel syndrome (possibly postinfective)
Aeromonas hydrophila	0–30%	Non-travel-related – inflammatory bowel disease, drugs, thortoxicosis, tumors, neuropeptides (carcinoid, gastrinoma), ischemic colitis
Parasites (*Giardia lamblia, Cryptosporidium, Cyclosporidium*)	Rare	
Norwalk	0–10%	

Adapted from Yung and Ruff (1994) by Wilson (1991).

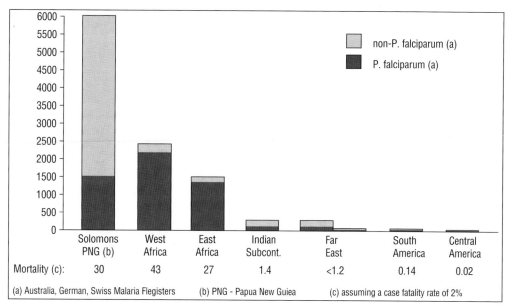

Figure 12.2: Morbidity and mortality in 100,000 nonimmune travelers exposed for 1 month without chemoprophylaxis. Reprinted with permission from Steffen et al. (2007).

ing chloroquine plus proguanil, and 14% of those taking mefloquine, with half of these neuropsychiatric (Hill, 2000).

Reports

Expedition History

The expedition's journal or log may be one of the most important records of the expedition. These records are not just for documentation or later study and research but can supply key data or potential explanations for medical or health events that occur after the expedition has returned. These notes could include such things as chronology, expedition situation reports, leader's notes, and perhaps documentation on any particularly noteworthy events. Noteworthy events could include exposure to known infectious, environmental, toxicological, or hazardous native fauna and flora.

Though 90% of infections acquired abroad will generally present themselves within 6 months, some infections acquired during the expedition, for example leprosy, filariasis, tuberculosis, onchocerciasis, and Chagas' disease, may not present for months or even years after exposure (Yung and Ruff, 1994). Relevant sections of the expedition journal should be made available to health care providers upon request. If there is a suspicion or concern regarding a communicable disease spreading in people either at home or abroad, then the expedition notes and documentation should be made available to the relevant public health officials to prevent further transmission of the disease.

Disease Reports

As mentioned, expeditions may come into contact with areas or peoples infrequently visited. Expedition

members may contract potentially contagious diseases, whether common, rare, or unknown. As a result, these diseases may pose a public health threat to communities where the returned expeditioners reside. Many national health authorities have disease reporting requirements. Annex 1 shows specific disease reporting requirements by the Centers for Disease Control in the United States and the Health Protection Agency in the United Kingdom.

In addition, the WHO, the international body with the mandate for global public health, has recently (2005) updated the international health regulations (IHR), following the recent global outbreak of the severe acute respiratory syndrome (SARS), which was imported to the developed world by travelers, as well as concerns regarding avian influenza in humans. The current IHR includes national reporting responsibilities for certain diseases as well as an obligation to report diseases that represent a "public health emergency of international concern." WHO has developed an algorithm to assist countries with this reporting requirement. Expeditions may return with a disease or case cluster that may need reporting to WHO, and expedition medical may find this algorithm useful to determine whether to alert national authorities.

SUMMARY

Expedition members can be considered travelers, though likely a highly selected group that often visits exotic locales or peoples. The primary responsibility of expedition medical officers is for the health of the expedition party. Expedition medical officers also have a public health responsibility to ensure that other populations both at home and abroad do not contract illnesses related to the expedition. Upon return home, expedition medical officers need to be alert to the physical, psychological, and emotional health of expedition members and be ready to guide or assist primary health care providers in evaluating postexpedition illness. Reports of significant medical events, both internal and external to the expedition, should be made available to individual team members and their medical providers as appropriate. Any medical interventions with local populations will need to be referred to competent health authority for follow-up. For reportable diseases, notification should be made to the relevant national health authorities where the expedition team member normally resides, and a courtesy report sent to health authorities where the expedition was likely to have contracted the illness.

LINKS

Centers for Disease Control, United States of America. *http://www.cdc.gov/travel/*. Accessed 31 Jan 2007.

Deployment Health Clinical Center PDHealth.mil was designed to assist clinicians in the delivery of postdeployment health care by fostering a trusting partnership between military men and women, veterans, their families, and their health care providers to ensure the highest quality care for those who make sacrifices in the world's most hazardous workplace (*http://www.pdhealth.mil/library/default.asp*, accessed 31 Jan 2007).

GeoSentinel, a worldwide communication and data collection network for the surveillance of travel related morbidity, was initiated in 1995 by the International Society of Travel Medicine (ISTM) and the Centers for Disease Control as a network of ISTM member travel/tropical medicine clinics. GeoSentinel is based on the concept that these clinics are ideally situated to effectively detect geographic and temporal trends in morbidity among travelers, immigrants and refugees (*http://www.istm.org/geosentinel/main.html*, accessed 31 Jan 2007).

GIDEON, a global infectious diseases database and the solution for diagnosis, treatment, and teaching of infectious diseases and microbiology, is a commercially available diagnostic program that can help in tabulating findings and providing differential diagnoses (*http://www.gideon.com*, accessed 31 Jan 2007).

Health Protection Agency (HPA). *http://www.hpa.org.uk/*.

World Health Organization (WHO), International Health Regulations (IHR). *http://www.who.int/csr/ihr/en/*. Accessed 24 Jan 2007.

ANNEX 1: REPORTABLE DISEASES

The Centers for Disease Control and Prevention (CDC) in the United States has the responsibility for the collection and publication of data concerning nationally notifiable diseases. The list of nationally notifiable diseases given here is revised periodically, by state health departments in collaboration. Reporting of nationally notifiable diseases to CDC by the states is voluntary and is currently mandated only at the state level. As such, the list varies slightly by state.

Acquired Immunodeficiency Syndrome (AIDS)

Anthrax

Arboviral neuroinvasive and nonneuroinvasive diseases

    California serogroup virus disease

    Eastern equine encephalitis virus disease

    Powassan virus disease

    St. Louis encephalitis virus disease

    West Nile virus disease

    Western equine encephalitis virus disease

Botulism

    Botulism, food-borne

    Botulism, infant

    Botulism, other (wound and unspecified)

Brucellosis

Chancroid

Chlamydia trachomatis, genital infections

Cholera

Coccidioidomycosis

Cryptosporidiosis

Cyclosporiasis

Diphtheria

Ehrlichiosis

    Ehrlichiosis, human granulocytic

    Ehrlichiosis, human monocytic

    Ehrlichiosis, human, other or unspecified agent

Giardiasis

Gonorrhea

Haemophilus influenzae, invasive disease

Hansen disease (leprosy)

Hantavirus pulmonary syndrome

Hemolytic uremic syndrome, postdiarrheal

    Hepatitis, viral, acute

Hepatitis A, acute

Hepatitis B, acute

Hepatitis B virus, perinatal infection

Hepatitis, C, acute

    Hepatitis, viral, chronic

Chronic Hepatitis B

Hepatitis C virus infection (past or present)

    HIV infection

    HIV infection, adult (> = 13 years)

    HIV infection, pediatric (< 13 years)

The event you experienced was: _____ **on:** _____

Below is a list of problems and complaints that people sometimes have in response to stressful life experiences. Please read each one carefully, put an "X" in the box to indicate how much you have been bothered by that problem *in the last month*.

	No response	Not at all (1)	A little bit (2)	Moderately (3)	Quite a bit (4)	Extremely (5)
1. Repeated, disturbing *memories, thoughts, or images* of a stressful experience from the past?						
2. Repeated, disturbing *dreams* of a stressful experience from the past?						
3. Suddenly *acting* or *feeling* as if a stressful experience *were happening* again (as if you were reliving it)?						
4. Feeling *very upset* when *something reminded* you of a stressful experience from the past?						
5. Having *physical reactions* (e.g., heart pounding, trouble breathing, or sweating) when *something reminded* you of a stressful experience from the past?						
6. Avoid *thinking about* or *talking about* a stressful experience from the past or avoid *having feelings* related to it?						
7. Avoid *activities* or *situations* because they *remind you* of a stressful experience from the past?						
8. Trouble *remembering important parts* of a stressful experience from the past?						
9. Loss of *interest in things that you used to enjoy?*						
10. Feeling *distant* or *cut* off from other people?						
11. Feeling *emotionally numb* or being unable to have loving feelings for those close to you?						
12. Feeling as if your *future* will somehow be *cut short?*						
13. Trouble *falling* or *staying asleep?*						
14. Feeling *irritable* or having *angry outbursts?*						
15. Having *difficulty concentrating?*						
16. Being *"super alert"* or watchful on guard?						
17. Feeling *jumpy* or easily startled?						

PCL-M for DSM-IV (11/1/94)

Influenza-associated pediatric mortality

Legionellosis

Listeriosis

Lyme disease

Malaria

Measles

Meningococcal disease

Mumps

Pertussis

Plague

Poliomyelitis, paralytic

Poliovirus infection, nonparalytic

Psittacosis

Q fever

Rabies

  Rabies, animal

  Rabies, human

Rocky Mountain spotted fever

Rubella

Rubella, congenital syndrome

Salmonellosis

Severe Acute Respiratory Syndrome–associated Co-ronavirus (SARS-CoV) disease

Shiga toxin-producing *Escherichia coli* (STEC)

Shigellosis

Smallpox

Streptococcal disease, invasive, Group A

Streptococcal toxic-shock syndrome

Streptococcus pneumoniae, drug-resistant, invasive disease

Streptococcus pneumoniae, invasive in children < 5 years

Syphilis

  Syphilis, primary

  Syphilis, secondary

  Syphilis, latent

  Syphilis, early latent

  Syphilis, late latent

  Syphilis, latent, unknown duration

  Neurosyphilis

  Syphilis, late, nonneurological

  Syphilitic stillbirth

Syphilis, congenital

Tetanus

Toxic-shock syndrome (other than Streptococcal)

Trichinellosis (Trichinosis)

Tuberculosis

Tularemia

Typhoid fever

Vancomycin–intermediate *Staphylococcus aureus* (VISA)

Vancomycin–resistant *Staphylococcus aureus* (VRSA)

Varicella (morbidity)

Varicella (deaths only)

Vibriosis

Yellow fever

The WHO revised the International Health Regulations, referred to as IHR (2005), which were unanimously adopted on 23 May 2005 by the World Health Assembly. These regulations entered into force on 15 June 2007. The broadened purpose and scope of the IHR (2005) are to "prevent, protect against, control and provide a public health response to the international spread of disease and which avoid unnecessary interference with international traffic and trade." According to the Health Protection Agency of the United Kingdom, the following diseases are notifiable (to local authority proper officers) under the Public Health (Infectious Diseases) Regulations 1988 (Reviewed 18 Jan 2006):

  Acute encephalitis

  Acute poliomyelitis

  Anthrax

  Cholera

  Diphtheria

Dysentery

Food poisoning

Leptospirosis

Malaria

Measles

Meningitis

  Meningococcal

  Pneumococcal

  Haemophilus influenzae

  Viral

  Other specified

  Unspecified

Meningococcal septicaemia (without meningitis)

Mumps

Ophthalmia neonatorum

Paratyphoid fever

Plague

Rabies

Relapsing fever

Rubella

Scarlet fever

Smallpox

Tetanus

Tuberculosis

Typhoid fever

Typhus fever

Viral hemorrhagic fever

Viral hepatitis

  Hepatitis A

  Hepatitis B

  Hepatitis C

  Other

Whooping cough

Yellow fever

Leprosy

SUGGESTED READINGS

American Psychiatric Association. *Diagnostic and Statistical Manual of Mental Disorders.* 4th ed. Arlington: American Psychiatric Association; 1994.

Anderson SR, Johnson CJ. Expedition health and safety: a risk assessment. *J R Soc Med.* 2000;93:557–62.

Antinori S, Galimberti L, Gianelli E, Calattini S, Piazza M, Morelli P, Moroni M, Galli M, Corbellino M. Prospective observational study of fever in hospitalized returning travelers and migrants from tropical areas, 1997–2001. *J Travel Med.* 2004;11:135–42.

Churchill DR, Chiodini PL, McAdam KP. Screening the returned traveller. *Br Med Bull.* 1993;49:465–74.

Cossar JH, Reid D, Fallon RJ, Bell EJ, Riding MH, Follett EA, Dow BC, Mitchell S, Grist NR. A cumulative review of studies on travellers, their experience of illness and the implications of these findings. *J Infect.* 1990;21:27–42.

Freedman DO, Weld LH, Kozarsky PE, Fisk T, Robins R, von Sonnenburg F, Keystone JS, Pandey P, Cetron MS. Spectrum of disease and relation to place of exposure among ill returned travelers. *N Engl J Med.* 2006;354:119–30.

Hill DR. Health problems in a large cohort of Americans traveling to developing countries. *J Travel Med.* 2006;7:259–66.

Hill DR, Ericsson CD, Pearson RD, Keystone JS, Freedman DO, Kozarsky PE, DuPont HL, Bia FJ, Fischer PR, Ryan ET. The practice of travel medicine: guidelines by the Infectious Diseases Society of America. *Clin Infect Dis.* 2006;43:1499–1539.

Horvath LL, Murray CK, and Dooley DP. Effect of maximizing a travel medicine clinic's prevention strategies. *J Travel Med.* 2005;12:332–7.

McIntosh IB, Reed JM, Power KG. The impact of travel acquired illness on the world traveller and family doctor and the need for pre-travel health education. *Scott Med J.* 1994;39:40–4.

Muentener P, Schlagenhauf P, Steffen R. Imported malaria (1985–95): trends and perspectives. *Bull World Health Organ.* 1999;77:560–6.

Mutsch M, Tavernini M, Marx A, Gregory V, Lin YP, Hay AJ, Tschopp A, Steffen R. Influenza virus infection in travelers to tropical and subtropical countries. *Clin Infect Dis.* 2005;40:1282–7.

Oliver DC. *Psychological Effects of Isolation and Confinement of a Winter-Over Group at McMurdo Station, Antarctica.*

In: Harrison AA, Clearwater YA, McKay CP, eds. *From Antarctica to Outer Space.* Berlin and Heidelberg: Springer-Verlag; 1991.

Pollard A, Clarke C. Deaths during mountaineering at extreme altitude. *Lancet.* 1988;1:1277.

Ryan ET, Wilson ME, Kain KC. Illness after international travel. *N Engl J Med.* 2002;347:505–16.

Shaw MT, Leggat PA, Weld LH, Williams ML, Cetron MS. Illness in returned travellers presenting at GeoSentinel sites in New Zealand. *Aust N Z J Public Health.* 2003;27:82–6.

Smithuis F, Shahmanesh M, Kyaw MK, Savran O, Lwin S, White NJ. Comparison of chloroquine, sulfadoxine/pyrimethamine, mefloquine and mefloquine-artesunate for the treatment of falciparum malaria in Kachin State, North Myanmar. *Trop Med Int Health.* 2004;9:1184–90.

Spira AM. Assessment of travellers who return home ill. *Lancet.* 2003;361:1459–69.

Steffen R, deBernardis C, Banos A. Travel epidemiology – a global perspective. *Int J Antimicrob Agents.* 2003;21:89–95.

Townes DA, Talbot TS, Wedmore IS, Billingsly R. Event medicine: injury and illness during an expedition-length adventure race. *J Emerg Med.* 2004;27:161–5.

Weathers F, Litz B, Herman D, Huska J, Keane T. The PTSD Checklist (PCL): Reliability, Validity, and Diagnostic Utility. Annual Convention of the International Society for Traumatic Stress Studies, San Antonio, TX; 1993.

White NJ. The treatment of malaria. *N Engl J Med.* 1996;335:800–6.

White NJ, Warrell DA. Dosage for malaria treatment. *Lancet.* 1996;348:1312.

Wilson ME. *A World Guide to Infections: Diseases, Distribution, Diagnosis.* New York: Oxford University Press; 1991.

Yung AP, Ruff TA. Travel medicine. 2. Upon return. *Med J Aust.* 1994;160:206–12.

13 | Tactical and Protective Medicine

Nelson Tang, MD, FACEP, Kevin B. Gerold, DO, JD, and Richard Carmona, MD, MPH, FACS

INTRODUCTION

Operational medical support is the provision of field medical care during high-risk, extended-duration, and mission-driven law enforcement operations, often rendered under functionally austere conditions. The goals of tactical medicine are to facilitate the success and the safety of law enforcement missions during all phases of a tactical or Special Weapons And Tactics (SWAT) operation through the delivery of preventative, urgent, and emergency medical care. The role of protective medicine is the similarly broad medical support of protective operations in which security and law enforcement personnel and resources are dedicated to the safety and physical well-being of an individual or group of individuals. There exists significant overlap both in the approach to and implementation of tactical and protective medicine. Both tactical and protective medicine methodologies intend to provide the best possible outcome for both the personnel and the mission and recognize that medical challenges emerging during a law enforcement operation present to commanders both a medical problem and a tactical problem.

HISTORICAL BACKGROUND

The principles employed by tactical medicine providers were initially developed by the military for small unit operations and continued to gain widespread acceptance in the civilian law enforcement community. The emerging need for tactical medical support followed closely the development and expansion of SWAT teams now commonly deployed by police departments and law enforcement agencies in the United States.

The need for these specialized tactical teams arose in response to the changing patterns of crime and violence in society and the need to provide an effective response to the criminal use of military-style weapons, the taking of hostages, and terrorist activities involving explosive, chemical, and biological agents. Despite better equipment, enhanced training, and improved organization and tactics, law enforcement fatalities in the line of duty have increased 21% since 1997. Were it not for widespread use of body armor worn by police officers, it is estimated that law enforcement fatalities would be double or triple what they are today.[1]

In 1989, representatives from law enforcement, emergency medicine, and prehospital Emergency Medical Services (EMS) began meeting to develop consensus on the provision of medical support to tactical teams.[2,3] In 1993, the National Tactical Officers Association (NTOA) issued a position statement in support of Tactical Emergency Medical Support (TEMS) emphasizing that, "the provision of TEMS has emerged as an important element of tactical law enforcement operation." The National Association of EMS Physicians issued a position paper in 2001 providing an overview of law enforcement special operations medical support.[4] In 2004, the American College of Emergency Physicians (ACEP) issued a position paper supporting the concept that TEMS is an essential component of law enforcement teams and "helps maintain a healthy and safer environment for both law enforcement and the public".[5]

Historically, protective methodologies were developed and utilized by law enforcement for the provision of physical security to political leaders and high-ranking government officials, typically referred to as "protectees" (Figure 13.1). One of the most widely recognized examples of executive protection is that of the U. S. Secret Service and its protective mission serving the president and vice president of the United States and their immediate families. Increasingly, the private sector has been similarly challenged to deploy protective measures for leaders of industry and commerce, popular sports and entertainment figures, as well as individuals of significant wealth and personal influence. The development and evolution of operational support for the protective mission has closely paralleled the enhancement of emergency medical capabilities in support of the law enforcement tactical mission.

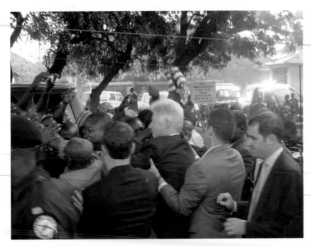

Figure 13.1. High-ranking government officials are often the focus of protective details. Here former President Clinton greets a crowd in Ghana. Photo courtesy of Gregory H. Bledsoe.

CURRENT PRACTICES

Specially trained tactical medicine teams now routinely support law enforcement operations throughout the United States by providing scene commanders with medical threat assessments and consultations, delivering immediate access to emergency medical care within the high-risk law enforcement perimeter and providing logistical support by promoting the safety and health of law enforcement personnel. Tactically trained paramedics, emergency medical technicians, nurses, physician assistants, and physicians achieve their objectives through mission preplanning, implementation of medically effective practices developed for law enforcement scenarios, and provision of a critical interface between law enforcement personnel and EMS. Extensive preparation for reasonably foreseeable injuries and illnesses

that typify law enforcement tactical operations and the exchange of experience and injury data between tactical law enforcement teams is a common approach. These efforts have ideally resulted in a reduction in the incidence of injury, illness, disability, and death and their associated personal and economic losses; a decrease in the exposure of law enforcement agencies to liability; and an increase in the safety of the general public at large.

Although organized and dedicated protective medicine is a relatively newer concept within the law enforcement special operations arena, the fundamental approach shares many commonalities with tactical medicine. Medical providers supporting protective operations are specifically trained in the logistics and methodologies of protection and serve both as an evaluative adjunct for threat assessments and mission preplanning and an immediate intervention mechanism in the event of medical contingencies.

Protective medicine also serves to promote the safety and health of law enforcement personnel dedicated to protection and acts as a functional liaison between the protective detail itself and EMS and hospitals when necessary. Protective operations are generally more likely to involve extended mobile operations, such as motorcades, and international deployments (Figure 13.2) that add logistical complexity to both anticipated medical needs and the availability of supportive resources.

Tactical and protective medical providers are increasingly viewed by law enforcement commanders as integral members of special operations teams and are often called upon to provide medical support within the perimeter of extended and large-scale events, high-risk warrant service, hostage or barricade incidents, civil disturbances, dignitary and executive protection missions, maritime and dive operations, and explosive ordnance

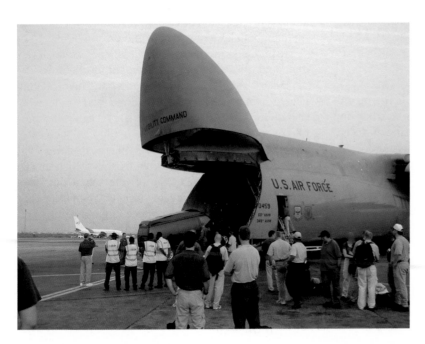

Figure 13.2. Protective medical units are at times called upon to function within highly complex logistical missions such as motorcades in international environments. Here a medical vehicle is unloaded from a military transport vessel en route to a governmental motorcade in Senegal. Photo courtesy of Gregory H. Bledsoe.

disposal. Their primary function during a mission is to provide broad medical oversight to operations including injury prevention, resource allocation, and rapid access to emergency medical care within the operation. During law enforcement operations, medical activities and casualty movements are a coordinated effort between the command post, operational team leaders, and the medical support element. Tactical and protective medicine physicians are often on-scene to ensure that local medical resources and EMS are properly staged, briefed, and ready to assist the operation, as circumstances require.

TACTICAL AND PROTECTIVE MEDICINE PROVIDERS

Tactical and protective medical support providers (emergency medical technicians, paramedics, nurses, physician assistants, and physicians) may have widely differing levels of training. Nevertheless, these providers are all highly skilled clinicians selected for their ability to work seamlessly as part of a team within the law enforcement culture and "chain of command." Once deemed eligible, candidates are required to undergo a rigorous physical, didactic, and practical skills training program requiring them to master both law enforcement and operational medical skills (Figure 13.3). Tactical and protective medical providers typically receive diverse training in combat casualty care, scene management, and extended operations support. Additionally, they have focused exposure to primary care, sports medicine, and occupational health concerns and must demonstrate proficiency in law enforcement team tactics, movements, weapon systems, communications, vehicle operations, and immediate action drills.

MISSION SUPPORT

The successful orientation of medical providers to tactical and protective medical support requires their

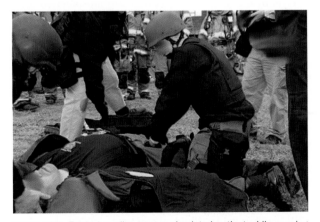

Figure 13.3. Tactical medics treat a simulated patient while wearing ballistic protection and full tactical gear as part of their tactical training. Photo courtesy of Kevin Gerold.

accepting the fundamental principle that the medical mission may be subordinate to the overall law enforcement mission. In contrast to EMS and hospital practices in which the driving priority is the health and welfare of the patient, the essential priority in a tactical or protective mission is the success of the overall law enforcement objective. In a tactical setting, the medical objective may represent a small part of the overall mission. When a casualty occurs during a tactical operation, medical providers may be directed to delay or modify medical care until the mission commander determines that rendering care will not jeopardize the overall mission. Similarly, the overriding principle that governs protective methodology is the single-minded focus on the safety and physical security of the protectee to whom all resources and efforts are to be directed.[6] As such, the institution of medical assessments or interventions are done solely at the discretion and direction of the protective detail leader in the context of potential needs for evacuation and escape in circumstances deemed to be a threat or attack.

THREAT ASSESSMENTS

A fundamental and common component of tactical and protective medical support is the mission preplan or medical threat assessment (MTA). An MTA is a prioritized acquisition of medically relevant information and data that may potentially impact the well-being and performance of law enforcement team members during the execution of the law enforcement mission. Factors generally considered during the preparation of an MTA include expected weather and environmental conditions that have the potential to affect human performance, suspected weapons threats, the nature and extent of local medical resources, local road conditions and terrain, animal or plant hazards, and the potential for exposure to hazardous materials such as chemical, biological, or radiation agents (Table 13.1).

Many law enforcement operations are conducted covertly or in secret. The preparation and execution of the MTA must occur in a manner that respects the needs of law enforcement to maintain the operational security (OPSEC) of the mission. Failures to maintain OPSEC during the preparation and staging of an operation can forfeit the element of surprise and allow opposing forces to defeat the mission plan, possibly resulting in otherwise preventable casualties or deaths.

When developing the MTA, tactical and protective medical providers should identify and implement a robust communication plan that will enable the medical support element to communicate with others involved in the operation and provide the ability to call for additional resources as needed. This includes identifying local telephone numbers for contacting police, fire, EMS, and hospitals; working radio frequencies for

Table 13.1. Key elements of an operational medical threat assessment

Location
Map coordinates (longitude and latitude)
Time zone(s)
Daylight hours (sunrise, sunset)
Weather conditions
Ambient temperatures, with extremes
Humidity
Wind patterns
Suspected weapons threats
Handguns
Long guns
Edged weapons
Booby traps
Explosive devices
Local medical resources
Hospitals
Emergency departments
Trauma centers
Burn centers
Veterinary services
Emergency services and public safety
EMS
Fire/rescue departments
Air medical resources, and landing zones
Antivenom banks
Local roads, traffic patterns, and terrain
Potential animal and plant hazards
Risks of exposure to hazardous materials
    (chemical, biological, or radiation agents)

all components of the operation; and cellular phone and direct-connect contact information of key personnel. The communication plan should include redundancy and back-up plans to implement in the event of primary communications failure.

If the MTA includes the use of a helicopter for medical evacuation, the plan must identify a suitable landing zone, the telephone numbers and radiofrequency contacts for the aircraft, and considerations of how expected weather conditions at the time of the mission might affect the ability to fly. Additionally, an effective MTA should determine whether it is appropriate to reduce aircraft response times by prestaging in proximity to the operation and consider how the weight and distance capabilities of the aircraft might affect the mission plan.

In addition to medical risks, most law enforcement special operations carry the additional risk of exposure to riot control agents such as oleoresin capsicum (OC) or "pepper spray" and orthochlorobenzylidene malononitrile (CS) or "tear gas," as well as the risk of fire associated with the deployment of distraction devices such as "flash-bangs." To mitigate these risks, the MTA should include plans for decontaminating casualties and tactical operators, separate from suspects, and have in place a fire suppression plan to deal with small fires should one occur. A decontamination plan might position a fire engine outside or in close proximity to the operation. A

fire suppression plan can include having the tactical entry team deploy with a fire extinguisher to put out a small fire. The best plan is always determined by the specific needs and circumstances of the overall operation.

TACTICAL CASUALTY COMBAT CARE

Tactical Combat Casualty Care (TCCC) originated as a project within Naval Special Warfare and was later continued by the U.S. Special Operations Command (SOCOM). TCCC modified civilian advanced life support principles for the provision of medical care during an effective hostile force encounter. These new combat trauma care guidelines combined advanced medical care with good small-unit tactics.[7] The three major goals of TCCC are to (1) treat the casualty, (2) prevent additional casualties, and (3) complete the mission. TCCC recognizes that good medicine is sometimes bad tactics and that bad tactics can cause a mission to fail. Its principles attempt to balance the need to treat casualties against the risks of providing treatment within the context of an ongoing operation (Figure 13.4). TCCC emphasizes that care provided by a wounded operator initially on his or her own behalf (self-aid) or that provided on his or her behalf by a nearby operator (buddy-aid) may determine life or death. This model of operational medical support is believed to increase the effectiveness and survivability of military and law enforcement operators during a hostile force encounter.

The treatment principles of TCCC were developed following the recognition that preventable deaths in combat scenarios occur from uncontrolled hemorrhage due to extremity wounds, tension pneumothorax, and airway obstruction from maxillofacial trauma. Tactical law enforcement operations conducted using weapons and tactics similar to those used by the military place operators at risk for injuries similar to those sustained during combat operations. With the exception of controlling life-threatening hemorrhage and correcting airway obstruction immediately, TCCC recognizes that the tactical objective of neutralizing an effective hostile threat generally takes precedence over providing medical care, including the provision of self-aid or buddy-aid. These principles have gained widespread acceptance throughout military forces and now increasing acceptance within the law enforcement community. TCCC divides the level of medical care provided during a hostile force encounter into three phases: care under fire (CUF), tactical field care (TFC), and combat casualty evacuation care (CASEVAC).

Care under Fire

CUF is the first phase of casualty care and is rendered initially while operators are actively engaged with a hostile force (Figure 13.3). The initial medical plan during CUF encourages the casualty to remain engaged in

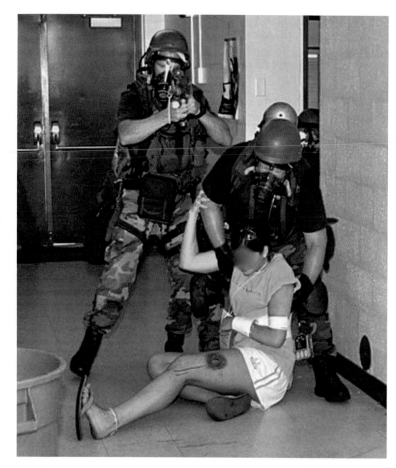

Figure 13.4. During tactical operations, medical care is deferred until casualties are removed from immediate hostile threats. Photo courtesy of Nelson Tang.

the operation if possible. If the casualty is armed, then he or she should return fire as necessary to assist with neutralizing the opposition force as quickly as possible. If under fire, he should also seek cover and concealment to protect himself from further injury. Other operators, when possible, should attempt to protect the casualty from sustaining additional wounds. Because uncontrolled hemorrhage from extremity wounds accounts for approximately 9% of all combat deaths and 60% of preventable deaths, the casualty or a nearby operator should render self- or buddy-aid to control life-threatening extremity hemorrhage, using a tourniquet if other means to stop the bleeding immediately and definitively are not possible under the circumstances. Attempts to control non-life-threatening hemorrhage should be deferred until the TFC phase.

Airway management while under fire is preferentially deferred until the TFC phase. CPR is usually contraindicated in the presence of an ongoing hostile threat except for cardiac arrest occurring in association with nontraumatic disorders such as electrocution, near-drowning, or hypothermia. Immobilizing the cervical spine during a hostile force encounter is reserved for casualties sustaining blunt force trauma resulting in neck pain or unconsciousness and when the danger to the medical provider does not exceed the potential benefit of performing spinal immobilization.[8] This is because effective immobilization of the cervical spine requires more than 5 minutes during which caregivers may be exposed to unnecessary risk during a hostile force encounter. Studies from Vietnam suggest that only 1.4% of casualties sustaining penetrating neck injuries will benefit from such immobilization.

Tactical Field Care

The TFC phase begins as soon as operators are no longer under an effective hostile threat. TFC is most often provided by trained medical providers. Assessment and treatment priorities include assessing the casualty for unrecognized hemorrhage and controlling all sources of bleeding. This is the first priority because uncontrolled hemorrhage is the leading cause of preventable death in a combat encounter. The second priority of TFC is airway management. Apnea is uncommon in survivable combat wounds so attention is directed toward establishing or maintaining an unobstructed airway using a chin lift or jaw thrust maneuvers, inserting a nasopharyngeal airway, and/or placing the casualty in a recovery position. Casualties with gunshot wounds to the face may require a surgical airway. Following unilateral blunt or penetrating chest trauma, casualties breathing spontaneously and in severe respiratory distress should undergo a needle decompression of the chest on the injured side for a presumptive diagnosis of tension pneumothorax. Sucking chest wounds that impair ventilation should be treated with an occlusive dressing and monitored for signs of a developing tension pneumothorax.

When possible, an intravenous saline lock (IV catheter without fluids attached) is placed in anticipation of the need to administer intravenous fluids or to administer analgesic medications. Hypotensive patients of average adult size with bleeding under control should receive 2 liters of isotonic crystalloid fluids. Casualties with uncontrolled bleeding into the chest or abdomen should generally not receive intravenous fluids unless they also exhibit signs of shock (i.e., no palpable radial pulse corresponding to a systolic blood pressure <90 mmHg) and/or a decreased mental status. In such cases, fluid resuscitation should continue only until mental status improves. The relative stability of hypotension and expected transport times to definitive care should be weighed against the possibility of inciting more vigorous hemorrhage with large fluid boluses that could theoretically "pop the clot" on thrombosed wounds. Pain may be treated with intravenous morphine or oral fentanyl "lollipops." Patients with grossly contaminated wounds, open fractures, or penetrating abdominal trauma or any patient in whom there will be a prolonged delay until definitive treatment should receive empiric intravenous antibiotics. When performing a complete medical examination (secondary survey), tactical medical providers should avoid the temptation to completely undress casualties in the field as this will increase the risk of hypothermia even in temperate climates. Removal of clothing should be limited to the degree necessary to expose known or suspected wounds.

Combat Casualty Evacuation Care

CASEVAC is the care rendered while the casualty is being evacuated by ambulance or helicopter to a trauma center. Additional medical personnel and equipment prestaged at a landing zone or a treatment area will assist in the care of the casualty at this point using local EMS guidelines. The operational tempo, the extent of the injury, and local practices generally determine whether the on-scene tactical medical provider accompanies an injured law enforcement operator to the hospital, acting as the patient's advocate as well as a liaison back to the operational command.

In the event that a person under protection is among the casualties of an attack, major elements of the protective operation will shift to the location of the receiving hospital or trauma center, thereby increasing dramatically the level of security in and around that location. In high-level protective operations, the detail will have designated specific hospitals or trauma centers that will be utilized in such situations and already have protective detail personnel preassigned and deployed to those facilities.

TACTICAL TRIAGE AND RAPID REMOTE ASSESSMENT

Triage is a French word meaning "to sort" and its primary purpose is to accomplish the greatest good for the largest number of casualties and permits the allocation of limited medical resources in the most efficient manner. Triage as it applies to tactical medical care means to prioritize casualties arising during a law enforcement operation. In an ongoing operation, the goal is to return key personnel to active duty as quickly as possible. There are many triage systems, but the one used most widely is the NATO Standard. The NATO Standard places casualties into one of four possible categories. Under this system, the highest treatment priority is IMMEDIATE, reserved for casualties needing an intervention within minutes to an hour in order to save a life, a limb, or eyesight and when there is a good chance of survival given the resources available. The second category is DELAYED, used for casualties requiring treatment that can wait for several hours. Examples include casualties with fractures or nonhemorrhagic wounds. The third category is MINIMAL, designated for casualties with minor medical problems that are unlikely to deteriorate if left untreated for as long as 24 hours. The final category is EXPECTANT, used for casualties that are so gravely ill or injured that their survival is considered unlikely, even with treatment. These patients are expected to die and are provided comfort measures to the extent possible.

A process for triaging patients into treatment categories begins by determining whether the injury scene is safe to enter and examine the casualties. In a tactical scenario, a special operations team may encounter casualties while still engaging a hostile opposition force, and circumstances may prohibit immediate access to medical care. Triage by medical practitioners under these conditions is often approached using a rapid and remote assessment methodology (RRAM).[9] When the scene is unsafe, this triage approach attempts to assess the casualty from a location of relative safety and provide critical treatment only when doing so can be accomplished without providing undue risk to the medical provider. The RAAM approach begins by gathering information about the casualty's condition without revealing to the opposition forces the tactical position or intent. Through the use of binoculars or night vision goggles, it is possible from a safe distance to determine if the patient is breathing, whether there is significant ongoing hemorrhage, and the existence of wounds incompatible with survival. Basic and/or advanced medical care is postponed until the casualty is repositioned to a safe location.

If the casualty is a law enforcement operator or an innocent civilian, efforts are made to direct the casualty, if able, to move to a position of safety where he or she is no longer exposed to the risk of further injury. When the tactical medical provider is able to communicate with the casualty, it may be possible to give instructions on how to initially provide self-care to the wounds, such as applying direct pressure or improvising a tourniquet. If the patient has an unstable injury or medical condition and the benefits to the casualty outweigh the risk to the medic under the circumstances, the law enforcement commander may authorize a rescue effort.

An approach similar to RRAM is used in tactical medicine to provide medical care to hostages, hostage takers, or barricaded subjects. During hostage or barricade situations, communication often occurs by telephone, public address system, or direct speech. Under these conditions, tactical medical providers can work closely with law enforcement hostage negotiators to collect medical intelligence on the condition of the hostages and hostage takers. This information is used to assist the on-scene commander with making strategic decisions regarding the operation. When necessary, and with the consent of the hostage takers, it is often possible to instruct hostages or their captors in the steps necessary to provide essential medical care.

REQUESTS FOR EVACUATION

Planning for a possible evacuation to a trauma center or other specialty medical care center begins with the threat assessment. Part of the medical threat assessment includes identifying modes of transporting patients taking into consideration time, distance, weather, and resources; developing possible routes for evacuation; securing radio channels and/or telephone contact numbers; and designating landing zones or collection points.

The need to evacuate a casualty is made by the operational commander based upon the assessments and recommendations of the tactical or protective medical providers. When making this decision, the commander takes into consideration multiple factors, including casualty condition, triage priority, and the overall tactical situation. To ensure that the request for evacuation contains all the necessary information, the military employs a standardized nine-element format (Table 13.2).

TACTICAL MEDICAL PROVIDER AS TEAM DOCTOR

As a basic force protection issue, the effectiveness of tactical and protective operations is critically dependent upon the health and safety of its manpower. In both the tactical and protection arenas, mission success is contingent upon law enforcement personnel who are

Table 13.2. Nine-line medevac request	
Line 1	**Landing zone or the location of casualty pickup.** Use map page and coordinates, latitude and longitude, a street address, or common landmarks.
Line 2	**Contact radiofrequency or telephone number and identifier.** The radio or telephone contact information allows the evacuation team to contact the requesting unit when they are in the area.
Line 3	**Evacuation priority.** The letter A (alpha) is used for urgent, B (bravo) for urgent/surgical, C (charlie) for priority, D (delta) for routine, and E (echo) for convenience. Each letter is preceded by the number of casualties in the category.
Line 4	**Requests for special equipment.** The letter A (alpha) signifies no special requests, B (bravo) requests a hoist, C (Charlie) requests extrication equipment, and D (delta) requests a mechanical ventilator. Alternatively, requests can be made by making a plain language request for special equipment.
Line 5	**Number of litter and ambulatory casualties.** This defines the number of litter and ambulatory casualties to enable evacuators to determine the number of vehicles or aircraft needed.
Line 6	**Evacuation site security.** This advises the evacuation team of possible hostile threats. The absence of an enemy is designated N; possible enemy, P; enemy in the area, E; and the need for an armed escort, X. In the absence of a threat, Line 6 can be used to provide a narrative of the casualties, wounds, or illness.
Line 7	**Designation of evacuation site.** This designates the markings used to designate the casualty transfer point, usually a landing zone. Designated colored panels, A; pyrotechnic devices, B; smoke, C; no designation, D; or other designation, E.
Line 8	**Casualty nationality and combat status, if appropriate.** U.S. military (A), U.S. civilian (B), non-U.S. military (C), non-U.S. civilian (D), or enemy prisoner (E).
Line 9	**NBC/terrain specifics.** Used to denote nuclear (N, november), biologic (B, bravo), or chemical (C, charlie) threats. Can also be used to designate terrain specifics relating to the patient transfer at the evacuation site and includes flat, sloped, or wooded terrain, or references to local landmarks or prominent terrain features.

fit, rested, hydrated, fed, and appropriately managed for both routine and unexpected medical conditions. Although the ability to provide combat casualty care during law enforcement operations is an essential component of operational medical support, the majority of care involves treating minor injuries and ailments that can affect the ability of those involved in the operation to function at peak performance.

Table 13.3. Common complaints during law enforcement operations

Headache
Dehydration
Seasonal allergies
Upper respiratory and sinus infections
Gastrointestinal upsets: heartburn, diarrhea
Insect bites and stings
Blisters
Dental pain
Contact dermatitis: poison ivy
Minor cuts, scratches, and abrasions
Musculoskeletal sprains and strains

Table 13.5. Water intake and work–rest–sleep cycles recommendations for hot conditions and heavy work

WBGT (°F)	WBGT (°C)	Water intake (L/hr)[a]	Hourly work–rest cycles (min)
< 82	< 28	0.75	40/20
82–84	28–29	1.0	30/30
85–87	29–30	1.0	30/30
88–89	31–32	1.0	20/40
≥ 90	≥ 32	1.0	10/50

[a]Do not exceed 1.5 qt/hr (L/hr) or 12 qt/day (L/day).
WBGT = wet bulb globe temperature
Adapted from FM 21-1, U.S. Department of the Army, Washington, DC

Law enforcement personnel within tactical and protective operations are generally younger, in top physical condition, and in good health. However, like professional athletes, operators must function at peak performance to perform their mission-critical tasks, which are often physically demanding and require the mental clarity to make split-second decisions. Tactical or protective medical providers work under the medical direction of an appropriately trained and experienced physician to tend to the global medical needs of law enforcement special operations team members. Less urgent or event minor medical ailments significant enough to potentially affect performance are often amenable to simple remedies, many of which are available "over the counter" (Table 13.3).

Following an initial evaluation and assessment of an operator's medical complaint, the medical provider should determine whether a delay in treatment could affect the operator adversely or degrade performance and impact the safety or success of the mission. In these circumstances, the medical provider should advise the commander as to how best to proceed. Minor complaints should be mitigated through the use of over-the-counter and prescription medications that alleviate symptoms without introducing side effects that might further degrade operational performance. Operators with atypical or worsening complaints suggest a more serious condition and warrant an immediate consultation with a physician.

Younger or less experienced law enforcement personnel are often less likely to seek advice or intervention for developing medical concerns. The relative inability to intervene early in this subgroup of operators makes

essential the need for vigilance and proactive interventions on the part of medical support personnel. Simple actions such as advocating hydration or ensuring safe food sources can significantly contribute to mission success by minimizing threats posed by performance degradation due to personnel illnesses (Table 13.4). During scenarios such as extended operations lasting more than 24 hours and overseas deployments, tactical and protective medical support may include establishing work–rest–sleep cycles, and preventing food-borne illness by ensuring that appropriate food, hydration, and sanitation facilities are available to sustain the operation (Table 13.5).

CONCLUSIONS

As the modern law enforcement mission continues to expand in both scope and complexity, special operations teams remain an essential adjunct to the command and control infrastructure. The tactical and protective missions are examples of specialized mission-driven functions developed by law enforcement in the United States to address and confront increasingly organized, armed, and hostile criminal elements. The operational medical support for tactical and protective operations is increasingly recognized as a critical component of these programs. As the law enforcement and homeland security missions develop and evolve, so will the demand for the thoughtful and proactive approach to medical services that are rendered in their support.

Table 13.4. Reducing foodborne illness during field operations

Use prepackaged food designed for field use
Enforce strict handwashing before meals
Prohibit the serving of food from unapproved sources
Keep hot foods hot, ≥140°F (60°C)
Keep cold foods cold, ≤40°F (4.5°C)

REFERENCES

1. Grossman D. Introduction: a new war at home: record crime and terrorism. In: *On Combat: The Psychology and Physiology of Deadly Conflict in War and in Peace.* PPCT Research Publications; 2004.
2. Rasumoff D. EMS at tactical law enforcement operations seminar a success. *Tactical Edge.* 1989;7:25–9.
3. Carmona R, Brennan K. Tactical emergency medical support conference (TEMS): a successful joint effort. *Tactical Edge.* 1990;8:7.

4 Heck JJ, Pierluisi G. Law enforcement special operations medical support. *Prehosp Emerg Care.* 2001;5(4):403–6.

5 American College of Emergency Physicians. Policy #400336. Dallas, TX. Approved June 2004. Available at: *http://www. acep.org/practres/aspx?id=29694.* Accessed November 2006.

6 Maniscalco PM, Dolan NJ. Dignitary protection. *Emerg Med Serv.* 2002;31(10):126–8.

7 Butler FK, Hagmann J, Butler EG. Tactical combat casualty care in special operations. *Milit Med.*1996;161(supp):1–16.

8 Arishita GI, Vayer JS, Bellamy RF. Cervical spine immobilization of penetrating neck wounds in a hostile environment. *J Trauma.* 1989;29:332–7.

9 Counter Narcotics Tactical Operations Medical Support (CONTOMS). A program of the Uniformed Services University of the Health Sciences, Department of Defense, Bethesda, Md.

14 | Hostile Geopolitical Environments

Michael J. VanRooyen, MD, MPH, FACEP

INTRODUCTION

Traveling and working in conflict areas or regions with significant political volatility requires a far more detailed understanding of the unique attributes of conflict areas. Civilians should only consider the prospect of traveling or working in an active war zone under well-defined circumstances, such as with a reputable relief organization or another organization that has significant logistical and security capability. This chapter focuses on two major themes: the complexities of traveling in hostile geopolitical environments and the unique features of providing medical services to populations affected by war.

Most physicians and medical personnel practice in relatively safe and stable environments, although some health care providers have chosen to work in conflict settings that have some degree of political instability and personal danger. To an inexperienced health worker, remote climates may seem inherently dangerous, but the opposite is often the case. Practicing in a rural setting in Somalia, for example, may be remote and relatively austere, but is likely to be safe and secure, while working in inner city Nairobi, Kenya, may be much more dangerous.

Judging whether a certain geographical region is dangerous requires significant knowledge of the unique political, economic, social, and cultural context. It's important to realize the relative risk of travel itself and the likely causes of mortality in travelers. The greatest killer of travelers is cardiovascular disease and accidental injuries, most commonly motor vehicle accidents. As this chapter reviews the unique risks to workers in hostile geopolitical environments, conflict settings, and war zones, it is important to keep in mind the more predictable risk of accidents and underlying health issues as the major threat to health in travelers.

That being said, there is very good evidence that health workers and humanitarians working in modern conflicts around the world have a significantly elevated risk of being killed or injured from violent causes. So how does one determine the degree of risk that accompanies any particular locale? The degree of danger is a complex and dynamic determination and cannot be adequately ascertained from media reports or State Department travel advisories. The risk of an adverse event while traveling is also closely linked to the traveler's own behaviors and abilities to adapt to the shifting political and security environment in regions that may be inherently dangerous due to military presence, differing ethnicity, and political volatility.

CHARACTERISTICS OF MODERN CONFLICTS

A number of locations frequented by civilian travelers and international workers are known to be relatively more dangerous that other places in the world. Modern conflict over the last two decades has increasingly victimized civilians and non-warring parties, including women and children, the elderly and vulnerable, as well as the local and foreign staff of humanitarian agencies who serve them. The conduct of war has changed considerably in the last decades in the following ways:

1. **Increase in violent regional ethnic conflicts:** As the Cold War era ended, the new world order quickly gave rise to a variety of ethnic tensions devoid of superpower arbitration. In the 1990s, civil conflicts erupted not only in the Balkans, Central Asia, and the Middle East but also throughout Africa. The world currently has at least 30 countries mired in serious conflict.[1] These conflicts are often intrastate struggles and often labeled (or mislabeled) as ethnic or religious wars. These contrast with previous international cross-border conflicts launched as "proxy" wars between the United States, the Soviet Union, and other superpowers and neocolonialists. The net result of modern civil conflict has been massive-scale refugee emergencies and public health disasters and an influx of foreign workers. Recent large-scale relief efforts include those in East Timor, Somalia, Sudan, Liberia, Sierra Leone, Guinea, Mozambique, Rwanda, Burundi, Democratic Republic of Congo, Chechnya, Colombia, Honduras, the Former Yugoslav Republics,

and northern Iraq. Emerging crises are predicted in several regions in Africa, the Middle East, Northern Caucasus, and central Asia.[2]

2. **Civilians as targets:** The crafting and promotion of the Geneva conventions and the promotion of standards in humanitarian law and codes of conduct in war have not stemmed the tide in human rights abuses and deliberate targeting of civilians in the past decades.[3] Indeed, civilian casualties resulting from regional conflicts or armed assault have increased compared to World War II or the Vietnam or Korean Conflicts. Today, for every armed combatant killed in a conflict, about ten civilians die, chiefly from communicable diseases and other preventable illnesses. In addition, civilians and foreigners can be targeted by combatants or used to advance a political or ideological agenda.

3. **Targeting of civilians based on nationality:** Despite diplomatic and ideological tensions, the international (nonmilitary) traveler in the pre-9/11 era could still live and work in politically tense situations like the Middle East in relative safety. In the post-9/11 era, and as wars in Afghanistan and Iraq rage on, it is increasingly difficult for Western workers to travel in several regions that are dominated by those ideologically opposed to Western involvement. Though the dynamics for this change are complicated and beyond the scope of this chapter, the net result is that an American traveling in the Palestinian Territories, Lebanon, Iran, Pakistan, and Afghanistan must take appropriate precautions for safety.

4. **Targeting aid workers:** The intentional targeting of civilian aid workers and the erosion of neutrality exemplifies this changing trend. Mani Sheik et al. analyzed 382 aid worker deaths from 1985 to 1998 and revealed an alarming fact; that most aid worker deaths (68%) were intentional and due to aggravated assault and murder, compared to the most commonly accepted risks of motor vehicle accidents, which was the second leading cause of death and accounted for only 17% of deaths.[4] Countries noted to be a significant risk to aid workers include Angola, Sudan, Rwanda, Afghanistan, Democratic Republic of Congo, Somalia, Burundi, the Former Yugoslavia, and regions in the Middle East, including Iraq.

5. **Restricted access to many regions:** Several regions are still quite restrictive in the number and types of travelers that are allowed in the country. Some of the most controlled areas include North Korea and Burma, with increasing restrictions to travel in Eritrea, Sudan (especially outside Khartoum), Chad, Zimbabwe, and several former Soviet states. Travel restrictions remain in effect (often for rather obtuse reasons) in Cuba and Iran, and travel to these regions may require special arrangements.

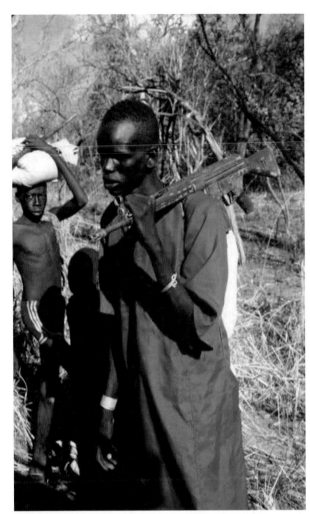

Figure 14.1. Boy soldier in Sudan. Photo courtesy of Michael J. VanRooyen.

6. **Modern combatants:** It is increasingly difficult to identify by sight local militias or combatants (Figure 14.1). "Soldiers" in a conflict may no longer wear uniforms to identify themselves as warring parties. The complexity of local conflicts and the ubiquity of weaponry lead to great difficulty in determining who is considered to be a combatant, and the lines between soldier and civilian are blurred. To the foreign traveler, this can mean that militia or combatants can be all around: in the market, in households, and on the road, and encounters may be unplanned and complicated.

DANGER BY GEOGRAPHY: THE WORLD'S MOST DANGEROUS PLACES

Some regions, in a general sense, are more dangerous than others. In his quirky, entertaining, and occasionally controversial book, *The World's Most Dangerous Places*, author Robert Young Pelton offers a list of some of the world's most difficult destinations.[5] Table 14.1 is a listing

Table 14.1. Dangerous destinations
Afghanistan ****
Algeria **
The Balkans (Croatia, Serbia, Kosovo) *
Chechnya *****
Colombia *****
Georgia **
Great Lakes region of Africa ****
India **
Iran *
Iraq ***** (changed from ***)
Israel/Palestine ****
Kurdistan **
Lebanon *** (changed from *)
Liberia *** (changed from *****)
Nepal **
North Korea *
Pakistan ***
Philippines ***
Russia **
South Africa ***
Sudan **** (changed from ***)
Yemen ***
Zimbabwe ***

of these with a five-star grading system for "dangerousness" with the author's editing based on current political changes.

TRAVEL TO HIGH-RISK AREAS AND HOSTILE ENVIRONMENTS

The decision to travel in a conflict or postconflict area or in a region that is subject to political or military turmoil is a serious one. If you must travel in an area where there has been a history of attacks on civilians, such as terrorism, kidnapping, or detention of foreigners, be sure to take the proper necessary precautions. The more complicated the destination, the more you need to make advance arrangements.

Many seasoned travelers working in conflict areas find it useful to register with the nearest U.S. embassy or consulate through the State Department's travel registration Web site.[11] Registering with the U.S. authorities can allow you to be contacted in the case of sudden political issues and can assist you in any evacuation or help track you in case of being trapped or being unable to move due to insecurity or military threat. Providing a detailed itinerary, copies of your passport and multiple contact numbers assist the consulate in locating you in an emergency.

When traveling to regions affected by conflict, it is important to have local contacts and resources in the region where you are traveling. Be cautious about discussing your itinerary with strangers and remain vague about personal matters, family, and finances. When traveling in regions with militia or in tense political climates, make an extra effort to ensure your personal security by

- Arranging for an alternate to your hotel or lodging, so if you are forced to flee, you have a safe haven.
- Establishing contact with someone local you can trust and keep their contact information handy. Make a special note of UN compounds, international organizations, and high-end hotels as possible destinations if you are in trouble.
- Remaining aware of people who are loitering around your hotel or who keep reappearing to assist you. Remain friendly, but be cautious about discussing personal matters, your itinerary, or your program.
- Leaving no personal or business papers in your hotel room and keeping copies of your documents in an alternate location.
- Avoiding predictable times and routes of travel and reporting any suspicious activity to local police and the nearest U.S. embassy or consulate.
- Being sure of the identity of visitors before taking rides or opening the door of your hotel room. Don't meet strangers at unknown or remote locations.
- Making a plan in the event that there is a bomb blast, gunfire, or sudden military activity in or around your hotel. Check exits and access routes in each place you stay.

HIGH-RISK SITUATIONS

When traveling to regions affected by conflict, it is important to get a sense of some traditionally dangerous situations and determine the details prior to encountering them. This will hold true for many regions that are experiencing political instability, and there are certain situations that should raise concern for any traveler. These include:

Checkpoints: Checkpoints and military barriers are notoriously high-risk places. Checkpoints manned with armed militia can be as simple as a local militia man in a ragtag uniform standing in the middle of the road to barricades, sandbags, and guard stations with organized militia. In general, checkpoints indicate an area of passage, often for civilians, into military-controlled areas. These areas are often the point of high tension, and if they can be avoided, it is better to do so. Many cannot be avoided, so a traveler should spend as little time as necessary in the vicinity of a checkpoint. Travelers should pay close attention to signs and instructions around a checkpoint and follow directions carefully, stopping when directed. Remain polite and business-like and have appropriate documents available. If questioned, remain calm and polite, and avoid sudden movements or erratic behavior.

Informal roadblocks: Informal roadblocks are quite different than official military checkpoints. Informal roadblocks are often set up by robbers or carjackers.

As will be discussed later, these should be avoided, and if they are encountered, it is advisable to either turn around or move beyond them as quickly as possible.

Demonstrations: Crowds and demonstrations are also high risk and should be avoided whenever possible. Driving through an agitated crowd as a foreigner is potentially dangerous, and if demonstrations are encountered, it is advisable to stop before entering the area and take an alternate route.

Weaponry: At least some of what defines a hostile environment for travelers and health workers is a place with a variety of weaponry. The most common weapon-related threat to the international tourist, health worker, or explorer is the gun, usually attached to someone who is willing to use it for ill gain. Guns are used to protect, intimidate, and create a threatening environment. Police, military, local militia, security personnel, and general gun ownership create a dangerous environment for travelers.

When traveling or working in a region that has armed combatants, there are some simple ways to avoid getting into trouble. Some basic recommendations follow:

Don't carry a gun: This may seem like simple logic, but a number of travelers who are working or recreating in exotic locations feel that they will be safer with a weapon. This logic is almost always false, and carrying a gun, as it turns out, is more likely to lead to an adverse event, even death.

Avoid places where you are in danger of being shot: This recommendation is also obvious, but certain locations within a country are notorious places for gun-related violence. These include large political gatherings, checkpoints, and border crossings. The less time spent in these locations, the more likely you will avoid being targeted or caught in the crossfire.

Avoid confrontation with local militia or thugs: This includes avoiding the areas previously described, as well as avoiding provoking military or paramilitary personnel by walking around past curfew, taking photos of guards or military installations, or displaying an attitude that is less than polite when being questioned by militia.

Avoid celebrations using guns: Bullets shot off in celebration can return to earth (or skull) at 500 feet per second. Celebrations in crowded areas, where those reveling in the moment are shooting guns up in the air, are a treacherous setting. Hundreds of people have been killed in many countries, including the United States. Three-quarters of these injuries are in the head, and many of these lead to death.

Stay low: In situations where there is shooting nearby, immediately drop to the floor or get down as low as possible and crawl to a sheltered location. Do not run and do not attempt to use a weapon unless you are trained and equipped. If it is necessary to move, crawl along the floor and find a place to hide, preferably near concrete walls or large solid objects. If there is gunfire within the building you are in, remember that bullets slide along flat surfaces and do not ricochet in laser-like angles. It is best to stay low and behind walls but not right up against a wall to avoid being hit.

LANDMINES AND UNEXPLODED ORDNANCE

Travelers to areas that have historically suffered from conflict should be aware of the very real threat of landmines and unexploded ordnance. This is especially the case in regions that are currently stable but historically have been contested in the recent past. There are 88 nations affected by landmines and unexploded ordnance (UXO) (Figure 14.2), and new victims in 71 countries since the turn of the century. Regions notorious for the presence of mines in areas frequented by civilians include Kosovo, Chechnya, China, Jordan, Ukraine, Mozambique, and the Balkans. Eighty-five percent of mine-related casualties occur in Afghanistan, Angola, and Cambodia, although details from Iraq are not accounted for in this figure.[6]

Mine Types

China, Russia, United States, Belarus, Ukraine, and Pakistan are the biggest producers (in that order) of the vast majority of the world's landmines. There are over 350 types of antipersonnel devices produced internationally, from large antitank mines to "toe-poppers" and small devices intended to maim, not kill. Mines, in general, are designed to injure, not kill, and to create terror and disrupt military targets by injuring soldiers. They can be detonated by direct pressure, vibration, or trip wires, sending high-velocity projectiles of metal, dirt, and debris into the tissue and bone of the victim. Mine types include those listed in Table 14.2.[7]

Avoiding Landmines

It is important that your expedition be aware of mine threats in regions where you will be traveling. You can take a number of steps in preparing to travel and in your activities while in-country to avoid mined areas.

- Get information on the country where you will be traveling. There are a number of good sites available to determine the regional risks of UXOs.
- Consult local officials if traveling or working in a mined region. Don't leave the paved areas of the road, not even to walk alongside the road to take a photo.

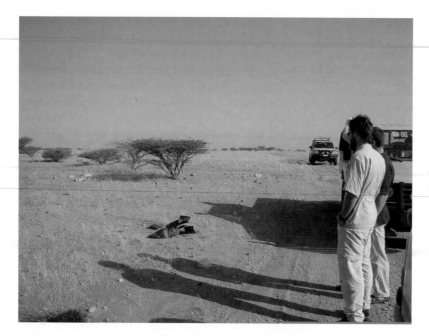

Figure 14.2. Unexploded ordinance in north-eastern Sudan. Photo courtesy of Gregory H. Bledsoe.

Table 14.2. Mine types

Scatter mines: Dropped by a plane or helicopter, scatter mines are small devices that may or may not explode on impact. These can look innocuous, even like toys, and are often the source of devastating injuries to children.

Antipersonnel mines: These are small, the size of a hockey puck, and designed to be buried close to the surface. They are often made of plastic, with the only metal components being a small pin or spring for the detonator, making them nearly impossible to detect with metal detectors. They are produced by China, the United States, and Italy, cost about a dollar, and can cause immediate amputations and devastating wounds. Larger antipersonnel mines can spray shrapnel over a larger area, injuring or maiming many people in its path.

Fragmentation mines: These include the well-known Claymore mines and mines on a stick that are designed to spray ball bearings or fragments over 50 m or more. Fragmentation mines can be detonated by trip wires and are used to protect perimeters.

Antitank mines: These large, plate-sized mines are used to disable and destroy military vehicles, such as tanks or armored personnel carriers. They are detonated by the weight of the vehicle or by remote control. These devices have grown in popularity and complexity over the course of the Iraq War, and variations are responsible for many road-side bombings.

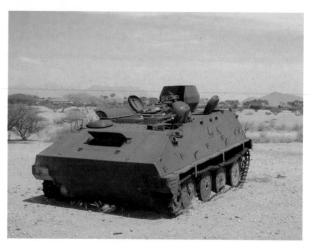

Figure 14.3. Stay on well–traveled paths and resist the urge to explore former military outposts or equipment. This armored military transport vehicle is an example of an item that should be recognized as a possible location of landmines or unexploded ordnances. Photo courtesy of Gregory H. Bledsoe.

- Stay on well-traveled roads and paths (Figure 14.3). Avoid being the first person or vehicle in a convoy that is going into a region that may be freshly mined. Follow behind larger vehicles, and allow them to be at least 100 m ahead of you.
- If you have a flack jacket and are working in a mined area, sit on it while driving.
- Never touch or handle suspicious items or devices, and do not pick up objects that appear to have a military function as souvenirs. Many tourists to prior conflict areas have been injured collecting souvenirs.

Antipersonnel landmines remain a threat to noncombatants despite a growing number of conventions aimed to ban them. Even though there are over 100 million landmines distributed across Asia, the Middle East, the Balkans, and South America, landmine production continues unabated by the world's superpowers. Someone is killed or injured by a landmine every 15–20 minutes, and destitute nations like Cambodia struggle with the burden of over 35,000 amputees.

Effects of Landmines on Populations and Health

Landmines represent both an immediate health risk and a delayed threat. Landmines have been deployed in over seventy countries. Of the 15,000 killed or injured annually,

Table 14.3. De-mining agencies
Commercial agencies Ronco Mine Tech International DynCorp
Humanitarian organizations HALO Trust (Hazardous Areas Life Support Organization) DEMIRA German mine clearance MAG (Mine Advisory Group) INTERSOS Response International DanChurchAid

80% are civilians. The epidemiology of landmine injuries is not known, but case fatality rates are very high.

Landmine injuries pose a major problem for health providers, who may be poorly equipped to manage the severe penetrating trauma, blast injury, and consequent infection and gangrene. Trauma due to mine injuries requires the need for high-level surgical services and can monopolize the curative health care resources.

Another major problem with landmines is that they outlast any conflict, and the removal of mines is both difficult and costly. De-mining programs exist in 41 nations, and new mines are being placed in contested areas every day. The reality of mines is that no one truly knows how many mines exist or where they are located. This creates significant economic, social, and psychological disruption in communities affected by landmines.

Ottawa Treaty and the ICBL

The 1997 Ottawa Treaty or the "Mine Ban Treaty," formally the Convention on the Prohibition of the Use, Stockpiling, Production and Transfer of Anti-Personnel Mines and on their Destruction, bans completely all antipersonnel landmines (AP-mines).[6] It has been signed by 155 countries since 1997. Forty nations have yet to sign, including China, Russia, India, and the United States, mainly because of a million landmines along the DMZ between North and South Korea. Only antipersonnel mines are covered. Mixed mines, antitank mines, remote-controlled Claymore mines, antihandling devices (booby-traps) are not within the treaty.

De-mining Agencies

De-mining agencies undertake the extremely difficult task of surveying, mapping, marking, and clearing. Major agencies include those listed in Table 14.3.[8]

KIDNAPPING AND HOSTAGE SITUATIONS

While the numbers of kidnappings are difficult to determine, the worldwide estimate for kidnappings is anywhere from 12,500 to 25,500. Most of these are businessmen, child custody cases, or politically motivated abductions. It is difficult to get a solid number because up to half of all kidnappings are not reported to the authorities.[9] Columbia boasts the greatest number of kidnapping, and it has become a regular source of revenue for terrorist networks like the FARC. It is estimated that ten people are kidnapped each day in Colombia. Other nations with high rates of kidnapping include Russia, the former Soviet States, and the Philippines.[9]

Being taken hostage, be it for political reasons or for economic reasons, is a terrifying occurrence. Each hostage situation is unique, and each requires a tailored approach by authorities. Regardless of the variations of a hostage situation, the U.S. government's position remains the same: The U.S. government will negotiate, but it will not make concessions. U.S. government officials will employ diplomatic processes and engage the resources of the host country to secure the safety and release of hostages.

The U.S. Department of State provides some advice to those who might find themselves in a possible hostage situation. Much of this advice is predicated on the notion that the most dangerous times for any hostage are upon abduction, when assailants are tense and anxious, and at any time there is a rescue attempt.[10] The State Department recommends taking the following actions in the event of a hostage situation:

- Do not struggle or make sudden or erratic moves.
- Avoid confrontation. Remain polite, calm, and follow instructions.
- Do not attempt to escape unless you are certain to be successful.
- If interrogated, be cooperative, but don't volunteer additional information.
- Prepare yourself for the long haul. Eat when you can, establish some form of routine, and try to establish rapport with your captors.
- Above all, remain resilient and keep a sense of optimism. Keep yourself mentally and physically healthy.

TERRORISM

Terrorism is defined by the U.S. government as "premeditated, politically motivated violence perpetrated against noncombatant targets by subnational groups or clandestine agents usually intended to influence an audience."[12] The use of the word "terrorist" is often contextual and has been expanded considerably to include many of the activities aimed at combating efforts of those doing the naming. Regardless of the application or misapplication of the term, terrorist activity, to the expatriate traveler, typically refers to acts that target those viewed as related to an occupying power or those nearby the target.

Terrorist activities may appear to be random and unpredictable, but there are several precautions that travelers can take to avoid such attacks. The first such protection is to avoid traveling to areas that are prone to terrorist acts in the first place and to avoid destinations that have a known record of terrorism, kidnapping, or politically motivated assaults on civilians. Other precautions include minimizing time spent in airports, shopping malls, large markets, nightclubs, and other places frequented by tourists.

WORKING IN A CONFLICT REGION

The chapter has thus far dealt with the nonmedical attributes of working in a conflict setting, with a particular focus on the foreign traveler. When considering working as a clinician in an active conflict setting, several considerations will impact the prioritization and provision of medical care. The most important consideration is understanding population-based vulnerability and the major determinants of health in displaced and war-affected populations. This may seem obvious, but for those who have not worked in a conflict setting, the concepts of vulnerability and the likely causes of illness may be very different than practicing at home. The remaining part of this chapter focuses on the unique considerations of health care provision in a conflict setting.

Humanitarian access: Humanitarian access and the significant difficulty in reaching populations in need is a prominent characteristic of working in conflict settings. Although the needs may be great, the ability of international aid organizations to provide services to civilian populations is severely restricted in many regions of the world. Organizations working in regions such as Chechnya, the Darfur region of Sudan, Iraq, and several other Middle Eastern nations are faced with extremely challenging logistical and security issues to simply move personnel and materials in and out of a region. In the Darfur region of western Sudan, the Sudanese government severely restricts the access of many aid organizations, effectively cutting off all aid to populations displaced in the Darfur conflict.

Scarcity of resources: In addition to difficulty in obtaining access to certain regions, relief workers providing health care in conflict areas are faced with ill-equipped, outdated, and often destroyed medical facilities, with very few options for adequate treatment. This requires a maximally flexible approach toward providing clinical services, and creativity in adapting to available resources. Support services, specialty care, and appropriate facilities and equipment are often lacking, as are familiar diagnostic resources and therapeutic options.

HUMAN VULNERABILITY AND HEALTH CONSIDERATIONS IN DISPLACEMENT

War and civil conflict create disruption of social order, economic collapse, and, in many cases, mass population displacement. Families, communities, and populations may be forced to migrate to find food, water, and shelter or to seek protection from persecution because of race, religion, politics, or nationality.

Refugees and Displaced Populations

By the start of 2006, the global refugee population had dropped from 9.5 million to 8.4 million – the lowest total since 1980, largely as a result of more than 6 million refugees (two-thirds of them Afghans) returning home over the past 4 years. In addition to the continuing return of Afghans, 2005 saw other major repatriations to Liberia, Burundi, Iraq, and Angola (all of which welcomed back more than 50,000 returnees during the course of the year).[12]

At the start of 2006, there were an estimated 23.7 million internally displaced people (IDP) worldwide. The United Nations High Commission for Refugees (UNHCR) assisted 6.6 million IDPs in 16 countries, a 22% jump compared to the previous year. The increase primarily reflected newly reported IDP situations in Iraq (1.2 million) and Somalia (400,000), and the number of IDPs of concern to UNHCR in the Darfur region of Sudan also rose.[13]

Refugees are people who, because of fear of persecution for reasons of race, religion, nationality, or membership in a particular social or political group, flee from their home country and seek protection across an international border.[14] UNHCR is mandated to guarantee protection for refugees as well as to find a long-term solution for their displacement, such as repatriation to the country of origin, integration into a neighboring country of asylum, or resettlement in a third country. Most displaced persons, however, are internally displaced persons. IDPs are forced to flee from their homes as a result of armed conflict, internal strife, violations of human rights, or disasters but remain within the borders of their country.

IDPs do not enjoy the same legal status for protection and for assistance simply because they did not cross their country's borders.

Refugees and IDPs display a number of vulnerabilities due to acute displacement, loss of livelihoods, and lack of shelter, sanitation, and proper nutrition. Displacement also leads to overcrowding, breakdown of sanitation, and spread of communicable diseases, as well as disruption of community traditions. Refugees are

Physiologically vulnerable: Those who lack access to basic needs, including health care (the malnourished, the sick, pregnant and lactating women, young children, and the elderly)

Socially vulnerable: Those who lack access to education and social support (female-headed households, unaccompanied minors, AIDS orphans, and the disabled)

Economically vulnerable: Those who lack sufficient income (the poorest)

Politically vulnerable: Those who lack autonomy and have no control over their situation (internally displaced persons, refugees, and ethnic minority groups)

HEALTH THREATS IN DISPLACED POPULATIONS

Population movements predispose to a variety of health problems including acute traumatic injuries secondary to assault, increased exposure to communicable diseases, and decompensation of chronic medical conditions and complications of social disruption.

Traumatic events, such as gunshot wounds, blast injuries, blunt trauma, and assault, lead to several transformational effects on a health care system, causing a major shift in the utilization of resources away from primary care and preventative health services toward surgical and emergency medical care, high consumption of resources, and high cost interventions. Trauma also disrupts communities and creates fear, paranoia, and movement of families to seek care for injuries and rehabilitation.

Despite the devastating effects of blunt and penetrating trauma on individuals, the public health consequences of war such as malnutrition, exposure to communicable diseases and lack of access to basic preventive health services such as immunizations, leads to far greater excess mortality than trauma or direct war-related injuries. Communicable diseases affecting neonates, children and malnourished populations occur disproportionately in displaced populations because of population migration into endemic regions, lack of sanitation, disruption of health care resources, and poor vector control.

Major infectious diseases affecting migratory and stressed populations include measles, acute respiratory infections, acute diarrheal illness, malaria, meningitis, and tuberculosis.

Measles

Measles is one of the leading causes of pediatric death in refugee camps, with reported case fatality rates as high as 30%. The displacement of large groups of people in Africa has led to major measles epidemics. Measles vaccination is the first priority in displaced populations with low immunization coverage (Figure 14.4). Mortality in measles is closely linked to malnutrition and vitamin A deficiency.

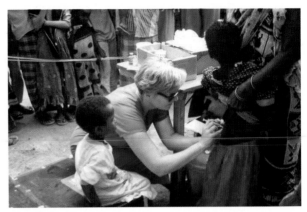

Figure 14.4. Immunization program among refugees in Somalia. Photo courtesy of Michael J. VanRooyen.

Acute Respiratory Infections

Acute respiratory infections (ARIs) are a major cause of death in displaced populations, especially in circumstances of major overcrowding. The establishment of ARI programs is an important priority in refugee camps, with appropriate health care expertise, case definitions, and antibiotic access.

Acute Diarrheal Illness

Diarrheal disease is the most lethal public health threat to displaced populations. Acute enteric illnesses such as cholera, shigella, *E. coli*, typhoid fever, or other infectious forms of diarrhea are strongly linked to population displacement and contaminated water supplies.

Cholera and shigella epidemics have occurred commonly in refugee camps in Somalia, Ethiopia, Sudan, Rwanda, and Zaire and have led to massive outbreaks with high case fatality rates. In Goma, a cholera outbreak among the nearly one million Rwandan refugees had an initial case fatality rate of 22%, which then declined to 3–5% as treatment centers were set up. About 50,000 refugees died in the first month of operation; over 90% of these deaths were due to diarrheal illness (cholera and shigella).

Malaria

Malaria, an acute febrile parasitic disease spread by the female *Anopheles* mosquito, is the most common disease in Africa, with high rates of morbidity and mortality among displaced persons where malaria is endemic. Malaria infects more than 100 million people a year and kills over a million per year, mainly in Africa. Malaria is a major threat among displaced populations, many of whom may have limited immunity and move into a region of high endemicity.

Meningitis

Meningococcal meningitis occurs in endemic areas along the "meningitis belt" (Figure 14.5) in sub-Saharan Africa. The disease is seasonal and has resulted in mass outbreaks with high case fatality rates in endemic areas with displaced populations and overcrowding. Immunization campaigns are often conducted before or during outbreaks in vulnerable populations.

Tuberculosis

Tuberculosis is a leading cause of preventable death among adults and is a major risk to displaced populations, particularly those with HIV/AIDS. Transient populations represent a particular risk, as treatment is complicated by difficulty in diagnosis and multiple drug resistance.

SEXUAL AND GENDER-BASED VIOLENCE IN CONFLICT

Gender-based violence perpetrated by combatants, occupying forces, and local militia has become a prominent and disturbing trend in many modern conflicts. An estimated 50,000 Muslim, Croatian, and Serbian women were raped during the conflict in the former Yugoslavia, and nearly ten times that number were raped and forced into sexual slavery during the genocide in Rwanda.[15] Rape, sexual slavery, and the

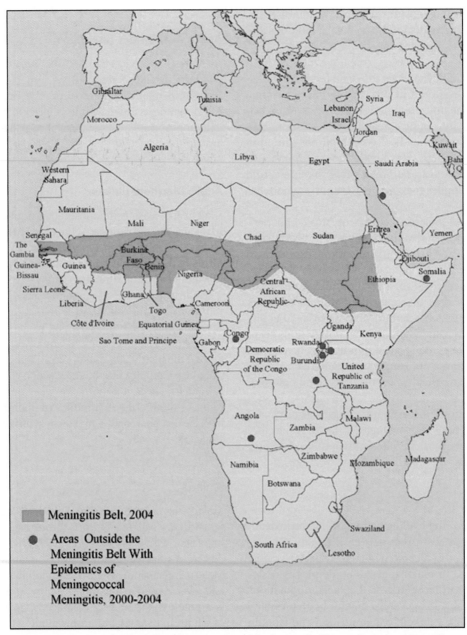

Figure 14.5. Meningitis belt in Africa. Photo courtesy of the Centers for Disease Control and Prevention.

deliberate targeting of both women and men for sexual abuse are both a human rights violation and major public health issue. Sexual violence creates profound physical and psychological trauma and has many long-term community consequences.

SUMMARY: TRAVELING AND WORKING IN A CONFLICT ZONE

International travelers, expeditions, and humanitarian organizations may venture into regions that are affected by war or political instability. Traveling to a conflict area or war zone is complex and requires detailed understanding of the political and military context and the potential for threats to personal security. It is essential to work with reputable agencies that have significant on-the-ground presence and understand the risks of the region. Significant advance preparation is required, and diligent attention to the details of personal security, situational awareness, and contingency planning is essential when traveling to countries or regions in the midst of, or the aftermath of, armed conflict.

REFERENCES

1 World Conflict List 2001. National Defense Council Foundation. Available at: *http://www.ndcf.org*. Accessed: January 2007.

2 The World at War. Available at: *http://www.globalsecurity.org/military/world/war/index.html*. Accessed: January 2007.

3 Guha-Sapir D, van Panhuis G, Gijsbert W. The importance of conflict-related mortality in civilian populations. *Lancet.* 2003;361 2126–8.

4 Shiek M, Guiterrez MI, Bolton P, Spiegel P, Thieren M, Burnham G. Deaths among humanitarian workers. *BMJ.* 2000;321(7254):166–8.

5 Pelton RY. *The World's Most Dangerous Places.* 5th ed. New York: HarperCollins; 2003.

6 International Campaign to Ban Landmines. Available at: *http://www.icbl.org/*.

7 Landmines. Available at: *http://www.globalsecurity.org/military/systems/munitions/landmines.htm*. Accessed: January 2007.

8 Landmine Monitor. Available at: *http://www.icbl.org/lm/research/mre/lm_2007_mre_background_and_terminology*. Accessed: January 2007.

9 Global list of kidnapping events. Available at: *http://www.mapreport.com/subtopics/c/k/html*. Accessed: January 2007.

10 U.S. Department of State. Crisis Preparedness. Available at: *http://travel.state.gov/travel/tips/emergencies/emergencies_1187.html*. Accessed: January 2007.

11 U.S. Department of State. Travel Registration. Available at: *https://travelregistration.state.gov/ibrs/*. Accessed: January 2007.

12 U.S. Department of State. Patterns of Global Terrorism. Available at: *http://www.state.gov/s/ct/rls/*. Accessed: January 2007.

13 United Nations High Commission for Refugees. Refugees by Numbers 2006 Edition. Available at: *http://www.unhcr.org/cgi-bin/texis/vtx/basics/opendoc.htm?tbl=BASICS&id=3b028097c*. Accessed: January 2007.

14 United Nations High Commission for Refugees. Introduction: international instruments defining the term "refugee." Available at: *http://www.hrea.org/learn/tutorials/refugees/Handbook/intro.htm*. Accessed: January 2007.

15 International Planned Parenthood Federation. Communicable disease threats in complex emergencies: salama article. GBV in conflict, numbers: Definitions: What is Gender-based violence? Available at: *www.ippfwhr.org*. Accessed: January 2007.

Richard S. Williams, MD, FACS, and Marc A. Shepanek, PhD

INTRODUCTION

The American Board of Preventive Medicine states that "Aerospace medicine focuses on the clinical care, research, and operational support of the health, safety, and performance of crewmembers and passengers of air and space vehicles, together with the support personnel who assist operation of such vehicles."[1] From inception, aerospace medicine has been an archetypical example of the practice of medicine attending the exploration of an extreme environment. The many physical and physiological risks attending atmospheric and space flight mandated intimate medical involvement early on. Aerospace medicine evolved as a unique specialty, blending preventive and occupational medicine with clinical diagnostic and therapeutic practice in a population of individuals whose overall health is often excellent. The traditional physician–patient relationship is highly modified, of necessity. The flight surgeon must measure the health of aerospace crew and support personnel by job qualification standards, with potentially profound career impact. At the same time, responsibility to maintain the health of these individuals and to protect the safety of the public must remain paramount. This produces potential conflicts of interest – aerospace crew members may be hesitant to seek medical attention for fear of medical disqualification, and flight surgeons must act in the best interest of crew health and public safety, even when personal relationships and concerns may make decisions and actions difficult. The flight surgeon–aircrew relationship is the most complex physician–patient relationship in all of medicine and requires a great deal of maturity and sound judgment for successful outcomes.

The exploration of extreme environments is accompanied by risks, many of which are unique to the environments in question. Aerospace medicine is, in a broad sense, very much a risk mitigation effort and is fundamental to the human exploration of all aerospace environments, from general aviation to space flight.

Understanding that aircraft and air travel have played such a pivotal role in the ongoing exploration of all extreme environments, aerospace medicine serves to help mitigate risks attending all exploration. In this chapter, we will trace the development of aerospace medicine as a medical specialty, consider its role in mitigation of key risks and risk areas attending exploration of the atmosphere and space, and examine trends and elements that will probably influence the future of the specialty, especially with respect to the commercialization of space flight and medical support of exploration beyond low earth orbit. Experiential vignettes, both hypothetical and actual, will be used to illustrate specific risk areas when practical. The chapter is written both from the perspective of a practitioner of aerospace medicine as well as that of a pilot.

HISTORY AND DEVELOPMENT

From the earliest flights of Montgolfier hot air balloons in the late eighteenth century, the unique risks attending exploration of the aerospace environment made themselves evident, and the disciplines that eventually coalesced into the specialty of aerospace medicine began to emerge. The first broadly public flight of a Montgolfier balloon at Versailles, France, a command performance for Louis XIV, marked the first aeronautical scientific experiment with animal subjects and the first aircraft accident investigation. The passengers on this first flight were a cock, a sheep, and a duck. When the balloon landed, the cock was found to have a damaged wing. The ensuing investigation revealed that the cock's injury was due to being kicked by the sheep, not to a risk inherent to flight. Human flights followed, with Jean-Françoise Pilatre de Rosier, the French physicist and physician, becoming history's first aviator on October 15, 1783, with a tethered balloon flight. Pilatre de Rosier later performed the first free balloon ascent with François Laurent Marquis d'Arlandes. Interestingly, de Rosier and his companion M. Romain became aviation's first human fatalities when they died in the fire that consumed their hybrid hot air and hydrogen balloon in an attempt to cross the English Channel.

Pilatre de Rosier was a scientist, and began the long tradition of scientific pursuit in atmospheric exploration. Early balloon flights began to systematically define some of the physiologic risks of flight, notably hypothermia and hypoxia, with increasing altitude. One of the most notable of these flights was conducted by Glaisher and Coxwell, who ascended to 31,000 ft. During this ascent, both aeronauts experienced profound hypothermia and hypoxia, and were almost incapacitated. Coxwell, with supreme effort, managed to grasp the valve cord with his teeth, releasing hydrogen and initiating descent, averting a tragic end to the flight.[2] Paul Bert, generally regarded as the "father of aerospace medicine," wrote the first textbook on the subject in 1878. He described altitude sickness, chronicled the balloon ascensions of many aeronauts of the day, and experimented extensively with animals and plants in low-pressure chambers of his own invention. He was particularly complimentary of Glaisher's aeronautical efforts, motivated by science.

Military leaders were quick to appreciate the tactical value of balloons, which were widely employed as aerial observation platforms in armies of the nineteenth century. The advent of powered flight, and the subsequent development of the airplane as a practical and somewhat reliable means of transportation, gave rise to new potential as weapons systems and platforms for modern warfare. In World War I, aircraft initially were used strictly for observation, a more mobile means for the traditional balloon mission. Pilots of passing observation aircraft began firing on one another with small arms, which led to the incorporation of machine guns integral to the aircraft. This opened up new horizons for the development of aerial combat techniques and tactics, based on aerobatic maneuvering. Fighter pilots began reporting symptoms of visual dimming or darkening, in association with aggressive turns or when recovering from a steep dive. This was the first identification of the symptom complex of tunnel vision and blackout associated with sustained acceleration environments, another of the many risks attending the aerospace environment. This risk, although now well understood, still presents a threat to modern-day fighter pilots as well as civilian aerobatic pilots.

Early in the First World War, aircraft accidents were disturbingly frequent, and losses in training accidents exceeded losses in combat. One of the preventive measures taken was to develop selection and qualification medical standards for pilots.[8] In the U.S. Army, Dr. Theodore C. Lyster led an effort to establish medical examining units for pilots and also to initiate efforts to begin research into the physiologic liabilities of flight. Accident rates improved, and this tradition of selection standards for air and space crews continues worldwide as a proven example of successful preventive intervention in protecting the health of aerospace crews.

The quest for higher performance in aircraft continued during the period between the wars. Another risk, that of spatial disorientation, had been identified by pilots attempting to operate in conditions of low visibility. Pilots entering clouds, fog, heavy precipitation, or other conditions of low visibility could rely only on their senses relative to the movement of the aircraft to maintain orientation. Highly experienced aviators attempted to employ these methods of "flying by the seat of the pants," which ultimately proved unreliable. Some pilots, finding themselves above an overcast, would spin the aircraft down through the clouds and hope to find clear weather beneath, rather than risk spatial disorientation and loss of control. The pioneering work of instrument flight by James Doolittle in the 1930s paved the way for routine aircraft operations in instrument meteorological conditions (IMC), but flight into adverse weather conditions by non-instrument-rated pilots remains one of the leading causes of fatal aircraft accidents today.

The interwar period also saw the earliest attempts to provide complex environmental control for aircraft cabins. Dr. Harry G. Armstrong was one of the pioneers in the study of aeromedical risks and mitigation efforts during this period. He established a research laboratory at Wright Field in Dayton, Ohio, and conducted research on hypoxia, carbon monoxide poisoning, decompression sickness, acceleration, and other important aeromedical risk areas. That laboratory continues in operation today, bearing his name. Another prominent aerospace medicine leader of the interwar period was Dr. Louis Bauer, who established the first School of Aviation Medicine in 1922 and developed the first physical standards for civilian pilots in 1926.

Pressurized cabins and pressure suits were developed during this period, but they were not widely employed in production aircraft. World War II was fought largely with unpressurized, high-performance aircraft operating at altitudes of 30,000 ft or higher. Many episodes of hypoxia were reported with failure of oxygen systems, and some aircraft and crews were lost to this physiologic risk. Cold injuries in the form of frostbite were common, as were cases of altitude-induced decompression sickness. Fighter aircraft operated at high speeds and were capable of sustaining acceleration environments for long periods of time during the course of aerial combat maneuvering. G-induced visual symptoms and even G-induced loss of consciousness (G-LOC) became operational considerations. The postwar period was characterized by development of successive generations of jet aircraft with ever increasing capabilities with regard to speed, service ceiling and maneuverability. This trend continues through the present, with development of the newest generation of superagile fighter aircraft.

Aerospace medicine has responded to and kept pace with the multiple risks attending flight as they expressed themselves through the years. Reliable cabin pressurization, the advent of pressure suits, better oxygen systems, G-protection garments integrated with aircraft systems, crew escape systems such as ejection seats, superior communications equipment integrated with conformal helmets, more intuitive presentation of flight instrument displays, impact attenuating aircraft seats, and effective restraint systems are a few of the developments attributable to aerospace medicine practitioners and associated engineering disciplines that routinely protect the health and safety of today's aircrews and passengers.

In the late 1940s, attention was drawn in earnest to the potential for human space flight. Dr. Hubertus Strughold, generally regarded as the "father of space medicine," was instrumental in establishing the department of Space Medicine within the U.S. Air Force School of Aerospace Medicine and in establishing space medicine as a discipline. His classical treatise, published in 1952, "Atmospheric Equivalence," related zones as one ascends in the atmosphere to physiological phenomena and consequences, portraying the transition to space as a continuum rather than as a set boundary. (See Figure 15.1.) Yuri Gagarin's orbital flight on April 12, 1961, followed by John Glenn's flight in February 1962 marked

the beginnings of human exploration of space, and the incredibly complex risks encountered beyond earth's atmosphere became reality. In addition to the hazards of launch and entry, vacuum, ionizing radiation, and extreme temperature changes, a suite of risks attending exposure to microgravity, the confinement of spacecraft, and orbital operations has emerged. These risks include cardiovascular deconditioning, reduction in circulating blood volume with orthostatic hypotension on return to earth, loss of bone mineral density, neurosensory adaptation, immune compromise, nutritional challenges, and the same behavioral health liabilities that attend all expeditions to isolated and extreme environments. These risks increase in degree with the duration of space flight missions.

Strict medical selection criteria were developed and applied to astronaut and cosmonaut selection at the inception of human space flight. These preventive measures have been extraordinarily effective in minimizing mission impact from medical concerns in both the Russian and U.S. space flight programs. No mission has been truncated or terminated due to health or medical concerns in the history of the U.S. space program. The Russians have foreshortened at least two *Salyut* space

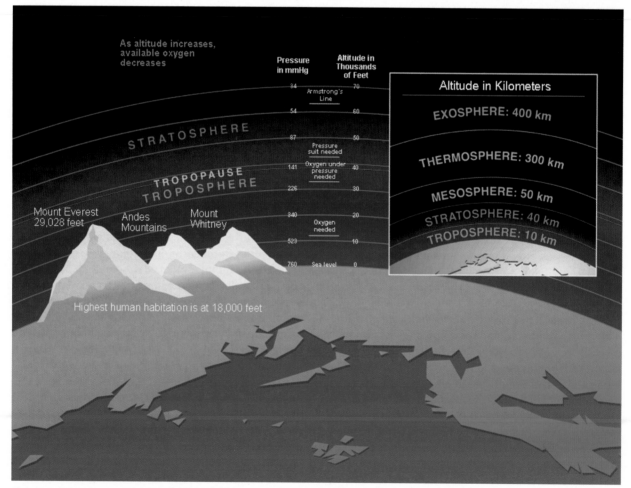

Figure 15.1. The atmosphere, with physiologically significant altitudes. Courtesy of NASA; adapted from the Aerospace Medical Association.

station missions due to medical concerns, but it must be noted that the Russian space flight experience is heavily weighted toward long-duration missions, increasing the exposure time in space and thus increasing the risk of untoward health or medical occurrence as a function of time.

Currently, International Space Station (ISS) operations are being conducted with full-time human habitation in low earth orbit. The ISS is managed by five major partner space agencies; the National Aeronautics and Space Agency (NASA), the Russian Space Agency (RSA), the European Space Agency (ESA), the Canadian Space Agency (CSA), and the Japanese Aerospace Exploration Agency (JAXA). The policy of strict crew medical selection and qualification standards continues. ISS medical selection and qualification standards are the product of international management groups consisting of physicians with expertise in space medicine from all partner agencies. The standards are periodically reviewed and updated, and are based on best available scientific evidence and clinical judgment. This international collaboration between nations of such different cultures is unprecedented, and proving highly successful to date.

Aerospace medicine, as practice and as a specialty, has evolved with exploration of the atmosphere and space. Since 1953, board certification in aerospace medicine has been available through the American Board of Preventive Medicine. There are currently four formal training programs in aerospace medicine in the United States. Two of these are military, sponsored by the U.S. Air Force and U.S. Navy. The other two are civilian, at the Wright State University in Dayton, Ohio, and the University of Texas Medical Branch at Galveston, Texas. The primary professional society of the field is the Aerospace Medical Association (AsMA), which counts among its members representatives from all fields related to aerospace medicine, life sciences, and human factors disciplines. There are proponents of creating additional or alternate formal credentialing means and processes for the discipline of space medicine. This, if pursued, must be done with care to avoid dividing an already very small specialty with a small constituency, beyond practicality.

AEROSPACE ENVIRONMENTS

The aerospace environment is arguably the most hostile, extreme environment humans have ever entered and explored. Earth's atmosphere is a thin veil of gas enveloping the planet to an altitude of about 90 km. The major components of the atmosphere, for practical purposes, are oxygen, which constitutes about 21% of the gases present, and nitrogen, which accounts for about 78%. About 1% of the atmosphere is made up of hydrogen, carbon dioxide, helium, and other gases. Water vapor is normally present in the atmosphere, and is expressed as relative humidity. Atmospheric humidity is directly dependent on temperature, with increasing amounts of water vapor possible with increasing temperatures. Atmospheric pressure reflects the actual weight of the column of air and varies at the surface based on prevalent meteorological conditions. During ascent, atmospheric pressure decreases. The relative percentages of gases stay constant during ascent in the atmosphere, but the partial pressure of oxygen lessens with ascent, making less oxygen physiologically available at higher altitudes (partial pressures of water vapor and carbon dioxide remain more or less constant in the alveoli at normal body temperatures). Temperature also falls with ascent, at a relatively constant rate, depending again on prevailing conditions. These properties of the atmosphere dictate physiologic limits with regard to respiration and pressure tolerance. The limit for altitude adaptation without supplemental oxygen is about 5,000–5,500 meters. At these altitudes, the risk of "mountain sickness," including high-altitude pulmonary edema (HAPE) and high-altitude cerebral edema (HACE) are realized. Supplemental oxygen can increase altitude tolerance, but eventually altitudes are reached where gas exchange in the alveoli becomes physically impossible (about 15 km), and oxygen must be supplied under pressure. At a barometric pressure of about 47 mm Hg (about 20,000 m), body fluid water vapor pressure and barometric pressure become equal, and gases evolve spontaneously in tissues. This condition is known as ebullism, and its presence denotes decompression at very high altitudes. The point in the atmosphere at which ebullism occurs has been termed the Armstrong Line. Cabin pressurization or pressure suits are mandatory at altitudes at and above this level. As altitude increases, available oxygen decreases.

Functionally, and from a physiological perspective, one has entered space at the Armstrong Line. Above this, the hazards usually associated with space begin to manifest. Radiation, in the form of cosmic radiation and solar particle radiation, becomes more of a risk as atmospheric shielding attenuates. As the atmosphere becomes less dense, aerodynamic surfaces become less effective, and aircraft control is compromised. By 200 km, one has entered the blackness of space. Ballistic flights to this altitude are characterized by a short period of microgravity, pending atmospheric reentry and descent. Cabin pressurization and integrity must be assured against hard vacuum. With continued expenditure of sufficient energy, orbit can be attained, and prolonged microgravity is experienced. Temperature extremes are great, and hazards from collisions with space debris and micrometeoroid damage are present. Staged flights beyond low earth orbit ensure entry into the most hazardous environment of all, with loss of particulate radiation trapping and attenuation by earth's magnetic fields, and loss of ability for expeditious return in case of untoward events.

AEROSPACE MEDICINE PRACTICE IN THE UNITED STATES

Aerospace medicine is practiced across several broad venues, in the civilian world and in government service. Military aerospace medicine is highly operational, focused on military mission success. In the military model, flight surgeons function both in the preventive and occupational roles and as the primary caregiver for their constituent populations, which include dependents of aircrew, air traffic controllers, and in some cases aircraft maintenance personnel. Military flight surgeons are, for the most part, assigned to military flying organizations and their professional lives are integrated into the operations of those organizations. In the process of integration, flight surgeons have the opportunity not only to work and fly with their aircrews, but to spend time with them in social settings. This, ideally, gives abundant opportunity for the development of mutual trust and respect, facilitating the willingness of aircrew to approach their flight surgeons with high regard and full disclosure. The commitment of recent years among aerospace medicine practitioners to function as aircrew advocates in the aeromedical certification process has been of great value to the flight surgeon–aircrew relationship. Aircrew selection and qualification standards are applied in the military setting. Aircrew who do not meet standards are carefully considered for waiver. The military waiver experience is extensive, and waivers are granted for continuing aeronautical duties if sound supporting aeromedical rationale exists.

Aerospace medicine practice in the civilian sector is markedly different in that Federal Aviation Administration (FAA) Aviation Medical Examiners (AMEs) do not, as a rule, function as caregivers for their aircrew populations. AMEs are responsible for applying the FAA aeromedical standards in their examinations of applicants for FAA medical certification. If no disqualifying conditions are identified by history or on examination, AMEs are authorized to issue medical certification. If disqualifying conditions are identified, medical certification decisions are deferred to FAA medical authorities. AMEs are encouraged to help applicants for medical certification obtain the required documentation to support consideration for special issuance, the FAA version of waiver. Like the military, the FAA special issuance experience is broad, and special issuances are readily granted in the face of sound aeromedical rationale and adequate workup. However, the primary duty of the FAA, and thus of the AME, is to protect the public health and safety. For this reason, aviation advocacy groups strongly recommend that aircrew not use AMEs for their primary caregivers. This arrangement is probably better for both aircrew and AMEs, to avoid potential conflicts of interest.

Aerospace and space medicine practice in NASA involves care of the astronauts, which is comprehensive and similar in principle to military practice. NASA also provides FAA AME services to NASA and some contractor aircrew. NASA aerospace medicine practice thus has features of both aeromedical certification systems. NASA flight surgeons are also strongly motivated as crew advocates, and the evidence base supporting the NASA waiver system with regard to human space flight is growing rapidly.

RISK AND PREVENTION

Aerospace medicine is an amalgam of preventive and occupational medicine practice, with the occasional need to treat illness and injury. The following sections will illustrate some of the most common areas of risk and health liability attending exploration of and operations in the aerospace environment. Most of these major risk areas have been associated with many fatalities through the years, and most still claim lives on occasion. Included are sections with broad discussions of health-related risk mitigation efforts currently employed in space, and discussions of the treatment capabilities for illness and injury in space. Experiential vignettes typical of some mishaps and "close calls" in the aerospace environment are used in some of these sections to illustrate risks from the aircrew perspective. These vignettes are representative of aerospace medical risks, but none of them are intended to be accurate renditions of specific, actual events.

Hypoxia

The crew of a four-engine Lockheed C-130 was conducting a night mission over the deserts of the southwest United States. Terrain elevation in the area of operations was about 5,000 ft, with mountains to 13,000 ft. The aircraft was operating at an altitude in excess of 30,000 ft. Pitch control was lost on one of the propellers, causing that engine to overspeed. The engine was shut down. Subsequently, a second engine developed mechanical problems and was shut down as well – a very unusual occurrence in a modern turboprop aircraft. The crew concentrated on maintaining altitude to ensure terrain clearance, and forgot that cabin pressurization in that model of C-130 was maintained by bleed air from the second engine that was shut down. Cabin pressure began to drop, and the cabin environment became hypoxic as well as hypobaric. Loss of cabin pressurization indication in that particular aircraft was a relatively small warning light on the instrument panel, which was not appreciated by the busy flight crew. The hypoxic cabin environment was eventually detected by the flight engineer, who recognized his own hypoxic symptoms, with which he was familiar from altitude chamber training. The crew donned oxygen masks and continued the flight to a successful precautionary landing.

This episode demonstrates several principles attending high-performance aircraft design and operation, and physiologic training for aircrew. Intimate knowledge of critical systems is essential to fully understand the implications of failures, especially in series. Cockpit displays, particularly caution and warning displays, should be sufficiently obvious to command attention – this is a discipline of cockpit ergonomics and human factors engineering. Finally, the utility of altitude chamber training, meant to familiarize aircrew with their personal symptoms of hypoxia, was clearly shown.

Hypoxia was one of the earliest risks described with exposure to high altitude. The Jesuit priest, Father Jose de Acosta, described acute altitude sickness and hypoxia during travels in the Andes in the sixteenth century. In mountain climbing, adaptation to relatively hypoxic environments is desirable. In aviation, we strive to normalize oxygen availability in the cockpit and do so through the administration of supplemental oxygen, under pressure if necessary, and through cabin pressurization or pressure suits. Hypoxia at the tissue level can be due to several causes, but in the aerospace environment it is generally due to reduced partial pressure of oxygen combined with reduced ambient pressure at the alveoli. Hypoxia is insidious in onset and can be difficult to appreciate. The first symptoms, with onset at altitudes at and below 3,000 meters, include drowsiness and impairment of color vision and visual acuity. Impaired thinking and intellectual abilities are constant features of hypoxia with ascent and worsen with altitude. Eventually, profound hypoxia is incapacitating and will lead to death if not corrected with supplemental oxygen. In the case of cabin decompression at altitudes above 14,000 meters, the time of useful consciousness becomes foreshortened, and incapacitation can be swift. The hazards posed by hypoxia require vigilance, and hypoxia will always remain a constant risk in the aerospace environment.

Spatial Disorientation

A relatively recently trained private pilot with limited flying experience, non-instrument-rated, planned a flight over 30 nautical miles of open water to an island destination at dusk. Visual meteorologic conditions prevailed at the time of the flight, but visibility was less than 5 miles in haze. At takeoff, the horizon was obvious and additional visual cues for orientation were provided by lights on the ground. The aircraft climbed to an altitude of 5,000 ft, and over water the horizon became obscured in haze. Sky blended with water from a visual perspective, and the flight essentially entered instrument meteorologic conditions. The pilot noticed he was tending to lose altitude, and attempted to pull up to climb. With this maneuver, he noticed that airspeed increased and the rate of altitude loss increased. The pilot then noticed his

artificial horizon indicated a turn to the right, and he attempted to level the wings. However, with this maneuver he strongly sensed he was in a left turn, and quickly returned the aircraft to his perception of wings level. The rate of altitude loss increased, and airspeed continued to increase. Thoroughly confused, he continued to aggressively pull up in an attempt to climb, but the rate of descent continued to increase, airspeed exceeded the structural limits of the aircraft and the rate of altitude loss exceeded 4,000 ft/min. Ambient noise from the high airspeed added to the confusion of the pilot, as well as centrifugal forces pushing him down into his seat. The pilot by this time could only continue his desperate attempt at pull out of what he perceived to be a steep dive. Tragically, the flight ended with impact in the water at well above 200 mph, in a steep right bank with total destruction of the aircraft and loss of all aboard. This episode represents one of the most common and deadly vestibular illusions, the graveyard spiral (Figure 15.2).

Orientation in flight is predominantly visual, but the vestibular system, auditory cues, and proprioception are also important contributors. In the absence of external visual cues in flight, the vestibular system gives the most powerful sensory input. The vestibular system consists of the otolith organs, which sense linear acceleration, and the semicircular canals, which sense angular motion. Vestibular sensation of angular motion depends on movement of fluid in the semicircular canals deflecting the hair cells of the cupola, which signals a turn to the central nervous system. If the angular motion persists, the fluid in the semicircular canals stabilizes, and hair cells of the cupola are no longer deflected. In fact, with cessation of the turn, a deflection of the hair cells in the opposite direction occurs, and a turn in the opposite direction is perceived. This explains the graveyard spiral phenomenon, properly known as the vestibulo-gyral illusion, which is an extraordinarily powerful vestibular illusion. There are several other vestibular and visual illusions possible in flight, some of which can be associated with total incapacitation of the pilot. All these illusions are dangerous, and all have caused fatal accidents.

Spatial disorientation remains a leading cause of aircraft accidents. In military aviation, more than 15% of accidents involve spatial disorientation, often with experienced pilots. The risk of spatial disorientation is reduced by increased proficiency in instrument flying and trust in the reliability of flight instruments in conditions of reduced visibility and loss of external visual cues.

Acceleration

An experienced general aviation aerobatic flight instructor was requested to provide instruction in basic aerobatics and upset recovery techniques to a private pilot. The first aerobatic introductory lesson was conducted in

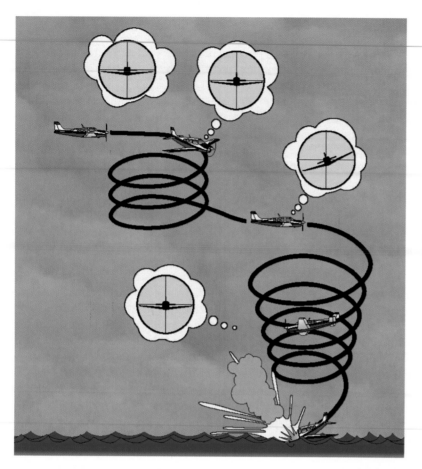

Figure 15.2. The graveyard spiral, one of the most dangerous vestibular illusions. Reference: original NASA artwork.

a Decathlon aircraft, in excellent visual meteorological conditions. The instructor demonstrated several aerobatic maneuvers, including a loop (an aerobatic maneuver in which the aircraft flies a vertical circle initiating from straight and level upright flight). The instructor handed control of the aircraft over to the student, who dove the aircraft to attain entry airspeed for a loop. The student pulled back vigorously on the stick, initiating the first half of the loop. On the back side, the student pulled back on the stick more aggressively and abruptly to come out of the loop, and the aircraft experienced over 5 G. The instructor became dimly aware of his name being called by the student, and gradually recognized that the aircraft was again in level flight. Although he had no memory of the event, the student informed him that he had lost consciousness and had been unconscious for the last 30 seconds. In addition, he had not responded to intercom calls for an additional 30 seconds. The flight was terminated and concluded with a successful landing.

This is a classic example of G-induced loss of consciousness. Although most episodes of G-LOC occur in high-performance military fighter aircraft, any aircraft that can sustain about 5 G for several seconds can produce conditions favorable for this phenomenon. Aerobatic instructors can be particularly at risk for this phenomenon if their students are unexpectedly aggressive in positive G maneuvers without warning. There have been many instances of G-LOC in military fighter and high-performance training aircraft, with loss of aircraft and fatality of crew. Episodes of G-LOC typically are associated with 20–30 seconds of unconsciousness, followed by another 20–40 seconds of relative incapacitation. Memory loss concerning the event is common, and pilots usually are unaware they have suffered an episode of G-LOC.

Sustained acceleration environments impose centrifugal forces on vehicles and their occupants. The vector of the forces determines the physiological effect. By convention, these vectors are named in accord with the three axes of physical space – x, y, and z – and quantitated in multiples of the force of gravity, G. Gx forces are exerted through the anterior-posterior plane of the human body. Gy forces are exerted laterally, and Gz forces are exerted in the vertical axis. *Positive Gz* forces are experienced head-to-foot, and negative Gz forces are experienced foot-to-head, in the reverse order. Gz forces are the most physiologically significant in the aerospace environment, with significant effects possible in both directions. Positive Gz forces are traditionally the most problematic, and have accounted for physiological incidents and fatal accidents in aviation. Positive Gz forces oppose cardiac output in perfusing the brain.

The central retinal artery is an exquisite indicator for cerebral perfusion pressure, as it ramifies on the retina at the same physical distance from the heart as do the vessels providing cerebral blood flow. In a positive Gz acceleration environment, retinal perfusion pressure, hence cerebral perfusion pressure, will be overcome in most individuals at about 5 positive Gz, resulting in a distinct symptom complex. Visual symptoms include loss of peripheral vision, followed by loss of vision entirely. Loss of consciousness follows shortly thereafter. Positive Gz tolerance varies between individuals, with shorter, more muscular individuals having greater resting Gz tolerance. Positive Gz tolerance can be improved by tensing peripheral musculature, straining against a partially closed glottis, changing the G force vector (semireclining seats), and wearing anti-G garments, which apply pressure against lower extremities, abdomen, and chest, with positive airway pressure, depending on design and complexity. All these measures increase G tolerance by increasing venous return to the heart and/or augmenting cardiac output to preserve cranial blood flow.

Military air combat tactics include 0 G maneuvers, employed to transiently increase airspeed, but usually negative Gz maneuvers are avoided. Negative Gz forces are generally encountered in advanced civilian aerobatics, where very short duration exposures can exceed 9 negative Gz. Negative Gz maneuvers are associated with physiological effects as well, the most significant of which involves sudden onset of a vertiginous disorder symptomatically very similar to benign paroxysmal positional vertigo (BPPV). This disorder, known among civilian aerobatic pilots as the "wobblies," is reported to be nearly incapacitating in its most severe expression. The etiology is unknown, but it is thought likely to be due to otoconia floating free in the otolith organs and migrating to the semicircular canals, where they can produce the false sensation of motion and resultant vertigo.

G forces pose a threat not only in atmospheric flight but in space flight as well. G tolerance is markedly reduced in returning space crews following adaptation to microgravity. By design, the primary G forces encountered in atmospheric reentry are in the x-axis, and efforts are made to keep the z-axis component at a minimum.

Decampression Sickness

A U-2 high-altitude reconnaissance aircraft departed from its base in northern California on a mission to overfly hostile areas for a reconnaissance mission. The aircraft was operating at about 70,000 ft, and its pilot was wearing a pressure suit with supplemental oxygen to maintain a relative cabin altitude of about 20,000 ft. While over the area of operations, the pilot became increasingly confused. He remained in radio contact with his base of operations, but his transmissions were characterized as almost childlike in nature. The pilot could not interpret his instruments, and only continued flying the aircraft by virtue of residual skill and experience. The diagnosis of central nervous system decompression sickness was strongly suspected. The pilot was "talked" through a diversion to the airspace of an allied county, where he was intercepted by allied fighter aircraft and led, with great difficulty, to a successful landing. Symptoms of profound confusion persisted after landing, and multiple recompressions were undertaken in a locally available hyperbaric chamber. The diagnosis of neurologic decompression sickness was confirmed by central nervous system imaging. Eventually, the pilot made a recovery, with return of normal thought and behavior (Figure 15.3).

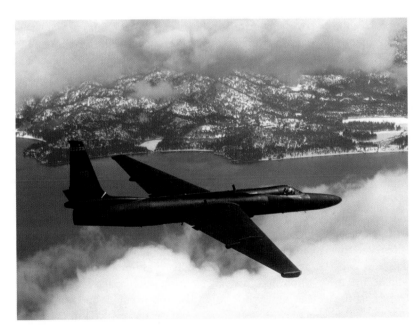

Figure 15.3. The U-2 aircraft. U-2 aircrew, despite the use of pressure suits, operate at effective cabin altitudes that place them at great risk of dysbarism.[9]

Altitude-related decompression sickness, the evolution of nitrogen bubbles in tissues, has been a risk of high-altitude operations for many years. During World War II, decompression sickness was encountered in bombing crews, who flew missions of 6–8 hours duration in unpressurized aircraft to altitude over 30,000 ft. routinely. Most of these cases were pain only, or type I decompression sickness (bends). Type II decompression sickness, either neurological or pulmonary, is more rare but immeasurably more serious in its potential for incapacitation, serious injury, or death. To protect against serious decompression sickness in aerospace environments, measures to optimize cabin altitude as much as possible are augmented by periods of prebreathing oxygen to reduce tissue nitrogen levels and decompression stress. Interestingly, and fortunately, the experience of decompression sickness in terrestrial altitude chambers and in atmospheric flight has not been reproduced in space flight extravehicular activities (EVA). EVA suit pressures range from 4.3 psi (about 24,000 ft cabin altitude) in U.S. systems, to 5.2 psi (about 18,000 ft cabin altitude) in Russian systems. Decompression sickness has not been reported during any Russian or U.S. EVA, probably due to a combination of effective pre-breathe protocols and the difficulty of separating bends pain from pain caused by the EVA suits themselves. However, the possibility that somehow the EVA environment affords some protection against decompression sickness cannot be entirely discounted.

Other, less life-threatening but still potentially serious examples of dysbarism are relatively common in atmospheric flight. Ear blocks, sinus blocks, and expansion of trapped gas under tooth fillings and in intestinal loops are examples of such episodes.

Human Factors

A commuter airliner was performing an approach to the New Haven, Connecticut, airport. Instrument meteorologic conditions prevailed at the time of the approach, with heavy fog. The aircraft was a Convair 340/440 commuter airliner, with twin turboprop engines. Minimum Descent Altitude (MDA), the altitude below which safe descent is not possible, was 380 ft. The captain intentionally descended below the MDA, and the aircraft crashed into three beach cottages about 29 ft above sea level on final approach. In the process, the captain disregarded the advice of the first officer that the MDA had been reached and descent was continuing.

This accident might have been avoided had there been better communication between the first officer and the captain, aided by a culture that encouraged the consideration of the opinions of junior officers by captains in aircraft operations. When this accident occurred, culture and company rules favored deference to the experience and authority of captains without question.

In intervening years, the value of coordinated crew input and management of the aircraft has resulted in specific training known as Cockpit Resource Management (CRM), later known as Crew Resource Management. Consideration of the opinions of all cockpit crew is considered a key feature of modern CRM training.

This example is illustrative of human habits, behaviors, limitations, strengths, and customs that constitute the broad range of human factors in the aerospace environment. The field of human factors is a discipline that actually represents a continuum. At one end of the continuum is human factors engineering, which deals with cockpit displays and their interpretation, cockpit ergonomics, and other considerations that may be addressed through engineering. At the other end of the continuum are considerations of human behavior and the consequences thereof. The field of human factors in the aerospace environment is incredibly complex and embraces such diverse professional disciplines as engineering and psychology. Consideration of human factors, and its constituent disciplines, has always been critical in the design and operation of manned air and space vehicles. In this age of advancing information technology and increasing dependence on automation, consideration of human factors and accommodating human operation and decision making in aircraft and spacecraft might be in jeopardy of losing emphasis in system design. It is hoped that the flexibility and adaptability of humans, demonstrated so often through the decades of atmospheric and space flight, will continue to be leveraged to advantage through active participation of the human factors disciplines in the design, engineering, and operations of air and space systems of the future.

Transportation of Ill and Injured Patients

Air transport of ill and injured patients has its roots, as do many medical advances, in the techniques of war. Helicopters were first used to transport injured combatants from the battlefield aid stations to field hospital facilities during the Korean War, with associated improvement in survival of battle injuries. The routine and aggressive use of more capable aircraft during the Vietnam War refined battlefield transport of wounded even further. The venerable UH-1 helicopter, and the crews that operated them, served with great and historic distinction in the extremely dangerous "dust off" medical evacuation mission of that conflict. Survival rates continued to improve. Theater medical evacuation using larger aircraft, such as the C-130 Hercules and the C-141 Starlifter, was also developed during this period. These aircraft, and subsequent military transport aircraft, were designed to accommodate medical evacuation systems. Air evacuation became a discipline of aerospace medicine and has undergone continual improvement and refinement since. Military air evacuation has evolved to the point where critical care can be delivered in flight, almost to fixed-base standards.

Civilian air transport of ill and injured patients has evolved as well, based on the techniques developed by the military. Civilian air ambulance services, using a variety of aircraft, operate worldwide, providing international air evacuation services. These aircraft are generally much less capable than military systems, but they still fill an important niche. Civilian helicopter air transport services are nearly ubiquitous in the United States. These systems emulate the military experience of providing air medical transport services initiating at the point of injury. Rapidity of transportation, coupled with emergency medical system services employed on civilian medical helicopters, continues to improve trauma survival rates nationwide.

Treatment of ill and injured patients on aircraft has always been difficult. Cramped spaces, noise, vibration, limitation of available electrical power, and poor lighting are a few of the challenges facing medical care in the aerospace environment. Technological advances in such areas as physiological monitoring, miniaturization, airway management, ventilatory support, drug delivery, and communications have facilitated and improved the quality of patient care during air transport.

Preventive Space Medicine

The extreme environment of space poses risks that cannot, at present, be completely mitigated. These risks can be grouped according to the agents of exposure: radiation, microgravity, and isolation and confinement.

Space radiation, for the most part, consists of solar particle radiation and galactic cosmic radiation (GCR). The constituents of solar particle radiation are mainly protons. Earth's magnetic field, the Van Allen belt, traps a great deal of solar particle radiation. Orbits that venture into the Van Allen belt expose crews to increased doses of radiation from trapped solar particles. GCR is composed of atomic nuclei, many of them heavy metal nuclei, traveling just below the speed of light. These heavy atomic nuclei act as atomic projectiles, disrupting chromosomal patterns in the tissues they traverse. The biological effects of space radiation are poorly understood, and predictions of radiation effect are almost exclusively based on data from gamma radiation exposures due to atomic bomb explosions during World War II. As a result, uncertainty factors are great. NASA-established space radiation dosage limitations are based on recommendations from the National Council on Radiation Protection and Measurements and currently restrict career exposure to the amount that will result in a 3% excess risk of fatal cancer development over a lifetime, with 95% confidence interval.

Aluminum spacecraft provide little protection against space radiation. In fact, GCR produces neutrons when interacting with aluminum, posing yet another radiation threat. More effective shielding materials, at present, are polyethylene foam and water. Sleep stations on the ISS shielded with polyethylene foam have reduced mission radiation doses significantly. Future spacecraft design, especially for those vehicles that venture beyond low earth orbit for long duration missions, should exploit the shielding properties of these and other materials to provide better protection for crew and equipment.

Exposure to microgravity results in a space adaptation syndrome that has been well recognized and described. One of the first effects is a particular form of space motion sickness with about a 70% attack rate. This can be incapacitating, but it can be successfully treated in most cases with parenteral promethazine.

Fluid shifts begin early on with exposure to microgravity, resulting in uniform distribution, which produces the "puffy" facial features associated with space flight. Intravascular volume decreases, and the cardiovascular and neurological systems adapt to the lack of gravity. Baroreceptors adapt to microgravity, and a decrease in cardiovascular conditioning occurs. Sensory and motor adaptation occurs, facilitating movement about the spacecraft environment in microgravity. There is loss of bone mineral density, especially in weight-bearing areas, and skeletal muscle mass and strength are gradually compromised. There is immune compromise manifested by virus shedding, but the clinical significance of this is at present unknown. There have been some isolated problems maintaining nutritional status, probably related to available food choices, but the potential for abnormalities of gastrointestinal absorption may also exist.

During the mission, these changes are adaptive. However, on return to earth, many of the changes become pathologic. Orthostatic hypotension (due to decreased circulating volume, cardiovascular deconditioning, and baroreceptor adaptation) and alterations in sensory and motor functions constitute the immediate untoward effects on return from space. These functions normalize over several days to weeks, depending on mission duration. Research has shown that resistive exercise during flight helps mitigate the risks of bone loss and muscle mass and strength compromise. For the most part, bone mineral density and muscle changes return to preflight levels over time, depending again on length of mission. Nutritional status and immune function compromise have also thus far proven transient.

Behavioral health liabilities in the isolated and confined environment of spacecraft have thus far not caused untoward mission impact, at least in the U.S. program. Behavioral health liabilities and risks may be expected to increase, however, with increasing mission duration and distance from earth. Behavioral health challenges consistent with those experienced in analogue expeditionary populations, especially in Antarctica, may arise in the setting of long duration exploration class missions beyond low earth orbit. Research regarding behavioral issues attending exploration class missions is being actively pursued by NASA in support of the United States' Vision for Space Exploration, which declares the intent of the United States to return to the moon and send human missions to Mars in the coming decades.

There have been ongoing concerns in the ISS program relative to overworking crews (during all mission phases) and stress induced by circadian shifting, mainly to accommodate the operations of arriving spacecraft. Crew fatigue was implicated in at least one accident during the MiR program, when an arriving automated supply vehicle collided with the station during manual docking procedures, causing partial spacecraft depressurization. Given the limited time available to complete all tasks aboard the spacecraft, crew fatigue will remain a concern for the foreseeable future.

NASA recently adopted a clearer occupational health approach to mitigating the health risks inherent to human space flight, in response to recommendations made by the Institute of Medicine. Fitness for duty and/ or exposure standards, based on best available scientific and clinical evidence and judgment, have been defined for the major human space flight health risk areas. These standards serve as declarations of acceptable health risk in human space flight. NASA is currently using these standards in defining biomedical research requirements as well.

Treatment of Illness and Injury in Space

Spacecraft are highly limited in space, power, and resupply capability. Space missions must be carefully planned due to the scarce resources available. Recognizing the limited ability to treat illness and injury during the course of low earth orbit missions, NASA has depended on preventive measures and strict astronaut selection and qualification medical standards to lessen the probability of illness and injury during flight. The Russian Space Program has followed much the same preventive philosophy. This tradition continues in medical management of the ISS, with recent development and adoption of international crew medical selection and qualification standards.

Based on analogue population data from polar and submarine experience and on the development of injury and illness in the active astronaut population on the ground, serious illness and injury of flight crew during a mission is expected to eventually occur over the operational lifetime of the ISS. Therefore, a limited ability to provide medical care, based on principles of telemedicine, is available on the ISS. This capability, comparable to that found in a general practice ambulatory care setting, is consistent with the NASA philosophy to stabilize and evacuate seriously ill and injured crewmembers from low earth orbit.

THE LONGITUDINAL STUDY OF ASTRONAUT HEALTH

The Longitudinal Study of Astronaut Health (LSAH) was formally established in 1992. Although much data, from as early as 1959, needed to be added retrospectively, currently the health data of over three hundred astronauts are included in this database spanning more than four decades of space missions. Information entered into the study emanates from routine medical examinations, pre- and postflight physicals, clinical events, and in-flight experimental data. In addition to the astronauts, over nine hundred Johnson Space Center employees, matched by age, sex, activity level, and body habitus with individual astronauts, are included as a control group. After retirement, former astronauts are offered a free annual physical, which is included in the database to help ascertain if there are any health differences between astronauts and the Earth bound cohort that evolve later in life.

Despite the breadth of the LSAH, there is as yet insufficient data available to fully understand the health effects of exposure to radiation, microgravity and the effects of isolation and confinement. Recently, however, analysis of data has begun to reveal scientifically quantifiable trends in the astronaut corp.

The overall fatality rate in the astronaut corps is striking, in part because of the loss of two space shuttles (*Challenger* and *Columbia*) and the *Apollo 1* fire. Serving as an astronaut is certainly one of the most dangerous occupations in modern, developed societies. The greatest health risk to the astronaut corps to date is catastrophic loss of space craft and crew.

Substantial impact on health is anticipated with exposure of crews to space radiation. In a comparison of cancer mortality rates in the astronaut population, the LSAH ground-based cohort, and the general population in the Texas gulf coast area, the astronauts had a higher age-specific risk of cancer mortality than the LSAH comparison group. This difference did not reach statistical significance. Both the astronauts and the LSAH control group participants had a lower age-specific cancer mortality risk than the general population. This may well be due to healthy worker effect, but there are as yet insufficient data to come to substantial conclusions on this subject, which bears further monitoring and evaluation.

A recently published study documents both an increased number and earlier onset of cataracts amongst astronauts who have been exposed to higher lens doses of space radiation versus those who have been exposed to lower lens doses of space radiation. Additional research in this area is anticipated, with the gathering of additional NASA data as well as data from military pilots involved in high-altitude flight.

The LSAH is one of NASA's most important data-gathering tools on the effect of space missions on human health. With limited access to space for a small cadre of individuals, the health data gathered from each member of the astronaut corps constitutes a critical evidence base for medical care, countermeasures development, preventive medicine, and engineering practices as well as a sound basis for biomedical research priorities. Expansion of the LSAH database and understanding emerging trends remains one of the highest priorities for NASA's medical infrastructure.

THE FUTURE OF AEROSPACE MEDICINE

Aerospace medicine has a definite and secure role in the support of military and NASA aerospace operations and in regulation of civilian aviation by the Federal Aviation Administration. There are areas of opportunity, however, for an expanded role for the specialty in the immediate and foreseeable future.

Recently, the FAA adopted a "sport pilot" rule, stipulating that pilots may independently fly light sport aircraft of no more than two seats, having certain configuration, weight, and performance characteristics without possessing current FAA medical certification. To operate such aircraft, pilots must not have been denied FAA medical certification, or if ever denied FAA medical certification for a disqualifying condition must have applied for and received medical certification as a special issuance. Pilots may then use their valid driver's license, issued by a U.S. jurisdiction, as evidence of medical qualification, employing the principle of medical self-certification applied by all pilots prior to every flight. As the sport pilot rule continues implementation, increasing numbers of pilots will exercise their privileges under these rules. Many of these pilots will be older individuals who have undergone special issuance in the past and do not want to continue meeting medical certification testing requirements annually in order to apply for continued FAA medical certification. There will be a role for aerospace medicine practitioners, familiar with medical qualifications necessary for safe operation of aircraft, in advising these aviators as to their personal suitability for continued aeronautical activities. This presumes most of these aviators will adhere to the principles of self medical certification and seek advice from aviation medical examiners should they have doubts about their medical status. It is hoped that these processes result in effective self-regulation by these pilots from a medical perspective.

Another opportunity for aerospace medicine practice is in the prospective "space tourism" business. Currently, a commercial enterprise has partnered with the Russian Federation in sponsoring space tourist visits to the International Space Station, launching and returning aboard *Soyuz* spacecraft. Other entrepreneurs and business leaders committed to developing commercial human space travel are in the advanced planning stages for excursions to the edge of space and for orbital operations. One of these designs is based on the successful *SpaceShipOne*

design of Burt Rutan. As space tourism develops and matures, applicants for travel will need to be medically screened for health conditions making space flight inadvisable. Companies engaging in space tourism would be well advised to engage medical consultants experienced in space medicine practice, to ensure individual clients are not subjected to inordinate medical risks and to treat health conditions that may accompany specific mission profiles.

A third area of developing aerospace medicine practice is in the translation of terrestrial medical care to space. As exploration class missions beyond low earth orbit are planned, the medical care systems for these missions must be more capable than those employed in low earth orbit. Such medical care systems will need to be essentially autonomous, with minimal store-and-forward type telemedicine consultation and support. The ethical considerations and methodologies for determining levels of care to offer in such exploration class missions are a source of interest for NASA at present. A synergy of advanced technologies such as artificial intelligence, nanotechnology, and biologically inspired technology will be employed to make space medical care systems lighter, smaller, and more efficient, with less power requirements. Technology, however, cannot as yet replace the human touch of a compassionate and capable physician. As such, an appropriately trained space medicine physician should accompany exploration class missions beyond low earth orbit, especially on Mars missions. The most suitable model for such a space medicine physician probably conforms to an earlier physician model that can be considered a "super generalist." Such a physician will be skilled in diagnosis and treatment of a wide spectrum of adult illnesses and will also have additional training in surgery and possess basic surgery skills, not unlike generalist physicians of decades ago practicing in rural environments. Physicians conforming to this model are currently employed with success in terrestrial extreme environments, such as Antarctic stations during winter-over expeditions. Thus, somewhat paradoxically, the future of aerospace medicine may well be found in traditions and practices of the past, combined with advanced technologies to produce effective diagnostic and treatment capability in the most highly resource constrained and extreme environment humans will ever explore.

REFERENCES

[1] American Board of Preventive Medicine. Available at: *http://www.abprevmed.org/aboutus.cfm.*

[2] DeHart RL, Davis JD, eds. *Fundamentals of Aerospace Medicine.* 3rd ed. Philadelphia: Lippincott Williams and Wilkins; 2002.

[3] Nicogossian AE, Huntoon CL, Pool SL, eds. *Space Physiology and Medicine.* 3rd ed. Philadelphia: Lea and Febiger; 1994.

4 Bendrick GA, et al. Prevalence of decompression sickness among U-2 pilots. *Aviat Space Environ Med.* 1996;67(3): 199–206.

5 Hamm PB, et al. Risk of cancer mortality among the longitudinal study of astronaut health (LSAH) participants. *Aviat Space Environ Med.* 1998;69(2):142–4.

6 Cucinotta FA, et al. Space radiation and cataracts in astronauts. *Radiation Res.* 2001;156(5 Pt 1):460–6.

7 Jennings RT, et al. Medical qualification of a commercial spaceflight participant: not your average astronaut. *Aviat Space Environ Med.* 2006;77(5):475–4.

8 Rayman, RB, et al. eds. *Clinical Aerospace Medicine*, 4th ed. New York: Professional Publishing Group, Ltd; 2006.

9 *http://www.af.mil/factsheets/factsheet_media.asp?fs ID=129.*

16 | Polar Medicine

Desmond Lugg, AM, MD, FACOM, FAFOEM, FACRRM, Dip. Polar. St., and
Jeff Ayton, MBBS, MPHTM, FRACGP, FACRRM, FACTM, AFFTM

The polar environment is hostile, dangerous and unfamiliar; cold, isolation, photoperiodicity, katabatic winds, and whiteout combine with the polar ice caps, crevassed glaciers, and ever-changing sea ice. Expedition medical practice in such regions is extreme, as all groups have had to travel great distances, are self-sustaining in that all medical supplies, equipment, and expertise must be available on the expedition, and complex logistics are required. Evacuation, if possible, is expensive, requires great effort, and can be dangerous.

Although Iceland and Greenland were discovered centuries before, it was not until the late 1500s that Davis, Frobisher, and Barents led expeditions to the Canadian Arctic, Greenland, and Spitsbergen. These were the stimuli for the many expeditions that followed. Magellan's discovery in 1520 of the straits that now bear his name and Cook's crossing of the Antarctic Circle in 1773 had a similar effect on the Antarctic. Initially, the motivation was exploration and discovery, but with time this changed to exploitation and science. The advent of commercial tourism and adventure travel over the past 50 years has seen a plethora of expeditions in the polar regions, bringing many more people of all ages and physical status. Such expeditions have been a catalyst for dramatic changes to medical support. Polar regions technology has made improvements in clothing, equipment, food, and shelter, but the environment is no less challenging than it was to the early explorers.

What are the polar regions? There are a number of definitions. These range from the high latitudes surrounding the North and South Poles, to the areas above the Arctic and Antarctic Circles (latitudes 66°33′N and S); the limit of the polar night and midnight sun. The most useful definition of the Arctic is the 10°C July isotherm that is based on climate and ecology and is essentially the tree line. Similarly, Antarctica is the lands and ice sheets below the Antarctic Convergence (Antarctic Polar Front), where the cold waters from the Antarctic region meet and sink beneath the warm waters from the middle latitudes.

CONTRASTS BETWEEN THE ARCTIC AND ANTARCTICA

The Arctic is a vast frozen sea, surrounded by frozen land on which no trees grow. In contrast, Antarctica is the coldest, highest, driest, windiest, and most isolated continent. The Antarctic continent is comprised of 98% continental ice sheet and 2% exposed, barren rock, surrounded by the Southern Ocean. This ocean freezes around the Antarctic continent and the resultant sea ice varies between 4 million square kilometers in austral summer to 20 million square kilometers in winter.

Although Antarctica is an icy continent, it has no land animals. The surrounding seas are populated by vast numbers of whales, seals, penguins, and seabirds; the seals haul out onto ice shelves and beach areas while the penguins and other birds nest on rock areas and ice shelves. The Arctic has no penguins, but it does have prolific bird life; sea mammals such as Beluga whales, Orca, polar bear, sea otter, seal and walrus; and land mammals including fox, caribou, reindeer, lemming, and musk ox. Dog teams are still present in the Arctic, but the last of the husky populations in Antarctica were removed in the early 1990s.

POPULATIONS

In addition to geographical and physical differences, the Arctic and Antarctic populations differ. The Arctic has had an indigenous population for millennia; today this group is estimated to have swelled to over four million with people who have migrated there and the itinerant population. The Antarctic has no indigenous population but for just over 100 years transient visitors have spent from days to several years at a time on the Antarctic continent. In 2006, 20 nations, all signatories to the Antarctic Treaty, operated 37 year-round scientific stations and 15 seasonal bases and traverses in support of scientific research. Around 1,000 scientists and support personnel spend the austral winter there; the number increases three- to fourfold in summer. Most of these are regarded as expeditions. During the same period in 2004–5, 28,000 tourists and adventure seekers visited Antarctica; many of these were on expeditions. They travel by ship, aircraft, and yachts to photograph and observe Antarctic landscapes, historical sites, and wildlife. In addition, they camp, climb mountains, ski, dive, skydive, parasail, kayak, and run marathons.

HISTORY OF POLAR EXPEDITION MEDICINE

The history of medicine in both polar regions is a most interesting one. A 200-year review was made of Antarctic medical practice (Lugg 1975a, 1975b). It begins with the primitive shipboard practice on Cook's ships and concludes with the modern era of permanent stations. Fortuine (1988, 1989) has written a series of reports of medical aspects of Arctic exploration. Fodstad et al. (1999) examined the roles of physicians and natural scientists in both the Arctic and Antarctica and reported that no significant Arctic voyage, particularly in the last 300 years, was made without a member of the group trained in the medical management of emergencies. Feeney (1997) has reviewed the role of food and nutrition in early polar exploration and highlights the fact that the success of expeditions depended on the quantity of their food and the quality of their nutrition. Nutritional disorders included scurvy and hypervitaminosis A. Advances in food preservation improved human survival. Although expeditions today rarely need to depend on wildlife as a food source, many of the lessons learned have application for present-day expeditioners.

EPIDEMIOLOGY

Table 16.1 lists the most common categories of illness and injury and visits to the doctors in the Australian National Antarctic Research Expeditions (ANARE) (now known as Australia's Antarctic Program (AAp) conducted by the Australian Antarctic Division) for the period 1989–2005. Annual summer and winter expeditions of personnel from the temperate and tropical regions have taken place since the late 1940s. This study using a computerized health register, records data on all health events requiring medical consultation at Australian Antarctic stations and field camps and on expedition ships (King, 1987; Sullivan & Gormly, 1999).

Table 16.2 lists the ten most common subcategories (ICD-9) of health events in the field setting for the period 1989–2005. Table 16.3 lists the most common medical procedures performed at all locations in the period 1989–2005. All stations have full sterile operating facilities maintained by one medical practitioner who is trained to perform emergency surgery (Lugg, 1993).

The epidemiology of polar expeditions will not discuss Arctic expeditions due to the presence of indigenous

Table 16.1. Most common categories of illness and injury on ANARE/AAp 1989–2005

World health organisation international classification of diseases (ICD-9-1975 revision) injury or illness categories	%
Injury and poisoning (800–999)	37.55
Supplementary contact with health services (V codes)	12.04
Diseases of the skin and subcutaneous tissue (680–709)	7.98
Diseases of the respiratory system (460–519)	7.11
Diseases of the nervous system and sense organs (320–389)	6.32
Infectious and parasitic disease (005–139)	6.09
Diseases of the musculoskeletal system and connective tissue (710–739)	5.98
Diseases of the digestive system (520–579)	5.89
Symptoms, signs and ill-defined conditions (780–799)	3.04
Mental disorders (290–319)	2.19
Other ICD-9 categories	5.81

Note: These health events occurring over a 17-year period were recorded by medical practitioners at all locations including ships, stations, and field.

Of note, supplementary V codes include routine midwinter and occupational health medical examinations. Interestingly, 40% of Health Events Classified as Mental Disorders ICD codes 290–319 were classified as disorders of sleep, commonly due to the prolonged austral summer daylight and the polar environment.

From Watzl R, Gormly P, Ayton J. ANARE Health Register. Australian Antarctic Division.

populations. However, it should be noted that an Arctic expedition's medical personnel may be called on to treat the local population in an emergency. Medical personnel on Antarctic expedition vessels and stations have been called upon to treat fishermen in emergencies (Ayton, 2005), but such occurrences are not included in the data presented here.

Reviewing all the Antarctic medical literature for the last 100 years reveals that trauma and accidents are the most common conditions (Lloyd, 1973; Lugg, 1973; Cattermole, 2001), although most are minor. Injuries can range from lacerations, abrasions, sprains and other musculoskeletal injuries to fractures, burns, and multiple injuries. Emergencies have included a ruptured intracranial aneurysm (Pardoe, 1965), breast cancer (Nielsen & Vollers, 2001), chest injuries, myocardial infarction (Taylor & Gormly, 1997; Ogle and Dunckel, 2002), acute abdomen (Podkolinski & Semmens, 1979; Priddy, 1985), a fractured cervical vertebrae, cold injuries (Sullivan, 1987; Taylor & Gormly, 1997), and a polio-like illness (Budd, 1962). After trauma, symptoms and ill-defined disease, such as insomnia (regarded as endemic in the 24-hour sunlight of summer), dyspepsia, and headaches rate high along with skin diseases and dental problems.

Table 16.2. The ten most common ICD-9 subcategories of health events occurring in the field on ANARE/AAp 1989–2005

ICD 9 code	Description of ICD-9 subcategory	Percentage
840–848	Sprains and strains of joints and adjacent muscles	29.5
920–924	Contusion with intact skin surface	9.3
991–995	Other and unspecified effects of external causes	7.1
726–729	Rheumatism, excluding the back	6.1
910–919	Superficial injury	5.9
880–887	Open wound of upper limb	4.1
873–879	Open wound of head, neck, and trunk	3.1
715–719	Arthropathies and related disorders	2.4
700–709	Other diseases of skin and subcutaneous tissue	2.1
958–959	Certain traumatic complications and unspecified injuries	1.8

Note: These comprise more than 70% of field health events recorded during the 17-year period. Of interest ICD 9 codes 991–995 include cold injuries mostly of trivial nature.
From Watzl R, Gormly P, Ayton J. *ANARE Health Register.* Australian Antarctic Division.

Table 16.3. Most common medical procedures performed on the ANARE/AAp 1989–2005 at all locations

Rank	Procedures: International classification of procedures in medicine (WHO 1978)	Percentage
1	8–19 Wound cleaning and dressing	10.8
2	3–94 Ultrasound therapy	7.5
3	8–30 Bandaging and sling support	5.1
4	9–30 Dental aid	4.9
5	4–35 Immunization against other viral and unspecified disease	4.6
6	4–12 Health examination related to employment	4.4
7	5–88 Incision and excision of skin and subcutaneous tissues	3.8
8	9–46 Passive exercise	3.7
9	9–45 Physical exercise	3.2
10	8–89 Pre- and postoperative procedures	3.1
11	2–25 Other physicochemical tests of urine	2.7
12	1–91 Collection of parasite or microorganism for diagnosis	2.6
13	5–89 Repair and reconstruction of skin and subcutaneous tissue	2.4
14	3–17 Radiography of upper limb	2.4
15	3–18 Radiography of lower limb	2.1
16	8–10 Removal of object	1.8
17	9–74 Counselling	1.6
18	8–11 Other removal of object	1.5
19	8–17 Evacuation by syringing or irrigation, insufflation	1.5
20	8–53 Other external manipulation or compression	1.2

This listing includes more than 70% of all procedures coded during the 17-year period.
From Watzl R, Gormly P, Ayton J. *ANARE Health Register.* Australian Antarctic Division.

Conditions related to the environment are of low incidence. Cold injury is uncommon, with most being recreational such as snowmobiling and skiing (Cattermole, 1999). Snow blindness and sunburn occur infrequently (Lugg, 1993). With changed attitudes to exposing skin to sunlight, the use of sunscreen, goggles protecting the eyes, and the presence of polar clothing covering most of the body, ozone depletion or the annual "ozone hole" is not thought to be a problem (Lugg & Roy, 1999). However with the long hours of polar sunlight, increased reflectivity from snow and water during austral and boreal summers, expeditioners should take measures to limit excessive UV exposures, which can potentially increase risk of skin cancers and eye damage.

In contrast, the polar winter environment has the potential for adverse effects relating to prolonged absence of sunlight and ultraviolet radiation exposures including vitamin D deficiency and chronobiology effects.

Diagnoses in Antarctica have included hepatitis, malaria, amoebic dysentery, pneumonia, anorexia nervosa, appendicitis, peptic ulcer, myocardial infarction, acute terminal ileitis, pyrexia of unknown origin, gout, and renal stones. Behavioral health disorders have low rates of occurrence in documented studies (Lugg, 1973; Palinkas et al., 2004; Lugg, 2005). It has been suggested that behavioral problems are underreported (Carlisle &

Shen, 2001), but many consider that much of this behavioral category are nonpathologic, adaptive mechanisms to the isolation and confinement. The role of alcohol in Antarctica reveals both positive and negative aspects (Carlisle & Shen, 2001). Alcohol abuse does occur, and alcohol has been implicated in accidents (Lugg, Gormly & King, 1978; Cattermole, 1997).

A review of women's health in Antarctica (Ayton, 2006) has shown there are similarities in the scope and context of day-to-day practice between rural and remote Australian and Antarctic medical practice. Pregnancies have been recorded on a number of national Antarctic expeditions and some on the Antarctic Peninsula have progressed to births. Difficulties in managing pregnancy in Antarctica are highlighted. Severe cases treated included a spontaneous first trimester miscarriage during the totally isolated winter months and hyperemesis gravidarum while crossing the Southern Ocean.

Over 1,000 persons have died in Antarctica, the majority perishing when the Spanish warship *San Telmo* was wrecked on Livingston Island in 1819, drowning hundreds, and when the Air New Zealand tourist flight crashed into Mount Erebus in 1979, killing 257. However, the mortality rate for Antarctica is low when compared with more densely populated regions.

Deaths in the "heroic era" such as those of Scott and his four colleagues, three members of the Ross Sea Party of Shackleton's Trans Antarctic Expedition 1914–17 and Mawson's two sledging companions on the Australasian Antarctic Expedition 1911–14, are the subject of many books and films. These contrast with the deaths of three skydivers near the South Pole in 1998, the death of a young woman from diabetes while traveling on a yacht in Antarctica waters in 2001, and a diving marine biologist killed by a leopard seal on the Antarctic Peninsula in 2003.

In September 2005, two Argentineans were lost in a crevasse while traveling between research bases in Antarctica. A week later, three of seven Chileans died when their vehicle fell into a crevasse. The Chilean rescuers were assisted by an Argentinean rescue team who had abandoned efforts to find the two Argentineans lost in the earlier accident.

Deaths on national expeditions have resulted from myocardial infarction, perforated gastric ulcer, appendicitis, cerebral hemorrhage, head injuries, alcohol poisoning, hypothermia, drowning, crush injuries, falls into crevasses, burns, pulmonary embolism, and carbon monoxide poisoning. Most national programs have had deaths; there were 18 fatalities in Australia's Antarctic program between 1947 and 2006. Aviation accidents have been the greatest cause of deaths in the U.S. Antarctic Program (Carlisle & Shen, 2001). Health risks are also present for those on cruise ships in Antarctica as the case report of a tourist death illustrates (Lamberth, 2001); the probable cause of the death was septic shock secondary to respiratory tract infection and suspected vertebral fracture.

HEALTH CARE ON EXPEDITIONS

A review of the epidemiology of Antarctic expeditions shows that there is no specific Antarctic disease. Medical practice in polar regions is no longer one of treating conditions resulting from the effects of the environment or due to isolation. With many of the people traveling on polar expeditions being highly mobile, exotic diseases contracted in temperate or tropical climates may surface on expeditions in both Antarctica and the Arctic, consistent with the sex and age of the individual. Antarctic

medicine is therefore the practice of medicine in Antarctic regions and not a specialty of Antarctic-specific disease states. However, Antarctic and Arctic expedition practice may take in many specialized medical areas such as altitude (the highest mountain in Antarctica is nearly 5,000 m), aviation, diving and hyperbaric, and shipboard and tourism medicine, as well as exposure and environmental medicine. All these specialties are referred to in specific chapters in this book.

HEALTH CARE SERVICES

Each group traveling to Antarctica, whether as a national researcher, tourist, or adventure seeker, must assess the risks to their particular group and develop health care services in response to the perceived needs. Anderson and Johnson (2000) studied 246 expeditions (known to the Expedition Advisory Centre of the Royal Geographical Society) retrospectively (26% were polar, desert, marine, and aquatic environments), and their findings suggested that health risks of participating in a well-planned expedition are similar to those encountered during normal active life. Norman (1991) found that there was a 1% risk of death to a participant in an Antarctic overwintering expedition. The factors to be taken into account when planning expedition health care are listed in Table 16.4. It is a lengthy list, but it does reflect the detailed planning necessary for the isolated and dangerous Antarctic environment. Such planning should also be performed for the Arctic.

Services range from multidisciplinary medical teams and modern medical suites and vast equipment and supplies at some national research stations to no medical or paramedical staff and basic equipment and supplies at others. Each should be self-sufficient because of the costs in both financial terms and the diversion of scientific and support personnel from their routine work at times of medical emergency. National programs have chosen different models of health care: civilian, military, contract, within the national polar organization, or a combination of these. Table 16.4 lists many of the determining factors, which include the number and skills of the medically trained staff, the degree of physical isolation, and the medical logistics capabilities, especially the ability to provide medical evacuation by ship or aircraft (Nielsen & Vollers, 2001; Ogle & Dunckel, 2002). As Ogle and Dunckel point out, the U.S. Antarctic Program has built its service around evacuation, and in the years 1993–6 had an evacuation rate of 1% (evacuations as a proportion of all clinic visits). In the years 1998–2001, 128 evacuations occurred, yielding a rate of 1.2%. The contrast in management of emergencies was highlighted in October 2005 when a case of appendicitis was evacuated from the Antarctic Peninsula to Punta Arenas, Chile, while on the same day another case on board an Antarctic icebreaker was successfully operated on in the ship's surgery.

Table 16.4. Factors to be taken into account when planning expedition health care for polar regions

1. Area of Arctic/Antarctica
   isolation factor, ship based, over flight, ice cap, sea ice, crevassing
2. Expedition personnel
   number, ages, sex, medical status
3. Length of stay
   summer, winter
4. Expedition program
   mountain climbing, trekking, aviation, diving, skiing, kayaking
5. Presence of medical practitioner, nurse, paramedical staff
6. Logistics
   weight/size restrictions, power, heating, food, water, clothing, equipment
7. Facilities
   tent, hut, warm and refrigerated storage, ablutions, toilet, rubbish
8. Communications
   satellite, telemedicine
9. Risk factors
   preventive medicine, risk–benefit ratio of every potential medical/surgical procedure, wildlife, carbon monoxide
10. Medevac capability
    plan to efficiently and effectively cover all contingencies
11. Level of medical care
    first-aid, perform sterile operations under anesthesia, diagnostic X-rays or ultrasound, medical supplies, equipment
    standard of predeparture screening (medical/dental)
12. Predeparture
    orientation, specialized training, first-aid, screening
13. Medicolegal
    indemnity, international patients, legal jurisdiction (Antarctic Treaty), medical insurance for all participants, medical evacuation insurance, search and rescue insurance

Each year the Antarctic Treaty System publishes details of operating stations, refuges, and the status of medical services. Most of these are not geared for major emergencies outside of their own sphere of operations and should not be relied on by those planning Antarctic expeditions. The Council of Managers of National Antarctic Programs (COMNAP) publishes an up-to-date Antarctic Flight Information Manual (AFIM) providing details of Antarctic air facilities and procedures. Information such as this is invaluable in planning.

Levinson and Ger (1998) have detailed the medical care and safety of tourists on tourist ships. Medical services for the younger, more adventurous tourists cater to traumatic injuries, whereas on traditional tourist ships, older passengers need support for age-related medical problems. Curry (2002) has reported that the International Association of Antarctic Tour Operations (IAATO), the voluntary self-regulating body for Antarctic tourism founded in 1991, is developing standards for its members' medical services.

Preventive medicine is arguably the most important factor and has been the cornerstone of "best practice" services in Antarctica, where logistic constraints prevent timely evacuation and resupply. Physicians in Antarctica who have been the sole medical providers consider that two-doctor teams are preferable. In addition to having a valuable second opinion, it also brings a wider range of skills and experience. However, few expeditions can afford the luxury of two doctors. Medevac capability is sought after by most expedition physicians, but without such capability, Antarctic health care providers must rely on their own skills, supplies, and equipment at hand, telemedicine, and lay assistance. Specialist advisers in the home country must know the doctor's skills and capabilities, as well as the limitations of facilities, pharmaceuticals, and equipment. Planning is very important, and the risk–benefit ratio of every potential procedure should be assessed.

PREDEPARTURE MEDICAL SCREENING

"The chief work of the surgeon of a polar expedition is done before the ship leaves." Thus wrote Macklin (1923) at the conclusion of Shackleton's *Quest* Expedition on which Shackleton died of a heart attack. Shackleton's preexisting health problems were known before the expedition. The dilemma faced in the "heroic era" is still present today. Nations practicing preventive medicine have a vigorous predeparture medical and dental screening, some having psychiatric and psychological assessment. This contrasts with many tourist operations (Levinson & Ger, 1998; Lamberth, 2001).

Guidelines for screening vary between groups, with the most rigorous rejecting persons with asthma, coronary artery disease, diabetes, epilepsy, and other chronic disease states, as well as those whose continuing good health depends on medication. Those who grant waivers must see that the expedition doctor is aware of the problems and the expedition has the available medical support to deal with a worsening condition, or there is comprehensive medical support and/or evacuation available at short notice. With the vagaries of Antarctic weather, and consequent unreliability of aircraft availability 24 hours a day 7 days a week, medical policy for polar expeditions is of utmost importance. Predeparture screening investigations vary between groups and may include blood donor screening (if a walking blood bank is part of the medical armamentarium), EKG (stress EKG for some above a certain age or risk profile), chest X-ray, and other laboratory tests.

SELECTION AND TRAINING OF MEDICAL STAFF

Ideally, a medical practitioner should accompany all groups and should have the skills and adequate predeparture training to manage all medical, surgical, and dental emergencies to the planned level of care. A doctor is a must for winter groups. Additional personnel should receive training in assisting the doctor should surgery, anesthesia, or sterile operating techniques be contemplated. If nurses or paramedics go instead of a doctor, they should be adequately briefed, trained, and involved in the planning for the expedition.

In selecting medical personnel, account must be taken of the likelihood and consequences of medical events and the needed medical skills. In addition, one must assess the personality and ability of the physician, nurse, or paramedic to deal with the demands of the medical practice with its basic nature in an isolated, extreme environment. If a doctor is taken, no one medical specialty is considered best. It is a combination of personal attributes for the environment as well as medical expertise and experience of the individual that is important – a true "super generalist."

Experience in a number of fields is desirable: obviously environmental medicine for cold injury, occupational medicine if research or construction is contemplated with the presence of scientific chemicals and building materials. Knowledge of food and nutrition and of public health is also important; food poisoning and contamination of potable water supplies occur (*Giardia* is present in both the Arctic and Antarctic), toilets must be established and in the case of Antarctica, all human waste and rubbish must be removed. If aviation and diving are part of the expedition, knowledge of these is useful. Medical handbooks and first-aid manuals specifically designed for polar regions are invaluable (Grant et al., 2005; Gormly, 2002). With many hazards confronting all groups, preventive aspects are important for all individuals. Those spending longer periods of time in isolation may need counseling and support on reentry into society.

One topic rarely discussed is what happens if the doctor, nurse, or paramedic becomes ill. This is important not only for the patient but also for the group. Such scenarios are illustrated by Rogozov's (1964) description of his self-operation for appendicitis and the highly publicized medical evacuations of doctors from the South Pole (Nielsen & Vollers, 2001; Ogle & Dunckel, 2002). Preventive principles have even been extended to predeparture prophylactic appendectomy for physicians (Lugg, 2000).

ORIENTATION AND MEDICAL TRAINING OF ALL PARTICIPANTS

All participants should be briefed on all aspects of the expedition including personal and field hygiene, what medical services are provided, the hazards and risks of the expedition, and safety. The need for each person to have the necessary immunizations, to take spare glasses or contact lenses, medicaments and sunscreen, and eye protection is paramount. The problems of the misting of glasses, dripping noses, the hobbling effect of polar clothing, the dangers of wearing metal-rimmed glasses and jewelry, and the need to carry spare socks and gloves on one's person should all be explained. If traveling to the Arctic, comment should be made of diseases such as rabies and other exotics in the dog population or wildlife. Ideally, all participants should be instructed in appropriate levels of first-aid.

If a doctor is present, then he or she will live and work with the group. The potential patients see their physician at close quarters as well as the nature and limitations of the medical system. This often puts stress on both the doctor and the patient. In most cases, this can be overcome by clear advice at the outset. Doctors, too, are well aware of perceptions of danger, risk taking, and outcomes in remote Antarctica (Burns & Sullivan, 2000). In addition, most expeditioners are very perspicacious patients (Plowright, 2000).

FACILITIES, EQUIPMENT, AND SUPPLIES

Each group should plan medical facilities, equipment and supplies with the policy determined and the perceived needs of that group. Small expeditions of short duration without a doctor obviously have different needs to those of a large wintering group with doctor and operating theater. Amundsen's Norwegian Antarctic Expedition (1910–12) had no doctor and the leader was obliged to take all the responsibility. He considered medical equipment important and described part of the main medical kit as "carefully chosen by a chemist in Christiania." The sledging medical kit used on the dash to the South Pole consisted of a "little traveling case of medicines," a dental forceps, and a beard clipper (Amundsen, 1912). A hundred years later with all the advances in medicine and technology, this would be inadequate. However, one must guard against taking sophisticated medical equipment that needs power that is not available or does not operate at the ambient temperatures found in the field. Each piece of equipment or drug must be carefully chosen as being necessary by physicians with experience in the conditions likely to be experienced. The field medical setting is not the emergency room in a major teaching hospital.

Care is needed in selection of pharmaceuticals both for prospective use, shelf life, and packaging, as freezing can break some liquid medicaments in glass. A review of the most common drugs used on expeditions detailed in the ANARE Health Register over the last 17 years show that simple analgesics (with or without codeine), nonsteroidal antinflammatories (NSAIDs) and first-line antimicrobials including oral and otic/ophthalmic were the most dispensed. Recent work by Priston et al. (2005) suggests many pharmaceuticals are less prone to break down and loss of efficacy than previously thought. One important principle in polar groups, whether at a fixed base or small field setting, is that the medical kit should be split into a main kit and a secondary one, which should always be stored away from the main. In this way, the group does have some medical supplies should the main kit be lost or destroyed. Useful advice on field kits is found in a number of polar medical manuals (Grant et al., 2005; Gormly, 2002).

TELEMEDICINE AND MEDICAL INFORMATICS

Medical communications have always been of utmost importance both within Antarctica and to the outside world, allowing physicians to advise patients remote in the field, as well as giving them access to the experience and expertise of medical specialists outside of the polar sphere. Communications were the cornerstone of many medical systems (Sullivan & Lugg, 1995). Simple, cheap, and effective solutions allowed data, clinical and microscopic photos, X-rays, and electrocardiograms to be transmitted from Antarctica to the countries of origin of expeditions for over 50 years (Taylor & Gormly, 1997; Hyer, 1999; Grant, 2004). Today with satellite systems, medical imaging and the transmission of medical and biomedical data are daily occurrences, even to and from a remote field party. Many groups have access to phone, fax, e-mail, and voice, video, and data circuits, as well as the World Wide Web. The system, in addition to providing clinical and peer support, has been innovative in giving doctors and paramedics access to medical databases and valuable information. Every expedition traveling to polar environs should investigate the use of telemedicine as an adjunct to its medical support.

MEDICOLEGAL

This is a complex issue for polar regions and far beyond the Good Samaritan principle and the extent of national expeditions providing medical care for nongovernmental activities (Carlisle & Shen, 2001). A number of countries have legislation covering areas of Antarctica (the so-called Frozen Claims of the Antarctic Treaty), but whether this pertains only to citizens of the claimant nation or beyond, probably will require legal testing in the courts.

RESEARCH

In Antarctic medicine, there has always been a close association between clinical practice and research. The prime responsibility of doctors is health care, and they are in a unique position to integrate clinical and evidence-based observation of their colleagues, especially during winter. The multidisciplinary research has centered on human interaction with the Antarctic environment (Lugg, 2000). For instance, the finding of an altered immune status in Antarctic wintering personnel has important health implications should viral disease occur,

even though it appears such subjects have normal antibody production (Shearer et al., 2001).

SPECIFIC POLAR MEDICAL PROBLEMS

Dehydration

In the ultradry polar environment, the fluid loss from the body may be greater than normal especially if intake is restricted due to inadequate melting of snow or ice for drinking water. One must not ignore thirst in polar regions but make sure that there is a sufficient daily fluid intake.

Cold Injury

Low temperatures, high winds, and blowing snow, which melts when it gets onto exposed skin or into warmer clothing, may cause both local cold injury (frostnip and frostbite) and/or general cold injury (hypothermia or exposure in which the body core temperature cools to dangerous levels). These injuries are covered in special chapters. Expeditions in polar regions should be cognizant of the management of all cold injury. Members should watch each other carefully (the "buddy system") for all cold injury and take rapid steps to treat. Hypothermia can be rapid such as falling into cold water or more insidious when clothing is inadequate or the victim has been injured, immobilized, or inactive. Sunburn may exacerbate hypothermia due to the radiation of heat from the burnt area. The aim of treatment is to restore body heat. In contrast, frostnip, often on the face but also on tips of fingers, a small waxy white patch of skin occurs rapidly and needs immediate application of heat in the form of a warm body part. Frostnip should not be rubbed.

Frostbite, the freezing of skin on deeper layers, is avoidable. Management is best accomplished by rapid rewarming in warm water (40°C) but this should only be carried out when there is no risk of refreezing. A patient can walk on a frostbitten limb but when thawed it is painful and useless. The treatment often continues for months, and this should be done in a hospital experienced in managing cold injury.

Sunburn

Sunburn can be particularly intense in the polar environment as the sun's UV rays may be reflected from the snow and daylight is prolonged in the summer. Prevention is best achieved with protective sunscreen regularly applied in addition to appropriate protective clothing.

Snowblindness

Dark glasses, goggles, or glacier glasses with adequate lens protection should be worn at all times in the field, complete with a cord around the neck to prevent loss.

These prevent snowblindness, which is a most painful and debilitating condition caused by UV burns to the eyes.

Polar Hands

Painful cracks in the skin around the nails and fingertips, caused by the cold, dry Antarctic environment, are called "polar hands." Moisturizers help, but skin tissue adhesives give a spontaneous result (Ayton, 1993).

Carbon Monoxide

Open-flamed stoves, gas heaters, and internal combustion engines must be handled with care in polar regions as they produce carbon monoxide, which is lethal. Snow may block ventilation or exhausts causing a buildup of the toxic gas.

Animal Bites

Animal bites in polar regions have a high rate of infection and contact with the large predators of both regions should be avoided. In the Arctic, the most notorious predator is the polar bear. Though relatively rare, this large carnivore has been implicated in a number of attacks on humans (Risholt et al., 1998). It is suspected that the polar bear interprets any object with color and movement as food and will therefore launch a predatory attack with seemingly little provocation (Dieter et al., 2001). Expeditioners in the Arctic should use extreme caution when traveling in polar bear territory and take the usual bear precautions such as the proper storage of attractants (food and/or garbage).

Even though there are no polar bears in the Antarctic, there have been reports of attacks by another large predator, the leopard seal, in this region with at least one fatality occurring in 2003. Leopard seals can grow to be 12 feet (3.4 m) in length and weigh in excess of 1,100 pounds (500 kg). They appear clumsy on land but are quick and agile swimmers. Current safety recommendations include exiting the Antarctic water when leopard seals are spotted and staying away from the edges of ice shelves as leopard seals are known to explode to the surface from under ice edges to attack prey. Explorer Gareth Wood was attacked in this fashion by a leopard seal during his 1985 South Pole expedition.

CONCLUSION

The remote, icy, and harsh polar regions, despite their many hazards, are beautiful, and those who go on expeditions there find them a stimulating and rewarding experience. Testimony to this is the number of people who return again and again.

ACKNOWLEDGMENTS

The assistance of Dr. Roland Watzl of the Polar Medicine Unit, Australian Antarctic Division, for analyzing the data from the health register is gratefully acknowledged. We are indebted to the many international polar doctors, psychologists, scientists, explorers, and expeditioners who gave, and continue to give invaluable information on medical aspects of polar expeditions.

SUGGESTED READINGS

Amundsen R. *The South Pole. An Account of the Norwegian Antarctic Expedition in the "Fram," 1910–1912*. London: John Murray; 1912.

Anderson SR, Johnson CJH. Expedition health and safety: a risk assessment. *J Roy Soc Med*. 2000;93:557–62.

Ayton JM. Spontaneous Skin Tissues Closed with Cyanoacrylate (Histoacryl Blue) Tissue Adhesive in Antarctica. *Arctic Med Res*. 1993;52:127–30.

Ayton JM. Medical emergency at sea. *Australian Antarctic Magazine*. 2005;8:26.

Ayton JM. Women's health in Antarctica. *ANZ J Obstet Gynecol*. 2006;8:16–18.

Budd GM. A polio-like illness in Antarctica. *Med J Aust*. 1962;1:483–6.

Burns R, Sullivan P. Perceptions of danger, risk taking and outcomes in a remote community. *Environment Behavior*. 2000;32:32–72.

Carlisle B, Shen B. Polar medicine. In: Auerback PS, ed. *Wilderness Medicine*, 4th ed. St. Louis: Mosby; 2001: 226–39.

Cattermole TJ. Snowmobile injuries in Antarctica 1989–1996. *Int J Circumpolar Health*. 1997;56:152–8.

Cattermole TJ. The epidemiology of cold injury in Antarctica. *Aviat Space Environ Med*. 1999;70:135–40.

Cattermole TJ. The incidence of injury with the British Antarctic Survey, 1986–1995. *Int J Circumpolar Health*. 2001;60:72–81.

Curry CM. Death in Antarctica. *Med J Aust*. 2002;176:451.

Dieter RA Jr, Dieter DL, Dieter RA 3rd, Forbes B. Bear mauling: a descriptive review. *Int J Circumpolar Health*. 2001;60(4):696–704.

Feeney RE. *Polar Journeys: The Role of Food and nutrition in Early Exploration*. Washington, DC, Fairbanks, AK: American Chemical Society, University of Alaska Press; 1997.

Fodstad H, Kondziolka D, Brophy BP, Roberts DW, Girvin JP. Arctic and Antarctic exploration including the contributions of physicians and effects of disease in the polar regions. *Neurosurg*. 1999;44:925–39.

Fortuine R. Medical aspects of arctic exploration 3. farthest north with the "Fram": Fridtjof Nansen (1893–1896). *Arctic Med Res*. 1988;47:92–5.

Fortuine R. Medical aspects of arctic exploration 7. the Northwest Passage at last: Roald Amundsen (1903–1906). *Arctic Med Res*. 1989;48:140–3.

Gormly PJ. *ANARE First Aid Manual*. 6th ed. with amendments. Kingston, Australia: Australian Antarctic Division; 2002.

Grant IC. Telemedicine in the British Antarctic Survey. *Int J Circumpolar Health*. 2004;63:356–64.

Grant IC, Cosgrove H, Thomson L, Guly H. Kurafid: *The British Antarctic Survey Medical Handbook*. 6th ed. Cambridge: British Antarctic Survey; 2005.

Hyer RN. Telemedical experiences at an Antarctic Station. *J Telemed Telecare*. 1999;5(Suppl 1):587–9.

King H. A new health register for Australian National Antarctic Research Expeditions. *Polar Rec.* 1987;23:719–20.

Lamberth PG. Death in Antarctica. *Med J Aust.* 2001;175:583–4.

Levinson JM, Ger E. *Safe Passage Questioned: Medical Care and Safety for the Polar Tourist.* Centreville, Md: Cornell Maritime Press; 1998.

Lloyd RM. Medical problems encountered on British Antarctic expeditions. In: Edholm OG, Gunderson EKE, eds. *Polar Human Biology.* London: Heinemann; 1973: 71–92.

Lugg DJ. Antarctic epidemiology – A survey of ANARE stations 1947–72. In: Edholm OG, Gunderson EKE, eds. *Polar Human Biology.* London: Heinemann; 1973: 93–104.

Lugg DJ. Antarctic medicine, 1775–1975. Part I. *Med J Aust.* 1975a;2:295–8.

Lugg DJ. Antarctic medicine, 1775–1975. Part II. *Med J Aust.* 1975b;2:335–7.

Lugg DJ. *Antarctica: Australia's Remote Medical Practice.* Kingston, Australia: Australian Antarctic Division; 1993.

Lugg DJ. Antarctic medicine. *JAMA.* 2000;283:2082–4.

Lugg DJ. Behavioral health in Antarctica: implications for long-duration space missions. *Aviat Space Environ Med.* 2005;76(6, Suppl):B89–93.

Lugg DJ, Gormly PJ, King H. SCAR Accident Survey: Australian results 1977–1985. *Polar Rec.* 1987;23:720–5.

Lugg DJ, Roy CR. UVB and health effects in Antarctica. *Polar Res.* 1999;18:353–9.

Macklin AH. Appendix V, Medical. In: Wild F, ed. *Shackleton's Last Voyage: The Story of the Quest.* London: Cassell; 1923: 352.

Nielsen J, Vollers M. *Ice Bound.* New York: Hyperion; 2001.

Norman JN. A Comparison of the patterns of illness and injury occurring on offshore structures in the northern North Sea and the stations of the British Antarctic Survey. *Arctic Med Res.* 1991;(Suppl 1):719–21.

Ogle JW, Dunckel GN. Clinical medicine: defibrillation and thrombolysis following a myocardial infarct in Antarctica. *Aviat Space Environ Med.* 2002;73:694–8.

Palinkas LA, Glogower F, Dembert M, Hansen K, Smullen R. Incidence of psychiatric disorders after extended residence in Antarctica. *Int J Circumpolar Health.* 2004;63:157–68.

Pardoe R. A ruptured intracranial aneurysm in Antarctica. *Med J Aust.* 1965;1:344–50.

Plowright RK. Crevasse fall in the Antarctic: a patient's perspective? *Med J Aust.* 2000;173:576–8.

Podkolinski MT, Semmens K. Intestinal haemorrhage in Antarctica: a multinational rescue operation. *Med J Aust.* 1979;2:275–7.

Priddy RE. An "acute abdomen" in Antarctica: the problems of diagnosis and management. *Med J Aust.* 1985;143:108–11.

Priston MJ, Grant IC, Hughes JM, Marquis PT. Pilot study on potential degradation of drug efficiency resulting from Antarctic storage, transport and field conditions. *Int J Circumpolar Health.* 2005;64:184–6.

Risholt T, Persen E, Solem OI. Man and polar bear in Svalbard: a solvable ecological conflict? *Int J Circumpolar Health.* 1998;(57 Suppl 1):532–4.

Rogozov LI. Self operation. *Soviet Antarctic Expedition Information Bull.* 1964;4:223.

Shearer WT, Lugg DJ, Rosenblatt HM, et al. Antibody responses to bacteriophage ØX-174 in humans exposed to the Antarctic winter-over model of space flight. *J Allergy Clin Immunol.* 2001;107:160–4.

Sullivan PG. Accidental hypothermia in Antarctica – an incident involving two cases of hypothermia and frostbite. *Med J Aust.* 1987;146:155–8.

Sullivan P, Gormly PJ. The Australian National Antarctic Research Expeditions (ANARE) health register. In: Peasley K, ed. *Proceedings of the National Centre for Classification in Health (NCCH),* 6th Annual Conference, Hobart, September 1999. Lidcombe, Australia: NCCH; 1999: 36–43.

Sullivan P, Lugg DJ. *Telemedicine between Australia and Antarctica: 1911–1995.* SAE Technical Paper 951616. Presented at: 25th International Conference on Environmental Systems, San Diego, Calif., Warrendale, Pa.: SAE; 1995.

Taylor D, Gormly P. Emergency medicine in Antarctica. *Emerg Med.* 1997;9:237–45.

World Health Organization. *International Classification of Diseases Ninth Revision 1975,* Vol,. 1 and 2. Geneva: WHO; 1997.

World Health Organization. *International Classification of Procedures in Medicine,* Vol,. 1 and 2. Geneva: WHO; 1978.

17 | Tropical Medicine for Expeditions

David M. Parenti, MD, MScCTM, and Peter J. Hotez, MD, PhD

GLOBAL BURDEN OF DISEASE

The major tropical infections of humans include malaria and other protozoan infections (e.g., amebiasis, human African trypanosomiasis, Chagas disease, and leishmaniasis), helminth infections (e.g., dracunculiasis, lymphatic filariasis, onchocerciasis, schistosomiasis, and soil-transmitted helminthiases), emerging arboviral (e.g., dengue and Japanese encephalitis), and hemorrhagic fever virus infections (e.g., Ebola and Marburg viruses), and specific bacterial infections (e.g., Buruli ulcer, leprosy, melioidosis, and trachoma).

As shown in Table 17.1, the tropical diseases represent some of the most common infections of humankind, with the three major soil-transmitted helminthiases (ascariasis, hookworm, and trichuriasis) exhibiting the greatest prevalence, followed by malaria, schistosomiasis, and lymphatic filariasis. Up to one-eighth of the world's population is infected with a tropical disease. The people at greatest risk for acquiring tropical diseases are the estimated 2.7 billion people who live on less than $2 per day. For the most part, the tropical diseases are diseases of poverty and are found almost exclusively in low- and middle-income countries of sub-Saharan Africa, Asia, and Latin America. In these regions, it is common for a single individual to be simultaneously afflicted with several tropical diseases. For instance, it would not be unusual for a school-aged child in Vietnam to be polyparasitized with all three major soil-transmitted helminths, while a pregnant woman in sub-Saharan Africa might be simultaneously infected with malaria, schistosomiasis, and hookworm.

The tropical diseases have a significant impact on the health and well-being of the world's poorest people living in the developing world. As shown in Table 17.2, the tropical diseases are major causes of global mortality – an estimated 2.1 million to 2.5 million people die annually from tropical diseases, a number that approximates the number of people who die annually from HIV/AIDS or tuberculosis. Most of the tropical disease-related deaths result from falciparum malaria. Approximately 90% of the estimated 1.2 million annual deaths from malaria occur in sub-Saharan Africa, and mostly in children younger than 5. Currently, malaria is Africa's leading cause of mortality in children younger than 5 (http://www.rbm.who.int), with approximately 3,000 young children dying from this condition each day.

Next to malaria, typhoid fever and schistosomiasis are the major causes of tropical disease-related death. Details on typhoid fever will be presented in Chapter 25. For schistosomiasis, many of these deaths result from the chronic renal complications of urinary schistosomiasis caused by *Schistosoma haematobium*. Amebiasis and chronic infections caused by the soil-transmitted helminths are also significant causes of death, as are the kinetoplastid infections, leishmaniasis, human African trypanosomiasis, and Chagas' disease. In contrast, some of the most notorious emerging hemorrhagic fever viral infections such as Ebola, Marburg, and Lassa are not considered significant causes of death worldwide. Although these illnesses present with dramatic and impressive symptoms, for the most part the hemorrhagic fevers tend to occur in very limited and focal outbreaks.

An examination of the deaths caused by tropical diseases does not provide a complete picture of their health impact. Equally important is the long-term disability resulting from these conditions. For instance, the major soil-transmitted helminth infections together with schistosomiasis are important causes of chronic anemia and inflammation among school-aged children and pregnant women and, as a result, cause significant impairments in childhood growth and development as well as bad pregnancy outcomes, including prematurity, low birth weight, and increased maternal mortality.[4,7] Similarly, tropical conditions such as lymphatic filariasis, leprosy, mucocutaneous leishmaniasis, onchocerciasis, and Buruli ulcer are disfiguring and disabling and impair worker productivity.[8,9] Since the early 1990s, the disability-adjusted life year or DALY has been used to measure the number of life years lost either from premature death or disability. The high childhood

Table 17.1. The major tropical diseases

Disease	Global prevalence	Population at risk	Regions of greatest prevalence
Ascariasis	807 million	4.2 billion	EAP, SSA, India, SAS, LAC
Trichuriasis	604 million	3.2 billion	SSA, EAP, LAC, India, SAS
Hookworm	576 million	3.2 billion	SSA, EAP, India, SAS, LAC
Malaria	300 million	2.6 billion	SSA, EAP, India, SAS, LAC
Schistosomiasis	200 million	0.6 billion	SSA, LAC
Lymphatic filariasis	120 million	1.3 billion	India, SAS, EAP, SSA
Trachoma	84 million	0.5 billion	SSA, MENA
Dengue	50 million	2.5 billion	EAP, LAC
Amebiasis	50 million (invasive disease)	Not determined	India, LAC, SAS, EAP, SSA
Taeniasis (*T. solium*)	50 million	Not determined	EAP, LAC, SSA
Food-borne trematodiases	40 million	Not determined	EAP
Onchocerciasis	18 million to 37 million	0.12 billion	SSA, LAC
Typhoid fever	16 million to 33 million	Not determined	EAP, India, SAS
Leishmaniasis	12 million	0.4 billion	India, SAS, SSA, LAC, CAR
Chagas' disease	9 million	0.025 billion	LAC
Loiasis	3–13 million	Not determined	SSA
Brucellosis	0.5 million	Not determined	MENA, CAR, India, EAP, SSA
Leprosy	0.4 million	Not determined	India, SAS, LAC, SSA
African trypanosomiasis	0.3 million	0.06 billion	SSA
Echinococcosis	0.3 million	Not determined	CAR, SSA, LAC
Yellow fever	0.2 million	Not determined	SSA, LAC
Japanese encephalitis	0.05 million	Not determined	EAP, SAS, India
Dracunculiasis	0.01 million	0.01 billion	SSA
Plague	0.002 million	Not determined	SSA, India, SAS, EAP
Cholera	Variable	Not determined	India, SAS, EAP, SSA, LAC
Rift Valley fever	Variable	Not determined	SSA, MENA
Crimean-Congo fever	Variable	Not determined	CAR, SAS, MENA, SSA
Leptospirosis	Not determined	Not determined	EAP, LAC, India, SAS, SSA
Murine typhus	Not determined	Not determined	EAP, SAS, MENA, SSA, LAC
Anthrax	Not determined	Not determined	MENA, EAP, SSA, LAC
Epidemic typhus	Not determined	Not determined	SSA, EAP, LAC
Mycetoma	Not determined	Not determined	SSA, LAC, MENA, India
Melioidosis	Not determined	Not determined	EAP
Buruli ulcer	Not determined	Not determined	SSA
Relapsing fever	Not determined	Not determined	SSA
Bartonellosis	Not determined	Not determined	LAC

EAP, East Asia and Pacific Islands; LAC, Latin America and Caribbean; MENA, Middle East and North Africa; CAR, Central Asia and Russian Federation; SAS, South Asia; SSA, sub-Saharan Africa.
Modified from Hotez et al.[1]

mortality resulting from malaria, together with chronic disabling features of many of the other tropical diseases account for the observation that the tropical diseases result in approximately 100 million DALYs lost annually (Table 17.3). This value exceeds the DALYs resulting from HIV/AIDS (84.5 million) or lower respiratory infections (91.3 million).

In addition to their health burden, the tropical diseases exert an enormous impact on the economic productivity of the developing world. These conditions not only occur in the setting of poverty, but because of their impact on child health, pregnancy outcome, and worker productivity, they also promote poverty.[4,9,10] Malaria has been shown to adversely affect the annual economic growth of sub-Saharan Africa, while the helminth infections together with trachoma diminish wage-earning capacity and worker productivity resulting in annual losses of at least tens of billions of dollars.[7] As a result,

tackling the tropical diseases represents an important target of the Millennium Development Goals (MDGs) for sustainable poverty reduction, especially MDG 6: *To combat HIV/AIDS, malaria, and other diseases.*[1,8]

The MDGs have provided a framework for launching several major multimillion dollar initiatives aimed at the control and elimination of the major tropical infections. For malaria, the G-8 nations have supported a Global Fund to Fight AIDS, Tuberculosis, and Malaria (*http://www.theglobalfund.org*), as well as the Roll Back Malaria (RBM) initiative (*http://www.rbm.whot.int*). This is in addition to a U.S.-based President's Malaria Initiative (PMI), and the Medicines for Malaria Venture (MMV). For helminth and trachoma control, the major public–private partnerships devoted to these conditions, including the Schistosomiasis Control Initiative (SCI), the International Trachoma Initiative (ITI), the Human Hookworm Vaccine Initiative, the Lymphatic

Table 17.2. Leading causes of death from tropical diseases

Disease	Estimated number of deaths	Reference
Malaria	1,207,000	Lopez et al., 2001[2]
Typhoid fever	216,000–600,000	Epstein and Hoffman, 2006[3]
Schistosomiasis	280,000	Hotez et al., 2006[4]
Amebiasis	100,000	Stauffer and Ravdin, 2003[5]
Hookworm infection	65,000	Hotez et al., 2006[4]
Ascariasis	60,000	Hotez et al., 2006[4]
Leishmaniasis	51,000	Lopez et al., 2001[2]
Human African trypanosomiasis	48,000	Lopez et al., 2001[2]
Yellow fever	30,000	Marfin et al., 2006[6]
Dengue	19,000	Lopez et al., 2001[2]
Chagas' disease	14,000	Lopez et al., 2001[2]
Japanese encephalitis	14,000	Lopez et al., 2001[2]
Trichuriasis	10,000	Hotez et al., 2006[4]
Leprosy	6,000	Lopez et al., 2001[2]
Total deaths	2,120,000–2,504,000	—

Filariasis Support Centre of the Liverpool School of Tropical Medicine, the Task Force for Child Survival and Development, Helen Keller International, and the Earth Institute at Columbia University, have joined in an alliance known as the Global Network for Neglected Tropical Diseases Control (GNNTDC). Together with the WHO, the African Programme for Onchocerciasis Control (APOC), the Carter Center, and the Global Alliance to Eliminate Lymphatic Filariasis, these organizations are coordinating tropical disease control and elimination efforts through mass drug administration. For this purpose, albendazole or mebendazole is being administered for the control of soil-transmitted helminth infections; ivermectin or diethylcarbamazine, for lymphatic filariasis and onchocerciasis; praziquantel for schistosomiasis; and azithromycin, for trachoma.[1,4,11] For LF and trachoma, there is additional optimism that these diseases could be eliminated (i.e., their transmission interrupted by 2020).

Because of the high rates of polyparasitism in sub-Saharan Africa and elsewhere,[11] a new effort is also underway to deliver these drugs together in a package of preventive chemotherapy (known as the rapid-impact package) in order to simultaneously target multiple so-called *neglected tropical diseases*, especially the soil-transmitted helminth infections, schistosomiasis, LF, onchocerciasis, and trachoma.[4,11] Many of the rapid impact drugs, such as albendazole, ivermectin, and azithromycin are currently donated by large pharmaceutical companies so that the package can be delivered at low cost, possibly as low as $0.40 per person.[11] Additional efforts are also underway to integrate malaria control measures comprised of bed nets, indoor residual spraying, and intermittent preventive therapy together with preventive chemotherapy for the neglected tropical diseases.[4] This would represent a massive global campaign to fight tropical diseases.[12]

THE MAJOR TROPICAL DISEASES OF EXPEDITIONS AND ADVENTURE TRAVELERS

This chapter considers the major tropical diseases likely to be encountered during an expedition, with an emphasis on the most common tropical infections of travelers including amebiasis, dengue, leptospirosis, malaria, schistosomiasis, and soil-transmitted helminth infections.[13, 14, 15] Here we also emphasize the possible routes of transmission that pose a special risk for expeditions and other travel adventurers (Table 17.4).

SOIL-TRANSMITTED TROPICAL DISEASES

The major soil-transmitted tropical diseases include leptospirosis, melioidosis, mycetoma, and the soil-transmitted helminth infections, also known as the intestinal nematode infections. Both leptospirosis and melioidosis are also considered waterborne infections.

Table 17.3. DALYS from tropical infections

Disease condition	DALYs
Malaria	46.5 million
Soil-transmitted helminth infections	39.0 million
Lymphatic filariasis and onchocerciasis	6.3 million
Schistosomiasis	4.5 million
Kinetoplastid infections	4.3 million
Trachoma and leprosy	2.5 million
Dengue and Japanese encephalitis	0.5 million
Total tropical diseases[a]	103.6 million

[a]DALY estimates do not include the diarrheal diseases, including typhoid fever, cholera, and amebiasis.
Modified from Hotez et. al.[4]

Leptospirosis

See discussion in section "Waterborne Tropical Diseases."

Table 17.4. The major tropical diseases classified by transmission route

Soil-transmitted tropical diseases
Leptospirosis
Melioidosis
Mycetoma and other fungal infections
Soil-transmitted helminthiases (ascariasis, hookworm, strongyloidiasis, toxocariasis, trichuriasis)

Food-borne tropical diseases
Enteric fever
Anthrax
Brucellosis
Food-borne trematodiases (clonorchiasis, fasciolopsiasis, opisthorchiasis, paragonimiasis)
Taeniasis and other tapeworm infections

Waterborne tropical diseases
Amebiasis
Buruli ulcer
Cholera and typhoid fever
Dracunculiasis
Leptospirosis
Melioidosis
Schistosomiasis

Person–person or animal–person direct contact
Anthrax
Brucellosis
Leprosy
Endemic treponematoses
Echinococcosis

Vector-borne tropical diseases
Mosquito
Malaria, yellow fever, dengue, Japanese encephalitis, filarial infections
Black fly
Onchocerciasis
Tabanid fly
Loiasis
Tsetse fly
African trypanosomiasis
Sandfly
Leishmaniasis, sandfly fever
Ticks
Rocky Mountain spotted fever, tick typhus, tick-borne relapsing fever
Lice
Epidemic typhus, louse-borne relapsing fever, bartonellosis
Fleas
Murine typhus, plague, bartonellosis
Mites
Scrub typhus, rickettsialpox
Reduviid bug
American trypanosomiasis

Melioidosis

Melioidosis is a serious gram-negative bacterial infection caused by *Burkholderia pseudomallei*, and an important cause of septicemia and mortality in Southeast Asia and northern Australia. Human infection usually occurs by inoculation or contamination of wounds (or mucosa) with soil or water, although in some cases infection can also occur via the aerosol route. The peak incidence occurs in individuals aged 40 to 60, with rice farmers in Southeast Asia and aboriginals in Australia representing high-risk groups.[16] There is a wide spectrum of clinical disease, with the most severe being septicemic melioidosis. Typically, this condition presents as a community-acquired sepsis with a one-week history of high fever, rigors, and weight loss. *Burholderia* septic shock has a mortality that approaches 100 percent. An important localized form of melioidosis occurs as a cavitating pneumonia, which resembles tuberculosis, or as a parotitis. Melioidosis is difficult to treat because the etiologic agent, *B. pseudomallei*, exhibits a high degree of intrinsic drug resistance.[16] When available, a new generation beta-lactam or carbapenems, such as meropenum, imipenem, or ceftazidime is used together with co-trimoxazole. Parenteral treatment is usually required for several weeks followed by oral therapy to prevent relapse.[16]

Mycetoma

Mycetoma is a condition of the foot or hand that occurs when soil saprophytes (often either fungi of the genus *Madurella* or bacteria such as *Nocardia spp.*) are introduced into human tissue with a contaminated foreign object such as a splinter or thorn. It occurs in tropical and subtropical regions worldwide, particularly among people who work outdoors.[17] Mycetoma typically begins as a painless nodule (most often on the sole of the foot) that increases in size. As expansion occurs sinus tracks open, which drain pus and grains. Infection in the skin and subcutaneous tissue can extend to the bones. On radiographs, there is evidence of cavities. A diagnosis is usually made on the basis of clinical evidence of a triad of painless swelling, sinuses, and grains.[18] Appropriate treatment requires initial identification of the etiologic agent. For infection caused by *Nocardia spp.* a combination of an aminoglycoside (e.g., streptomycin sulfate or amikacin) and co-trimoxazole is often used, whereas for fungal mycetoma several agents have been used with success including ketoconazole and itraconazole.[18] Long-term therapy is usually required.

Soil-Transmitted Helminth Infections

The soil-transmitted helminth (STH) infections caused by intestinal nematodes are transmitted through contact with viable parasite eggs (e.g., ascariasis and trichuriasis) or larvae (e.g., hookworm infection and strongyloidiasis) that live in the warm and moist soil of low- and middle-income countries in the tropics.[19] In these regions, eggs and larvae are almost ubiquitous in the soil accounting for the observation that hundreds of millions of people are infected with STH infections. The greatest number of cases of STH infections currently occurs in sub-Saharan

Africa, Asia, and the tropical regions of the Americas. Poverty is a key element for ensuring high levels of transmission, most likely because propagation of the parasite life cycle requires human feces containing parasite eggs to be deposited on the soil rather than in areas with latrines and other sanitary measures in place. Another key element is the link between STH transmission and rural surroundings. STH infections, especially hookworm, occur predominantly in areas of intense agriculture in the setting of promiscuous defecation. However, ascariasis and trichuriasis have also been well described in extremely poor urban areas such as the slums of large cities in developing countries.[20] Two other important STH infections are zoonoses. Toxocariasis is the major cause of visceral and ocular larva migrans and results from the accidental ingestion of canine roundworm eggs, while cysticercosis is platyhelminth infection that results from the accidental ingestion of eggs from the pork tapeworm, *Taenia solium*.

Generally speaking, the STH infections are not considered serious infections of adult travelers and individuals participating in expeditions. More than any other group, school-aged children are considered the most susceptible to high-worm burdens leading to serious disease (e.g., intestinal obstruction for heavy *ASCARIS* infections, colitis and dysentery for heavy *Trichuris* infections, and severe anemia and malnutrition for heavy hookworm infections).[19] These conditions occur mostly in children from poor families who are chronically exposed to eggs and larvae in the environment. The behavioral or physiologic basis for children experiencing heavy worm burdens compared to other groups is unknown.

Among short-term travelers who are susceptible to STH infections are military personnel who are engaged either in combat or training with extensive exposure on the ground and who do not have access to adequate sanitation. For instance, following the U.S. invasion of Grenada in 1983, a large percentage of troops from several army units noted signs and symptoms consistent with STH infections including abdominal pain and eosinophilia. Subsequently, hookworm infection was confirmed in thirty-five soldiers and there was one confirmed case of strongyloidiasis.[21] Eosinophilia is a common finding in STH and other human helminth infections in which parasitic larval stages migrate through the tissues.[22] This can persist for several weeks or longer, and it is not unusual to see eosinophilia among refugees, military personnel, and other travelers returning from hookworm-endemic regions.[23,24] In such individuals, it is important to rule out infection caused by *Strongyloides stercoralis*, which can persist for years through a process known as autoinfection.[25] There are well-documented cases of *Strongyloides* hyperinfection occurring years or even decades following return from an endemic region, especially following the administration of corticosteroids for the treatment of neoplasms or autoimmune disorders.[26]

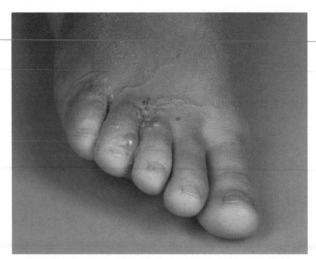

Figure 17.1. Cutaneous larvae migrans. Photo courtesy of J. Dick MacLean, McGill University Centre for Tropical Diseases.

The diagnosis of an STH infection is established by a fecal examination looking for the presence of parasite eggs. Because each female STH produces thousands of eggs per day, a single examination is usually sufficient to establish a diagnosis of ascariasis, trichuriasis, and hookworm infection. Exceptions include human strongyloidiasis for which multiple fecal exams must be obtained in order to identify first-stage larvae, together with an enzyme-linked immunosorbent assay (ELISA)-based serologic assay,[25] and toxocariasis, which also requires an ELISA-based serologic assay. Except for strongyloidiasis, albendazole or mebendazole are the treatments of choice for the major STH infections.[19] Because albendazole is metabolized to a derivative that achieves a high volume of distribution in the tissues, this agent is the recommended treatment for toxocariasis. Ivermectin is the treatment of choice for strongyloidiasis[25,26].

Cutaneous larva migrans (CLM) (Figure 17.1) is a common condition among travelers and participants in expeditions, particularly in coastal areas where zoonotic hookworm larvae may be present in the sandy soils of beaches contaminated with dog and cat feces. CLM occurs most commonly when infective larvae of the hookworm *Ancylostoma braziliense* burrow into the skin at the site of entry and then migrate laterally in the epidermis. This results in serpiginous tracks appearing on the feet, hands, abdomen, and buttocks.[27] Oral albendazole or ivermectin are the treatments of choice, although topical thiabendazole can also be used.

FOOD-BORNE TROPICAL DISEASES

Enteric Fever

Enteric fever is a systemic illness caused by the invasive pathogens *Salmonella* serotype *typhi* or *paratyphi*. As with other organisms from the genus *Salmonella*, the *typhi* and *paratyphi* serotypes are distributed worldwide in areas of poor sanitation and unsafe water supplies and are transmitted by the fecal–oral route from contaminated food or water. The inoculum size is estimated to be approximately 10^7–10^9 organisms, and this has been verified in animal models and human volunteer studies of typhoid vaccines. Unlike other *Salmonella* infections, *S. typhi* and *S. paratyphi* infections are confined to humans.

After they are ingested, the organisms multiply in the gastrointestinal tract, particularly in the small bowel. *S. typhi* does not cause mucosal damage, but it does multiply in Peyer's patches, regional lymph nodes and subsequently disseminates to the bloodstream. Organisms can seed other body sites, particularly the reticuloendothelial system (liver, spleen), and rarely may seed the central nervous system and other organs.

Enteric fever presents as an acute febrile illness with symptoms of fever, headache, fatigue, nausea, and vomiting. Diarrhea may be present early in the course of illness but has usually resolved by the time patients seek medical attention. Illness with *S. paratyphi* may be less severe than that caused by *S. typhi*. Initial examination often reveals a relative bradycardia or pulse–temperature dissociation. An evanescent macular rash (rose spots) is notable in 10–15% of patients with enteric fever. Hepatomegaly and splenomegaly are seen in 50 and 35%, respectively. Lymphadenopathy is less common. Severe enteric fever is also associated with significant alterations in mental status with confusion, prostration, and coma. Mortality from enteric fever may be as high as 30% in acutely ill hospitalized patients. Some individuals may remain persistent carriers, especially in those with underlying gallbladder disease.

Diagnosis is made by recovery of *S. typhi* or *S. paratyphi* in culture of blood, urine, or stool. Bone marrow and small intestinal aspirates give perhaps the highest yields. Serologic tests such as the Widal test or febrile agglutinins are less specific, particularly if there has been prior immunization.

Treatment of enteric fever is dependent on antimicrobial sensitivity. Resistance to doxycycline, trimethoprim/sulfamethoxazole, and chloramphenicol (multidrug resistance) is quite common. Recent emergence of ciprofloxacin (and other fluoroquinolones) resistance in Southeast Asia and the Indian subcontinent has also developed. Some isolates appear sensitive to ciprofloxacin on Kirby Bauer testing but have increased minimum inhibitory concentrations. Nalidixic acid resistance seems to be the best marker to identify these strains, which in some series may represent up to 50% of isolates.[86] These resistant strains are best treated with ceftriaxone or cefotaxime.

Two preparations of *S. typhi* vaccine are currently available, an oral live-attenuated Ty21a vaccine and a capsular Vi polysaccharide vaccine.[87] Efficacy rates range from 65 to 95%, with the variance related to the degree of water contamination and the inoculum size in the region of exposure. For example, the efficacy of the oral Ty21a vaccine was 95% in Alexandria, Egypt,[88] but only 66% in Santiago, Chile.[89] The oral vaccine is given on alternate days for four doses, needs refrigeration, and cannot be taken with concomitant oral antibiotics. It should theoretically not be administered in pregnancy or to immunocompromised hosts. Both vaccines are well tolerated. Either vaccine should be administered several weeks prior to departure to allow for the development of immunity, and booster immunization should be given every 3 years.

Brucellosis

Brucellosis is a chronic granulomatous infection cased by intracellular bacteria of the genus *Brucella*, especially *Brucella melitensis* in developing countries where goats are the principal reservoir. In the United States, brucellosis is a zoonosis from cattle, caused by *B. abortus*. Brucellosis is one of the most common zoonoses, and annually there are more than 500,000 new cases worldwide.[28] Currently, Syria has the highest annual incidence, but the infection is common elsewhere in the Middle East, with large numbers of cases observed in Turkey, Oman, Saudi Arabia, the United Arab Emirates, and Jordan.[28] High incidence rates of brucellosis also occur in the Central Asian republics of the former Soviet Union, Mongolia, China, and India, as well as North Africa.[28] In Latin America, high rates of infection occur in Mexico, Peru, and Argentina.[28] Brucellosis also occurs in sub-Saharan Africa, but there is very little known about its incidence there.

In developing countries, brucellosis classically occurs following ingestion of contaminated dairy products, including nonpasteurized goat milk and cheese. It is believed that hard cheese, yogurt, and sour milk are less hazardous,[29] possibly because the acids produced during fermentation are bactericidal. Human infection results in fever, which can be spiking and accompanied by rigors, and often with malodorous perspiration (29). Anemia and leukopenia are common. Bacteremia is frequently present and often accompanied by lymphadenopathy and hepatosplenomegaly. In its chronic form, arthritis is extremely common. Peripheral arthritis is the most common and typically involves the knees, hips, ankles, and wrists, while sacroiliitis is the second most common form of arthritis, followed by spondylitis.[29] In men, epididymo-orchitis is common, and brucellosis in pregnancy is associated with poor fetal outcome. Other complications can include hepatitis, meningitis, and endocarditis.

Brucellosis is diagnosed by isolating the bacterium from the blood or bone marrow, although the sensitivity of recovering the organism is not always high. Serum agglutination is still used, with titers above 1:160 considered diagnostic in an appropriate clinical setting,[29] with newer ELISA and PCR (polymerase chain reaction) techniques under development and early clinical use. Antibiotic treatment requires agents that exhibit activity in an intracellular environment.[29] The World Health Organization recommends use of doxycycline for a period of 6 weeks in combination with either streptomycin (for 2–3 weeks) or rifampin (for 6 weeks). Because doxycycline is contraindicated in pregnancy and in young children, rifampin is the drug of choice, possibly in combination with either an aminoglycoside or trimethoprim/sulfamethoxazole.

Food-borne Trematodiases

The major human food-borne trematode infections include clonorchiasis and opisthorchiasis (liver fluke), fascioliasis (liver fluke), fasciolopsiasis (intestinal fluke), and paragonimiasis (lung fluke). Approximately 20 million people are infected with liver flukes. Clonorchiasis caused by *Clonorchis sinensis* occurs in China, Korea, and Southeast Asia, while opisthorchiasis caused by *Opisthorchis viverrini* occurs predominantly in Thailand, and *O. felineus* occurs in Russia. Transmission occurs by ingestion of uncooked fish. Chronic heavy infections result in abdominal pain, liver enlargement, and weight loss, as well as recurrent ascending cholangitis. There is also an epidemiological association between chronic liver fluke infections and cholangiocarcinoma. Fascioliasis is endemic to parts of Latin America, Africa, the Middle East, and South Asia.

Paragonimiasis also occurs in approximately 20 million people, with the greatest number of cases in China, Taiwan, Korea, and the Philippines where it is caused predominantly by *Paragonimus westermani*. Transmission occurs by ingestion of uncooked crab or crayfish. Pleuropulmonary paragonimiasis from *P. westermani* infection is associated with cough, chest pain, and hemoptysis. *P. skrjabini* also occurs in East Asia and is associated with larva migrans, whereas *P. mexicanus* causes pulmonary infection in Peru and Ecuador, and *P. uterobilateralis* and *P. africanus* are prevalent in Cameroon.

Fasciolopsiasis is caused by *Fasciolopsis buski* and is endemic to East Asia, as well as India and Bangladesh. Transmission occurs by ingestion of uncooked aquatic vegetation and results in enteritis. Most fluke infections are treated with praziquantel, with the exception of fascioliasis for which the drug of choice is triclabendazole.

Taeniasis

Human tapeworm infections caused by *Taenia solium* and *T. saginata* occur through ingestion of uncooked or undercooked contaminated pork and beef, respectively. Although the adult tapeworms grow to enormous lengths, up to 2–4 meters, in the human gut, they

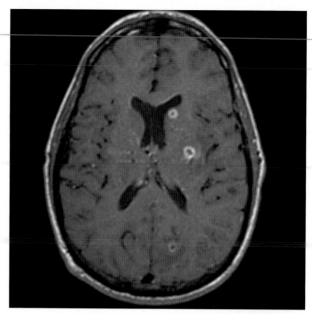

Figure 17.2. Neurocystocercosis. Photo courtesy of David Parenti.

cause minimal symptoms, either acutely or chronically. *T. solium* infection is found in developing countries wherever humans live in proximity with pigs, particularly in East Asia, Africa, and Latin America. Far more severe are the consequences that arise when humans serve as accidental intermediate hosts and ingest *T. solium* eggs transmitted by fecal–oral contact from tapeworm-infected carriers. Onchospheres liberated from the ingested eggs invade the muscles and brain where they cause remarkably little inflammation while viable. However, after the parasites die and degenerate they lose their antigen-masking abilities, and the resulting host inflammation sets off a seizure focus. The exact clinical manifestations of neurocystocercosis (Figure 17.2) are a function of the individual differences in the number, size, and topography of the cysts in the brain,[30] however, classically the patient presents with epilepsy.

Diagnosis is usually made through neuroimaging by either MRI or CT, with confirmation by a positive serology. The enzyme-linked immunotransfer blot has a high specificity, although the sensitivity is low in patients with only a single brain cyst. In an optimal setting, the treatment of complex neurocystocercosis with subarachnoid or ventricular lesions requires a multidisciplinary approach involving both medical and surgical specialists. A single parenchymal cyst is typically managed medically with anticonvulsants and corticosteroids; the role of antiparasitic therapy with albendazole or praziquantel is controversial because it is believed that the larval parasite might already be dying or dead.

Typhoid Fever

See previous discussion in section "Enteric Fever."

WATERBORNE TROPICAL DISEASES

Fenwick[31] estimates that approximately 15% of the world's population lives in areas of so-called *water stress* (i.e., impoverished areas where people conduct a daily struggle for access to safe and clean water for drinking, cooking, and washing). Adding even further to water stress in many developing regions of the world are large water resource development projects such as dams including the Gezira Scheme in Sudan, the High Dam on the Nile at Aswan, and dams on the Senegal and Volta Rivers, which have done much to promote the emergence of waterborne tropical diseases, especially schistosomiasis.[31] There are concerns that the Three Gorges Dam in China could create a similar situation.[32,33]

Amebiasis

Our knowledge about the actual number of people infected each year with invasive amebiasis is confused because of recent evidence that the organism formerly known as *Entamoeba histolytica* has been reclassified into three morphologically identical amebae: *E. histolytica*, the etiologic agent of classical amebiasis, and two nonpathogenic amebae, *E. dispar* and *E. moshkovskii*.[34] Invasive disease caused by *E. histolytica* is one of the most common tropical diseases in returning travelers. Asymptomatic colonization can occur with *E. histolytica* infection, although this usually occurs from *E. dispar* infection.

The two major disease syndromes caused by *E. histolytica* are intestinal and extraintestinal amebiasis. Intestinal amebiasis is characterized by amebic dysentery and colitis. Amebic colitis presents with a history of several weeks of gradually worsening abdominal pain and tenderness, diarrhea, and bloody stools.[34] About half of these patients exhibit weight loss, although fever occurs in only about 10%. The most common manifestation of extraintestinal amebiasis is amebic liver abscess (Figure 17.3), which occurs more commonly in males. Classical signs and symptoms of amebic liver abscess include fever, right upper quadrant pain, elevated transaminases, and leukocytosis. Many such patients do not have a history of amebic colitis and they may not have amebae present on stool examination.[34] Increasingly, specific diagnostic tests are replacing the classical methods of microscopic examination of feces and liver aspirates. These include a stool antigen detection test (a commercial test is available from TechLab, Inc., Blacksburg, VA) for intestinal amebiasis, and an indirect hemeagglutination (IHA) test for antiamebic antibody, together with liver imaging (e.g., ultrasound, CT, and MRI) in patients with amebic liver abscess.[34] Invasive amebiasis should be treated with metronidazole together with a luminal agent.

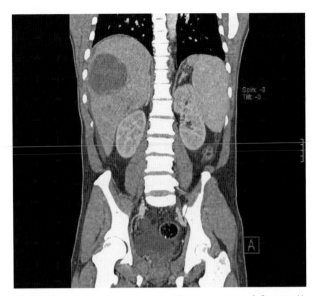

Figure 17.3. Amebic liver abscess. Photo courtesy of Gregory H. Bledsoe.

Buruli Ulcer

Buruli ulcer (Figure 17.4) is a cutaneous infection that occurs predominantly among children living in humid rural tropical areas of sub-Saharan Africa (especially West Africa) and elsewhere.[35] The infection is caused by *Mycobacterium ulcerans*, which produces a toxin called mycolactone that results in tissue necrosis and produces a painless but large and highly disfiguring ulcer, usually on the limbs. It is believed that humans come into contact with the organism in water, possibly in association with biofilms on the surface of aquatic insects.[35] A diagnosis of Buruli ulcer is established through laboratory culture of *M. ulcerans* or staining for acid-fast bacilli. Recently, a PCR test has been developed. Treatment has traditionally required surgical excision of visibly affected tissue, but because of high relapse rates there is now a trend to also examine the role of antibiotics such as rifampin together with an aminoglycoside (e.g., streptomycin or amikacin).[35]

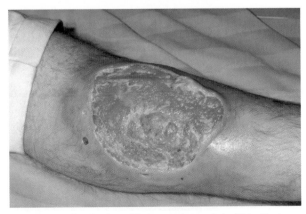

Figure 17.4. Buruli ulcer. Photo courtesy of J. Dick MacLean, McGill University Centre for Tropical Diseases.

Cholera

See discussion in Chapter 25.

Dracunculiasis

Prior to the 1980s, guinea worm infection was a major waterborne scourge of sub-Saharan Africa, the Middle East, and India. The infection is associated with the presence of a large nematode, *Dracunculus medinensis*, living in the subcutaneous tissues of the extremities (Figure 17.5). Adult female *D. medinensis* can grow to a length of 1 m, which produces a disfiguring ulcer in order to allow its progeny exit out of the body and into water. The ulcer and the secondary infection that accompany chronic infection cause incapacity and lost economic productivity.[31] Through an aggressive campaign led by the World Health Organization and the Carter Center global efforts are in place to filter water for removal of the *Cyclops* intermediate host together with health education efforts. As a result, the infection has been nearly eradicated, and today, fewer than 16,000 cases remain, mostly in Sudan, Ghana, and Nigeria.[31] At this current pace, the global eradication of guinea worm infection is forecasted within the coming decade.

Leptospirosis

Leptospirosis is a bacterial zoonotic disease caused by indirect contact with water or soil contaminated with urine from animals, especially rodents, infected with *Leptospira spp.* The infection is found throughout regions of the tropics and subtropics with heavy rainfall (e.g., sub-Saharan Africa, Central and South America, India, China, and Southeast Asia), where it is commonly associated with water-related activities and occupations.[36,37] Urban epidemics also occur,[14] particularly in slums and other pockets of urban poverty. Even though leptospirosis may be the world's most common zoonosis, the disease is vastly underreported.[14] The disease is considered an

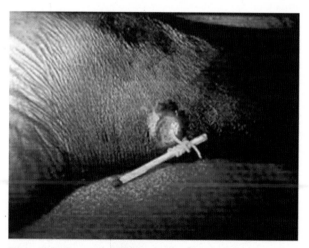

Figure 17.5. Emergent guinea worm wrapped around a matchstick. Photo courtesy of Herman Zaiman.

important hazard for adventure travelers; for instance, it was found among athletes returning home from the 2000 EcoChallenge in Malaysian Borneo,[38] and it was a significant problem associated with contaminated surface waters in Hawaii.[14]

Two distinct syndromes result from leptospirosis. The first is a mild febrile illness associated with high fever, chills, headache, and conjunctival suffusion. This phase is followed by the appearance of leptospira in the urine sometimes accompanied by rash, uveitis, and aseptic meningitis. A second form of the illness is known as icteric leptospirosis (also known as Weil's disease), a hemorrhagic illness associated with liver dysfunction or failure and jaundice, renal insufficiency, myocarditis, shock, and thrombocytopenia. Pulmonary hemorrhage is also emerging as an important yet previously unrealized clinical feature.[14] Icteric leptospirosis has a high mortality. Because most laboratories do not have the capability of culturing leptospira from urine and other fluids, it is more common to diagnose the illness by a serological agglutination test. Treatment requires antibiotics early in the illness either with doxycycline, penicillin, or cephalosporin.[39] Jarisch-Herxheimer-type reactions are commonly seen after initiating treatment.[37] Supportive measures including intensive care monitoring are often required for icteric leptospirosis. To better track this disease, there have been calls for the development of an international registry of cases.[14]

Schistosomiasis

Schistosomiasis is the most important waterborne helminth infection of humans and a major tropical disease of the adventure traveler. Approximately 180 million to 200 million cases occur worldwide, resulting in approximately 280,000 deaths annually. *Schistosoma haematobium* is the cause of urinary schistosomiasis and the predominant schistosome of sub-Saharan Africa; *S. mansoni* causes intestinal and hepatic schistosomiasis, mostly occurring in Africa and Brazil; and *S. japonicum* causes intestinal and hepatic schistosomiasis in China and the Philippines. *S. mekongi* and *S. intercalatum* are minor schistosomes of Southeast Asia and Africa, respectively. The infection occurs by contact with the cercarial stages (which can cause a cercarial dermatitis known as "swimmers' itch") in fresh water where appropriate snail intermediate hosts live. Both acute and chronic forms of schistosomiasis have been described.

Acute Schistosomiasis

Also known as Katayama fever, acute schistosomiasis is a disease that resembles serum sickness. The illness typically begins within 2–12 weeks following initial contact with cercariae, and coincides with the deposition of eggs into host tissues.[33] The condition is characterized by fever, hepatosplenomegaly, lymphadenopathy, interstitial pneumonitis, and eosinophilia, occurring with the highest frequency from infection by either *Schistosoma japonicum* or *S. mansoni*. Symptoms include fever and chills, cough, and headache.[40] This condition is particularly important for the adventure traveler because it occurs most commonly in new visitors to an endemic region, especially Africa. Swimming in Lake Malawi, Lake Kariba, and the Zambezi River has notoriety as an important risk factor for acute schistosomiasis among travelers.[33] Death can result from heavy infections. Transverse myelitis and other signs and symptoms of central nervous system egg deposition have also been described.[33] Diagnosis of Katayama fever is a challenge because schistosome eggs may not yet appear in the feces until after the peak onset of symptoms. For this reason, it is necessary to have a high index of suspicion to obtain serologic testing in order to establish a firm diagnosis.

Chronic Intestinal and Hepatic Schistosomiasis

Chronic *S. mansoni* and *S. japonicum* are major causes of intestinal fibrosis and hepatosplenomegaly. The greatest worm burdens occur among school-aged children and adolescents, peaking in the 15- to 20-year-old age group.[40] Symptoms include colicky hypogastric pain, and diarrhea with blood in the feces.[33] Hepatosplenomegaly and intestinal fibrosis occur because of granulomatous inflammation surrounding eggs in the intestine and liver. Chronic heavy infections among pediatric populations result in physical and intellectual growth retardation. For that reason, mass drug administration with praziquantel has been recommended for school-aged children living in endemic regions.[41]

Chronic Urinary Schistosomiasis

Chronic *S. haematobium* infection is a major cause of hematuria and bladder fibrosis. Long-term infection can produce an obstructive uropathy leading to renal failure or squamous cell carcinoma of the bladder. In women, *S. haematobium* commonly causes vulval and perineal disease, which can also facilitate the transmission of HIV/AIDS.[33] Like *S. mansoni* and *S. japonicum* infections, chronic pediatric infections with *S. haematobium* also result in physical and intellectual growth retardation. A diagnosis of schistosomiasis is based on the detection of schistosome eggs in either the feces (*S. mansoni* and *S. japonicum*) or urine (*S. haematobium*). Praziquantel is the treatment of choice, and reexamination is recommended one month after treatment.[33]

PERSON–PERSON OR ANIMAL–PERSON DIRECT CONTACT

Anthrax

Anthrax is caused by a gram-positive spore forming bacillus, *Bacillus anthracis*. The infection is transmitted by spores that are long-lived and relatively resistant to

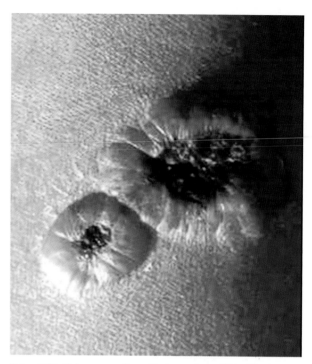

Figure 17.6. Cutaneous anthrax. Photo courtesy of Brian Ward, McGill University Centre for Tropical Diseases.

heat and chemical agents. Two toxins, edema factor and lethal factor, are important in pathogenesis. The anthrax spores are usually found in soil or animal hides. Human infection occurs most often following exposure to animal hides or other products, or by ingestion of contaminated meat. Farmers, veterinarians, and butchers are at particular risk. *B. anthracis* usually enters un-intact skin. After an incubation of from 1–12 days, a small papule begins and then progresses to a vesicle and then to a necrotic ulcer with a black eschar (Figure 17.6).[42,43] The lesion is usually painless and is frequently associated with substantial surrounding edema. Systemic symptoms include fever, malaise, headache, and regional lymphadenopathy. The mortality untreated is 20%.

Anthrax can also occur by ingestion of contaminated meat.[44] This form leads to ulcerated lesions in the oral cavity and gastrointestinal tract. Cervical and submandibular lymph node swelling is noted, again with substantial surrounding edema. Abdominal pain, gastrointestinal hemorrhage, and rarely intestinal obstruction develop. In this form, the mortality may reach 60%. Inhalational anthrax usually occurs in an industrial setting where spore aerosolization can take place. This has also been seen following inhalation associated with a bioterrorism event. The mortality of inhalational anthrax is 80%.

The diagnosis of anthrax is made by isolating the organism from standard aerobic culture. The laboratory should be alerted about the possibility of anthrax as a clinical diagnosis. Treatment has been successful with doxycycline, ciprofloxacin, and penicillin.[42] Rifampin may also be helpful to decrease toxin production in severe disease. Prolonged antibiotic prophylaxis has also been used for inhalational exposures. An inactivated vaccine made from adsorbed culture filtrate is relatively effective. It is not widely available and takes 18 months to complete the primary immunization series.[45]

Leprosy

Leprosy is a chronic granulomatous infection caused by *Mycobacterium leprae*. It multiplies slowly and affects cooler tissues such as skin, peripheral nerves, eyes, and testes. It is probably transmitted person-to-person; humans and the nine-banded armadillo are the only known reservoirs. Leprosy is found worldwide, particularly in developing countries. It is estimated that there are approximately 400,000 cases worldwide, but this reflects a dramatic decrease from the 5 million cases in 1985, and is reflective of the World Health Assembly's elimination program.[1,7] There are still pockets of high endemnicity in some areas of Angola, Brazil, Central African Republic, Democratic Republic of Congo, India, Madagascar, Mozambique, Nepal, and Tanzania (*http://www.who.int/lep/en*). Although only 6,000 deaths from leprosy occur each year, there is substantial morbidity, disfigurement, social isolation, and loss of productivity.[7]

The incubation period for leprosy is estimated to be 5 years or more, and the nature of the illness is dependent on the individual's immune response to the bacterium. Paucibacillary disease (indeterminate, tuberculoid, borderline tuberculoid) is characterized by an active granulomatous response with limited numbers (≤ 5) of mycobacteria in skin smears or biopsies, and reflects a competent cell-mediated immune response.[43,46] In multibacillary disease (borderline, borderline lepromatous, lepromatous), there is an ineffective immune response with large numbers of organisms packed into macrophage vesicles. In this form, skin smears demonstrate more organisms (> 5), and organisms may be detected in nasal secretions and bone marrow.

The typical skin lesion in paucibacillary disease is an anesthetic hypopigmented macule, of varying size that can occur on any skin surface.[43,46] There may be one or several lesions identified by close inspection. In this form, there may also be isolated involvement of cutaneous nerves such as the dorsalis pedis, lateral peroneal, and greater auricular nerves, which may be palpable. Rarely acute inflammatory reactions involving motor nerves can lead to paralysis, and this is somewhat more common after initiation of therapy (reversal reaction). In multibacillary disease, the lesions are nodular, teeming with bacteria, and widely distributed. Bacilli can also be found in cutaneous nerves leading to sensory loss in the hands and feet. This insensitivity, seen in both paucibacillary and multibacillary disease, leads to repeated trauma, infection, and subsequent loss of digits or limbs.

The diagnosis of leprosy is made by Fite-stained skin smears or skin biopsies that demonstrate the organism. The organism has been cultured in mouse foot pads or armadillos. Since 1981, treatment has consisted of multidrug therapy (MDT) with dapsone, rifampin, and clofazimine.[46] Since 1995, the WHO has provided free MDT for all patients in the world, initially through the Nippon Foundation and since 2000 through the Novartis Foundation for Sustainable Development (*http://www.who.int/mediacentre/factsheets/fs101/en*). Paucibacillary patients are treated for 6 months, and in the United States may be treated with dapsone and rifampin only. Multibacillary patients are treated for 12 months with all three drugs. Drug resistance has not been established. Surgical intervention may be necessary to acutely decompress swollen motor nerves or to treat infection or other disabilities. The Bacille Camette-Guerin vaccine has been tried for prevention in multiple clinical trials, but at best it is only partially protective.[7]

Endemic Treponematoses

The human treponemal (spirochetal) infections include yaws (*T. pallidum pertenue*), pinta (*T. carateum*), bejel or endemic syphilis (*T. pallidum endemicum*), and venereal syphilis (*T. pallidum pallidum*).[47,48] The global burden is estimated to be approximately 25 million cases, the majority of which occur in sub-Saharan Africa and Asia. These subspecies are morphologically indistinguishable and appear as corkscrew-shaped rods on darkfield examination of skin lesions. They cannot be grown in vitro and must be injected into rabbit testes for growth. Although they have somewhat different geographical distributions and clinical presentations, they may not be distinguished by serologic testing. Transmission is person-to-person. All of the treponemal infections begin with a primary lesion, followed by secondary dissemination of the organism to other areas of skin, periosteum and bone. Late or tertiary disease involving skin and bone can also occur. Treatment is with penicillin, tetracycline, or erythromycin.

Yaws is a disfiguring childhood infection that occurs in warm, humid tropical regions of Africa,[43,47,48] Central America, the Caribbean, and the equatorial islands of Southeast Asia. It is endemic in areas where hygiene is poor and large areas of the body surface are exposed. The causative organism, *T. pallidum pertenue*, is transmitted to traumatized skin by direct personal contact or contact with wound exudates. The primary lesion or "mother yaw" appears as a papule that enlarges over a period of several months. Secondary lesions are large and nodular in character, and painful lesions often involve the palms and soles. Painful bony lesions causing dactylitis or periostitis may also occur. In late stages, destructive mucocutaneous lesions of the face can be quite disfiguring (gangosa). Treatment of case contacts, and entire populations in endemic areas, are important control strategies (*http://www.searo.who.int/en/Section10/Section2134_10824.htm*).

Pinta is a disease of young adults in the Americas caused by *T. carateum*.[43,47] Its current distribution is in southern Mexico and the Amazon River basin. It also begins as a primary papule on the face or extremities. As the lesion enlarges over several months, it transforms into an irregular bluish-brown, scaly plaque, up to 10 cm in diameter. Secondary lesions may occur at multiple skin sites, occasionally with lymph node enlargement. In the late stages, the lesions become hyperkeratotic and hypopigmented, but there is no bony involvement. A single dose of benzathine penicillin G, 2.4 million units intramuscularly is curative.

Bejel or endemic syphilis, caused by *T. pallidum endemicum*, is a disease of children living in arid regions among nomadic families on the Arabian Peninsula and on the southern border of the Sahara desert.[43,47] The initial lesions are mucous patches in the oral cavity. Dissemination leads to moist papules at multiple skin sites, especially in the axillae and skin folds, and can involve the palms and soles. In late stage disease, mucocutaneous and bony involvement is more common than with yaws.

Echinococcosis

Cystic echinococcosis or hydatid disease is a zoonosis caused by *Echinococcus granulosus*. An estimated 285,000 cases occur worldwide, with the greatest increase in cases seen in Eastern Europe and the former Soviet republics.[49] Hydatid disease, like many neglected tropical diseases, is a condition of impoverished people, and not commonly seen among travelers or among expedition adventurers. Infection is acquired by ingesting *E. granulosus* eggs through fecal–oral contact from dogs, which serve as the definitive host. The infection is often asymptomatic. However, when hydatid cysts become large enough, usually either in the liver (Figure 17.7) or lung, they can cause right upper quadrant pain, nausea, and

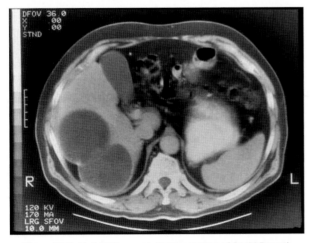

Figure 17.7. Hydatid liver cyst. Photo courtesy of David Parenti.

vomiting, or cough, dyspnea, and hemoptysis, respectively. Treatment requires an interdisciplinary approach sometimes involving both medical management with the drug albendazole and/or surgical management with percutaneous puncture (using sonographic guidance), aspiration of the cyst contents, injection of a scolicidal agent, and re-aspiration (PAIR).

VECTOR-BORNE TRANSMISSION

The "tropical medicine niche," or those infections prevalent in a given area, is frequently dependent on the microclimate and the availability of the vector adapted to the transmission of that particular pathogen. Vector-borne illness is distributed throughout the developing world, particularly in tropical climates. Seasonality may be evident, particularly for mosquito-borne illness. Breeding of mosquitoes and hence transmission of mosquito-borne illness may be influenced by rainfall, temperature, and altitude. Specific ecological locations for other vectors include the forest canopy (Chrysops fly, loiasis), fast moving streams or rivers (black fly, onchocerciasis), or savanna (tsetse fly, trypanosomiasis). Essential to the control of vector-borne transmission is control of the vector itself, either on an environmental level or on a personal level with the use of insect repellents and protective clothing or bed nets.

Mosquitoes

Mosquitoes are the vector for transmission of a variety of infectious diseases of public health importance. These infections include protozoan infections (malaria), helminths (lymphatic filariasis) and Flavivirus infections (yellow fever, dengue, Japanese encephalitis, West Nile virus). There is a wide range of species specificity for the individual pathogens, and different species preferentially grow in specific ecological niches. The *Anopheles* mosquito is the sole transmitter of all four species of malaria, *Culex* transmits Japanese encephalitis, and *Aedes* mosquitoes can transmit dengue, yellow fever, and other viruses. Lymphatic filariasis is primarily transmitted by *Culex* mosquitoes, but can also be transmitted by *Anopheles* and *Aedes* species. Mosquito eggs are deposited in water where subsequent development to larvae, pupae, and adults occurs. Each species of mosquito breeds in a specific ecological niche, whether it be a stagnant pool, saltwater marsh, or a container containing small amounts of water. Modification of the environment to control specific vectors therefore requires a thorough understanding of vector ecology and biology. See Chapter 26 for a thorough discussion of malaria.

Yellow Fever

Transmission of yellow fever continues throughout the tropics of sub-Saharan Africa and South America, with an estimated 200,000 cases each year and an estimated

30,000 deaths.[50] Transmission of yellow fever tends to occur during periods of peak rainfall, in both an urban and a sylvatic (jungle) form, where monkeys are the primary reservoir.[51,53] In Africa, transmission occurs in moist savanna and tropical zones in West and Central Africa (> 30 countries) including recent outbreaks in Cote d'Ivoire, Guinea, Mali, and southern Sudan.[54] Transmission is highest during the rainy season, and can occur in urban areas as well. The major vector of urban yellow fever, *Aedes aegypti*, has become increasingly prevalent in urban areas. In Latin America, the majority of sylvatic yellow fever transmission occurs in the countries comprising the Amazon River basin: Brazil, Bolivia, Peru, Ecuador, Colombia, and Venezuela. Transmission occurs when non-immune hosts enter the forest or are in close proximity.

Transmission in urban areas is by *Aedes aegypti*, where peridomestic containers (e.g., flower pots, tires, water collection containers) collect water and provide optimal breeding sites. Other *Aedes* and "tree-hole breeding" *Haemagogus* mosquitoes transmit yellow fever in forest areas. Extensive control programs have substantially decreased transmission in urban areas. The Centers for Disease Control and Prevention (CDC) has designated certain countries as yellow fever endemic zones, and travel to (and sometimes through) these areas may necessitate immunization.[50]

The hallmarks of yellow fever are hepatitis, a hemorrhagic diathesis, and renal disease.[53] After injection of the virus during the blood meal of the mosquito, there is an incubation period of 3–6 days. In some individuals, infection may be asymptomatic or cause only mild disease (5–50%). The syndrome begins with the abrupt onset of fever, headache, and myalgias. It progresses to abdominal pain, nausea and vomiting, and severe lethargy, prostration, and altered mental status. Infection subsequently leads to jaundice, coagulopathy, severe dehydration and hypotension, and renal failure. Bleeding may occur in the gastrointestinal tract, skin, kidney, and multiple other organs. There is currently only supportive therapy, and mortality of the full blown syndrome may be as high as 35–50%. Laboratory features include leukopenia, elevated transaminases and bilirubin, disseminated intravascular coagulation, and proteinuria and renal failure. Direct person-to-person transmission does not occur in contrast to other hemorrhagic fever viruses, and there has been no evidence for chronic hepatitis following recovery. The diagnosis is made serologically using a variety of tests such as the IgM-capture ELISA.[53]

A live-attenuated vaccine for yellow fever (17D–204 strain) was first licensed in the United States in 1953 and is manufactured in embryonated hens' eggs (see Chapter 4).[50–52,55,56] The vaccine is almost 100% effective, with booster doses required every 10 years. Yellow fever vaccine is recommended for individuals traveling to yellow fever endemic areas. Many countries will also require immunization for entry if you have previously traveled through a yellow fever endemic country. Vaccine is administered at CDC-approved yellow fever vaccination centers, where a yellow immunization card is issued stamped with the official stamp. If not adequately immunized, the traveler risks quarantine for 2 weeks in the destination airport or immunization on site. Those with a significant contraindication to immunization may obtain a waiver letter by their physician stating this, and this is usually sufficient. The CDC also recommends obtaining a waiver from the embassy or consulate as well. As it is a live virus vaccine, immunocompromised hosts and pregnant women may be immunized if the risks of acquiring yellow fever outweigh the risks of the vaccine. Those with significant impairment of the immune response may not develop adequate immunologic responses. As it is made in embryonated eggs, those with severe egg allergies should not be immunized.

Dengue

Dengue fever or "breakbone fever" is a common tropical viral illness caused by the dengue virus. Four immunologically distinct dengue viruses (types 1–4) make up the dengue virus group, a member of the Flavivirus family. The distribution of dengue closely approximates that of the major vector *Aedes aegypti*, although *Aedes albopictus* has become an increasingly important vector in the western hemisphere.[51,57]

The incubation period is 3–8 days, and illness begins with the abrupt onset of fever, chills, headache, and back pain.[57] A transient maculopapular rash may be seen in the first 1–2 days. The individual then develops severe musculoskeletal pain involving bones and joints, so-called "breakbone fever." There may also be gastrointestinal or respiratory symptoms, anorexia, and malaise. On physical examination, the rash may be evident, with lymphadenopathy, and relative bradycardia. Leukopenia and elevated transaminases may be present as well. The rash may reappear on the third to fifth days.

A minority of patients with dengue fever may go on to develop the dengue hemorrhagic fever (DHF) syndrome. This occurs more commonly in children than adults and results from prior exposure to one dengue serotype and subsequent exposure to a heterologous strain. DHF is manifested by a coagulopathy and marked capillary-leak syndrome leading to bleeding in multiple organ systems. Illness may progress to altered mental status, shock, and death, and the mortality of the DHF syndrome may reach 50%.

Diagnosis of dengue is made by a variety of serologic tests including the IgM-capture ELISA. Dengue vaccines have been in development for many years but are not commercially available.[55] Prevention is based on vector control programs and the use of insect repellants for travelers to endemic areas.

Japanese Encephalitis

Japanese (B) encephalitis is distributed widely throughout Asia, with an estimated 30,000–50,000 cases annually, and 14,000 deaths.[51,58] The illness has recently increased in incidence in East Asia and the Pacific Islands, with introduction into Australia in 1995 and 1998. Aquatic birds and pigs are major reservoir and amplifying hosts, and the highest prevalence of Japanese encephalitis is in areas where commercial pig farming is common. Seasonal transmission is noted from July to September in more temperate areas but occurs year-round in tropical areas. *Culex tritaeniorhynchus* group mosquitoes are the prime vectors, and flooded rice paddies provide an ideal breeding ground for some species. The risk to standard travelers is estimated to be 1/150,000 person-months of exposure.

Less than 1% of infections result in clinical illness, although older adults apparently have a higher susceptibility to neurovirulence.[56,58] Following transmission by a feeding mosquito, viral replication occurs in regional lymph nodes, followed by viremia and dissemination to multiple organs including the CNS. CNS lesions are distributed throughout the CNS including brainstem, cerebellum, and cerebral cortex. The incubation period is 4–14 days followed by a prodromal phase of fever, malaise, headache, and abdominal pain. Subsequently encephalitis develops over several days, manifested by altered level of consciousness, behavioral changes, ataxia, motor weakness, and seizures. Involuntary movements and extrapyramidal signs are not infrequent.

Laboratory abnormalities include elevation of the WBC and mild transaminase elevation. Cerebral spinal fluid (CSF) pleocytosis is present usually with a lymphocyte predominance. Mortality may be as high as 35% in areas without sophisticated supportive medical services. Long-term neurologic and psychiatric complications are common, developing in an estimated 10–75%. Diagnosis is made by identification of IgM antibody in the CSF.

An inactivated Japanese encephalitis vaccine (see Chapter 4) made from infected mouse brains was licensed in Asia in 1956 and in a number of countries such as Japan, Korea, Taiwan, and China has greatly reduced the incidence of disease.[55,56,58,59] In nonendemic situations, the vaccine is administered subcutaneously on days 0, 7, and 21 (or 0, 7, 14), and 80% will seroconvert after just two immunizations. Booster doses may be administered 2 or more years after the primary series. The decision to immunize is based on location of residence, type of activities, and the possibility of travel to high-risk areas. Adverse effects include local reactions such as pain, redness, or swelling at the vaccine site in 20%, or systemic effects including fever, headache, malaise, and rash in 10%. An alternative live-attenuated vaccine is currently being used in China.

Filarial Infections

Several filiarial species infect man and may be transmitted by different vectors. *Onchocerca volvulus* is transmitted by the simulid or black flies; *Loa loa*, by the *Chrysop* fly; and the agents of lymphatic filariasis, *Wuchereria bancrofti* and *Brugia malayi*, by mosquitoes. Lymphatic filariasis affects over 120 million people in over eighty countries and is a substantial cause of morbidity and loss of economic productivity.[1,4,60,61] Endemic areas for transmission of lymphatic filariasis are located in sub-Saharan Africa, Latin America (Guyana, Brazil, Suriname), Asia, and the Pacific. *W. bancrofti* is worldwide in distribution (90% of cases) and is transmitted by *Culex*, *Anopheles*, and *Aedes* mosquitoes; *B. malayi* (10% of cases) is confined primarily to East and South Asia and is transmitted by species of *Mansonia* and *Anopheles*. The microfilariae are adapted to circulate in the bloodstream when the vectors are most likely to bite. In the case of periodic *W. bancrofti* infection, vectors bite at nighttime, and this is when parasitemia is most likely to occur; in subperiodic *W. bancrofti* or *B. malayi* infection the parasitemia is less variable throughout the day.

Bancroftian Filariasis

Following the injection of infective third-stage larvae by the infected mosquito, worms mature to adults in lymph nodes, particularly in the inguinal region.[62] There lymphatic obstruction eventually leads to severe lymphedema or "elephantiasis" and often hydrocele. This process gradually takes place over months or years and generally requires continued reinfection. It is for this reason that the disease is infrequent in short-term travelers and most commonly seen in individuals living long-term in endemic areas. Severe lymphedema can result, often with superimposed bacterial infections, leading to substantial disability. The adults mate and produce microfilariae, which are a source for continual infection of mosquitoes and a means to make a diagnosis.

Examination of direct or concentrated smears of blood collected during the nighttime or evening demonstrates the characteristic sheathed microfilariae with terminal nuclei not extending to the tip of the tail (*W. bancrofti*) or widely spaced subterminal nuclei (*B. malayi*). Filtration or centrifugation (Knott's) techniques, antigen detection assays, and PCR may also be helpful in circumstances with low parasitemia.[61] Serologic testing using the ICT card (ICT Diagnostics) is also useful particularly in field settings.

Treatment of lymphatic filariasis is most effective in elimination of microfilariae, as adult worms are relatively treatment-resistant.[61,62] Diethylcarbamazine (DEC) and ivermectin (Stromectol, Mectizan) have both been used in individual patients. DEC is given in increasing doses for the first 4 days (14 days total administration) to help reduce the likelihood of treatment-related encephalitis. Ivermectin can be administered as a single dose.

For mass drug administration (MDA) in endemic areas, yearly administration of DEC or ivermectin has contributed to a significant reduction in circulating microfilariae and clinical manifestations.[60] In 1998, Merck expanded the Mectizan Donation Program to provide ivermectin to areas of sub-Saharan Africa also infected with lymphatic filariasis. In 2005, 42 million treatments were approved for distribution to Africa and Yemen through this program, the Global Programme to Eliminate Lymphatic Filariasis.[63] Recent studies have suggested that coadministration of doxycycline, which eradicates *Wohlbachia* bacterial endosymbionts from adult female worms, can greatly extend the period of amicrofilaremia.[60] Prevention focuses on vector control by elimination of mosquito larvae, personal protective measures such as bed nets and insect repellents, and yearly mass treatment of at-risk populations

Black Fly: Onchocerciasis

Onchocerciasis, or river blindness, is a filarial infection caused by *Onchocerca volvulus*. It is distributed throughout west and central Africa, and in areas of Latin America. The black fly, *Simulium damnosum*, is the only vector. Black flies lay eggs along the banks of fast flowing streams, and the density of onchocercal infection is directly proportional to the proximity of these streams. It is this association that has led to its description as "river blindness."

It is estimated that 99% of the 18 million to 37 million people infected with onchocerciasis reside in thirty countries in sub-Saharan Africa.[64] Approximately 1.5 million people have developed visual impairment, and 600,000, blindness. Onchocerciasis is especially prevalent in Cote d'Ivoire, Senegal, Niger, and Cameroon. In Latin America, the disease is found in Venezuela, Colombia, Brazil, Ecuador, Guatemala, and Mexico.

The infectious third-stage larvae are injected by the bite of the fly. These migrate in the subcutaneous space and after several months develop into adult worms. These form nodular lesions, often up to several centimeters in size, and are predominately located over bony prominences such as the hip and scapula.[64] Microfilariae are produced after mating of male and female worms, and the microfilariae are responsible for the attendant symptoms and pathology. The microfilariae circulate through the skin where they incite an inflammatory response comprised of lymphocytes, eosinophils, and fibroblasts, which then leads to dermal fibrosis. Microfilariae also localize to the eye where the cornea is the prime site of involvement, often leading to keratitis, corneal scarring, and blindness.

The diagnosis of onchocerciasis is made by demonstrating microfilariae in "skin snips" (Figure 17.8) or skin biopsies.[64] Skin snips can be performed using a beveled needle and scalpel. The skin fragments are placed under

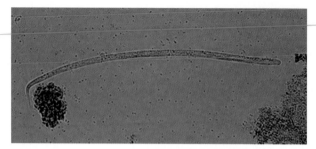

Figure 17.8. Microfilaria of *Onchocerca volvulus*, obtained by skin snip. Photo courtesy of Centers for Disease Control and Prevention.

a coverslip with saline and observed for the movement of microfilariae out of the skin fragment into the surrounding fluid. Microfilariae can also sometimes be demonstrated in the anterior chamber of the eye by slip lamp examination. ELISA and western blot have been used for serologic diagnosis.

Infections are manifested by the development of a diffuse pruritic papular rash involving the trunk and extremities. Chronic infection may lead to lichenification from inflammation and excoriation. Nodules may be apparent in chronic infection located over the bony prominences, but they are less common in acute infection and would be unlikely in travelers or expatriates. In Latin America nodules are often located in the suboccipital region. Ocular disease tends to occur in chronic infection as well, associated with substantial worm burden. Keratitis is the most common manifestation, but uveitis and retinitis may also occur.

Treatment can be accomplished with DEC or ivermectin.[64] There is frequently an exacerbation of the skin rash in response to initial treatment, called the Mazzotti reaction. This may be treated symptomatically with diphenhydramine or corticosteroids. At one time, nodule removal was used in an attempt to decrease worm burden and ameliorate the sequelae of high level microfilariae production. Doxycycline has been shown to eradicate *Wohlbachia* bacterial endosymbionts from adult female worms as well and can also extend the period of amicrofilaremia.[60,65]

Control programs have focused on vector control and mass chemotherapy. Vector control has implemented larvicide spraying and larval habitat management. Relocation of villages from highly endemic riverine areas is a less satisfactory and marginally effective approach. In 1987, The Mectizan Donation Program was initiated by Merck to provide free ivermectin to areas with endemic onchocerciasis. Over 470 million treatments have been provided for mass treatment programs since 1988.[63]

Tabanid Fly: Loiasis

The Tabanid fly or deerfly is the vector for another filarial infection, loiasis. Infection with *Loa loa* is distributed primarily in west and central Africa, particularly the Congo

River basin, and in the rainforest areas of Sudan, Gabon, Angola, and the Democratic Republic of the Congo.[66,67] An estimated 9–70% of individuals in endemic areas are infected. The *Chrysops* fly is the prime vector and is located in forest canopies, and transmission occurs in Africa preferentially where these areas exist. The *Chrysops* fly is a daytime biting vector, and this parasite exhibits daytime periodicity.

After the host is infected, the adult worms migrate throughout the subcutaneous space. The hallmark of loiasis is the presence of subcutaneous swellings, particularly in the distal extremities, so-called Calabar or fugitive swellings. These are felt to be an allergic response to live or dying worms. Adult worms may also migrate in the subconjunctival space where they may be readily visible, much to the dismay of affected patients.

Eosinophilia in loiasis is common and may be as high as 50–70%.[66, 67] Diagnosis is made by examination of direct or concentrated blood smears collected during the daytime hours. Characteristic sheathed microfilariae with terminal nuclei extending to the tip of the tail are demonstrated on smear. Serologic testing may be helpful when microfilaremia is low, but there may also be cross-reactivity with other filarial parasites. Nested-PCR has also been recently developed for diagnosis.

DEC and ivermectin are only microfilaricida and have both been used in the treatment of loiasis with success; however, treatment frequently needs to be periodically repeated.[66] As in lymphatic filariasis, DEC is given in increasing doses for the first 4 days (21 days total administration) to help reduce the likelihood of treatment-related encephalitis. This has also been seen with ivermectin therapy, particularly in patients with high parasitemia.[67] Surgical removal of subconjunctival worms has also been effective. Prevention via vector control has been difficult given the distribution and habits (outdoor biting) of the *Chrysops* fly. Weekly DEC, at a dose of 300 mg q week, has been useful in the prophylactic setting.

Tsetse Fly: African Trypanosomiasis

African trypanosomiasis (sleeping sickness), caused by *Trypanosoma brucei*, is transmitted by the tsetse fly (*Glossina*). In east Africa (*T. b. rhodesiense*) the illness is more acute and virulent in nature, often leading to acute meningoencephalitis. In west and central Africa, the disease is more subacute (*T. b. gambiense*), with gradual change in level of alertness, behavior, and memory.

T. b. rhodesiense (Figure 17.9), the etiology of "Rhodesian" trypanosomiasis is transmitted in savanna areas of eastern and southern Africa, especially southeastern Uganda, Tanzania, Mozambique, and Zambia.[68,69] Here antelope and cattle are the main reservoirs. Disease in cattle is an important obstacle to economic development. *Glossina morsitans* group are the prime vectors. An

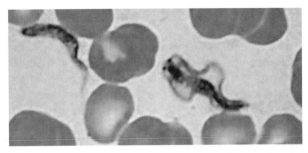

Figure 17.9. Blood smear from a patient who had returned to the United States after visiting Africa. Trypomastigote of *Trypanosoma brucei rhodesiense* is seen. Photo courtesy of Centers for Disease Control and Prevention.

eschar often develops at the site of the tsetse fly bite and is where the initial inoculation occurs. In west and central Africa, "riverine" tsetse flies of the *G. palpalis* group are the main vectors, and they breed in the dense vegetation near rivers and forests. Biting occurs frequently at water sites during the dry season. Current areas of endemnicity are the Congo, southern Sudan, northern Angola and northwestern Uganda. In the early stage of *T. b. gambiense*, infection lymphadenopathy, particularly in the posterior cervical and occipital locations, is an early diagnostic sign (Winterbottom's sign). After several months, patients progress to chronic meningoencephalitis.

Anemia, thrombocytopenia, and hypergammaglobulinemia are common. Definitive diagnosis is made by demonstration of characteristic flagellated trypomastigotes in blood (*T. b. rhodesiense*), CSF (*T. b. rhodesiense*, *T. b. gambiense*), or lymph node aspirate (*T. b. gambiense*).[68] All patients should have a lumbar puncture, with > 5 cells/mm^3 suggesting the presence of CNS disease. Morula or Mott cells can be demonstrated in CSF of both forms of African trypanosomiasis. Serologic testing (ELISA) and PCR may also be helpful. The Card Agglutination Test for Trypanosomiasis (CATT) is a field serologic test that is useful only for *T. b. gambiense* infection.

Pentamidine is the drug of choice for early *T. b. gambiense* infection, given intravenously (preferably) or intramuscularly at 4 mg/kg/day for a total of 7 days.[68,69] It does not penetrate the CNS well enough to be effective treatment for late stage disease. No evidence for resistance has been documented. For neurologic disease, eflornithine, given intravenously every 6 hours for 14 days, is effective. The oral form does not have good bioavailability. The high cost of eflornithine precludes its use in most endemic countries. Melarsoprol, a trivalent arsenical compound, is effective for late stage Gambian trypanosomiasis. Dosing is determined by the degree of CSF pleocytosis. A shortened treatment course of 10 days has recently been shown to be effective.[68,70,71] Side effects are substantial. A reactive encephalopathy with coma and seizures occurs in 4–8% with late stage disease, can develop rapidly, and has 60% mortality. Concurrent administration of corticosteroids is routinely used with melarsoprol therapy, as they substantially decrease the incidence of encephalopathy and improve mortality as well. Other complications include peripheral neuropathy (10%), phlebitis, and fever.

Early-stage *T. b. rhodesiense* infection is treated with suramin, a naphthylurea derivative, and it appears to have better efficacy in this setting than pentamidine.[68] Melarsoprol is the treatment of choice for late-stage disease, as eflornithine has not been proven effective. Encephalopathy is more common and overall mortality during treatment is 5–10%. Dose escalation of melarsoprol may help prevent this side effect. Drugs may be obtained through the Parasitic Disease Drug Service of the CDC (404-639-3670).

Sandfly (Midges, Phlebotomine Flies)

Leishmaniasis

Leishmania are protozoa of the order Kinetoplastida for which man is an incidental host. The organisms are located intracellularly within macrophages in the skin and reticuloendothelial system. They contain a self-replicating organelle called the kinetoplast, which contributes to flagellar development. This organelle is readily seen on stained smears of skin lesions or reticuloendothelial tissue. Several species of *Leishmania* have been identified as causes of cutaneous, mucocutaneous, or visceral disease. Isolates were formerly classified based on clinical manifestations, geographic origin, and ecological characteristics. Subgenera designations may be given depending on where development occurs in the sandfly gut: subgenus *Leishmania* (pyloric and midgut), or subgenus *Viannia* (hindgut). Traditionally, species have been divided into "old world" (*L. (L.) donovani, L. (L.) infantum, L. (L.) major, (L.) L. (L.) tropica, L. (L.) aethiopica*) and "new world" species (*L. (L.) chagasi, L. (L.) mexicana, L. (L.) amazonensis, L. (V.) braziliensis, L. (V.) panamensis, L. (V.) guyanensis*). More recently analysis of nuclear and kinetoplast DNA has formed the basis for species identification and taxonomy.[72]

Leishmania are transmitted by infected sandflies (phlebotomine flies) of the genus *Phlebotomus* (old world) or *Lutzomyia* (new world). They are small in size (2–3 mm) and can easily pass through bed nets and screens. Humans (India, Sudan), canines (Mediterranean basin, Middle East, China, South America), or rodents (Sudan) are the typical reservoir hosts.[73] The geographic distribution of leishmaniasis is determined by the availability of the sandfly vector and the animal reservoir, and transmission occurs when man is in proximity to both the vector and reservoir hosts.

The flagellated promastigote moves from the midgut to the proboscis and is transmitted by the bite of the feeding female sandfly. After the host is inoculated, the promastigote invades reticuloendothelial cells (primarily macrophages) and transforms into the amastigote form. Here asexual multiplication occurs in phagosomes, and the parasite evades the host immune response through complex mechanisms.[74] Immunologic protection is primarily cell–mediated in origin, and immunodeficiencies demonstrating cellular defects, such as HIV, have been associated with an increased incidence of visceral leishmaniasis.

Visceral leishmaniasis is caused by the *L. donovani* complex (*L. donovani, L. infantum, L. chagasi*) and is manifested by fever, weight loss, lymphadenopathy, massive splenomegaly and hepatomegaly, and pancytopenia.[73] Recently during the Gulf War conflict, U.S. soldiers developed visceral disease from *Leishmania tropica*, a species classically associated with cutaneous disease.[75]

Cutaneous leishmaniasis (Figure 17.10) begins as a papular or nodular lesion that then ulcerates ("oriental sore").[74,76] These are frequently single in number and located on exposed body areas such as the extremities and face. The lesions then ulcerate, and although many self-heal, they may become chronic, nonhealing ulcers.

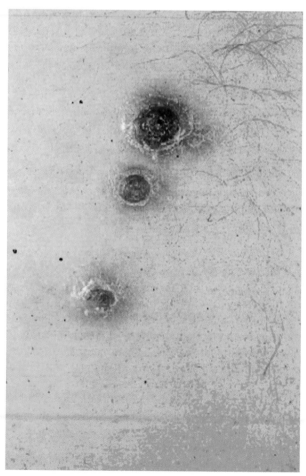

Figure 17.10. Cutaneous leishmaniasis. Photo courtesy of J. Dick MacLean, McGill University Centre for Tropical Diseases.

Diffuse cutaneous leishmaniasis (DCL) is a form associated with multiple skin lesions with substantial parasite burden and a generalized lack of immune responsiveness to the pathogen. This has been particularly noted in Ethiopia (*L. aethiopica*) and in regions of South America (*L. (L.) amazonensis*), and whether there is a genetic predisposition to this form is unclear. Mucocutaneous disease, sometimes leading to destruction of the palate and nasal septum (espundia), is seen primarily in Central and South America and is caused by species of the *Viannia* subgenus such as *L. (V.) braziliensis*.

Visceral leishmaniasis is associated with significant pancytopenia and polyclonal hypergammaglobulinemia. Definitive diagnosis is made by demonstration of organisms with characteristic kinetoplasts on Giemsa-stained smears of biopsies of skin or reticuloendothelial tissue (spleen, bone marrow, liver).[73,74,76] Splenic aspiration has proven relatively safe and provides the highest diagnostic yield for visceral disease. Parasite numbers are highest for visceral leishmaniasis and diffuse cutaneous leishmaniasis. The organism can also be cultured, but this requires the use of specific biphasic (NNN) media, and the organisms may take from 1 to 3 weeks to grow. This is not available in most diagnostic laboratories. PCR may also be useful in diagnosis.

Treatment of leishmaniasis is complex, may vary geographically, and is often associated with adverse effects.[73,74] Amphotericin B has been the best tolerated agent for visceral disease and has been used as amphotericin B deoxycholate or as a newer lipid-associated formulation. Pentavalent antimony compounds [sodium stibogluconate (Pentostam) or meglumine antimoniate (Glucantime)] have been used extensively in the past but resistance has developed and the drugs cause significant hepatic and cardiac toxicity. Recently, miltefosine (hexadecylphosphocholine) has also been used orally with some success for both visceral and cutaneous disease,[77] even in resistant cases. Cutaneous leishmaniasis has also been effectively treated with local heat, intralesional antimony, and oral fluconazole. Immunocompromised hosts should be treated with systemic therapy. Prevention involves environmental measures such as elimination of rodent colonies, insecticide-spraying programs in focal areas, and personal application of mosquito repellants. Vaccine development is still in the early stages.

Sandfly Fever

Sandfly fever (pappataci fever, phlebotomus fever) is a self-limited viral illness caused by several viruses of the phlebotomus fever serogroup of the *Phlebovirus* genus in the family *Bunyaviridae*. The viruses are endemic in countries that border the Mediterranean but are also found in Africa, Central Asia, and the Americas. The serogroups are named for the regions in which they predominate: Naples, Sicilian, Toscana, Punta Toro. Sandflies are the necessary vectors (*Phlebotomus papatasi*, *P. perniciosus*, *Lutzomyia trapidoi*). Humans or sandflies may be a reservoir, and the viruses may be passed to new generations of sandflies by the transovarial route. Outbreaks have commonly occurred when nonimmune military populations enter an endemic region.

Many infections are mild or asymptomatic. Symptoms begin abruptly after a 3–6 day incubation period, with fever, malaise, headache, retroorbital pain, and photophobia. Nausea and vomiting may also develop, but there is no rash. The acute febrile illness lasts several days and may take 1–2 weeks to completely resolve. Toscana virus has tropism for the central nervous system and can cause both aseptic meningitis and encephalitis.[78]

The CBC frequently demonstrates leukopenia. In CNS disease associated with the Toscana virus there is CSF pleocytosis and elevated protein. Diagnosis is made serologically or by detection of Toscana virus in the CSF by nested or RT-PCR.[78] There is no proven therapy, although ribavirin may be useful in more severe disease. Residual insecticide spraying has been a successful public health strategy. Adult midges are small and readily pass through bed nets and screens, although these may be an effective preventative if permethrin-impregnated.

Ticks

Ticks are responsible for transmission of a variety of infections including *Rickettsia* (Rocky Mountain spotted fever, tick typhus), bacteria (Lyme disease, tick-borne relapsing fever), viruses (hemorrhagic fever), and protozoa (babesiosis). Disease transmission occurs from the bites of both hard (*Dermacenter*, *Ixodes*, *Amblyomma*) and soft (*Argasid*, *Ornithodoros*) ticks. Often there is transovarial and transstadial transmission to maintain the tick reservoir, and usually the nymphal stages as well as adults may be vectors. Ticks are usually encountered in wooded or scrubland areas, where animal reservoirs are also located. Ticks are long-lived, and vector control is often impractical. Control measures are directed toward personal measures such as protective clothing, insect repellants, habitat avoidance, and personal examination with early tick removal.

Rocky Mountain Spotted Fever

Rocky Mountain spotted fever (RMSF) is caused by *Rickettsia rickettsii*.[79] It is transmitted through the bite of nymphal and adult ticks of several species such as *Dermacenter andersoni* (wood tick, eastern United States), *D. variablis* (dog tick, west-central United States), and *Amblyomma americanum* (Lone Star tick, Oklahoma, Texas). Transmission of RMSF occurs in the eastern and west-central United States in several states including North Carolina, South Carolina, Oklahoma, Arkansas, and Missouri. The disease is also distributed throughout

Latin America, particularly in areas of Brazil, Colombia, Costa Rica, Panama, and Mexico.

After inoculation into the host, the organisms multiply in the reticuloendothelial system as well as endothelial cells, leading to a vasculitis involving multiple organs.[79] After an incubation of 5–10 days, illness begins with fever, rash, and severe headache. The rash begins on the extremities, initially often involving the palms and soles, and spreads to the trunk. It is usually maculopapular at the outset, but it may become petechial, hemorrhagic, or necrotizing, especially late in the illness. Central nervous system complications include meningoencephalitis manifested by altered mental status, seizures, or coma.

Diagnosis of RMSF is usually made serologically using indirect immunofluorescence (IFA) or ELISA, with demonstration of IgM antibody or a fourfold rise or fall in IgG titer as diagnostic. Leukopenia, thrombocytopenia, and disseminated intravascular coagulation are often associated findings. CNS disease is accompanied by CSF pleocytosis, usually a mix of polymorphonuclear neutrophils (PMNs) and mononuclear cells, and often is associated with hyponatremia due to inappropriate ADH secretion (SIADH). Immunofluorescence of skin biopsy specimens can also be diagnostic.

Tetracycline (doxycycline) is the treatment of choice for adults with RMSF. In children (≤ 12 years old), chloramphenicol has been traditionally used because of tetracycline interference with dental and bony development. Other agents (fluoroquinolones, rifampin) have demonstrated activity in tissue culture or animal models but have not been used extensively in humans.

Tick Typhus

Tick typhus (African, Siberian, or Queensland tick typhus or boutonneuse fever) is caused by a variety of species of *Rickettsia*.[79] The etiologic agents vary geographically and some are listed below:

African tick typhus	*R. conorii, R. africae*
Siberian tick typhus	*R. sibirica*
Queensland tick typhus	*R. australis*

The pathogenesis of this disease is similar to that of RMSF, although the illness is milder. Not infrequently there is a black eschar at the site of the tick bite (Figure 17.11) and a diffuse maculopapular rash. Fever, fatigue, and headache are also associated features. CNS involvement is rare. Diagnosis is generally made clinically, and can be supported by serologic testing. Treatment is with tetracycline (doxycycline) as noted for RMSF above.

Tick-borne Relapsing Fever

Tick-borne relapsing fever is caused by several spirochetal organisms in the genus *Borrelia*: *B. duttoni*, *B. hispanica*, *B. persica*, and *B. hermsii*.[80] Transmission

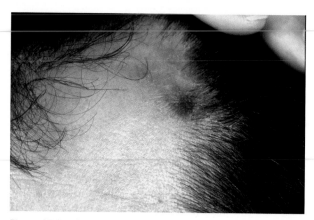

Figure 17.11. Queensland tick typhus. Photo courtesy of J. Dick MacLean, McGill University Centre for Tropical Diseases.

occurs via the bite of soft or Argasid ticks of the genus *Ornithodoros*. Distribution occurs throughout Africa, Asia, and Latin America. Various rodents are the reservoir hosts, except in East Africa where humans are the prime reservoir. The spirochete is transmitted to man through salivary secretions by the bite of the infected tick.

The incubation period is from 4–18 days. There is the abrupt onset of fever, rigors, headache, and fatigue, with the illness building in severity over the first few days. The illness then takes on a relapsing nature, with intervals of about 7 days in between febrile episodes. Each subsequent episode is shorter and milder than the initial attack. Physical findings include conjunctival injection, a petechial rash, and hepatosplenomegaly.

Extracellular spirochetes 5–20 μm in length can be detected on peripheral blood smear. The WBC count is normal to elevated with band forms, and there is often associated thrombocytopenia. Elevated transaminases and DIC are also noted. Treatment is with single doses of tetracycline or erythromycin, or with two intramuscular doses of procaine penicillin. Some patients will develop a Jarisch-Herxheimer reaction with the initiation of treatment.

Lice

Human lice (*Pediculus humanus*) are endemic worldwide and are especially prevalent in areas of crowding (Figure 17.12). They are frequently exchanged person-to-person in this setting. The principal diseases for which they are vectors are epidemic typhus (*Rickettsia prowazekii*), louse-borne relapsing fever (LBRF, *Borrelia recurrentis*), and trench fever (*Bartonella quintana*). In these infections, the organisms multiply in the gastrointestinal tract of the louse; then louse feces contaminate the bite wound leading to transmission.

Epidemic Typhus

Rickettsia prowazekii is the etiologic agent of endemic or louse-borne typhus. Transmission of epidemic typhus is more common in the winter months, as crowding is

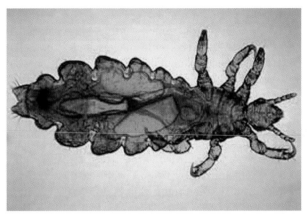

Figure 17.12. Adult female louse. Photo courtesy of Centers for Disease Control and Prevention.

enhanced during colder weather. It was a common problem in U.S. troops in World War I. Transmission may occur in the setting of refugee camps in particular. Epidemic typhus is most prevalent in regions of Africa (Ethiopia, Burundi, Rwanda, Lesotho), Asia (Afghanistan, Pakistan), northern China, and Latin America (Mexico, Guatemala, the Andean countries), especially in areas of civil unrest and where large encampments of refugees are located. Man is the only reservoir.

Disease manifestations are similar to those of RMSF, with fever, malaise, and headache, although rash may be less common. In severe cases, the rash becomes hemorrhagic or purpuric. CNS manifestations may become apparent with obtundation and coma. As with the other rickettsial infections, the diagnosis is made serologically and tetracycline is the treatment of choice. Prevention includes overall improvement in living conditions, fumigation of contaminated clothing and population-wide treatment with doxycycline. Chemoprophylaxis with doxycycline has also been shown to be effective.

Louse-borne Relapsing Fever

Louse-borne relapsing fever, caused by *Borrelia recurrentis*, is also transmitted by lice in areas with crowding and poor living conditions.[80] Endemic areas are located in a variety of developing countries in Africa, (particularly Ethiopia), Asia, and Latin America. Humans are the only reservoir. The spirochete multiplies in the gastrointestinal tract of the human body louse, *Pediculus humanus*. The organism is passed in the fecal material of the louse and contaminates the bite wound.

After an incubation period of 4–18 days, a febrile illness begins with headache, malaise, nausea, and vomiting. There is the abrupt onset of fever, rigors, headache, and fatigue, with the illness building in severity over the first few days. The first episode lasts approximately 6 days and is followed by an asymptomatic interval of about 9 days, and then a final 2–3 days of recurrent illness. Physical findings include conjunctival injection, a petechial rash, and hepatosplenomegaly.

Untreated the mortality may be as high as 40%. Diagnosis is confirmed by demonstration of spirochetal organisms in Giemsa-stained peripheral blood films. Culture of the organism is difficult except in a research setting, but *Borrelia* DNA may be demonstrated in peripheral blood by PCR. As with tick-borne relapsing fever, treatment is with doxycycline, erythromycin, or penicillin. Chemoprophylaxis with doxycycline may be indicated for relief workers entering high-risk settings.

Bartonella quintana

Bartonella quintana, the agent of trench fever, is a louse-borne pathogen with a human reservoir host.[81] It is reemerging as an infection among homeless populations in the United States and Europe, and like epidemic typhus, has occurred in refugee populations in Africa. The organism multiplies in the louse intestine, is excreted in the feces, and is subsequently scratched into the wound. *B. quintana* causes a wide spectrum of illness, including trench fever, chronic bacteremia, endocarditis, and bacillary angiomatosis.

Trench fever is manifested by recurrent fever, headache, shin pain, and dizziness, occurring in 4–6 day cycles, each with decreasing intensity.[81] It may take 4–6 weeks before there is complete recovery. As with *B. bacilliformis*, a chronic bacteremia may develop, and prevalence may be as high as 14% in some populations. *B. quintana* endocarditis is a cause of "culture-negative" endocarditis and may infect a previously normal heart valve. Bacillary angiomatosis is an illness characterized by disseminated vascular skin lesions, occurring particularly in individuals with HIV infection. It can also be caused by *B. henselae*.

Diagnosis can be made serologically by indirect immunofluorescence. The organism can be recovered from blood, but this is a laborious process often taking from 2–6 weeks. Subculturing in shell vials or the lysis centrifugation method may increase yields. Immunohistochemistry and PCR may allow detection of *B. quintana* in tissue and blood. Treatment is with doxycycline, with gentamicin added in combination for more severe disease. Bacillary angiomatosis can be treated with erythromycin.

Fleas

Fleas are common pests of domestic animals, rodents, and man. Several diverse illnesses may be transmitted by fleas in specific epidemiologic settings.

Murine Typhus

Murine typhus is a rickettsial illness caused by *Rickettsia typhi*. Mice and small rodents are the reservoir hosts, and transmission to man occurs when there is close proximity to these reservoir hosts. Murine typhus is widely distributed in both tropical and temperate climates. Serological surveys in patients with acute undifferentiated febrile illness frequently reveal infections with *R. typhi*. Fleas expose the host by defecation following feeding with contamination of the bite site. The typhus illness has many of the features of rickettsial illness as described previously, with fever, headache, and rash. Leukopenia and occasionally thrombocytopenia are noted, as well as elevated transaminases. A diagnosis can be made with the characteristic clinical findings in the appropriate epidemiologic setting. Serologic tests may be helpful to confirm the diagnosis. Treatment with doxycycline is similar to the other rickettsial illnesses as described previously.

Plague

Yersinia pestis, the agent of plague, is transmitted by the rat flea *Xenopsylla cheopis*. Wild rodents are the main reservoir hosts, but the disease may spread to peridomestic rodents as well. Endemic areas for plague are in more temperate climates and at higher elevations. Areas of potential exposure would include rural regions of Southeast Asia (Vietnam, Myanmar), Africa (Tanzania, Democratic Republic of the Congo, Madagascar) and Latin America (Brazil, Peru, Bolivia). Recent outbreaks have occurred in the Democratic Republic of the Congo and Algeria.

Fleas become infected with *Y. pestis* and develop intestinal obstruction. Vomited material subsequently contaminates the bite site and leads to infection. Infection with *Y. pestis* typically leads to the bubonic form of the illness. The illness is manifested by fever, chills, myalgias, prostration, and gastrointestinal symptoms.[43] There is enlargement and suppuration of regional lymph nodes. Rarely inhalation of aerosolized plague bacilli can lead to a pneumonic form, associated with pneumonia, septicemia, and respiratory failure. Terminal-staining Gram-negative coccobacilli can be demonstrated on lymph node aspiration or organisms can be recovered by standard aerobic cultures. Treatment is with tetracyclines, aminoglycosides, and fluoroquinolones.

A formalin-inactivated vaccine (Greer Laboratories, Inc.) was developed in the early 1900s, is not widely available, and requires three immunizations over 6 months. Chemoprophylaxis with doxycycline has been proven effective in preventing infection during exposure in high-risk settings.

Bartonellosis

There are three major species that cause infection in man: *Bartonella bacilliformis* (Oroya fever and verruga peruana), *B. henselae* (cat scratch disease, bacillary angiomatosis), and *B. quintana* (trench fever). The flea is the vector for *B. bacilliformis* and *B. henselae*; *B. quintana* is louse-borne.

Bartonella bacilliformis

B. bacilliformis is a small, motile, Gram-negative coccobacillus. It infects erythrocytes and endothelial cells. It has been postulated that humans with chronic low grade bacteremia or vascular verrucous lesions are an important reservoir host.[82] It was initially believed that flies of the phlebotomine genus *Lutzomyia* were vectors of *B. bacilliformis*, but more recently fleas have been implicated for this and other *Bartonella* species (*B. henselae*). The verrucous form of the disease may also be transmitted by ticks. The disease is endemic in the Andean mountain valleys of Peru, Ecuador, and Colombia.

Bartonellosis is most common in children younger than 10 years of age, and there appears to be the development of acquired immunity. The bacteremic form of the illness is called Oroya fever or Carrion's disease.[82] The initial acute bacteremic phase is manifested by fever, chills, myalgias, headache, and malaise and may begin abruptly or more insidiously. Central nervous system involvement may lead to altered consciousness and death. In severe disease, there is dehydration, shock, and DIC. Salmonellosis is a frequent complication. In survivors, the disease may last as long as 3–4 weeks, with gradual convalescence.

After the acute stage of the disease, the organism leaves the bloodstream and localizes to endothelial cells in the skin and subcutaneous tissue. This leads to vascular proliferation and the development of vascular, "verrucous" skin lesions, verruga peruana.[43,82] As many as 50% of patients may go on to develop verrucous disease. Lesions begin as small, round mobile subcutaneous nodules and progress to skin papules and then more vascular verrucous lesions. They are located predominately on the face and extensor surfaces and are warm and tender. The verrucous lesions may bleed following trauma or become secondarily infected. When healed, the lesions appear as hypopigmented macules with a surrounding zone of hyperpigmentation.

Reticulocytosis (up to 50%) is seen and in severe disease almost all erythrocytes may be infected, with up to 20 bacilli/RBC. Hemolysis occurs, principally from removal of deformed erythrocytes by the liver and spleen. During the acute phase of the illness a clinical diagnosis is confirmed by demonstration of intraerythrocytic bacilli on Giemsa- or Wright-stained blood film (sensitivity 30–40%) and the organisms can be recovered by aerobic blood culture. Bacilli can also be demonstrated in biopsies of skin lesions. Serologic testing by immunofluorescence and PCR has been developed but is not widely available.

A variety of antibiotics including penicillin, tetracycline, quinolones, streptomycin, and chloramphenicol have been useful clinically. In vitro sensitivity testing is generally not available. Chloramphenicol also has the advantage of being effective against salmonellosis, a common complication. Chronic verrucous disease responds less well to the above antibiotics but may be helped by rifampin therapy.

Bartonella henselae

B. henselae, the agent of cat scratch disease, is also felt to be flea-transmitted.[83] It was previously thought to be transmitted by the scratch or bite of infected cats, but in as many as 40% of cases, no prior bite or scratch injury was identified, and of course cats have fleas. This illness is predominately seen in temperate climates. It is manifested initially by a primary lesion then followed by fever and localized lymphadenopathy, predominately in the neck and axilla. The nodes become suppurative or necrotizing, have a characteristic pathology, and may drain spontaneously. Lymphadenopathy may resolve spontaneously within several months.

A small percentage of patients develop systemic involvement, including infection of the liver, spleen, bone, and CNS.

The diagnosis is made by the appropriate clinical setting, characteristic pathologic findings, or the demonstration of organisms on methenamine silver or Warthin-Starry stain. *B. henselae* can also be recovered by culture of lymph nodes or demonstrated by PCR, and indirect fluorescent antibody and PCR-based testing have been developed. Treatment is with doxycycline, trimethoprim/sulfamethoxazole, or fluoroquinolones.

Bartonella quintana

See previous discussion in section "Lice."

Trombiculid Mites

Scrub Typhus

Larval trombiculid mites or chiggers are the vector of transmission of scrub typhus or "tsutsugamushi" fever. *Orientia (Rickettsia) tsutsugamushi* is the etiologic agent and is transmitted by the bite of the mite. It is found in East and Southeast Asia (China, Vietnam, the Philippines, Indonesia, India, North Australia) and is transmitted in a number of ecosystems, including rainforest, mountain, and coastline areas. It was an important illness in U.S. troops in both World War II and the Vietnam War.

There is often an eschar that develops at the site of the initial bite as with other rickettsial illnesses, with subsequent development of a diffuse maculopapular rash, fever, and headache. There may be regional lymphadenopathy, and decreased hearing and tinnitus occur in 30%. A diagnosis can be made clinically after exposure in the appropriate epidemiologic setting or by serologic testing. The differential diagnosis also includes dengue and other rickettsial infections. Treatment is similar to the rickettsial illnesses described previously. Weekly

chemoprophylaxis with doxycycline is effective in high-risk populations.

Rickettsialpox

Rickettsialpox is a mite-borne disease caused by *Rickettsia akari*. It differs from other rickettsial illness in that the character of the rash is vesicular rather than maculopapular. It has been described in the United States (particularly in New York City and Baltimore), Eastern Europe, Korea, and South Africa.[84] Peridomestic mice are the reservoir, and the mouse mite (*Liponyssoides sanguineus*) is the vector.

After a 7-day incubation period, there is an initial lesion at the bite site. It begins as a papule, which then becomes a vesicle and then a black eschar. Several days later a more diffuse rash with the same characteristics develops, with sparing of the palms and soles. Fever and headache are associated features, and there may be regional lymphadenopathy.

Diagnosis can be made serologically, but immunohistochemistry and nested-PCR of skin biopsies have also proven useful for diagnosis.[84] Treatment with doxycycline is similar to other rickettsial infections.

Reduviid or Triatomine Bugs

Reduviid bugs (triatomine bug, assassin bug, kissing bug) such as *Rodnius prolixus* and *Triatoma infestans* are the principal vectors for *Trypanosoma cruzi*, the causative agent of American trypanosomiasis or Chagas' disease. There are an estimated 11,000,000 cases of Chagas' disease in the Americas, with transmission in the southwestern United States, Mexico, and Central and South America.[69,85] The reduviid bugs live in dark crevices in the interior walls of substandard housing. The bugs are nocturnal feeders, coming out of their hiding places to feed on sleeping hosts. The infective trypomastigote stage is passed through postprandial defecation at the bite site (Figure 17.13), which can occur on skin or mucous membranes (e.g., conjunctiva). Transmission has also occurred in utero and through blood transfusion or organ transplantation. Seroprevalence estimates in endemic areas have varied from 1–2% in Mexico, to as high as 20% in highly endemic areas in Bolivia and Argentina. A variety of wild and domestic mammals have been identified as reservoirs.

An initial papulonodular lesion (chagoma) is noted after a 1–2 week incubation period in 50% of patients, and conjunctival or periorbital edema (Romaña's sign) may be seen if the site of inoculation is the conjunctiva.[69,85] There may be a febrile illness during acute infection that resolves in several days. The chagoma may resolve over several weeks and leave a hyperpigmented scar. Rarely acute myocarditis or meningoencephalitis may develop. Organisms disseminate to multiple organs,

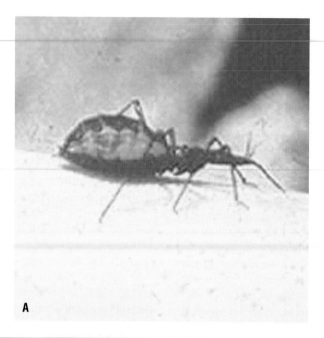

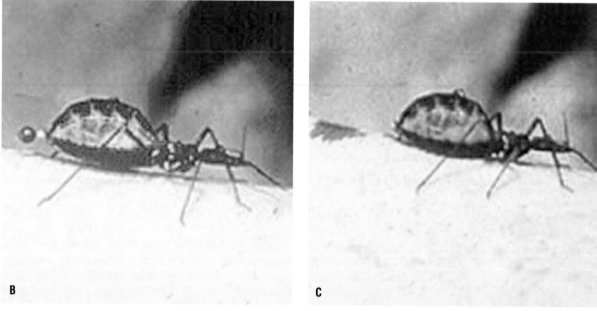

Figure 17.13. The reduviid (or triatomine bug), the vector for *Trypanosoma cruzi*, defecating in the bite wound of its victim. Photo courtesy of Centers for Disease Control and Prevention.

with subsequent pathologic damage to the heart and smooth muscle of the esophagus and colon. The chronic manifestations of Chagas' disease may take years to develop and consist of muscular fibrosis leading to cardiomegaly, megaesophagus, or megacolon.

Diagnosis of acute Chagas' disease is made by demonstrating intracellular parasites on blood film examination. In chronic disease, the parasitemia has resolved so the diagnosis is made serologically by a variety of tests including ELISA, IHA, and IFA. PCR-based testing has also been successful in a number of recent studies. Cardiomegaly, megaesophagus, or megacolon can be diagnosed radiographically.

Treatment of Chagas' disease is far from satisfactory.[69,85] Acute Chagas' disease can be treated with nifurtimox, a nitrofuran derivative, given orally with weight-based dosing for 90–120 days. Eradication of parasitemia can be expected in 70%. Nifurtimox causes abdominal pain, nausea, and vomiting and may also lead to insomnia, paresthesias, muscle twitching, and seizures. Advanced disease can be treated as well, with benznidazole, a nitroimidazole derivative, orally for 60 days, but due to the presence of fibrosis, there may be no change in clinical symptoms. Some data suggests that even patients with late stage disease may benefit from therapy. Rash, peripheral neuropathy, and granulocytopenia are potential adverse effects. Both drugs are available from the Parasitic Disease Drug Service of the CDC (404-639-3670).

Prevention is focused on improving housing conditions and eliminating potential habitats for reduviid bugs and residual insecticide spraying. Screening of blood transfusions and donor organs has also been helpful.

SUMMARY

The global burden of infectious disease is staggering, with the majority of illness occurring in poor developing countries with limited diagnostic and therapeutic resources. Not only is there substantial mortality from such diseases as malaria, HIV, and tuberculosis, but there is considerable morbidity with a reduction in DALYs. For the adventurer, exposure to these more unusual infections is determined by geographic location and the nature and degree of exposure in primitive settings. Limiting potential exposure, whether it be by securing a safe water supply or avoiding potential vectors, is critical for prevention.

REFERENCES

1. Hotez PJ, Fenwick A, Kumaresan J, Molyneux D, Ehrlich Sachs S, Sachs J, Savioli L. The control of the neglected tropical diseases. *N Engl J Med.* 2007; 357:1018–27.

2. Lopez AD, Mathers CD, Ezzati M, Jamison DT, Murray CJL. Annex 3B: deaths by cause, sex, age, and region, 2001 and Annex 3C: DALYs (3,0) by cause, sex, age, and region, 2001. In: *Global Burden of Disease and Risk Factors.* Disease Control Priorities Project. New York: The World Bank and Oxford University Press; 2001: 126–233.

3. Epstein JE, Hoffman SL. Typhoid fever. In: *Tropical Infectious Diseases, Principles, Pathogens, & Practice,* Volume 1. London: Churchill Livingstone Elsevier; 2006: 220–40.

4. Hotez PJ, Molyneux DH, Fenwick A, Ottesen E, Ehrlich Sachs S, Sachs JD. Incorporating a rapid impact package for neglected tropical diseases with programs for HIV/AIDS, tuberculosis, and malaria. *PLoS Medicine.* 2006;3:e102.

5. Stauffer W, Ravdin JI. *Entamoeba histolytica*: an update. *Curr Opin Infect Dis.* 2003;16:479–85.

6. Marfin AA, Barwick Eidex R, Monath TP. Yellow fever. In: *Tropical Infectious Diseases, Principles, Pathogens, & Practice,* Volume 1. London: Churchill Livingstone Elsevier; 2006: 797–812.

7. Hotez PJ, Ferris MT. The antipoverty vaccines. *Vaccine.* 2006;24:5787–99.

8. Hotez PJ. The "biblical diseases" and U.S. vaccine diplomacy. *Brown World Affairs J.* 2006;2:247–58.

9. Hotez PJ, Ottesen E, Fenwick A, Molyneux D. The neglected tropical diseases: the ancient afflictions of stigma and poverty and the prospects for their control and elimination. *Adv Exp Med Biol.* 2006;582:23–33.

10. Hotez PJ, Bundy DAP, Beegle, K, Brooker S, DeSilva N, Montresor A, Engles D, Drake L, Chitsulo L, Michaud C, Bethony JM, Oliveira R, Xiao SH, Fenwick A, Savioli L. Helminth infections. In: *Disease Control Priorities in Developing Countries.* 2nd ed. New York: The World Bank and Oxford University Press; 2001: 2006.

11. Molyneux DH, Hotez PJ, Fenwick A. "Rapid impact" interventions: how a policy of integrated control for Africa's neglected tropical diseases could benefit the poor. *PLoS Med.* 2005; 2:e336.

12. Sachs JD, Hotez PJ. Stepping up the fight against tropical diseases. *Science.* 2006;211:1521.

13. Ansart S, Perez L, Vergely O, Danis M, Bricaire F, Caumes E. Illnesses in travelers returning from the tropics: a prospective study of 622 patients. *J Travel Med.* 2005;12:312–18.

14. Cachay ER, Vinetz JM. A global research agenda for leptospirosis. *J Postgrad Med.* 2005;51:174–8.

15. Boggild AK, Yohanna S, Keystone JS, Kain KC. Prospective analysis of parasitic infections in Canadian travelers and immigrants. *J Travel Med.* 2006;13:138–44.

16. Dance DAB. Melioidosis. In: *Tropical Infectious Diseases, Principles, Pathogens, & Practice,* Volume 1. London: Churchill Livingstone Elsevier; 2006: 381–8.

17. Ahmed AO, van Leeuwen W, Fahal A, van de Sande W, Verbrugh H, van Belkum A. Mycetoma caused by *Madurella mycetomatis*: a neglected infectious burden. *Lancet Infect Dis.* 2004;4:566–74.

18. Mahgoub E-S. Mycetoma. In: *Tropical Infectious Diseases, Principles, Pathogens, & Practice,* Volume 1. London: Churchill Livingstone Elsevier; 2006: 892–7.

19. Bethony J, Brooker S, Albonico M, Geiger S, Loukas A, Diemert D, Hotez PJ. Soil-transmitted helminth infections: ascariasis, trichuriasis, and hookworm. *Lancet.* 2006; 367:1521–32.

20. Hotez PJ, Bethony J, Bottazzi ME, Brooker S, Diemert D, Loukas A. New technologies for the control of human hookworm infection. *Trends Parasitol.* 2006;22:327–31.

21. Kelly PW, Takafuji ET, Wiener H, Milhous W, Miller R, Thompson NJ, Schantz P, Miller RN. An outbreak of hookworm infection associated with military operations in Grenada. *Military Med.* 1989;54:55–9.

22. Hotez, P, Brooker S, Bethony J, Bottazzi M, Loukas A, Xiao S. Hookworm infection. *New Engl J Med.* 2004;51:799–807.

23. Berke R, Wagshol LE, Sullivan G. Incidence of intestinal parasites in Vietnam veterans: eosinophilia a guide to diagnosis. *Am J Gasteroenterol.* 1972;57:63–7.

24. Nutman TB, Ottesen EA, Ieng S, Samuels J, Kimball E, Lutkoski M, Zierdt WS, Gam A, Neva FA. Eosinophilia in Southeast Asian refugees: evaluation at a referral center. *J Infect Dis.* 1987;155:309–13.

25. Neusch R, Zimmerli L, Stockli R, Gyr N, Christoph Hatz FR. Imported strongyloidiasis: a longitudinal analysis of 31 cases. *J Travel Med.* 2005;12:80–4.

26. Keiser PB, Nutman TB. *Strongyloides stercoralis* in the immunocompromised population. *Clin Microbiol Rev.* 2004;17:208–17.

27. Blackwell V, Vega-Lopez F. Cutaneous larva migrans: clinical features and management of 44 cases presenting in the returning traveler. *Br J Dermatol.* 2001;145:434–7.

28. Pappas G, Papadimitriou P, Akritidis N, Christou L, Tsianos EV. The new global map of human brucellosis. *Lancet Infect Dis.* 2006;6:91–9.

29. Pappas G, Akritidis N, Bosilkovski M, Tsianos E. Brucellosis. *N Engl J Med.* 2005;352:2325–36.

30. Garcia HH, Gonzalez AE, Evans CAW, Gilman RH, for the Cysticercosis Working Group in Peru. *Taenia solium* cysticercosis. *Lancet.* 2003;361:547–56.

[31] Fenwick A. Waterborne infectious diseases – could they be consigned to history? *Science*. 2006;313:1077–81.

[32] Hotez PJ, Feng Z, Xu LQ, Chen MG, Xiao SH, Liu SX, Blair D, McManus DP, David GM. Emerging and reemerging helminthiases and the public health of China. *Emerg Infect Dis*. 1997;3:303–10.

[33] Ross AGP, Bartley PB, Sleigh AC, Olds GR, Li YS, Williams GM, McManus DP. Schistosomiasis. *N Engl J Med*. 2002;346:1212–20.

[34] Petri WA, Singh UP. Enteric amebiasis. In: *Tropical Infectious Diseases, Principles, Pathogens, & Practice*, Volume 2. London: Churchill Livingstone Elsevier; 2006: 967–90.

[35] Wansbrough-Jones M, Phillips R. Buruli ulcer: emerging from obscurity. *Lancet*. 2006;367:1849–58.

[36] John TJ. The prevention and control of human leptospirosis. *Postgrad Med*. 2005;51:205–9.

[37] Shieh W-J, Edwards C, Levett PN, Zaki SR. Leptospirosis. In: *Tropical Infectious Diseases, Principles, Pathogens, & Practice*, Volume 1. London: Churchill Livingstone Elsevier; 2006: 511–18.

[38] Sejvar J, Bancroft E, Winthrop K, Bettinger J, Bajani M, Bragg S, Shutt K, Kaiser R, Marano M, Popovic T, Tappero J, Ashford D, Mascola L, Vugia D, Perkins B, Rosenstein N. Leptospirosis in eco-challenge athletes, Malaysian Borneo, 2000. *Emerg Infect Dis*. 2003;9:702–7.

[39] Kobayashi Y. Human leptospirosis: management and prognosis. *J Postgrad Med*. 2005;51:201–4.

[40] King CH. Schistosomiasis. In: *Tropical Infectious Diseases, Principles, Pathogens, & Practice*, Volume 2. London: Churchill Livingstone Elsevier; 2006: 1341–8.

[41] World Health Organization. 2005. *Deworming for Health and Development*, Report of the third global meeting of the partners for parasite control, Geneva, November 29–30, 2004.

[42] Godyn JJ, Reyes L, Siderits R, Hazra A. Cutaneous anthrax: conservative or surgical treatment? *Adv Skin Wound Care*. 2005;18:146–50.

[43] Lupi O, Madkan V, Tyring SK. Tropical dermatology: bacterial tropical diseases. *J Am Acad Dermatol*. 2006;54:559–78.

[44] Beatty ME, Ashford DA, Griffin PM, Tauxe RV, Sobel J. Gastrointestinal anthrax: review of the literature. *Arch Intern Med*. 2003;163:2527–31.

[45] Grabenstein JD. Anthrax vaccine: a review. *Immunol All Clin North Am*. 2003;23;713–30.

[46] Meyers W. Leprosy. In: Strickland GT, ed. *Hunter's Tropical Medicine and Emerging Infectious Diseases*. 8th ed. Philadelphia: W. B. Saunders; 2000: 513–23.

[47] Perine PL, Bell TA. Syphilis and the endemic treponematoses. In: Strickland GT, ed. *Hunter's Tropical Medicine and Emerging Infectious Diseases*. 8th ed. Philadelphia: W. B. Saunders; 2000: 354–64.

[48] Farnsworth N, Rosen T. Endemic treponematoses: review and update. *Clin Dermatol*. 2006;24:181–90.

[49] Budke CM, Deplazes P, Togerson PR. Global socioeconomic impact of cystic echinococcosis. *Emerg Infect Dis*. 2006;12: 296–303.

[50] Centers for Disease Control and Prevention. *Health Information for International Travel* (the Yellow Book) 2005–2006. Atlanta: DHHS.

[51] Peterson LR, Marfin AA. Shifting epidemiology of flaviviridae. *J Travel Med*. 2005;12(Suppl 1):S3–S11.

[52] Monath TP, Cetron MS. Prevention of yellow fever in persons traveling to the tropics. *Clin Infect Dis*. 2002;34:1369–78.

[53] Tsai T. Yellow fever. In: Strickland GT, ed. *Hunter's Tropical Medicine and Emerging Infectious Diseases*. 8th ed. Philadelphia: W. B. Saunders; 2000: 272–5.

[54] World Health Organization. Yellow fever situation in Africa and South America, 2005. *Weekly Epidemiologic Record*. 2006;81:317–24.

[55] Pugachev KV, Guirakhoo F, Monath TP. New developments in Flavivirus vaccines with special attention to yellow fever. *Curr Opin Infect Dis*. 2005;18:387–94.

[56] Marfin AA, Eidex RS, Kosarsky PE, Cetron MS. Yellow fever and Japanese encephalitis vaccines: indications and complications. *Infect Dis Clin North Am*. 2005;19:151–68.

[57] Wilder-Smith A, Schwartz E. Dengue in travelers. *New Engl J Med*. 2005;353:924–32.

[58] Mackenzie JS, Gubler DJ, Peterson LR. Emerging flaviviruses: the spread and resurgence of Japanese encephalitis, West Nile and dengue viruses. *Nat Med*. 2004;10(Suppl 12):S98–S109.

[59] Centers for Disease Control and Prevention. Inactivated Japanese encephalitis virus vaccine recommendations of the Advisory Committee on Immunization Practices (ACIP). *MMWR*. 1993;42(RR-01):1–15.

[60] Molyneaux DH, Bradley M, Hoerauf A, Kyelem D, Taylor MJ. Mass drug treatment for lymphatic filariasis and onchocerciasis. *Trends Parasitol*. 2003;19;516–22.

[61] Melrose WD. Lymphatic filariasis: new insights into an old disease. *Int J Parasitol*. 2002;32:947–60.

[62] King CL, Freedman DO. Filariasis. In: Strickland GT, ed. *Hunter's Tropical Medicine and Emerging Infectious Diseases*. 8th ed. Philadelphia: W. B. Saunders; 2000: 740–52.

[63] Alleman MM, Twum-Danso NAY, Thylefors BI. The Mectizan donation program – highlights from 2005. *Filaria J*. 2006;5:11–21.

[64] Udall DN. Recent updates on onchocerciasis: diagnosis and treatment. *Clin Infect Dis*. 2007;44:53–60.

[65] Hoerauf A, Mand S, Adjei O, Fleischer B. Buttner DW. Depletion of *Wolbachia* endobacteria in *Onchocerca volvulus* by doxycycline and microfilaridermia after ivermectin treatment. *Lancet*. 2001;31:96–8.

[66] Klion A. Loiasis. In: Strickland GT, ed. *Hunter's Tropical Medicine and Emerging Infectious Diseases*. 8th ed. Philadelphia: W. B. Saunders; 2000: 754–6.

[67] Boussinesq M. Loiasis. *Ann Trop Med Parasitol*. 2006;100:715–31.

[68] Pepin J. African trypanosomiasis. In: Strickland GT, ed. *Hunter's Tropical Medicine and Emerging Infectious Diseases*. 8th ed. Philadelphia: W. B. Saunders; 2000: 643–53.

[69] Barrett MP, Burchmore RJ, Stich A, Lazzari JO, Frasch AC, Cazzulo JJ, Krishna S. The trypanosomiases. *Lancet*. 2003;362:1469–80.

[70] Pepin J, Mpia B. Randomized controlled trial of three regimens of melarsoprol in the treatment of *Trypanosoma brucei gambiense trypanosomiasis*. *Trans Roy Soc Trop Med Hyg*. 2006;100:437–41.

[71] Schmid C, Richer M, Bilenge CM, Josenado T, Chappuis F, Manthelot CR, Nagouma A, Doua F, Asumu PF, Simarro PP, Burri C. Effectiveness of a 10-day melarsoprol schedule for the treatment of late-stage human African trypanosomiasis: confirmation from a multinational study (IMPAMEL II). *J Infect Dis*. 2005;191:1922–31.

[72] McMahon, Pratt D, Alexander J. Does the leishmania major paradigm of pathogenesis and protection hold for New World cutaneous leishmaniasis or the visceral disease? *Immunol Rev*. 2004;201:206–24.

73 Magill AJ. Leishmaniasis. In: Strickland GT, ed. *Hunter's Trop-ical Medicine and Emerging Infectious Diseases*. 8th ed. Phila-delphia: W. B. Saunders; 2000: 665–87.

74 Murray HW, Berman JD, Davies CR, Saravia NG. Advances in leishmaniasis. *Lancet*. 2005;366:1561–77.

75 Hyams KC, Riddle J, Trump DH, Graham JT. Endemic infec-tious diseases and biological warfare during the Gulf War: a decade of analysis and final concerns. *Am J Trop Med Hyg*. 2001;65:664–70.

76 Magill AJ. Cutaneous leishmaniasis in the returning traveler. *Infect Dis Clin North Am*. 2005;19:241–66.

77 Soto J, Soto P. Miltefosine: oral treatment of leishmaniasis. *Expert Rev Anti Infect Ther*. 2006;4:177–85.

78 Charrel RN, Gallian P, Navarro-Mari JM, Nicoletti L, Papa A, Sanchez-Seco MP, Tenorio A, de Lamballerie X. Emergence of Toscana virus in Europe. 2005;11:1657–63.

79 Parola P, Paddock CD, Raoult D. Tick-borne rickettsioses throughout the world: emerging diseases challenging old concepts. *Clin Microbiol Rev*. 2005;18:719–56.

80 Butler T. Relapsing fever. In: Strickland GT, ed. *Hunter's Tropi-cal Medicine and Emerging Infectious Diseases*. 8th ed. Phila-delphia: W. B. Saunders; 2000: 448–52.

81 Foucault C, Brouqui P, Raoult D. *Bartonella quintana* characteristics and clinical management. *Emerg Inf Dis*. 2006;12:217–23.

82 Laughlin L. Bartonellosis. In: Strickland GT. ed. *Hunter's Tropical Medicine and Emerging Infectious Diseases*. 8th ed. Philadelphia: W. B. Saunders; 2000: 394–8.

83 Massei F, Gori L, Macchia P, Maggiore G. The expanded spec-trum of bartonellosis in children. *Infect Dis Clin North Am*. 2005;19:691–711.

84 Paddock CD, Zaki SR, Koss T, Singleton J, Sumner JW, Con-nor JA, Eremeeva ME, Dasch GA, Cherry B, Childs JE. Rickettsialpox in New York City: a persistent urban zoonosis. *Ann N Y Acad Sci*. 2003;990:36–44.

85 Magill AJ, Reed SG. American trypanosomiasis. In: Strick-land GT, ed. *Hunter's Tropical Medicine and Emerging Infec-tious Diseases*. 8th ed. Philadelphia: W. B. Saunders; 2000: 653–65.

86 Ahmed D, D'Costa LT, Alam K, Nair GB, Hossain MA. Multidrug-resistant *Salmonella enterica serovar typhi* isolates with high-level resistance to ciprofloxacin in Dhaka, Bangladesh. *Antimicrob Agents Chemother*. 2006;50: 3516–17.

87 CDC. Typhoid immunization: recommendations of the Advisory Committee on Immunization Practices (ACIP). *MMWR*. 1994;RR14:1–14.

88 Wahdan MH, Serie C, Cerisier Y, Sallam S, Germanier R. A controlled field trial of live *Salmonella typhi* strain Ty 21a oral vaccine against typhoid: three-year results. *J Infect Dis*. 1982;145:292–5.

89 Levine MM, Ferreccio C, Black RE, Germanier R. Large-scale field trial of Ty21a live oral typhoid vaccine in enteric-coated capsule formulation. *Lancet*. 1987;1(8541):1049–52.

R. W. Bill Hamilton, PhD, and Noel E. Sloan, MD

INTRODUCTION

Subterranean environments are some of the most diverse and extreme of all wilderness destinations. Subterranean medicine, strictly speaking, is that grouping of medical skills that pertains to medical care of patients below the earth's surface, or in caves. The hazards in caves make them most challenging to deal with from medical and rescue viewpoints, with some obvious and some very unique hazards.

This chapter is an overview of providing medical care in these unique subterranean environments. The goal of this chapter is to introduce the uninitiated medical provider to the unique aspects of subterranean medicine and working in underground environments. Aspects of environmental hazards, cave diving, cave rescue, and the cave medical kit are covered.

SUBTERRANEAN ENVIRONMENTAL HAZARDS

The subterranean environment is unique. Medical providers working underground are not guaranteed basic support that the typical provider takes for granted. When working in a cave or other underground location, a lack of natural lighting, dampness – sometimes even partial submersion – constant exposure to mud and other debris, cold temperatures, and possibly long periods of isolation all factor into the equation.

In addition to handling these general considerations, medics who enter subterranean locations should be aware of more specific threats including the risk of histoplasmosis, exposure to rabies through infected bat populations, hypothermia, falls, and the proper handling of waste.

Histoplasmosis

Histoplasmosis is a disease caused by the spore-forming fungus, *Histoplasma capsulatum*. Cavers – often referred to as spelunkers – are exposed to histoplasmosis when they disturb soil that is contaminated with bat guano containing these spores, or are exposed directly to infected bat guano. Unlike birds, which propagate the spread of the disease by fertilizing *Histoplasma*-containing soil with their droppings, bats can become infected by the disease so even fresh bat guano is potentially infectious (*http://www.cdc.gov*). According to the Centers for Disease Control and Prevention (CDC), *H. capsulatum* has been described on every continent except Antarctica. In the United States, it is most often found around the river valleys of the Ohio River and Mississippi River in the southeastern and central states.

Histoplasmosis is not often a threat to the general traveler, but for those who choose to mount expeditions in caves, it presents a very real risk. Although the exact rates of infection among spelunkers is not known, it is generally thought that the disease is underreported due to the mild symptoms and a lack of recognition of most cases by clinicians. While there are multiple reports of histoplasmosis involving cave explorers in the medical literature, two striking examples are the fifty-one individuals of two separate tour groups who were infected while exploring a cave in Costa Rica (Lyon et al., 2004), and the eighteen individuals who presented with acute pulmonary histoplasmosis after visiting caves during the 1994 National Speleological Society Convention in Texas (Ashford et al., 1999).

Over 90% of histoplasmosis cases are either asymptomatic or present as a mild malaise with mild respiratory symptoms after 3–17 days of incubation. Often the symptoms are so mild that the patient assumes he has caught a mild cold, or may barely even notice the symptoms at all. In most cases, symptoms of histoplasmosis dissipate after 2–3 weeks without intervention. A few cases of acute pulmonary histoplasmosis present with the patient experiencing a nonproductive cough, high fever, weakness, and pleuritic chest pain. In 5% of acute pulmonary histoplasmosis, pericarditis develops that is associated with pericardial rubs that can often be heard on physical exam.

In patients with underlying lung disease, a chronic form of histoplasmosis can be seen. Furthermore, a disseminated form of histoplasmosis can occur in patients who are immunocompromised and is fatal if left untreated. There is also an ocular syndrome that is seen in endemic areas that is presumed to be caused by *Histoplasma*, although most patients with this diagnosis are asymptomatic.

Diagnosis is made by serology and cultures. Chest radiography is most often normal but hilar lymphadenopathy, patchy infiltrates, a nodular or miliary pattern in diffuse pulmonary cases, and, rarely, cavitations can be seen. Most cases are self-limited and do not require medical intervention. However, in cases that are systemic, prolonged, or involve immunocompromised patients, therapy is recommended. Itraconazole is the treatment of choice for mild to moderate cases while Amphotericin B is the first-line therapy for severe infections (Kauffman, 2007).

Prevention of histoplasmosis includes avoiding caves or specific areas within caves that are known harborers of the disease and educating expedition members to avoid bat guano and contaminated soils and to wash their hands upon exiting a cave. Loose fitting masks are not effective in preventing spore inspiration, so the National Institute for Occupational Safety and Health now recommends that workers with occupational exposure to *Histoplasma* be fitted with sealed masks when working in these environments (*http://www.cdc.gov/niosh/docs/2005-109/2005-109c.html*). Studies have not been conducted to determine whether masks would prevent histoplasmosis among spelunkers, and based on surveys few of those who participate in caving have ever worn a mask (Ashford et al., 1999). Using antifungals to prophylax spelunkers who are entering caves known to contain *Histoplasma* has not been studied (Ashford et al., 1999).

Rabies

Although in developing countries dogs are the most common transmitter of rabies to humans, bats are still a significant reservoir of the disease and a definite threat to transmit rabies to expeditioners. Because of this, the CDC now recommends that those individuals who have significant occupational or recreational exposure to potentially rabid animals, including bats, receive the rabies vaccination (*http://www.cdc.gov*). Spelunkers and other expedition participants who will be spending time around bat populations – especially if this time is spent in developing countries or away from proper medical facilities – should consider receiving the rabies vaccine.

Rabies is an almost universally fatal viral disease. Only six people have survived a documented case of rabies infection and only one of these has survived in the United States since 1980 (Willoughby et al., 2005). Each year in the United States one or two people die from rabies in

spite of intensive medical care. Most of these patients are diagnosed with bat variant rabies virus (*http://www.cdc. gov*). (See Figure 18.1.)

Current recommendations require that any expeditioner who is bitten, scratched, or had mucous membranes exposed to the bat's saliva receive immediate postexposure prophylaxis. This prophylaxis consists of a single dose (20 IU/kg) of human rabies immunoglobin (HRIG) and a full regimen of the rabies vaccine given on days 0, 3, 7, 14, and 28. As much of the HRIG should be infiltrated around the wound as possible – even if the would is sutured – with the remainder injected intramuscularly. The first dose of one of the three commercially available rabies vaccines should be injected intramuscularly at a site distant from the HRIG (Weber et al., 2004). Individuals who have been immunized to rabies prior to exposure still need a vaccine booster on days 0 and 3 although HRIG can be withheld.

Although most bats do not harbor rabies, spelunkers should make it a habit to avoid contact with bats. Since there have been documented cases of rabies

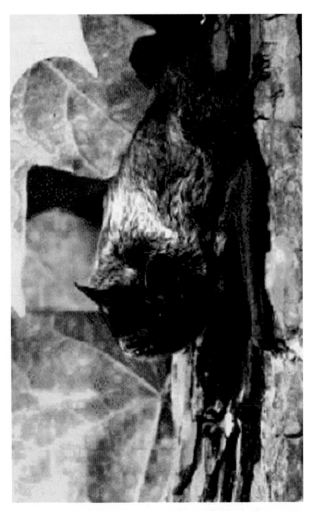

Figure 18.1. Silver-haired bat, Lasionycteris noctivagans, often associated with human rabies infections in the United States. Photo courtesy of Centers for Disease Control and Prevention.

transmission without significant bat contact – mostly in patients who awoke to find a bat in their house but had no recollection of a bite and no injury attributable to the animal – individuals who handle or have other contact with a bat should seek the advice of public health authorities regarding postexposure prophylaxis. Possible exposure to rabies is considered a medical emergency and any expedition participant who is bitten by a bat should have his or her wounds thoroughly cleaned with soapy water (or other virucidal agent) and be immediately evacuated to a medical facility to receive postexposure prophylaxis.

Cold

The cave environment produces an exceptional thermal stress with constant, cool temperatures and wet conditions. Long exposure to wet cold can cause a drop in body temperature and subsequent symptoms. The development of hypothermia over time may be subtle and not noticed until symptoms become significant. As temperature is lowered, an individual will begin to develop incoordination and eventually considerable cognitive deficits if not warmed.

To help prevent the onset of hypothermia in a cave environment, expedition members should dress appropriately with water-repelling outer garments (Figure 18.2) and layered undergarments. Team members must maintain vigilance to monitor their colleagues for signs of hypothermia. Mild hypothermia can be treated with external rewarming and the removal of any wet clothes from the patient's skin. However, if a team member begins to develop signs of moderate to severe hypothermia including a loss of alertness, incoordination, or cognitive impairment, they should be escorted out of the cave environment for proper evaluation and rewarming. A more thorough discussion of hypothermia and its treatment occurs in Chapter 31.

Noxious Gases and Hypoxia

Although a rare problem, bad air can be a serious hazard when encountered. Caves are normally well ventilated (mines may not be) but airbells – separated by sumps filled with water – can be unsafe to breathe. Certain types of limestone can create an atmosphere rich in CO_2, and sometimes iron ore can remove oxygen. CO_2, being heavier than air, can collect in low spots. Unnatural gases such as propane and gasoline can stay in caves for years and may be found 20 miles from a source such as leaking gas tanks.

Occasionally, a cave may have decaying vegetation that acts to remove oxygen and replace it with carbon dioxide. Pockets of air that contain low oxygen and high carbon dioxide can pose hazards for spelunkers. An example of how this might cause death in a seasoned explorer is the case of an experienced diver who surfaced in an airbell within a cave, became unconscious, and drowned (Bozanic, 2000).

Entanglements and Falls

Being entangled can appear to be a simple problem, but it is one of the most serious threats to a caver. The trapped caver is at risk of hypothermia as well as injuries such as compression nerve injuries, venous stasis, and thromboembolism. If a caver remains hung in an entangled harness for an extended period of time, symptoms of post-reperfusion syndrome – such as hypotension and bradyarrhythmias – may develop when he is extracted from the entanglement. This post-reperfusion syndrome can easily be confused with other

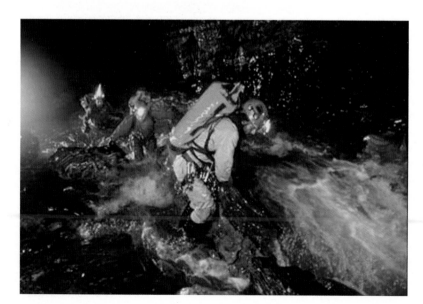

Figure 18.2. Expeditioners in caves must wear appropriate clothing to prevent hypothermia. Photo courtesy of William Stone.

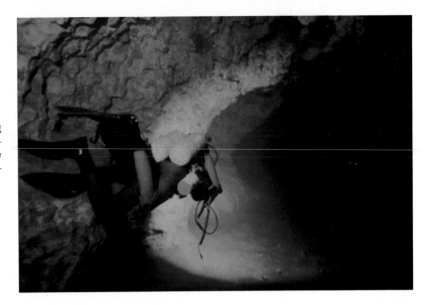

Figure 18.3. Cave diving can be challenging even for the experienced practitioner and expeditioners involved in exploring underwater cave systems need sophisticated training to maintain safety. Photo courtesy of William Stone.

simultaneous issues such as hypothermia or exhaustion.

Along with entanglements, falls are a constant threat in the cave environment. The floor of most caves is damp and cluttered with debris that causes footing to be suspect. In extreme cave expeditions, the technical skill an explorer must achieve to scale obstacles rivals elite mountaineering. Cave expedition members involved in extreme exploration are often well-versed in climbing up and rappelling down lines, and spend a significant amount of time around steep precipices and drops. The opportunity for falls is significant and any cave medical officer must be prepared to stabilize a patient who has suffered significant trauma during a fall.

Handling Water and Waste

The normal pattern for handling waste underground is for potable water to be carried in and waste carried out. For multiday penetrations, expeditions will sometimes use water found in caves after it has been properly treated. Camp latrines must be located a significant distance from the campsite and away from any food or water sources. Some cave expeditions have carried waterproof biohazard bags during travel to facilitate the transport of waste out of the cave environment (Stone and am Ende, 2002).

CAVE DIVING

Cave diving (Figures 18.3 and 18.4) may be needed to get through a sump in an otherwise dry cave. Navigating an underwater cave requires a high level of training and rigid adherence to preformulated protocols. Cave diving by divers not specifically trained for the activity has proven to be extremely dangerous, but with the right

care it can be carried out with acceptable safety (Farr, 2003).

The cave diving environment poses specific challenges to the diver. Lines are laid to aid with navigation and the cave diver must be very aware not to stir up silt that can cause a visual blackout. The extreme isolation of cave environments necessitates redundancy of every necessary piece of diving equipment. For example, cave divers should be certain to have at least three reliable sources of light on their person at all times. In extremely technical cave diving expeditions, divers enter the water with entire dive systems that are redundant. In addition, it must be ensured that all equipment is protected from the abrasive surfaces of the cave and configured for the tight confines of the cave environment.

While most traditional scuba equipment is based on the open-circuit model, modern expedition cave diving rarely uses open-circuit equipment and relies more often on rebreathing technologies. Rebreathers offer a convenient solution to the weight and bulk problems encountered with tanks housing a gas. However, rebreathers come with increased cost and complexity, and divers using these systems must have specialized training to maintain safety.

An example of rebreather technology applied to expedition cave diving is the series of Cis-Lunar rebreathers designed and built by Dr. William Stone. Dr. Stone designed the Cis-Lunar rebreather with the goal of using the technology to explore and map the Huautla cave system in Mexico, which he chronicled in his book, *Beyond the Deep: The Deadly Descent into the World's Most Treacherous Cave* (Stone and am Ende, 2002). The Huautla expedition (Figure 18.5) demonstrated the extremes of expedition cave diving including the political wrangling to get permission to enter the cave, the logistical difficulty of preparing for and entering the cave, and

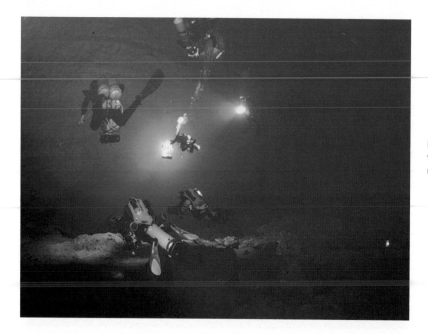

Figure 18.4. A properly trained and outfitted team helps increase dive safety in cave environments. Photo courtesy of William Stone.

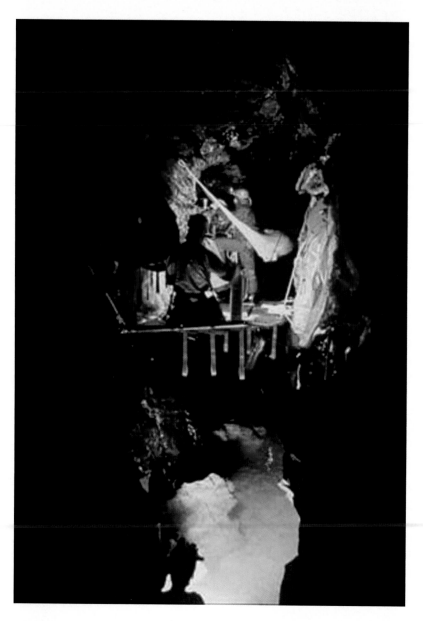

Figure 18.5. Members of the Huautla expedition set up camp 1,300 meters below the surface of the earth. Photo courtesy of William Stone.

eventually the handling of unexpected and calamitous events while far away from any support.

It should be noted that many locations for cave diving are situated at altitudes significantly above sea level (Egi et al., 2003; Stone et al., 2002). At these dive sites, the elevations are high enough that normal surface-based decompression tables cannot be used without modification. Decompression tables developed specifically for diving at elevations above sea level include the altitude tables in the Canadian Defense and Civil Institute of Environmental Medicine (DCIEM) manual and the altitude tables of the British Sub-Aqua Club. A thorough and reliable set of tables are those prepared by Professor Bühlmann of Switzerland (Bühlmann, 1984; 1995). In addition, there are a number of methods of adapting regular tables for use at altitude including the Cross Corrections, presented and critiqued by Bell and Borgwardt in 1976 (Bell and Borgwardt, 1976).

Both individuals and diving gauges must adjust to altitude prior to diving. An explorer who has just arrived from sea level with a sea level gas loading cannot use altitude decompression tables at face value until equilibrated with the pressure at the dive site's elevation. This equilibration results in a loss of dissolved nitrogen in the body and may take up to 24 hours. It is important that gauges be zeroed at the dive altitude prior to exploring a cave above sea level, as they may work differently at higher elevations (Wienke, 1993; Lippmann and Mitchell, 2005).

Many resources for training in cave diving are available including some excellent texts and training programs. One well-known source is the book *Caverns Measureless to Man* by Sheck Exley, which is credited with having had a major role in decreasing the extremely high cave diving fatality rate in Florida. Formal certification programs in cave diving are offered by the National Association of Cave Divers (NACD) and the National Speleological Society–Cave Diving Section (NSS–CDS).

CAVE RESCUE

In areas where there is a lot of caving activity, there will likely be established cave rescue teams. The most important and effective care is that administered immediately by the victim's companions so members of cave expeditions should be properly trained in first-aid. More advanced care begins with the Initial Response Team, consisting of a paramedic and two or more experienced cavers familiar with the cave containing the patient. Medical assessment and stabilization begin at once, while other cavers and rescue personnel begin route preparation for evacuation. Rescue teams without proper cave rescue training may place the patient and themselves at undue risk. The medical person in charge of the medical evacuation must have cave experience and prompt evacuation is of major importance.

Cooperation between rescue agencies and cavers is essential to achieve the most optimal rescue outcome, and it works best if this relationship exists before it is needed. Likewise, a medical protocol should be part of the expedition planning, and a prepackaged cave-ready trauma pack and litter should be on hand.

Patient Packaging

One of the greatest sources of delay in evacuation is in preparing the patient. This delay can be minimized by having a prepackaged kit, which should contain patient monitoring devices, a vapor barrier, exposure bag, head/face protection, 1-inch tubular webbing (two 20-foot pieces), rigid cervical collar, splints, and padding. Where conditions permit, a short spine board (Kendrick Extraction Device, KED, or Oregon Spine Splint) or even a litter could be carried along. Essentials of patient packaging include stabilizing injuries, treating or preventing hypothermia, protection from further injury, easy patient access, adequate immobilization for rigorous transport, and patient comfort. Protect the eyes of the patient by either taping the eyelids shut or providing goggles.

Cave passage may include waterfalls, deep pools, mud, vertical drops, low crawlways, and narrow crevices. Litter availability, patient condition, and the underground environment must be considered in planning patient transport. A preplan includes an optimal litter for the specific cave, but evacuation should not be delayed to wait for a litter. Patients with spine or pelvic fractures will require immobilization with at least a short spine board. For the rescue situation two basic litter systems can solve most cave rescue problems, the combination of a Sked Stretcher and/or an Oregon Spine Splint. The Sked is semirigid, made of a 3/16-inch polyethylene sheet that can be rolled up and weighs only 12 pounds. The Oregon Spine Splint is a compact short backboard and might well be carried along. The combination is easily transportable. For a large cave, the Ferno-Washington model 71 is excellent, and it is best for vertical evacuation.

Initial Management

The initial management of an injured caver begins with situation and patient assessment, including patient location, environmental hazards to both patient and rescuers, obstacles to the evacuation, time estimates, and consideration of rescuer fatigue. If the patient's location is not known, rescuers may stage outside the cave until the victim is found. On arrival at the rescue site, hazards should be inspected, including such things as perched rocks, unstable breakdown, inadequate riggings, and ongoing patient heat loss from water or waterfall spray. Electric head lamps for all personnel are mandatory. Rescuer fatigue must be monitored. While traveling to the patient, obstacles should be evaluated. Clear delays from things like pits, water obstacles, and tight and twisting passages determine medical management, packaging, and safe litter movement. The time required for rescue influences the degree of medical intervention at the site.

Airway Management

Airway compromise is expected in patients who are unconscious or have facial fractures or chest trauma. The alert patient might develop breathing difficulties from positioning, packaging, or tight passageways. Airway obstruction can occur from dislodged rock or mud, water, vomitus, blood, or saliva. The patient with his arms packaged is particularly vulnerable. The airway should be inspected, and a suction device (100-ml syringe with large tip and tubing extension) should be available at the head of the litter. Monitoring can be done by watching chest movements, listening to breath sounds, and feeling expired breath with the hand. An unconscious patient's tongue can sometimes occlude the airway. Airway aids may be needed to improve or maintain the airway. A nasal airway may be more easily tolerated than an oral airway but placement may cause a nosebleed that can cause increased distress. The Laryngeal Mask Airway (LMA) is a possible choice for maintaining the airway. The routine use of oxygen has not generally been practiced in cave rescue, largely because of the weight of the tanks and most cavers are healthy and can tolerate the lower blood oxygen levels associated with general trauma.

Intravenous Fluids and Medications

An intravenous line should be established early, before patient packaging, for drug and fluid infusion. This should be done for seemingly stable patients if they have to face a long evacuation. Blood samples should be drawn and sent with the patient to the hospital. Solutions should be in plastic bags, and during administration these can be pressurized with a blood pressure bulb, dedicated pump, or a spring clamp. All air should be removed from the bag and tubing. Fluids should be heated to body temperature, in a pan of warm water or inside clothing of other team members. Warmed bags placed next to the patient can provide warmth and are accessible. Maintain an even flow to keep the line open, with rate determined by the situation. Wrap excess tubing around the bag.

Catheterization

A variety of conditions necessitate the use of a Foley catheter. Urine output helps assess a severely traumatized patient. A hypothermic patient may have consider-able urine flow as a result of cold diuresis. Any patient packaged for a long evacuation will need to void, preferably without disturbing the packaging.

Monitoring

For monitoring blood pressure the cuff is permanently attached, with a Diasyst (molded rubber stethoscope pad) or a stethoscope head with 3 feet of tubing taped to the arm or leg. The best cuff design has a long hose with a detachable combination sphygmomanometer, making blood pressure and pulse rate available despite packaging. The ear pieces can be removed and stowed when not being used. The remote probe of an indoor–outdoor thermometer can be used for esophageal, rectal, or urine temperature to provide a true core temperature. As mentioned previously, it may be difficult to rewarm a patient in the cave environment, but insulation against further heat loss makes good sense. An inexpensive pulse oximeter is light and can provide valuable data.

CAVE MEDICAL KIT

Ambulance and most wilderness medical kits are not appropriate for caves. The cave trauma kit should be equipped for common caving injuries and be compact and indestructible. Multiuse items are attractive. Kits should be sealed with contents visible, with packs in clear containers like freezer bottles. In addition to the splints mentioned previously in the "Patient Packaging" section, the following can be fit into a single pack.

Assessment and Monitoring

The cave medical kits should include treatment flow sheets, cards, pencils, a BP cuff, a stethoscope with detachable head, a hypothermia thermometer (e.g., Radio Shack indoor–outdoor electronic), scissors, and tape.

Airway Management

For airway management, the cave medical kit should include a suction device (e.g., 100-ml large tip syringe), oropharyngeal airways, three-blade laryngoscope, two wire-reinforced endotracheal tubes (5 mm will provide adequate airway and will pass nasally with minimal trauma; 7 mm is good for oral approach), #4 Laryngeal Mask Airway, ventilation bag and mask, nasal decongestant spray, 2% lidocaine lubricant, nasogastric suction tube (18F), cricothyrotomy kit, and tape.

Intravenous Equipment

Venous prep set (Betadine skin prep pads, 20- and 18-ga venous catheters, tourniquet, tape). Blood specimen set (tubes for blood count, electrolytes, glucose, blood-type crossmatching), IV administration tubing sets, 4 ea 5 ml syringes with attached needles, IV fluids.

Wound Care

For wound care, the cave medical kit should include dressings, sterile gloves, antiseptic (Betadine solution), clear waterproof breathable wound cover (e.g., OP-Site), heavy trauma dressing (surgical 6 × 9 inch), 2 ea elastic (Ace) bandages (4 and 6 inch), gauze rolls Kerlix (4 and 6 inch), 4 × 4 inch squares, sealant dressings (Xeroform gauze), two rolls of 3-inch tape, Space Blanket, and splinting material (Polysplint, air splint).

Medications

The cave medical kit should include the following medications: four doses of IV broad spectrum antibiotics, Decadron 100-mg vial, mannitol 20% 400-ml bag, IV Valium, Dilantin, dextrose 50% injection, analgesic (acetaminophen), codeine, Ketorolac 4 ea 30-mg IM, sodium bicarbonate 8.4% injection, Narcan, Marcaine 0.5% solution, syringes with needles, alcohol wipe pads, Foley urine catheter kit (16F), rigid cervical extraction collar.

SUMMARY

Subterranean environments are extreme environments by definition and offer those who enter their realm a host of unique opportunities. However, they can be unforgiving to those who are careless or unprepared, and individuals should receive formal training before entering caves, and especially before attempting cave diving. The medical professional must be aware of the environmental hazards unique to subterranean environments and how best to treat and evacuate patients from within these often difficult locations.

SUGGESTED READINGS

Ashford DA, Hajjeh RA, Kelley MF, Kaufman L, Hutwagner L, McNeil MM. Outbreak of Histoplasmosis among cavers attending the national speleological society annual convention, Texas, 1994. *Am J Trop Med Hyg.* 60(6);1999: 899–903.

Bell RI, Borgwardt RE. 1976 Mar. The theory of high-altitude corrections to the U.S. Navy standard decompression tables: the cross corrections. *Undersea Biomed Res.* 1976;3(1):1–23.

Bozanic JE. Cave diving fatalities in 2000. *Underwater Speleol.* 2000;28(2):6–8.

British Sub-Aqua Club. 1990. The BS-AC '88 decompression tables, levels 1 to 4. South Wirral, Cheshire, UK: British Sub-Aqua Club.

Bühlmann AA. *Decompression: Decompression Sickness.* Berlin: Springer-Verlag; 1984.

Bühlmann AA. *Tauchmedizin. Barotrauma. Gasembolie. Dekompression, Dekompressions-krankheit, Dekompressionscomputer.* 4 Auflage. Berlin: Springer-Verlag; 1995. (In German)

Cousteau JY. Working for weeks on the sea floor. *National Geographic.* 1966;129:498–537.

DCIEM. *DCIEM Diving Manual.* Parts 1 & 2. DCIEM No. 86-R-35. North York, Ontario, Canada: DCIEM, Department of National Defence, Canada; 1992.

Egi SM, Gürmen NM, Aydin S. Field trials of no-decompression stop limits for diving at 3500 m. *Aviat Space Environ Med.* 2003;74(3):228–35.

Farr, M. *Darkness Beckons: The History and Development of Cave Diving.* 2nd ed. Crickhowell, Wales, UK: Farrworld; 2003.

Kauffman CA. Histoplasmosis: a clinical and laboratory update. *Clin Microbiol Rev.* 2007;20(1):115–32.

Lippmann J, Mitchell S. *Deeper into Diving.* Melbourne, Australia: JL Publications; 2005.

Lyon GM, Bravo AV, Espino A, Lindsley MD, Gutierrez RE, Rodriguez I, Corella A, Carrillo F, McNeil MM, Warnock DW, Hajjeh RA. Histoplasmosis associated with exploring a bat-inhabited cave in Costa Rica, 1998–1999. *Am J Trop Med Hyg.* 2004;70(4): 438–42.

Stone W, am Ende B, with Paulsen M. *Beyond the Deep: The Deadly Descent into the World's Most Treacherous Cave.* New York: Warner Books; 2002.

Weber DJ, Wohl DA, Rutala WA. Rabies. In: Tintinalli JE, Kelen GD, Stapczynski JS, eds. *Emergency Medicine: A Comprehensive Study Guide.* 6th ed. New York: McGraw-Hill, Health Professions Division; 2004.

Wienke BR. *Diving above Sea Level.* Flagstaff, AZ: Best; 1993.

Willoughby RE Jr, Tieves KS, Hoffman GM, Ghanayem NS, Amlie-Lefond CM, Schwabe MJ, Chusid MJ, Rupprecht CE. Survival after treatment of rabies with induction of coma. *N Engl J Med.* 2005;352(24):2508–14.

Luanne Freer, MD, and Peter H. Hackett, MD

The medical officer on a high-altitude expedition will be consulted about the prevention and treatment of high-altitude medical problems, as well as the effects of altitude on preexisting medical conditions and fitness for travel to these demanding destinations. Although there have been numerous recent advances in the field of high-altitude medicine, significant morbidity and mortality persist (Table 19.1), and it is essential to better prepare and educate the at-risk population. In this chapter, we review basic physiology of altitude ascent, recognition and management of high-altitude medical problems, altitude effects on chronic medical conditions, and suggested components of a high-altitude medical kit. The reader is also referred to a recent publication for a more detailed review (Hackett and Roach, 2007). See Table 19.2 for online resources. For discussions about children and pregnancy at altitude, see Chapter 9, and for treatment of other conditions that commonly occur on cold weather expeditions (ultraviolet keratitis, hypothermia, frostbite and other cold injuries), please see Chapters 16 on polar medicine, 31 on environmental injuries, and 36 on the eye.

DEFINITIONS

At high altitude (1,500–3,500 m), decreased exercise performance and increased ventilation (lower arterial PCO_2) develop due to diminished inspired oxygen. Arterial PO_2 is significantly diminished, but saturation levels (SaO_2) remain 90% or greater. Because of the large number of tourists who are frequenting ski resort and adventure destinations and pursuing rapid ascents to 2,500–3,500 m, high-altitude illness is common in this range (Tables 19.1 and 19.3).

At very high altitude (3,500–5,500 m) maximum arterial oxygen saturation drops under 90% as the arterial PO_2 values fall below 60 torr (Table 19.3). During exercise, sleep, and with high-altitude pulmonary edema or other acute lung illnesses, extreme hypoxemia is not uncommon. HAPE and HACE occur most commonly in this range.

At extreme altitude (over 5,500 m) physiologic deterioration overcomes adaptation and marked hypoxemia, hypocapnia, and alkalosis develop. Progressive deterioration of physiologic function eventually outstrips acclimatization. Because the body is unable to permanently acclimatize in "the death zone," no long-term human habitation exists above 5,500 m. A well-planned acclimatization schedule is necessary when ascending to extreme altitude; abrupt ascent without supplemental oxygen for other than brief exposures will result in severe altitude illness and possibly death.

THE HIGH-ALTITUDE ENVIRONMENT

Increasing altitude results in a logarithmic drop in barometric pressure. Therefore, the partial pressure of oxygen (21% of barometric pressure) also decreases, and humans suffer the primary insult of high altitude, hypoxia. Barometric pressure is half its sea level value at 8,500 m, and on the summit of Mt. Everest (8,848 m) climbers effectively breathe only 28% of the inspired pressure of oxygen they enjoy at sea level (Table 19.3).

Polar expeditioners suffer even greater hypoxia because barometric pressure at high altitude drops with increasing distance from the equator. In addition to the role of latitude, weather and temperature fluctuations may have substantial influence on pressure–altitude relationships, and seasonally, pressure is lower in winter than in summer. For example a low-pressure trough can reduce pressure 10 torr in one night on Mt. McKinley, making climbers awaken "physiologically higher" by 200 m. Therefore, hypoxia is directly related to barometric pressure, and not solely to geographic altitude (West, 1984).

Increasing altitude is directly associated with drop in temperature (on average, 6.5°C per +1,000 m), and the combined effects of cold and hypoxia provoke both cold injuries and high-altitude pulmonary edema. Glacial sun reflection can cause intense heat radiation, and we have observed temperatures of 52°C in tents on Mt. Everest. Expedition medical officers need to be aware that heat

Table 19.1. Incidence of Altitude Illness in Various Groups

Study group	Number at risk per year	Sleeping altitude (m)	Maximum altitude reached (m)	Average rate of ascent[a]	Percent with AMS	Percent with HAPE and/ or HACE	Reference
Western State Visitors	30 million	~2,000 ~2,500 ~≥3,000	3,500	1–2	18–20 22 27–42	0.01	Honigman, Theis, et al. (1993)
Mt. Everest Trekkers	6,000	3,000– 5,200	5,500	1–2 (fly in) 10–13 (walk in)	47 23 30–50	1.6 0.05	Hackett, Rennie, et al. (1976) Murdoch (1995)
Mt. McKinley Climbers	1,200	3,000– 5,300	6,194	3–7	30	2–3	Hackett (1986)
Mt. Rainier Climbers	10,000	3,000	4,392	1–2	67	—	Larson, Roach, et al. (1982)
Mt. Rosa, Swiss Alps	—[b]	2,850 4,559	2,850 4,559	1–2 2–3	7 27	— 5	Maggiorini, Buhler, et al. (1990) Maggiorini, Buhler, et al. (1990); Cremona, Asnaghi, et al. (1999); Schneider, Bernasch, et al. (2002)
Indian Soldiers	Unknown	3,000– 5,500	5,500	1–2	†	2.3–15.5	Singh, Kapila, et al. (1965); Singh, Khanna, et al. (1969)
Aconcagua Climbers	4,200	3,300– 5,800	6,962	2–8	39 (LLS > 4)	2.2	Pesce, Leal, et al. (2005)

AMS, Acute mountain sickness; HAPE, high-altitude pulmonary edema; HACE, high-altitude cerebral edema.
[a]Days to sleeping altitude from low altitude.
[b]Reliable estimate unavailable.
With permission from Hackett and Roach (2007).

Table 19.2. Online information resources on altitude illness

International Society for Mountain Medicine http://www.ismmed.org	Detailed practical information on altitude illness available for both physicians and nonphysicians. Includes diagnostic criteria for AMS, HACE, and HAPE, as well as AMS scoring tools for adults children. An "ask the experts" section is available for difficult cases.
The High Altitude Medicine Guide http://www.high-altitude-medicine.com	Information on altitude illness and other health issues for travelers and their physicians. Has a practical tutorial on field hyperbaric treatment, and comparisons of the various portable hyperbaric bags.
eMedicine http://www.emedicine.com/ emerg/environmental.htm	Written in a brief, easy-to-review format; targeted at physicians. The cerebral and pulmonary syndromes of altitude illness are covered in separate "chapters."
Everest Base Camp Medical Clinic http://www.EverestER.org	Information on sidebars for laypeople traveling to high altitude. Updates on altitude and mountaineering news and research. "Ask the Doc" section for special questions.
Web MD http://www.webmd.com	Separate consumer and physician sections, and extensive medical info for consumers. Online chat rooms cover various topics including altitude illness and travel medicine.
ICAR-MEDCOM http://www.mountainmedicine.org/ mmed/icarmedcom/papers.html	A collection of articles on medical management of mountaineering emergencies, including a suggested alpine medical kit. Presented by the International Commission for Mountain Emergency Medicine
Wilderness Medical Society http://www.wms.org	Complete archives of Wilderness and Environmental Medicine and the prior Journal of Wilderness Medicine. Archives are open, but the current issue is only accessible to subscribers and WMS members.

Table 19.3. Altitude conversion: barometric pressure, estimated partial pressure of inspired oxygen, and the equivalent oxygen concentration at sea level[a]

Altitude (m)	Altitude (ft)	Barometric pressure, P_B	Estimated partial pressure of inspired oxygen, P_IO_2	Equivalent oxygen concentration at sea level, F_IO_2 at SL
Sea level	0.0	759.6	149.1	0.209
1,000	3,281	678.7	132.2	0.185
2,000	6,562	604.5	116.7	0.164
3,000	9,843	536.9	102.5	0.144
4,000	13,123	475.4	89.7	0.126
5,000	16,404	419.7	78.0	0.109
6,000	19,685	369.4	67.5	0.095
7,000	22,966	324.2	58.0	0.081
8,000	26,247	283.7	49.5	0.069
9,000	29,528	247.5	42.0	0.059
10,000	32,808	215.2	35.2	0.049

[a]Barometric pressure is approximated by the equation $P_B =$ Exp(6.6328 − (0.1112 * Altitude − (0.00149 * (Altitude^2))), where Altitude = Terrestrial altitude in (meters/1,000 or km). P_IO_2 is calculated as the P_B − 47(Water vapor pressure at body temperature) * Fraction of O_2 in inspired air. The equivalent F_IO_2 at sea level for a given altitude is calculated as P_IO_2/ (760 − 47). Substituting ambient P_B for 760 in the equation allows similar calculations for F_IO_2 at different altitudes.

exhaustion can go unrecognized in traditionally cold high-altitude environments.

Extreme altitudes are sometimes referred to as high-altitude deserts because water is usually sparse and can be obtained only by melting snow or ice. When combined with increased insensible water loss from rapid respiration and skin evaporation, water scarcity commonly results in debilitating dehydration. Summarily, high-altitude environments impose many stresses, some of which contribute to or may be confused with the effects of hypoxia.

ALTITUDE ACCLIMATIZATION

Rapid ascent from sea level to the summit of Mt. Everest (8,848 m) causes unconsciousness within minutes and death shortly thereafter. Acclimatization explains the fact that climbers ascending Mt. Everest over a period of weeks, even without supplemental oxygen, have experienced only minor symptoms of illness. This acclimatization process, by which individuals gradually adjust to hypoxia and enhance survival and performance, is essential for survival at extreme altitude and for comfort and well-being at lesser altitudes. Adaptation to altitude results in improved cellular oxygen delivery and improved tolerance of hypoxia. Severity of hypoxic stress, exposure rate, and individual physiology determine whether an altitude sojourner successfully acclimatizes or is overwhelmed. There is substantial variability in an individual's ability to acclimatize, no doubt reflecting genetic

polymorphisms, since the tendency to acclimatize well or to become ill is consistent on repeated exposure if rate of ascent and altitude gained are similar. Initial acclimatization (first 4–5 days) protects against altitude illness and improves sleep and longer term acclimatization (weeks) primarily improves aerobic exercise capacity.

ALTITUDE PHYSIOLOGY

With altitude exposure, increased ventilation reduces alveolar carbon dioxide, raising alveolar oxygen and resulting in improved oxygen delivery. This adaptation begins at elevations as low as 1,500 m and occurs within minutes to hours of high-altitude exposure. Sensing arterial hypoxemia, the carotid body signals the medulla respiratory center to increase ventilation. This hypoxic ventilatory response (HVR) is genetically determined but can be influenced by extrinsic factors such as use of respiratory depressants and fragmented sleep, which is common on expeditions. Metabolic agitants, such as caffeine and coca, and respiratory stimulants, such as progesterone and almitrine, increase HVR. Acetazolamide, a respiratory stimulant, acts directly on the central respiratory center rather than on the carotid body. Physical conditioning does not alter HVR, but studies show that a good ventilatory response enhances acclimatization and performance. Very low HVR may contribute to illness (see "Acute Mountain Sickness" and "High-Altitude Pulmonary Edema").

As ventilation increases, resulting alkalosis acts as a braking mechanism in the medulla, limiting further increases in ventilation. Within 1–2 days, the kidneys compensate for the alkalosis by excreting bicarbonate and adjusting the pH toward normal, allowing further ventilation increase. Ventilation continues to increase slowly, reaching a maximum only after 4–7 days at the same altitude. Plasma bicarbonate concentrations continue to decline, and ventilation increases with additional ascent. Individuals with lower oxygen saturation at altitude have higher serum bicarbonate values; whether the kidney limits acclimatization or whether this reflects poor respiratory drive is unclear. Acetazolamide rapidly facilitates the acute acclimatization process (see "AMS Prevention").

Altitude ascent is accompanied by increased sympathetic activity causing an initial mild increase in blood pressure, moderate increase in heart rate and cardiac output, and increase in venous tone. The bicarbonate diuresis, a fluid shift from the intravascular space, and suppression of aldosterone all result in decreased plasma volume and lower stroke volume. As the body acclimatizes, the resting heart rate returns to near sea level values, except at extremely high altitude. As the limits of hypoxic acclimatization are approached, maximum and resting heart rates converge. Probably partly because of a reduction in myocardial oxygen demand from reduced maximal heart rate and cardiac output, there are no reports of myocardial ischemia at extremely high altitude in otherwise healthy persons.

Pulmonary vascular resistance increases almost immediately on ascent to high altitude because of hypoxic pulmonary vasoconstriction and results in increased pulmonary artery pressure. Mild pulmonary hypertension is augmented quickly by exertion, and pulmonary pressures may reach systemic values, especially in those with a previous history of high-altitude pulmonary edema.

Cerebral oxygen delivery is the product of arterial oxygen content and cerebral blood flow (CBF) and depends on the net balance between hypoxic vasodilation and hypocapnia-induced vasoconstriction. CBF increases, despite hypocapnia, when PaO_2 is less than 60 torr (altitude over 2,800 m), but this response is quite variable. Generally, cerebral metabolism is well maintained with moderate hypoxia.

Erythropoietin is secreted and stimulates bone marrow production of red blood cells in response to hypoxemia. This adaptation to altitude is detectable within 2 hours of ascent when the hormone first appears, and nucleated immature red blood cells can be found on a peripheral blood smear within days, with new red blood cells in circulation within 4–5 days. Over a period of weeks to months, the degree of hypoxemia causes a proportional red blood cell mass to increase. Iron supplementation can be crucial, especially for females; women who supplement iron intake at high altitude approach the hematocrit values of their male cohorts.

The early increase in hemoglobin concentration after ascent is due to hemoconcentration secondary to diminished plasma volume, rather than a true increase in red blood cell mass. This results in a higher effective hemoglobin concentration at the cost of decreased blood volume, a trade-off that might impair exercise performance. Longer term acclimatization increases both plasma volume and red blood cell mass, increasing total blood volume. Overshoot of the hematopoietic stimulation at altitude can cause polycythemia, which may actually impair oxygen transport because of increased blood viscosity. The ideal hematocrit for high-altitude performance is unknown, but it is probably less than 55%.

At altitude, the oxygen dissociation curve plays a crucial role in improving oxygen transport. SaO_2% is well maintained up to 3,000 m, despite a significant decrease in arterial PO_2, but above 3,000 m, small changes in arterial PO_2 result in large changes in oxygen saturation. Recall that oxygen saturation determines arterial oxygen transport, but the PO_2 determines diffusion of that oxygen from capillary to cell.

In vitro right shift in the position of the oxyhemoglobin dissociation curve at high altitude (a shift favoring release of oxygen from the blood to the tissues) was first demonstrated in 1936. An increase in 2,3-diphosphoglycerate (2,3-DPG), which is proportional to the severity of hypoxemia, is responsible for this shift. In vivo, however, this is offset by alkalosis, and at moderate altitude little net change occurs in the position of the oxygen dissociation curve. On the other hand, the marked alkalosis of extreme hyperventilation, as measured on the summit and simulated summit of Mt. Everest (PCO_2 8–10 torr, pH greater than 7.6), shifts the oxygen–hemoglobin dissociation curve to the left, which facilitates oxygen–hemoglobin binding in the lung, raises SaO_2%, and is thought to be advantageous.

SLEEP AT HIGH ALTITUDE

Disturbed sleep is common at high altitude, and its cause is multifactorial. As altitude increases, nearly all subjects complain of disturbed sleep, and a restful night is exceedingly uncommon at extreme altitudes. In general, sleep shifts from deeper to lighter sleep, and arousals are more frequent and more time is spent awake. Periodic breathing appears to play only a minor role in altering sleep architecture at high altitude. Predisposing factors to problem sleep such as obesity may explain a degree of susceptibility to both deranged sleep and sleep-disordered breathing in some individuals (Ge et al., 2005). Although deranged sleep is a frequent complaint in high-altitude visitors, it seems to have little relation to susceptibility to altitude illness or other serious problems. Symptomatic treatment that avoids respiratory depression is safe.

Periodic Breathing

Periodic breathing at altitude is most common in early and light sleep and may occur during wakefulness when drowsy. Sleep patterns are characterized by hyperpnea followed by apnea (Figure 19.1) and are caused by a battle for control of breathing between the peripheral chemoreceptors (carotid body) and the central respiratory center. The hyperpneic phase results in alkalosis, which acts on the central respiratory center, resulting in apnea. During apnea, SaO_2% decreases, carbon dioxide increases, and the carotid body is stimulated, causing a recurrent hyperpnea and apnea cycle. Periodic breathing may lessen with acclimatization but does not disappear, especially over 5,000 m. Periodic breathing has not been implicated in the causation of high-altitude illness, although nocturnal oxygen desaturation has.

Acetazolamide, 125 mg at bedtime, diminishes periodic breathing and awakenings, improves oxygenation and sleep quality, is a safe agent to use as a sleeping aid, and has the added benefit of diminishing AMS symptoms. Diphenhydramine (Benadryl, 50–75 mg) or the short-acting benzodiazepines such as triazolam (Halcion, 0.125–0.25 mg), and temazepam (Restoril, 15 mg) may be useful as well. Caution is advised for the use of any agent that might reduce ventilation at high altitude,

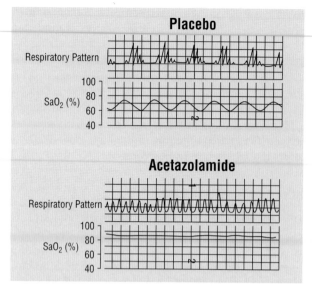

Figure 19.1. Respiratory patterns and arterial oxygen saturation (SaO₂) with placebo and acetazolamide in two sleep studies of a subject at 4,200 m. Note pattern of hyperpnea followed by apnea during placebo treatment, which is changed with acetazolamide. Modified from Hackett, Roach, et al. (1987).

but some studies have suggested that low-dose benzodiazepines may be safely used in this situation. Bradwell and colleagues (Bradwell, Coote, et al., 1987) showed that acetazolamide (500 mg slow-release orally) given with temazepam (10 mg orally) improved sleep and maintained SaO₂%, counteracting a 20% decrease in SaO₂% when temazepam was given alone. The non-benzodiazepine hypnotic, zolpidem (Ambien, 10 mg) was shown to improve sleep at 4,000 m without adversely affecting ventilation (Beaumont, Goldenberg, et al., 1996).

NEUROLOGIC SYNDROMES AT ALTITUDE

Altitude-related neurologic syndromes evolve due to both nervous system sensitivity to hypoxia, and effects of compensatory mechanisms. Although brain ATP production and metabolism remain intact during hypoxia, neurotransmitter synthesis is sensitive to hypoxia, and impaired synthesis of neurotransmitters accounts for symptoms of acute cerebral hypoxia as well as cognitive defects at high altitude. Compensatory cerebral vasodilation at altitude appears to play a role in causing altitude headache, and is also a contributor to the development of acute mountain sickness (AMS) and high-altitude cerebral edema (HACE). However, much of the pathophysiology of AMS and HACE remains a mystery. Focal neurologic deficits without cerebral edema are also difficult to explain; cerebral artery spasm and watershed hypoxia have both been invoked.

ACUTE CEREBRAL HYPOXIA

Acute, profound hypoxia, although of greatest interest in aviation medicine, may also occur on ground when ascent is too rapid or when hypoxia abruptly worsens. Carbon monoxide poisoning, pulmonary edema, sudden overexertion, sleep apnea, or a failed oxygen delivery system may rapidly exaggerate hypoxemia. Immediate administration of oxygen, rapid pressurization or descent, or correction of an underlying cause, such as relief of apnea, removal of a carbon monoxide source, repair of an oxygen delivery system, or cessation of overexertion can reverse or improve symptoms.

High-Altitude Headache

The first unpleasant symptom after altitude exposure is commonly headache; it is sometimes the only symptom. Headache may or may not be the harbinger of AMS, which is defined as the presence of headache plus at least one of four other symptoms, in the setting of an acute altitude gain (Roach, Bärtsch, et al. 1993). The typical high-altitude headache (HAH) is bilateral, generalized, dull, exacerbated by exertion or movement, often occurring at night, and resolved within 24 hours. (These headaches have some features of increased intracranial pressure.) Literature suggests that HAH can be prevented with the use of nonsteroidal antiinflammatory drugs (Broome, Stoneham, et al., 1994; Burtscher, Likar, et al., 1998) and acetaminophen (Harris, Wenzel, et al., 2003) as well as the drugs commonly used for prophylaxis of AMS, acetazolamide, and dexamethasone. Oxygen is often immediately effective for HAH (within 10 minutes) in subjects with and without AMS, indicating a rapidly reversible mechanism of the headache.

Acute Mountain Sickness

The incidence and severity of AMS depend on the rate of ascent and the altitude attained (especially the sleeping altitude), duration of altitude exposure, level of exertion, recent altitude exposure, and inherent physiologic (genetic) susceptibility. For example, AMS is more common on Mt. Rainier because of the typical rapid ascent, while high-altitude pulmonary or cerebral edema is uncommon because of the short stay (less than 36 hours). Individuals with previous susceptibility to AMS have twice the incidence of AMS compared to nonsusceptibles, and this is independent of rate of ascent (Schneider, Bernasch, et al., 2002). The specific factor that is the basis for inherent susceptibility is still unknown and is likely genetic. Age has an influence on incidence, with those older than 50 years old somewhat less vulnerable (Silber, Sonnenberg, et al., 2003), and no study has ever shown the older to be more susceptible. Women apparently have the same or a slightly greater incidence of AMS. There is no demonstrated connection between AMS and the menstrual cycle. Most studies show no relationship between physical fitness and susceptibility to AMS, but obesity seems to increase the odds of developing AMS. Smoking does not increase risk of AMS, nor does use of oral contraceptives. In summary, the most important variables related to AMS susceptibly are genetic predisposition, altitude of residence, rate of ascent, and prior recent altitude exposure.

The diagnosis of AMS is based on the setting, symptoms, physical findings, and exclusion of other illnesses. The history is typically rapid ascent of an unacclimatized person to 2,500 m or higher from altitudes below 1,500 m. For partially acclimatized persons, abrupt ascent to a higher altitude, overexertion, use of respiratory depressants, and perhaps onset of infectious illness are common contributing factors.

The cardinal symptom of early AMS is headache, followed in incidence by fatigue, dizziness, and anorexia (Honigman, Theis, et al., 1993). The headache is described above (see "High-Altitude Headache"). A good appetite is rare in AMS, and nausea is common. Symptoms are familiar to those who have suffered an alcohol hangover. Frequent awakening may fragment sleep, and periodic breathing often produces a feeling of suffocation. Although sleep disorder is nearly universal at high altitude, also affecting those without AMS, these symptoms may be exaggerated during AMS. Those with AMS commonly complain of a deep inner chill, unlike mere exposure to cold temperature, accompanied by facial pallor. Other symptoms may include vomiting, dyspnea on exertion, and irritability. Lassitude can be disabling, with the victim too apathetic to contribute to his or her own basic needs.

Pulmonary symptoms vary considerably. Everyone experiences dyspnea on exertion at high altitude; it may be difficult to distinguish normal from abnormal. Dyspnea at rest is distinctly abnormal, however, and is an important warning symptom for HAPE rather than AMS.

Specific physical findings are lacking in mild AMS. A higher heart rate has been noted in those with AMS, but Singh and associates (Singh, Khanna, et al., 1969) noted bradycardia (heart rate less than 66 beats/min) in two-thirds of 1975 soldiers with AMS. Blood pressure is normal, but postural hypotension may be present. A slight increased body temperature with AMS may be present, but is not diagnostic. Peripheral oxygen saturation as measured by pulse oximetry correlated poorly with presence of AMS during rapid ascent (O'Connor, Dubowitz, et al., 2004) but was related to AMS during trekking (Basnyat, Lemaster, et al., 1999). SaO$_2$ at altitude on Denali was predictive of developing AMS upon further ascent (Roach, Greene, et al., 1998). Overall, pulse oximetry is of limited usefulness in diagnosis of AMS. Funduscopic examination reveals venous tortuosity and dilation; retinal hemorrhages may or may not be present and are not diagnostic; they are more common in AMS than non-AMS subjects at 4243 m (Hackett and Rennie, 1979). Absence of the normal altitude diuresis, evidenced by lack of increased urine output and retention of fluid, is an early finding in AMS, although not always present.

More obvious physical findings develop if AMS progresses to HACE. Typically, with onset of HACE, the victim wants to be left alone, lassitude progresses to inability to perform perfunctory activities such as eating and dressing, ataxia develops, and finally, changes in consciousness appear, with confusion, disorientation, and impaired judgment. Coma may ensue within 24 hours of the onset of ataxia. Ataxia and confusion are the most useful signs for recognizing the progression from AMS to HACE; all persons proceeding to high altitudes should be aware of this fact. It is clinically useful to classify AMS as mild or moderate to severe on the basis of symptoms (Table 19.4). Importantly, AMS can herald the beginning of life-threatening cerebral edema.

Differential Diagnosis of AMS

Because of the nonspecific nature of the symptoms and absence of specific signs, AMS is commonly confused with other conditions. Alternative diagnoses include viral flu-like illness, hangover, exhaustion, dehydration, or medication or drug effect. Unlike an infectious illness, uncomplicated AMS is not associated with fever and myalgia. Hangover is excluded by the history. Exhaustion may cause lassitude, weakness, irritability, and headache and may therefore be difficult to distinguish from AMS. Dehydration, which causes weakness, decreased urine output, headache, and nausea, is commonly confused with AMS. Treatment with rehydration helps to differentiate the two, since AMS is not improved by fluid administration alone. Hypothermia may manifest as ataxia and mental changes, which are absent in uncomplicated AMS. Sleeping medication can cause ataxia and mental changes, and soporifics may also precipitate high-altitude illness because of increased hypoxemia during sleep. Migraine may be very difficult to distinguish from AMS. A trial of recompression therapy, oxygen breathing, or actual descent can be helpful to discriminate these other conditions from AMS.

Carbon Monoxide

It should be noted that carbon monoxide (CO) exposure is a risk of high-altitude expeditions and increases the risk of AMS. Tents and shelters in high-altitude environments are generally designed to be light, small, and windproof, which can be a hazard for carbon monoxide poisoning. Melting snow for drinking water and cooking inside these structures during storms can be particularly dangerous. Hypoxia at altitude can add to the effects of even mild carbon monoxide poisoning because even small amounts of carboxyhemoglobin can produce symptoms of poisoning. Reduced oxyhemoglobin caused by carbon monoxide increases hypoxic stress, rendering a person at

Table 19.4. Clinical classification of AMS

	HAH	Mild AMS	Moderate to severe AMS	HACE
Symptoms	Headache only	Headache + 1 more symptom: (nausea/vomiting; fatigue/lassitude; dizziness or difficulty sleeping) All symptoms of mild severity	Headache + 1 or more symptoms (nausea/vomiting; fatigue/ lassitude; dizziness or difficulty sleeping) Symptoms of moderate to severe intensity	+/- Headache Worsening of symptoms seen in moderate to severe AMS
LL-AMS score[a]	1–3, headache only	2–4	5–15	
Physical signs	None	None	None	Ataxia Altered mental status
Findings	None	None	Antidiuresis Slight increase T° Slight desaturation Widened A-a gradient Elevated ICP White matter edema (CT, MRI)	HAPE common: +chest x-ray, rales, dyspnea at rest Elevated ICP White matter edema (CT, MRI)
Pathophysiology[b]	Unknown; cerebral vasodilatation, trigeminovascular system[a]?	Unknown; same as HAH?	Vasogenic edema	Advanced vasogenic cerebral edema

[a] The self-report Lake Louise AMS score.
[b] See Figure 19.2.
From Hackett and Roach (2007).

a "physiologically higher" altitude, which may precipitate AMS. Immediate removal of the victim from the source of carbon monoxide and forced hyperventilation, preferably with supplemental oxygen, can rapidly reverse mild to moderate carbon monoxide poisoning.

Natural Course of Acute Mountain Sickness

The course of AMS varies with beginning altitude, rate of ascent, and severity of symptoms (Figure 19.2). Symptoms may begin as early as within 2 hours after arrival but rarely if ever start after 36 hours at a given altitude. Symptoms resolve with acclimatization, usually over the next 24–48 hours. The more rapid the ascent, and the higher the altitude, the more likely the symptoms will appear sooner and be worse. Singh and associates (Singh, Khanna, et al., 1969) followed AMS in soldiers airlifted from low altitude to between 3,300 and 5,500 m; incapacitating AMS lasted 2–5 days, but 40% still had symptoms after one week and 13% after one month. A small percentage of those with AMS (8% at 4,243 m) (Hackett and Rennie, 1976) go on to develop cerebral edema, especially if ascent continues in spite of illness. Persistent anorexia, nausea, and headache may afflict climbers at extreme altitude for weeks and can be considered a form of persistent AMS.

AMS Treatment

Treatment of AMS is based on the severity of illness at presentation and often depends on logistics, terrain, and experience of the caregiver. Treatment in the early stages of illness is easier and more successful, so early diagnosis is key (Box 19.1). Ascent in the presence of symptoms is contraindicated, and victims must be carefully monitored for progression of illness. Worsening symptoms despite an extra 24 hours of acclimatization or treatment should invoke descent. The two indications for immediate descent are neurologic findings (ataxia or change in consciousness) and pulmonary edema.

Mild AMS can be treated without medication by halting the ascent and waiting for acclimatization to improve, which can take from 12 to 96 hours. Acetazolamide (250 mg twice a day orally, or as a single dose) speeds acclimatization and terminates the illness if given early (Grissom, Roach, et al., 1992). Symptomatic therapy includes analgesics such as aspirin (500 or 650 mg), acetaminophen (650–1,000 mg), ibuprofen or other nonsteroidal antiinflammatory drugs, or codeine (30 mg) for headache. Antiemetics such as promethazine (25–50 mg by suppository or ingestion) or ondansetron (4 mg sublingual or oral) are useful for nausea and vomiting. Persons with AMS should avoid alcohol and other

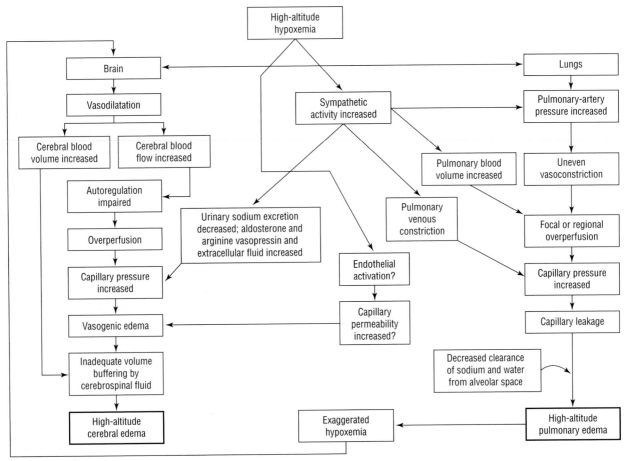

Figure 19.2. Proposed pathophysiological process of high-altitude illness. At high altitudes, hypoxemia can lead to overperfusion, elevated capillary pressure, and leakage from the cerebral and pulmonary microcirculation. Increased sympathetic activity has a central role in this process, and increased permeability of capillaries as a result of endothelial activation (inflammation) may also have a role. With permission from Hackett and Roach (2001).

respiratory depressants because of the danger of exaggerated hypoxemia during sleep.

Descent to an altitude lower than where symptoms began effectively reverses most symptoms of AMS; descending 500–1,000 m is usually sufficient. Physical exertion should be minimized, and low flow oxygen is particularly effective during sleep. Hyperbaric chambers, which simulate descent, have been used to treat AMS and aid acclimatization. They are effective and require no supplemental oxygen. Lightweight (less than 7 kg) fabric pressure bags inflated by manual air pumps are used by many mountaineering expeditions and in mountain clinics (Figure 19.3). An inflation of 2 psi is roughly equivalent to a drop in altitude of 1,600 m; the exact equivalent depends on initial altitude. A few hours of pressurization result in symptomatic improvement and can be an effective temporizing measure while awaiting descent or the benefit of medical therapy.

Studies have found dexamethasone to be effective for treatment of all degrees of AMS. Hackett and colleagues (Hackett, Roach, et al., 1988) used 4 mg orally or intramuscularly every 6 hours, and Ferrazzini and associates (Ferrazzini, Maggiorini, et al., 1987) gave 8 mg initially, followed by 4 mg every 6 hours. It is important to note that while both studies reported marked improvement within 12 hours, symptoms sometimes return or increase when dexamethasone is discontinued after 24 hours. Clinicians debate whether the use of dexamethasone should also require descent. In our opinion, dexamethasone use should be limited to fewer than 48 hours, in order to minimize side effects. This generally provides sufficient time to descend, or to better acclimatize, with or without acetazolamide. The mechanism of action of dexamethasone is unknown; it does not affect oxygen saturation, fluid balance, or periodic breathing. It does block the action of vascular endothelial growth factor (VEGF), diminishes the interaction of endothelium and leukocytes thus reducing inflammation, and may also reduce cerebral blood flow. Dexamethasone seems to not improve acclimatization because symptoms recur when the drug is withdrawn. Therefore, an argument could be made for using dexamethasone to relieve symptoms and acetazolamide to speed acclimatization.

Box 19.1. Field treatment of high-altitude illness

High-altitude headache and mild acute mountain sickness

> Stop ascent, rest, and acclimatize at same altitude
> Acetazolamide, 125–250 mg bid, to speed acclimatization
> Symptomatic treatment as necessary with analgesics and antiemetics
> Or descend 500 m or more

Moderate to severe acute mountain sickness

> Low-flow oxygen, if available
> Acetazolamide, 125 to 250 mg bid, with or without dexamethasone, 4 mg po, IM, or IV q6h
> Hyperbaric therapy
> *Or* immediate descent

High-altitude cerebral edema

> Immediate descent or evacuation
> Oxygen, 2–4 L/min
> Dexamethasone, 4 mg po, IM, or IV q6h
> Hyperbaric therapy if descent is delayed

High-altitude pulmonary edema

> Minimize exertion and keep warm
> Oxygen, 4–6 L/min until improving, then 2–4 L/min
> At moderate altitudes in mild/moderate disease, oxygen may be adequate alone
> If oxygen/descent not available or limited:
> Nifedipine, 10 mg po q4h by titration to response, or 10 mg po once, followed by 30 mg extended release q12 to 24h
> Consider inhaled beta-agonist (salbutamol or albuterol 2 puffs every 3–4 hours)
> Consider sildenafil 50 mg every 8 hours in lieu of nifedipine
> Consider acetazolamide 250 mg every 12 hours
> Consider dexamethasone 4 mg every 6 hours if cerebral dysfunction present, or for cerebral protection from severe hypoxemia
> Hyperbaric therapy
> *And/or* immediate descent

AMS Prevention

Slow and measured ascent is the surest and safest method of prevention, although particularly susceptible individuals may still become ill. Current recommendations for persons without altitude experience are to avoid abrupt ascent to sleeping altitudes greater than 3,000 m and to spend two or three nights at 2,500–3,000 m before going higher, with an extra night for acclimatization every 600–900 m if continuing ascent. Abrupt increases of more than 600 m in sleeping altitude should be avoided when over 2,500 m. If feeling well, day trips to higher altitude, with a return to lower altitude for sleep, aid acclimatization. Genetically resistant persons will be able to ascend more quickly. Alcohol and sedative-hypnotics should be avoided the first two nights at high altitude. Whether a high carbohydrate diet reduces AMS

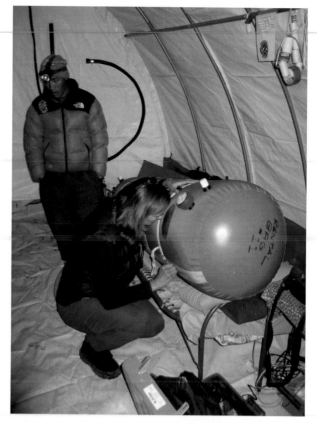

Figure 19.3. A fabric hyperbaric pressure bag being used at the Everest Base Camp Medical Clinic (5,350 m) for treatment of severe altitude illness. 2-psi pressure is equivalent to a drop of approximately 1600 m in altitude. Photo courtesy Luanne Freer.

is uncertain. Exertion early in altitude exposure contributes to altitude illness, whereas limited exercise seems to aid acclimatization. Because altitude exposure in the previous weeks is protective, a faster rate of ascent may then be possible.

Acetazolamide is the clear drug of choice for AMS prophylaxis. The drug, a carbonic anhydrase (CA) inhibitor, slows the hydration of carbon dioxide:

$$CO_2 + H_2O \overset{CA}{<==>} H_2CO_3 \overset{CA}{<==>} H^+ + HCO^3$$

By inhibiting renal carbonic anhydrase, acetazolamide reduces reabsorption of bicarbonate and sodium and causes a bicarbonate diuresis and metabolic acidosis starting within 1 hour after ingestion. This rapidly enhances ventilatory acclimatization, increasing oxygenation. Importantly, the drug maintains oxygenation during sleep and prevents periods of extreme hypoxemia (Figure 19.1). Acetazolamide's diuretic action counteracts the fluid retention of AMS; it also diminishes nocturnal antidiuretic hormone (ADH) secretion and decreases cerebrospinal fluid (CSF) production and volume and possibly CSF pressure. It is unclear which of these effects is most important in preventing AMS, but acetazolamide is approximately 75% effective in preventing AMS in persons rapidly transported to altitudes of 3,000–4,500 m (Ellsworth, Meyer, et al., 1991). Indications for acetazolamide prophylaxis include rapid ascent (1 day or less) to altitudes over 3,000 m; a rapid gain in sleeping altitude, such as moving camp from 4,000 to 5,000 m in a day; and a past history of AMS or HAPE. The ideal dose of acetazolamide for prevention is debatable; many studies have shown that 250 mg two to three times a day is effective, as well as 500 mg in sustained action capsule taken every 24 hours. To reduce side effects such as paresthesiae, clinicians suggest smaller doses (125 mg twice a day), and recent studies show the lower to dose to be effective (Basnyat, Gertsch, et al., 2003) Renal carbonic anhydrase is blocked at 5 mg/kg/day, and because this seems to be the important effect for preventing AMS, this is probably the ideal dose, both in children and adults; adjusting the dose for body weight might provide the best effect with the least side effects. Suggested duration of medication use varies; standard advice is to start 24 hours before ascent, and most authors recommend continuing for at least the first two days at high altitude (longer if there is a continuing gain in altitude). Acetazolamide can also be taken episodically, to speed acclimatization at any point while gaining altitude, or to treat mild AMS; there is no rebound when discontinued.

Use of acetazolamide is associated with high incidence of side effects, most notably peripheral paresthesiae and polyuria, and less commonly nausea, drowsiness, impotence, and myopia. Because it inhibits the instant hydration of carbon dioxide on the tongue, acetazolamide allows carbon dioxide to be tasted and can ruin the flavor of carbonated beverages. Acetazolamide, a sulfonamide drug, is usually tolerated well by persons with a history of sulfa antibiotic allergy; approximately 10% may have an allergic reaction (Strom, Schinnar, et al., 2003). It is best avoided in persons with a history of anaphylaxis to either sulfa or penicillin. Many experts recommend a trial dose of the medication before the altitude sojourn to determine drug tolerance. Although the usual allergic reaction consists of a rash starting a few days after ingestion, anaphylaxis to acetazolamide can occur.

Dexamethasone effectively prevents AMS at doses of 2 mg every 6 hours or 4 mg every 12 hours in sedentary subjects, (Johnson, Rock, et al., 1984) but for exercising subjects at or above 4,000 m, 4 mg every 6 hours may be necessary to prevent AMS. (Rock, Johnson, et al., 1989) The combination of acetazolamide and dexamethasone is superior to dexamethasone alone. (Zell and Goodman, 1988) Because of potential serious side effects and the rebound phenomenon, dexamethasone is best reserved for treatment rather than for prevention of AMS, or used for prophylaxis when necessary in persons intolerant of or allergic to acetazolamide.

Studies using ginkgo biloba for AMS prevention have shown inconsistent results. Four studies had positive results, ranging from 100 to 50% reduction in AMS when given either 5 days or 1 day before ascent (Roncin, Schwartz, et al., 1996; Maakestad, Leadbetter et al., 2001; Gertsch, Seto, et al., 2002; Moraga, Flores, et al., 2003). Three studies were negative, two of which were follow-up studies by investigators with positive results previously. Conflicting results can possibly be explained by differences in dosing, duration of pretreatment, and varying rates of ascent, but most likely, they are due to differences in preparations of ginkgo. Ginkgo biloba is a complicated plant extract whose active ingredient in terms of preventing AMS is unknown. Even in the "standardized" preparations (24% flavonoids and 6% turpene ginkolides), the amounts of specific chemicals can vary considerably. Until the active ingredient is discovered and standardized, results with ginkgo will continue to be mixed. Meanwhile, because the product is very safe, nonprescription, and inexpensive and can be helpful, it is reasonable to consider its use, especially in acetazolamide-intolerant subjects.

HIGH-ALTITUDE CEREBRAL EDEMA

High-altitude cerebral edema (HACE) is an uncommon altitude illness occurring in those with AMS or HAPE, and is fatal if untreated. Although occurrence is most common over 3,000 m, it has been reported as low as 2,100 m (Dickinson, 1979) and may develop in 0.5–1% in unselected high-altitude visitors, and in 3.4% of those with AMS (Bärtsch and Roach, 2001; Hackett and Roach, 2004) HACE occurs in 13–20% of persons with HAPE, and in up to 50% of those who die from HAPE (Hackett and Roach, 2004). Pure cerebral edema, without pulmonary edema, is uncommon. Data are insufficient to draw any conclusions regarding effects of gender, age, preexisting illness, or genetics on susceptibility to HACE. Clinically and pathophysiologically, advanced AMS and HACE are similar so that a distinction between them is inherently blurred.

The hallmarks of HACE are ataxic gait, severe lassitude, and altered consciousness, including confusion, impaired mentation, drowsiness, stupor, and coma. Headache, nausea, and vomiting are frequent but not always present. Hallucinations, cranial nerve palsy, hemiparesis, hemiplegia, seizures, and focal neurologic signs have also been reported, and retinal hemorrhages are common but not diagnostic. The progression from mild AMS to unconsciousness may develop in as little as 12 hours but usually requires 1–3 days; HACE can develop more quickly in those with HAPE. Computerized tomography may show compression of sulci and flattening of gyri, and attenuation of signal more in the white matter than gray matter. MRI is more revealing, with a characteristic high T-2 signal in the white matter, especially the splenium of the corpus callosum, and most evident on diffusion-weighted images (Hackett, Yarnell, et al., 1998; Wong, Turner, et al., 2004).

The pathophysiology of HACE is a progression of the same mechanism as advanced AMS, a vasogenic edema. Whereas the brain edema of reversible HACE is most likely vasogenic, as the spectrum shifts to severe, end-stage HACE, then gray matter (presumably cytotoxic) edema develops as well, resulting in brain herniation and death. Decreased cerebral blood flow and ischemia result from increased intracranial pressure. Focal neurologic signs caused by brainstem distortion and extraaxial compression, as in third and sixth cranial nerve palsies, may develop, making cerebral edema difficult to differentiate from primary cerebrovascular events. The most common clinical presentation, however, is change in consciousness associated with ataxia, without focal signs.

HACE Treatment

Because HACE is uncommon and usually occurs in remote locations, there are no controlled HACE treatment trials. Successful treatment requires early recognition, and at the first sign of ataxia or change in consciousness, descent should be initiated, dexamethasone (4–8 mg intravenously, intramuscularly, or orally initially, followed by 4 mg every 6 hours) administered, and oxygen (2–4 L/min by vented mask or nasal cannula) applied if available (Box 19.1). Oxygen should be titrated to maintain SaO_2 at greater than 90%. In unconscious patients, routine coma care should be employed with appropriate airway management and bladder drainage. Simulated descent with use of a portable hyperbaric chamber may be lifesaving but should not delay an actual descent. Attempting to decrease intracranial pressure by intubation and hyperventilation is a reasonable approach, although these patients are already alkalotic, and overhyperventilation could result in disastrous cerebral ischemia. Loop diuretics such as furosemide (40–80 mg) or bumetanide (1–2 mg) may reduce brain hydration and have been used successfully, but an adequate intravascular volume to maintain perfusion pressure is critical. Hypertonic solutions of saline, mannitol, or oral glycerol have been suggested, but they rarely are used in the field. Controlled studies are lacking, but empirically the response to steroids and oxygen seems excellent if they are given early in the course of the illness and disappointing if they are not started until the victim is unconscious. Coma may persist for days, even after evacuation to low altitude, but other causes of coma must be considered and ruled out by appropriate evaluation. The average time to full recovery from HACE is 2.4 weeks, with a range of 1 day to 6 weeks. Sequelae lasting weeks are common; longer term follow-up has been limited, but presumed permanent impairment has been reported (Hackett and Roach, 2004). Prevention of HACE is the same as for AMS and HAPE.

FOCAL NEUROLOGIC CONDITIONS WITHOUT AMS OR CEREBRAL EDEMA

Transient focal neurologic signs that develop at altitude but not with preceding AMS suggest migraine, cerebrovascular spasm, transient ischemic attack, local hypoxia without loss of perfusion (watershed effect), or focal edema. Cortical blindness was reported by Hackett and colleagues (Hackett, Roach, et al., 1987) who treated six cases of transient blindness in climbers or trekkers with intact pupillary reflexes, indicating a cortical process. Treatment with breathing of either carbon dioxide (a potent cerebral vasodilator) or oxygen resulted in prompt relief, suggesting that the blindness was due to inadequate regional circulation or oxygenation; descent affected relief more slowly. Other conditions that could be attributed to spasm or "transient ischemic attack" have included transient hemiplegia or hemiparesis, transient global amnesia, unilateral paresthesiae, aphasia, and scotoma (Cauchy, Larmignat, et al., 2002; Basnyat, Wu, et al., 2004). The true mechanism of these focal findings is unknown and may be multifactorial.

The occurrence of stroke in a young, fit person at high altitude is uncommon but a number of case reports have described climbers with resultant permanent dysfunction. Cerebral venous thrombosis presents insidiously, and diagnosis is often delayed (Torgovicky, Azaria, et al., 2005). Altitude-related polycythemia, dehydration, and increased intracranial pressure if AMS is present, increased cerebrovenous pressure, cerebrovascular spasm, and coagulation abnormalities all may contribute to development of stroke. Stroke may be confused with HACE. Neurologic symptoms, especially focal abnormalities without AMS or HAPE that persist despite treatment with oxygen, steroids, and descent, suggest a cerebrovascular event and mandate comprehensive evaluation after evacuation to definitive care.

Treatment of stroke is supportive, and oxygen and steroids may be worthwhile to treat any AMS or HACE component. Persons with transient ischemic attacks at high altitude should be started on aspirin therapy and proceed to a lower altitude. Oxygen may quickly abort cerebrovascular spasms and will improve watershed hypoxic events. When oxygen is not available, rebreathing to raise alveolar PCO_2 may be helpful through increasing cerebral blood flow.

COGNITIVE CHANGES AT HIGH ALTITUDE

Mild cognitive changes at high altitude are well recognized and may be related to hypoxia's effect on specific neurotransmitters. In the serotonin synthesis pathway, tryptophan hydroxylase has a high requirement for oxygen (K_m = 37 torr). Tyrosine hydroxylase, in the dopamine pathway, is also oxygen-sensitive. A decrease in acetylcholine activity during hypoxia might explain lassitude at altitude. Increased dietary tyrosine reduces mood changes and symptoms of environmental stress in subjects at simulated altitude. Further work with neurotransmitter agonists and antagonists will help shed light on their role in cognitive dysfunction at altitude and could lead to new pharmacological approaches to improve neurologic function.

HIGH-ALTITUDE PULMONARY EDEMA

HAPE is the most common cause of death related to high altitude and is completely and easily reversed if recognized early and treated properly. HAPE was likely misdiagnosed for centuries, as evidenced by frequent reports of young, vigorous men suddenly dying of "pneumonia" within days of arriving at high altitude. It was not until Hultgren (Hultgren and Spickard, 1960; Hultgren, Lopez, et al., 1964) and Houston (Houston, 1960) that the English-speaking world became aware of high-altitude pulmonary edema, a noncardiogenic edema.

The factors determining development of HAPE include individual susceptibility, rate of ascent, altitude reached, degree of cold, physical exertion, and certain underlying medical conditions. The incidence varies from less than 1 in 10,000 skiers at moderate altitude in Colorado to 1 in 50 climbers on Mt. McKinley (6,194 m) and up to 6% of mountaineers in the Alps ascending rapidly to 4559 m (Table 19.1). Individuals with a previous episode of HAPE had a 60% attack rate when they went to 4,559 m in 36 hours, but with a slower ascent, some of the same individuals were able to climb over 7,000 m without developing HAPE (Bärtsch, 1999). Although HAPE occurs in both sexes, it is somewhat less common in women. Whether all persons are capable of developing HAPE (with a very rapid ascent to a sufficiently high altitude and with heavy exercise) is arguable (Bärtsch, Mairbaurl, et al., 2005). Even well-acclimatized individuals with a sudden push to a higher altitude can succumb to HAPE, but a population of HAPE-susceptible persons with unique physiological characteristics has been described. Victims are frequently young, fit males who ascend rapidly from sea level and may not have previously suffered HAPE even with repeated altitude exposures; this ascent may have been faster than previously. HAPE usually occurs within the first 4 days of ascent to higher altitudes (above 2,500 m), most commonly on the second night. Decreased exercise performance and increased recovery time from exercise are the earliest indications of HAPE; victims notice fatigue, weakness, and dyspnea on exertion, especially when walking uphill. Signs of AMS, such as headache, anorexia, and lassitude, are present about 50% of the time. A persistent dry cough develops, and nailbeds and lips become cyanotic. The condition typically worsens at night, and tachycardia and tachypnea develop at rest. Dyspnea at rest and audible congestion in the chest herald the development of a serious condition.

HAPE may strike abruptly, especially in a sedentary person who may not notice the early stages. Orthopnea is uncommon (7%). Pink or blood-tinged, frothy sputum is a very late finding. Severe hypoxemia may produce cerebral edema with mental changes, ataxia, decreased level of consciousness, and coma.

Elevated temperature of up to 38.5°C is common. Tachycardia correlates with respiratory rate and severity of illness. Râles may be unilateral or bilateral and usually originate from the right middle lobe. Concomitant respiratory infection is sometimes present.

Hemodynamic measurements show elevated pulmonary artery pressure and pulmonary vascular resistance, low to normal pulmonary wedge pressure, and low to normal cardiac output and systemic arterial blood pressure. Echocardiography demonstrates high pulmonary artery pressure, tricuspid regurgitation, normal left ventricular systolic function, somewhat abnormal diastolic function, and variable right-sided heart findings of increased atrial and ventricular size.

In HAPE, elevation of the peripheral white blood cell count is common, but rarely is it above 14,000 cells/ml^3. The serum concentration of creatine phosphokinase (CPK) is increased; most of the rise in CPK has been attributed to skeletal muscle damage. B-type natriuretic peptide (BNP) values may or may not be elevated. Arterial blood gas studies are unnecessary if noninvasive pulse oximetry is available to measure arterial oxygenation; values in HAPE subjects at 4,300 m ranged from 40 to 70%, with a mean of 56 ± 8% (Schoene, Swenson, et al., 1988).

The radiographic findings in HAPE are consistent with noncardiogenic pulmonary edema, with generally normal heart size and left atrial size and no evidence of pulmonary venous prominence. The pulmonary arteries increase in diameter (Vock, Brutsche, et al., 1991). Infiltrates are commonly described as fluffy and patchy with areas of aeration between infiltrates and in a peripheral location rather than central. Infiltrates may be unilateral or bilateral, with a predilection for the right middle lung field, which corresponds to the usual area of râles. Pleural effusion is rare. The X-ray findings generally correlate with the severity of the illness and degree of hypoxemia.

Clearing of infiltrates is generally rapid once treatment is initiated. Depending on severity, complete clearing may take from one to several days. Infiltrates are likely to persist longer if the patient remains at high altitude, even if confined to bed and receiving oxygen therapy. Radiographs taken within 24–48 hours of return to low altitude may still be able to confirm diagnosis of HAPE.

In contrast to HACE, the physiology of HAPE has been the subject of intense study and ultimately provides us with more insight into the causes and treatment of the disease. Excessive pulmonary artery pressure (PAP) is the sine qua non of HAPE; no cases of HAPE have been reported without pulmonary hypertension. The degree of hypoxic pulmonary vascular response (HPVR) varies widely and is most likely an inherent trait. Persons who are HAPE-susceptible have a greater increase in PAP than those who are not susceptible. Although other factors, such as the vigor of the ventilatory response and subsequent alveolar PO_2 may help determine the ultimate degree of pulmonary hypertension, HPVR appears to be the dominant factor. Because all persons with HAPE have excessive pulmonary hypertension, but not all those with excessive pulmonary hypertension have HAPE, it appears that pulmonary hypertension is a necessary factor but in itself is not the cause of HAPE.

Hultgren suggested that, in those who develop HAPE, the hypoxic pulmonary vasoconstriction is uneven and that delicate microcirculation in unconstricted (relatively dilated) areas is subjected to high pressure and flow, leading to leakage (edema). HAPE's rapid reversibility and response to vasodilators are consistent with this mechanism. When hydrostatic pressure is reduced, alveolar fluid is quickly reabsorbed.

Other factors contributing to increased hydrostatic pressure, such as exercise or a high salt load with subsequent hypervolemia, also may play a role in HAPE. In fact, the authors have several times observed onset of HAPE after a large salt intake. Some studies have also suggested a role for pulmonary venous constriction, which would contribute to increased capillary hydrostatic pressure.

The end result of overperfusion and increased capillary pressure (Maggiorini, Melot et al. 2001) is distension, increased filtration of fluid, and even rupture of the capillary–alveolar membrane, termed stress failure, with subsequent leakage of cells and proteins.

Individuals who contract HAPE appear to have an impaired ability to clear alveolar fluid, with lower activity of the epithelial sodium channel (ENaC) and reduced ability to transport sodium across the epithelium back into the interstitial space (Sartori, Duplain et al., 2004). In addition, epithelial sodium transport is diminished by hypoxia per se, so that those with already impaired function become more impaired at altitude.

As in AMS, control of ventilation may play a role in the pathophysiology of HAPE. Those with HAPE have a lower hypoxic ventilatory response (HVR) than persons who acclimatize well, but not all persons with a low HVR become ill; low HVR may play a permissive, rather than causative, role in the development of HAPE. A brisk HVR, and therefore a large increase in ventilation, appears to be protective. Hypoventilators at altitude are more hypoxemic and presumably suffer greater pulmonary hypertension, and a low HVR may permit episodes of extreme hypoxemia during sleep. Supporting this concept is the frequency with which the onset of HAPE occurs during sleep, especially in persons who have ingested sleep medications. In addition, a HAPE victim

with a low HVR does not mount an adequate ventilatory response to the severe hypoxemia of the illness and may suffer further ventilatory depression through CNS suppression (hypoxic ventilatory depression). Such persons, when given oxygen, show a paradoxical increase in ventilation. Despite the correlation of HAPE with low HVR, its value as a sea level predictor is poor.

Persons susceptible to HAPE (HAPE-s) have abnormal endothelial function, as evidenced by reduced nitric oxide (NO) synthesis during hypoxia, and during HAPE, and higher levels of endothelin, a potent pulmonary vasoconstrictor. The importance of reduced NO is reinforced by studies showing improvement in pulmonary hemodynamics when either NO or a PDE-5 inhibitor, sildenafil or tadalafil was given to HAPE subjects (Anand, Prasad, et al. 1998; Maggiorini, Brunner-LaRocca, et al., 2006).

Gene polymorphisms coding for the angiotensin receptor and endothelial nitric oxide distinguish those who are prone to develop HAPE. In the near future, single nucleotide polymorphism scanning techniques as well as RNA gene expression techniques will be used to explore the genetic contributions to high-altitude physiology and pathophysiology. The search for a genetic basis of HAPE susceptibility continues.

HAPE Treatment

Treatment choices for HAPE depend on severity of illness and logistics, and early recognition is the key to a successful outcome, as with all high-altitude illnesses (Box 19.1). On expedition, where oxygen may be limited or unavailable, persons with HAPE may need to be urgently evacuated to lower altitude. However, because exertion augments pulmonary hypertension and hypoxemia, and cold augments PAP, exertion must be minimized and the victim should be kept warm. If HAPE is diagnosed early, recovery may be rapid with a descent of only 500–1,000 m, and the victim may be able to reascend slowly 2 or 3 days later. In high-altitude locations with oxygen supplies, bed rest with supplemental oxygen may suffice, but severe HAPE may require high-flow oxygen (4 L/min or more) for more than 24 hours. Hyperbaric therapy with the fabric pressure bag can help conserve oxygen supplies. Administration of oxygen immediately reduces pulmonary artery pressure, heart rate, respiratory rate, and symptoms. When descent is not possible, oxygen (or a hyperbaric bag) can be lifesaving. Delivery of oxygen to the HAPE victim, by airdrop if necessary, should be of highest priority if descent is slow or delayed, as waiting for a helicopter or rescue team has too often proved fatal. The use of a mask providing pressure (resistance) on expiration (EPAP) was shown to improve gas exchange in HAPE, and this may be useful as a temporizing measure (Schoene, Roach, et al., 1985). The same is accomplished with pursed-lip breathing.

Medications that reduce pulmonary blood volume, PAP, and pulmonary vascular resistance are physiologically rational to use when oxygen is not available, descent is delayed, or symptoms are severe. Nifedipine (30 mg slow release every 12–24 hours or 10 mg orally repeated as necessary) effectively reduces pulmonary vascular resistance and PAP during HAPE, and slightly improves arterial oxygenation (Oelz, Maggiorini, et al., 1989). Nitric oxide, a potent pulmonary vasodilator, improves hemodynamics in HAPE (Anand, Prasad, et al., 1998) but is rarely available, and in any event is usually given with oxygen. The PDE-5 inhibitors, which increase c-GMP to produce pulmonary vasodilation during hypoxia, have shown value for prevention of HAPE (Maggiorini, Brunner-LaRocca, et al., 2006), and although not yet studied for treatment, their use would be rational; studies of these agents for HAPE treatment are forthcoming. Whether these agents will prove to be more effective than nifedipine for treatment is unknown. A theoretical advantage is that the PDE-5 inhibitors produce less systemic vasodilation.

The therapeutic potential of beta-2 adrenergic agonists has been evaluated in some experimental models that are relevant for HAPE. In hydrostatic pulmonary edema, beta-agonists can accelerate the resolution of alveolar edema experimentally. In the presence of acute lung injury, beta-2 adrenergic agonists have been reported to augment the rate of alveolar epithelial fluid transport in rats with moderate lung injury from hyperoxia by about 50% above basal levels. Theoretically, beta-2 agonists may also augment surfactant secretion, decrease lung endothelial permeability, and decrease airway resistance and therefore are useful for treatment of HAPE. More experimental studies are needed to test the potential efficacy of beta-2 agonists in HAPE, but one might argue that use of beta-2 adrenergic agonists is a safe therapy because aerosolized beta-agonists are easily used, familiar to patients and practitioners and well tolerated, with minimal hemodynamic side effects.

After evacuation of the victim to a lower altitude, hospitalization may be warranted for severe cases. Treatment consists of bed rest and oxygen titrated to maintain SaO_2% greater than 90%. Rapid recovery is the rule, and antibiotics are indicated for infection when present. Occasionally, pulmonary artery catheterization or Doppler echocardiography is necessary to differentiate cardiogenic from high-altitude pulmonary edema. A HAPE victim demonstrating unusual susceptibility, such as onset of HAPE despite adequate acclimatization, or onset below 2,750 m, might require further investigation, such as echocardiography, to rule out an intracardiac shunt. Patients are advised to resume normal activities gradually and are warned that they may require up to 2 weeks to recover complete strength. An episode of HAPE is not a contraindication to subsequent high-altitude

exposure, but education to ensure proper preventive measures and recognition of early symptoms is critical.

HAPE Prevention

The preventive measures previously described for AMS also apply to HAPE (Box 19.1). Because exertion may contribute to onset of HAPE, especially at moderate altitude, prudence dictates not overexerting for the first 2 days after ascent. Clinical experience suggests that acetazolamide prevents HAPE in persons with a history of recurrent episodes; recent animal and human studies show that acetazolamide blocks hypoxic pulmonary hypertension, thus supporting this practice. Clinical trials of acetazolamide for prevention of HAPE are pending. Nifedipine (20 mg slow release every 8 hours) prevents HAPE in subjects with a history of repeated episodes (Bärtsch, Maggiorini, et al., 1991); it should be carried by susceptible individuals and started at the first signs of HAPE or, for an abrupt ascent, started when leaving low altitude. The PDE-5 inhibitors sildenafil and tadalafil effectively block hypoxic pulmonary hypertension and therefore will prevent HAPE (Maggiorini, Brunner-LaRocca, et al., 2006), but the optimal dose has not been established. [Regimens for sildenafil have varied from a single dose of 50 or 100 mg just prior to exposure for acute studies (Ghofrani, Reichenberger, et al., 2004; Ricart, Maristany, et al., 2005) to 40 mg tid for 2–6 days at altitude (Perimenis, 2005; Richalet, Gratadour, et al., 2005) and for tadalafil 10 mg every 12 hours while ascending. (Maggiorini, Brunner-LaRocca, et al., 2006).] Dexamethasone, 8 mg every 12 hours while ascending for 2 days, was as effective as tadalafil in reducing PAP in a small study of susceptible subjects, and was 100% effective in preventing HAPE (Maggiorini, Brunner-LaRocca, et al., 2006). A clinical study indicated that use of an inhaled lipid-soluble beta-2 agonist reduced the incidence of high-altitude pulmonary edema by 50% in patients with a prior history of HAPE (Sartori, Allemann, et al., 2002).

In summary, there are now a number of effective agents for prevention of HAPE, and choice of agent depends upon safety, cost, effectiveness and the individual patient. Based on current evidence, salmeterol, nifedipine, tadalafil, and dexamethasone are useful and reasonable. Nifedipine is less costly than tadalafil but carries the risk of hypotension. Dexamethasone has the significant advantage of also preventing AMS, unlike the other agents, but also produces more potentially serious side effects. Salmeterol does not appear to be as effective as the other medications. If further clinical trials with acetazolamide show it to be as effective as tadalafil and dexamethasone, these authors would suggest it, since acetazolamide is the only agent that speeds acclimatization, while it also prevents AMS and periodic breathing and improves nocturnal oxygen saturation.

REENTRY PULMONARY EDEMA

HAPE develops on reascent from a trip to low altitude in some long-term altitude residents, and authors have suggested that the incidence of HAPE on reascent may be higher than that during initial ascent by flatlanders, although data on true incidence are difficult to obtain. Children and adolescents are more susceptible than adults. Severinghaus has postulated that increased muscularization of pulmonary arterioles that develops with chronic high-altitude exposure generates an inordinately high pulmonary artery pressure on reascent, causing the edema. Whether this occurs in expeditioners is unclear. Climbers have certainly developed HAPE after being high on a mountain, descending to base camp or lower, and then reascending to their previous high altitude or higher. The stay at lower altitude may be as short as 2–3 days. However, the reascent is often faster, sometimes skipping lower camps, and other variables such as temperature and load carried are often different. Therefore, such episodes may not represent "classic" reentry HAPE. Common wisdom, however, is to reascend cautiously after a stay of a few days or more at a lower altitude. Pending systematic study of this issue, this approach seems reasonable.

HIGH-ALTITUDE DETERIORATION

Above 5,500 m, deterioration outstrips the ability to acclimatize, and this deterioration is more rapid the higher one goes above the maximum point of acclimatization. The death zone (above 8,000 m) is so named because deterioration is so rapid that, without supplemental oxygen, death can occur in a matter of days. Life-preserving tasks such as melting snow for water may become too difficult and death may result from dehydration, starvation, hypothermia, and especially neurologic and psychiatric dysfunction.

Loss of body mass is a prominent feature of high-altitude deterioration. Weight is progressively lost due to combined anorexia and malabsorption during expeditions to extreme high altitude. Climbers on the 1953 British Mt. Everest Expedition lost 14–20 kg, and nearly 30 years later, despite improvement in food and cooking techniques, climbers on the American Medical Research Expedition to Mt. Everest still lost an average of 6 kg (Boyer and Blume, 1984). At very high altitudes, an increase in caloric intake may not be sufficient to completely counteract the severe anorexia and weight loss as other mechanisms may come into play.

High-Altitude Syncope

A problem limited to the acute acclimatization period, syncope within the first 24 hours of arrival occurs occasionally at moderate altitude (Nicholas and O'Meara, 1993) and is not observed in mountaineers at higher altitudes. The mechanism for high-altitude syncope is an unstable cardiovascular control system, a form of neurohumoral (or neurocardiogenic) syncope (Freitas, Costa, et al., 1996). An unstable state of cerebral autoregulation may also play a role. Syncopal events tend to be random, seldom occur a second time, and not predict ensuing high-altitude illness. Preexisting cardiovascular disease is not a factor in most cases. Postprandial state and alcohol ingestion seem to be contributing factors.

THROMBOSIS: COAGULATION AND PLATELET CHANGES

Autopsy findings of widespread thrombi in the brain and lungs after altitude death, and an impression that thrombosis is greater at altitude have led to many investigations of the clotting mechanism at high altitude. Even though changes in platelets and coagulation have been observed in animals and humans on ascent to high altitude, these occur with very rapid ascent and are generally found in vitro. In vivo studies using typical ascent profiles up to 4,500 m in the mountains, and higher in chambers, have generally not found changes in coagulation and fibrinolysis (Grover and Bärtsch, 2001). Although higher incidence of thrombosis in soldiers and others at extreme altitude can be attributed to dehydration, polycythemia, and forced inactivity, there is some evidence of enhanced fibrin formation with stay of a few weeks over 5,000 m.

Does ascent to altitude result in thrombosis in persons with familial thrombophilia? Such cases have been reported (Boulos, Kouroukis, et al., 1999; Basnyat, Graham, et al., 2001), but cause and effect cannot be established. In addition, persons with a history of deep vein thrombosis or pulmonary embolus wonder if they are at increased risk at high altitude, as do women on hormonal contraceptives; unfortunately, the literature does not provide guidance for these individuals. Some experts empirically recommend an aspirin a day during altitude exposure for such patients, and this seems to be safe advice.

PERIPHERAL EDEMA

Edema of the face, hands, and ankles at high altitude is common, especially in females. The incidence of peripheral edema in trekkers at 4,200 m was 18% overall (28% in females, 14% in males, 7% in asymptomatic trekkers, and 27% in those with AMS) (Hackett and Rennie, 1979). Not a serious clinical problem in and of itself, edema can be bothersome, and its presence demands at least a cursory examination for pulmonary and cerebral edema. In the absence of AMS, peripheral edema is effectively treated with a diuretic. Treatment of accompanying AMS by descent or medical therapy also results in diuresis and resolution of peripheral edema. The mechanism is presumably similar to fluid retention in AMS, but it may also be merely due to exercise.

Immunosuppression

Infections are common at high altitude, slow to resolve, and often resistant to antibiotics. On the American Medical Research Expedition to Mt. Everest in 1981, serious skin and soft tissue infections developed. "Nearly every accidental wound, no matter how small, suppurated for a period of time and subsequently healed slowly" (Sarnquist, 1983). Most high-altitude expeditions report similar problems.

Healthy individuals are probably more susceptible to infections at high altitude because of impaired T lymphocyte function; this is consistent with previous Russian studies in humans and animals. In contrast, B cells and active immunity are not impaired, so resistance to viruses may not be impaired, while susceptibility to bacterial infection is increased. The degree of altitude-related immunosuppression is similar to that seen with trauma, burns, emotional depression, and space flight, and the mechanism may be related, at least in part, to release of adrenocorticotropic hormone, cortisone, and beta-endorphins, all of which modulate the immune response. In addition, intense ultraviolet exposure, an integral feature of high-altitude expeditions, has also been shown to impair immunity. Persons with serious infections at high altitude may need oxygen or descent for effective treatment.

HIGH-ALTITUDE PHARYNGITIS AND BRONCHITIS

Sore throat, chronic cough, and bronchitis are extremely common in persons who spend more than 2 weeks at extreme altitude (over 5,500 m) (Litch and Tuggy, 1998; Mason, Barry, et al., 1999). Acute hypoxia directly lowers the cough threshold, thus exacerbating high altitude cough, but other factors are at play. At altitude, sore throat and cough usually appear without fever or chills, myalgia, lymphadenopathy, exudate, or other signs of infection. The increase in ventilation, especially with exercise, forces obligate mouth breathing at altitude, bypassing the warming and moisturizing action of the nasal mucous membranes and sinuses. Movement of large volumes of dry, cold air across the pharyngeal mucosa can cause marked dehydration, irritation, and pain, similar to pharyngitis. Vasomotor rhinitis, quite common in cold temperatures, aggravates this condition by necessitating mouth breathing during sleep. For this reason, decongestant nasal spray is one of the most coveted items in an expedition medical kit. Other countermeasures include forced hydration, hard candies, lozenges, and steam inhalation.

Severe cough with resultant rib fracture can be a disabling and expedition-ending consequence of high altitude. Purulent sputum is common, and response to antibiotics is poor; most victims resign themselves to taking medications such as codeine and do not expect or get a cure until descent. Although an infectious etiology is possible, experimental evidence suggests that respiratory heat loss results in purulent sputum and sufficient airway irritation to cause persistent cough. This is supported by the beneficial effect of steam inhalation and lack of response to antibiotics. Many climbers find that a thin balaclava, porous enough for breathing, traps some moisture and heat and effectively prevents or ameliorates the problem.

THE EYE AT ALTITUDE

Altitude-associated ocular disorders have been addressed in several recent review articles (Butler, 1999; Cinal, Yasar, et al., 1999; Mader and Tabin, 2003; Butler, 2007), and we discuss the more common problems here. Those eye problems not directly related to altitude exposure are discussed in Chapter 36.

The hypoxic hypobaria of altitude causes retinal blood flow to increase by 128% after 4 days at 5,300 m (Frayser, Houston, et al., 1971). Observable changes ensue in otherwise asymptomatic patients, including an increase in diameter and tortuosity of retinal vessels and optic disk hyperemia.

The cornea receives most of its oxygen supply from the surrounding atmosphere, so it may suffer hypoxic dysfunction even if the inspired gas mix is not hypoxic, for example, in climbers breathing supplemental oxygen.

High-Altitude Retinal Hemorrhage

A review of the literature finds many reports of retinal hemorrhages in mountain climbers described as high-altitude retinal hemorrhages (HARH) or as part of the more inclusive term "altitude retinopathy" (see Figure 19.4). One study reported an incidence of HARH of 29% in Mt. Everest climbers (Butler, Harris, et al., 1992), and another reported a 56% incidence of HARH at an altitude of 5,360 m (McFadden, Houston, et al., 1981). Hackett and Rennie described HARH in 4% of 140 trekkers examined at 4,243 m and found a significant correlation of retinal hemorrhages with AMS (Hackett and Rennie, 1979). Differences in the incidence of HARH for exposures at similar altitudes is likely due to factors including differences in ascent itinerary, individual exertion or comorbidities, and examination techniques among others.

Although the majority of HARH are not symptomatic, in some cases they result in a loss of visual acuity or paracentral scotoma. Permanent visual deficits are uncommon but have been reported, and HARH that results in decreased visual acuity should be a contraindication to further ascent. Experts recommend that

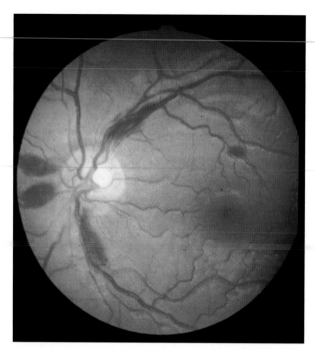

Figure 19.4. Photo of high-altitude retinal hemorrhage. Photo courtesy Peter Hackett.

evacuation of individuals with decreases in visual function resulting from HARH (in the absence of high-altitude cerebral edema or high-altitude pulmonary) be considered nonemergent unless reexamination indicates a progressive deterioration of vision or increasingly severe retinopathy. HARH resolves over a period of 2–8 weeks after the altitude exposure is terminated.

Intraocular Gas Bubbles at Altitude

Intraocular gases are frequently used to provide internal tamponade during and after vitreoretinal surgery and the resulting expansion of the bubble can lead to a rapid rise in intraocular pressure. Therefore, the presence of an intraocular gas bubble presents a hazard for anyone exposed to a hypobaric environment such as ascent to altitude on a mountaineering expedition.

Fang reported a case of a 46-year-old man who ascended to an altitude of 1,900 m after vitreoretinal surgery with a residual perfluoropropane bubble in his right eye. He noted a sensation of fullness in his right eye accompanied by loss of vision and when he returned to sea level, his intraocular pressure was 54 mmHg. The etiology of this vision loss was believed to be central retinal artery occlusion caused by expansion of intraocular gas during mountain travel (Fang and Huang, 2002).

Cortical Blindness at High Altitude

Hackett (Hackett, Roach, et al., 1987) reported six cases of cortical blindness at high altitude; these victims were found to have intact pupillary reflexes and not to have

a primary ophthalmologic process. See section "Neurologic Syndromes at Altitude" for further discussion.

Ocular Motility

One author reported convergence insufficiency in women with altitude illness (Kramar, Drinkwater, et al., 1983), and another noted occasional lateral gaze palsy and other focal neurologic deficits, often in the absence of other symptoms of AMS or HACE (Basnyat, Wu, et al., 2004). Rennie and Morrissey (1975) reported a person with nystagmus at altitude that was associated with ataxia and intention tremor. Ocular motility abnormalities mandate a careful examination for high-altitude cerebral edema or other signs of CVA or TIA. Oxygen, descent, rebreathing to increase CO_2, or steroids may be indicated based on the most likely diagnosis. As mentioned earlier, focal neurologic deficits should not be attributed to altitude illness and require a careful evaluation.

Contact Lenses in Mountaineering

Contact lenses may be used successfully at high altitude (Butler, 2007), but use of contact lenses at altitude during trekking or mountaineering entails several considerations beyond those encountered in normal use. In general, overnight use of extended-wear contact lenses is not recommended because of the associated increased incidence of microbial keratitis. Even soft contact lenses decrease the oxygen available to the cornea, and lid closure during sleep further accentuates corneal hypoxia. Routine nightly contact lens removal, however, can be difficult in a mountaineering setting and practicing acceptable lens hygiene during an expedition is difficult. Wearers who leave lenses in a fluid filled case at night may awaken to find the solution and lenses frozen solid.

Guidelines for military personnel using contact lenses in austere environments have been developed and apply to the expedition setting (Butler, 1999): Please see Chapter 36 for further discussion.

The decision to wear contact lenses while mountaineering should be made carefully; microbial keratitis and ultraviolet keratitis, among other potential complications, leave experts recommending a good pair of prescription glacier glasses, or laser refractive surgery might be a more reasonable alternative than contact lenses as a long-term solution to the refractive needs of mountaineers.

Refractive Changes at Altitude after Refractive Surgery

Individuals with previous radial keratotomy (RK) may experience an acute hyperopic shift with altitude exposure, and this has been observed at altitudes as low as

2,744 m. Further studies on subjects who had undergone RK or photorefractive keratectomy (PRK) and had a 72-hour exposure at 4,299 m revealed a progressive hyperopic shift associated with flattened keratometry (Mader, 1996). Those who had undergone PRK experienced no change in their refractive state, but peripheral corneal thickening was seen in both groups, and refraction, keratometry, and pachymetry all returned to baseline after return to sea level. Strong evidence suggests that the effect of altitude exposures on post-RK eyes is caused by hypoxia rather than by hypobarism. The same changes are induced by exposing the eyes to nitrogen in special goggles, so that the hypoxia is limited to the cornea, further illustrating that breathing a normoxic inspired gas mix will not protect against the development of hypoxic corneal changes.

Altitude-related hyperopic shift in post-RK patients depends on the postoperative refractive state (undercorrected patients may actually have their vision improve) and the individual's baseline accommodative capacity. There exists compelling evidence for myopic mountaineers that PRK instead of RK is the refractive surgical procedure of choice (Mader and Tabin, 2003). Individuals who have undergone RK and plan altitude exposure of 2,744 m or more while mountaineering should bring multiple glasses with increasing plus lens power. The altitude at which RK is performed also affects the surgical outcome. RK done at altitude (1,753 m) produces more of a hyperopic shift than the same procedure done at sea level (Dimmig and Tabin, 2003).

The most commonly performed laser refractive surgery at present is laser in situ keratomileusis (LASIK). Recent studies have examined the effects of altitude exposure on individuals who have had this procedure, and the authors' conclusion was that LASIK may be a good choice for individuals involved in high-altitude activities, but those achieving extreme altitudes of 7,927 m (26,000 ft) and above should be aware of possible fluctuation of vision (Dimmig and Tabin, 2003) with myopic shifts that resolve after return to sea level. Climbers who do not ascend beyond moderate altitudes should not experience a post-LASIK refractive shift.

Glaucoma at Altitude

Individuals who have mild, well-controlled glaucoma may suffer adverse effects at altitude if they are being treated with topical beta-blockers because these drugs may produce systemic side effects of lethargy and exercise intolerance that may be exacerbated at altitude (Mader and Tabin, 2003). Physicians should consider alternative choices for topical therapy in persons who will be traveling to significant altitude. Hypoxia at altitude may also worsen glaucomatous optic neuropathy, and those effects may persist on descent (Mader and Tabin, 2003).

Ultraviolet Keratitis

See Chapter 36.

COMMON MEDICAL CONDITIONS AND HIGH ALTITUDE

Expeditioners with certain preexisting illnesses might be at risk for adverse effects upon ascent to high altitude, either because of exacerbation of their illnesses or because these illnesses might impact acclimatization and susceptibility to altitude illness (Box 19.2). Although altitude-related research on these groups is limited, some literature provides guidance for the common problems that follow. We assume that persons with moderate to severe lung and cardiovascular disease will not be on an expedition, and we therefore limit our discussion to the more likely conditions to be encountered by the expedition doctor. For a more complete review, see Hackett (2001).

Asthma

Literature suggests that asthmatics do well at moderate altitude, both residents and sojourners, primarily because of decreased allergens and pollution (Hackett, 2001), and high altitude as a treatment for asthma has been popular in Europe for many decades. The effect of a high-altitude environment may approach the effects of high doses of inhaled steroids (Cogo, Fischer, et al., 2004). However, because altitude exposure often includes exercise (and cold), asthmatics with exercise-induced bronchospasm, rather than allergic asthma, might have increased problems at altitude. In a study of asthmatic high-altitude trekkers, risk factors for an asthma attack at altitude were use of inhaled bronchodilators more than three times a week prior to travel and intensive physical exertion during the trek (Golan, Onn, et al., 2002). In one study of 31 ski-mountaineers in cold temperatures and exercising heavily above 3000 m, 16 developed exercise-induced bronchospasm (EIB, decrease in peak flow of > 10%) (Durand, Kippelen, et al., 2005). Interestingly, only four had a previous diagnosis of EIB. This study suggests that half of the people in such circumstances can develop bronchospasm. Therefore, even in those without a history of EIB, beta-agonists, or even inhaled steroids should be considered mountaineers who develop bronchospasm with exertion.

Persons with asthma ascending to high altitude should be advised to undertake travel only after achieving maximum function before ascent, to continue on their usual medications, including steroids, and to carry steroids and bronchodilators with them in the event of an exacerbation. Because airway heat loss can be a trigger for bronchospasm, the use of an airway-warming mask might be helpful but is unproven. In summary, although

Box 19.2. Advisability of exposure to high and very high altitude for common conditions (without supplemental oxygen)

Probably no extra risk
Young and old
Fit and unfit
Mild obesity
Diabetes
Asthma
Low-risk pregnancy
Controlled hypertension
Controlled seizure disorder
Stable psychiatric disorders
Neoplastic diseases
Inflammatory conditions
Mild COPD
After coronary artery bypass grafting (without angina)

Caution
Moderate COPD
Asymptomatic pulmonary hypertension
Compensated congestive heart failure (CHF)
Morbid obesity
Sleep apnea syndromes
Troublesome arrhythmias
Stable angina/coronary artery disease
High-risk pregnancy
Sickle cell trait
Cerebrovascular diseases
Any cause for restricted pulmonary circulation
Seizure disorder (not on medication)
Radial keratotomy

Contraindicated
Sickle cell anemia (with history of crises)
Severe COPD
Symptomatic pulmonary hypertension
Uncompensated CHF

From Hackett and Roach (2007).

caution and adequate preparation are necessary, asthma is not a contraindication to high-altitude travel.

Pulmonary Vascular Disorders

Because of the danger of HAPE, preexisting pulmonary hypertension (of any etiology) is at least a relative contraindication to high-altitude exposure. Hypoxic pulmonary vasoconstriction will most likely exaggerate preexisting pulmonary hypertension and could lead to greater symptomatology in those with congenital cardiac defects, primary pulmonary hypertension (PPH), unilateral absent pulmonary artery, granulomatous mediastinitis, and restrictive lung diseases, all of which have been associated with high-altitude pulmonary edema (Hackett, 2001). Other conditions warranting caution include bronchopulmonary dysplasia, recurrent

pulmonary emboli, mitral stenosis, kyphoscoliosis, and scleroderma. Whether pulmonary hypertension is primary or secondary, expeditioners should be made aware of the potential hazards of high altitude, including HAPE. A mean PAP of greater than 30 mmHg is a useful threshold for caution (or oxygen) on ascent to altitude (Cogo, Fischer, et al., 2004).

Sleep Apnea, Sleep Disordered Breathing

Climbers with snoring, sleep apnea syndrome, and sleep disordered breathing (SDB) who become mildly hypoxemic at sea level may become severely hypoxemic at high altitude, and this could contribute to high-altitude illness and aggravate attendant problems such as polycythemia, pulmonary hypertension, cardiac arrhythmia, or insomnia. The scant research available has shown that obstructive sleep apnea tends to improve at altitude, while central apnea can become worse. Because central sleep apnea responds well to acetazolamide, and because obstructive apnea tends to convert to central apnea at altitude, an argument can be made to use acetazolamide in these persons. We feel that expeditioners with sleep-disordered breathing should have pulse oximetry during sleep, at least spot checks, and that supplemental oxygen should be considered for those who markedly desaturate despite acetazolamide.

Cardiovascular Conditions

Hypertension

Most studies of altitude ascent effects on blood pressure report a slight increase in blood pressure, associated with increased catecholamine activity and increased sympathetic activity. However, some individuals appear to have a pathologic response upon induction to high altitude, with a much higher change. After a period of at least a few months at altitude, down-regulation of adrenergic receptors results in attenuation of the initial blood pressure elevation, and long-term high-altitude residents have lower blood pressure than their sea level counterparts (Hultgren, 1979; Roca-Cusachs, 1995). Chronic altitude exposure has also been shown to inhibit progression of hypertension (Mirrakhimov and Winslow, 1996).

Studies on the effect of short-term altitude exposure on preexisting hypertension have generated mixed results; in general, the response in hypertensives is similar to those without hypertension (i.e., a small increase in blood pressure, with an exaggerated response in some individuals). The greater the hypoxic stress (the higher the altitude), the greater the change in blood pressures, and altitudes less than 3,000 m seem to result in little if any change (Hackett 2001).

Experts recommend patients who take antihypertensive treatment continue their medications while at high altitude. But because some persons may unpredictably become markedly hypertensive on altitude exposure, blood pressure monitoring should be considered, especially in those with labile hypertension or those who become symptomatic at altitude. Hypertension in short-term high-altitude sojourners, for the most part, should be considered transient and should not be treated because it rarely reaches dangerously high levels and will resolve on descent. As large number of hypertensive patients visit ski resorts and trek at high altitude, however, the occasional person with an exaggerated response will require treatment. Because the mechanism appears to be increased alpha-adrenergic activity, an alpha-blocker might be the best choice of therapy for these individuals. However, these agents can be difficult to use, and a calcium-channel blocker, ACE inhibitor, or a thiazide may be more practical. There is no evidence to date to suggest that hypertensive patients are more likely to develop high-altitude illnesses. Even though it requires some caution and monitoring, hypertension is not a contraindication to high-altitude exposure.

Arteriosclerotic Heart Disease

Increased myocardial vascularity may be an adaptation to life-long residence at high altitude that offers some protection from coronary artery disease, and the effect of acute, transient exposure to high altitude on the healthy heart appears to be benign. Research indicates that the healthy heart tolerates even extreme hypoxia quite well; this could partly be due to the marked reduction in maximal exercise with increasing altitude, which reduces maximal heart rate and myocardial oxygen demand, and also due to the increased coronary blood flow. A person with coronary artery disease (CAD), however, may not have the same adaptive capacities, as diseased coronary arteries might have limited ability to vasodilate and might actually constrict, due to unopposed sympathetic activation.

Surprisingly little literature is available to help the physician advise patients with existing CAD proposing a high-altitude expedition. In the United States, no evidence from state or county mortality statistics suggests an increased prevalence of acute coronary events in visitors to high-altitude locations; in contrast are data from Austria claiming a higher rate of sudden cardiac death in the mountains, compared to the overall risk of sudden cardiac death (Burtscher, Philadelphy, et al., 1993). However, the altitudes were rather low (1,000–2,100 m), and no increased risk was evident in men who participated regularly in sports. The authors suggested that abrupt onset of exercise in sedentary men combined with altitude stress might induce cardiac sudden death, but whether altitude contributed at all is unclear.

The slight increase in heart rate and blood pressure on initial ascent to altitude might exacerbate angina in those with otherwise stable coronary artery disease. One study evaluated men with stable exercise-induced angina by exercise treadmill test at 1,600 m, and within the first hour of arrival at 3,100 m (Morgan, Alexander, et al., 1990). Cardiac work was slightly higher for a given workload at high altitude compared to low altitude, and as a result, the onset of angina was at a slightly lower workload. They found that a heart rate of 70–85% of the rate that produced ischemia at low altitude was associated with angina-free exercise at 3,100 m, and they suggested that angina patients at altitude adjust their activity level based on heart rate, at least on the day of arrival. Other experts conclude that well-compensated sea level CAD patients do well at a moderate altitude after a few days of acclimatization, but that the acute angina threshold may be lower and activity should be reduced (Levine, Zuckerman, et al., 1997).

Although no dangerous arrhythmias have ever been reported in high-altitude studies, persons with troublesome or high-grade arrhythmia have not been studied at high altitude. Anecdotally, atrial fibrillation is sometimes aggravated or induced by acute ascent. Prudent advice to patients whose arrhythmias are well controlled on medication should be to continue the medication at altitude, whereas those with poorly controlled arrhythmias might do better to avoid a visit to high altitude.

Advising persons with CAD or who have a high likelihood of CAD about altitude exposure should be based on evidence that the stress of high altitude on the coronary circulation appears to be minimal at rest, but significant in conjunction with exercise. Ideally, no one with known CAD or even risk factors for CAD should undertake unaccustomed exercise at any altitude, and especially at high altitude. Therefore, advising an exercise program at sea level prior to exercising at altitude is prudent, and risk stratification that is commonly used at sea level can be applied for providing advice for high altitude. Using the standard recommendations, asymptomatic males older than age 50 with no risk factors require no testing. For asymptomatic males older than age 50 with risk factors, an exercise test is recommended to determine risk status prior to exercising at high altitude, followed by further evaluation as indicated. Patients with previous myocardial infarction (MI), bypass surgery, or angioplasty are considered high risk only if they have a strongly positive exercise treadmill test. High-risk patients may require coronary angiography to establish appropriate management. Noninvasive multislice computed tomography for CAD risk stratification may hold promise for use as an effective and sensitive screening tool for preexpedition evaluation (Hoffman, Shi, et al., 2005).

Obesity

The literature on altitude effects on obese patients is sparse, but a small study suggested a slight increased susceptibility to AMS in mildly obese men (Ge, Chase, et al., 2005), possibly due to lower nocturnal oxygen saturation that was present despite greater than normal hypoxic and hypercapnic chemosensitivity (Ge, 2003). Another study of men with metabolic syndrome (obesity, hypertension, diabetes, and hyperlipidemia) during a 3-week stay at 1,700 m found normal altitude responses, and a loss of body fat (Gunga, Fries, et al., 2003). Altitude has been suggested as a treatment for obesity.

Sickle Cell Disease

Sickle cell crisis is a well-recognized complication of high-altitude exposure. Even the modest altitude of a pressurized aircraft (1,500–2,000 m) induces acute vasoocclusive crisis in 20% of persons with hemoglobin SC and sickle-thalassemia genetic configuration (Hackett, 2001). High-altitude exposure may precipitate the first vasoocclusive crisis in persons previously unaware of their condition. Persons with sickle cell anemia and a history of vasoocclusive crises are advised to avoid altitudes over 1,800 m unless they are taking supplemental oxygen. Some authors have suggested that nonblack persons with the trait may be at greater risk for splenic syndrome at high altitude than are individuals of African descent. Treatment of splenic syndrome consists of intravenous hydration, oxygen, and removal to a lower altitude. The overall incidence of problems in persons with the trait is low, however, and no special precaution other than recognition of the splenic syndrome is recommended. The U.S. Army, for example, does not consider soldiers with the trait unfit for duty at high altitude. An expedition doctor, however, must consider splenic crisis in any member at high altitude with left upper quadrant pain.

Pregnancy

Based on the available research, it is prudent to recommend that only women with normal, low-risk pregnancy undertake a sojourn to altitude. For these women, exposure to an altitude at which SaO_2 will remain above 85% most of the time (up to 3,000 m altitude) appears to pose no risk of harm, but further study is needed to place these recommendations on a more solid scientific footing (Hackett, 2001). Risk stratification with the use of ultrasound may be useful to rule out the more common complications prior to travel. It is not the altitude per se that determines whether a fetus becomes stressed, but rather the maternal (and fetal) arterial oxygen transport. A woman with high-altitude pulmonary edema at 2,500 m, for example, is much more hypoxemic than a healthy woman at 5,000 m. Therefore, a strategy for preventing altitude illness, especially pulmonary edema,

must be explained and implemented. Consideration of a high-altitude sojourn in the developing world, or in a wilderness setting, raises other issues that may be more important than the modest hypoxia.

Chronic Altitude Illness

It is beyond the scope of this text to discuss the treatment of the various chronic altitude syndromes that may affect long-term residents and natives of high-altitude communities. Any expedition physician may be called on to render medical care to local communities in high-altitude villages and should be prepared to recognize and advise treatment for chronic altitude conditions such as chronic mountain sickness and high-altitude pulmonary hypertension among others. Excellent consensus recommendations for chronic altitude problems have recently been published (Leon-Velarde, Maggiorini, et al., 2005).

HIGH-ALTITUDE MEDICAL KITS

Please see Chapter 3 for a complete discussion of composition of expedition medical kits. Additional special equipment that should be considered for inclusion in any high-altitude expedition is listed below:

- Portable hyperbaric chamber (see Box 19.3 for list of suppliers)
- Oxygen cylinders or oxygen concentrator
- Medications: Acetazolamide tablets
- Dexamethasone tablets and injectable
- Nifedipine capsules
- Sildenafil or tadalafil tablets
- Inhaled salmeterol and salbutamol

Box 19-3. Portable hyperbaric chamber suppliers

CERTEC Bag from CERTEC (*http://www.certec.eu.com/*)

GAMOW Bag from Chinook Medical Gear (*http://www.chinookmed.com/*)

Portable Altitude Chamber (PAC Bag) from TREKSAFE (*http://www.treksafe.com.au/*)

SUMMARY

High-altitude expeditions are becoming more common and a variety of individuals are venturing to high altitudes. The expedition physician needs to be able to recognize common high-altitude ailments in order to ensure that the team's time at altitude is a safe and enjoyable one.

SUGGESTED READINGS

Anand S, Prasad B, et al. Effects of inhaled nitric oxide and oxygen in high-altitude pulmonary edema. *Circulation.* 1998;98:2441–5.

Bärtsch P. High altitude pulmonary edema. *Med Sci Sports Exerc.* 1999;31(1 Suppl): S23–7.

Bärtsch P, Maggiorini M, et al. Prevention of high-altitude pulmonary edema by nifedipine. *N Engl J Med.* 1991;325: 1284–9.

Bärtsch P, Mairbaurl H, et al. Physiological aspects of high-altitude pulmonary edema. *J Appl Physiol.* 2005;98(3): 1101–10.

Bärtsch, P, Roach RC. Acute mountain sickness and high-altitude cerebral edema. In: Hornbein TF, Schoene RB, eds. *High Altitude: An Exploration of Human Adaptation.* New York: Marcel Dekker; 2001: 731–76.

Basnyat B, Gertsch JH, et al. Efficacy of low-dose acetazolamide (125 mg BID) for the prophylaxis of acute mountain sickness: a prospective, double-blind, randomized, placebo-controlled trial. *High Alt Med Biol.* 2003;4(1):45–52.

Basnyat B, Graham L, et al. A language barrier, abdominal pain, and double vision. *Lancet.* 2001;357(9273):2022.

Basnyat B, Lemaster J, et al. Everest or bust: a cross sectional, epidemiological study of acute mountain sickness at 4243 meters in the Himalayas. *Aviat Space Environ Med.* 1999;70(9):867–73.

Basnyat B, Wu T, et al. Neurological conditions at altitude that fall outside the usual definition of altitude sickness. *High Alt Med Biol.* 2005;5(2):171–9.

Beaumont M, Goldenberg F, et al. Effect of zolpidem on sleep and ventilatory patterns at simulated altitude of 4,000 meters. *Am J Respir Crit Care Med.* 1996;153:1864–9.

Boulos P, Kouroukis C, et al. Superior sagittal sinus thrombosis occurring at high altitude associated with protein C deficiency." *Acta Haematol.* 1999;102:104–6.

Boyer SJ, Blume FD. Weight loss and changes in body composition at high altitude. *J Appl Physiol.* 1984;57:1580–5.

Bradwell AR, Coote JH, et al. The effect of temazepam and diamox on nocturnal hypoxia at altitude (Abstract). In: Sutton JR, Houston CS, Coates G, eds. *Hypoxia and Cold.* New York: Praeger; 1987: 543.

Broome JR, Stoneham MD, et al. High altitude headache: treatment with ibuprofen. *Aviat Space Environ Med.* 1994;65(1):19–20.

Burtscher M, Likar R, et al. Aspirin for prophylaxis against headache at high altitudes: randomised, double blind, placebo controlled trial. *BMJ.* 1998;316(7137):1057–8.

Burtscher M, Philadelphy M, et al. Sudden cardiac death during mountain hiking and downhill skiing. *N Engl J Med.* 1993;329:1738–9.

Butler F. The eye in the wilderness. In: Auerbach P, ed. *Wilderness Medicine.* St. Louis: C. V. Mosby; 2007.

Butler FK Jr. The eye at altitude. *Int Ophthalmol Clin.* 1999;39(2):59–78.

Butler FK, Harris DJ, et al. Altitude retinopathy on Mount Everest, 1989. *Ophthalmology.* 1992;99(5):739–46.

Cauchy E, Larmignat P, et al. Transient neurological disorders during a simulated ascent of Mount Everest. *Aviat Space Environ Med.* 2002;73(12):1224–9.

Cinal A, Yasar T, et al. A comparative study on the effect of radial keratotomy in patients who live at sea level and high altitude. *Eye.* 1999;13(Pt 3a):339–44.

Cogo A, Fischer R, et al. Respiratory diseases and high altitude. *High Alt Med Biol.* 2004;5(4):435–44.

Cremona G, Asnaghi R, et al. High altitude pulmonary edema at 4559 m: a population study (Abstract). In: Roach RC, Wagner PD, Hackett PH, eds. *Hypoxia: Into the Next Millennium.* New York: Plenum/Kluwer Academic Publishing; 1999: 474, 375.

Dickinson J. Severe acute mountain sickness. *Postgrad Med.* 1979;55:454–8.

Dimmig J, Tabin G. The ascent of Mount Everest following laser in situ keratomileusis. *J Refract Surg.* 2003;19:48.

Durand F, Kippelen P, et al. Undiagnosed exercise-induced bronchoconstriction in ski-mountaineers. *Int J Sports Med.* 2005;26(3):233–7.

Ellsworth AJ, Meyer EF, et al. Acetazolamide or dexamethasone use versus placebo to prevent acute mountain sickness on Mount Rainier. *West J Med.* 1991;154(3):289–93.

Fang IM, Huang JS. Central retinal artery occlusion caused by expansion of intraocular gas at high altitude. *Am J Ophthalmol.* 2002;134(4):603–5.

Ferrazzini G, Maggiorini M, et al. Successful treatment of acute mountain sickness with dexamethasone. *BMJ.* 1987;294:1380–2.

Frayser R, Houston CS, et al. The response of the retinal circulation to altitude. *Arch Intern Med.* 1971;127:708–11.

Freitas J, Costa O, et al. High altitude-related neurocardiogenic syncope." *Am J Cardiol.* 1996;77:1021.

Ge RL, Chase PJ, et al. Obesity: associations with acute mountain sickness. *Ann Intern Med.* 2003;139(4):253–7.

Ge RL, Stone JA, Levine BD, Babb TG. Exaggerated respiratory chemosensitivity and association with SaO_2 level at 3568 m in obesity. *Respir Physiol Neurobiol.* 2005;146(1):47–54.

Gertsch JH, Seto TB, et al. Ginkgo biloba for the prevention of severe acute mountain sickness (AMS) starting one day before rapid ascent. *High Alt Med Biol.* 2002;3(1):29–37.

Ghofrani HA, Reichenberger F, et al. Sildenafil increased exercise capacity during hypoxia at low altitudes and at Mount Everest base camp: a randomized, double-blind, placebo-controlled crossover trial. *Ann Intern Med.* 2004;141(3):169–77.

Golan Y, Onn A, et al. Asthma in adventure travelers: a prospective study evaluating the occurrence and risk factors for acute exacerbations. *Arch Intern Med.* 2002;162(21):2421–6.

Grissom CK, Roach RC, et al. Acetazolamide in the treatment of acute mountain sickness: clinical efficacy and effect on gas exchange. *Ann Intern Med.* 1992;116(6):461–5.

Grover R, Bärtsch P. Blood. In: Hornbein T, Schoene R, eds. *High Altitude: An Exploration of Human Adaptation.* New York: Marcel Dekker; 2001.

Gunga HC, Fries D, et al. Austrian Moderate Altitude Study (AMAS 2000) – fluid shifts, erythropoiesis, and angiogenesis in patients with metabolic syndrome at moderate altitude (congruent with 1700 m). *Eur J Appl Physiol.* 2003;88(6): 497–505.

Hackett, PH. High altitude and common medical conditions. In: Hornbein T, Schoene R, eds. *High Altitude: An Exploration of Human Adaptation.* New York: Dekker; 2001: 161, 839–86.

Hackett PH, Roach RC. High-altitude illness. *N Engl J Med.* 2001;345:107–14.

Hackett PH. The Denali Medical Research Project, 1982–1985. *Am Alpine J.* 1986;28(60):129.

Hackett PH, Rennie D. The incidence, importance, and prophylaxis of acute mountain sickness. *Lancet.* 1976;2(7996): 1149–55.

Hackett PH, Rennie ID. Rales, peripheral edema, retinal hemorrhage and acute mountain sickness. *Am J Med.* 1979;67: 214–18.

Hackett PH, Roach RC. High-altitude medicine. In: Auerbach P, ed. *Wilderness Medicine.* St. Louis: C. V. Mosby; 2007.

Hackett PH, Roach RC. High altitude cerebral edema. *High Alt Med Biol.* 2004;5(3).

Hackett PH, Roach RC, et al. Respiratory stimulants and sleep periodic breathing at high altitude. Almitrine versus acetazolamide. *Am Rev Respir Dis.* 1987;135: 896–8.

Hackett PH, Roach RC, et al. Cortical blindness in high altitude climbers and trekkers – a report on six cases (Abstract). In: Sutton JR, Houston CS, Coates G, eds. *Hypoxia and Cold.* New York: Praeger; 1987: 536.

Hackett PH, Roach RC, et al. Dexamethasone for prevention and treatment of acute mountain sickness. *Aviat Space Environ Med.* 1988;59(10):950–4.

Hackett PH, Yarnell PR, et al. High-altitude cerebral edema evaluated with magnetic resonance imaging: clinical correlation and pathophysiology. *JAMA.* 1998;280(22):1920–5.

Harris NS, Wenzel RP, et al. High altitude headache: efficacy of acetaminophen vs. ibuprofen in a randomized, controlled trial. *J Emerg Med.* 2003;24(4):383–7.

Hoffman M, Shi H, et al. Noninvasive coronary angiography with multislice computed tomography. *JAMA.* 2005;293: 2471–8.

Honigman B, Theis MK, et al. Acute mountain sickness in a general tourist population at moderate altitudes. *Ann Intern Med.* 1993;118:587–92.

Houston CS. Acute pulmonary edema of high altitude. *N Engl J Med.* 1960;263:478–80.

Hultgren H, Spickard W. Medical experiences in Peru. *Stanford Med Bull.* 1960;18:76–95.

Hultgren HN. Reduction of systemic arterial blood pressure at high altitude. *Adv Cardiol.* 1979;5:49–55.

Hultgren HN, Lopez CE, et al. Physiologic studies of pulmonary edema at high altitude. *Circulation.* 1964;29:393–408.

Johnson TS, Rock PB, et al. Prevention of acute mountain sickness by dexamethasone. *N Engl J Med.* 1984;310:683–6.

Kramar PO, Drinkwater BL, et al. Ocular functions and incidence of acute mountain sickness in women at altitude. *Aviat Space Environ Med.* 1983;54:116–20.

Larson EB, Roach RC, et al. Acute mountain sickness and acetazolamide: clinical efficacy and effect on ventilation. *JAMA.* 1982;288:328–32.

Leon-Velarde F, Maggiorini M, et al. Consensus statement on chronic and subacute high altitude diseases. *High Alt Med Biol.* 2005;6(2):147–57.

Levine BD, Zuckerman JH, et al. Effect of high-altitude exposure in the elderly: the Tenth Mountain Division study. *Circulation.* 1997;96(4):1224–32.

Litch JA, Tuggy M. Cough induced stress fracture and arthropathy of the ribs at extreme altitude. *Int J Sports Med.* 1998;19(3):220–2.

Maakestad K, Leadbetter G, et al. Ginkgo biloba reduces incidence and severity of acute mountain sickness. *Wild Environ Med.* 2001;12(1):51.

Mader T. Refractive changes during a 72 hour exposure to high altitude after refractive surgery. *Ophthalmology.* 1996;103:1188.

Mader T, Tabin G. Going to high altitude with preexisting ocular conditions. *High Alt Med Biol.* 2003;4:419.

Maggiorini M, Brunner-LaRocca H, et al. Both tadalafil and dexamethasone may reduce the incidence of high-altitude pulmonary edema; a randomized trial. *Ann Intern Med.* 2006;145:497–506.

Maggiorini M, Buhler B, et al. Prevalence of acute mountain sickness in the Swiss Alps. *BMJ.* 1990;301:853–4.

Maggiorini M, Melot C, et al. High-altitude pulmonary edema is initially caused by an increase in capillary pressure. *Circulation.* 2001;103(16):2078–83.

Mason NP, Barry PW, et al. Cough frequency and cough receptor sensitivity to citric acid challenge during a simulated ascent to extreme altitude. *Eur Respir J.* 1999;13(3):508–13.

McFadden DM, Houston CS, et al. High altitude retinopathy. *JAMA.* 1981;245:581–6.

Mirrakhimov M, Winslow R. The cardiovascular system at high altitude. In: Fregly M, Blatteis C, eds. *Section 4: Environmental Physiology, Vol. 2.* Oxford: Oxford University Press (American Physiological Society); 1996: 1241–57.

Moraga F, Flores A, et al. Ginkgo biloba decreases acute mountain sickness at 3700m. *High Alt Med Biol.* 2003;3:453.

Morgan BJ, Alexander JK, et al. The patient with coronary heart disease at altitude: observations during acute exposure to 3100 meters. *J Wilderness Med.* 1990;1: 147–53.

Murdoch DR. Symptoms of infection and altitude illness among hikers in the Mount Everest region of Nepal. *Aviat Space Environ Med.* 1995;66(2):148–51.

Nicholas RA, O'Meara PD. High-altitude syncope: history repeats itself. *JAMA.* 1993;269:587.

O'Connor T, Dubowitz G, et al. Pulse oximetry in the diagnosis of acute mountain sickness. *High Alt Med Biol.* 2004;5(3): 341–8.

Oelz O, Maggiorini M, et al. Nifedipine for high altitude pulmonary edema. *Lancet.* 1989;2:1241–4.

Perimenis P. Sildenafil for the treatment of altitude-induced hypoxaemia. *Expert Opin Pharmacother.* 2005;6(5):835–7.

Pesce C, Leal C, et al. Determinants of acute mountain sickness and success on Mount Aconcagua (6962 m). *High Alt Med Biol.* 2005;6(2):158–66.

Rennie ID, Morrissey J. Retinal changes in Himalayan climbers. *Arch Ophthalmol.* 1975;93:395–400.

Ricart A, Maristany J, et al. Effects of sildenafil on the human response to acute hypoxia and exercise. *High Alt Med Biol.* 2005;6(1):43–9.

Richalet JP, Gratadour P, et al. Sildenafil inhibits altitude-induced hypoxemia and pulmonary hypertension. *Am J Respir Crit Care Med.* 2005;171(3):275–81.

Roach RC, Bärtsch P, et al. The Lake Louise acute mountain sickness scoring system. In: Sutton, JR, Houston CS, Coates G, eds. *Hypoxia and Molecular Medicine.* Burlington, VT: Queen City Press; 1993: 272–4.

Roach RC, Greene ER, et al. Arterial oxygen saturation for prediction of acute mountain sickness. *Aviat Space Environ Med.* 1998;69(12):1182–5.

Roca-Cusachs A. Pattern of blood pressure among high and low altitude residents of southern Arabia. *J Hum Hypertens.* 1995;9(4):293.

Rock PB, Johnson TS, et al. Dexamethasone as prophylaxis for acute mountain sickness. Effect of dose level. *Chest.* 1989;95:568–73.

Roncin JP, Schwartz F, et al. EGb 761 in control of acute mountain sickness and vascular reactivity to cold exposure. *Aviat Space Environ Med.* 1996;67(5):445–52.

Sarnquist FH. Physicians on Mount Everest: a clinical account of the 1981 American medical research expedition to Everest. *West J Med.* 1983;139:480–5.

Sartori C, Allemann Y, et al. Salmeterol for the prevention of high-altitude pulmonary edema. *N Engl J Med.* 2002;346(21): 1631–6.

Sartori C, Duplain H, et al. High altitude impairs nasal transepithelial sodium transport in HAPE-prone subjects. *Eur Respir J.* 2004;23(6):916–20.

Schneider M, Bernasch D, et al. Acute mountain sickness: influence of susceptibility, preexposure, and ascent rate. *Med Sci Sports Exerc.* 2002;34(12):1886–91.

Schoene RB, Roach RC, et al. High altitude pulmonary edema and exercise at 4400 meters on Mt. McKinley: effect of expiratory positive airway pressure. *Chest.* 1985;87: 330–3.

Schoene RB, Swenson ER, et al. The lung at high altitude: bronchoalveolar lavage in acute mountain sickness and pulmonary edema. *J Appl Physiol.* 1988;64:2605–13.

Silber E, Sonnenberg P, et al. Clinical features of headache at altitude: a prospective study. *Neurology.* 2003;60(7): 1167–71.

Singh I, Kapila CC, et al. High altitude pulmonary oedema. *Lancet.* 1965;1:229–34.

Singh I, Khanna PK, et al. Acute mountain sickness. *N Engl J Med.* 1969;280(4):175–84.

Strom BL, Schinnar R, et al. Absence of cross-reactivity between sulfonamide antibiotics and sulfonamide nonantibiotics. *N Engl J Med.* 2003;349(17):1628–35.

Torgovicky R, Azaria B, et al. Sinus vein thrombosis following exposure to simulated high altitude. *Aviat Space Environ Med.* 2005;76(2):144–6.

Vock P, Brutsche MH, et al. Variable radiomorphologic data of high altitude pulmonary edema. Features from 60 patients. *Chest.* 1991;100(5):1306–11.

West JB. "Oxygenless" climbs and barometric pressure. *Am Alpine J.* 1984;226:126–33.

Wong SH, Turner H, et al. Reversible abnormalities of DWI in high-altitude cerebral edema. *Neurology.* 2004;62(2): 335–6.

Zell SC, Goodman PH. Acetazolamide and dexamethasone in the prevention of acute mountain sickness. *West J Med.* 1998;148:541–5.

Joyce M. Johnson, DO

INTRODUCTION

Explorations at sea differ from those on land. A ship at sea is a self-contained community that must provide all the services needed by those aboard, including medical care. Though most expeditions actually require relatively few medical services, proper planning is necessary to ensure that the appropriate services, including emergency care, are available when needed. In addition to actual medical treatment, public health and preventive services are also essential to a safe and rewarding venture. The early planning stages of the expedition should be used to begin to identify the needed resources. The specifics will vary with the characteristics of the expedition. The success of the expedition in fulfilling its mission is often dependent upon adequately addressing these health issues *prior* to leaving shore.

The first section addresses the variables that determine the health care needs underway, and how those needs can be met. The next section discusses several medical conditions that are relatively common on seagoing expeditions. The last section addresses safety, public health, and personal health behaviors. Proper predeployment planning and careful attention to health concerns underway are key to a successful seagoing expedition.

PREDICTING AND ADDRESSING HEALTH CARE NEEDS AFLOAT

As the expedition leader begins the early planning process, questions are asked such as: What pharmaceuticals should we bring? and What vaccinations do we need? Unfortunately these questions don't have standard answers applicable to every expedition. As part of the initial planning, the expedition leader, in consultation with the expedition health provider (if there is one) should begin considering the medical needs the expedition may have, and then to make plans to address them. This section focuses on these concerns.

Predicting Medical Needs Underway

Each expedition has different characteristics which determine the specific health care requirements. These characteristics can also be used to guide the operational risk management assessment of the entire mission. Some of these variables are shown in Table 20.1.

Prediction of the health care needs underway is very difficult. Even with an expedition party of two or three, if one uses his or her imagination, nearly any medical problem is possible. However, the reality is that some medical problems are more likely than others. For example, if the expedition includes members who are new to the ocean, some members will get seasick in rough seas. There is always the risk of "man overboard" and related hypothermia and near-drowning. If the expedition involves completing dangerous evolutions with specialized equipment or gear, there may be a traumatic accident.

No matter now long or short the list of possible or probable medical problems underway, the realities of the environment must always be considered. The boat or ship is at sea, and the sea can become rough, and the weather, unpredictable. The expedition party is a long way from any established medical care facilities. It can take days to reach a shore-side clinic or hospital. The medical care at most foreign ports is not the same as the expedition members may receive at home. These are the realities of an expedition at sea. Each member of the expedition party should fully understand and accept this. Each member of the expedition party should have realistic expectations about the medical care that can be provided at sea. Each member should be fully aware of the personal risks they take by participating in the expedition. Further, they should fully understand the complications and time needed to get a sick or injured person to a shore facility and recognize that facility will not be the same as a hospital in their hometown.

Those aboard ship include crew and expedition members and may also include friends, other passengers, and others who may join the cruise en route such as local

Table 20.1. Expedition variables that determine health requirements
Description of potential expedition "patients" Number in expedition party Other potential patients (crew, family, friends, etc.) Demographics: age, gender Preexisting medical conditions (if known) Will any women aboard be pregnant? Patient expectations
Variables affecting potential patient need Duration of cruise Mission and unique risks of mission Physical requirements and stresses of mission Other factors specific to the vessel or mission
Existing availability of medical care afloat Existing shipboard capabilities Capabilities of crew Understanding of crew role in caring for expedition members Expedition-provided medical care – first-aid, health provider?
Accessibility and availability of medical care ashore Have ashore "consultation" resources been identified? Communications (cell phone, Internet, radio, etc.) with shore-side specialty consultants for shipboard treatment Clinical information to be communicated to shore-side consultants for shipboard treatment Considerations of patient condition and transport to shore medical facilities – closest or "most capable"? Time and distance to closest shore medical facilities (changes throughout cruise) Availability of medical care at closest port Perceived quality of care at closest port Time and distance to "most capable" medical facility Medevac options? Decision – closest facility or transport to more distant facility?

Table 20.2. Predeployment medical screening: policy questions
How will a sick team member affect the expedition's mission? How will the rigors and isolation of the expedition affect the well-being and overall prognosis of a sick team member? Is predeployment medical screening necessary? If so, who does the screening apply to? (Expedition members, family members or guests, etc.) Are specific forms, diagnostic procedures, lab tests required? Is a pregnancy test indicated? Is dental screening, or the requirement to complete needed dental work indicated? Who pays for the screening – expedition or member? Who reviews the medical history and/or physical exam screening data? Who has the authority to make the medically based go/no go decision? Is there a waiver or appeal process? Does the American with Disabilities Act or other law apply?

scientists, philanthropists, or venture capitalists supporting the expedition. Any person afloat may have new medical problems underway, but medical emergencies are often due to preexisting health issues. Predeployment medical screening is one approach to minimizing medical needs underway. If people with significant preexisting conditions are prevented from participation, and if the expedition team is healthy when the expedition begins, there will likely be fewer medical problems underway. Table 20.2 lists several questions that are useful in determining whether predeployment screening is advantageous for a particular expedition.

Various options exist for predeployment medical screening. At the "minimal" end of options, the expedition member can sign a simple statement that he or she is in good health. At the "maximal" end of the range of options is for a physical exam and related lab tests to be done by the "expedition physician," who would then interpret the medical data and make the go/no go medical recommendations. If a dental screening (and/or requirement to complete needed dental treatment) is indicated, this, too, will require an evaluation by expedition staff.

Table 20.3 provides additional information on predeployment screening options.

Even though the realities of the underway expedition are that medical care has limited availability and accessibility, the expedition leader and physician (if there is one) have responsibilities to the expedition party. Table 20.4 provides a general list of medical problems and capabilities that should be considered. However, it should be fully recognized that treatment of most of these will be limited to the most basic first-aid underway. For example, in most situations, management of an extremity fracture would be limited to splinting, pain management, and transport. For a laceration, efforts would focus on controlling bleeding, and then, depending upon the location and extent of the injury and proximity to reliable shore-side medical care; wound closure and suturing aboard could be considered. Transport to shore-side care may also be advisable. If CPR is started, all should recognize that it cannot be continued for days – the time it may take to get the patient to definitive care on shore. There should be no expectation that the boat or ship will provide any type of definitive care for serious injuries or illnesses. Depending upon the acute natural history of a medical problem and the distance (in time) to get a patient to a shore facility, stabilization and transport may be a stretch goal as well.

In summary, though the medical problems underway can be serious and life-threatening, the tools to address them are few as measured by today's standards of tertiary care. However, the physician or other designated health provider should be knowledgeable about basic first-aid and simple emergency medicine practices, as well as the use of the contents of the ship's medicine chest. There should be full competency in advanced first-aid and basic medical techniques. These can be lifesaving in many situations. However, when the injury or disease is

Table 20.3. Types of predeployment medical screening

Type of predeployment screening	Advantages	Disadvantages
None	Easy, no cost to expedition or member	Will not identify significant health issues
Expedition member signs statement of "good health" possibly to include disclaimer and liability waiver	Easy, no cost to expedition or member Requires member to consider health conditions and expedition demands Provides at least minimal evidence of no serious medical conditions No expedition physician review needed	Expedition member may not fully disclose all health issues No physician input to statement
Member's personal physician signs "good health" statement	Easy, little or no cost Requires personal physician to relate member's health to expedition demands Physician likely knows patient's condition	Requires no physical exam or other specific evaluation Physician may not be objective – may do what patient wants
Member completes medical history form Member's personal physician reviews medical history form and completes designated (perhaps age-related) exam	Physician knows patient and has medical records/history Provides standardized history and physical exam Provides more objective health data	Costly to member – not covered by health insurance Costly and cumbersome to expedition leader Requires expedition physician or someone else to evaluate exam Requires standards or guidelines since used for go/no go decision Appeal process needed Physician may side with patient
Member completes medical history form Expedition physician reviews medical history form and completes designated physical exam	Objective data from physical Physician knowledgeable about expedition requirements Expedition physician completes consistent standardized exam Expedition leader/physician can set the guidelines/standards	Expensive – must pay physician for physical Logistics difficult – members must see same physician Physician does not know patient or medical history Requires standards or guidelines Appeal process needed
Dental exam and/or requirement to complete needed dental work	Minimizes dental emergencies afloat	Can be very expensive to participant who may need a lot of dental work

severe, the risk of permanent disability or death is high. Those aboard the vessel should recognize and accept the limitations and realities of medical care throughout the expedition.

Meeting Medical Needs Underway

When an explorer, passenger, or crew member becomes sick or injured underway, the initial medical care is provided by the ship's master or designee, or expedition personnel. Shore consultation via radio or e-mail often augments shipboard assets. In some situations, it becomes necessary to transport the patient to shore – either to the closest facility or to a more comprehensive facility back home.

If the ship is under the jurisdiction of the U.S. Coast Guard, the ship's owner and master have responsibilities to provide certain minimal levels of health care.[1,2,3] The ship's master generally delegates this responsibility to a crew member who has completed a week or more of medical training.

The expedition members should expect no more than basic first-aid from the ship's crew. Small boats and even large ships under foreign domain are under different regulations and may have no medical resources. In chartering the boat or ship, it is useful to ask about the specifics of medical capabilities aboard. However, even with this, it is generally best for the expedition leader to assume there won't be any significant medical care capabilities aboard. With few exceptions (such as an "expedition" added on to a tourist cruise ship), the expedition leader should plan to provide for the anticipated medical needs.

In this context, the expedition leader must decide whether to employ a physician, nurse practitioner, emergency medical technician (EMT), or other health provider for the expedition. Table 20.5 identifies some criteria used to make this decision.

In selecting a health provider, consider physicians, nurse practitioners, and possibly other health professionals who have the basic clinical skills. Primary care physicians and family nurse practitioners are well trained in basic medical care. If a physician is preferred for the expedition, recognize that physicians have different specialties and different areas of professional expertise, many of whom have had little recent experience

Table 20.4. Medical problems and capabilities to consider

Basic life support and CPR (short term)
Pain management
Emergency trauma care/stabilization
Treatment of hemorrhage, bandaging, splinting
Burn treatment
Shock recognition and management
General injuries – abrasions, lacerations, avulsion, puncture
 wounds, fishhooks
Fractures, dislocations, sprains
Bandaging and splinting
Head injuries
Injuries to the eye, ear, and throat
Chest injuries
Allergies and anaphylactic reactions
Abdominal injuries
Chest pain, heart disease, including acute exacerbations
 such as heart attack
Environmental emergencies
Dehydration
Hyperthermia
Heat exhaustion
Hypothermia
Frostbite
Drowning and near drowning
Diving accidents
Substance abuse including withdrawal syndromes
Patient assessment and management
Psychiatric conditions and serious behavioral problems

in primary care or emergency medicine, especially in remote and isolated areas without the luxury of lab, X-ray, or other diagnostic support, and with limited treatment options.

The expedition leader should recruit a health provider who meshes well with the expedition mission and crew. The health provider should expect that some extra

Table 20.5. Is a health provider needed as part of the expedition party?

What are the expedition's projected medical needs based on
 the expedition's characteristics (e.g., party size, isolation
 of cruise such as distance from shore facilities, nature of
 complex and potentially dangerous evolutions, etc.)?
What are the ship's inherent medical capabilities?
What are the first-aid and other clinical skills of the other
 expedition members? (EMT? nurse? other?)
Do the finances of the expedition allow for a practitioner?
 Is a volunteer available (such as the spouse of a party
 member)?
What clinical skills are needed? What level of practitioner
 is needed (e.g., general practice or emergency physician,
 nurse practitioner, EMT)?
Can the vessel and expedition generally accommodate an
 additional party member (e.g., health provider)? What are
 the costs and trade-offs of including a health provider on
 the expedition?
If a health provider is not included in the expedition party,
 what arrangements will be made for clinical coverage?
Overall, what are the risks and benefits of not having and
 having a health provider in the expedition party?

formal or informal training will be needed before the expedition. For example, a surgeon may need a refresher in managing hypothermia and drowning. An internist may need a review of suturing a minor wound. When the ship embarks, the health provider's abilities should complement the projected medical needs of the expedition, and the medicine chest should support those needs. Ideally, the health provider will have had extensive travel and expedition experience at sea and will be able to acclimate to the rigors of shipboard life.

If the expedition party includes a physician, nurse practitioner, or other health care provider, the expedition leader and health care provider should discuss and agree on the expected level of medical care. Any necessary medical supplies, equipment, pharmaceuticals and other resources should be provided by the expedition leader. Issues of licensure and malpractice insurance should also be addressed because they usually are state specific and cover specific clinic sites. The provider should confirm that he or she is licensed to practice in the jurisdiction of the expedition, and that his or her malpractice insurance is in effect.

The expedition members should also have realistic expectations about what the physician or nurse practitioner will be able to do. The medical platform will be the boat or ship and will be limited to what is available. In reality, on nearly all expeditions, the provider will be able to do little more than advanced first-aid and abbreviated emergency medicine. However, when "definitive care" (quality shore hospital) is several days away, the provider's role in stabilizing and transporting the patient can be critical, and can be lifesaving.

Shore-Side Medical Consultation and Transport to Care

Should a major emergency occur, shore-side medical consultation will be necessary. Several university and commercial-based organizations provide specialty consultation to remote areas. It is useful to identify one of these specialty consultant services, and to make initial contacts, before the expedition begins. Payment schedules can be fee-for-service or on a "per capita" retainer basis for the duration of the expedition. Alternatively, informal arrangements can be made with physicians known back home. Making some type of arrangements for specialty consultation before the ship leaves home port is helpful, because, during an emergency, the limited time and resources can be used to obtain help for the patient, not merely to try to find a consultant.

The effectiveness of on-shore specialty consultant services is dependent upon the ship-to-shore communication. Though much expanded in recent years, e-mail, cell phone, and radio communication may not be reliable in all locations. Nevertheless, there is a general expectation that expert consultation will be

Table 20.6. Components of a medical chart entry	
Patient data	**Comments**
Patient's name	Write patient's name on top of each paper.
Date	Current date should be noted.
Time	Current time should be on every entry.
Demographics	General description – age, gender, other relevant information.
Chief complaint and its history	What the problem is and how it happened.
Relevant medical and family history such as similar problem in past	Any past medical history that may be related should be included. If the patient is unconscious, ask family member or other expedition member.
Any related hospitalizations, surgeries, etc.	
Current medications	May be necessary to look in cabin to get list of current medications.
Subjective findings	General observations such as patient alert and eating; not very alert; appears to be in pain; etc.
Objective findings	Includes vital signs and other findings from physical exam.
Assessment	Diagnosis (if known) and how serious it seems.
Plan	May not yet be determined; reason for consult is to develop plan.
Consultation	Details about any outside consultation.

Box 20.1. Sample patient description to present to shore-side consultant

This 35-year-old woman presents with a chief complaint of "I fell down the ladder and I can't walk because my ankle hurts." About an hour ago, patient was going down the ladder, holding a large fish, taking it to the galley. As the fish began to slip out of her hands, she moved to catch the fish and fell down the ladder, landing with her weight on a twisted left ankle. She is complaining of ankle pain.

Patient is a long distance runner with no past surgeries or serious foot injuries. She is on no medications.

Patient is complaining of severe pain in her left ankle.

Patient is in acute distress, writhing in pain clenching her foot with occasional screams for help. The seas are getting rougher, and the ship is rocking, which seems to be increasing her pain with every movement.

Her vital signs have been stable over the last hour – pulse 70–80 beats/min (she says her usual resting pulse is 60); temp is 98.6, respirations are 10–12 per minute. No blood pressure cuff is aboard ship.

The patient's foot has been stabilized with a splint. There is no evidence of blood or broken skin. However, the foot is in an odd position and is angulated.

The assessment is the ankle appears to be broken.

We are seeking consultation on a plan to proceed. We are 3 days from the nearest port, and it is only a small town without our customary standards of medical care.

sought (via e-mail, cell phone, or radio) should there be a medical emergency on board.

Electronic ship-to-shore specialty consultation has medical challenges, and the onshore consultant should be aware of the diagnostic and treatment limitations aboard ship. The consultant should not expect any X-ray, lab, or other diagnostic or treatment data. On a noisy ship, even heart sounds may be difficult to hear clearly. Information from the physical examination, perhaps coupled with some medical history, becomes the only patient information that can be transmitted back to the shore-side consultants.

A physician or other health provider will know what clinical data are important and will be able to obtain the information and communicate with the shore-side consultant. However, if there is no clinician aboard, this becomes more difficult, especially recognizing the emergency nature of the situation and the realities of individual crisis response.

Most important for a lay first-aid responder is to collect the necessary clinical data. As these data are collected, they should be written down in something resembling a medical record. Vital signs should be charted as they are taken – the critical nature of the patient determines

how frequently this should be – whether every 15 minutes or every hour or several hours. Each chart entry, whether prepared by a health professional or lay first-aid responder, should have the elements outlined in Table 20.6.[4]

Patient transport to shore providers is sometimes needed. In a case like the one in Box 20.1, the shore-side consultant would likely confirm what the expedition leader had already suspected – the patient appears to have a complex fracture and requires "immediate" medical care. What "immediate" means will depend upon the various options available. The ankle may be further stabilized, the patient medicated for pain, and the options for medical care assessed.

In most cases, the decision to transport is not clear. Table 20.7 provides a list of variables that contribute to the decision about whether to transport the patient to shore. A decision to transport to shore can be difficult as it often adversely impacts the entire expedition – it results in delays and unanticipated port calls. Further, the shore-based care may be of unpredictable quality, and it can take some time to arrange and to actually transport the patient. Further, most shore-side overseas providers will require payment before services are rendered, and some type of arrangement must be made for this transfer of funds. Should the expedition member not have these funds, the decisions become even more complex. (Many expedition leaders require team members

Table 20.7. Determining whether to transport patient to shore medical services

Patient's condition

Is there risk of loss of life, limb, or function?

Can patient be treated underway?

Can patient be stabilized for transport to closest facility?

Can patient's condition likely be treated at closest shore facility?

Should patient be treated at the closest shore facility or evacuated elsewhere?

Can patient be stabilized for transport to a more distant facility?

How long will patient remain stable?

What is likelihood of patient's condition suddenly deteriorating?

What is patient's preference for location of treatment?

Shore services

What is the availability and perceived quality of closest shore services?

What is the accessibility of quality shore services?

Closest shore services or more distant facilities?

How long would it take to get to provider?

What is impact on expedition of diverting to shore?

Are there physical risks to the crew or ship in going to shore?

What are payment arrangements? (Expect to pay before services are provided.)

What are the options for transport?

Table 20.8. Traveler medical resources

International SOS: *http://www.internationalsos.com*

MEDEX: *http://www.medexassist.com*

International Association for Medical Assistant to Travelers (IAMAT): *www.iamat.org*

Travel Health Online: *http://www.tripprep.com/scripts*

International Society of Travel Medicine: *http://www.istm.org*

American Society of Tropical Medicine and Hygiene: *http://www.astmh.org*

American Citizens Services and Crisis Management: *http://travel.state.gov/travel/overseas_whoweare.html*

to purchase travel medical insurance that includes both medical services and emergency transport. This greatly simplifies the decisions around providing treatment in case of emergency.)

When an expedition member becomes ill, a decision on where to treat must be made. If the illness is minor, it can be treated by the ship's crew or expedition medical providers. This shipboard care can be augmented by consultation with shore-side experts. In some situations, it becomes necessary to transport the patient off the ship for care – either to a local shore facility or back to the home port. Though often necessary, this can be a time-consuming and financially costly approach.

Several resources are available to travelers. Various organizations specialize in locating health providers for travelers and providing other related services. The time to contact these organizations is *before* the expedition begins and *before* they are needed. During an emergency is not the time to begin thinking about the need for additional assistance. The expedition leader should have a definite plan about the resources to be utilized in case of medical emergency. The Web sites of some travel assistance organizations are listed in Table 20.8.[5–11]

Though patient transport to a shore-side facility (either the closest or the most capable) may be desired, the patient still requires care while these arrangements are being *made*. The limited shipboard medical resources often lead to reliance on the closest shore-side facilities.

Though many shore-side facilities can provide the appropriate medical care, for large or extended expeditions, it can be useful to do some pretravel homework, especially for overseas travel. Small, isolated ports may offer little more than the first-aid available aboard ship. Larger cities overseas often have several hospitals, but because of limited requirements for licensing and accreditation, the differences among hospital facilities in remote locations tend to be greater than the differences among U.S. hospitals. For example, a large city may have a public hospital, several private hospitals, and perhaps even an "American" hospital or U.S. military hospital. (The U.S. military hospital will usually see retired U.S. uniformed service members with a proper identification card, especially if they are enrolled in TriCare in the United States.) A quick check of these hospitals beforehand can identify the preferred site for care. For some emergent problems, such as a heart attack, the first available medical facility may provide the patient with the best opportunity for survival. In some geographic regions, especially for certain medical emergencies such as surgical treatment of a complex femur or tibia–fibula (leg bones) fracture, none of the local hospitals may seem adequate. International SOS and other groups have developed lists of preferred hospitals around the world. They can also arrange, though often at significant expense, extraction from the site and transport to the United States or other desired medical treatment location. Travel insurance is available to help cover these costs. (For more information, refer to Chapter 11.)

The distance between patients at sea and facilities ashore can be greater than geography suggests. In order for a patient to be seen ashore, transport is needed, which is generally a lengthy and complex evolution. There is no fast and easy way to transport a patient to shore from the middle of the ocean. The range of most helicopters is limited to about 150 miles. Further, a landing pad is needed to extract the patient from the ship, except in the direst of emergencies (such as a search and rescue mission using a complicated system of hoists and baskets to bring a patient into the helicopter). Estimates to transport a patient from sea to a shore-side medical facility should usually be measured in days rather than hours. If a ship is 2 days from shore, it will take about 3 days to get to medical care, assuming that care is available at the closest shore location. When the patient requires additional transport once on shore, additional time (a day or more) should be added. Getting a patient from ship to medical care on shore can be a long (and costly) process that can significantly impact the expedition's mission if the ship is forced to deviate from its planned course. The complexity of these arrangements and the time they take can be reduced if an international organization specializing in patient transport is involved early. This generally benefits both the patient and the entire expedition.

The Ship's Medicine Chest

The ship's medicine chest includes medications, supplies, and equipment that may be needed underway, or on any land portions of the expedition. The concept of the ship's medicine chest dates to the eighteenth century or before. By 1790, the new colonial government enacted legislation requiring merchant ships of above a minimum weight to carry a medicine chest. Though initially there was little guidance about the exact contents of the chest, several books have been written over the centuries to address this. For over a century the Marine Hospital Service and then the U.S. Public Health Service have published books such as *The Ship's Medicine Chest and Medical Aid at Sea* to fill this void.[12–15]

The ship's owner and master are required, if under the jurisdiction of the U.S. Coast Guard, to have some medical supplies aboard. They are primarily for the crew but can also be used by others aboard. They are usually limited to basic first-aid supplies and a few over-the-counter pharmaceuticals.

If the vessel is a small boat or a ship registered outside the United States, the ship's master may have even fewer medical supplies aboard. In any case, it is difficult to predict exactly what these might be or their quantity or condition. Thus, the expedition leader or physician (if there is one) may choose to provide all their own medications and supplies.

If the expedition includes many people or has members with any unique health risks, it is wise for the expedition's leader/physician to bring a separate cache. The contents of the expedition's medicine chest should be consistent with the projected medical needs and capabilities of the expedition.

No matter how complete the ship's medicine chest, expedition members should not expect that it will have their routine medications. Every expedition member should be fully informed, long before the expedition begins, about the necessity to bring a personal supply of medications. To ensure the medications can transit customs at various immigration sites, it is generally best for over-the-counter and prescription medications to be transported in their original labeled containers.

It can be difficult for the expedition leader or physician to know what supplies and medications to bring. Except for the largest ships, it is generally best to assume that no supplies will be available and to transport all that will likely be needed. The ship generally has some location identified as a sickbay, though it may have few supplies and little or no equipment. Once aboard, the supplies and medications should be stored in a locked area with limited access. Narcotics, if aboard, require even more specialized storage and tracking.

As discussed earlier, the specific supplies and medications needed depend upon the nature of the expedition. The ship's medicine chest can be divided into equipment, supplies, and medications. Tables 20.9, 20.10, 20.11, and 20.12 provide guidelines for developing the ship's medicine chest.[15,16]

If there is an expedition physician, the minimal diagnostic medical equipment is that which is customary in the physician's "little black bag." This is the basic equipment needed to do a general physical examination as well as a systems-oriented examination related to a specific chief complaint. Most physicians are knowledgeable about the use of these items. In most cases, the physician can provide this equipment if asked.

Several surgical instruments such as tweezers and forceps can also be useful. However, in today's world of disposable supplies, most medical instruments will be part of disposable sterile kits. This will alleviate concerns about sterility and will ensure that all of the instruments and supplies needed for a given function, such as suturing, are together.

The basic medical equipment listed in Table 20.9 is needed for basic examinations. Individual physicians

Table 20.9. Medical equipment in doctor's black bag and its use

Medical equipment	Primary use
Stethoscope	Listening to heart, lungs, abdomen
Oto-ophthalmoscope (with batteries)	Examining eyes, ears, nose, and throat
Sphygmomanometer (blood pressure cuff)	Taking blood pressure
Percussion hammer	Checking reflexes
Tuning fork	Checking vibratory sense, hearing
Thermometer	Measuring temperature
Pulse oxymeter	Measure peripheral oxygen level
PDA programmed with various medical books	Quick medical reference
Miscellaneous instruments such as scissors, tweezers, forceps	Minor activities not requiring sterile field
Miscellaneous items for neurological and other exams such as penlight, sharp/dull object; watch	Neurologic exam

Table 20.10. Consumable supplies and disposable trays

Bandages, dressings and related items
Band-Aids
Compress and bandage (4 × 4s, etc.)
"Telfa" or other nonstick bandage pads
Elastic bandage (Ace bandage)
Surgical tape
"Steri-strips"
Alcohol wipes
Povidine iodine solution
Hydrogen peroxide
Rubbing (isopropyl) alcohol
Nonlatex gloves
Surgical masks

Supply sets or trays
Supplies for suturing – disposable suture kit with sterile
   gloves; suturing anesthetic and needle/syringe for
   administering
Supplies for intravenous fluids (IVs) – several bags of half
   normal saline or other as preferred; several sets of IV
   tubing sets
Disposable Foley catheter set
Dental supplies and equipment as appropriate

Table 20.11. Over-the-counter medications and products

Medication/product	Primary indication
Meclazine, Dramamine	Seasickness
Aspirin	Pain, inflammation, fever
Acetaminophen	Pain, fever
Nonsteroidal antiinflammatory (e.g., ibuprofen)	Pain, inflammation
Topical steroid	Skin lesions
Antibiotic ointment	Prevent infection when skin broken (cut)
Burn treatment ointment	Treat burns
Imodium	Diarrhea
Milk of Magnesia	Constipation
Sunscreen	Prevent sunburns
Insect repellent with DEET	Prevent insect bites
Iodine or chlorine water purification pills/products	Disinfection of drinking water if necessary
Oral rehydration salts	Dehydration, especially from nausea, vomiting, and diarrhea

Table 20.12. Classes of medication

Prescription medication	Primary indication
Analgesic (nonsteroidal antiinflammatory, salicylic acid, acetaminophen)	Headaches, minor pain (some are also effective for inflammation and fever)
Antipyretic (salicylic acid, acetaminophen)	Fever
Oral antibiotic (one or more broad spectrum) (doxycycline, azithromycin)	Bacterial infections such as upper respiratory infections and *Salmonella*
Ciprofloxacin, levofloxacin, or other quinolone	Urinary tract and other infections
Oral steroid mutidose packet	Acute allergic reaction; "hives"
Nitroglyercin (other cardiac meds as indicated)	Chest pain
EpiPen or similar	Anaphylactic type reaction
Opthalmic antibiotic	Eye infection
Fluconazole (1 dose/treatment)	*Candida albicans* (vaginal)
Clotrimazole, topical	Skin fungal infections
Valium, intravenous	Treatment of seizures
Benzodiazepine – long acting	Treatment of alcohol withdrawal
Local anesthetic (injectable) for suturing	Anesthetic for suturing
Oral rehydration (first treatment); antibiotics, primarily fluoroquinolones, such as ciprofloxacin or norfloxacin	Treatment of diarrhea Oral rehydration best option Antibiotics may be needed
Antimotility agent such as loperamide or diphenoxylate	Antimotility agents rarely indicated for "traveler's diarrhea"; should not be used if high fever or blood in stool; provides only symptomatic treatment and may delay actual resolution of infection
Dental medications	As appropriate

may make a few modifications to that list. Further, if the scope of medical capabilities expands beyond basic first-aid, and if the ship has adequate space and other support, additional supplies and equipment can be added to the list. However, each additional instrument should have a specific purpose and be selected in response to a specific significant risk. The physician should be involved in selecting the equipment and should be well versed in its use. It is counterproductive to add even

one piece of medical equipment "just in case" some remotely possible and highly unlikely event may occur, especially if no one is skilled in its use. Any pieces of medical equipment should be carefully chosen to respond to a specific identified risk, and also that someone aboard can effectively use it.

The expedition leader/physician should make certain that appropriate consumable medical supplies are aboard. Most of these are to care for minor trauma. The exact numbers of each become a function of the scope of the mission (duration, number on board, geography of sail). The physician may have preferences for one brand or type over another. The specifics are not as important as ensuring that enough supplies are aboard to manage the usual cuts and scrapes while underway and providing a first-aid response to a more serious laceration. More items will be included on a larger ship with more space and a larger expedition team. Only a few of these items might be practical on a crowded ship or smaller boat. The quantity of each depends upon the projected need. Table 20.10 provides some guidelines on consumable supplies and disposable trays.[4,15,16]

Over-the-counter (OTC) medications are another essential that sometimes cause controversy. Expedition members are routinely instructed to bring whatever OTCs they will need. However, this is rarely done. It is generally easiest to bring at least a small supply of these items for the group to share. Even though they are OTCs, it is advisable for the physician or other assigned person to dispense them as needed. This will help ensure they are available for all to use throughout the expedition. Also, note the items listed in Table 20.11 (along with the supplies listed in Table 20.10) can usually be replenished in port.[4,15–17]

Some prescription medications are useful to have aboard if there is a physician to prescribe them. The general classes of medications are listed in Table 20.12. The physician should select the medication, dose, and number of tablets to bring based on his prediction of need.[4,15,16,18] Note that many pharmaceutical products that require a prescription in the United States can be purchased over-the-counter in foreign ports. However, it is generally better to bring the medications on the expedition.

Basic medical supplies and equipment should be available, the specifics dependent upon the scope of the expedition. Of extreme importance is that someone aboard is familiar with each of the items in the medicine chest and trained to use them. This is especially important if a physician is aboard. Conversely, prescription medications should not be included if no licensed practitioner to prescribe them is aboard.

SHIP HEALTH: UNDERWAY MEDICAL CONCERNS

Life aboard ship is conducive to several types of medical problems. Motion sickness or "seasickness" due to the movement of the boat or ship is probably the most common. Drowning and near drowning – also referred to as submersion injury – are also genuine threats to any waterborne expedition. The body's response to temperature extremes – both cold and hot – are also risks. Dehydration is a common, but preventable, ailment when underway. Burns are a constant threat underway. Trauma and the resultant need for wound care are common. Substance abuse is an often hidden problem, but alertness is critical because even alcohol withdrawal can result in fatal seizures. Acute and painful dental problems, though often preventable with comprehensive dental care before the voyage, are still a threat to any expedition. These conditions are discussed in this chapter.

Motion Sickness Including Seasickness

Seasickness, a type of motion sickness, is very common among those new to shipboard life, even in calm seas. When the seas get rough (Figure 20.1), almost everyone suffers at least minor levels of seasickness. It usually begins with nausea, which in Greek actually means seasickness.[19–22]

The body has several mechanisms to sense motion and position – the eyes, ears, and proprioceptors (in

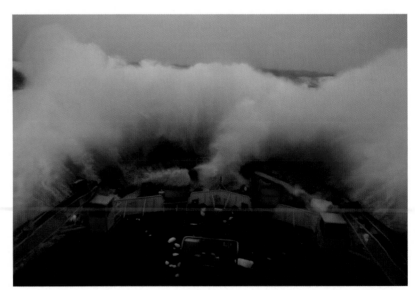

Figure 20.1. Even experienced sailors can experience seasickness on rough seas. Photo courtesy of Hanne Zak.

muscles, joints, skin, etc.). The eyes send visual clues to the brain that often relate to a reference point, such as the horizon, to determine motion. The inner ears' vestibular system also recognizes motion – semicircular canals detect rotation and the otolith organs recognize vertical movement. The skin, joints, and other tissues recognize miniscule changes in pressure, such as the increased pressure on the feet to keep balance when a ship is rocking back and forth. Ideally, each of these sensors sends the same signal to the brain. Trouble arises when the messages are different.

On a boat, one may feel fine on deck where the body's cues are consistent – the eyes, ears, and proprioceptors sense the same motion. However, if one goes below deck to a small cabin or to the head (latrine) where there are no visual cues about motion, but the inner ear and proprioceptors continue to sense motion, sickness often results.

Seasickness is a common problem, and can affect even the most experienced sailors if the boat is small or the sea is rough. Motion sickness should not cause shame. Astronauts are also affected by it, and the space shuttle's zero-gravity toilet has a special setting for "vomit."

Incidentally, physical motion isn't necessary for motion sickness. It can result from watching a movie. The eyes "sense" motion but the ears and proprioceptors do not. This body sensation can be used as part of the movie's "excitement." This response rarely happens if the same movie is on a small-screen television because the eyes can also sense that the room around the screen is not moving, so the body is not tricked into visually sensing any motion.

Motion sickness includes fairly predictable symptoms. The first is slight nausea. This may be accompanied by a cold sweat, flushing or drop in blood pressure, and general fatigue. Vomiting is the usual last step. The vomiting of motion sickness does not relieve the nausea, which differs from some other causes of vomiting.

Behaviors as well as medications can prevent motion sickness. The goal of behavioral approaches is to ensure that all signals going to the brain about the body's motion and position are sending the same message. In a boat or ship, the least motion is generally in the middle of the ship at the water level. The more expensive outer births with port holes may actually have more motion and be less advantageous. On a small boat, being on deck and watching the horizon is beneficial. (In a car, sitting in the front seat to see the horizon often helps. Being the driver so that you can even feel the slight maneuvers in the steering wheel helps even more. In an airplane, the window seats in front of the wings are best – they have the least motion and also allow one to look outside.) Even just being distracted from the nauseous feelings can help.

Since medications can prevent, but not treat, motion sickness, it is important to use them before the trip begins. Both oral medications and patches are available

Table 20.13. Medications used to prevent seasickness and other forms of motion sickness	
Product	**General information**
Dimenhydrinate	Oral, approved for children; can cause complications in persons with asthma, heart disease, urinary retention (such as from an enlarged prostate), glaucoma. Causes drowsiness.
Diphenydramine	Oral, approved for children; can cause complications in persons with asthma, heart disease, urinary retention (such as from an enlarged prostate), glaucoma. Causes drowsiness.
Meclizine	Not for use in children; can cause complications in persons with asthma, glaucoma, and urinary obstruction. Causes drowsiness.
Promethazine	Not for use in children; can cause complications in persons with asthma, glaucoma, and urinary obstruction. Causes drowsiness. Reduces nausea more than vomiting.
Scopolamine	Not for use in children; can cause complications with urinary obstruction, glaucoma, as well as liver and kidney disease; can have emotional/cognitive effects including decreased memory, attention, alertness with effects on judgment; available both in oral and skin patch forms.
Ginger	Herbal preparation with little scientific data available on dosing, contraindications, and side effects.

over-the-counter and by prescription. Only a couple of these medications are safe for children. During the pre-expedition travel medical appointment, motion sickness medication should be discussed. For longer voyages, some find the scopolamine skin patch to be preferable. (In the United States, this is a prescription-only product.) Note motion sickness medications adversely affect alertness and attention. These side effects must be recognized when considering use by those operating a ship or boat. These medications also interact with the central nervous system depressant effects of alcohol, and alcohol should be avoided when they are taken. There is anecdotal evidence that the herb, ginger, also helps to prevent motion sickness. It can be taken in various forms, including chewing candied ginger. Note that some medications to prevent vomiting (metoclopramide and prochlorpemazine) are usually ineffective for preventing the nausea and vomiting of motion sickness.

Table 20.13 lists the available medications to prevent motion sickness. Note that most should be taken at least an hour before the ship leaves shore. After motion sickness begins, it is very difficult to control, and thus prevention is advisable. For the explorer with little afloat experience, it is advisable to begin the journey with prophylactic medication. The medication can then be slowly discontinued (by increasing intervals between doses) as the cruise continues.

On a long expedition at sea, motion sickness is bound to be a problem for at least some expedition members. Table 20.14 outlines some common first-aid approaches that may be helpful.

In summary, motion sickness is an expected occurrence aboard a boat or ship. Those aboard can manage and often prevent it by following some behavioral guidelines. Medication is also available, but it must be taken before there are any signs of seasickness. The nervous system depressant side effects of the medications must also be considered because the drowsiness and other complications can be very dangerous for those operating the vessel.

Drowning and Near-Drowning

Drowning and near-drowning (more recently referred to as submersion injury) are constant threats around the water. Waters frequently have unexpected currents or eddies that can pull even the best swimmer under. In the course of daily activities, a passenger or crew member can go overboard. This risk is greater on an expedition on a small boat, in turbulent and high seas, or with rough weather, especially at night or when visibility is reduced. Children and adolescents may not be aware of the risks of the water or being underway and may not recognize the dangerousness of their behavior. Understanding the

Table 20.15. Drowning-related terminology

Term	Description
Submersion	Head and body are both under water.
Immersion	Head is above water, body is under water.
Near-drowning (submersion injury)	Water aspirated in airways during submersion or immersion; treatment required.
Drowning	Death due to water aspiration in airways.
Cold shock response (initial immersion)	Rapid skin cooling – gasp response – can't hold breath - hyperventilation. Gasp causes drowning if head underwater.
Impaired performance (short-term immersion)	Skin cooling – peripheral vasoconstriction – increased cardiac output, heart rate, blood pressure – myocardial ischemia – arrhythmias – sudden death. Survive cold shock response – muscle and soft tissue cooling – decreased neuromuscular activity – loss of motor control, especially of hands then can't hold rescue line or save self; drowning results from inability to save self or inhaled water.
Hypothermia (long-term immersion)	Immersion 30 minutes or more – heat lost from body – core temperature decreases – hypothermia results

mechanisms of drowning and near-drowning can help to prevent them and to appropriately respond should an emergency arise.

Several terms are helpful to understand drowning and near-drowning, as shown in Table 20.15.[15,23,24]

Submersion injuries can starve the brain and other body tissues of oxygen. Thus, the most important step in treating near drowning is to treat hypoxia and to reoxygenate the patient. This should be done after checking to make certain the airway is clear. The steps in treating a near drowning or submersion injury patient are shown in Table 20.16.

The essential goal of treating near-drowning is to reoxygenate the patient, and to prevent permanent brain damage. Constant vigilance around water and immediate recognition of anyone in distress are critical. In plan-

Table 20.14. First-aid for seasickness and other motion sickness

First-aid approach	Comments
Try to stay outside on deck.	Look at the horizon; try to maintain constant visual and proprioceptive cues.
Stay hydrated – drink water, noncaffeinated beverages.	Do not drink caffeinated beverages or alcohol because both are diuretics and will decrease hydration; can also cause gastrointestinal irritation.
Stay away from noxious fumes including cigarette smoke and ship exhaust.	Fumes will increase nausea.
Salty, dry crackers sometimes help.	Some find salty foods helpful.
Stay away from others who are seasick, especially if they are vomiting.	The odor of other's vomit can stimulate vomiting.
Mental distractions are helpful.	Verbal games and other activities that distract from thoughts of motion sickness are useful.
Don't read or do activities that change visual cues away from the ship's motion.	Goal is to keep eye, ear, and proprioceptive cues consistent

Table 20.16. Treatment of near-drowning

Remove victim from water
Assess breathing and pulse
Clear airway of water, vomit, other objects
CPR if needed
Administer oxygen
Defibrillate if necessary

ning for a catastrophe aboard ship such as fire, which necessitates abandonment of the ship, recognize that rescue efforts must include appropriate treatment of near-drowning.

Cold-Related Illness

Immersion in cold water lowers the body temperature when the body fails to compensate for the loss of heat to the surrounding water (see Chapter 31 on environmental extremes). Though hypothermia is considered "mild" down to a body temperature just above 90°F, there are still significant symptoms – shivering, loss of grip strength, and slowed thinking. The victim does not think clearly and is unable to try to save him- or herself. The loss of grip strength further complicates the victim's ability to cooperate with the rescuer. When the patient's core body temperature drops below 90°F, the patient can become confused or unconscious, often with cardiac arrhythmias that can lead to death. Below 82°F, vital signs become difficult to measure and cardiac arrest becomes more probable.[15,24,25]

Hypothermia can occur in most deep waters. If the water temperature is colder than 77°F, hypothermia is a risk. Except for certain tropical regions, salt water temperatures are generally colder than this.

When exposed to cold water, the body undergoes a series of reactions that are listed in Table 20.17.

Treating a patient in hypothermia is complex. A patient with mild hypothermia is conscious, and treatment includes continued monitoring and recording of vital signs, removal of cold, wet clothing and other gear, and insulating the patient with warm blankets. Use caution in giving any liquids because, should the patient vomit, aspiration can result.

A patient with more severe hypothermia is very difficult to manage. While one person is taking vital signs, another should be contacting the previously identified shore-side medical consultation service. Keep the patient as still as possible (to minimize cardiac arrhythmias), and do not provide any fluids (to prevent aspiration). Try to gently rewarm the patient. Warm blankets, hot water bottles (use care not to burn the patient), or lying next to the patient in a sleeping bag should be tried. A warm IV (105°F, which is slightly less than lukewarm) can be used. Invasive procedures such as warm water gastric lavage, bladder lavage, and peritoneal lavage can be used if equipment and proper support are available. Be alert for cardiac arrest, respiratory arrest, and vomiting (with risk of aspiration). Because of the fragile state of the chilled heart and the propensity for arrhythmias, coupled with the patient's hypothermia and slowed metabolism, cardiac drugs are metabolized very slowly and can be toxic even in small dosages. Constant consultation while monitoring and treating the patient is essential.

Table 20.17. Sequential responses to cold water exposure
How cold water exposure leads to death
Immersion or submersion in cold water
Decrease in skin temperature
Cold-shock reflex
Increases in heart rate, respiratory rate, blood flow, and blood pressure to try to maintain body temperature
Efforts to maintain body temperature fail; body temperature declines
Metabolism increases and shivering begins to maintain body temperature
Extremities cool rapidly
Loss of manual dexterity, strength
Body cools more
Shivering ceases, body processes slow – heart rate and blood pressure drop, thinking slows
Loss of consciousness
Death by drowning (if submerged) or cardiac arrest

Though water immersion is the most common cause of hypothermia underway, the air environment on deck can also lead to problems. It is a myth that drinking alcohol can "warm" the body. Never use alcohol if there is a threat of being chilled. Alcohol dilates the peripheral blood vessels, causing warm blood to go to the arms, fingers, feet, and toes. When more warm blood is in the periphery, more calories of heat are lost, and the net result is that the body is cooled.

Some voyages are to very cold climates, where preparation for cold weather is customary. However, even in warmer areas, after the sun sets, evenings aboard ship can get cool, especially with a breeze. Further, storms can come up and unexpectedly bring rain. The crew and expedition team can get cold and wet undergoing maneuvers to try to protect the ship. Though this rarely develops into full blown hypothermia in a healthy person, caution should be used – cold damp clothes should be replaced with warm dry ones. Warm clothing, appropriate for the weather, is important. Older persons and those with other medical problems are more susceptible to hypothermia. If someone seems to be "out of it" and the weather is cool and the person is wet, suspect hypothermia and act promptly to reverse.

Heat-Related Illness

Life aboard a ship offers many heat-related risks (see Chapter 31 on environmental extremes), from the exhausting heat of the engine room to the often exhilarating heat of the sun on deck. The body has many internal controls to regulate temperature when exposed to heat. Perspiration is well recognized – the body secretes water and salts through the skin, and the process of evaporation cools the body's surface. The vascular system is another temperature regulator because of the heat calories circulating blood holds. Blood vessels constantly dilate and constrict to move blood between the body's core and periphery to regulate the body's heat exchange with the ambient air. In response to heat, and in an effort to cool the body, the blood vessels in the periphery dilate so that more blood goes to the body's surface resulting in more heat exchange with the ambient environment. Note that the body is most sensitive to heat when the humidity is high because of decreased evaporation of perspiration. Still air, in contrast to a light breeze, also reduces evaporation and increases heat effects. Heavy clothes are a third contributor to decreased evaporation and cooling.

Attention to some basic concepts can prevent most heat-related illness. Try to avoid hot areas and direct sunlight. If they can't be avoided, try to minimize time and exposure. Wear appropriate clothing – lightweight "breathable" clothing that provides sun protection yet allows for evaporation of perspiration is best. Light-colored cotton fabrics work well as do some of the specially designed synthetics. Wear a brimmed hat. Monitor and moderate exertion, and take frequent breaks. Pay attention to fluid intake and output (perspiration and urine), and remain hydrated. Water should be the primary hydration fluid; alcohol and caffeinated beverages should be avoided because of their diuretic effects.

However, even with the various thermal regulation mechanisms and best preventive behaviors, the human body is very sensitive to heat, especially when coupled with dehydration. Heat injury can be a medical emergency – it can be life-threatening. The American Red Cross and others[24,25] generally group heat-related illness into three categories: heat cramps, heat exhaustion, and heat stroke as shown in Table 20.18. These are on a continuum, and a minor heat reaction can rapidly progress to life-threatening illness.

Some persons are at increased risk for heat-related illness. In a shipboard environment, those doing the most strenuous labor are at highest risk. The strenuous activity generates heat, and the body must dissipate that heat. Medications including some antihistamines and antidepressants also increase the risk. Children and the elderly, especially those in generally poor physical condition may be less able to regulate temperature.

Early recognition is the key to managing heat-related illnesses. Heat cramps are recognized by the associated

Table 20.18. Types of heat-related illness

Cause	Signs and symptoms	Approach to treatment
Heat cramps		
Strenuous activity Increased perspiration Fluid and electrolyte imbalance	Painful muscle cramps Calves of legs, abdomen affected Body temperature generally elevated Sweating Increased heart rate Thirst	Move patient to cooler place if possible Gently stretch cramping muscles Slowly replace fluid and electrolytes if patient is conscious and not expected to vomit Try to gently cool body – remove heavy clothing, cover with damp sheets or towels
Heat exhaustion		
Strenuous activity Perspiration Perspiration does not evaporate enough to cool body (hot, humid environment, heavy clothes, etc.) Body does not cool	Increased temperature Signs of dehydration Increased heart rate Shallow breathing Nausea, vomiting Headache Confused, easily agitated Not rational	Move patient to cooler place Cool body by removing heavy clothing, cover with damp sheets or towels If conscious and not expected to vomit, slowly give fluids and electrolytes *Watch for signs of shock*
Heat stroke – This is a life-threatening EMERGENCY		
Body loses ability to control temperature Temperature reaches dangerously high levels Enzymes and other body processes affected by high temperature Brain damage Multiorgan failure Death	Core body temperature above 104°F Dry mouth, signs of dehydration Altered consciousness; may be unconscious May have seizures Confusion/mental status changes Seizures Vomiting (can aspirate) Fast, weak pulse Fast, shallow breathing Multiorgan failure (kidneys, liver, blood clotting (DIC), muscles, etc.)	*Immediately* get medical consultation Cold packs on wrists, ankles, armpits, neck IV hydrate patient Wrap in cool wet sheet Fan patient May need to treat renal failure and other complications

pain. Heat exhaustion may go unrecognized and can quickly develop into life-threatening heat stroke. It is critical that all aboard the expedition are able to recognize heat-related illness, in either him- or herself or a shipmate. When any signs of heat-related illness are identified, it is critical to stop strenuous activity and move to a cooler location out of the sun. The expedition's culture must accept this without causing embarrassment, ridicule, or a sense of failure. Early recognition and response, however, can prevent a shipmate's death.

Dehydration

Dehydration occurs when the body loses more fluid than it takes in. Electrolytes (including sodium and potassium) are also generally lost. Underway, the usual causes of dehydration relate to increased perspiration. Up to 6 cups of fluid per hour can be lost while working in hot environments. Motion sickness (with nausea causing decreased interest in consuming fluids, and overt vomiting), and diarrhea (usually water- or food-borne illness) can also cause dehydration (Table 20.19). Up to 3% of body weight can be lost. This amount of fluid, especially when coupled with the balance of electrolytes, is not readily replaced.[21,25]

The diagnosis of dehydration is made based on the patient's history (such as vomiting), coupled with physical signs and symptoms as shown in Table 20.20. An effective way to assess dehydration underway is to assess several physical parameters. The heart rate increases as the heart tries to pump the decreased blood volume where it is needed. Urine output decreases. On average, urine output should be between 1½ to 3 tablespoons per hour. The urine should be light yellow. If there is concern about dehydration, collect a urine sample. Very dark yellow urine suggests dehydration (though it can also be caused by other problems such as liver disease). Also, ask the patient to only urinate in a container and, over time, measure and record the amount. If there is a blood pressure cuff aboard, take the blood pressure lying, sitting down, and standing, each about a minute apart. If the patient is dehydrated, there will be a positional drop in blood pressure from lying to sitting down to standing.

Table 20.20. Signs and symptoms of dehydration
Increased heart rate
Increased respiratory rate
Decreased urine output
Concentrated urine (dark color, high specific gravity)
Postural hypotension
Dry mouth
Feeling thirsty, want to drink
Headache
Fatigue, lethargy
Muscle weakness
Muscle cramping
Abdominal cramping
Feeling dizzy when standing; fainting
Changes in cognition and judgment
Seizures
Changes in consciousness including coma
Shock
Death

If there is no blood pressure cuff, ask the patient to lie down for several minutes, then sit up for a minute, and then stand. If the patient feels dizzy this suggests dehydration because there is not enough blood volume to adequately supply the brain, and a dizzy feeling results. (Make sure that the patient does not collapse or fall.)

Treatment of dehydration focuses on reducing ongoing fluid loss and adding fluids. If the dehydration is due to heat exposure, the patient should be moved to a more comfortable temperature if possible. If vomiting and/or diarrhea are the cause, they should be treated. Fluid replacement is the essential treatment. Most dehydration can be treated with oral fluids. Rarely, intravenous fluids will be necessary. Even with nausea, vomiting, or diarrhea, fluids are often best tolerated if sipped slowly, but continuously. Otherwise, fluids should be taken more rapidly.

Water is the most important replacement fluid. Because electrolytes have also been lost, they should be replaced. Commercial sports drinks work well, or a special solution can be made from the recipe given in Table 20.21. For shipboard use, bringing a plastic carton of powdered sports drink is convenient because the salts and sugars are precombined, the drink has a pleasant

Table 20.19. Dehydration causes underway
Prolonged work in hot area such as engine room
Sun and heat exposure (such as on deck)
Excessive perspiration
Motion sickness, nausea
Vomiting
Diarrhea
Decreased fluid intake
Alcohol, caffeine, or other diuretics can magnify
Medical problems such as diabetic ketoacidosis

Table 20.21. Recipe for oral rehydration solution
1½ tablespoons sugar
½ teaspoon table salt
¾ teaspoon baking soda
¼ teaspoon potassium-based salt substitute
1 quart/liter of water
Flavoring (powdered drink mix, lemon juice) (if this has sugar or salts, adjust accordingly)

Note: Absorption will be increased if the water used to cook rice, potatoes, or pasta is substituted for the plain water. The sugar components of these starchy waters combine with the electrolytes and facilitate absorption.

flavor, and the plastic container requires little space for storage and is waterproof.

Treatment of dehydration with oral fluids is generally successful. However, if the patient is unable to tolerate oral liquids, or the underlying cause of the dehydration cannot be controlled, intravenous fluids and shore consultation may be considered.

Burns

The skin and tissue damage of a burn can be due to heat, radiation including sunlight, chemicals, and electricity. All are threats aboard ship.

Whatever their cause, burns are generally classified into three groups – first, second and third degree as shown in Table 20.22.[26,27]

The location of the burn also affects its impact. Inhalation of hot gases (steam) or chemicals can burn the respiratory tract resulting in serious injury that may not be visible. Further, the damaged tissue can swell blocking off the airway. Burns to the eye cause scarring, damage the cornea, and can result in blindness. Even skin burns, when at the joints, can affect mobility. Burns to the tender skin of the face or genitals can be especially deforming.

The size of the area burned is another measure of seriousness. Larger areas result in more fluid and electrolyte imbalances, and more chance of infection and other complications. When seeking consultation for a burn patient, an approximation of surface area affected is important to relay. The well-known "rule of nines" can be used to approximate the surface area of the burn. In adults, the head and neck comprise 9% of the surface area, each arm 9%, each leg 18%, the front and back of the trunk, each 18%, and the genitalia 1%.[25]

Aboard ship, heat-related burns are the most common. Removing the source of the heat, and continuing to cool the affected area in cold running water, often reduces the burn damage. Heat-related burns can be "moist" or "dry." Moist burns, due to steam or hot liquids can be very dangerous because of the amount of "heat" (kilocalories) trapped in the moisture does the damage. The extent of the damage may not be apparent at first.

Sunburn is common, yet preventable, underway. Sunburn is possible, summer or winter, sunny day or cloudy. On voyages close to the equator, the sun's rays are most direct, and damage can be faster and more severe than in the home environment. Expedition members should be especially cautious at the beginning of the voyage, when they are not used to the sun, and may be distracted by other, more exciting activities. Vigilance with sunburn prevention is critical – sunscreen, brimmed hats, long light-colored loose clothing, and the like. With an hour or two of direct sun exposure, second degree burns can result. Sunglasses are essential to protect the eyes because reflection from the water can be especially damaging when on deck for days at a time. In a shipboard environment, sunburn can easily become infected when the blisters break, and result in complications that can incapacitate the exploration member.

The shipboard environment includes a range of toxic chemicals. Chemical burns can be very serious especially if the chemical is not immediately removed from the skin. Most chemicals should be thoroughly washed off with running water. It is important not to abrade the skin while washing as this will only deepen the damage. It can take 30 or more minutes of running water to remove the chemical.

Electrical burns not only affect the skin, but can also affect the electrical conduction of the heart and result

Table 20.22. Classification and treatment of burns

Category of burn	Skin damage	Appearance	Immediate treatment approach
First degree	Outer layer of skin (epidermis) affected	Red, swollen, and painful	Cool with cold water Dry dressing or silver sulfadiazine or antibiotic dressing
Second degree	Middle layer of skin (dermis) affected	Blisters Red, swollen, and painful	Do not debride blisters Clean Bandage; silver sulfadiazine or other dressing; change frequently to prevent infection Elevate to reduce swelling
Third degree	Deep layers of skin and possibly other tissues affected Blood vessels, nerves, and hair follicles damaged	Deep skin damage Not painful – nerves are deadened Skin does not "blanch" – vessels damaged	Try to assess amount of damage and body area burned Seek immediate shore-side consultation Clean and bandage burn with silver sulfadiazine or other dressing; change several times daily Manage fluids; patients easily dehydrated; IV if possible, elevate to reduce swelling

in immediate cardiac arrhythmias or arrest or cardiac arrhythmias. Further, because the electricity is conducted into the body, deep organ damage can result. This is difficult to both recognize and treat. Electrical burns may seem minor and superficial, yet they can result in serious hidden damage.

Though burn patients are often recognized shortly after the event, the burn can progressively damage tissues for 24 hours or more. This is especially true for inhalation burns, moist burns, chemical burns, and sunburn. A burn patient requires continual monitoring. Burns result in fluid loss from blistering lesions and other fluid changes. Fluid and electrolyte management can be very challenging. Patients with serious burns – deep burns, burns over large body areas, or burns to sensitive areas (eyes, genitalia, respiratory system) – require more sophisticated medical care than most shipboard environments can provide. Immediate shore consultation, and most likely evacuation, will be required.

Wound Care

Cuts, abrasions, lacerations, and puncture wounds are a risk of seagoing life. Imbedded fishhooks are probably the most classic, but all aspects of life underway can lead to wounds. Fortunately most wounds are relatively minor and can be managed with simple first-aid, others can be treated with steri-strips or a few sutures, while a few are life-threatening. This section will address some of the basics of wound care underway.[15,16]

The usual assumption is that most wounds are fairly obvious – blood is coming from a new break in the skin, and there is some type of recent trauma history such as a fall or puncture wound. However, the seriousness of the injury can be very difficult to determine. Assessing for cervical spine injury, internal injuries, head trauma, and fractures can be forgotten while attending to a profusely bleeding wound. If the injury is serious, the patient may be in shock. The patient should be treated for shock while controlling the bleeding and managing the ABCs (airway, breathing, circulation).

Controlling bleeding is key in the management of wounds. Most bleeding can be controlled by applying pressure to the wound. However, do not apply so much pressure as to stop circulation to the extremity past the wound. If bleeding cannot be controlled, a tourniquet can be applied. However, this can result in loss of the limb and requires *immediate* medical intervention at a shore facility.

Minor wounds can be cared for aboard ship. Serious or infected wounds often require immediate medical evacuation and care. Serious or infected wounds can be life-threatening.

The first step in wound care is to assess and evaluate the wound, including the cause. (See Tables 20.23 and 20.24.) Some wounds appear to be relatively minor

Table 20.23. General steps to wound care

Action to take	Comments
Assess patient. Assume cervical spine injury until proven otherwise.	Examine for "hidden" injuries – look for signs of cervical spine injury, head trauma, internal injuries, fractures, etc. Treat for shock if necessary.
Stop bleeding.	Pressure to area; avoid use of tourniquet if at all possible to avoid loss of limb.
Irrigate wound thoroughly.	Preferable to use sterile water for irrigation; if none available, then any potable water can be used.
Bandage wound.	Compression bandage can also help decrease bleeding.
Splint if useful to decrease mobility if possible fracture.	Minimize movement if fracture suspected.
Some large wounds require suturing.	Steri-strips are often a good alternative to suturing when underway.
Administer tetanus toxoid if necessary.	May wait until shore; predeployment tetanus vaccine is helpful.
Consider antibiotics.	Antibiotic use dependent upon severity of wound and contamination.
Determine if outside consultation is needed.	Obtain consult via radio.

but can mask serious injuries such as cervical spine fractures, internal injuries, head injuries, and even broken long bones. When you see a patient with any type of wound or injury, it is important to determine what happened and assess the patient for further "hidden" injuries. This is often the most challenging part of patient care in an emergency situation.

When caring for any wound or other malady with apparent blood or body fluids, it is critical to the safety of the health care provider to follow "universal precautions." Universal precautions are the procedures the health care provider should use in treating patients to avoid contact with (and thus infection from) human tissues, blood, and other body fluids. The basic approach is to avoid contact with any potentially infectious body tissue or liquid. This assumes the patient may have a transmittable disease. All patients are treated the same, whether or not there is a blood-borne infection such as HIV/AIDS or hepatitis B or C. Because all patients are treated the same, it is not always necessary for the health care provider to know whether the patient can transmit a blood-borne infection.

The Centers for Disease Control and Prevention Web site contains complete information on universal precautions for the health care provider (*http://www.CDC.gov*). The first step in universal precautions is to wear gloves when handling blood or body fluids. (Due to the number of people with latex allergies, it is best

Table 20.24. Types of wounds		
Type of wound	Characteristics	Treatment
Puncture wound	Foreign body punctures skin	Remove foreign body if possible; cleanse thoroughly
Abrasion	Surface of skin is rubbed off	Cleanse; if small, allow to air dry uncovered; bandage loosely if large; keep clean; these will ooze
Avulsion	Tear of skin	Cleanse; close wound and bandage
Contusion	A blow or bump that bruises the soft tissue without penetrating the skin; results in black-and-blue area	Can ice the area immediately
Laceration	Cut in skin	Cleanse and reposition edges; hold in place with steri-strips or sutures
Burns	Injury to skin and deeper tissues from hot temperature	Treatment varies with severity; severe burns cause fluid imbalances and require sophisticated hospital treatment; prevention of infection is also critical

Note: Wounds with extensive bleeding, wounds resulting in shock or loss of consciousness, and other serious wounds require immediate evacuation to a medical facility.

for the ship's medicine chest to have latex-free gloves.) Masks and protective eyewear are also appropriate when there may be splash of blood. Any type of protective eyewear will suffice underway – eye glasses or sunglasses work well. In a hospital setting, gowns are often worn. Aboard ship, one can examine their clothes after completing treatment – if they are blood stained, they can be carefully washed and treated with chlorine bleach (recognizing that this will fade the color of the garment). Of most importance is to use extreme caution during procedures to avoid needle sticks and other exposures to blood and body fluids. Needle stick injuries are much easier to get underway with the rocking and rolling of the vessel.

If any skin areas of the health care provider are splashed with blood or body fluids they should be gently washed with soap and water. It is important not to abrade the skin because the skin is a protective barrier. Should there be a serious exposure, such as a needle stick, seek immediate shore consultation, preferably with a U.S.-based provider so that a decision can be made about beginning prophylaxis, especially if the patient is at high-risk for HIV.

After providing medical care, the treatment area should be observed for any splashes of blood or other body fluids. The treatment area should be disinfected with a solution made from one part chlorine bleach and ten parts water.

An embedded fishhook is a common puncture wound at sea. Fishhooks are relatively easy to remove if the barbs have not penetrated skin. With a forceps or tweezers, grab the hook, and bring it back through the skin in reverse of the way it entered. However, if the barbs have penetrated the skin, the challenge is much greater. One method of removing the hook is to push the hook through the skin in the same direction it entered. When the barb is exposed, it can be cut off and the fishhook

extracted. Depending upon the size and location of the fishhook, however, this technique can cause significant damage. A second technique is to slide an 18g needle down the hook to cover the barb of the hook with the needle bevel. Once covered, the barb can be disengaged and the hook removed. A third way to remove a fishhook is to wrap string around the hook and to put downward pressure in the direction opposite the barb. Once the barb is disengaged, the string can be pulled to slide the hook out of the wound. It should be noted, though, that if embedded deeply or near a vital structure (i.e., the eye or within the neck), it is best to stabilize the fishhook and transport the patient to a facility with a surgical capability to remove it.

Standard recommendations are to give a patient a tetanus shot if they have a seriously contaminated wound. Because this cannot be done underway, it is extremely important that all members of the expedition have current tetanus vaccinations. The recommendation is to receive a booster shot every 10 years, and then to receive an additional vaccination if you have a serious contaminated puncture or other penetrating wound. When tetanus vaccine is indicated but not available, patients may be prophylaxed with penicillin (if not allergic to penicillin).

Substance Abuse

Substance abuse is the use of substances – illegal drugs, prescription medications, and products such as glue and other inhalants and alcohol – in ways that interfere with one's life. Underway this can include intoxication that interferes with one's ability to safely navigate and operate the vessel, to concentrate and perform the missions of the expedition, and in general to carry on with routine daily activities. Substance abuse can lead to serious illness, dependency (with withdrawal), and death. Death may be due to acute or chronic affects. Drugs of abuse may be swallowed, inhaled, snorted, injected, or even absorbed through the skin and mucous membranes.[15,28,29]

Table 20.25 identifies the major substance abuse diagnoses.[29]

Alcohol is the most widely abused drug underway. Alcohol use has been a factor in many drownings, tragic ship collisions, and other mishaps at sea. It is the responsibility of everyone aboard – crew and expedition members alike – to promote and practice responsible attitudes toward alcohol use. Those in command of the vessel and the expedition leadership are ultimately responsible for reinforcing responsible alcohol use and not tolerating illegal drug use. Intoxication from alcohol and drugs can endanger the entire crew and expedition party. It is important to recognize the signs and symptoms of substance use disorders and to intervene to maintain the safety of all aboard.

Ethyl alcohol, also known as grain alcohol or ethanol, is the active ingredient in alcoholic beverages such as beer, wine, and hard liquors. When underway, if ethanol is not available, some people are tempted to drink other chemically related substances, which can be poisonous and deadly. Denatured alcohol, used for industrial purposes, is ethanol that has been mixed with other chemicals to make it poisonous to drink. It smells like the usual drinking alcohol, but has been made poisonous (to avoid beverage taxes since the product is not meant to be consumed). Denatured alcohol has many uses aboard ship and is fairly common. Everyone aboard should be educated that this is highly poisonous and should *never* be a substitute for consumable grade grain

alcohol. Another poisonous alcohol is methyl alcohol, also called wood alcohol or methanol, and is used as a fuel and solvent. Even in small quantities, it causes liver damage, blindness, and death. Isopropyl alcohol, or "rubbing alcohol" is commonly found in sickbays. It, too, is poisonous if consumed. Education is critical to prevent chemical poisoning aboard ship, especially when beverage alcohol is not available to a person dependent upon it (see Chapter 30 for more information on treatment of poisonings).

Though routinely consumed, alcohol use can be deadly underway. Alcohol can kill when it is taken with other CNS depressants such as some "sleeping pills," tranquilizers, and motion sickness medications. The use of alcohol predisposes one to fatal accidents – underway this can be serious – falls down ladders, man overboard, or collisions while boat driving. The impaired judgment associated with alcohol use can lead to fights, murder, or suicide. Fortunately, most often recreational alcohol use is relatively harmless. The expedition leader should always be alert to the difference between casual social drinking and dangerous, even life-threatening alcohol consumption. Also, in port, drinking is common and can lead to a host of problems including fights, falls, traffic accidents, and lapses in judgment with unsafe sex (and resultant HIV/AIDS and other sexually transmitted diseases).

The *Diagnostic and Statistical Manual – IV-TR*[29] by the American Psychiatric Association identifies a range of alcohol-induced disorders including dependence, abuse, intoxication, withdrawal, intoxication delirium, and withdrawal delirium. Alcohol can also induce dementia and amnesic, psychotic, mood, anxiety, and sleep disorders as well as sexual dysfunction. Alcohol intoxication, alcohol withdrawal, and alcohol dependence will be discussed because of their relevance to an underway expedition.

Alcohol Intoxication

Alcohol intoxication, at lower blood alcohol levels, is self-limiting as long as the person stops drinking. However, with as little as one drink reflexes are impaired, and activities such as boat driving and working with machinery are dangerous. For the safety of the expedition members, the expedition leader should ensure that the crew is not under the influence of alcohol at any time when they are on duty.

As alcohol levels increase with more drinking, there is poor control of muscles, reduced coordination, double vision, flushing of the face, bloodshot eyes, and vomiting. Behavior varies greatly. It is hard to predict what an intoxicated person will do next. There may be profuse crying or unexplained euphoria. Moods can change rapidly. Dangerous fights can result.

Alcohol is metabolized by the body at a constant rate – about one drink per hour – regardless of activity.

Table 20.25. Substance abuse diagnoses	
Diagnosis	**Signs and symptoms**
Intoxication	Inappropriate behavior, impaired judgment, physical changes like slurred speech, unsteady gait, poor attention
Abuse	Use of drug that causes problems at work, at home, or with relationships with others
Tolerance	Requires increasing amounts for the same effect
Physical dependence	Body requires drug to prevent withdrawal symptoms
Psychological dependence	Craving for drug
Withdrawal	Physical symptoms when drug use stops in dependent person; patient can have life-threatening seizures
Withdrawal delirium or delirium tremens	DTs – serious, life-threatening alcohol withdrawal with a change in consciousness or cognition; patient can have life-threatening seizures

(One drink is a 12-ounce beer, 4-ounce glass of wine, or 1 ounce of hard liquor.) Black coffee or a cold shower may make an intoxicated person feel better, but their reaction times are not changed – they remain slowed and impaired. It is impossible to "walk off" excess liquor or intoxication. Performance remains subpar.

Serious intoxication results when a large amount of alcoholic beverage is taken over a relatively short period of time or for a longer period of time when alcohol intake exceeds alcohol metabolism and excretion. Memory is commonly lost for the events while intoxicated. Symptoms are drowsiness that can progress rapidly to coma; slow snoring with noisy breathing; blueness of the face, lips, and fingernail beds; involuntary passage of urine or feces; dilated pupils; and rapid weak pulse.

An unarouseable patient is a medical emergency, and consultation and medical evacuation may be necessary. Information that is useful to communicate to the medical consultant is the patient's vital signs, information on the amount of alcohol consumed and the time frame, and other medical problems. Be aware that the signs and symptoms of drunken stupor are similar to other medical emergencies such as intoxication from prescription or illegal drugs, other poisonings, stroke, brain injury, hypoglycemia, and diabetic coma. Never assume that a patient's altered mental status is simply caused by alcohol. For example, a person may have an odor of alcohol on the breath and also be in a diabetic coma or may have fallen and have a serious head injury.

Stupor or coma always requires immediate treatment, no matter what the cause, though the specific treatment varies, dependent upon the cause. Note that alcohol can be a fatal combination with other central nervous system depressant drugs such as the benzodiazepines. Remember that accidents, falls, and fights are commonly associated with drunkenness, so the head should be checked for signs of injury, and the pupils of the eyes should be checked for equality of size and moderate dilation (in serious head injury and stroke, the pupils may be unequal and nonreactive to light); the patient's temperature should be recorded. The individual's shipmates should be questioned on whether the patient might have taken drugs (either prescription or illegal drugs), been injured, or overexposed to fumes and poisons. Also, try to determine how much alcohol the person may have consumed and over what time period. Personal effects should be checked for medications and other drugs if indicated. Accurately diagnosing the cause(s) of the stupor is key to successful treatment. A rapid and appropriate response can prevent an unnecessary and tragic death.

Immediate treatment of the stupor or coma is the ABCs – airway, breathing, and circulation. Another person should concurrently *obtain medical consultation by radio* and provide as much information about the patient's condition and possible causes of the stupor. Continue to monitor vital signs and the patient's general condition. Keep an ongoing written log of the patient's condition, vital signs, and any treatment. Keep the patient lying on the side to reduce the chances of aspiration in case there is vomiting. The specific treatment is dependent upon the cause(s) of the stupor or coma such as trauma, alcohol, or diabetes. Treatment must address all the interacting factors. Further, though not the mission of the expedition, if alcohol is the cause, the patient should be referred for long-term alcohol treatment in the home port.

Alcohol Withdrawal

Alcohol withdrawal occurs when a physiologically dependent person abruptly stops drinking alcohol. Physiologic dependence can develop after prolonged and heavy drinking. For example, consider an expedition member who drinks alcohol regularly when at home before the expedition. When this person goes to sea on the expedition and suddenly stops drinking, he or she may experience withdrawal within several days. Alternatively, the patient could be drinking at the beginning of the expedition and then run out of liquor. Withdrawal can occur at any time during an expedition. *Alcohol withdrawal can be a life-threatening emergency.*

The *Diagnostic and Statistical Manual-IV-TR*[29] identifies symptoms characteristic of withdrawal. These include increased sweating and pulse (greater than 100 beats/min), hand tremor, insomnia, nausea or vomiting, hallucinations or illusions, agitation, anxiety, and grand mal seizures. The patient is distressed by the symptoms. Alcohol withdrawal is diagnosed when the symptoms are due to the cessation of alcohol and not due to another medical or psychiatric disorder.

Alcohol withdrawal can advance to withdrawal delirium, called delirium tremens or "DTs" DTs include a disturbance of consciousness and a change in cognition. DTs usually occur within 24–72 hours of stopping alcohol intake; however, they may occur as much as a week after. *DTs are a life-threatening emergency requiring complex medical treatment. To prevent serious DTs, any alcohol withdrawal symptoms require early pharmacologic treatment (with benzodiazepines) and immediate medical consultation by radio.* (If benzodiazepines are not available, alcohol withdrawal can be treated with alcohol, in amounts that are just enough to decrease symptoms. Make certain the patient is conscious and does not aspirate.)

A delirious patient should never be left alone. Even when the symptoms appear mild, constant observation is required. An accurate and ongoing written record should be kept of the patient's condition, including vital signs and urinary output. Treatment should be symptomatic. The patient's recent history should be reviewed carefully to determine the cause of the delirium. In addition to alcohol withdrawal, there may be a co-occurring head injury or another medical problem. Medial advice by radio should be obtained and followed.

In treating impending (and actual DTs), medium- to long-acting benzodiazepines are used to "substitute" for the body's dependence on alcohol. When withdrawal symptoms are first observed, prompt treatment should begin with a drug such as oral chlordiazepoxide or diazepam. This should control the minor symptoms and, if properly managed under medical direction, should prevent the severe withdrawal symptoms of delirium tremens, including seizures. Keep a running chart of the patient's condition and care provided, including vital signs, medications given, and other relevant information. When the patient is stable, the benzodiazepine dosage should be tapered over several days, while the vital signs and condition are closely monitored. Tapering, rather than sudden stopping, is important to prevent further complications such as benzodiazepine withdrawal seizures.

Patients in withdrawal are easily agitated and very uncomfortable. Reassurance and a careful explanation of procedures are important. The patient may experience nightmares, illusions, and hallucinations. Placing the patient in a well-lit room in the presence of others is often helpful. Isolation and restraints will only further agitate the patient. Vital signs should be taken at least every 4 hours; more often if unstable. Written charting of the patient's condition and interventions (including all vital signs) is important so that any changes are quickly noticed. Any changes can be warning signs that the patient's condition is worsening.

If the patient is not stabilized after 24 hours of treatment with a benzodiazepine, look for other medical complications requiring immediate intervention. Continue to seek radio consultation.

Seizures, historically called rum fits, also accompany alcohol withdrawal. They can be treated with intravenous benzodiazepines. Administer low doses slowly and carefully to avoid respiratory depression, respiratory arrest and death. Continue radio consultation for assistance with medical management. Very rarely are restraints necessary. If restraints are used, careful medical records should be maintained explaining why they are used, and providing regular, about every 15-minutes, notes on the patient's condition. Restraints should only be used if no other intervention will prevent danger to the patient or others; a patient in restraints requires close and continual one-on-one monitoring. Never leave a person in restraints alone.

Alcohol Dependence and Alcohol Abuse

Alcohol dependence and abuse are sometimes called alcoholism. Alcohol dependence may include tolerance, withdrawal, and the inability to reduce use, even when it interferes with other parts of one's life. Alcohol abuse occurs when alcohol use interferes with work, school, home life, and relationships with others, and it may also include alcohol-related legal problems.

Problem drinkers have varying degrees and patterns of alcohol use. Some alcohol abusers go on periodic sprees or binges, but between these they drink little or no alcohol. Others may drink regularly every day for long periods. Alcohol causes various problems both aboard ship and while ashore. Alcohol is a common contributor to fights and arguments. Chronic alcohol abuse causes many medical problems and is especially damaging to the liver, brain, and nervous system.

Treatment of alcohol dependence and abuse requires long-term formal intervention, which exceeds the care provided during the expedition. However, prevention of alcohol incidents requires senior leadership throughout the expedition. It also requires effective management of any problems as they occur. The expedition's culture (and that of the ship) should expect (and demand) responsible alcohol behavior.

Other Drugs of Abuse

A range of chemicals can be abused – illicit drugs, prescription drugs, and shipboard chemicals, especially those with an organic solvent base. They can be consumed as a solid or liquid, sniffed, inhaled, snorted, smoked, inserted rectally, or applied to the skin. Symptoms of intoxication and withdrawal vary with different chemicals. When drug dependence occurs, both tolerance (more drugs are needed for the same effect) and withdrawal symptoms can present.

Suspect drug abuse when there are changes in behavior. The behavior changes are dependent upon the drug taken. A person on hallucinogens may see and hear things that are not there. Other drugs are stimulants or depressants. Some behavioral changes may actually first appear to be positive. For example, with amphetamine use, a usually bored sleepy withdrawn person may be more alert and even improve his or her performance. Conversely, a nervous, high-strung individual on barbiturates may be more cooperative and easier to manage.

Signs that suggest drug abuse include sudden and dramatic changes in discipline and job performance. Drug abusers may display unusual activity or inactivity as well as sudden and irrational flare-ups involving strong emotion or temper. There may be an increase in arguments. Personal appearance may decline – often a drug abuser becomes indifferent to his appearance.

Expedition members may not know each other well before the expedition. Some may bring drugs aboard, others may purchase them at port, or they may also be provided by the crew. The expedition leader, ideally in conjunction with the ship's master, should clearly communicate the inappropriateness and dangers of drug use during the expedition. A drug-intoxicated expedition member who falls overboard and drowns is a real tragedy.

Dental Care

Dental emergencies, though rarely life-threatening, can significantly impair mission accomplishment.

Table 20.26. Considerations for an oral evaluation

Characteristic	Description of finding
Location or quadrant of pain	Upper right, upper left, lower right, lower left
Onset	Sudden or gradual
Duration	Length of time – hours, days, weeks
Type of pain	Sharp, dull, throbbing, etc.
Factors that initiate or increase pain	Sensitivity to hot, cold, sweets, pressure (mastication/ chewing)
Swelling	Location, size, description
Bleeding	Yes or no
Vital signs (temperature, blood pressure, pulse)	Stable? Within normal limits?
Localized or systemic?	Is only the oral cavity involved? Does patient appear septic?
Patient's general condition	Stable, deteriorating, emergent

Table 20.27. Dental analgesics, antibiotics, and rinses

Class of drug	Specific pharmaceuticals
Oral analgesics	Ibuprofen, 400 mg
	Acetaminophen, 650 mg
	Acetylsalicylic acid, 650 mg
	Acetaminophen with codeine
Oral antibiotics	Penicillin, V 500 mg QID for 10 days
	Clindamycin, 300 mg QID for 10 days
Rinses	Chlorhexidine rinse
	Warm salt-water rinse

A patient with a dental emergency is in excruciating pain, and time generally only makes it worse. Eventually, the nerve and root of the tooth will die, and the pain may begin to resolve some. However, when the initial pain begins to resolve, an infection with its corresponding abscess may begin, resulting again in serious pain.[15,30]

When underway, one shouldn't expect the ship's master to have any dental expertise. Similarly, physicians are rarely trained to provide any dental care, including tooth extractions.

The best way to avoid dental emergencies is to require that all expedition members have a dental exam, coupled with completion of all recommended dental work, before the expedition departs. In cases where teeth are in poor repair, this can cost thousands of dollars. This may not be a popular recommendation among team members. However, this is a situation where the ones who complain most, are the ones who need it the most.

Even with the best prevention, dental problems underway can and do occur. Pain is the most common presentation of a dental problem. First, efforts should be made to identify the cause of the pain. Many problems present as "tooth pain," but they are actually medical conditions that can respond to medical treatment that may be available aboard ship. Examples of some medical problems that present as dental problems include sinusitis, neuralgias, ear infections, and temporomandibular joint dysfunction.

Evaluation of oral pain should be done in a systematic way. Table 20.26 provides guidance for the oral evaluation. This can be used in describing the problem via e-mail or voice communication to a shore-side consulting dentist. These characteristics are helpful in making the differential diagnosis and developing an emergency treatment plan.

When a dental emergency occurs underway, and far from competent dental care, it must be managed with the available resources. The first step is to examine the area that the patient identifies as the problem, recognizing that it is often difficult to accurately localize a dental problem. The actual problem may be the tooth or gum area adjacent to that identified by the patient. Examine the entire quadrant, or even the entire mouth, before determining the specific area needing treatment.

Once the dental problem is localized, it should be carefully examined and described. The severity of the problem should be determined. This is approximated by physical evaluation of the oral cavity combined with a subjective assessment of the patient's pain and general condition. From this, a treatment plan can be developed. Frequently, the treatment plan will include cleansing the area, treating pain, and treating any infection with antibiotics. Table 20.27 identifies commonly used medications for dental pain as well as antibiotics that are used for oral problems.

When a patient complains of a dental problem, it is important to respond promptly. Dental problems can rapidly cause excruciating pain. The infection that often causes or accompanies dental disease, if untreated, can spread beyond the oral cavity and result in systemic illness that can sometimes be life-threatening. Even if a dental problem isn't life-threatening, it can seriously impact the expedition's mission. It can be the reason to change the ship's course – so that a patient can receive treatment on shore. In the interest of the patient and the expedition, it is important to prevent dental emergencies through good dental care prior to deployment and then quickly responding to any dental problems once underway.

PREVENTION: SAFETY AND PUBLIC HEALTH CONCERNS

Prevention is an important focus during an expedition at sea. Prevention includes safety activities, public health concerns, and individual behavior. The vessel's safety features and sanitation practices are keys to preventing injury and illness aboard. A travel medicine consultation that includes predeployment vaccinations and education about healthy behaviors underway can significantly reduce the need for medical care during an expedition. Attention to safety and public health will help ensure an effective expedition that meets its mission goals.

The Vessel

Chartering and contracting for a boat or ship is one of the expedition leader's most important tasks for an underway expedition. The safety of the boat or ship is critical to a successful expedition.

For some projects, boats are contracted for a day at a time – for a specific component of the expedition. These boats don't go far from shore, generally carry relatively few people, and the safety concerns are somewhat less than for an expedition where one lives aboard for a period of days or weeks.

Commercial vessels that are registered in the United States must meet U.S. Coast Guard standards, which help to ensure their seaworthiness. Internationally, there are various other groups with established operations and personnel safety standards. Examples of these are compliance with the International Maritime Organization (IMO) and the International Convention for the Safety of Life at Sea (SOLAS) standards. If a boat or ship is being chartered for more than a day trip, compliance is essential to ensure the vessel and crew meet minimum safety and other standards. Vessels that lack certification of compliance with one of these or similar standards may not be seaworthy and could lead to an expedition disaster.

Even when vessels are certified, it is advisable to give them a quick look over before chartering. Table 20.28 identifies some of the areas to survey.

Once aboard and underway, it is critical that each expedition member participate in an initial safety brief,

Table 20.28. Informal vessel inspection

Informal vessel inspection criteria	Description
Overall condition	General cleanliness; minor repairs appear to be done; general appearance shows that owner/master takes pride in vehicle's condition.
Observe operations	Observe operators approach dock. Check for accuracy and organization of approach. Does crew appear to be a competent cohesive team?
Firefighting supplies	Working fire extinguishers that are loaded, within expiration date, and accessible; other fire equipment as appropriate.
Personal protective gear	Life jackets, in good condition for all aboard; easily accessible; also, if ship will go above or below 32° latitude, exposure suits; gear appropriate for passenger number and size/age.
Flares and other pyrotechnics	Flares should be within date and functional.
Radio transmitters, strobes, flashlights, etc.	Workable condition with new accessible batteries.
Lifeboats, life rafts	Equipment and plan necessary to abandon ship.
English-speaking crew member	At least one crew member who speaks English, or speaks the predominate language of the expedition party; it's also helpful if at least one member of the crew speaks the predominate language ashore.
Bilge pump	Working bilge pump to remove water that the vessel takes on.
Radio communication	UHF radio in good repair and functioning.
Global Marine Distress Single Sideband (GMDSS), Radio Common Carrier (RCC), etc.	Effective communication system such as GMDSS communication system in good repair and functioning; shipboard capability to patch through to the United States so that medical or other safety consultation can be obtained in real time
First-aid kit	Check availability, accessibility, and contents.
Abandon ship/emergency gear bag	Check availability, accessibility, and contents.
Galley sanitation, handwashing facilities, heads (toilets)	Check general sanitation; prevention of diarrhea and other diseases requires clean galley, handwashing facilities, and clean heads with handwashing sinks, soap, paper towels; also a culture among crew to use them.
Other safety equipment/gear/supplies; assess	Miscellaneous items appropriate for the location and duration of cruise such as EPIRB, AM/FM battery-powered radio, and simple general safety interest and preparedness things like green dye markers, signal mirrors, hand compass.
Crew	Observe crew. Does crew work together or are conflicts apparent? Assess morale. Note the working environment; it will be the expedition's environment, too.
Drills	Plan in place for regular drills including crew and passengers for fire, abandon ship, etc.

Table 20.29. Sample safety drills
Personal flotation devices (life jackets)
Other personal protective equipment
Abandon ship evolution
Mustering to lifeboats, life rafts
Survival skills aboard life rafts
Fire drills
Man overboard evolutions
Rough sea and bad weather precautions

followed by a series of specific-emergency briefs. The general safety brief is the initial orientation to the vessel. Emergency procedures in case of fire should be addressed. The "man overboard" procedure should also be discussed. Information on personal protective gear including life jackets – location aboard ship and special features such as lights, whistles, and dye should be included. Life jackets should be appropriate for the size of the passenger and age, if children. The procedures for an abandon ship evolution should be discussed including information on mustering, assignment of lifeboats or life rafts, and other related information. The vessel may have other special rules (such as where smoking is allowed), policies, procedures, and features that warrant a safety explanation. Though safety briefs sometimes seem elementary and of less importance than the mission of the expedition, they are critical in helping to ensure a safe expedition and an appropriate response should an emergency aboard occur.

After the ship is underway, there is usually unscheduled time that is convenient for safety drills. These can be an expansion (or practicing) of the earlier safety briefs as listed in Table 20.29. The drills require some planning, generally between the expedition leader and master. However, should there be an emergency, appropriate response learned from these drills can prove lifesaving.

These safety drills are important and can be planned so that they are a fun learning experience. They also provide an opportunity for the expedition members and crew to work together as a team.

Safety should be a paramount consideration on any seagoing expedition. Full expedition party participation in safety briefs and drills is critical to help ensure the safety of all during a real emergency. The expedition leader should provide his or her full support (and often initiation) of these activities. The expedition leader, and ship's master and crew, should have "safety first" as their motto.

Shipboard Sanitation

Shipboard sanitation is an essential component to a safe and healthy expedition. Ideally, the expedition leader will be able to inspect the ship before chartering. Unfortunately, this may not be possible. However, estab-

lishing requirements for ship sanitation should be part of the contracting process.

The ship's sanitation areas include food preparation, potable water, handwashing (including "head"), garbage storage, and pest management.

Food Sanitation

Food is one of the most important aspects of the expedition, from both morale and health perspectives. While underway, the expedition party has no place to eat except the ship's galley. Tasty and nutritious food will significantly improve the overall team spirits. However, if the food is contaminated because of poor selection, improper storage, or preparation, the expedition members will get sick with diarrhea or other gastrointestinal diseases and impede mission fulfillment.[16,21,31,32]

The expedition leader should ensure that the food aboard the ship is safe to eat. Special attention should be given to the sources of meats, poultry, and seafood; origins of raw fruits and vegetables; refrigeration of perishable foods and leftovers; and general galley sanitation.

Food sanitation includes several factors, as outlined in Table 20.30.

Throughout the cruise, the expedition leader should spend time in the galley area observing the cooking sanitation practices. Efforts should be made to educate the galley crew and others aboard to modify behaviors as needed to ensure a safe food supply. A direct, but diplomatic and friendly approach, may be more effective than more rigid and hostile communications. Galley staff must always wash hands after toileting to prevent diarrhea and other oral–fecal transmitted disease. Handwashing facilities must be available for, and used by, everyone aboard.

If there is any doubt about the ship's food safety, the extra precautions (Table 20.31) should be followed. These precautions are also advisable when eating ashore in unknown areas.

Potable Water

Throughout history, safe drinking water has been an essential maritime requirement. European ports including Antwerp, Belgium, and Amsterdam, Netherlands, gained prominence early when seagoers learned to trust the port's safe water supply. Today, water is an equally important element to a successful expedition. Contaminated water can be a cause of significant disease during the expedition. Potable drinking water is essential.

Some boats and ships have onboard desalination facilities. These should be in operable condition, and their capacity should be appropriate for the number of people aboard.

Care should be used to ensure that water obtained in foreign ports is potable, and safe to drink. Potable

Table 20.30. Components of food sanitation aboard ship	
Food preparation	**Components**
Food handler	Good personal hygiene; handwashing; knowledge about safe food handling and appropriate technique; wear gloves; don't work if sick, especially if diarrhea
Galley and equipment	Clean and sanitary; good lighting
Food selection and procurement	Purchase food that is not contaminated; choose menu carefully (no lettuce in many areas), caution with unpeeled fruits and vegetables
Food storage	Refrigerate until used; keep hot food hot until served; use caution when storing and serving leftovers; store dried goods tightly covered and away from rodents and insects
Food preparation	Don't cross contaminate food prep areas (raw meat, poultry, fish and other foods); wash raw fruits and vegetables in potable water before cooking or serving (consider washing in a bleach–water solution if produce is to be eaten raw)
Cooking	Cook meats to well done; cook or peel fruits and vegetables
Serving food	Serve hot food hot; cold food cold
Galley water supply	Potable water with no back-siphonage
Clean-up	Wash dishes in hot soapy water; discard all cooking waste immediately; clean all food-prep areas especially if used to cut raw meat, poultry or fish

water tanks and hoses should be appropriately cleaned, sanitized, and maintained. They should only be used for potable water. Larger ships should have water-testing capabilities aboard. If the potable water system becomes contaminated, such as from pumping in contaminated water from port, sanitizing the pipes, hoses, and rest of the plumbing system is a major job. Caution in bringing on board potable water is essential.

If the ship has potable and nonpotable water sources, they should be clearly separated and not interchanged. Nonpotable water may be used for activities such as bathing and flush toilets. Plumbing systems should be designed to prevent backflow, especially between potable water and sewerage systems. Hoses should be clearly labeled and not interchanged.

If there is any doubt about potable water aboard ship, especially when "fresh" water is newly obtained in foreign ports, it may be advisable to use bottled water for drinking if methods for testing the water are not available.

Table 20.31. Precautions: foods to eat and foods to avoid
Usually safe foods
Dry food such as bread and cereal
Packaged food
Hot, freshly cooked food – meats, vegetables, rice, pasta
Cold *pasteurized* milk
Fruits you peel yourself (bananas, oranges, etc.)
Foods to avoid
Do not eat fruit or vegetables salads that have been handled by people who may not have clean hands – cutting potatoes in potato salad, peeling and cutting pineapple, etc.
Eat hot food hot, and cold food cold. (Be especially careful eating ship's leftovers or at buffets ashore.)
Eat meat, poultry, and fish that have been fully cooked.
Generally avoid "street food" and food stored and prepared without refrigeration.
Do not eat food washed in contaminated water.
Do not eat lettuce salad.
Remove lettuce if it is in a sandwich.
Don't eat vegetables if sewerage irrigation.
Other safe food tips
Food is only as clean as the people who prepare it.
The people who prepare the food are only as clean as the bathrooms they use.
Do food service workers and other crew members have a place to wash their hands, and do they actually wash them?

Safe drinking water is essential for any cruise. The expedition leader should make certain the ship's master takes appropriate precautions to ensure a safe water supply.

General precautions (Table 20.32) are advisable if there is any question about the ship's water supply being potable. Many of the same precautions should be followed when going to shore in areas with questionable water supplies.

Table 20.32. "Don't drink the water" – what It *really* means
Know the source of drinking water on the ship or on land.
Obtain only potable water in foreign ports.
Afloat, boil or halogenate (chlorine, iodine) drinking water if necessary.
Afloat, filter water if necessary.
Drink only potable water aboard; drink bottled water ashore.
Ashore, make sure bottled water is sealed (that is isn't refilled with tap water).
Carbonated beverages (*without ice*) are safe if in original containers.
Drink all beverages in original, sealed containers.
Ashore, beware of orange drink – made with local tap water but served in soda bottles; this is not carbonated.
Ashore, *do not drink* iced tea, lemonade, etc., that could be made with tap water; it is okay afloat if made with potable water.
• *Do not use ice*, or drink anything that has had ice in it (the bacteria are not killed by freezing).
• Use only potable or bottled water to brush teeth and rinse toothbrush.

Handwashing and "Head" Facilities

About a third to half of all travelers to developing countries develops some type of diarrheal disease. Some are self-limited, while others are more serious. Extreme care with food and water is necessary to prevent them. However, many food-borne outbreaks can be traced to inadequate handwashing practices.[21]

Everyone aboard requires access to handwashing facilities, especially after toileting. It is critical that all food service personnel thoroughly wash their hands after toileting, before and after handling foods, especially raw meats, poultry, and fish.

If someone in the group develops diarrhea or other gastrointestinal disease, extreme consistent precautions must be taken to prevent transmission among others in the group. Most important is handwashing. The sick team member must thoroughly wash his or her hands after going to the bathroom – this may mean using a series of two or three "baby wipes" if no other facility is available. Some type of isolation can be helpful – consider having the sick person in a single berth or have several sick people share a berth, so they don't spread disease to healthy roommates. Use extreme caution when handling anything fecally stained such as clothing items and bed linens. Also, note toilet paper is often put in a container, not flushed. Bathroom surfaces (doors, light switches, faucets, etc.) may be contaminated. Preventing oral–fecal contamination requires extreme vigilance to prevent disease transmission. Handwashing after toileting, before preparing food, and before eating is essential, especially when living in confined environments such as a boat or ship.

Traveler's diarrhea and other enteric illnesses are spread by oral–fecal contamination. The usual route is someone not washing his or her hands after defecating. A microscopic amount of fecal contamination can spread disease to an entire expedition party. Handwashing by everyone, crew and expedition party alike, is critical.

Some boats don't have adequate handwashing facilities. If this is the case, it is imperative to augment them. Boxes of disposable wet towels (such as baby wipes) should be left in a convenient place near each toilet. Similar arrangements should be made for galley staff handwashing. Liquid hand sanitizers are helpful but should not be relied upon if there is any particulate matter on the hands. Also, they are only useful if used according to directions, which generally means about 30 seconds of wet rubbing or scrubbing. Always clean hands before putting anything in your mouth.

Table 20.33 outlines some basic handwashing hygiene.

Garbage

Because most boats and ships are fairly crowded, the management of garbage is critical. Trash should be

Table 20.33. Handwashing is the best prevention
Tap water may not be available for handwashing.
Wash hands before eating.
Bring alcohol wipes or baby wipes.
Bring hand sanitizer; use according to directions.
Always wash your hands after going to the bathroom.
Try to ensure the crew washes their hands as well.
Always wash your hands before eating or putting anything in your mouth.
A box of baby wipes might be good for the group to share to wash hands before meals.
If someone aboard gets diarrhea, use extra precautions; they must be *very careful and always* wash their hands.
Avoid contaminating environmental surfaces with fecal material (faucets, door knobs, toilet flush handles, etc.).
Sanitize any contaminated areas with a 10% bleach and water solution.

tightly covered. It must be stored so as not to attract rats or insects when the vessel docks. Liquid and solid waste should be disposed of consistent with environmental laws.

Pest Management

Keeping ships pest-free is an ongoing process. Limiting food to galley areas helps prevent a food source for pests throughout the vessel. Further, care should be taken that food and other items brought aboard are not contaminated. Proper storage of foodstuffs in the galley also helps to prevent pest infestation.

Ships can easily be infested with rats and various insects including mosquitoes, flies, bedbugs, lice, ticks, and cockroaches. Managing and eliminating these pests contributes to a pleasant and healthy expedition.

Rats, mice, and other vermin contribute to destruction of food and other items aboard ship, as well as spreading disease. Some countries require a certificate that the ship is rat-free. It is much easier to prevent rats aboard than it is to get rid of them after they infest. Good sanitation, especially with food, is a beginning. Rat guards will also help keep rats from boarding when docked. At the first sign of rats, trapping and poisoning will help to keep the problem from growing.

Maintaining an insect-free ship is also important to the comfort of the expedition members. Some insects, such as mosquitoes, spread diseases including malaria, West Nile virus, and yellow fever. Mosquito netting over sleeping areas may be needed in some ports. Flies and roaches also spread disease. Lice, bedbugs, and fleas can bite and caused various skin ailments. Other insects such as mites, silverfish, and beetles will infest food and other items. Continual surveillance and immediate response is needed to manage insects on the vessel.[33]

Personal Health – Pre-Deployment, Afloat, and Ashore

Predeployment Medical Preparation: "Travel Medicine"

"Travel medicine" is a relatively new medical specialty focusing on the medical services needed before embarking on an expedition, whether it is by sea, air, or land. With the increase in international travel, many travel medicine clinics have been established to provide basic consultation prior to travel and follow-up medical care.

Prior to many expeditions by sea, it is recommended or required that participants receive certain vaccines, take antimalarials, or take other precautions. It is generally preferable for the expedition leader/physician to make recommendations, though these decisions can also be left to each individual. In any case, the traveler will likely have to schedule an appointment with a public health clinic, travel medicine physician, or family physician. The plan should also include educating participants in the basic prevention behaviors recommended for any traveler to the areas visited – such as care with food and water to prevent diarrhea and other gastrointestinal disease.

The pretravel medical consultation should be scheduled at least 2 months before travel to ensure adequate time between, and sequencing of, vaccines. The consultation includes a review of the risks of the travel areas. Information on these can also be found on the Centers for Disease Control and Prevention travel Web site at *http://www.cdc.gov/travel/*.[21,34] This provides an overview of common diseases of travel, along with recommendations for vaccinations, antimalarials, and other travel precautions, including country-specific information. The Web site is updated regularly as recommendations change, such as the development of chloroquine-resistant malaria in yet another area.

When most people think of travel medicine they think of "shots." The specific vaccinations recommended for travel depend upon the geographic location, type of travel (remote areas or urban areas with good sanitation), demographics of the traveler (age, gender, pregnancy status), and other factors. However, it is important for all travelers to be current with the Center for Disease Control and Prevention's vaccination schedule.[22] Separate recommendations have been developed for children, based on age. Table 20.34 provides a list of commonly recommended vaccines.

The initial recommendation for most foreign travel is to be "current" on the generally recommended vaccinations. For some of these, such as influenza, an annual vaccination is needed. For others, such as measles or mumps, after the initial series is complete, no further vaccinations are required. For others, such as polio, after the childhood series, a one-time adult booster dose is

Table 20.34. List of commonly recommended vaccines in the united states

Adult recommended vaccines
Diphtheria
Hepatitis A
Hepatitis B
Human papillomavirus
Influenza
Measles
Meningococcal
Mumps
Pertussis
Pneumococcal
Polio (injected not oral)
Rubella
Tetanus
Varicella

Pediatric recommended vaccines
Diphtheria
Haemophilius influenzae, type b
Hepatitis A
Hepatitis B
Inactivated poliovirus
Influenza
Measles
Meningococcal
Mumps
Pertussis
Pneumococcal
Polio
Rubella
Tetanus
Varicella

Note: For both the adult and pediatric vaccines, some are only recommended for certain age groups or genders. For the complete vaccine recommendations, see the CDC Web site at *http://www.cdc.gov/travel/*.

often recommended before travel to a polio-endemic area. Each traveler should review his or her vaccination history [ideally recorded on a yellow World Health Organization Vaccination Card][19,25] and specific travel plans with a health provider to determine the most appropriate pretravel vaccines for their individual circumstance.

In addition to the routine vaccines, additional vaccines may be recommended for travel to certain areas depending upon one's activities. Yellow fever vaccine may be required when travel is anticipated to yellow fever endemic areas. Rarely, cholera vaccine may be required if one has just left a country with a cholera epidemic. Because cholera vaccine is not very effective, it is generally given only if required by a specific country for transit across specific country borders. Note the vaccine is no longer available in the United States, and any requirement for cholera vaccine is rare today. If the water supply is unpredictable, typhoid vaccine may be recommended. As another example, for extended travel to cities where rabies is endemic among local dogs, rabies vaccine may

Table 20.35. Vaccines specifically recommended for some foreign travel
Cholera (rarely recommended)
Polio (adult booster)
Rabies
Rotavirus
Typhoid, oral or intramuscular injection
Yellow fever

be recommended. Table 20.35 lists vaccines that may be recommended for foreign travel to some areas.[21,34]

Malaria prophylaxis is another essential in many areas. When ashore in many tropical areas, one of the most life-threatening yet preventable diseases of traveler's is malaria. Malaria is always a serious disease, and it can be a deadly disease. Malaria is from mosquito bites, and the mosquitoes usually bite between dusk and dawn. Prevention of malaria and other insect-borne diseases including yellow fever, viral encephalitis, West Nile virus, and others begins with protection from mosquito and other insect bites. Wear long pants, long sleeved shirts, and hats. Hats with netting are available. Sleep under insect netting if needed. Use mosquito repellent – DEET. (Do not use DEET on wounds or broken skin; use care not get into your mouth; do not swallow it; and wash off when not needed.) Also, use a flying insect spray if mosquitoes are in your berth; pyrethroid insecticides are most effective.

Antimalarial medications differ and should be selected primarily based on the geographic area of travel because the parasite in different geographic areas has developed varying susceptibilities and resistance to antimalarial products. (See Table 20.36.) The malaria parasite in many parts of the world has developed resistance to one or more commonly used antimalarials. Thus, it is critical to choose the medication according to area to be visited. Different antimalarials have various dosing schedules – daily or weekly. Note that most medications should be taken a few days to a week prior to travel and should be continued about 4–6 weeks afterwards, even if there are no symptoms of disease. This extended course of drug helps prevent symptomatic infection from parasites that might still be in the liver. Antimalarials can interact with other drugs the patient is taking; some should be avoided in patients with certain enzyme deficiencies, and some have other special applications.[21,34]

Table 20.36. Malaria treatment options
Chloroquine phosphate (Aralen and generics)
Doxycycline
Hydroxychloroquine sulfate (Plaquenil)
Malarone (atovaquone and proguanil)
Mefloquine (Lariam and generic)
Primaquine

What to Bring

Packing for an expedition afloat can be challenging because only the items brought aboard will be available during the cruise, and storage space is often very limited. Careful packing is essential. Knowledge about weather and sea conditions is helpful.

Table 20.37 provides a list of items essential for most sea expeditions. The specifics vary with the location, season, purpose, and duration of the expedition and the expedition member's role. For example, an expedition member working sails may need different gear than one who is less physically involved on the voyage.

In packing for your trip, bring all prescription and over-the-counter medications you may need. Pack them in their original containers. "Baggies" of miscellaneous pills may be easy to carry, but they may look suspicious to customs officials and result in delay, confiscation, or worse.

Bring clothing appropriate to the weather. Bring clothes that will protect from the sun, wind, and other weather conditions. Remember the outside decks can be cool at night, even in otherwise warm tropical areas. Shoes are especially important. Soles should be non-skid and designed to prevent slipping. Wet floors and rough seas are conducive to dangerous falls, and proper shoes can be very helpful. Shoes should be comfortable because they will be worn during most waking hours. Sandals may not provide adequate support in rough seas. Bring at least one extra pair of shoes, and prepare for them to get wet.

Bring eyeglasses even if you plan to wear contact lenses. Sometimes the environmental conditions favor wearing glasses. Sunglasses are also important.

Careful packing is key to a fun and productive expedition. The expedition leader will likely provide a suggested list of items. Use care to bring what is needed but not to overpack because storage areas are small and cramped. Many clothes will be washed by hand, so synthetic fast drying fabrics are often preferred to natural fibers such as cotton and wool. A few hours spent in a quality outdoor clothing and supply store can be extremely helpful. For something as simple as a waterproof jacket, there is a range of options and prices. Learn about the options before deciding to get the cheapest, most expensive, or something in between. Features vary, and different items are designed with specific purposes in mind.

General Travel Precautions

Though high-adventure travelers frequently want to believe they are "exempt" from local disease, they must take the same precautions as any traveler to prevent traveler's diarrhea, malaria, and other travel-related illness.

Swimming should be avoided in areas with contaminated water. In many parts of the world, it is commonplace to discharge raw sewerage into the closest water.

Table 20.37. Packing for an underway expedition

Item	Comments
Expedition supplies	Paper, pens, books, log books, laptop computer, cell phone (if in receiving area), etc.
Eyeglasses, contact lenses, sunglasses	Extra pair of eyeglasses even if generally wear contact lenses; adequate numbers of contact lenses and cleaning solutions (daily disposable lenses work well); prescription/nonprescription sunglasses
Gloves	Lightweight warm weather gloves that permit manual dexterity; warmer gloves if needed
Hat	Wide-brimmed to protect from sun; fleece to keep head warm at night and with cold winds
Headlamp	A high-quality, long-life headlamp is invaluable for night work and just maneuvering through the ship
Hearing protection	During some operations, hearing protection is needed to prevent hearing loss; also, hearing protection may facilitate sleep on a noisy boat or ship
Packaged foods	Airtight containers are best for favorite "health food" and/or "junk food"
Pants	Long pants to protect from sun; cotton or "wicking" synthetic fabrics; warm weather gear; shorts
Personal supplies	Medications, cosmetics, shaving supplies, personal journal, pleasure books, etc.
Raingear	High-quality lightweight raingear that "breathes"; waterproof jacket with hood and waterproof pants
Shirts	Long-sleeve light-colored cotton shirts to protect from sun; some "wicking" synthetic fibers also work well
Shoes, socks	Comfortable, low heels, nonslip soles (check to see if soles must be white to protect decks from black marks) Socks to minimize leather allergies and resultant itching
Travel essentials	Passport, vaccination record, money (including small U.S. bills), traveler's checks or other access to additional funds, camera with adequate memory (may not be able to download pictures during expedition), addresses/e-mail addresses/phone numbers, etc.
Warm weather gear	The outside deck can be cold at night or in rough weather; bring upper and lower layers of fleece and other "wicking" fabrics that dry quickly; heavy parka may be indicated
Windproof jacket	Wicking windproof jacket is very useful to protect from night breezes and winds

Do not swim in stagnant fresh water such as lakes. Rivers are often equally contaminated. Ocean water may be a little cleaner, but recognize that in many areas raw sewerage and solid wastes are dumped directly into the ocean. In some areas, due to cost and custom, swimming pool water may not be adequately chlorinated. If you choose to swim, make certain not to drink water when swimming. Also, keep contaminated water out of eyes; be especially careful if wearing contact lenses. Many recommend avoiding swimming in anything but ocean water, and then only in areas distant from sewerage dumping.

When ashore, use care in motor vehicles. Many travelers are seriously injured or killed each year in motor vehicle accidents. In many areas, motor vehicle accidents provide the greatest risk of injury while traveling. If you are the driver, learn local traffic customs *before* getting behind the wheel. Cars rarely have seatbelts, but wear them if available. Driving laws and their enforcement vary, especially as related to drinking alcohol and driving. Always know your drivers and, when possible, the vehicles. Many vehicles have poor brakes, burned out lights, and other safety hazards. The slopes and curves of roads – inclines and declines, and twists around hills and mountains – may be greater than usual. Driving and riding at night, especially in mountainous areas, should be avoided when possible. Bicycles, motor scooters, and motorcycles can be especially dangerous, even when wearing a helmet and other protective gear. When a pedestrian, learn to expect the unexpected while crossing streets, especially when cars drive on the side opposite to home.

Don't be too ambitious in estimating how far you can drive in a day – animals on the road, blocked roads due to local markets or celebrations, unexpected road conditions, and other factors can delay the trip. Ships leave port at the designated time, and missing the ship can be expensive and embarrassing. In many areas it can be very difficult to catch up with the ship later.

When ashore, remember that animals spread many diseases. Many mammals carry tapeworms and other intestinal parasites that can easily be spread to humans. Some countries have endemic rabies. Rabies is almost universally fatal in humans. Avoid approaching homeless domestic dogs, especially if they are in groups or packs. Even if not rabid, these animals can have unpredictable behavior and bite even the friendliest of tourists. Avoid all wild animals. If you are bitten by any animal, report it *immediately*; you may need a series of rabies vaccinations. The sooner you are vaccinated, the likelier you will survive.

Sexually Transmitted Diseases

Various diseases are sexually transmitted – HIV/AIDS, hepatitis B and C, syphilis, gonorrhea, and others. Though following the U.S. "safe sex" practices can significantly reduce the risk of disease transmission, there is still risk of infection. Make certain to think ahead and use good judgment and not act impulsively. Port areas may offer new experiences to expedition members. Alcohol can affect judgment and increase impulsive sexual behavior.[15]

SUGGESTED READINGS

American Psychiatric Association. *Diagnostic and Statistical Manual of Mental Disorders, Fourth Edition, Text Revised (DSM-IV-TR).* Arlington, VA: American Psychiatric Association; 2000.

Auerbach, P., ed. *Wilderness Medicine.* 4th ed. Bellerose, NY: Mosby Saunders; 2001.

Auerbach PS, Donner HJ, Weiss EA. *Field Guide to Wilderness Medicine.* 2nd ed. Bellerose, NY: Mosby Saunders; 2003.

Barkauskas V, Baumann L, Darling-Fisher C. *Health and Physical Assessment.* 3rd ed. Bellerose, NY: Mosby Saunders; 2001.

Beer M, Porter RS, Jones TV. *Merck Manual of Diagnosis and Therapy.* 18th ed. Whitehouse Station, NJ: Merck Research Labs; 2006.

Bledsoe BE, Porter RS, Cherry RA. *Intermediate Emergency Care: Principles and Practice.* Upper Saddle River, NJ: Pearson Education Publishers; 2003.

Bonewit-West K. *Clinical Procedures for Medical Assistants.* 6th ed. Bellerose, NY: Mosby Saunders; 2006.

Currance PL, Clements B, Bronstein AC. *Emergency Care for Hazardous Materials Exposure.* 3rd rev. ed. Bellerose, NY: Mosby Saunders; 2006.

Dorlands Pocket Medical Dictionary. 27th ed. Bellerose, NY: Mosby Saunders; 2004.

Estes M. *Health Assessment and Physical Assessment.* 3rd ed. Stamford, CT: Thomson Learning; 2005.

Hemann D. *Control of Communicable Diseases Manual.* 18th ed. Washington, DC: American Public Health Association; 2004.

Mandell GL, ed. *Principles and Practice of Infectious Disease.* 6th ed. Philadelphia: Mosby Saunders; 2004.

Phinney DJ, Halstead J. *Delmar's Dental Assisting: A Comprehensive Approach.* 2nd ed. Stamford, CT: Thomson Learning; 2003.

Salvato JA, Nemerow NL, Agardy FJ. *Environmental Engineering.* Hoboken, NJ: John Wiley & Sons; 2003.

Saunders CE, Ho MT. *Current Emergency Diagnosis and Treatment.* 4th ed. New York: McGraw Hill; 1992.

Skinner HB. *Current Diagnosis and Treatment in Orthopedics.* 3rd ed. New York: McGraw Hill; 2003.

Skinner HB. *Current Diagnosis and Treatment in Orthopedics.* 4th ed. New York: McGraw Hill; 2006.

True B, Dreisbach R. *Dreisbach's Handbook of Poisoning Prevention, Diagnosis and Treatment.* 13th ed. Lancashire, UK: Parthenon Publishing Group; 2002.

USEFUL WEB SITES

Useful Government Web Sites

http://www.cdc.gov The Centers for Disease Control and Prevention, Department of Health and Human Services, is recognized as the lead federal agency for protecting the health and safety of people – at home and abroad. Key areas on the site include Traveler's Health, Health Topics A–Z, and CDC Publications. This Web site provides the most current information on malaria prophylaxis and other aspects of traveler's health.

http://www.cdc.gov/nip This is the federal Web site for the National Immunization Program of the Centers for Disease Control and Prevention. It provides the latest vaccination recommendations for adults and children.

http://www.bt.cdc.gov/ This Centers for Disease Control and Prevention Web site is dedicated to public health emergency preparedness and response information.

http://www.uscg.mil/hq/g-m/nvic/ The U.S. Coast Guard Web site has extensive information on boating safety, health requirements for Coast Guard approved vessels, and other relevant information.

Other Useful Web Sites

http://www.merck.com/pubs/mmanual/ The *Merck Manual* is an excellent all-in-one reference that provides exceptional breadth of medical information in one volume. Various medical conditions along with diagnostic and treatment information are provided. This is an online version of the often-used book.

http://www.pdr.net PDR.net is an online version of the *Physicians' Desk Reference.* It provides drug information for essentially all marketed prescription drugs. Formulation, indication, and dosing range information are provided.

http://www.rxlist.com/ RX List is the Internet Drug Index. It lists over 4,500 popular medications with descriptions understandable to consumers. It also has a link to *Taber's Medical Encyclopedia.*

http://www.medem.com/MedLB/medlib_entry.cfm Medem's Medical Library represents a range of patient education information including diseases, conditions, therapies, and health strategies.

http://familydoctor.org/ This Web site from the American Academy of Family Physicians offers a range of health information. It also includes facts on common medicines, including possible interactions, facts on common herbal remedies and dietary supplements, and advice on what you can treat at home (or aboard ship) and when a physician's expertise is needed.

http://www.health.harvard.edu/ This Web site sponsored by Harvard Health Publications provides access to newsletters on a range of topics.

REFERENCES

[1] 46 CFR Parts 1–40 (references U.S. Coast Guard)

[2] Standards of Competence for Seafarers Designated to Provide Elementary First Aid, U.S. Coast Guard, as amended

[3] Standards of Training, Certification and Watchkeeping for Seafarers (STCW), 1978 and as amended.

[4] U.S. Navy Bureau of Medicine. *Hospital Corpsman Sickcall Screener's Handbook,* Great Lakes, MI: Naval Hospital; 1999.

[5] *http://www.internationalsos.com*

[6] *http://www.medexassist.com*

[7] *http://www.iamat.org*

[8] *http://www.tripprep.com/scripts*

[9] *http://www.istm.org*

[10] *http://www.astmh.org*

[11] *http://travel.state.gov/travel/overseas_whoweare.html*

[12] Marine Hospital Service. *Handbook for the Ship's Medicine Chest.* Washington, DC: Marine Hospital Service; 1881 (1st ed.), 1904 (2nd rev. ed.), 1929 (3rd ed.).

[13] U.S. Public Health Service. *The Ship's Medicine Chest and First Aid at Sea.* Washington, DC: U.S. Government; 1947, 1955 (reprinted and revised), 1978 (rev.).

[14] Duffy JC, ed. *The Ship's Medicine Chest and Medical Aid at Sea.* Washington, DC: U.S. Public Health Service; 1984.

[15] Johnson JM, ed. *The Ship's Medicine Chest and Medical Aid at Sea.* Washington, DC: U.S. Public Health Service; 2003.

[16] World Health Organization. *International Medical Guide for Ships.* Geneva, Switzerland: World Health Organization; 1988 (2nd ed., reprinted 2002).

[17] PDR Staff. *Physicians' Desk Reference for Nonprescription Drugs, Dietary Supplements, and Herbs.* Montvale, NJ: Medical Economics; 2007 (28th ed.)

[18] PDR Staff. *Physician's Desk Reference.* Montvale, NJ: Medical Economics; 2007 (61st ed).

[19] Johnson JM. Motion sickness. *Military Officer.* April 2007.

[20] Benson, AJ, Motion Sickness. In Pandolf KB, Burr RE, ed. *Med Medical Aspects of Harsh Environments, Vol 1*, Washington, DC: Borden Institute; 2002.

[21] Centers for Disease Control and Prevention. *Health Information for International Travel 2005–2006.* Atlanta: U.S. Department of Health and Human Services; 2005.

[22] *http://www.CDC.gov*

[23] Wittmers LE, Savage MV. Cold water immersion. In: Pandolf KB and Burr RE, eds. *Medical Aspects of Harsh Environments, Vol 1.* Washington, DC: Borden Institute; 2001.

[24] Auerbach PS, Donner HJ, Weiss EA. *Field Guide to Wilderness Medicine.* 2nd ed. Bellerose, NY: Mosby Saunders; 2003.

[25] Beers, MH, ed. *The Merck Manual of Diagnosis and Therapy.* Whitehouse Station, NJ: Merck Research Laboratories; 2006.

[26] Field Medicine Service School. Burn Casualties. In: *Student Handbook.* Camp Pendleton, CA: Field Medicine Service School; 1999.

[27] Bergman R. Burns (by Degree). In: *Anatomy of First Aid: A Case Study Approach, Anatomy Atlases.* Iowa City: The University of Iowa; 2004.

[28] Ray O, Ksir C. *Drugs, Society and Human Behavior.* St. Louis: Mosby-Year Book; 1993.

[29] American Psychiatric Association. *Diagnostic and Statistical Manual of Mental Disorders Text Revision – DSM-IV-TR.* Arlington, VA: American Psychiatric Association; 2000.

[30] Phinney DJ, Halstead J. *Delmar's Dental Assisting: A Comprehensive Approach.* 2nd ed. Stamford, CT: Thomson Learning; 2003.

[31] American Medical Association. *Diagnosis and Management of Foodborne Illnesses: A Primer for Physicians and Other Health Care Professionals, 15 volumes.* Chicago: American Medical Association; 2004.

[32] Johnson, JM, Calderwood, JA. Healthy travels. *Military Officer.* June 2005.

[33] Armed Forces Pest Management Board. *Technical Guide No. 36 Personal Protective Measures Against Insects and Other Arthropods of Military Significance.* Aberdeen Proving Ground, MD: U.S. Army Center for Health Promotion and Preventive Medicine.

[34] *http://www.cdc.gov/travel/*

ACKNOWLEDGEMENTS

Special thanks to James Caldevwood for his contributions to this chapter.

21 | Event Medicine

David A. Townes, MD, MPH, DTM&H

INTRODUCTION

Historically, participation in expeditions was limited to explorers, scientists, the very wealthy, and the occasional free thinker or lost soul brought along for logistical support. During the past several decades, there has been a dramatic shift in this demographic with participation no longer the purview of a privileged few. Today, individuals of all ages, from a wide variety of cultural, professional, and socioeconomic backgrounds regularly participate in expeditions and "expedition-type" activities. Several factors have contributed to this change. Development and advances in equipment have increased participation in such activities as backcountry skiing and snowboarding, flat and whitewater kayaking and rafting, mountain biking, mountaineering, orienteering, rock climbing, scuba diving, and trekking. In addition, safe, efficient and affordable travel has extended participation in these activities to the far reaches of the globe. Combined with economic prosperity, these factors have helped fuel the multibillion dollar adventure travel industry providing easy access to expedition and expedition-type activities for a large number of individuals.

During the past several decades, there has also been growth in the popularity of endurance events including marathons, triathlons, multiday bicycle rides, ultra-marathons, and ultra-triathlons. Increased participation in these activities has resulted in a larger number of events being held each year with greater diversity in the type of events held.

More recently, the growing popularity of adventure travel, endurance events, and expedition-type activities has given rise to "expedition-type events" that combine aspects of all of these. Adventure racing or multisporting is perhaps the most popular and fastest growing example.

Due to their large scale and competitive nature, expedition-type events are unique within event and expedition medicine. Unfortunately, there is little information available, and no formal guidelines to assist in the provision of medical support for these events.

Expedition-length adventure races provide an ideal example for discussion of medical support for expedition-type events.

This chapter introduces the development of a *medical support plan* for expedition-type events utilizing expedition-length adventure races as the primary example. Injuries and illness associated with participation in these events are highlighted and some of the common challenges and controversies associated with the provision of medical support for them are discussed. The information should prove useful for those charged with the provision of medical care for expedition-type events.

EXPEDITION-LENGTH ADVENTURE RACES

Expedition-length adventure races are competitive team events that require athletes perform multiple disciplines such as caving, flat and white water boating, hiking, horseback riding, mountain biking, mountaineering, navigation/orienteering, technical climbing/ropes skills, trail running, and trekking on courses that cover hundreds of miles. Teams commonly consist of four individuals with at least one member of each sex. They race together with all team members completing each discipline along the course. Adventure races are categorized by duration into expedition length (> 36 hours), long (12–36 hours), intermediate (6–12 hours), and sprint (< 6 hours).

Background

The first well-organized, large expedition-length adventure races include the Coast-to-Coast, started in New Zealand in 1980 and the Alaska Wilderness Classic started in 1983. Other events soon followed including New Zealand's well-known Raid Gauloises in 1989 and Southern Traverse in 1991. In 1995, expedition-length adventure racing first gained widespread exposure in the United States through The Eco-Challenge. More recently, the sport has been brought even more into the American mainstream through network television coverage of the Primal Quest, which began in 2002 in Telluride, Colorado.

In the spirit of true expeditions, most expedition-length adventure races do not have a set route. While there are checkpoints and transition areas (where teams change disciplines) that teams must pass through, each team must find a route between these points. They are provided basic maps and the Universal Transverse Mercator (UTM) coordinates for each checkpoint and transition area. Teams choose their route based on a variety of factors including weather conditions, temperature, time of day or night, and the skills of the team. For example, one team may decide to go around a ridge while another may opt to go over it. In addition, teams race continually and must strategize if and when to rest. The lack of both a predetermined route and built-in rest periods has important implications for the provision of medical support for these events.

While on the course, teams are governed by the "rules of travel." This set of instructions dictates many aspects of the race including required safety equipment for each discipline, where and when a team may travel on paved roads or existing trails, and mandated "dark zones" prohibiting certain types of travel at night in the interest of safety, such as white-water boating. The rules of travel also govern certain aspects related to the provision of medical care for participants including the use of medications and performance-enhancing substances, specifying penalties for utilization of medical resources during the race, and outlining criteria for medical withdrawal from the event.

A team is penalized for a breech of the rules of travel. The penalty for a minor infraction such as travel on an unapproved section of trail might include additional hours added to the team's total time at the completion of the race. The penalty for a major infraction such as not wearing a personal flotation device during a water section of the course might be disqualification of the team from the event.

Upon completion of the event, all penalties are allocated and the team with the fastest total time is declared the winner. In most large events, prize money is awarded to the top teams.

MEDICAL SUPPORT FOR MASS GATHERINGS

Mass gatherings have been defined both as events with > 1,000 participants and those with > 25,000 participants.[7,26] For the provision of medical support, events are divided into four categories, classes, or types. In category I events, spectators are essentially immobile for the duration of the event. Stadium sporting events and concerts are common examples. In category II events, spectators are mobile and may or may not actively participate in the event. Examples include golf tournaments, Carnival and Mardi Gras celebrations, and state fairs. Charity walks, bicycle rides, marathons, and triathlons are examples of category III events characterized by a large geographic area and participants often outnumbering spectators.[28] Category IV events, including adventure races and other expedition-type events, occur in rough and often remote terrain where precise location of participants is at times unknown, communication is limited, and technical search and rescue may be required with prolonged transport time to definitive care.[41,42] Category IV events tend to have the smallest number of participants and rarely meet the definition of a mass gathering.

There have been only a small number of investigations of medical support for category IV events.[4,5,13,25,40,42,43] The majority have focused on the frequency and type of injury and illness treated, the rate of utilization of on-site medical services, and the rate of transfer to local care facilities for category I, II, and IIII events. These investigations do, however, provide important information for the development of a medical support plan for a category IV event. Many of these investigations are anecdotal and descriptive. Several describe some of the factors that influence the type and frequency of injury and illness encountered and offer some general guidelines for the delivery of care at mass gatherings. There is, however, no universally accepted standard of care for emergency medical services at mass gatherings.[2,7,32,35]

In general, the incidence of significant medical emergencies at mass gatherings appears to be small. Relatively minor injury and illness accounts for the majority of medical encounters. In one investigation, mild respiratory illness, heat-related injuries, sunburn, blisters, and headache accounted for 75% of medical encounters. Acute exacerbation of asthma is the most common reason to require acute medical intervention.[3]

The relationship between event attendance and utilization of on-site medical services is unclear. Overall utilization of on-site medical services increased with attendance; however, *rate* of utilization did not increase and in some cases decreased with larger attendance.[2,8,46] The overall utilization rate of on-site medical services varies between 0.14 and 90 patients per 1,000 participants. For the majority of events, the utilization rate varied between 0.5 and 2 patients per 1,000 participants.[2,7,35]

Several factors influence the rate of utilization of on-site medical services including type and duration of the event, weather, availability of alcohol and drugs, and demographics of the crowd including average age, density, and mood. These factors also influence the type of medical care delivered.[2,3,26] One should expect to encounter a larger number of medical problems related to drug and alcohol use when these are readily available such as during rock concerts.[2,26] In contrast, one might expect to encounter less intoxication but more cardiac-related problems during a Papal visit.[22]

Temperature and relative humidity appear to have a major impact on utilization of on-site medical resources at mass gatherings. While both are associated with an increase in demand for on-site medical services, humidity has a larger impact. Not surprisingly, the availability of water influenced the incidence of dehydration and heat illness.[2,7,22] It is thus essential to consider the likely temperature and humidity during any event and plan accordingly.

Provision of medical support for events and mass gatherings begins with development of a medical support plan.[8,20,22] In one investigation, nine key elements of this process were identified: attendance or crowd size, personnel, medical triage and facilities, communication, transportation, medical records, public information and education, mutual aid, and data collection.[20] The basic goals are to provide rapid access and triage, stabilize and transport seriously injured or ill patients, and provide on-site care for minor complaints.[7] Early planning and good communication are critical in this process.[44]

The medical support plan should be based on *anticipation of need* beginning with an estimation of both the number and type of medical encounters in both the best- and worst-case scenarios. As previously described, a number of factors influence utilization of medical resources that should be considered. If available, a review of utilization of on-site medical resources for prior, similar events may prove very helpful.[22]

Even though there are no universally accepted standards for the location and staffing of on-site medical facilities at mass gatherings, some general guidelines have been proposed. One guideline for placement of Advanced Life Support (ALS) providers sets a goal of providing ALS care within 5 minutes for all participants under all conditions.[35] Another sets a goal of basic first-aid in 4 minutes, ALS care in 8 minutes, and evacuation to a medical facility within 30 minutes.[32] A guideline for staffing recommends a minimum two-person team consisting of registered nurses, emergency medical technicians, and/or paramedics for every 10,000 attendants.[8,20]

Many of the general findings of investigations of category I, II, and III events are helpful in development of a medical support plan for category IV events including the basic influence of attendance, weather, and basic demographics on utilization of medical resources. Caution should be applied however when calculating *utilization rates* for category IV events. Due to their extreme nature, utilization rates tend to be significantly higher for category IV events.[25]

MEDICAL SUPPORT PLAN DEVELOPMENT

Similar to other types of events, the provision of on-site medical care for expedition-type events begins with development of a medical support plan under the direction of the medical director. Depending on complexity, this might begin months to years prior to the event. Ideally, the medical director should be a physician, paramedic, emergency medical technician, nurse, or other medical professional with prior experience as a medical director for similar events. Their primary responsibility should be the health and safety of the participants. In this capacity, they will serve as care provider, planner, adviser, educator, and liaison with the community.[16]

For expedition-type events, the goal of the medical support plan should be to provide definitive treatment for minor illness and injury and to provide initial stabilization and facilitate transfer for more severe illness and injury.[42] The medical support plan should be comprehensive, outlining all aspects of medical support including listing personnel, supplies, and equipment, outlining communication, treatment and transfer protocols, assigning penalties for receiving medical care, and establishing indications for medical withdrawal from the event.

Development of a medical support plan begins with a careful review of the course, its location, local flora and fauna, the disciplines required, the time of year, and the environmental conditions including altitude, precipitation, temperature, and humidity. In this way, the occurrence and type of injury, illness, endemic disease, environmental emergencies such as dehydration, heat and cold illness, and altitude illness can be roughly predicted.

Expedition-type events often occur in very remote, sparsely populated, rugged wilderness terrain where there are inherent difficulties in communication, travel, and general logistics. The medical director must also be familiar with the availability and capability of local emergency medical services (EMS), local health care facilities, and the local search and rescue (SAR) system. It is often unrealistic to assume local EMS, health care facilities, and SAR will be able to handle the potential increased burden imposed by the event.

After considering all of these variables, the medical support plan should be based on *anticipation of need* in both the worst- and best-case scenarios. It is also important to review any available literature of medical support for similar events. In the case of expedition-length adventure races, the literature suggests that medical providers should be prepared to treat a wide variety of injury and illness.[13,43]

Injury and Illness

Injury and illness are common during adventure races. Fortunately, most injuries are minor, and relatively few result in withdrawal from an event.[4,40,43] In one investigation, 73% of adventure race participants reported an injury during the prior 18 months.[13] Acute injuries were reported in 44% of advanced, 35% of intermediate, and 19% of beginner racers and chronic injuries in 59, 54, and 56%, respectively.[13] The overall percentage of participants reporting injuries is comparable with participants in orienteering and standard triathlons;

however, acute injuries are considerably more common during adventure races. Interestingly, up to 90% of participants in ultra-endurance triathlons reported injuries.[13]

The majority of acute injuries reported by adventure race participants involve the skin and soft tissues.[4,13,43] The most common sites of acute injury were the lower extremities, the arm/shoulder, and the lower back.[13] Mountain biking and foot travel over unstable and uneven terrain during adventure races may in part account for these findings.

The 2002 Primal Quest expedition-length adventure race was held in July in Telluride, Colorado. During the event, 243 medical encounters and 302 distinct injuries and illnesses were reported among the 248 participants. Skin and soft tissue injuries accounted for 48% for all injuries and illnesses. Blisters on the feet were the single most common reason to utilize on-site medical care (32.8%).[43] A complete list of injuries and illness by type, number, and frequency are shown in Table 21.1.

Overall, there were 179 (59%) injuries and 123 (41%) illnesses reported. Of the 28 athletes who withdrew for medical reasons, 60% were due to illness, and 40% were due to injury. The most common medical reasons to withdraw were respiratory illness including upper respiratory infection (URI), bronchitis, and reactive airway disease/asthma (32.1%) followed by dehydration (25.0%), altitude illness (14.3%), skin and soft tissue problems (14.3%), orthopedic problems (10.7%), and genitourinary problems (3.6%).[43] During Australia's Winter Classic, a 2-day event, 21% of participants developed symptoms consistent with exposure but reactive airway disease/asthma in the setting of a viral respiratory infection accounted for the only medical withdrawal from the 2-day wilderness multisport event.[4]

Respiratory problems including reactive airway disease/asthma appear to be relatively common during adventure races. Several investigations suggest this may be partially explained by changes in respiratory function in adventure race participants. In one investigation, oxygen saturation (SaO_2), forced expiratory volume in 1 second (FEV1), and forced vital capacity (FVC) were measured before, at 45-minute intervals during, and after a wilderness multisport endurance event two consecutive years. Both FEV1 and FVC declined from the normal baseline observed at the start. The FEV1 declined 25 and 22% and the FVC declined 14 and 22%, respectively, for the two years. The change in SaO_2 was less dramatic.[31] In a similar investigation of FEV1 and FVC in 25 adventure race participants, the mean FEV1 declined 15.1%, and the mean FVC declined 13.0% between the start and finish of the race. The decrease in FEV1 and FVC was greater than 10% in 14 (56%) of the participants and greater than 20% in 7 (28%).[30] Similar findings have been described in other endurance athletes, but the decline has been less significant.[18,23,24] Possible explanations for the changes in respiratory function observed during adventure races include development of bronchospasm, airway inflammation, muscle fatigue, and pulmonary edema. The exact etiology is unclear.

Altitude illness has been observed during adventure races. During the 2002 Primal Quest, the incidence of altitude illness requiring medical treatment was 14.1%. Almost all of the cases were acute mountain sickness (AMS) (13.3%) with only 0.81% cases of high-altitude pulmonary edema.[40] This is not surprising because races often include sections at altitude. In addition, it has been suggested that exercise at altitude may exacerbate AMS.[29]

The role of altitude in exacerbating or alleviating reactive airway disease/asthma during adventure races is unclear because asthma has been observed to improve at high altitude. Possible explanations for this improvement include the reduction in pollen and pollution and the increase in cortisol levels at high altitude.[1,6] Further investigations may lead to better understanding of reactive airway disease/asthma and altitude illness in adventure race participants.

Dehydration and Hyponatremia

Hyponatremia is a recognized complication of participation in endurance events. The majority of investigations of hyponatremia has been in marathon and triathlon participants. Hyponatremia is also an important potential complication of participation in expedition-type events, and medical staff for these events should be able to recognize the signs and symptoms and be familiar with treatment of this condition.

Hyponatremia, defined as serum sodium of less than 135 mEq/L, may result in malaise, disorientation, hyperreflexia, nausea, and fatigue. Severe cases may result in seizures, stupor, coma, and death. It occurs when free water intake exceeds free water loss. While there is some debate about the exact etiology of exercise-associated

Table 21.1. Injuries and illness during the Primal Quest (2002) by type, number, and frequency

Type of injury/ illness	No. of cases (n = 302)	Percentage of cases
Skin/soft tissue	145	48.0
Respiratory	55	18.2
Altitude (AMS/HAPE)	36	11.9
Orthopedic	29	9.6
Dehydration	21	7.0
Gastrointestinal	6	2.0
HEENT	5	1.7
Genitourinary	3	1.0
Other	2	1.0

From Townes DA, Talbot TS, Wedmore IS, Billingsly R. Event medicine: injury and illness during an expedition-length adventure race. *J Emerg Med.* 2004;27:161–5.

hyponatremia, it is thought to occur in two distinct ways during endurance events. First, hyponatremia results from net water gain during exercise secondarily associated with sodium loss via sweat.[19] Second, hyponatremia results when there is salt depletion due to massive sweat losses associated with net dehydration.[19] In fact, hyponatremia occurs both in the setting of *dehydration* and *overhydration*.[36] Dehydration with hyponatremia is rare in races lasting less than 4 hours but becomes more common in races lasting longer than 8 hours.[19]

In the literature, there are several case reports of hyponatremia in marathon and triathlon participants including seizures in a triathlete with serum sodium of 116 mEq/L and rapid neurological deterioration and encephalopathy in an ultra-marathon runner.[15,37,39]

During the Hawaii Ironman Triathlon, dehydration was the most common reason to receive on-site medical care with hyponatremia the most common electrolyte disturbance.[19]

In a study of serum sodium concentration in 605 triathlon participants in New Zealand, 58 (18%) were found to be hyponatremic of which 18 were symptomatic and 11 were severely hyponatremic defined as having serum sodium of less than 130 mmol/L. In addition, weight change during the event was calculated to determine the relationship between hydration status and hyponatremia. An inverse relationship between postrace serum sodium concentration and weight change during the event was found, indicating athletes with hypernatremia were dehydrated but athletes with *severe* hyponatremia were generally overhydrated. The relationship between hydration status and *mild* hyponatremia was less clear as some athletes with mild hyponatremia were dehydrated, while others were overhydrated. It appears that mild hyponatremia may result from fluid overload, large salt losses via sweat, or a combination of the two.[36]

For members of the medical team, it may be difficult to determine if an athlete suffers from dehydration, hyponatremia, or both because the clinical presentation of these conditions during endurance events may be similar. It is important that members of the medical team be familiar with the recognition and treatment of both dehydration and hyponatremia. In addition, they should be able to provide education and general guidelines for participants to reduce the incidence of dehydration and hyponatremia.

General recommendations to reduce the incidence of dehydration and hyponatremia include intake of 1/2 liter of fluid for each pound lost during an event and use of some form of sodium replacement (1 g/hr) in events lasting longer than 4 hours. It is recommended that athletes acclimatize to hot and humid environments for approximately 1 week and increase their salt intake by 10–25 g/day. Intravenous fluid recommendations include the use of 5% dextrose in normal saline for races

longer than 4 hours and either 5% dextrose in normal saline or 5% dextrose in 1/2 normal saline for races shorter than 4 hours.[19] Another study of marathon participants suggests replacement of sodium at rate of 20 mEq/hr and potassium at 8 mEq/hr to maintain normal blood levels.[27]

Endemic Disease

Because adventure races and other expedition-type events are held throughout the world, participants may be exposed to a wide variety of endemic disease. Both isolated cases and widespread infections have been reported.

The largest outbreak of endemic disease associated with an adventure race was leptospirosis during Eco-Challeng-Sabah held in Malaysian Borneo in 2000.[9,10,33,38] After the event, 189 of the 304 athletes were contacted of which 80 met the case definition for leptospirosis. This bacterial zoonotic infection is characterized by fever, chills, myalgias, headache, conjunctival suffusion, abdominal pain, vomiting, diarrhea, and rash. Domestic and wild animals serve as a reservoir and shed the organism in their urine, contaminating soil and water. The incubation period ranges from 2 to 30 days but most illness occurs in 5–14 days. Further investigation of the Borneo outbreak identified kayaking and swimming in the Segama River, swallowing water from the Segama River, and spelunking (caving) as possible risk factors. Only swimming in the Segama River was independently associated with illness.[33]

Initial treatment of mild disease includes tetracycline; however, the illness may progress to aseptic meningitis, jaundice, renal failure, hepatic failure, and hemorrhage. Severe illness should be treated with IV penicillin. Weil's disease is the leptospirosis syndrome of fever, meningismus, and renal and hepatic failure. In Malaysian Borneo, of the 20 athletes who reported taking doxycycline for prophylaxis of malaria and/or leptospirosis, 4 (20%) developed symptoms. When compared with those not taking doxycycline, adjusting for exposure, doxycycline was protective; however, the difference was not significant.[33] Leptospirosis infections have also occurred in participants in an adventure race in Guam, triathlons in Illinois and Wisconsin, and white-water rafting in Costa Rica.[11,12,17]

Other examples of endemic disease infection include an athlete who sustained a wound that was infected with a third-stage larva of the New World screwworm fly, *Cochliomyia hominivorax*, during a race in the Para jungle region of Brazil in 2001, and 13 French athletes who contracted African tick-bite fever during the 1997 Raid Gauloises held in Lesotho and Natal, South Africa. Myiasis by invasive species like the screwworm may result in severe pain, extensive tissue damage, and death as the larvae have powerful oral hooks that can invade cartilage and bone.[34] African tick-bite fever is a rickettsial infection caused by *Rickettsia africae* and transmitted by *Amblyomma* ticks. The signs and symptoms of African tick-bite fever include headache, multiple inoculation scars, regional lymphadenopathy, and rash.[14]

Given the potential for adventure race participants to become ill, it is essential that the medical director be familiar with endemic diseases for a particular event given its location, the time of year, and the current environmental conditions.

Major Trauma

Even though the incidence of major trauma during adventure races is relatively low, it has resulted in significant injury and death.[21] Due to the potential morbidity and mortality associated with major trauma, the medical support plan should include specific protocols for initial stabilization, treatment, and evacuation of severely injured participants. This should be developed in close conjunction with local EMS and SAR including necessary equipment, supplies, and personnel. It may be necessary for the race organization to provide full-time paramedic-staffed ALS ambulances, helicopters, and other rescue vehicles requiring a significant financial commitment. For smaller events, even litters and Gamow chambers may represent a significant expense. The importance of appropriate resources cannot be overemphasized, and the medical director should insist on them even though they may go unused. It may be cost-effective to "leapfrog" certain limited resources from one location to another during the event. The location and movement of these resources during the event should be clearly outlined in the medical support plan prior to the start of the event. This should be done conservatively and with enough flexibility that, as the event progresses, there is minimal or no chance a limited resource will be required in more than one location. If this cannot be ensured, duplication of that resource is required.

For most events, through careful review of the course and required disciplines, it is possible to estimate the type and amount of environmental injury and illness that will require treatment. This should be reflected in the medical support plan. For example, if the course includes sections at high altitude, there should be a protocol for the treatment of altitude illness including indications for oxygen, medications such as dexamethasone, and the location and use of a Gamow chamber.

Foot Care

Foot problems, particularly blisters, are the single most common reason to seek medical care during adventure race (Figure 21.1). In one investigation, blisters on the feet accounted for 53% of all medical encounters.[43] The medical director should anticipate treating a

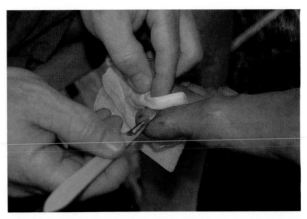

Figure 21.1. Foot problems, particularly blisters, are the single most common reason to seek medical care during adventure races. Photo courtesy of David A. Townes.

large number of foot-related problems. This should be reflected in the medical support plan. Foot care supplies should be plentiful and the members of the medical team should have a basic understanding of foot and blister care. Ideally, the medical team should include providers with specific expertise in foot and blister care.

A large number of techniques are utilized in the prevention and treatment of blisters. One text dedicated to the subject includes 159 different ways to prevent blisters.[45] Common techniques utilized by adventure race participants include duct tape, antiperspirants, petroleum jelly, and multiple newer products designed specifically for blister prevention. Susceptibility to blisters will vary from individual to individual and no single method will work for all athletes. Some athletes will remain blister free with little effort, whereas others will suffer from blisters no matter what measures are taken.

Some general recommendations can be made in the treatment of blisters. The key is that treatment of blisters begins before they form. All blisters begin as "hot spots," and treatment should begin as soon as the hot spot is identified. A delay of even an hour may significantly worsen the situation. Initial treatment may be with tape or any one of the many blister products on the market. After a blister develops, the decision to drain it is controversial, and there is no uniformly agreed-upon practice. Blisters provide a natural sterile dressing and it may not be necessary to drain them unless they are infected. It may however be necessary to drain blisters to allow proper adherence of a dressing especially if the athlete plans to continue in the race. Draining can be performed with any sterile sharp object such as a needle, blade, scissors, or nail clippers. The recommended technique is making a small hole in the blister to drain the fluid leaving the overlying skin in place. The area should be cleaned and dressed with tape or a blister care product. The athlete should be instructed to monitor all blisters closely for infection. Specific techniques for blister and foot care are discussed in Chapter 38.

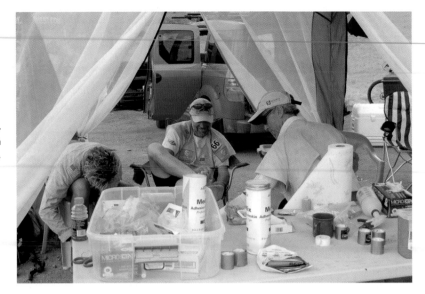

Figure 21.2. At self-care blister stations, members of the medical team provide athletes with blister care supplies and basic instructions. Photo courtesy of David A. Townes.

One strategy is to set up "self-care blister stations" where athletes are provided with blister care supplies and basic instruction by members of the medical team but are responsible for their own blister care (Figure 21.2). This reduces potential "burnout" of medical team members created by large numbers of athletes requiring blister care.

Even with the best planning, the wide variety and variability of adventure races and expedition-type events make it impossible to precisely predict the injury and illness pattern for any one event. There may even be significant differences in one event from year to year. During the Primal Quest in 2002, a large number of participants developed shortness of breath requiring treatment with beta-agonists, whereas very few athletes required beta-agonists the following year. Prior to both events, only a few athletes reported a history of exercise-induced asthma. In contrast, during Primal Quest 2003, poison ivy on the course left prednisone in short supply, whereas it went unused in 2002.

Equipment and Supplies

An important part of the medical support plan is a list of all medical supplies and equipment. This list should be available at each medical station so that personnel are not looking for items that are not available and an inventory can be maintained (Figure 21.3). A sample list of supplies is shown in Table 21.2. This is intended to serve as an example; substitutions, adjustments, additions, and subtractions should be made for each individual event.

Supplies should be consistently organized in durable carts and containers at each medical station. This allows personnel to move from one medical station to another and easily locate supplies. It is helpful to package individual supplies in clear plastic bags with labels

to aid in organization especially when carts and containers are moved on the course over rough terrain. The basic organization of the supplies should be consistent from station to station with some adjustment in the *amount* of supplies at each medical station. For example, foot care supplies will be in higher demand at the medical station after a long trek than after a kayaking section.

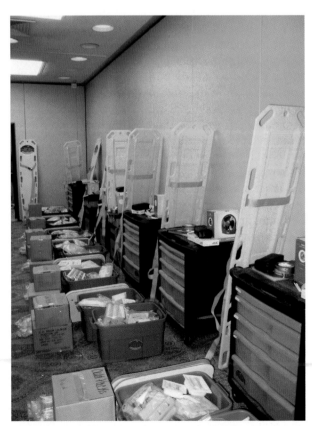

Figure 21.3. Supplies should be consistently organized in durable containers at each medical station. Photo courtesy of David A. Townes.

Personnel

On-site medical personnel must be able to recognize and initiate treatment for routine injury and illness, major and minor trauma, environmental conditions, and endemic diseases. Essential skills include assessing patients, establishing intravenous access, administering fluids and medications, and packaging patients for transfer or evacuation. Additional useful skills include expertise in foot care and wilderness and event medicine. Minimum staffing of each medical station should include an individual or individuals with excellent patient assessment skills and the ability to establish intravenous access and administer fluids and medications. The compliment of personnel might include physicians, paramedics, emergency medical technicians, physician's assistants, nurse practitioners, and wilderness first responders.

Medical care is administered at each "transition area" where racers change from one discipline to another and at designated checkpoints where it is anticipated that medical care may be required. On a 400-mile-long course, for example, there may be 10 medical stations.

In remote locations where local EMS response may be prolonged, the medical support plan should also provide for ALS staffed ambulance and helicopter support. As discussed, this may require a major financial commitment by event management. The helicopter used for general transportation and media may also serve to transport medical personnel and evacuate ill and injured participants.

Injury and Illness Classification

The medical support plan should include a protocol for efficient communication about any medical emergency on the course. This should allow race participants and staff to accurately and quickly communicate the type and severity of the situation to provide medical personnel with the information necessary to respond appropriately. The need to relay information quickly is especially important when communication is inconsistent or unreliable.

One example utilizes a simple, three-tiered classification when notifying race and medical personnel of an emergency. Athletes are instructed to first provide their team number and the emergency classification number. Class I emergencies require no evacuation, and the athlete proceeds to the nearest medical station for evaluation and treatment. Class II emergencies require nonemergent evacuation of the athlete. An example is an ankle injury that prevents further progress along the course. Class III emergencies require immediate evacuation of an athlete with a potentially life-threatening injury such as a head injury. If communication permits, athletes can then provide additional information.

Table 21.2. Suggested medical equipment and supplies

General
Alcohol pad
Blanket
Cotton swab
Examination glove (S/M/L)
Flashlight/batteries
Hand cleaner/sterilizer
Instant cold pack
Iodine swab
Portable bed/cot
Sharp/needle box
Sphygmomanometer
Stethoscope
Syringes/needle (3cc/22G/1")
Tape (various sizes)
Thermometer (oral/rectal)
Tongue depressor
Trauma shears
Utility towel

Medications – injection
Benadryl
D50
Epinephrine
Ketorolac
Lidocaine (1–2%)
Promethazine

Medications – inhaled
Albuterol

Medications – oral
Acetaminophen
Antihistamine
Hurricaine gel®
NSAID
Antidiarrheal
Prednisone
Sudafed®

Medications – topical
Antibiotic ointment
2% xylocaine jelly
Hydrocortisone cream
Ophthalmic antibiotic

IVF
Angiocatheter (18 ga/22 ga)
Fluid – 9% NaCl (1 L)
IV starter kit
Tubing kit

Wound
Bandage (various sizes)
Dressing (4 × 4, roll gauze)
Masks with eye shield
Needle for irrigation
NS for irrigation (500 cc)
Sterile gloves
Steri-strips®
Suture kit
Suture (3.0, 6.0)
Forceps
Wound glue

Foot care
Coban™ self-adhesive wrap
Elastikon™ tape

(Continued)

Table 21.2. *(Continued)*

Hypafix® tape
Leukotape®
Moleskin
New skin

Orthopedic
Elastic bandage
Cardboard splint
Finger splint
SAM® splint

Respiratory
Ambu bag
Laryngoscope/blades
ETT (various sizes)
Nebulization pipe
Oxygen mask
Oxygen tank
Oxygen tank regulator
Oxygen tubing

Trauma/transport
14-g angiocatheter
Backboard
Cervical collar
Head immobilizer
Strap kit

Miscellaneous
Duct tape
Fans/water sprayer
Foley catheter
Nasal pack (packing)
Pregnancy test kit

Townes DA. Strategies for Medical Support for Adventure Racing. *Sports Medicine.* 2005;35(7):557–64.

EMS and SAR

Another essential part of the medical support plan is to identify and list local ground and air ambulance services, search and rescue services, care facilities, hospitals, and trauma centers (and their capabilities) for each location along the course. Expedition-length adventure races and other expedition-type events may cover multiple hospital, trauma center, and EMS and SAR jurisdictions. This information should be readily available at each medical station including the location and contact information for these resources specific to that medical station. This should include a description of the medical station location that will be familiar to local providers. This allows medical personnel without local knowledge to quickly and accurately communicate with local services. For example, "Pleasant Bay Camp Ground off Route 28" may provide better information to local officials compared to "Medical Tent 6." It should also list if there is an emergency network such as 911 (in the United States) and if it can by accessed with an out-of-area cellular phone.

The medical director should contact members of the local medical, EMS, and SAR community early in the development of the medical support plan. If possible, a member of the local EMS community should be identified to act as a liaison between the race and the local medical community. During the event, this individual may help determine what EMS, SAR service, or care facility should be utilized for a particular situation.

Logistics

Basic logistics including the location and transport of equipment and supplies and scheduling of personnel often present the biggest challenge in providing medical support for adventure races and expedition-type events. This is a very dynamic process, as medical stations will open as the fastest teams reach them and remain open until the slowest teams have passed. Even with the best planning, it is impossible to predict the exact timing prior to the event. It is important to schedule personnel and equipment with enough flexibility to allow for this uncertainty.

Communication

Expedition-type events take place in rugged terrain and remote locations where communication among athletes, race and medical staff, and EMS and SAR personnel can be difficult and unreliable. It is an essential and often challenging component for providing medical support for expedition-type events especially in the event of an emergency when communication between race participants and medical personnel is especially important.

Common communication options including cellular phones, satellite phones, and radios all have advantages and disadvantages, and the best modality will depend on the individual situation. Cellular phones offer widespread availability and direct, private, person-to-person communication but are limited by network availability making them useless in many situations. Satellite phones offer better coverage, but they are expensive, relatively large and heavy, and unreliable under certain conditions. To minimize the chance of dropped calls, they require the caller to remain in one place with an unobstructed view of the sky, limiting their utility in certain locations including in canyons, under a forest canopy, and in moving vehicles. In contrast, radios are generally readily available and offer reliable coverage in a variety of conditions. Disadvantages of radios include the lack of privacy of communication that is particularly important for medical personnel and the need for battery dependent repeaters to cover large areas.

Global positioning system (GPS) technology has been utilized in adventure races and expedition-type events for tracking of participants. This technology has revolutionized the localization of teams in emergency situations.

During some expedition-length adventure races, teams carry units that combine a GPS tracking unit with either a radio or satellite phone (Competitio, Inc., Montreal, Quebec, Canada). In the event of an emergency, teams utilize the radio or satellite phone to notify race officials. Through GPS tracking, their exact location can be determined almost immediately.

The best communication system will depend on the individual event. In the majority of situations, no single communication modality will provide uninterrupted, private, and reliable communication over the entire course. Multiples such as cellular phones or radios as a primary modality with satellite phone back-up modalities are often utilized. In all situations, technology may fail and the medical support plan should include parameters for that eventuality.

PENALTIES FOR ACCEPTANCE OF MEDICAL CARE

One area of potential controversy in the provision of medical support for adventure races and other competitive expedition-type events involves penalties for acceptance of medical support during the event. Should the acceptance of medical care during the event result in removal or disqualification from the event? What level of medical support is acceptable while still allowing the individual to continue participation in the event? For example, if the acceptance of intravenous fluids (IVF) results in disqualification, athletes may push themselves too hard in an attempt to remain in the event. In contrast, if the administration of IVF is without penalty, racers may request them at every opportunity to gain a competitive advantage. For the acceptance of medical care during the event, guidelines should be established that emphasize safety yet allow for fair competition. This may be very challenging. An example of one such guideline for the administration of IVF is listed in Table 21.3. This IVF Rule has been used during several large expedition-length adventure races. As more events are held, these guidelines may be further refined.

Table 21.3. IVF rule used during Primal Quest (2002–2004, 2006)

1. Athletes who receive up to 2 liters of IVF are automatically penalized 4 hours with the penalty period beginning upon the completion of the last liter of fluid.
2. All athletes who require IVF must be evaluated and medically cleared by the race medical director or his or her designee prior to returning to the race. Return to the race will occur only after the 4-hour penalty has been served.
3. Athletes requiring more than 2 liters of IVF at one time (one medical station) or any amount of IVF at more than one time (multiple medical stations) will be automatically disqualified from the event.

From: Townes DA. *Medical Support Plan: Primal Quest 2006.* Unpublished.

MEDICAL DISQUALIFICATION

Another area of potential conflict arises when an individual wishes to continue to participate in an event when the medical team determines that further participation is unsafe. For the participant, completion of the event may represent a life-long dream or personal goal and have required a significant commitment of time and financial resources. It is understandable that he or she would want to continue to participate, and the medical team and event organizers must balance this with the health and safety of both the individual and the other participants in the event.

The author has found that it is often possible to resolve or diffuse these conflicts without incident. One strategy medical personnel may utilize is to explain their concerns to the other members of the individual's team including teammates and support crew because they know the individual well and have his or her best interest in mind. They will often support the opinion of the medical team and help convince their ill or injured teammate that withdrawing from the event is appropriate and acceptable. It may also be the case that these individuals recognize their teammate cannot continue but are unable or unwilling to convince the teammate to stop. The team may rely on the medical team for assistance. At the start of the event, it should be clearly explained to all participants that the medical director has final say on whether an athlete is able to continue the race and that his or her decision will be based solely on maintaining the health and safety of all event participants and staff. In the end, heath and safety should determine the course of action.

LEGAL CONSIDERATIONS

In the development of a medical support plan for any event, licensing, liability, and insurance coverage for medical personnel must be addressed. As events are held throughout the world, there will be variability in the necessary requirements, and no single set of standards will be applicable to each situation. It is important to understand and adhere to the requirements for a specific location. It may be necessary for the race organization and medical director to solicit expert legal advice in this matter.

In addition to basic licensing and liability, other issues should be considered. What, if any, is the liability difference for volunteer and paid medical staff? Are medical personnel covered under the general liability policy of the event or do they require additional coverage? What is the validity and implications of the liability waiver signed by event participants? Do all medical personnel need to be licensed, or can they practice under the license of the medical director? If licensing is required, what constitutes the practice of medicine? Does a volunteer medic need to be licensed to apply a dressing to a blister? What additional measures are required if narcotics or other controlled substances are included in the medical kit? The answers to these questions will depend on the laws that govern the location of the event and are beyond the scope of this chapter.

CONCLUSION

Expedition-type events including wilderness and endurance events continue to push the limits of human performance. These category IV events represent a new and exciting area of expedition, event, and wilderness medicine. The provision of medical support for these events is both exciting and challenging. Even though there is currently limited information to assist in this task, a growing body of literature is dedicated to this endeavor. It is the hope that as more events are held, the provision of medical support for them will continue to evolve. With continued efforts by dedicated medical personnel, accurate and effective guidelines should be developed and refined to ensure the health and safety of these athletes and thus the success of future events.

REFERENCES

1. Allegra L, Cogo A, Legnani D, Diano PL, Fasano V, Negretto GG. High altitude exposure reduces bronchial responsiveness to hypo-osmolar aerosol in lowland asthmatics. *Eur Respir J.* 1995;8:1842–6.
2. Arbon P. The development of conceptual models for mass-gathering health. *Prehosp Diast Med.* 2004;19:208–12.
3. Arbon P, Bridgewater FH, Smith C. Mass gathering medicine: a predictive model for patient presentation and transport rates. *Prehosp Diast Med.* 2001;16:150–8.
4. Borland ML, Rogers IR. Injury and illness in a wilderness multisport endurance event. *Wilderness Environ Med.* 1997;8:82–8.
5. Burdick TE, Brozen R. Wilderness event medicine. *Wilderness Eviron Med.* 2003;14:236–9.
6. Cogo A, Basnyat B, Legnani D, Allegra L. Bronchial asthma and airway hyperresponsiveness at high altitude. *Respiration.* 1997;64:444–9.
7. De Lorenzo RA. Mass gathering medicine: a review. *Prehosp Diast Med.* 1997;12:68–72.
8. De Lorenzo RA, Gray BC, Bennett PC, et al. Effect of crowd size on patient volume at a large, multipurpose, indoor stadium. *J Emerg Med.* 1989;7:379–84.
9. Department of Health and Human Services, Centers for Disease Control and Prevention. Update; outbreak of acute febrile illness among athletes participating in Eco-Challenge-Sabah 2000 – Borneo, Malaysia, 2000. *JAMA.* 2001;285:728–30.
10. Department of Health and Human Services, Centers for Disease Control and Prevention. Update; outbreak of acute febrile illness among athletes participating in Eco-Challenge-Sabah 2000 – Borneo, Malaysia, 2000. *MMWR Morb Mortal Wkly Rep.* 2001;19:21–4.
11. Department of Health and Human Services, Centers for Disease Control and Prevention. Update: leptospirosis and unexplained acute febrile illness among athletes participating in triathlons – Illinois and Wisconsin, 1998. *MMWR Morb Mortal Wkly Rep.* 1998;47:673–6.
12. Department of Health and Human Services, Centers for Disease Control and Prevention. Outbreak of leptospirosis among white-water rafters – Costa Rica, 1996. *MMWR Morb Mortal Wkly Rep.* 1997;46:577–9.
13. Fordham S, Garbutt G, Lopes P. Epidemiology of injuries in adventure racing athletes. *Br J Sports Med.* 2004;38:300–3.
14. Fournier PE, Roux V, Caumes E, Donzel M, Raoult D. Outbreak of *Rickettsia agricae* infections in participants of an adventure race in South Africa. *Clin Infect Dis.* 1998;27:316–23.
15. Frizzell RT, Lang GH, Lowance DC, Lathan SR. Hyponatremia and ultramarathon running. *JAMA.* 1986;255:772–4.
16. Gonzalez D. Medical coverage of endurance events. *Prim Care.* 1991;18:867–87.
17. Haddock RL, Gilmore JW, Pimentel F. A leptospirosis outbreak on Guam associated with an athletic event. *Pac Health Dialog.* 2002;9:186–9.
18. Hill NS, Jacoby C, Farber FW. Effect of an endurance triathlon on pulmonary function. *Med Sci Sorts Exerc.* 1991;21:1260–4.
19. Hiller DB. Dehydration and hyponatremia during triathlons. *Med Sci Sports Exerc.* 1989;21:S219-21.
20. Hnatow DA, Gordon DJ. Medical planning for mass gatherings: a retrospective review of the San Antonio Papal Mass. *Prehosp Disast Med.* 1991;6:443–50.
21. Jhung L. Fateful journey. *Adventure Sports.* November/December 2004: 24–34.
22. Leonard RB. Medical support for mass gatherings. *Emerg Med Clin North Am.* 1996;14:383–97.
23. Mahler DA, Lake J. Lung function after marathon running at warm and cold ambient temperatures. *Am Rev Respir Dis.* 1981;124:154–7.
24. Mahler DA, Lake J. Pulmonary dysfunction in ultramarathon runners. *Yale J Biol Med.* 1981;54:243–8.
25. McLaughlin KA, Townes DA, Wedmore IS, Billingsley RT, Listrom CD, Iverson LD. Pattern of injury and illness during expedition-length adventure races. *Wilderness Environ Med.* 2006;17:158–61.
26. Milsten AM, Maguire BJ, Bissell RA, Seaman KG. Mass-gathering medical care: a review of the literature. *Prehosp Diast Med.* 2002;17:151–62.
27. Newmark SR, Toppo FR, Adams G. Fluid and electrolyte replacement in the ultramarathon runner. *Am J Sports Med.* 1991;19:389–91.
28. Norberg M. EMS and mass gatherings. *Emerg Med Serv.* 1990;19:46–51, 54–6, 91.
29. Roach RC, Maes D, Sandoval D, et al. Exercise exacerbates acute mountain sickness at simulated high altitude. *J Appl Physiol.* 2000;88:581–5.
30. Rogers IR, Inglis S, Speedy D, Hillman D, Noffsinger B, Jacobs I. Changes in respiratory function during a wilderness multisport endurance competition. *Wilderness Environ Med.* 2001;12:13–16.
31. Rogers IR, Speedy D, Hillman D, Noffinger B, Inglis S. Respiratory function changes in a wilderness multisport endurance competition; a prospective case study. *Wilderness Environ Med.* 2002;13:135–9.
32. Saunders AB, Criss E, et al. Effect of crowd size on patient volume at a large, multipurpose, indoor stadium: an analysis of medical care at mass gatherings. *Ann Emerg Med.* 1986;15:515–19.

33 Sejvar J, Bancroft E, Winthrop, et al., for the Eco-Challenge Investigation Team. Leptospirosis in "Eco-Challenge" athletes, Malaysian Borneo, 2000. *Emerg Infect Dis.* 2003;9: 702–7.

34 Seppanen M, Virolainen-Julkunen A, Kakko I, Vilkmaa P, Meri S. Myiasis during adventure sports race. *Emerg Infect Dis.* 2004;10:137–9.

35 Spaite DW, Criss EA, Valenzuela TD, et al. A new model for providing prehospital medical care in large stadiums. *Ann Emerg Med.* 1988;17:825–8.

36 Speedy DB, Noakes TD, Rogers IR, et al. Hyponatremia in ultradistance triathletes. *Med Sci Sports Exerc.* 1999;31: 809–15.

37 Speedy DB, Rogers I, Safih S, Foley B. Hyponatremia and seizures in an ultradistance triathlete. *J Emerg Med.* 2000;18: 41–4.

38 Stone SC, McNutt E. Update; outbreak of acute febrile illness among athletes participating in Eco-Challenge-Sabah 2000 – Borneo, Malaysia, 2000. *Ann Emerg Med.* 2001; 38:83–4.

39 Surgenor S, Uphold RE. Acute hyponatremia in ultra-endurance athletes. *Am J Emerg Med.* 1994;12:441–4.

40 Talbot TS, Townes DA, Wedmore IS. To air is human: altitude illness during an expedition length adventure race. *Wilderness Environ Med.* 2004;15:90–4.

41 Townes DA. Event medicine; medical support for adventure racing. *Wilderness Medicine.* 2003;20:7–8.

42 Townes DA. Wilderness medicine; strategies for provision of medical support for adventure racing. *Sports Med.* 2005;35:557–64.

43 Townes DA, Talbot TS, Wedmore IS, Billingsly R. Event medicine: injury and illness during an expedition-length adventure race. *J Emerg Med.* 2004;27:161–5.

44 Whipkey RR, Paris PM, Stewart RD. Emergency care for mass gatherings. *Postgrad Med.* 1984;76:44–52.

45 Vonhof J. *Fixing your Feet: Prevention and Treatments for Athletes.* 3rd ed. Berkeley, Calif.: Wilderness Press; 2004.

46 Zeitz KM, Schneider DA, Jarrett D, Zeitz CJ. Mass gathering events: retrospective analysis of patient presentations over seven years. *Prehosp Diast Med.* 2002;17:147–150.

22 Telemedicine in Evolution
Implications for Expeditionary Medicine

William P. Wiesmann, MD (COL, USA, Ret.), M. Nicole Draghic, and L. Alex Pranger

INTRODUCTION

According to the Travel Industry Association of America, 31 million adults have taken a rigorous adventure trip in the past 5 years. Even though the vast majority of these travelers return unscathed from these trips, the climatic and environmental conditions coupled with the exertive nature of an expedition pose a serious risk of injury and/or illness. Because many of these adventures take place in both remote and rugged locations, without the presence of a trained medical specialist, telemedicine can offer an adjunctive bridge to treatment.

In its simplest form, telemedicine is a basic telephone call. This is a key point to remember, as much of the sophisticated technological infrastructure commonly associated with telemedicine will generally not be available to an expedition. *Telemedicine* is commonly defined as the use of electronic communication and information technologies to provide or support clinical care at a distance (Department of Commerce, 1997).

A broader concept is that of *telehealth*, which is defined as the use of electronic information and telecommunications technologies to support long-distance clinical health care, patient and professional health-related education, public health and health administration (Department of Health and Human Services, 2001).

This chapter is designed to provide an overview of telemedicine applications adaptable to the needs of expedition medicine. The complex legal issues associated with telemedicine will not be addressed due to the disparate geography of expeditionary medicine and the difficulty in interpreting numerous international laws regarding this subject. For the purposes of this chapter, the person diagnosing and treating an injury will generally refer to another member of the expedition working with consultations by communications links and using diagnostic tools where appropriate to care for the injured party.

HISTORY

Telemedicine is as old as the telephone itself. One of the earliest documented telemedicine applications appears to be in 1905 when Willem Einthoven uses a telephone cable to transmit electrocardiograms from the hospital to his laboratory 1.5 km away. On March 22, 1905, the first "telecardiogram" is recorded from a generally healthy man. The high amplitude of the R waves received is attributed to the subject's exertion just prior to the measurement when he cycled from laboratory to hospital for the recording (Jenkins & Gerred, 1996).

In 1955, The Nebraska Medical Center received a sizable grant to create a closed circuit television (CCTV) link between itself and the Norfolk State Hospital. Over a distance of 112 miles, this link was used primarily for specialists and general practitioners to consult and for educational purposes; however, they also experimented with group therapy (Brown, 1995).

The true power and reach of telemedicine was demonstrated with a program that started in 1967 linking Logan Airport with the Massachusetts General Hospital. A nurse practitioner was stationed 24 hours a day at the clinic in Logan Airport with the doctor, other than during peak travel periods, located 2.7 miles away. The doctor interacted with the patient by means of a two-way microwave video and communications link to a 17-inch television monitor. This link was also able to transmit microscope images from blood samples to the doctor. The design of this system was such that other than the telepresence of the doctor, the normal clinical setting was reproduced. The nurse assisted as necessary in performing the physical exam. The conclusions after treating 1,000 patients (some by the nurse, some by a physician in person, and some by telediagnosis) was that the patients were clearly satisfied with the telediagnosis transaction (Murphy, 1974). Only 2% of the cases evaluated were not suited to telediagnosis, much of this attributed to the state of electronic technology at the time. The effect of this study was to demonstrate the greater availability and efficiency of a scarce resource such as the doctor by interacting remotely with the patient.

In 1971, the National Library of Medicine's Lister Hill National Center for Biomedical Communication used NASA Applied Technology Satellites in a field trial to determine if the health care of 26 villages in Alaska could be improved with video consultations. This one-way, black-and-white video and bidirectional audio communication link was workable, but it could not be used to support emergency medical care, as satellite transmission times were scheduled (Brown, 1995).

During the Mercury (1961–3) mission, biosensors were incorporated into the astronauts' flight suits. Ground crew analyzed data via telemetry and voice communications and conducted private medical consultations with the astronauts. In 1974, a NASA-sponsored study was conducted to determine the minimum requirements for a television system for telediagnosis.

NASA constantly monitored physiologic data of the early astronauts throughout the Mercury, Gemini, and Apollo programs. A flight surgeon was on hand for the duration of the missions, working to keep the flight crew in the best of all possible health. Although shuttle missions no longer monitor the crew 24 hours a day, medical data are frequently taken onboard and transmitted to the mission control center for evaluation.

Many other telemedicine programs and studies have been conducted, but the worldwide explosion of the Internet has made medical information available to almost anyone, at any time. With this infrastructure in place, in many cases the cost for rolling out a telemedicine program has been reduced from being prohibitively expensive to a minor cost. Likewise, the increase in capabilities in combination with the decrease in price and size of computers and other electronics has improved the quality of diagnostic instrumentation.

TELEMEDICINE SUCCESSES

Telemedicine reduces the distance between patient and provider to improve the quality and accessibility of health care. The development of large-scale telemedicine networks is becoming an integral part of modern health care. One of the prime areas where telemedicine has significantly impacted health care is through the remote management of chronic disease, particularly for patients who live in isolated and/or medically underserved areas.

Not only are chronic diseases costly to manage, a myriad of factors may impact management, as these diseases often have associated secondary illnesses and conditions and are further complicated by noncompliance with treatment recommendations due to depression and other psychosocial or behavioral factors.

Increased medical costs are the result of not only acute complications but also a higher incidence of chronic care services. Medical monitoring via telemedicine techniques has contributed to improved health care by diverting the onset of acute complications through targeted intervention and has helped enhance preventive care practices.

THE UNIQUE NATURE OF EXPEDITIONARY MEDICINE

In the commercial and industrialized world, much of the focus of telemedicine and telehealth has been to achieve cost reductions, either through more effective home or clinic monitoring of chronic care to reduce expensive hospitalizations or by making more efficient use of medical personnel. For example, a rural clinic that might see one or two patients a day is not an effective location from which to base a full-time physician, whereas a nurse located at the clinic, linked with a physician at a major medical center, is viewed as a better distribution of health care dollars.

Most expeditions are carried out, by definition, in remote environments where telecommunications capabilities may be limited. This necessitates the use of alternative sources of communication that involve satellite transmissions, local cellular networks, and radio communication, all of which can be variable and lack sufficient bandwidth to perform the high-resolution imaging and data analysis necessary to make more complex diagnoses and triage decisions. This is also compounded by the fact that on large expeditions, particularly without the infrastructure of a large ship or brick and mortar facilities that can house diagnostic equipment such as MRI, CT scanners, X-ray machines or other more sophisticated diagnostic equipment, the application of high-bandwidth telemedicine is relatively limited. Additionally, there is generally a lack of treatment facilities or capabilities in expeditionary environments, such as surgical interventions, intensive care facilities, continuous care monitoring capabilities for chronic illness, intravenous imaging, or the ability to deliver or make diagnostic and therapeutic decisions based on high-end Western medical practice standards of care. Ultimately, the data are mostly restricted to utilization and to support triage decisions. And finally, because of time constraints, often times the patient could be transported much quicker than a telemedicine decision or a therapeutic intervention could occur in a local environment.

Severe injuries may require air evacuation to a medical facility; depending on location and medical condition, medevac can well exceed $10,000. The U.S. Department of State provides a list of travel insurance and evacuation companies on their Web site: *http://travel.state.gov/travel/tips/health/health_1185.html#insurance*.

Recreational Expeditions

Travel to scenic or wilderness reserves may appear to be less physically daunting in comparison to other forms of adventure travel, but the risks of injury and disease remain a constant peril. Travelers cannot rely on staffed or medically trained and equipped ranger stations or similar aid, especially in a remote area.

Tour Expeditions

Organized tours generally limit the number of travelers in respect to the type of expedition and are led by professional guides. However, the level of medical experience and first-aid qualifications and available communication equipment is variable to the organization and location, and most corporate tours assume no responsibility regarding provision of medical care or evacuation.

Institutional Expeditions

Excursions directed by organizations may or may not have a physician as part of the team. Because these expeditions often combine adventure with scientific exploration, they may have a longer duration, involve more rigorous physical activities, and/or may only be able to support minimal gear, as travelers may be limited to what they can carry.

Regardless of the type of expedition, a careful review of medical history prior to a trip is prudent. The following questions summarize some key health considerations:

Any preexisting medical problems?

Any significant medical issues on previous travel?

Past surgical history (e.g., recent surgery)?

When was most recent dental examination?

What are current medications?

Any allergies (to medications and foods)?

Pregnant?

What is level of fitness compared to proposed activities?

Any known epidemiology of disease and injury for the region of travel?

THE MILITARY EXPERIENCE WITH TELEMEDICINE

Telemedicine in Action

The U.S. military has wrestled for years to improve far-forward care on the battlefield. To meet wartime and deployment needs, military health service support is organized into five echelons of care, ranging from initial care (Echelon I) to definitive care, including full rehabilitative care and tertiary-level care (Echelon V). The introduction of telemedicine in remote environments has been most valuable in specific locations such as Echelon II or III support hospitals utilizing high-bandwidth links to relay data to off-site specialists for the care and management of chronic illness and other nonacute decisions. The application in acute care battlefield trauma has been a large lesson in the difficulty of administering telehealth or the projection of health care through telemedicine in this environment. Again, the difficulties are the bandwidth requirements to make adequate diagnoses, the time involved, and the inadequate or limited care capabilities.

The use of telemedicine in Iraq and Afghanistan has been hindered by a lack of satellite bandwidth to accommodate the high-tech tools. However, telemedicine has been successfully used to diagnose soldiers suffering from leishmaniasis, a parasitic disease carried by sandflies. Left untreated, some forms of the disease can cause organ damage. Digital images of infected skin have been sent to dermatologists in the United States for review, and recommended treatments have been relayed using e-mail. Medics have also used text messages to communicate with medical personnel about injured soldiers.

In recent experiences in the Middle East, the U.S. military has solved most of this problem by improved care and management training of far-forward medics and support personnel, far-forward deployment of surgeons with surgical capabilities closer to the time of the casualties, improved and more intelligent care of casualties shortly after injury, including wise and improved use of tourniquets, hemostatic dressings, aggressive use of blood transfusions, fracture stabilization, and close-in cache or field surgical support hospitals have all resulted in improved survival in this very severe expeditionary environment. Previous dreams of enhancing or equipping medics with cameras or communication systems to obtain advice regarding the acute management of trauma, particularly battlefield trauma at the time of injury have been largely supplanted by these techniques. Indeed, at one time, the development of robotic surgical capability (Figure 22.1) to manage battlefield trauma was envisioned. This has been largely succeeded by improvements in far-forward care, stabilization and management of trauma patients by trained medical personnel, the far-forward placement of surgical units close to the time of injury, and more rapid and careful evacuation capabilities. Indeed, what's been learned from Operation Iraqi Freedom has taught many good lessons that will have important implications for expeditionary medicine for years to come.

Current telesurgery tools are dependent on satellite communication and streaming video delivered via high-speed Internet. The U.S. military has supported the development of surgical robot systems to allow surgeons to operate on wounded soldiers in the battlefield, such as the daVinci telesurgery system. With the daVinci system, surgeons operate while sitting at a computer terminal to control a robot. The daVinci robot has three arms; one arm has a pair of miniature cameras that produce a 3D image viewable by the surgeon on a monitor, the other two perform the operation through tiny incisions 8 mm wide. A key consideration with the device, aside from the expense, is the great deal of data generated by the video that must be transmitted and processed during the operation. In remote locations, satellite signals are

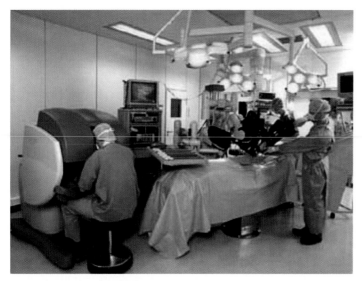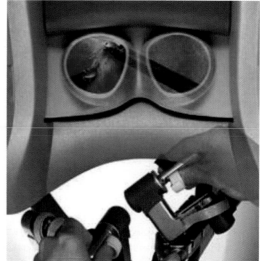

Figure 22.1. The daVinci telesurgery system manufactured by Intuitive Surgical System, Sunnyvale, Calif.

not always reliable and can result in delays that make surgery difficult. Table 22.1 summarizes the challenges and advantages of telemedicine in the U.S. military.

Telemedicine at Home

Telemedicine can provide diagnostic and consultation services through the application of high-bandwidth Internet like communication platforms that transfer and store data easily across wide geographic distances and into isolated communities. These communication services are designed to assist local health care providers in the management of complex and routine cases rather than replace local providers. Most physicians utilize telemedicine for physician-to-physician consultation, educational resources, and transfer of patient records. These interactions certainly impact patient care, but they do not directly involve the patient. Telemedicine offers the promise of helping to standardize health care and improve patient accessibility, and it could reduce or stabilize health care costs resulting from expensive acute treatments for patients with chronic illnesses.

The development of large-scale telemedicine networks is becoming an integral part of modern health care. One of the prime areas where telemedicine can impact health care is through the remote management of chronic disease, particularly for patients who live in isolated and/or medically underserved areas. A home telemedical monitoring system for these patients serves to recognize minor fluctuations and trends in health status and allows for rapid medical intervention, thereby preventing or reducing the length and number of disease-related hospitalizations.

It is the responsibility of the U.S. military to care not only for the soldiers in field but also for their families at home. TRICARE, the health care plan for the Uniformed Services, serves more then 9.2 million beneficiaries worldwide. Owing to the large numbers and geographically diverse families, TRICARE has been very active in evaluating telemedicine applications. TRICARE has employed telemonitoring for chronic illness such as asthma; for ear, nose, and throat examinations; for neurologic and psychiatric evaluations; and to reduce travel costs and time away from the unit, as well as to reduce the number of emergency room visits.

The Remote Access to Medical Specialists-Maui Test Bed (RAMS-MT) program was initiated in 1999 as an 18-month digital medicine test bed sponsored by the U.S. Army, Medical Research and Materiel Command to test and evaluate if remote monitoring of diabetic patients would improve their overall health management. The unique geography of the Hawaiian Islands isolates many established communities from high-quality medical care, diagnostics, and follow-up medical infrastructure. Because the high death rates for diabetes among Hawaiian Islanders may in part be due to this geographical isolation, a home monitoring system was developed to facilitate early intervention. The monitoring system used in this study was a modified version of the Interactive Home Care Monitoring System, developed by a 1999–2000 Harvey Mudd College student Engineering

Table 22.1. Telemedicine in the U.S. military

Benefits	Disadvantages
Reduces unnecessary evacuations	Limited use
Better use of limited specialists in the military	Bandwidth requirements
Diagnose infections	Turn-around consult time
Facilitates referrals	Lack of technical capability
	Potential confidentiality issues in deployment zones
	Not for urgent care

Clinic team sponsored by CIMIT, the Center for Innovative Medicine and Technology in Boston.

The system was designed to measure, record, store, and trend weight, blood pressure, oxygen saturation, heart rate and rhythm, and blood glucose. Patient data are entered into a secure database via residential phone lines, with an average transmission time well under 1 minute.

The system recognizes minor fluctuations in health status and allows for rapid medical intervention, immediately alerting the physician if physiological data are outside of a doctor-specified range, thereby preventing or reducing the length and number of disease-related hospitalizations.

The Challenge of Delivering Health Care during Space Flight – Telemedicine When Evacuation Is Not an Option

Key to the success of any of NASA's operations is effective, reliable monitoring of not only personnel but also equipment and spacecraft. The effect of microgravity on astronauts' health is a constant concern, as is the maintenance and operation of the shuttle itself. Understandably, NASA has embraced the use of telemedicine to alleviate the extreme distance between the shuttle and the ground control station.

Telemedicine has enabled the ground crew to monitor health parameters such as muscle atrophy, cardiovascular and pulmonary health, immune system alterations, and radiation levels to not only evaluate changes in status and consult with on-flight medical personnel to determine optimal treatment but also to provide trending data on the effects of space flight.

NASA, however, faces a very unique problem with its telemedicine needs. Whereas it may be difficult for an expedition to evacuate personnel after initial diagnosis and treatment for advanced medical attention, this option will not always be available to NASA. A planned man-mission to Mars could take as long as 4 years for a round-trip journey, and it will not be possible to cancel the mission for medical evacuations. Therefore, NASA's unique expedition environment necessitates the supply of a wider array of medical devices to cover a broader range of potential medical conditions. NASA is also able to afford greater training in medical procedures and devices for expeditionary personnel. In fact, 10 of the 137 members of the astronaut corps in 2001 (Mitka, 2001) were physicians, and for a long duration mission, it is likely that at least one member, probably more, would be medical doctors.

One need not be in space, however, to have difficulties with medical evacuations. This problem can be exemplified by the experience of Dr. Jerri Nielsen. In March of 1999, she was the only physician on a 1-year posting to the South Pole. After she discovered a lump in her breast, it was nearly 2 months before equipment could be air-dropped so she could perform a biopsy. After video-linked conferencing and microscopy confirmed the cancer, Dr. Nielsen administered her own chemotherapy injections. It was not until October that weather conditions allowed for her evacuation (Gidey, 2004).

How These Lessons Apply

Expedition medicine and combat casualty care share a number of unique challenges not found in the well-populated civilian sector including extended periods between injury and definitive care, limited medical expertise of providers, lack of external power sources, physical demands, and weight, size, and portability considerations.

The U.S. Army medical care responsibilities on the battlefield include challenging requirements of diagnosing and treating seriously ill penetrating injuries and other battle-associated injuries in very short periods of time. This task is often performed by medics or individuals with less than EMT training who are often tasked with not only treating single serious casualties, but also multiple casualties simultaneously. The diagnostic capabilities for these individuals are minimal, and traditional medical tools to validate such common but lethal occurrences of pneumothorax, hemopericardium, fractures, alterations in mental status, and cardiovascular and pulmonary status are rudimentary at best. Indeed, the simple operation of a stethoscope is rendered almost impossible in any environment outside a hospital situation due to extraneous noise and confusing sounds. The relatively short training periods and the level of education possessed by most battlefield EMTs or medics training are inadequate to interpret some vital signs data or patterns of vital signs data that could be consistent with detrimental outcomes and ameliorated by early and aggressive treatment.

TELEMEDICINE VERSUS LOCAL DECISION MAKING

Ultimately, the application of telemedicine or telehealth might be best and more intelligently thought of as a more careful application of electronic sensors and devices to not only monitor illness after it has occurred but also to predict complications, illness, and reactions to environment in the patient's health prior to the onset of an irreversible medical catastrophe. This would have limited use in preventing occurrences such as fractures or acute illness due to unexpected physical injury, but it does have a number of exciting applications including predicting and preventing serious and irreversible consequences of altitude sickness, hyperbaric illness, dehydration, heat stroke, heat shock, and secondary expression of emergency conditions manifested in an expeditionary environment such as acute myocardial infarction, pulmonary edema, stroke, metabolic abnormalities, and the management of acute infectious illness.

Indeed, the whole focus of the U.S. Army toward the management of expeditionary forces has been to develop and rely on the concept of a personal status

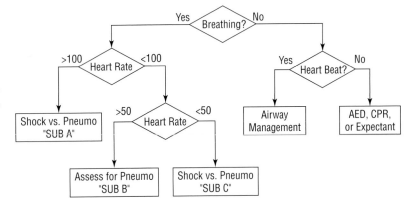

Figure 22.2. BioGlove algorithm: hemorrhagic shock and pneumothorax (Blanchard et al., 2001a).

monitor to constantly evaluate the health and physical ability of soldiers to operate in particular physical environments as well as to provide direction regarding triage after injury, preventative care and maintenance of normal body physio-homeostasis, and, to a large degree, to provide some predictive value to prevent irreversible injury.

As microelectronics, microprocessors, and other electronic systems become smaller, lighter, and more capable of doing more complicated computations in real time, it is not unreasonable to envision a small, wearable medical device capable of predicting a number of afflictions that expeditionary individuals could commonly be exposed to in very harsh environments. Faster processors, greater memory capacity, and more sophisticated algorithms are constantly enhancing the abilities of fielded medical devices to operate with greater accuracy, less training , and eventually, automated diagnosis and treatment. This would, in many ways, supplement the need for real-time, high-bandwidth telemedicine capabilities because many of these illnesses and conditions could be prevented with these interventional devices, and the capability of smart microprocessors with adapted or intelligent algorithms could direct

preventative measures to the individual or individuals caring for an injured person to rationally and intelligently reverse a medical trend or intervene at a time before a condition became irreversible.

An analogous consideration would be the environment to which firefighters are exposed almost continuously – high thermal environments that require acute physical exertion, often at a time when individuals are wearing extremely heavy personal protective gear and have limited air supplies to operate in extremely hostile environments. Firefighters are often exposed to great physical stress, thermal stress, and rapid dehydration, which in some cases can unmask underlying medical conditions that have been previously unknown, such as myocardial ischemia and respiratory problems.

The military has recognized that the future of battlefield medicine will require greater diagnostic and decision-making capabilities to be bestowed upon the devices themselves. The battlefield is not conducive to use or dependence upon communications links, and the limited medical training that soldiers have necessitates that the devices pick up the slack to offer greater capabilities without greater burden. These series of algorithms (Figures 22.2–22.6) described below (Blanchard

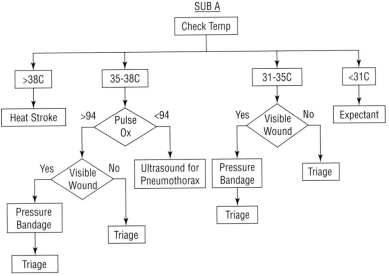

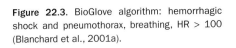

Figure 22.3. BioGlove algorithm: hemorrhagic shock and pneumothorax, breathing, HR > 100 (Blanchard et al., 2001a).

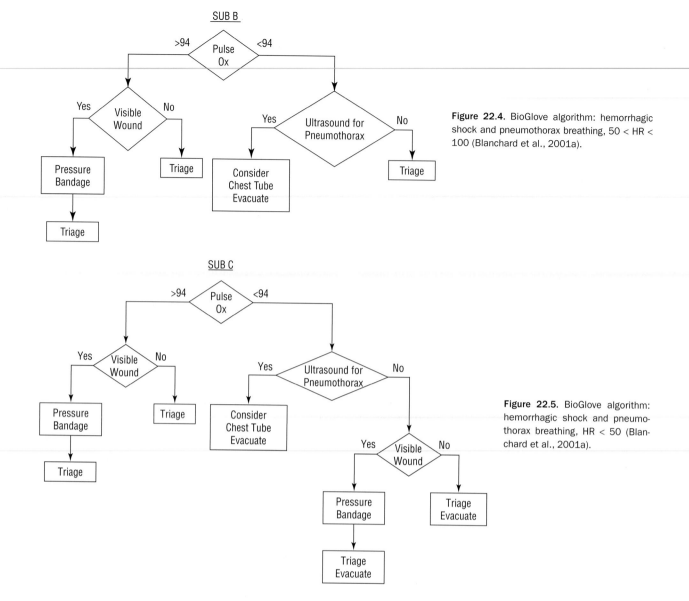

Figure 22.4. BioGlove algorithm: hemorrhagic shock and pneumothorax breathing, 50 < HR < 100 (Blanchard et al., 2001a).

Figure 22.5. BioGlove algorithm: hemorrhagic shock and pneumothorax breathing, HR < 50 (Blanchard et al., 2001a).

Patient with Known/Suspected Head Injury
Evident Head Wound/Altered

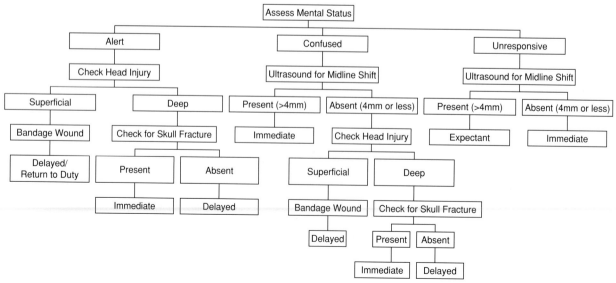

Figure 22.6. BioGlove algorithm: head injury (Blanchard et al., 2001b).

et al., 2001a, 2001b), while following common medical practices, are established as examples of a means of empowering medics with greater diagnostic and triage capabilities. These algorithms would be implemented into the medical devices themselves or into diagnostics tools such as the "data glove."

For expeditionists, sensors designed to measure bodily response to high temperature, humidity, and associated syndromes could be used to determine signals of potential life-threatening events, such as hyperthermia, cardiovascular collapse due to dehydration, hypothermia (during rainstorms), and altered physiologic performance. These are characteristics that can be quantified, identified, and trend-analyzed to prevent an event, modify behavior, and provide greater protection by alerting wearers of potential life-threatening conditions resulting from these conditions.

SELECTING A TELEMEDICINE PLATFORM

Threat Assessment, Needs, and Trade-Offs

A successful expedition must start with careful, meticulous planning. The following series of questions can be used as a starting point for determining the medical care needs (clinical or telehealth) of your journey.

Where are you planning to go?

The selection of the location will have a significant influence on the types of medical risks the expedition will be subject to, which in turn will influence the types of medical equipment to be taken. However, in addition to medical risks, the environment itself will dictate whether or not some types of medical or communications equipment and power sources will even function, or if special precautions or modifications are required for the equipment to remain functional when needed.

What injuries might happen (in general or specific to the activities of the expedition)?

Physical injuries due to a fall or other mishap remain a constant possibility in any expedition. However, higher levels of physical exertion, particularly on a long expedition, increase the likelihood of injury. The environment, including its remoteness, weather conditions, indigenous animals, insects, or foliage that may cause health threats, should also be carefully considered.

What diseases and other medical conditions could occur (in general or specific to the geographic region of travel)?

Personal injury resulting from physical activity can occur regardless of the region. The Centers for Disease Control and Prevention (CDC) and the World Health Organization (WHO) provide a wealth of information on their Web sites including endemic diseases and recommended or mandatory vaccines.

What chronic medical conditions do members of the expedition have?

Conditions associated with chronic illness, such as cardiovascular disease, hepatitis, and diabetes, can be exacerbated due to climate, temperature, and elevation.

What level of medical training will the members of my expedition have?

There is very little point in bringing medical treatment equipment that no one knows how to use. Although it is possible to be trained in the operation of some equipment "on-the-fly," it is much more practical to spend the time learning the proper operation of the instrument prior to departure.

Some skills and capabilities cannot be transferred through communications links. If the only place a treatment can be practically performed is in some form of formal care facility, there is little value to the expedition to bringing that equipment along, with the exception that there may be some value in "staging" the equipment nearby to a facility that might not have the equipment but would have personnel capable of operating it.

Cross training is also important because it is always possible that the person trained to diagnose and treat an injury might be the one to sustain it. Very few expeditions wish to be caught in circumstances similar to those of Dr. Jerri Nielsen, the sole physician stationed at the National Science Foundation's Amundsen-Scott research station (Gidey, 2004). Dr. Nielsen needed to train a welder to perform her biopsy. Due to the extreme weather conditions at the South Pole, Dr. Nielsen was unable to evacuate for several months. Detailed information was sent via e-mail to help diagnosis and treat her cancer; her subsequent chemotherapy was conducted via video-conferencing until the weather relented and allowed for transport off the station. While this is obviously an extreme example, it underscores the importance of appropriate training and equipment.

Will we have power necessary to operate telemedicine instrumentation and communications hardware when necessary?

The team should plan for unpredictable circumstances encountered during an expedition, such as weather delays, and pack back-up batteries, satellite phones, and GPS equipment.

What are the size, weight, cost, and technology export limitations of the expedition?

These parameters will be unique to each expedition and dependant upon such factors as location, duration of trip, number and expertise of team, etc.

How much monitoring is necessary?

The type of medical monitoring and communications devices the expedition will be interested in will be highly influenced by the number of devices likely to be operated. For systems only used during acute medical care (a hopefully infrequent event), the expedition may be better off with more manual devices with data manually entered into the communications device or verbally expressed to the medical consultant. However, systems designed to constantly monitor and/or archive expedition members' physiologic data (even when not injured) will be much more elaborate in both design and operational requirements.

Expeditions often operate in environments of extreme temperatures and other environmental conditions. It may take some time for expedition members to adjust to the new environment before some of the more strenuous activities of the expedition should be taken on. Thus, it may be advisable to regularly monitor otherwise uninjured expedition members as a part of an acclimation study and to use the analysis of the resulting data to know when expedition members have properly acclimated.

Conditions Likely to Occur during an Expedition That May Benefit from Telemedicine for Diagnosis and/or Treatment

As it is difficult to predict who will develop altitude sickness and persons often deny symptoms, telemedicine tools could be used to monitor acclimation to altitude or the onset of high-altitude cerebral edema (HACE) or high-altitude pulmonary edema (HAPE), decompression sickness in scuba divers, or the onset of heat stress and heat shock in tropical environments.

Telemedicine physician consultations for diagnostics and treatment recommendations could help determine the severity of the following conditions as well as the optimal course of therapy.

High-altitude sickness

Diving medicine

Heat stress and heat shock

Thermal injury

Muscular skeletal injuries

CNS and spinal cord trauma

Penetrating trauma and blunt trauma

Hemorrhage and cardiovascular shock

Acute infectious diseases

Insect and snake envenomation, anaphylaxis

Medical Devices

The basic complement of general medical diagnostic tools will also be necessary. A thermometer, blood pressure cuff, and stethoscope form the most basic core of medical diagnostic tools. These devices do not need to have built-in communication links or even be electronic so long as the operator is properly trained. The information gathered by these devices can simply be relayed orally over the phone to a consulting physician.

Although it will always be necessary to balance the size, weight, power, and other factors in the selection of equipment, the following devices are highly recommended for their ability to provide important information to an on-scene or remote caregiver or to provide critical treatment options:

Thermometer (manual or electronic)

Blood pressure monitor (self-operating or manual inflate cuff)

Pulse oximeter

Digital camera with close up or macro mode

Automated emergency defibrillator (AED)

ECG monitor (if the AED does not provide this)

Mechanical ventilation (bag valve mask or portable ventilator)

Portable ultrasound (requires proper training)

Communications Equipment

Going all the way back to basics, the first tool of the trade is some form of communication link. This could be a cell phone having adequate coverage in the expedition's operating region, a satellite phone , or a radio system

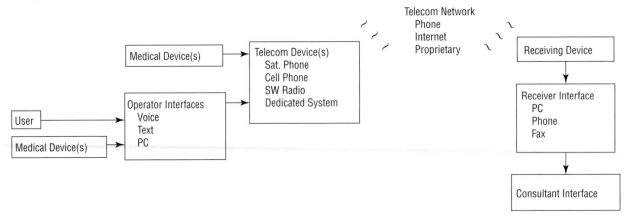

Figure 22.7. The structure of a telemedicine network.

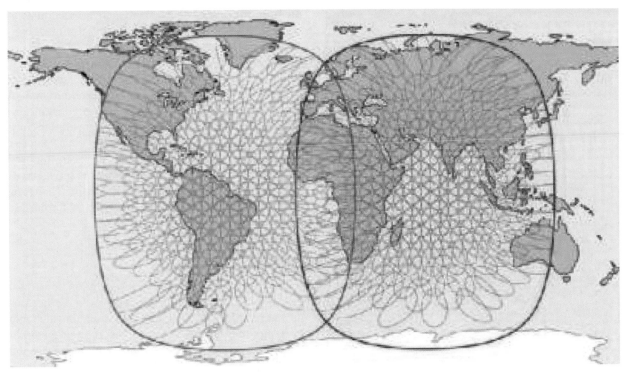

Figure 22.8. Inmarsat BGAN coverage map.

(e.g., HAM radio or a dedicated radio transmitter and receiver connected to a base of operations).

Numerous varieties of specific hardware instruments can be used to connect to these communications networks (Figure 22.7). It is necessary for the expedition planners to match the hardware, communications network, user interfaces, and medical devices to the needs of the expedition.

Several wireless satellite communications systems (Figures 22.8 and 22.9) have the capability to provide data services (usually through the Internet to a connected computer) in addition to voice services. Additional factors to be considered will be the bandwidth of the data connection, which will be influenced by the type of equipment, the location of the expedition, the weather conditions, and the cost and capabilities of the service

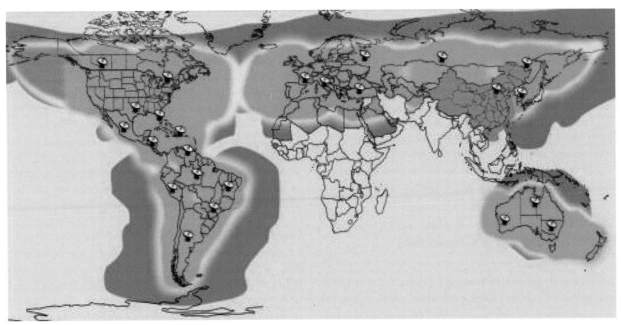

Figure 22.9. Globalstar coverage map.

Table 22.2. Communication data rates

System	Data rate		Interface
Inmarsat KVH/CapSat)	600	bps	RS-232
Globalstar	7620	bps	RS-232
Inmarsat 252	9600	bps	RS-232
Iridium	10	kbps	RS-232
Dial-up-modem	*56*	*kbps*	*RS-232, PCI card*
Inmarsat C33	58	kpbs	RS-232
GSM/GPRS phone	114	kbps	USB, Bluetooth
ThurayaDSL	144	kbps	Ethernet
EDGE data network	237	kbps	USB, Bluetooth
Inmarsat F55	320	kbps	ISDN, RS-232, USB, Ethernet
Inmarsat BGAN	492	kbps	USB, Ethernet, WiFi
Inmarsat F77	640	kbps	ISDN, RS-232, USB, Ethernet
DSL (low)	720	kbps	USB, Ethernet, WiFi
DSL (high)	1500	kbps	USB, Ethernet, WiFi
Cable modem	3000	kbps	USB, Ethernet, WiFi
Fiber optic	20	mbps	USB, Ethernet, WiFi

Note: These are maximum data rates and are rarely achieved. Entries in *italics* are for reference and are generally not suited to an expedition's telemedicine needs.

provider. If any of the equipment to be used requires a real-time connection, the bandwidth must be at least the size required by the device to function properly. For large scanned images, such as X-rays, the bandwidth will determine how long it takes for the image(s) to be transmitted through the system. Bear in mind that the longer it takes, the greater risk there is for a loss of the connection signal, which could terminate or corrupt the data transmission (Table 22.2).

One additional piece of equipment to consider would be the type of computer to be used for communicating with the data network and/or electronic medical devices. One platform that may warrant consideration is the One Laptop Per Child (OLPC) (*http://laptop.org*) or other similar devices. These durable, low cost, small, and highly portable systems in conjunction with its solar or human power source may prove to be ideally suited to the needs of a remote expedition.

Engineering Challenges in Expedition Telemedicine

Telemedicine directed toward expedition medicine faces numerous engineering challenges. Any devices used during an expedition must not only be highly accurate and sensitive and capable of withstanding body stresses and pressures during wear by highly active individuals in extreme environmental conditions but also must consider the size, weight, storage, and power requirements. Wearable (body-worn) sensors must be ergonomically consistent with the environment and associated activity. Other technical issues include battery power, duty cycle of the instrument, and data collection storage and transfer.

Table 22.3 summarizes the average data rates of common devices used in telemedicine.

In addition to the limitations of medical care imposed by an expedition, it is equally problematic to service medical devices and communications equipment. Therefore, back-ups and spare parts may be necessary for devices critical to the success of the expedition.

Training

Without the proper training in its operation, a medical device or communications system is almost useless. As a normal logistics precaution, it would be advisable to ensure that at least two members of the expedition are properly trained in the operation of each device the expedition brings. Training becomes even more important when manually operated systems are selected in lieu of highly automated systems.

The Other End

Services

As important to the expedition as having the proper tools for gathering and transmitting medical data is the issue of who will be at the other end of the telephone reviewing and analyzing the data. In the most ideal case, this may be a physician or service that has had the opportunity to examine the expedition members prior to their departure and will have a complete copy of the necessary medical records at hand, reducing the need to retransmit them.

A growing number of internationally based services will, for a relatively low cost, evaluate medical data sent by e-mail and provide a diagnosis. ARC Telediagnosis of India (*http://www.arctelediagnosis.com*), for example, can provide a diagnosis within hours for as little as $35 but would not charge if the data provided could not be used to lead to a diagnosis.

However, with all such services, it should be ensured, prior to actually needing the service, that the mechanisms to use and pay for the service are in place.

Legal Issues

Legal issues surrounding telemedicine are constantly improving and adapting to meet the needs of this new field, but much still remains to be done. Many states offer reciprocity to physicians practicing telemedicine; however, many counties have not yet adapted their legal structure wherein a physician in the United States can

Table 22.3. Data rates of typical devices used in telemedicine	
Digital device	**Data rate required**
Digital blood pressure monitor (sphygmomanometer)	<10 kilobits of data per second (kbps) (required transmission rates)
Digital thermometer	<10 kb of data (required transmission rates)
Digital audio stethoscope and integrated electrocardiogram	<10 kb of data (required transmission rates)
Ultrasound, angiogram	256 kilobytes (KB) (image size)
Magnetic resonance image	384 KB (image size)
Scanned X-ray	1.8 megabytes (MB) (image size)
Digital radiography	6 MB (image size)
Mammogram 24 MB (image size)	24 MB (image size)
Compressed and full motion video (e.g., nasopharyngoscope, ophthalmoscope, proctoscope, episcope, ENT scope)	384 kbps to 1.544 Mb/s (speed)
A clear voice communication	8 kbps
Videoconferencing with voice	1.5 Mbps (30 fps)
Videoconferencing (minimum)	256 kbps (12 fps) (Wacher, 2000)

provide a diagnosis and treatment plan for an expedition located elsewhere without violating the laws of that location.

In addition to legal issues surrounding the provider of the medical consultation, there are also numerous legal issues with the patient's medical privacy. The Health and Insurance Portability and Accountability Act (HIPAA, PL 104–191) establishes rules for electronic transmission and privacy of medical data and records (Wacher, 2001). Patient consent for the exchange of information and the secure treatment of the information are the two issues most relevant to telemedicine. Disclosure consent forms should be executed with all expedition members prior to departure because it may not be possible to execute consent following the injury or medical condition.

An expedition should be sure to check the legal issues involving telemedicine for their planned destination.

The Simpler, the Better

As previously discussed, telemedicine offers many potential benefits to an expedition; however, there is a natural tendency to "tech it up" when simpler diagnostic tools, with data relayed to a consultant over a phone or radio may be all that is required and necessary.

One additional item, often overlooked in planning for an expedition, is to collect the medical records of the expedition members so that their history is readily available to the nearest care available. These records could be simple paper files. The records may also be kept with a service that could fax the records as needed to your designated location. However, an additional effective means for keeping the records, and having them readily available, would be to store them on a secure Web site accessible when needed, and/or to store them on a USB thumb/flash/jump drive that could readily be accessed

from any available computer. When storing such records, it is important to keep the files in a readily accessible file format such as html, PDF, and jpg images to minimize the risk that the care provider may not be able to open or read the files.

Alternatively, a rugged laptop computer equipped with a built-in Web camera, microphone, and WI-FI, similar to the OLPC model, could be another valuable method to transfer medical data and receive medical support. Because these models are designed for use in locations where power is often scarce and equipped with a pull-cord charger or solar panel to recharge, they could be suitable for expedition medicine applications.

THE FUTURE OF TELEMEDICINE

Technology evolves quickly, particularly in the fields of sensors and data processing. As such, listing here specific devices for an expedition to carry may not be relevant by the time of the expedition. However, the devices themselves will fall into one of the following categories. There will be a class of products designed for constant or occasional monitoring of otherwise healthy personnel for the purpose of predicting and preventing injuries and illness. There will be a class of devices and system designed to diagnose the acute onset of injuries or illness. These devices may go even further by providing guidance on suggested treatment and, in the case of multiple injured personnel, triage the treatment and evacuation priority. The final class of devices will be those used for the treatment of injuries and medical conditions. Over time, these devices will become increasingly smart and automated. They will require less training to operate, optimize treatment for the patent, and reduce the need for telecommunications links.

Constant Monitoring – Preventative

Concepts of telemedicine, including sensors, smart personal assistants, and electronic data collection, have been routinely applied to chronic illness management such as diabetes, hypertension, and heart disease to support early detection of changes in patient status. In addition to the plethora of medical device monitoring applications, a number of noninvasive telemedicine based monitoring systems have been developed to support industry.

Although the following examples have been developed for initial use for other market groups, they have applications to expedition monitoring. There are certain variables relating to performance and environment that could be predictive in terms of high-altitude sickness and associated syndromes in expeditionists, physiologic markers such as hypoxia, altered respiratory function in low-oxygen environments, hypothermia, cardiovascular collapse due to dehydration, high-altitude pulmonary edema, high-altitude cerebral edema, cardiac ischemia, and altered physiologic performance. These characteristics can be quantified, identified, and trend-analyzed to prevent events, modify behavior, and provide greater protection.

Most expeditionists are young, healthy, and active and, therefore, do not undergo medical screening prior to an excursion, but physical and environmental stressors experienced by explorers during expeditions has similar relevance and could greatly benefit from careful physiologic monitoring. Data obtained from unobtrusive body-worn physiologic monitors could provide prognostic data that might prevent further stress or injury and even identify individuals at unusual risk prior to irreversible damage.

Disaster Network Monitor

Currently there is no effective systematic tracking and monitoring for the health care and location of displaced evacuees following a natural disaster or a regional medical quarantine.

After Hurricane Katrina, thousands of refugees housed in temporary, disparate shelters urgently required medical care. Medical issues ranged from chronic disease, to postdisaster infections including wound infections, complicated by unsanitary and overcrowded conditions of makeshift shelters as well as the lack of clean water, scheduled prescribed medicine, food, and electricity. Many of the hospitals were forced to close; patients waited days for treatment by volunteer medical staff. Additionally, the disaster itself and evacuation/rescue attempts left many families separated and unaware of the locations of other members, greatly adding to the mental stress for refugees.

The critical health issues following this disaster were sanitation and hygiene, water safety, infection control, and surveillance, issues compounded by lack of access to care. The lingering effects of the disaster mandated treating patients without laboratory/radiological tests, with limited medicines and potable water, and access to specialists. Additionally, shelters are not frequently staffed with public health experts or physicians, which complicates adequate surveillance and collection of health data not only for infectious disease threats and environmental illness but also for the management of chronic illness.

The Katrina disaster exposed the difficulties in providing adequate health care response to displaced populations. Telemedicine, adapted to utilize minimal power reserves and equipment, could provide an excellent adjunct to the management of mass casualty and disaster medicine.

The Real Time Mass Casualty Accountability System (Figure 22.10) is a prototype system to track and monitor patient location and vital statistics. This system is designed for quick deployment and setup, with the capability to monitor and triage large numbers of patients over a wide geographic region without significant power resupply. The system will accommodate both disaster situations, where the patients may be concentrated at one or more shelter sites, and quarantine, where patients may remain in their individual homes or current locations.

The device will have three inputs: an ECG reading, a temperature reading, and a heart rate reading. Data from the physiological sensors will be stored and analyzed

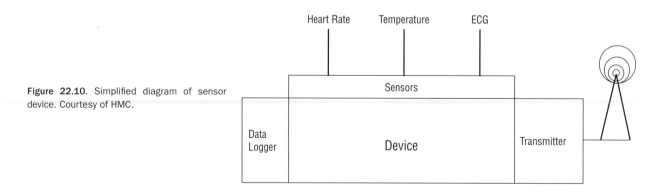

Figure 22.10. Simplified diagram of sensor device. Courtesy of HMC.

internally for transmission. To conserve power, the device will not transmit continuously; however, when a deviation is detected, data will be transmitted more frequently.

This research effort is sponsored by the Center for Integration of Medicine and Innovative Technology, Massachusetts General Hospital, Boston, through a 2006–7 Harvey Mudd College student Engineering Clinic project.

Oximetry/Hydration

Currently it is very difficult to actively monitor individuals working in high-risk situations. Each year thousands of lives are lost or individuals are seriously injured working in hostile or difficult environments where, often times, physiologic and medical risk is unknown until it's too late to perform necessary preventive or medical care.

As an example, structural firefighting involves extreme aerobic effort and muscular exertion in heat while wearing heavy, thermoprotective, waterproof clothing. The consequences of working to a state of collapse due to exertional heat stress or an intervening medical condition such as myocardial ischemia are increased because of the intrinsic hazards of the fire ground. Poor visibility from smoke and darkness, inadequate and ineffective voice communications, instability of burning structures, and evolving fire conditions all contribute to making timely rescue of incapacitated firefighters more difficult. In the United States, thousands of firefighters are injured and roughly 100 die in the line of duty each year. Half of the deaths are attributed to heart attack and other forms of physiologic stress.

One such device, a variation on an oximetry monitor, is designed to mitigate this risk by identifying working firefighters who have exhausted their physiologic compensatory mechanisms and cannot safely continue to work (Figure 22.11). This device is focused on correlating changes in oximetry data gathered from sensors integrated into self-contained breathing apparatus (SCBA) face pieces with a statement of volitional fatigue in firefighters, to allow a firefighter to exit the hazard zone without assistance. Pulse oximeter sensors, which are integrated into the respiratory protection gear, track changes to warn of potential physiologic collapse.

In this example (Figure 22.12), the data collected from a firefighter who became symptomatically fatigued and was unable to complete an experiment protocol showed a marked downward deflection that occurred just prior to a self-indication for a need to stop the test and rest.

Such systems would relate to the potential telemedicine needs of an expedition, particularly if some activities or some individual members of the expedition would benefit from continuous monitoring. Even this specific system, designed to monitor persons who work in high-heat environments, wear protective equipment making heat dissipation difficult, and engage in rigorous physical activity may directly relate to monitoring needs for the expedition.

Diagnostic and Triage

Data Glove

The digital diagnostic glove is one of several similar experimental prototype diagnostic ensembles under development by the military or their subcontractors (Figure 22.13). This device is worn by a battlefield medic on a hand and connected to a body-worn computer system. A medic can use this device to gather information on multiple patients in the field and track their progress – even during hazardous conditions such as heavy fire. This system links to a series of critical diagnostic sensors and arrays, comparing the "normal" values and ranges against those continuously read for each vital sign measured, and recognizes signals, patterns, and critical vital

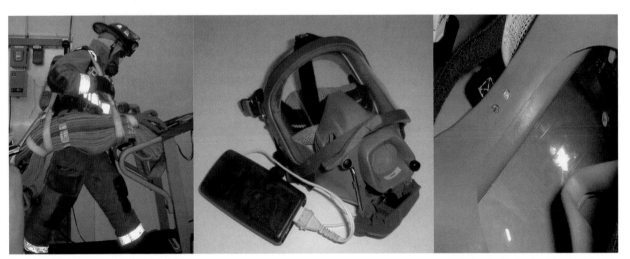

Figure 22.11. Continuous data monitoring of firefighters through oximetry. Courtesy Sekos, Inc.

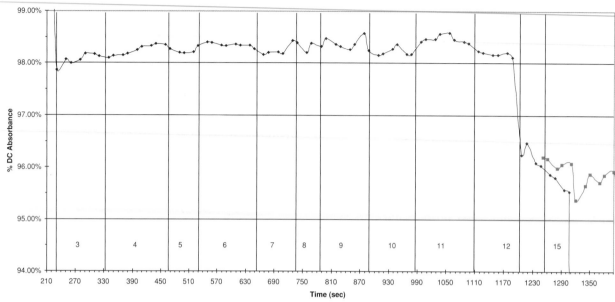

Figure 22.12. Mean absorption minima (MAM) tracing of firefighter who was subjected to a protocol of exercise and heat stress and became symptomatic during the protocol and needed to exit the test for rest and rehabilitation. The vertical bar (at 1,205 seconds) shown in activity 12 indicates the time stamp marking the subject's self-report that they could not continue.

signs' changes and responses to therapy. Alarms alert the user or standby personnel to unsafe and life-threatening conditions. The sensor systems employed in this single device include temperature and pulse oximetry, blood pressure, respiration, and heart rate. Data reporting is performed using radiotelemetry transmission to a solid-state instrument. This type of device can temporarily or permanently record and store the biological data for later diagnosis or for real-time or automatic retrieval.

Medic Triage Assist

The Medic Triage Assist is a working prototype consisting of an integrated sensor array to measure physiological parameters in real time, software to analyze the data

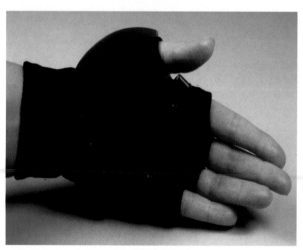

Figure 22.13. Digital data glove.

and output the most probable diagnosis and treatment, and user interface displaying the most probable diagnosis. Sensors outfitted include a thermistor, three-lead EKG, and pulse oximetry. Processing capability facilitates simultaneous data-capture from all sensors; data are output into a single serial stream, yet the data from each individual sensor are distinguishable from the others.

EEMMA/SonoSite

Portable ultrasound systems, such as SonoSite, perform high-quality examinations and allow for quick examinations to diagnosis trauma injuries; however, a radiologist or other trained specialist must interpret the images displayed on the screen.

The extended electromagnetic medical advisor (EEMMA) is a portable prehospital diagnostic tool to evaluate and triage casualties. EEMMA is a fusion of ultrasonic (US) interrogation, which is conducted over a narrow frequency band, with extended electromagnetic radiation (EM) interrogation, which operates over a wide frequency range. Using these two technologies together increases the yield from testing. For example, US interrogation does not identify free blood as accurately as EM interrogation does; however, US interrogation provides a more precise injury location estimate. EEMMA will, therefore, be better able to effectively capture and measure physical parameters in order to more accurately and noninvasively provide diagnosis.

The dual sensor unit, the EMUS 1 (Figure 22.14), employs both an electromagnetic sensor and an ultrasound transducer. Sensor data output will permit the user to diagnose several conditions common in battlefield

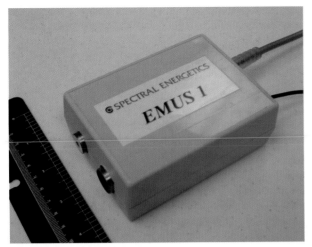

Figure 22.14. The EMUS 1 system for diagnostic assessment. Courtesy Spectral Energetics, Inc.

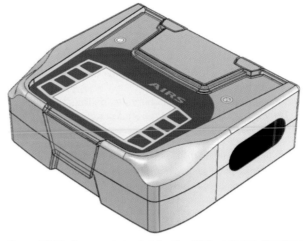

Figure 22.16. A concept drawing for the AIRS ventilator. Courtesy Automedx, Inc.

and emergency situations including brain injury, pneumothorax, and compartment syndrome.

The system can then be used to approximate the location and quantity of blood in an internal hemorrhage or to diagnose conditions such as compartment syndrome and pneumothorax. Preliminary measurements demonstrating blood detection are included. (See Figure 22.15.)

Therapeutic

AIRS

Automated Individualized Respiratory Support (AIRS) (Figure 22.16) is a small, rugged, battery-operated emergency transport ventilator developed by AutoMedx, Inc. (Germantown, Md) for the U.S. military. This ventilator can be stored for long periods of time and then

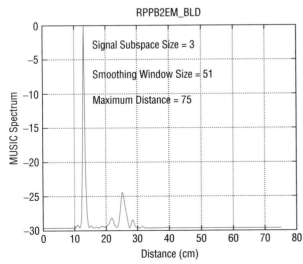

Figure 22.15. The EMUS 1 data used to detect the presence of blood, approximately 12 cm from the antenna (direct contact with the patient's body is not required). Courtesy Spectral Energetics, Inc.

quickly deployed by a relatively unskilled first responder. This device is designed for simple operation with minimal training requirements yet offers the specificity demanded from more highly trained personnel. The AIRS allows a medic or combat lifesaver with limited training to provide targeted ventilatory support in a hostile or remote environment, while also accommodating the requirements of an advanced practitioner where more skilled and advanced medical care are available.

SUMMARY

Due to both climates and activities, expedition travelers face a variety of potentially serious illnesses and injuries. Medical management during remote expeditions is largely confined to care rendered by fellow travelers and, as such, is limited by the level of medical training and available equipment contained in a first-aid bag. Telemedicine can help overcome some of these restrictions.

Advancements in telemedicine equipment, such as reduced size and cost, and ease of portability and use will aid in the progression and adoption of telemedicine in expeditions as these items become closer and more prevalent to the consumer marketplace. Technology is constantly evolving, resulting in the development of components such as faster and better communication links and smaller faster and smarter processors. These developments offer the possibility of shifting the expeditionary medical decision process to include intelligent sensors rather than sole dependence on communication links that may be tenuous and do not offer the direct ability to treat the patient. Ultimately, expedition travelers will come to depend on both enhanced communications, with real-time monitoring and decision-assist capabilities that far exceed what has customarily been considered possible with traditional applications of telemedicine.

SUGGESTED READINGS

Aldrich EF, Eisenberg HM, Saydjari C, Foulkes MA, Jane JA, Marshall LF, Young H, Marmarou A. Predictors of mortality in severely head-injured patients with civilian gunshot wounds: a report from the NIH traumatic coma data bank. *Surgical Neurol.* 1992;38:418–23.

American College of Surgeons: Committee on Trauma. *Advanced Trauma Life Support for Doctors: Student Course Manual.* Chicago; 1997:87–107.

Blanchard J, Lee E, Martens J, Wiesmann W, Nicholson K, Yun C, Ling G, *Bioglove Algorithm: Hemorrhagic Shock and Pneumothorax.* Bethesda, Md: Uniformed Services University, Neurotrauma Research Group; 2001a.

Blanchard J, Jarell A, Lee E, Martens J, Wiesmann W, Nicholson K, Yun C, Ling G. *Bioglove Algorithm: Hemorrhagic Head Injury.* Bethesda, Md: Uniformed Services University, Neurotrauma Research Group; 2001b.

Bjornstad H, Smith G, Storstein L, et al. Electrocardiographic and echocardiographic findings in top athletes, athletic students and sedentary controls. *Cardiology.* 1993;82(1):66–74.

Brown N. A Brief History of Telemedicine. Telemedicine Information Exchange. Available at: *http://tie.telemed.org.* Accessed May 30, 1995.

DeLurgio DB, Barbour A. Palpitations and tachycardia. *Cardiology in Primary Care.* 2000;57–64.

Department of Commerce. *Telemedicine Report to Congress;,* 1997.

Department of Health and Human Services. *Telemedicine Report to Congress;* 2001.

Dulchavsky SA, Schwarz KL, Kirkpatrick AW, Billica RD, Williams DR, Diebel LN, Campbell MR, Sargysan AE, Hamilton DR. Prospective evaluation of thoracic ultrasound in the detection of pneumothorax. *J Trauma.* 2001;50(2):201–5.

El-Bakry AK, Channa AB, Bakhamees H, Turkistani A, Seraj MA. Heat exhaustion during mass pilgrimage – is there a diagnostic role for pulse oximetry? *Resuscitation.* 1996;31:121–6.

Erickson RS, Kirklin SK. Comparison of ear-based, bladder, oral, and axillary methods for core temperature measurement. *Critical Care Med.* 1993;21(10):1528–34.

Gentilello LM. Advances in the management of hypothermia. *Horizons Trauma Surg.* 1995;75(2):243–56.

Gidey, Y. Doctor speaks about 1999 cancer scare at South Pole. *Durango Herald* and *Antarctical News Archive.* August 24, 2004.

Giesbrecht GG. Cold stress, near drowning and accidental hypothermia: a review. *Aviation, Space, and Environmental Med.* 2000;71(7):733–52.

Jenkins D, Gerred S. A (not so) brief history of electrocardiography. Available at: *http://www.ecglibrary.com/ecghist.html,* 1996 (updated 2006).

Loane M, Wootton R. A review of guidelines and standards for telemedicine. *J Telemed Telecare.* 2002;8(2):63–71.

Luce JM. Respiratory monitoring in critical care. *Goldman: Cecil Textbook of Medicine.* 21st ed. Philadelphia: W. B. Sanders; 2000: 485–9.

Marshal, LF, Toole BM, Bowers SA. The National Traumatic Coma Data Bank: part 2: patients who talk and deteriorate: implications for treatment. *J Neurosurg.* 1983;59:285–8.

Marshall LF, Gautille T, Klauber MR, et al. The outcome of severe closed head injury. *J Neurosurg.* 1991;75:S28–36.

McCallum JE, LoDolce D, Boehnke M. CT scan in intraventricular hemorrhage: correlation of clinical findings with computerized tomographic scans of the brain. *Neurosurg.* 1978;3(1):22–5.

Mitka M. Physician-astronauts have pioneered during two decades of shuttle flights. *JAMA.* 2001;286:291–92.

Murphy RLH, Bird KT, Telediagnosis: a new community health resource. *AJPH.* 1974;64(2):113–19.

Pavlik G, Bachl N, Wollein W, et al. Resting echocardiographic parameters after cessation of regular endurance training. *International J Sports Med.* 1986;7(4):226–31.

Riechers R. Extended Electromagnetic Medic Assist Contract Summary Report. Spectral Energetics, Inc. September 2006.

Rutherford EJ, Fusco MA, Nunn CR, et al. Hypothermia in critically ill trauma patients. *Injury.* 1998;29(8):605–8.

Servadei F, Nasi MT, Cremonini AM, Giuliani G, Cenni P, Nanni A. Importance of a reliable admission Glasgow coma scale score for determining the need for evacuation of posttraumatic subdural hematomas: a prospective study of 65 patients. *J Trauma.* 1998;44(5):868–73.

Simon HB. Hyperthermia. *N Eng J Med.* 1993;329(7):483–7.

Valadka AB, Gopinath SP, Robertson CS. Midline shift after severe head injury: pathophysiologic implications. *J Trauma.* 2000;49(1):1–10.

Wacher G. Telecommunication, Linking Providers and Patients. Telemedicine Information Exchange. June 2000.

Wacher G. HIPAA's Privacy Rule Summarized: What Does it Mean for Telemedicine. Telemedicine Information Exchange. February 2001.

Wiesmann WP, Pranger LA, Bogucki MS. Integrated Physiologic Sensor System; Patent Number 6,199,550. March 13, 2001.

Wiesmann WP, Pranger LA, Bogucki MS. Method and Apparatus for Noninvasive Physiologic Monitoring; Patent Application: 60/363600, March 12, 2002.

Wiesmann WP, Pranger LA, Bogucki MS. Integrated Physiologic Sensor System; Patent Number 6,606,993. August 19, 2003.

Wiesmann WP, Pranger LA, Bogucki MS, Integrated Physiologic Sensor System; Patent Number 6,934,571. August 23, 2005.

Yoder E. Disorders due to heat and cold. In: Goldman, ed. *Cecil Textbook of Medicine.* 21st ed. Philadelphia: W. B. Saunders; 2000: 513–15.

Young B, Rapp RP, Norton JA, Haack D, Tibbs PA, Bean JR. Early prediction of outcome in head-injured patients. *J Neurosurg.* 1981;54:300–3.

23 | Dive Medicine

Craig Cook, MD

INTRODUCTION

The underwater world holds the largest unexplored expanses on our planet and naturally invites those with the curiosity and determination to undertake the challenge. Shipwrecks, cave exploration, scientific surveys have always provided the impetus for exploration and discovery and continue to provide new opportunities. New technology and resources serve to open up to divers previously inaccessible areas that were not possible only a few years ago. Privately organized expeditions on the scale of public and academic efforts have become increasingly common and will continue to become more prevalent (Figure 23.1).

This expansion in undersea exploration continues to push into some of the most remote areas that are far from any support bases. Individuals and expeditions undertaking such ambitious plans face unique challenges that must be addressed to ensure the success of their mission. Planning and preparation are essential in this success and must be approached with this in mind. In remote locations, there is little tolerance for poor planning compared to those areas with greater accessibility and resources.

The undersea environment imposes unique physical environmental changes on the physiology of the human body, which need to be recognized in order to prevent injury. The increased ambient pressure at depth causes changes in gas behavior in our tissues and organs. Encounters with marine creatures may result in injury or envenomation. The management and avoidance of potential adverse consequences of these may be different in remote locations and need to be anticipated.

It is important that the diver understand these differences and how to deal with them should they appear. This will be the underlying theme in this chapter. While the basic tenants of diving medicine and physiology are unchanged, it is the approach, management, and treatment of these issues that may vary in remote locations.

DIVING PHYSICS

All changes in human physiology underwater are caused by the physical gas laws as a result of the pressure of the water column. The weight of seawater is 0.445 pounds per square inch (psi) per foot of depth, while that of fresh water is 0.432 psi. For example, at a depth of 33 ft (101 kPa), the water pressure is 14.7 psi. This is sometimes referred to as *gauge pressure* or the difference between the pressure being measured and atmospheric. The weight of the atmosphere will need to be added to this and is also calculated to be 14.7 psi at sea level. Thus, at 66 ft (202 kPa) a diver will be subject to two atmospheres of water pressure plus atmospheric, totaling three atmospheres. Water pressure plus atmospheric is referred to as atmospheres absolute or ATA.

The increased ambient pressure a diver experiences at depth will result in changes internally in any air- or gas-filled cavities. *Boyle's law* states that the volume of a gas is inversely proportional to its pressure when temperature is held constant (Figure 23.2). At 33 ft, a diver will have his or her lung volume compressed to half of its surface volume. To regain its original volume at this depth, twice the number of gas molecules will be needed to fill this compressed space. Returning to the surface while holding one's breath would result in expansion of the lungs to twice the surface volume and could potentially result in rupture of lung tissue and fatal air embolism (Figure 23.3). Similarly, the increased pressure being imposed on the tympanic membrane separating the ambient pressure in the external ear from the air-filled cavity of the middle ear, can result in barotrauma or rupture of this membrane if the pressure in the middle ear is not equalized on descent.

Dalton's law states that the total pressure of a gas mixture is proportional to the individual pressures of each component gas (Figure 23.2). Using this formula, we can find the total gas pressure, partial pressure of a component gas, or the fraction or percentage of the

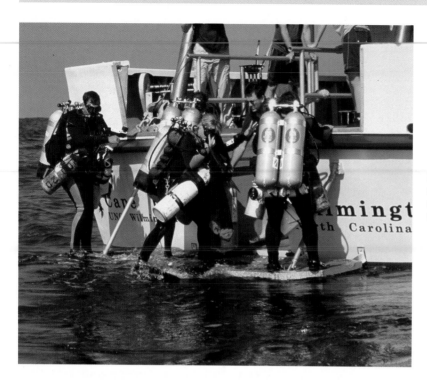

Figure 23.1. Divers wearing double tanks with side-mounted decompression gas preparing for a dive on the *USS Monitor*. Photo courtesy of Craig Cook.

Boyle's Law	PV = K
Dalton's Law	Ptotal = ppGas1 + ppGas2 + ppGas3 (etc.)
Henry's Law	Vg = ppGas x Gas solubility Coefficient

Figure 23.2. The gas laws primarily responsible for the physiologic changes underwater, where *P* is pressure, *pp* is partial pressure, *V* is volume, and *K* a constant.

component gas. This becomes critical in understanding when the partial pressure of oxygen becomes toxic or incapable of sustaining life or determining how deep a diver can descend breathing a particular oxygen mixture.

Henry's law states the quantity of a gas that can dissolve in a liquid is directly proportional to its partial pressure and solubility (Figure 23.2). For example, the increased partial pressure of nitrogen at depth forces nitrogen to be absorbed in tissue in larger amounts dependent on depth and time. This becomes the limiting factor on how long a diver can remain at depth in order to avoid decompression illness.

These physical laws not only determine how a dive can be performed but also can play an effect in diving injuries. If a diver understands these laws and mechanisms, then he will be in the best position to be able to prevent an injury from occurring.

BAROTRAUMA

Barotrauma refers to the changing effects of pressure (both increasing and decreasing) in causing injury to a tissue or organ. These can range from the very common such as middle ear barotraumas to life-threatening such as lung barotrauma causing an arterial gas embolism; any gas-containing space may be affected. By far the most common problems affecting divers are those of the ear.

Ear Concerns

The ear has been traditionally divided into three separate compartments that allow transmission of sound from the environment to be converted into an electrophysiologic signal that can be transmitted to the brain (Figure 23.4). The outer ear begins at the eternal ear canal and ends at the tympanic membrane (TM) or ear drum and functions as a passage for auditory transmission. The middle ear is a closed space surrounded by bone on all sides except for its external side, which is composed of the tympanic membrane separating it from the outer ear. Inside the middle ear space are the boney ossicles connecting the TM with the oval window of the inner ear, which allow the transmission and amplification of sound to the inner ear. The inner ear is composed of a bony-membranous structure called the cochlea, which contains specialized cells for conversion of the sound into an electrical signal before it is relayed to the brainstem auditory nuclei. Also part of the inner ear is the semicircular canals and the utricle and saccule, which are specialized organs essential for balance and equilibrium.

All three structures may be affected by barotrauma though the middle and inner ear are the most common.

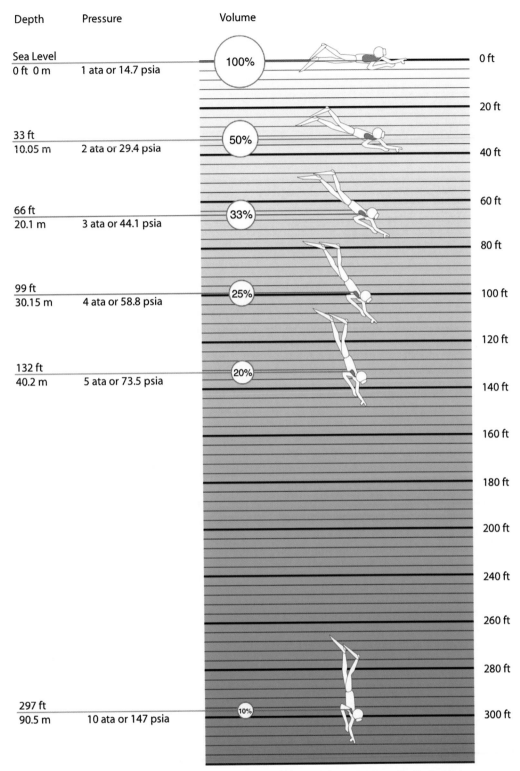

Depth	Pressure	Volume
Sea Level		100%	0 ft
0 ft 0 m	1 ata or 14.7 psia		
			20 ft
33 ft		50%	
10.05 m	2 ata or 29.4 psia		40 ft
			60 ft
66 ft		33%	
20.1 m	3 ata or 44.1 psia		80 ft
99 ft		25%	100 ft
30.15 m	4 ata or 58.8 psia		
			120 ft
132 ft		20%	
40.2 m	5 ata or 73.5 psia		140 ft
			160 ft
			180 ft
			200 ft
			240 ft
			260 ft
			280 ft
297 ft		10%	
90.5 m	10 ata or 147 psia		300 ft

Figure 23.3. The relation between gas volume in a diver's lungs and pressure according to Boyle's law.

External Ear

Though the external ear may be traumatized by a free diver using ear plugs for example, the most common concern among divers is infection and inflammation from otitis externa. Referred to also as swimmer's ear, it presents as an itchy, painful affliction due to incomplete drying of the external ear canal after immersion. The ear canal is lined with squamous epithelial cells, which secrete the various oils and water-soluble fatty acids that comprise cerumen and function to keep the canal slightly acidic and bacteriostatic. When this lining becomes wet and macerated, this protective function is lost, and the

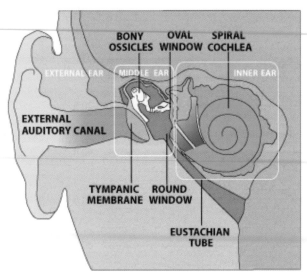

Figure 23.4. Anatomy of the ear showing structures that can be potentially affected by pressure changes and barotrauma.

canal becomes more alkaline forming a medium conducive to such bacterial species as *Proteus mirabilis* and *Pseudomonas*. This usually results in the canal lining becoming tender, swollen, and inflamed. In severe cases, the canal itself may close shut with the potential for abscess formation, though this is uncommon.

Treatment consists of staying out of the water and using drops of a drying acid-alcohol solution, such as 5% acetic acid and 60% isopropyl alcohol, applied four times a day. These serve to dry the external canal and also to convert the alkaline environment back to an acid one. Antibiotics or steroid suspension such as cortisporin otic suspension or ciprofloxacin otic suspension may be required in moderate or severe cases. In individuals where there is suspicion of a tympanic membrane perforation, the suspension is prescribed rather than the solution.

Otitis externa is a serious concern in saturation habitats and commercial diving due to repetitive dives and exposure to a humid surface environment, which can compromise the working ability of the divers. This can be prevented by using an acid-alcohol combination or Domeboro's solution applied after every dive.[1]

Middle Ear

Middle ear barotrauma is by far the most common of all dysbaric disorders and is probably responsible for the majority of all lost diving opportunities. It is composed of a bony space separated from the external ear by the TM and lined with mucosal epithelium. It communicates with the oropharynx through the eustachian tube, which is also lined with respiratory epithelium. The eustachian tube normally remains closed except for swallowing but can also be opened by gently blowing against a closed glottis and pinched nose. This is commonly though incorrectly referred to as a Valsalva maneuver and serves to equalize pressure in the middle ear with the outside ambient pressure.

A diver descending in the water column will experience increased pressure against the TM causing it to push into the middle ear space. The middle ear becomes negative due to the decreased volume according to Boyle's law. The diver would then equalize this pressure by performing one of the equalization maneuvers, and the middle ear pressure would return to ambient pressure. Problems arise when the eustachian tube becomes blocked or cannot open due to inflammation or mechanical reasons. Continued descent under this circumstance will cause the TM to continue to be pushed inward into the middle ear with eventual rupture occurring at depths from 10 to 40 ft.[2] Poor clearing techniques and/or repeated diving can result in traumatizing the epithelium lining of the middle ear and eustachian tube with edema, swelling, and even hemorrhages further interfering with equalization. Eventually clearing becomes impossible and diving activities have to be ceased. Symptoms range from ear discomfort and fullness in mild middle ear barotrauma to pain, hearing loss, and possible vertigo upon rupture of the TM. With moderate to severe barotrauma, a reverse squeeze can occur when the middle ear has equalized at depth but on ascent the eustachian tube remains closed resulting in gas expanding in the middle ear with potential rupture of the TM outward. Reverse squeeze is a serious consequence of forced equalization and a lesson well known to divers who have been "trapped" at 15 ft and unable to ascend.

Treatment of middle ear barotrauma consists of stopping all diving activity and allowing eustachian tube and middle ear trauma to heal. This may take anywhere from a few days to over a week. Diving should not be resumed until all symptoms have subsided and the diver can easily autoinflate (clear) his or her ears without difficulty. Systemic and topical decongestants such as pseudoephedrine (60 mg one hour prior to diving) may be useful for prevention in some individuals, but it should not be used routinely in place of good equalization techniques (Table 23.1).[3] In cases of suspected

Table 23.1. Techniques that can be used to decrease the risk of middle and inner ear barotrauma
Avoidance of ear barotrauma
Begin equalization as soon as submerged
Descend even slower than you may think you need to
Clear continuously; do not wait until ear pressure is experienced
Descend feet first and use descent line if possible
Look up, neck extension may stretch and open the eustachian tubes
Avoid forceful Valsalva maneuvers, use gentle efforts
If ear discomfort is experienced, stop and ascend until discomfort eases and try clearing again
Never force a descent if still experiencing difficulty clearing
Do not dive with an upper respiratory infection
Some authorities recommend avoiding milk products (may increase mucous production), alcohol, and tobacco

tympanic membrane perforation, systemic antibiotics such as amoxicillin (especially in cases of contaminated water) are usually administered, and the ear is kept dry. The diver will need to be examined by a physician as soon as possible.

Inner Ear Barotrauma

Barotrauma of the inner ear is less common than middle ear problems, but it is potentially more serious. The mechanism is similar with difficulty in clearing and using a forceful Valsalva maneuver. This pressure may be transmitted through the cerebral spinal fluid (CSF) and back into the inner ear perilymph forcing a rupture of either the round or oval window into the middle ear resulting in a perilymph fistula.[4] The diver experiences sudden pain, dizziness, vertigo, and commonly nausea and vomiting. The vertigo may be extreme and disorienting, and with nausea and vomiting could, in severe cases, lead to drowning. Treatment consists of bed rest, head elevation, and avoidance of straining. Symptoms can be relieved with small doses of steroids and benzodiazepines. The diver will need to be seen by an otolaryngology specialist as soon as possible. Usually the rupture will close spontaneously, but in some cases surgical exploration and closure is necessary. Traditionally, further diving was prohibited due to a risk of further hearing loss or damage to the vestibular apparatus, but some cases have been allowed to return to diving.

Inner ear barotrauma can be difficult to differentiate from inner ear decompression sickness (DCS) because the symptoms can be similar. The treatments are different however, with inner ear barotraumas being treated conservatively while inner ear DCS is an emergency requiring immediate recompression in a chamber. The diving profile is very useful in sorting this out. Symptoms appearing at the beginning of a dive during descent usually point to barotrauma while inner ear DCS usually presents on ascent or on the surface after a deep dive using mixed gas though an increasing number of cases are being seen in recreational divers (Table 23.2).[5]

Table 23.2. Factors that may help in the differentiation of inner ear barotrauma from inner ear decompression sickness

Differentiating inner ear barotrauma from inner ear DCS

Usually a history of ear pain and difficulty clearing during descent with inner ear barotrauma

Onset of symptoms during ascent or shortly after surfacing suspicious for inner ear DCS

Decompression diving typically using mixed gas with inner ear DCS compared to shallow or no-stop diving with inner ear barotrauma

Often evidence of barotrauma on otologic exam with inner ear barotrauma

Often other symptoms of DCS present in cases of inner ear DCS

Sinus Barotrauma

The paranasal sinuses are four paired air-filled spaces located in the maxillary, ethmoid, frontal, and sphenoid bones comprising the skull. These spaces are lined by epithelial mucosa and communicate with the nasal passage through various small ostia or openings. If during descent, an ostia becomes occluded due to inflammation, infection, or mechanical reasons then the pressure in the sinus is unable to equilibrate with the outside ambient pressure with resulting pain. The resulting traumatized mucosal layer becomes swollen and edematous with varying degrees of hemorrhage into the mucosa or sinus space. Upon ascending, pain can reoccur when the ostia becomes blocked due to edema or debris. With eventual equalization, it is common to notice blood and mucus from the sinus in the face mask. Persistent sinus pain while diving usually involves an infection, chronic irritation, allergy, or mechanical etiology such as a sinus or nasal polyp. Topical nasal spray such as oxymetazoline or systemic decongestants such as pseudoephedrine may be helpful. Should symptoms become more troublesome, the diver should be referred to a physician.

Pulmonary Barotrauma

The consequences of pulmonary barotrauma (PBT) are the most serious of all pressure-related (dysbaric) accidents. These commonly result from an inexperienced or panicked diver making a rapid ascent while holding his or her breath. Unfortunately, PBT and resultant arterial gas embolism along with ischemic heart disease account for the majority of diving deaths.

Alveolar gas that is prevented from escaping due to breath holding or air trapping expands during ascent and may rupture into the perivascular spaces. Relatively small transpulmonic pressures of 60–70 mmHg can cause alveolar rupture producing PBT from only 1–2 meter ascents.[6] Interestingly, studies looking at pulmonary function found PBT to be associated with restrictive lung function rather than an obstructive pattern, probably due to the potential for tears to develop from the decreased compliance.[7]

From the perivascular space, the gas volume may produce mediastinal emphysema, subcutaneous emphysema, pneumothorax, or an arterial gas embolism. Symptoms from mediastinal emphysema range from mild discomfort to voice changes, cough, or difficulty swallowing; mild cases may even be asymptomatic. Gas trekking further up the perivascular tree may manifest as subcutaneous emphysema. Small areas of swelling in the upper chest above the clavicles and neck may be seen and palpated as crepitus. All patients should be examined and watched closely for other associated signs of decompression sickness since these commonly coexist if there has been a gas load incurred during the dive. One hundred percent oxygen should be administered and the patient transported to a medical facility and observed if no other signs or symptoms are found.[8]

A pneumothorax will result from gas rupture through the visceral pleura. Symptoms such as pleuritic pain and shortness of breath (dyspnea) are dependent on the percentage of lung collapse. Fortunately, this manifestation is uncommon and appears in less than 10% of PBT. If it is necessary to recompress a patient with a pneumothorax, preparations for emergency placement of a chest tube should be made due to the possibility of a tension pneumothorax during ascent.

Avoidance of PBT centers on a slow controlled ascent, avoiding diving with any pulmonary infections that could predispose to air trapping and avoiding heavy exertion close to the surface at maximal lung volumes.

Arterial Gas Embolism

The most feared complication of PBT is arterial gas embolism. Ruptured alveoli allow gas to enter traumatized vessels where it is passed to the left heart and into the arterial circulation with system embolization. Bubble emboli may distribute throughout the body as evidenced by biochemical markers.[9] The brain is the most common organ clinically affected with this presentation being referred to as cerebral air embolism (CAGE).

Once in the cerebral circulation, the bubble eventually lodges in a small vessel branch where local ischemia results. Depending on the bubble size and other factors, the bubble may eventually pass through the circulation and be absorbed. During this transit, there will invariably be endothelial damage caused by the bubble passage followed by an inflammatory response.

Interestingly, it is rare that frank infarction develops as seen in stroke syndromes.

One of the sentinel features of CAGE is its abrupt onset, with the majority of cases presenting with loss of consciousness, confusion, convulsions, and other serious neurologic symptoms within 5–10 minutes of surfacing (Table 23.3).[10] Such a presentation is generally considered to be air embolism until proven otherwise. Often, spontaneous improvement will be seen with partial or complete resolution of symptoms. This may reflect bubble passage through the circulation with reestablish-

Table 23.3. Most common presenting signs and symptoms in cases of arterial gas embolism	
Stupor and confusion	24
Coma with convulsions	18
Coma without convulsions	22
Unilateral motor changes	14
Visual disturbances	9
Vertigo	8
Unilateral sensory changes	8
Bilateral sensory changes	8
Collapse	4

ment of blood flow. A small subset present in cardiac arrest is difficult to resuscitate, and it is speculated that this may reflect a massive gas load filling the vascular tree.[11]

Most of the descriptions of CAGE are from submarine escape trainees where there was no gas load accumulated. Except in specific situations, most divers will have acquired a gas load with arterial gas embolism (AGE), complicating the presentation. In addition, many cases are also near drowning cases adding additional morbidity. Despite these complicating factors, a diver presenting with collapse immediately after surfacing should be considered to have an AGE component.

Fortunately, treatment is the same both for AGE and DCS, requiring immediate surface oxygen and transport to a recompression chamber. Early recommendations of a head down position in order to prevent an air lock in the ventricle have been revised. Due to potential increases in cerebral pressure and edema, it is now recommended that the diver be placed supine or in the recovery position. Treatment is discussed in more detail later in the chapter.

PHYSIOLOGIC LIMITS OF GASES

Normal gas components that are physiologic at sea level will produce tissue injury and death at specific partial pressures underwater. Nitrogen and carbon dioxide will cause harmful effects based on their concentration, while the toxic effect of oxygen is dependent on both the concentration and time duration. Recognition and awareness of these limits are essential for safe diving, and contributing factors must be understood.

Oxygen Toxicity

The implementation of undersea warfare and use of closed circuit oxygen rebreathers led to the discovery that oxygen was toxic after specific exposures.[12] Despite the known ranges and establishment of partial pressure limits, there are still a number of deaths each year among technical and recreational divers from oxygen toxicity. Oxygen enriched air (nitrox) has experienced a tremendous increase in use by recreational divers due to its reduced decompression requirements and increased bottom time.

At increased partial pressures, oxygen is known to produce toxic molecules known as free radicals that can produce cell damage and death. In the diver, these present in the form of central nervous system (CNS) and pulmonary symptoms. Additional organs such as the eyes and kidneys have been described but are uncommon.

CNS toxicity is the most dangerous, producing sudden onset seizures with little or no warning. Underwater, such a seizure will usually result in the loss of the diver's mouthpiece, drowning, and death. A brief prodro-

Table 23.4. Symptoms of oxygen toxicity
Convulsions
Lip twitching
Visual symptoms
Auditory hallucinations
Vertigo
Nausea
Irritability – behavioral changes
Dizziness
Tingling – paresthesias
Breathing difficulties

Table 23.5. Oxygen limits for diving and life support in atmospheres absolute

ATA	Designated oxygen limits
2.8	100% O_2 U.S. Navy Table 6
2.0	U.S. Navy exceptional military operations
1.6	U.S. Navy normal working operations
1.4	Recreational diving limits
0.5	Maximal saturation exposure
0.35	Normal saturation exposure
0.21	Normal air
0.16	Minor signs of hypoxia
0.10	Serious signs of hypoxia

mal symptom may or may not precede the seizure. The more common symptoms consist of visual or auditory changes, facial muscle twitching, tingling, anxiety, confusion, and nausea, among others (Table 23.4). These symptoms show an almost random distribution across exposures illustrating that oxygen tolerance does not occur and showing tremendous individual variability. (Figure 23.5).

A lowered seizure threshold has been shown to occur with exercise and carbon dioxide retention. Unfortunately, a great degree of variability among individuals makes seizure prediction impossible. As a result, most certification agencies have established a conservative limit at 1.4 ATA oxygen partial pressure for 150 minutes single exposure (Table 23.5). It must be emphasized that higher partial pressures have been utilized, but these are in military operations where increased levels of risk were required or for therapy under resting conditions in a dry hyperbaric chamber. Some divers are tempted to utilize a higher partial pressure while decompressing, but this practice should be discouraged. Most seizures and deaths are due to inadvertent usage of the wrong O_2 mix at depth or too high a partial pressure during decompression.

Similar to CNS toxicity, pulmonary toxicity has a dose/time relationship resulting in free radical damage to alveolar and endothelial cells. An oxygen partial pressure of below 0.55 ATA has been shown to be tolerated indefinitely. Symptoms range from cough and vague chest discomfort to severe substernal burning and dyspnea at rest. Spirometric studies reveal a decreased vital capacity, FEV1 and lung compliance. To track the potential for pulmonary damage, the Unit Pulmonary Toxicity Dose (UPTD) was introduced.[13] The time exposure is multiplied by an oxygen partial pressure constant to give the UPTD dose, which can then be correlated to vital capacity decrements. Most diving computers using nitrox or mixed gas algorithms will compute UPTD dosing automatically. Unless there is an extreme exposure requiring hyperbaric treatment, pulmonary toxicity is usually not an issue in recreational diving.

Hyperbaric oxygen also has been shown to produce several types of visual changes. The most concerning is a type of progressive myopia that has affected technical divers using closed circuit rebreathers.[14] In most of these cases, the diver utilized a high set point of 1.3 ATA during long dives over several days. In many cases, these changes can be reversible, but in some divers these have been permanent.

Nitrogen Narcosis

More appropriately defined as inert gas narcosis, the narcotic-like effects of nitrogen under pressure are well known to divers. The effects are first apparent at 100 ft (30.5 meters of seawater or msw) and are thought to be caused by the effects of increased nitrogen partial pressure on neuronal synapses possibly in the polysynaptic regions of the reticular activating system. Studies have shown mental slowing and impairment in memory, computational skills, and judgment. Fine motor skills have also shown to be affected.[15]

Divers often report that adaptation occurs, but this is probably due to learning and subjective opinion since

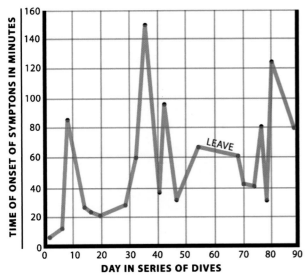

Figure 23.5. A graph of multiple oxygen exposures showing the tremendous variation in time before onset of oxygen toxicity.

performance testing does not support this. A slight departure in expected routine or an emergency can result in serious impairment. At deeper depths breathing air, the diver is truly at risk, and at depths greater than 300 ft (91.4 msw), severe impairment including unconsciousness has been observed. It is important then, that measures be taken to ensure a gas mix that will minimize narcosis. Divers who state that they have unique tolerance to narcosis are not to be believed and must adhere to standard guidelines. Most certification agencies recommend an equivalent narcotic depth of no deeper than 130 ft when using mixed gas.

Carbon Dioxide

In contrast to oxygen and nitrogen, carbon dioxide (CO_2) is produced by cellular metabolism and maintained within a narrow physiologic range until it is exhaled via the lungs. Increased amounts of CO_2 can be eliminated by hyperventilation until the buffering and pulmonary mechanisms become overwhelmed. At a CO_2 level of 3%, a doubling of respiratory minute volume will be observed, which continues upward in a linear manner with dyspnea first being noticed. Performance impairment is noted at 4–6% and at 10–15% the subject becomes severely impaired (Table 23.6). Finally, at concentrations of greater than 15–20% there is loss of consciousness and convulsions.[16]

Elevated CO_2 can be produced by increased dead space in the breathing apparatus, increased work of breathing, gas supply contamination, failure of the CO_2 absorbent mechanisms in closed or semiclosed rebreathers, or failure to provide adequate ventilation in surface-supplied helmet diving. The most common of these are in the use of rebreathers and work of breathing.

Divers using rebreathers are well trained in the recognition and management of CO_2 breakthrough. There are often no warning signs, and the first indication of toxicity has been loss of consciousness or seizures. Meticulous attention must be paid to absorbent packing, which should be promptly discarded when exhausted at the end of the recommended scrubber life.

It is known that CO_2 will become elevated during exertion at deep depths as a result of increased gas density and work of breathing.[17] A number of unexplained deaths could possibly be attributed to this mechanism.

It has also been recognized for some time that there are individuals who, despite being in excellent physical condition, retain CO_2. These individuals experience no increased dyspnea and may be at risk when there is potential for CO_2 elevation from the mechanisms just discussed.

Finally, it is known that CO_2 has effects on other gases. Seizure threshold for oxygen toxicity is lowered in hypercarbia and the effects of nitrogen narcosis increase. There is also an increased risk of DCS due to perfusion changes from elevated CO_2. There are other sources of breathing gas contamination in addition to CO_2 such as carbon monoxide and interior rust in a scuba cylinder leading to unconsciousness underwater and must be watched for.

DECOMPRESSION SICKNESS

Since the first divers ventured beneath the water breathing gas under pressure, it was quickly noticed that spending too long a time at depth produced symptoms of what was later determined to be decompression sickness (DCS). Now every dive is planned and executed by the diver in order to avoid DCS. The diving tables that dictate how long a diver can remain at depth have undergone a steady evolution in safety and reliability. These algorithms have been incorporated into small, wrist-worn, compact computers or integrated with the pressure gauge console, which display a minute by minute update of the diver's decompression state and obligations (Figure 23.6).

Despite these advances, the risk of decompression sickness remains, and the disease is still poorly understood. The incidence of DCS varies considerably in regard to the type of diving performed and ranges from 1.0 cases per 10,000 dives in the recreational community to as high as 28 cases per 10,000 in challenging

Table 23.6. Carbon dioxide concentrations and physiologic effects	
Carbon dioxide concentration	Physiologic effects
0–4%	None
4–6%	Shortness of breath
6–10%	Confusion
10–15%	Loss of consciousness
15–20%	Convulsions

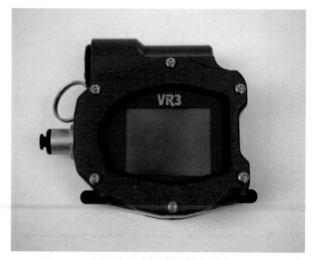

Figure 23.6. Decompression computer. This wrist-worn computer is able to calculate mixed gas decompression tables as well as fixed set point calculations for closed circuit rebreathers. Photo courtesy of VR Technology Limited.

conditions.[18,19] Interestingly, the DCS incidence in commercial diving in the North Sea has remained at virtually zero over the last few years – an example of how attention to operational safety can impact the outcome. Still, the concern remains on how a diver can reduce his and the team's risk for developing DCS.

Divers involved in expedition diving have an additional concern and motivation in planning to keep their risks as low as possible because they are frequently involved in deeper depths and longer exposures. A case of DCS requiring treatment could mean abandonment of the project in order to get an injured diver to treatment facilities that may be a considerable distance from the dive site. In many areas of the world, there are no readily accessible recompression chambers. As a result, it is critical that the diving medical officer (DMO) or equivalent have well-planned protocols to both reduce the risk and undertake treatment options.

Etiology of DCS

Though many aspects of DCS are poorly understood and debated, it is generally agreed that gas bubbles initiate the process. Once under pressure, gas is absorbed into tissues proportional to time and depth. Upon ascent, this increased quantity of gas passes back out of the tissues into the blood stream and into the pulmonary alveoli where it is exhaled. As long as the ambient water pressure does not significantly exceed the tissue pressure, the gas stays in solution and is slowly eliminated. If however, this relationship is exceeded, gas may come out of solution as bubbles.[20]

The continual refinement of decompression tables centers on preventing bubble formation or, in newer theories, the recognition that some bubbles may form and incorporating them into the decompression algorithm.[21] Another recent approach centers on the realization that decompression sickness can be modeled as a statistical or probabilistic event.[22] The result is that at each depth there is a finite amount of time that the diver can spend at depth and still be able to ascend directly to the surface (no-decompression limits). After this time has been exceeded, the diver must spend time off-gassing at defined decompression stops below the surface (Figure 23.7).

Despite these measures, bubbles may form and cause a varied collection of symptoms referred to as decompression sickness.

Classification

One of the best illustrations of the poor understanding of decompression sickness is that debate still continues as to how to describe the terminology even today. Traditionally, DCS as been subdivided into groups based on severity and location referred to as type I and type II DCS.[23] Type I encompasses generally mild cases such

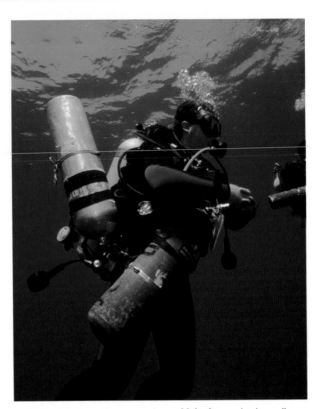

Figure 23.7. Diver decompression at 20 ft after a mixed gas dive. Photo courtsey of Craig Cook.

as limb or periarticular pain, nonspecific constitutional symptoms, or an isolated rash. Type II refers to more serious symptoms such as paralysis, other serious neurological deficits, or pulmonary symptoms (Figure 23.8 and Table 23.7).

The difficulty has been that attempts to couple a mechanism to the location and presentation have been

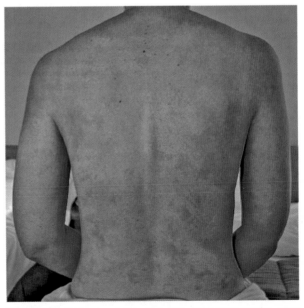

Figure 23.8. Cutis marmorata. This rash often accompanies more serious symptoms of decompression illness. Photo courtesy of Paul Cianci.

Table 23.7. Classification of decompression illness	
Type I (mild DCS)	**Type II (serious or neurologic)**
Limb pain only	Any neurologic symptoms such
Mild rash	as paresthesias or paralysis
Fatigue	Cardiopulmonary (chokes)

Note: This classification is problematic as these symptoms frequently coexist and may progress from pain only to neurologic symptoms rapidly. Pain in the thoracic distribution (girdle pain) and cutis marmorata while classified as Type I or mild, are often early harbingers of serious disease.

are collectively refereed to now as decompression illness or DCI. Finally, in spite of these diagnostic and classification difficulties, treatment will be generally the same regardless of the causative mechanism except in special circumstances.

Pathophysiology

Despite these controversies, it is generally agreed that DCS begins with a bubble obstructing an arterial vessel, either internally or by external compression, producing localized ischemia and injury. The location of bubbles in limb and periarticular locations remains controversial, and theories have ranged from intraarticular gas to bubbles obstructing blood flow in the bone marrow.[26] In neurologic DCS, bubbles have been shown to affect the spinal cord, cerebral matter, and the peripheral nerves. Severe presentations are typically thought to affect multiple areas of the spinal cord and reflect the diversity of symptoms such as combined motor and sensory symptoms. It is unusual for symptoms to take on a dermatomal pattern, and suspicion should be redirected to other causes.

problematic. Further complicating these issues has been the classification itself, which has been seen as hindering the understanding of the disease and its treatment. This has led to proposals for a revised description that more accurately reflects the disease itself.[24] Unfortunately, even though it is useful in some areas, it has its own limitations, and the older classification continues to be used.

Another confounding issue is difficulty in assigning the origin of arterial gas bubbles in the cerebral circulation to either arterial gas embolism from pulmonary barotrauma or to decompression sickness. In cases of AGE where a diver is observed to make a fast ascent to the surface from a shallow depth and minimal gas load, this diagnosis may be reasonably determined. In other situations where there has been time spent at depth, this differentiation becomes virtually impossible to undertake. In fact, it has been shown that these two mechanisms can coexist and produce a worse outcome.[25] In either case, the signs and symptoms are often the same, except for the immediate loss of consciousness seen at the surface in AGE cases. As a result, both DCS and AGE

There is debate about whether bubbles travel as emboli in the blood stream until they impact in a small vessel or whether they arise in the tissues themselves (autochthonous bubbles).[27,28] Another theory postulates that bubbles in the epidural venous plexus obstruct circulation and slow down off-gassing and result in bubble formation and infarction of the spinal cord.[29]

Whatever the etiology, the obstruction and resultant vessel wall endothelial damage heralds a second phase of tissue injury due to inflammatory mechanisms such as leukocyte migration and platelet and compliment activation.[30,31] This second phase of injury probably begins

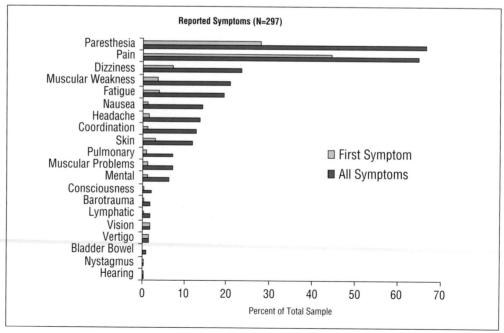

Figure 23.9. Reported symptoms in divers with decompression illness reported to Divers Alert Network in 2003.

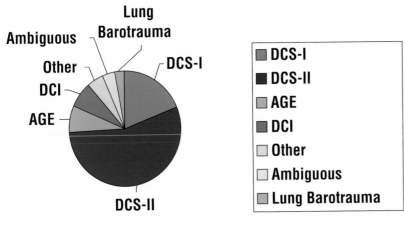

Figure 23.10. Distribution of cases as reported to Divers Alert Network in 2003. From DAN, *Decompression Illness, Diving Fatalities and Project Dive Exploration*. Durham, NC. Divers Alert Network; 2005.

soon after the bubble resolves and may last for days afterward. It has been shown that hyperbaric oxygen is successful in treating this inflammatory phase and probably accounts for the reason that many individuals with decompression sickness improve despite long delays to treatment, during which time it would be expected that the bubble would have been absorbed.

It should be emphasized that any delay to treatment allows the inflammatory process and ischemia to proceed and will impact on successful treatment.

Manifestations

Decompression sickness is currently classified as either type I DCS (mild) or type II (serious or neurologic). Type I DCS encompasses mild symptoms such as musculoskeletal pain, rash, and constitutional symptoms such as fatigue, dizziness, headache, nausea, and vomiting. Type II DCS presents as neurologic symptoms such as numbness or tingling in an extremity, motor or bladder weakness, gait disturbances, ataxia, and speech or hearing difficulties.[32]

Cardiopulmonary symptoms such as shortness of breath, cough, hemoptysis, and palpitations are also considered type II in nature. Inner ear decompression sickness (IEDCS) is also classified as type II and is usually seen on deep dives using mixed gas. Symptoms present during ascent or shortly after surfacing and consist of vertigo, nausea, and vomiting. Finally, specific manifestations such as girdle pain and rash known as cutis marmorata have been historically associated with serious outcomes and are also classified as type II. It should be noted that this particular rash usually exists in association with other symptoms compared to the more common erythematous rash seen in type I presentations that often are isolated occurrences and spontaneously resolve without treatment (Figure 23.8).

The most common presenting symptoms are pain and numbness seen in 44 and 28%, respectively, while type II is the most common classification at approximately 60% of all cases of DCS (Figures 23.9 and 23.10). The diving incident database maintained at Divers Alert

Network (DAN) recently introduced a perceived severity index ranging from the most severe symptoms to least severe and serves to illustrate the spectrum of presentation (Table 23.8).[33]

Table 23.8. Perceived severity index according to classification of symptoms of decompression illness developed by Divers Alert Network	
Perceived severity index	Reported signs or symptoms
Serious neurologic	Bladder or bowel dysfunction
	Altered coordination, difficulty walking, gait
	Altered consciousness
	Altered hearing, tinnitus, vertigo
	Difficulty talking, altered mental status, memory, mood,
	Orientation or personality
	Altered reflexes
	Weakness, partial weakness involving one side of the body
	Motor weakness, paraplegia, muscular weakness
	Decreased strength
	Altered vision
Cardiopulmonary	Cardiovascular irregularities, irregular heartbeat, palpitations
	Pulmonary irregularities, cough, coughing up blood from lungs, shortness of breath, respiratory distress, voice change
Mild neurologic	Paresthesias, numbness, numbness and tingling, tingling sensation, twitching
Pain	Pain, ache, cramps, discomfort, joint pain, pressure,
	Sharp pain, spasm, stiffness
Lymphatic/skin	Lymphatic irregularities, swelling, skin irregularities
	Burning of skin, itching, marbling, rash
Constitutional	Dizziness
	Fatigue
	Headache
	Nausea and/or vomiting
	Chills, perspiration, heaviness, heavy load, lightheadedness
	Malaise, restlessness

Most symptoms of DCS present within 2 hours of surfacing, and any symptoms presenting later than 24 hours are likely due to another etiology and not DCS. Latency of symptom onset correlates with injury severity – the more severe the case, the quicker the symptom onset. For example, weakness and confusion usually appear within 10 minutes of surfacing, while pain and sensory deficits had a median onset time of approximately 90 minutes.

A common thread in the initial presentation of DCS is the potential for evolution. It is quite common for a mild localized pain to evolve over time into a more serious presentation such as sensory disturbances, motor weakness, or even hemiparesis. It is essential that a diver initially presenting with symptoms of DCS be monitored closely with frequent neurologic exams in order to be aware of any possible deterioration. It is unlikely that any further clinical deterioration will occur after 24 hours.

TREATMENT

With respect to oxygen administration and chamber recompression, the primary goal of treatment centers is to accelerate off-gassing, decrease bubble size, and restore tissue blood flow. The reduction in bubble size occurs by increasing the oxygen gradients for off-gassing called the oxygen window (Figure 23.11).[34] The mechanical effects on bubble volume and radius reduction are due to Boyle's law. Additionally, hyperbaric oxygen will

slow down and reverse the biochemical and inflammatory changes that occurred as result of bubble injury.

Emergency treatment begins with a thorough physical and neurologic exam. The dive profile must be looked at to determine the gas load accumulated and other factors such as ascent rate and risk for pulmonary barotrauma that may produce arterialized bubbles. Often the greatest challenge is to determine if DCS is actually present, especially with pain only symptoms. Many divers have undergone chamber recompression only to be finally diagnosed with a musculoskeletal strain or other nondecompression etiology.

The diver must immediately be placed on surface oxygen with a tight fitting mask in order to achieve as high an oxygen concentration as possible. It has been shown that prompt institution of surface O_2 can lead to a reduction in residual deficits as opposed to delayed or omitted surface oxygen. Diving medical and safety officers should make sure that the supply of oxygen is sufficient for a long evacuation. Currently available are small portable surface oxygen rebreathers that can dramatically reduce the oxygen utilization while maintaining a high oxygen concentration (Figure 23.12). Alternatively, with the increasing popularity of closed circuit oxygen rebreathers, these also can be easily utilized for surface oxygen administration. It is common for symptoms to regress or even disappear with surface oxygen. It should

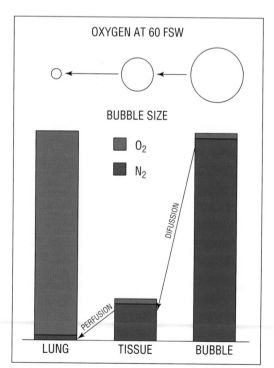

Figure 23.11. The oxygen window. The lungs contain almost 100% oxygen during treatment, which accelerates the nitrogen removal from a bubble thus shrinking it.

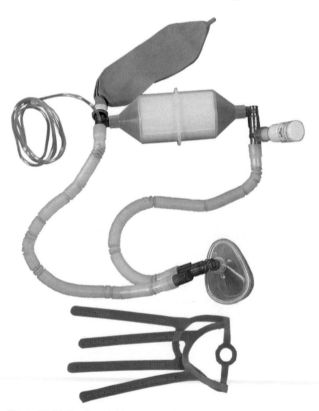

Figure 23.12. Small portable oxygen rebreathers developed by Divers Alert Network. The carbon dioxide absorbent is in the container centered in the hoses. It offers duration of 6 hr versus 2 hr using a demand regulator and E-cylinder. Photo courtesy of Divers Alert Network.

not, however, lead to canceled plans for chamber recompression as symptoms may quickly reappear.

Definitive treatment remains recompression in a hyperbaric chamber (Figure 23.13). Over the years a number of specialized treatment tables have emerged targeted at specific decompression and arterial gas embolism presentations. Today, the majority of chamber facilities provide treatment using the U.S. Navy's treatment Table 6.[35] This table provides a total run time of 3 hr on alternating oxygen and air at 60 ft (18 msw) and 30 ft (9 msw) (Figure 23.14). There have been and still are deeper treatment tables that have their advocates, but most facilities today use Table 6.[36] The advantage of the U.S. Navy Table 6 is its operational ease of use with less risk to chamber attendants and observers and proven efficacy. Multiplace chambers have traditionally been

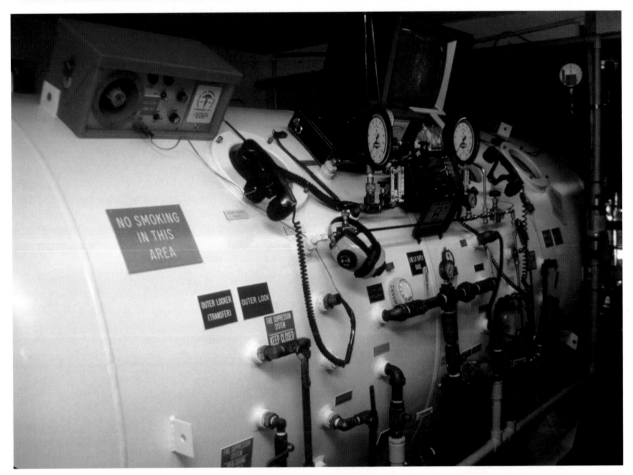

Figure 23.13. Standard multiplace chamber capable of locking in attendants. Photo Courtesy of Craig Cook.

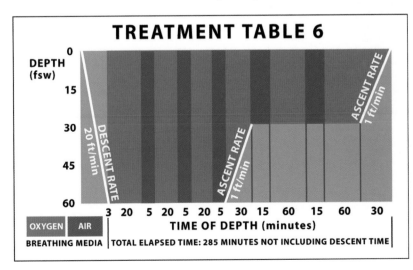

Figure 23.14. U.S. Navy Table 6. The standard recompression table used in treating decompression illness today.

used, but single-patient monoplace chambers have been shown to be able to treat an injured diver if a multiplace chamber is not readily assessable.[37]

Finally, the option exists for an expedition to have a lightweight portable hyperbaric chamber on site. This type of fully collapsible and easily transported composite chamber is capable of administering a Table 6 (Figure 23.15). It can be broken down into two cases weighing a total of 120 pounds. In remote locations, this would be the optimal choice short of a shipboard multiplace chamber. The disadvantages are that it is a monoplace chamber with no room for an attendant. Therefore, if the diver is unconscious or semiconscious, there is no way to monitor the vital signs or airway.

IN-WATER RECOMPRESSION

In remote areas, there may not be an accessible chamber. This may be due either to the fact that the nearest chamber facility may be thousands of miles away or although the chamber is physically available, it may not be operational due to lack of parts, staff, or expertise. Furthermore, in international settings, the time to organize and effect an air ambulance transport has been shown to average 22 hours before the diver arrives at the facility.[38]

In-water recompression using oxygen has been advocated in those situations when long delays would be incurred in reaching an established chamber. It should be noted that this is still a hotly debated topic, and many authorities continue to advocate surface oxygen until transport is available despite any delay. Nevertheless, the method has a number of advantages, particularly in an expedition setting. First, it allows for immediate treatment avoiding a potentially lengthy delay, which has been shown to be directly correlated to permanent neurologic residua.[39,40] Second, an expedition would likely have the equipment, such as sufficient oxygen supply, plus the expertise and training to administer the treatment, and the diver undergoing the treatment would have this same familiarity with equipment and procedure. Finally, the treatment could be undertaken and completed during the period that emergency evacuation is being arranged, and hence no delay in transport to a treatment facility.

The disadvantages to in-water recompression are, among others, placing the injured diver back in a marine environment, the potential for oxygen toxicity and hypothermia, and equipment or operational errors. It becomes critical for an expedition that intends to use this method to plan and train its members thoroughly in order to avoid these issues. The single most important key to the success of this method is the ability to rapidly place the diver back in the water as soon as symptoms become apparent. Animal studies have shown dramatic recoveries from DCS when recompressed within 30 minutes despite a heavy gas load.[41] It becomes imperative that members of the dive team understand that prompt reporting of symptoms is crucial in order to avoid delays due to denial that can reduce the chance of complete resolution of symptoms.

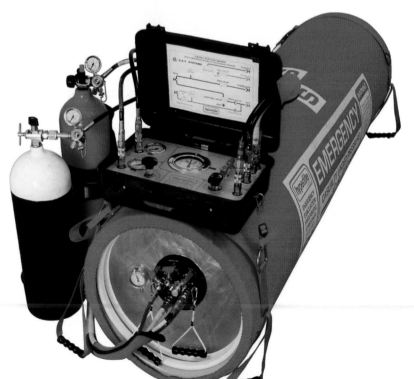

Figure 23.15. Portable Kevlar hyperbaric chamber capable of pressurization to 2.1 ATA. Photo courtesy of SOS Hyperlite UK.

The treatment protocol requires the diver be placed back in the water at a depth of 30 ft (9 m) on a secure shot line while wearing a full face mask and breathing 100% oxygen accompanied by a tender. The full-face mask ensures that in the case of an oxygen seizure he will not aspirate water and drown. The protocol prescribes approximately 30 min at 30 ft (or 60 min in severe cases) followed by a gradual 1 ft every 4 min ascent rate and can be extended according to symptoms (Table 23.9).

It is speculated that by immediate recompression, gas bubbles are being treated thereby limiting vessel endothelial damage as opposed to treating the inflammatory effects and tissue ischemia seen after long delays.

This method has proven successful among commercial spearfishers and divers in the South Pacific where it has been utilized extensively.[42,43]

ADJUNCTIVE TREATMENT

Since most cases of DCS have some degree of intravascular hypovolemia, fluid administration is necessary. Isotonic intravenous fluids such as lactated Ringer's solution would be optimal. Intravenous glucose containing solutions should not be administered due to the vulnerability of potentially viable nerve tissue. If IV fluids are not available, oral rehydration should be encouraged. Sport drinks such as Gatorade contain optimal concentrations of electrolytes and glucose and would be superior to other fluids in speed of rehydration. One liter during the first hour and continued to maintain a urine output of 1–2 cc/kg/hr or a clear appearance. Monitoring the urine output will also alert the practitioner to any signs of bladder dysfunction from spinal cord damage. A urinary catheter would be needed in those cases.

There have been many investigations into other adjuvant treatments for DCS but unfortunately none have emerged as recommended at this time. Corticosteroids have not proved beneficial nor have anticoagulants such as aspirin or heparin due to the danger of hemorrhage at the site of injury. Individuals at risk for deep vein thrombosis present as special cases where the risk benefit ratio must be considered in deciding whether to administer low-dose anticoagulants.

Intravenous lidocaine has been proposed to offer some benefit in treatment, but further investigation is needed. Nonsteroidal antiinflammatory agents (NSAIDs) are useful for patient comfort and should not be withheld.[44]

FLYING AFTER DIVING

In cases of treated DCS, it is recommended that the divers wait an additional 3 days after treatment before flying. In cases of emergency evacuations, aircraft that can be pressurized to sea level would be preferred such as the C-130 or Learjet. Other commercial aircraft are pressurized to 8,000 ft. It has been shown that too soon an exposure to the reduced barometric pressure and oxygen concentration in flight can lead to a reoccurrence of symptoms.

The regular guidelines for all divers flying after diving have recently been revised and include waiting at least 18 hr before flying after repetitive multiday dives.[45] For a single no decompression dive, it is recommended a diver wait a minimum of 12 hr before flying (Table 23.10). As with decompression tables, these guidelines are based on limited data, and rare cases of DCS can still occur despite adherence to these guidelines; accordingly, the longer the wait before flying, the less the risk.

FITNESS TO DIVE

A number of medical conditions are considered to be disqualifying for diving (Table 23.11). These are screened

---

Table 23.9. Australian underwater oxygen table (RAN 82) for in-water recompression

Method
1. The patient accompanied by an attendant, is lowered on a shot rope to 30 ft breathing 100% oxygen.
2. Ascent is commenced after 30 min in mild cases, or 60 min in severe cases, if improvement has occurred. These times may be extended to 60 and 90 min. respectively if there is no improvement.

Depth [ft (m)]	Elapsed time Mild	Elapsed time Serious	Rate of ascent
30 (9)	0030–0100	0100–0130	
26 (8)	0042–0112	0112–0142	
23 (7)	0054–0124	0124–0154	
20 (6)	0106–0136	0136–0206	4 min/ft
16 (5)	0118–0148	0148–0218	(12 min/m)
13 (4)	0130–0200	0200–0230	
10 (3)	0142–0212	0212–0242	
6 (2)	0154–0224	0224–0254	
3 (1)	0206–0236	0236–0306	

3. Ascent is at the rate of 3 ft every 12 min.
4. If symptoms recur, remain at depth a further 30 min before continuing ascent.
5. If oxygen supply is exhausted, return to the surface rather than breathe air.
6. After surfacing, the patient should be given 1 hour on oxygen, 1 hour off, for an additional 12 hr.

Equipment
Full-face mask with demand valve and surface supply system.
Adequate supply of 100% oxygen for patient and air for attendant.
Wet suit for thermal protection
Shot with at least 30 ft of rope (a seat or harness may be rigged to the rope)
Some form of communication system between patient, attendant, and surface.

Note: Total table time is 2 hr 6 min for mild cases or 2 hr 36 min for serious cases.
Source: Edmonds C, Lowery C, Pennefather J. *Diving and Subaquatic Medicine.* Oxford: Butterworth-Heinemann; 1992.

Table 23.10. Current recommendations for flying after diving

Flying after diving recommendations

1. For a single no-decompression dive, a minimum preflight surface interval of 12 hr is suggested.
2. For multiple dives per day or multiple days of diving, a minimum preflight surface interval of 18 hr is suggested.
3. For dives requiring decompression stops, there is little evidence on which to base a recommendation, but a preflight surface interval substantially longer than 18 hr appears prudent.
4. These recommendations apply to air dives followed by flights at cabin altitudes of 2,000 to 8,000 ft (610 to 2,438 m).
5. These recommendations are for recreational divers who do not have symptoms of decompression sickness.

Source: Sheffield P, Vann R, eds. *DAN Flying after Diving Workshop Proceedings.* Durham, NC: Divers Alert Network; 2004.

Table 23.11. A partial list of medical contraindications to diving

Recent intraocular gas-vitrectomy
Psychosis/acute depression
Seizures
Transient ischemic attack
Recent head injury
Acute stroke
Ischemic coronary artery disease
Valvular heart disease
Cardiac arrhythmias
Implantable cardiac defibrillator
Acute asthma
Spontaneous pneumothorax
Insulin dependant diabetes
Pregnancy

for during the certification process, but as divers age, new medical conditions may develop. It is also known that, despite recommendations otherwise, many recreational divers with medical problems dive. In expedition diving, owing to the remoteness and frequent potential for adverse and strenuous diving conditions, this may increase the risk of injury. It is important then that particular attention be paid by the diving medical officer and each of the diving members of the team to the consequences of individual health issues. Medical records of each diver and team member should be in the possession of the diving medical officer on site.

The diving medical officer should obtain the medical history of all members of the expedition for review. If there are questions regarding any health issues, there will be time for referral and consultation. A physical conditioning plan should be undertaken for all members as

a way to both determine and ensure optimal physical endurance and strength. The following are conditions that have the potential to produce the greatest risk to team members and should be considered carefully.

It is generally agreed that pregnancy is a contraindication to diving. The concerns are the potential risk of teratogenic effects on the fetus from gas emboli and oxygen toxicity. Unfortunately, there is a general lack of supporting evidence from the limited studies available. One survey covering women who dived during pregnancy showed an increase in congenital abnormalities such as cardiac defects and hand absence.[46] Due to the presence of the fetal circulation, any bubbles present would have access to the cerebral and coronary vessels. Despite the limited data available, it is clear that the risk of fetal injury is real and, although small, does not warrant diving during pregnancy especially considering the guilt that would be experienced should a congenital defect or fetal death occur. On the other hand, a woman who dives early in her first trimester before discovering she is pregnant should be reassured that the risk probably is no higher than other generally contraindicated behaviors such as smoking, excessive caffeine ingestion, or air travel.

Coronary artery disease is second only to drowning as the leading cause of diving fatalities in divers older than 35 and should be looked for carefully.[47] Risk factors should be identified and assessed for further testing, such as a cardiac stress test. Valvular heart disease and a history of cardiac rhythm disturbances are also considered disqualifying. The recent association of a patent foramen ovale and decompression illness has generated as yet unresolved questions as to the management of this issue. Patent foramen ovale (PFO) is the remnant of the fetal circulation consisting of a small opening between the right and left heart present in roughly a third of all individuals. The concern is that under certain conditions such as a cough or Valsalva maneuver, venous bubbles could pass through a PFO into the arterial side of the circulation and embolize either the brain or spinal cord. Several studies have demonstrated an association between a PFO and type II DCS.[48] This has been projected to be an almost twofold increase in DCS incidence.[49] However, because the overall incidence of DCS is very low, this still represents a very small risk considering the number of divers that have a PFO. Generalized screening for a PFO is not currently recommended, but may be useful in a diver who has experienced undeserved DCS. In these cases, if a PFO is present, counseling with options ranging from no diving to conservative profiles can be presented. Another option is closure of the PFO by way of the several intracardiac percutaneous devices now available.

Active lung disease, either restrictive or obstructive including a history of lung blebs or spontaneous pneumothorax, has been associated with cases of arterial gas embolism, and these individuals have been disqualified from diving. Asthma was traditionally considered an absolute contraindication to certification and diving. Over the last decade, this view has moderated, and some divers with well-controlled asthma have been allowed to dive if they are symptom free and meet other requirements.[50] On the other hand, a diver who requires the use of a rescue inhaler or who has made a recent trip to the emergency department for treatment should not be allowed to dive.

In addition to asthma, insulin dependent diabetics were also traditionally excluded from diving. Several studies have now shown that well-motivated and monitored diabetics can dive without a significant risk of hypoglycemia underwater.[51,52] However, these studies involved recreational divers in tropical conditions and may not be representative of other diving scenarios. Other medical conditions considered absolutely disqualifying for diving include seizure disorders due to the potential for loss of consciousness underwater and drowning.

Again, it must be emphasized these recent revisions concerning asthmatics and diabetics are only in the recreation diving population and military and commercial operations still prohibit diving. Other medical issues are best considered on a case-by-case basis between the diving medical officer or a diving physician and the diver. A careful examination and awareness of all potential heath issues of the team members will contribute greatly to the safety and success of the expedition.

SEARCH AND RESCUE PROCEDURES AND THE LOST DIVER

Due to unexpected events, it is not uncommon for a diver to be separated from the team or support vessel. In most circumstances, this amounts only to an inconvenience for those involved. In some situations, however, this may evolve into a serious problem for members of the expedition team if contact with the diver remains lost. This may occur during a decompression stop that had to be done off the designated ascent line while free in the water column during which time a diver could conceivably drift miles from the support vessel before surfacing. Many other reasons, usually related to weather and sea conditions, could precipitate such an event.

The potential seriousness of such a situation is increased in remote locations where resources for search and rescue (SAR) are either limited or nonexistent. It is therefore imperative that team members carry signaling devices that will aid in their recovery. It is also important that a plan for search and rescue be understood and agreed to by members of the expedition.

When it is known that a diver is lost, definite actions need to be undertaken depending on how far the diver

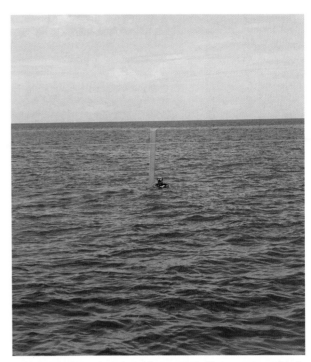

Figure 23.16. Diver deploying safety sausage. Photo courtesy of Craig Cook.

may have drifted from the support boat. These can be separated into two phases based on whether the diver can be spotted by use of his or her personal signaling devices. If formal SAR procedures need to be instituted, such as activation of an emergency position indicating radio beacon (EPIRB) or personal locator beacon (PLB).

Close Proximity Location Measures

If a diver can see the support vessel, the likelihood will be that eventually the vessel will be able to locate the diver. Various signaling devices can be used that will increase the odds of being seen. The safety sausage has become the standard for daylight location (Figure 23.16). This device is a long colored plastic tube that can be inflated by a regulator creating a 3–6 ft long cylinder that can be easily seen from a distance. It is compact and can be easily rolled up and placed in a buoyancy compensator pocket.

The signal mirror is another standard signaling device that can be easily carried. Divers should be familiar with aiming the mirror in order to increase the chances of being seen since a misdirected aim may not be noticed. If used correctly this device may be visible at longer distances than a safety sausage (Figure 23.17).

Another device that has been recently introduced is the green laser (Figure 23.18). This has been shown to be effective in daylight also when aimed properly and may be the preferred method for signaling in darkness.

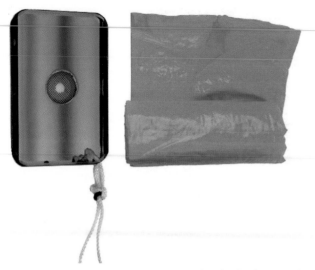

Figure 23.17. Signal mirror (left) can be seen for 10 miles from search aircraft. Safety sausage (right) is easily carried and the primary location device utilized by divers. Photo courtesy of Craig Cook.

It is compact and easily carried. Other signaling devices for nighttime use are small strobe lights available from a number of manufacturers.

Distant Location Measures

A diver who has drifted out of visual signaling range will need to be located by formal SAR efforts by third parties who must be notified. A greater likelihood of a prompt recovery can be ensured if an EPIRB or PBL is carried and deployed. The PLB is a small radio receiver that is able to transmit a coded GPS 406-MHz 5-W signal to both polar and geostationary satellites operated under the COSPAR-SARSAT international agreement (Figure 23.18). This signal is transmitted to the U.S. mission control center (USMCC), which then notifies the appropriate geographic rescue coordination center (RCC).

In this manner, a diver activating his or her unit can be pinpointed to within 100 m within minutes. Older PLBs or EPIRBs that do not contain a GPS chip, will have a 3- to 5-mile location radius and up to a 3-hour lag time due to polar orbiting satellite passes. If the team has international communication capability such as satellite phone, it can contact the USMCC or RCC directly and obtain the diver's GPS coordinates. The advantage to this method is that a diver can be quickly located and retrieved with minimal resource utilization. The disadvantage is that the SARSAT system becomes activated with potential deployment of SAR resources and therefore activation of a PBL or EPIRB should not be done casually. In circumstance where the expedition support vessel is unable to pick up the diver themselves then usual SAR procedures such as air deployment of SAR units would be undertaken.

Another method of locating a lost diver is to use a small marine radio, which the diver carries in a

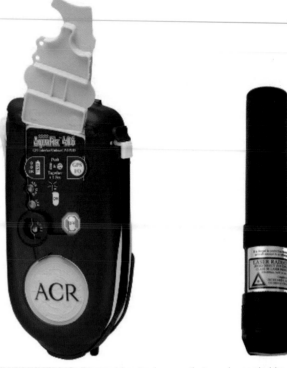

Figure 23.18. Left. Personal locator beacon that can be carried by a diver. Courtesy of ACR electronics. Right. Green signal laser. Courtesy of Greatland Lasers.

pressure-proof container (Figure 23.19). In most cases, the diver will be within several miles of the support vessel and will still be able to see it. Using the radio, the diver can communicate his or position relative to the vessel, which can then change course accordingly. The advantage here is that the SARSAT system does not need to be activated and the vessel is notified early before a longer separation distance occurs.

Finally, the location and contact information of SAR units in the expedition area should be obtained. These should be contacted or visited and the expedition mission discussed including procedures for SAR and medical evacuation of injured personnel.

CONCLUSION

The underwater environment produces a unique set of physical effects on the human body. These physiologic changes need to be understood in order to ensure an optimal safe diving experience. Each of these areas discussed should be reviewed by the team members and diving safety or medical officer with the emphasis and relation on the diving profiles that will be utilized, environmental conditions, and team member's health and age status. Potential points of risk can be identified and methods implemented to reduce the risk in these areas. Attention to these areas should begin preexpedition and continue daily on site.

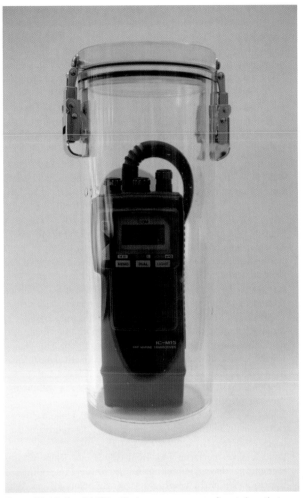

Figure 23.19. Small VHF radio in a pressure proof container that can be carried on the diver. Photo courtesy of Craig Cook.

Planning, preparation, anticipation, and avoidance are the key processes that can be utilized to ensure minimal risk and optimal success for the expedition goals. Careful adherence to these areas with an emphasis on prevention and safety will ensure a successful effort.

REFERENCES

1 Ott MC, Lundy LB. Otitis externa prophylaxis in saturation diving habitats. *Undersea Hyper Med.* 2003;30(Suppl):222.

2 Farmer JC. Otologic and paranasal sinus problems in diving. In: Bennett PB, Elliot DN, eds. *The Physiology and Medicine of Diving.* San Pedro, Calif: Best; 1982: 517–518.

3 Brown M, Jones J, Krohmer J. Pseudoephedrine for the prevention of barotitis media: a controlled clinical trial in underwater divers. *Ann Emerg Med.* 1992;21:849–52.

4 Pullen FW. Otolaryngological aspects of diving. In: *Insights in Otolaryngology.* St. Louis: Mosby; 1990: 22–3.

5 Smerz RW. A descriptive epidemiological analysis of isolated inner ear decompression illness in recreational divers in Hawaii. *SPUMS J.* 2007;37:2–9.

6 Malhoutra MC, Wright HC. Arterial air embolism during decompression and its prevention. *Proc Roy Soc B.* 1960;154:418–27.

7 Colebatch HJ, Smith MM, Ng CK. Increased elastic recoil as a determinant of pulmonary barotrauma in divers. *Resp Physiol.* 1976;26:55–64.

8 Kindwall E. *Hyperbaric Medicine Practice.* Flagstaff, Ariz: Best; 1995.

9 Smith RM, Neuman TS. Abdominal biochemistries in association with arterial gas embolism. *J Emerg Med.* 1997; 15: 285–9.

10 Edmonds C, Lowery C, Pennefather J. *Diving and Subaquatic Medicine.* 3rd ed. Oxford: Butterworth-Hinemann; 1992:103.

11 Neuman TS. Arterial gas embolism and pulmonary barotrauma. In: Brubakk AO, Neuman TS, eds. *Bennett and Elliott's Physiology and Medicine of Diving.* Toronto: Saunders; 2003: 568–71.

12 Donald K. *Oxygen and the Diver.* Welshpool: The Spa; 1992.

13 Bardin LH, Lambertson CJ. *A Quantitative Method for Calculating Pulmonary Toxicity: Use of the "Unit Pulmonary Dose" (UPTD).* Institute for Environmental Medicine Report. Philadelphia: University of Pennsylvania Press; 1970.

14 Butler FK, White E, Twa M. Hyperoxic myopia in a closed-circuit mixed-gas scuba diver. *Undersea Hyper Med.* 1999;26: 41–5.

15 Bennett PB, Rostain JC. Inert gas narcosis. In: Brubakk AO, Neuman TS, eds. *Bennett and Elliott's Physiology and Medicine of Diving.* Toronto: Saunders; 2003: 300–4.

16 Clark JM, Thom SR. Toxicity of oxygen, carbon dioxide, and carbon monoxide. In: Bove, ed. *Bove and Davis' Diving Medicine.* Philadelphia: Saunders; 2004: 246–8.

17 Forkner IF, Pollack NW, Frieberger JJ, et al. Effect of inspired po2 on hemodynamics and gas exchange during immersed exercise at 122 fsw. *Undersea Hyper Med.* 2006.

18 Vann RD, Denoble PJ, Uguccioni DM, et al. Incidence of Decompression sickness (DCS) in four recreational diving population samples. *Undersea Hyper Med.* 2004; 31(Suppl):304.

19 Ladd G, Stephan V, Stevens L. New method for counting recreational scuba dives establishes risk of death and DCI injury. *Undersea Hyper Med.* 2002; 29(Suppl):93.

20 Boycott AE, Damant GCC, Haldane JS. The prevention of compressed-air illness. *J Hyg.* 1908;8:342–3.

21 Weinke BR. Tissue gas exchange models and decompression computations: a review. *Undersea Biomed Res.* 1988;15(6): 53–89.

22 Weathersby PK, Homer LD, Flyn ET. On the likelihood of decompression sickness. *J Appl Physiol.* 1984;57:815–25.

23 Golding F, Griffiths P, Hempleman HV, et al. Decompression sickness during construction of the Dartford Tunnel. *Br J Ind Med.* 1960;17:167–80.

24 Francis TJR, Smith DJ, eds. *Describing Decompression Illness: The Forty-second Undersea and Hyperbaric Medical Society Workshop.* Bethesda, Md: Undersea and Hyperbaric Medical Society; 1991.

25 Neuman TS, Bove AA. Combined arterial gas embolism and decompression sickness following no-stop dives. *Undersea Biomed Res.* 1990;17(5):429–36.

26 Strauss MB. A mechanism for explaining the pathogenesis of pain only (limb) bends. *Undersea Biomed Res.* 1990;17(Suppl):57.

27 Francis TJR. A current view of the pathogenesis of spinal cord decompression sickness in an historical perspective. In: *The Physiological Basis of Decompression: The Thirty-Eighth Undersea and Hyperbaric Workshop.* Bethesda, Md: Undersea and Hyperbaric Medical Society; 1989.

28 Francis TJR, Pezeshkpour GH, Dukta AJ, et al. Is there a role for the autochthonous bubble in the pathogenesis of spinal cord decompression sickness? *J Neuropathol Exp Neurol.* 1988;47(4):475–87.

29 Haymaker W, Johnston AD. Pathology of decompression sickness. *Milit Med.* 1955;117:285–306.

30 Frances TJR, Gorman DF. Pathogenesis of the decompression disorders. In: Bennett PB, Elliott DH, eds. *The Physiology and Medicine of Diving.* London: W. B. Saunders; 1993:454–80.

31 Martin JD, Beck G, Treat JR. Leukocyte sequestration as a consequence of decompression sickness. *Undersea Hyper Med.* 1999;26(Suppl.):58.

32 Edmonds C, Lowery C, Pennefather J. *Diving and Subaquatic Medicine.* 3rd ed. Oxford: Butterworth-Hinemann; 1992.

33 Vann RD, Freiberger JJ, Caruso JL. *Annual Diving Report 2006 Edition.* Durham, NC: Divers Alert Network; 2006.

34 Benhnke AR. The isobaric (oxygen window) principle of decompression. Transcripts of the third annual conference of the Marine Technology Society, San Diego; 1967.

35 Dunford RG, Hampson NB. Use of USN Table 6A for the treatment of arterial gas embolism in divers in the United States. *Undersea Hyper Med.* 2001;28(Suppl.):49.

36 Smerz RD, Overlock RK, Nakayama H. Hawaiian deep treatments: efficiency and outcomes 1983–2003. *Undersea Hyper Med.* 2005;32:363–73.

37 Cianci P, Green B. Delayed treatment of decompression illness with monoplace tables. *Undersea Hyperb Med.* 1997;24(Suppl.):33.

38 Wachholz CJ, Terjung HC, Frieberger JJ, et al. Time required to organize and effect air ambulance transport in 99 DCI cases referred to DAN Travelassist. *Undersea Hyper Med.* 2001;28(Suppl.):72.

39 Benton PJ, Pitkin AD. Acute neurological DCI; the importance of rapid treatment. *Undersea Hyper Med.* 1999;26(Suppl.):57.

40 Smith LA, Hardman JL, Beckman EL. Immediate in water recompression – does it make a difference in the pathology of the central nervous system decompression sickness? *Undersea Hyper Med.* 1994;21(Suppl.):23–4.

41 Brubakk AO, Krossnes B, Hjelde A, et al. Organ injury after "treatment" of gas bubbles in the pig. *Undersea Hyper Med.* 2000;27(Suppl.):37.

42 Farm FP, Hayashi EM, Beckman EL. Diving and decompression sickness treatment practices among Hawaii's fisherman. Sea Grant Technical Paper UHIHI-SEAGRANT-TP-86—01. Honolulu: University of Hawaii; 1986.

43 Farm FP, Hayashi EM, Beckman EL. Treatment of decompression sickness Hawaiian style. In: Kay E, Spencer MP, eds. *In-Water Recompression.* Kinsington, Md: Undersea and Hyperbaric Medical Society; 1998:17–20.

44 Moon RE, ed. *Adjunctive Therapy in Decompression Illness.* Report of the Decompression Illness Adjunctive Therapy Committee of the Undersea and Hyperbaric Medical Society. Kensington, Md: Undersea and Hyperbaric Medical Society; 2003.

45 Sheffield P, Vann R, eds. *DAN Flying after Diving Workshop Proceedings.* Durham, NC: Divers Alert Network; 2004.

46 Bolton ME. Scuba diving and fetal well-being: a survey of 208 women. *Undersea Biomed Res.* 1980:7;183–9.

47 Caruso JL, Uguccioni DM, Dovenbarger JA, et al. Fatalities related to cardiovascular disease in the recreational diving population. *Undersea Hyper Med.* 1997;24(Suppl.):26.

48 Moon RE, Camporesi EM, Kisslo JA. Patent foramen ovale and decompression sickness in divers. *Lancet.* 1989;1:513–14.

49 Bove AA. Risk of decompression sickness with patent foramen ovale. *Undersea Hyper Med.* 1998;25:175–8.

50 Neuman TS, Bove AA, O'Conner R, et al. Asthma and diving. *Ann Allergy.* 1994:73;344–50.

51 Dear Gde L, Pollock NW, Uguccioni DM, et al. Plasma glucose responses in recreational divers with insulin-requiring diabetes. *Undersea Hyper Med.* 2004;31:291–301.

52 Pollock NW, Uguccioni DM, Dear Gde L, eds. Diabetes and recreational diving: guidelines for the future. Proceedings of the Undersea and Hyperbaric Medical Society/Divers Alert Network, 2006 June 19 Workshop. Durham, NC: Divers Alert Network; 2005.

24 | General Medical

J. Lee Jenkins, MD, MSc, Edbert B. Hsu, MD, MPH, Italo Subbaro, DO, MBA
Kisha Moore, BA, MBBS, MRCS(Ed), and Alex Vu, DO, MPH

INTRODUCTION

The majority of this text is dedicated to medical problems that are encountered during expeditions typically in remote, extreme, and politically unstable environments. In reality, many of the medical problems that arise during expeditions are less "exotic" and medical personnel should be prepared to treat a wide variety of more "common" medical problems as well.

When common medical problems do occur, they may represent new, acute illness or exacerbation of chronic disease. In either case, due to limited resources, during an expedition, evaluation and treatment may differ from that offered in traditional care settings. It is thus important to understand when on-site treatment may be appropriate and when evacuation of an ill or injured individual is necessary.

A comprehensive discussion of all possible medical problems that might occur during an expedition is beyond the scope of any single text. Rather, this chapter discusses some of the more common medical problems that could occur during expeditions and that may be treated by on-site medical personnel. In addition, several less common medical problems that are not covered elsewhere in the text are included. Medical problems such as myocardial infarction that may be relatively common but often require evacuation and treatment beyond the scope of on-site medical personnel are not included.

ALLERGIC REACTIONS

During an expedition, it is likely that individuals will be exposed to allergens different from those in their home region. Allergic reactions range from very mild to life-threatening, including allergic rhinitis, sinusitis, reactive airway disease, urticaria, angioedema, and anaphylaxis.

Allergic rhinitis often presents as sneezing, watery rhinorrhea, and nasal congestion. It may be accompanied by itchy, red, watery eyes consistent with allergic conjunctivitis. These symptoms may present after exposure to allergens outside such as pollen or fungi or inside from dust mites or animal dander. Symptoms will likely be worse in warmer months in conjunction with pollination and fungi growth. It may be beneficial to be aware of the botany of the region of travel and possible allergens that may be expected.

Mild symptoms may be treated with a first- or second-generation oral antihistamine or nasal corticosteroid. First-generation oral antihistamines have significant side effects including drowsiness, dry mouth, and altered mental and physical performance. Moderate symptoms may benefit from a second-generation oral antihistamine, a nasal corticosteroid, and the addition of a leukotriene-receptor antagonist such as montelukast. Ophthalmic preparations of antihistamines and mast-cell stabilizers are also available for allergic conjunctivitis.

Other manifestations of allergic reactions include urticaria or hives that are papules or wheals that are nonpitting, edematous, pruritic, erythematous, raised, circular, or annular, and range in size from millimeters to several centimeters. They tend to occur on the extremities and trunk and are usually transient, with crops of hives appearing and resolving spontaneously in a matter of hours.

Angioedema is similar to urticaria but involves the deep dermis and subcutaneous tissue as a result of vascular leakage. It is generally transient, lasting 24–48 hours, and is rarely pruritic. Angioedema lesions may occur anywhere on the body but commonly involve highly vascular areas such as the lips, oropharynx, and periorbital region. Angioedema may also occur in nonallergic settings including in response to cold, vibration, or certain medications.

Initial treatment for mild allergic reactions includes the administration of diphenhydramine with or without oral corticosteroids. Ranitidine or cimetidine may also be given. The delayed onset of action of corticosteroids prevents their use as a first-line agent; however, they may be useful to prevent a protracted or biphasic allergic response.

Anaphylaxis, the most severe form of Type 1 hypersensitivity, can broadly be defined as a life-threatening allergic reaction that results in IgE-mediated mast cell and basophile degranulation. Causative agents for anaphylaxis typically include foods (peanuts), drugs (penicillin, cephalosporins, insulin, NSAIDs), insect stings and bites, and other exposures such as antivenin or aquatic proteins. It is a life-threatening emergency requiring immediate treatment.

Anaphylactoid reactions may be clinically identical, but they are non-IgE mediated. Anaphylactoid reactions may result from drugs (vancomycin, opiates) or physical stimuli such as exercise or cold.

Anaphylaxis often occurs soon after contact with the allergen. Manifestations include hives, pruritus, flushing, and swollen lips and tongue. Gastrointestinal symptoms including cramping, abdominal pain, and vomiting are also seen. In addition, dyspnea, bronchospasm, wheezing, and stridor may result in respiratory compromise. In severe cases, respiratory failure and hypotension may occur leading to shock, hypoxia, altered mental status, end organ damage, and death.

Epinephrine is the first-line treatment for anaphylaxis. It is usually given intramuscularly (IM) or subcutaneously (SQ). IM injection in the anterior thigh has been recommended over SQ because it results in a higher level of plasma epinephrine. Intravenous (IV) epinephrine may be used for severe hypotension unresponsive to SQ and IM administration. Large volumes of IV fluids may be needed in severe reactions with hypotension. The patient should be placed in a recumbent position with the lower extremities elevated to increase venous return, stroke volume, and cardiac output. In addition, high-flow oxygen should be given to any patients experiencing dyspnea or hypoxemia. Albuterol may be useful in the treatment of associated bronchospasm.

Prednisone may be given either IV or orally (PO). Patients who experience anaphylaxis while on beta-blockers may be given glucagon (IM, IV, SQ) if symptoms are refractory to epinephrine. Extra caution must be taken when giving glucagon because it may cause emesis.

If possible, patients with anaphylaxis should be immediately evacuated to the closest care facility.

BLOOD-BORNE PATHOGENS

Expedition participants are at risk of exposure to blood-borne pathogens particularly when the mission of the expedition includes the delivery of heath care. Hepatitis B virus (HBV), hepatitis C virus (HCV), and human immunodeficiency virus (HIV) are the most important of these pathogens.

For any potential exposure, an assessment of the risk to the individual must be made and the need for postexposure prophylaxis (PEP) determined. This can be challenging even in an ideal setting and potentially extremely difficult during an expedition.

A protocol should be established prior to the expedition for blood-borne pathogen exposure. It is important to consider the overall risk to the expedition participants and the availability of drugs for PEP in area or country of the expedition. If the drugs are not readily available, they should be included in the medical supplies for the expedition. It is important to consider if the individual will receive an entire course of PEP on-site or just an initial course and the remaining drugs delivered to the expedition or the individual evacuated for further treatment.

Pathogens including hepatitis B and C and HIV may be transmitted by exposure to body fluids during provision of medical care and through engaging in consensual or nonconsensual sexual activity, sharing of needles, getting a tattoo, receiving blood transfusions, or having medical or dental procedures. Percutaneous exposures including needle sticks should be treated immediately by washing the area and surrounding skin with hot water and preferably a virocidal–germicidal soap.

If the HBV, HCV, or HIV status of the source patient is known, the decision to administer PEP may be fairly straightforward. Unfortunately, the status of the source patient is often unknown, significantly complicating the decision to administer PEP. In these cases, multiple factors must be considered including the type of exposure (on intact skin, mucous membranes, compromised skin, or percutaneous), the amount of exposure (a scratch, a few drops, a major splash, or a deep puncture with a large-bore hollow needle), the body fluid involved (blood, seminal fluid, vaginal fluid, or normally sterile fluid or tissue), and the risk characteristics of the source patient.

Exposure through sexual contact and sharing of needles carries a higher risk of transmission than through delivery of medical care, and the threshold to treat should thus be lowered in these cases.

Hepatitis B and C Viruses

Vaccination against hepatitis B virus is safe, effective, and generally readily available. It is highly recommended that anyone who is potentially at risk of exposure to HBV including through the delivery of medical care receive a full series of one of the two hepatitis B vaccines currently available. This is discussed in greater detail in Chapter 4.

In an ideal setting, after a potential exposure to HBV, if the source patient known HBs Ag–, no treatment is necessary. If the source patient is known HBs Ag+ or unknown but high risk, treatment will depend on the immunization status of the individual. If the individual's anti-HBs titer is ≥10 milli-International units per mL, then no treatment is indicated. If the anti-HBs titer is <10 milli-International units per mL, then hepatitis B immunoglobulin (HBIG) and hepatitis B vaccine should be administered.

No prophylaxis is recommended for potential exposure to hepatitis C, but these individuals should be monitored closely for infection as early treatment may reduce progression to chronic hepatitis.

Human Immunodeficiency Virus

PEP for HIV exposure should be based on current protocols. Common protocols include a two-drug basic regime and a three-drug expanded regime. Choice of basic or expanded regime should be based on risk assessment. Although there are potential advantages of treating all patients with the expanded regime, the associated additional side effects increase the chance of discontinuation prior to completion, and there is some evidence that a full basic regime is better than a discontinued expanded one.

Protocols change in response to several factors including pharmacologic developments and the epidemiology of HIV, but current protocols often include nucleoside reverse transcriptase inhibitors (NRTIs), nonnucleoside reverse transcriptase inhibitors (NNRTIs), and protease inhibitors (PIs). It is important to obtain up-to-date information prior to the development of a PEP protocol.

When choosing PEP medications, other factors may need to be considered. For example, efavirenz should not be used during pregnancy or if there is a potential for pregnancy. In addition, it is important to consider what medications the source patient is taking or has taken in the past. Ideally, PEP should include alternative drugs to reduce the risk of resistance and increase the likelihood of susceptibility.

DEEP VEIN THROMBOSIS AND PULMONARY EMBOLISM

Deep vein thrombosis (DVT) and subsequent pulmonary embolism (PE) are potential complications of expeditions due to the lower extremity immobilization associated with prolonged travel.

Signs of deep vein thrombosis of the lower extremities are inconsistent but may include swelling, tenderness, erythema, and palpable veins. Signs and symptoms of pulmonary embolus include sudden onset of dyspnea, tachypnea, pleuritic chest pain, and tachycardia. Physical examination may reveal blood pressure that may be low, normal, or high; hypoxemia; fever; a pleural rub; rales; and right heart dysfunction.

Patients with suspected DVT or PE should be transferred to a health care facility for further evaluation and treatment. Treatment includes aspirin, oxygen, and low-molecular-weight heparin (enoxaparin) or heparin. Thrombolytics such as tissue plasminogen activator (tPA) should be considered in severely compromised patients.

ELECTRICAL INJURIES

Electrical injuries may occur in a variety of settings including contact with power lines or general household current and lightning strikes. The intensity of current is measured in volts and categorized as direct current (DC) or alternating current (AC). Direct current flows constantly in the same direction. Examples include the current generated by batteries, automobile electrical systems, high-tension power lines, and lightning. Direct current tends to cause a single muscle contraction often strong enough to force the person away from the current's source. In contrast, alternating current, such as the current available through household wall sockets, changes direction periodically. Alternating current often prevents the person from releasing his or her grip on the current's source resulting in prolonged exposure.

Electrical injuries are classified into low and high voltage. Anything over about 500–1,000 volts is considered high voltage. Typical household electricity has 110–230 volts, whereas high-tension power lines have more than 100,000 volts. Lightning strikes may produce 10 million volts or more. High voltage causes more severe injury than low voltage and is more likely to cause internal damage. High voltage can arc through the air up to several feet depending on the voltage and simply coming too close to a high-voltage line without direct contact may result in injury.

The path that the current takes through the body determines which tissues are affected. Tissues differ in susceptibility to electrical damage. For example, nerves, blood vessels, and muscle tend to be more easily damaged than bone and tendon. The most common entry point for electricity is the hand, and the second most common the head. The most common exit point is the foot. A current that travels from arm to arm or from arm to leg may go through the heart and is thus much more dangerous than a current that travels between a leg and the ground. A current that travels through the head may affect the brain. If the current travels close to the eyes, it may lead to cataracts, which can develop within days of the injury or years later.

A minor shock may cause muscle pain and may trigger mild muscle contractions or startle a person, causing a fall. Severe shocks can cause arrhythmias, ranging from inconsequential to ventricular fibrillation. Severe shocks can also trigger powerful muscle contractions sufficient to throw a person to the ground or to cause joint dislocations, fractures, and other blunt injuries.

Often, the main symptom of an electrical injury is a skin burn, although not all electrical injuries cause external damage. High-voltage injuries may cause massive internal burns. If muscle damage is extensive, a limb may swell so much that its arteries become compressed, cutting off blood supply to the limb.

If an electrical injury does occur, scene safety should always be considered first. The person must be separated from the current's source in the safest manner possible. No one should touch the person until the current has been shut off, particularly if high-voltage lines are involved. High-voltage and low-voltage lines are difficult to distinguish, especially outdoors.

The person should be evaluated for both electrical injury and trauma that may have occurred as a result. They should be kept warm, and intravenous fluids should be administered for volume replacement if needed. If the injury is severe or if it is suspected that electricity passed through the chest, evacuation may be necessary to obtain an electrocardiogram (ECG) and monitor the individual for arrhythmias for 24–48 hours. If the person appears otherwise well, mild burns may be treated with bacitracin and sterile dressings. Any substantial injury including moderate to severe burns, however, should be transported to the nearest health care facility.

Lightning Strikes

Most lightning strikes occur in the equatorial belt from South America to Africa, Southeast Asia, and northern Australia. Lightning strikes may be classified as direct strikes, side flash (or splashes), and ground strikes.

Direct strikes cause maximum injury because the entire charge of the lightning passes through or over the person's body. Because of the short duration of contact during a lightning strike, often not enough voltage is transferred to break the insulating effect of the skin; therefore, the charge typically passes along the surface of the body in a process known as flashover causing less damage than a direct strike. Side flash occurs when lightning jumps from the primary strike area to the victim. A ground strike occurs when the charge hits the ground in proximity to the victim. In this instance, if a potential difference exists between the victim's legs, the current enters the body through one leg and exits through the other. This is known as step voltage.

As discussed previously, the extent of injury depends on a number of variables including amperage, voltage, current pathway, length of contact, resistance of the body, and the victim's relationship to discharging electrical fields.

Individuals struck by lightning with minimal resulting injury often report loss of consciousness, amnesia, confusion, tingling, and numerous other nonspecific symptoms. Lightning burns in these individuals are rare and invariably superficial and have little or no deep tissue damaging effects.

More severe lightning injuries may cause seizures, respiratory arrest, or cardiac standstill, which may spontaneously resolve with resumption of normal cardiac activity. The signs and symptoms are similar to mild injury except superficial burns are much more common. In addition, these patients may suffer lifelong sleep disorders, paresthesias, and increased irritability. Three-quarters of survivors from lightning strikes will have prolonged effects and morbidity.

Patients with severe lightning injury usually present with cardiopulmonary arrest. Survival is rare in this group unless a bystander expeditiously begins CPR. The most common cause of death from lightning strike is cardiac arrest after acute arrhythmias at the scene of the incident.

EPISTAXIS

Epistaxis is a common problem in expedition participants particularly in certain environmental conditions including low humidity, cold, and high altitude. It may also occur in the setting of trauma or infection. The use of aspirin, nonsteroidal antiinflammatory drugs, and blood thinning medications such as warfarin may exacerbate the problem.

Epistaxis may be divided anatomically into anterior and posterior. The vast majority of nosebleeds are anterior arising from the nasal septum.

The initial approach to management of anterior nosebleeds includes application of direct pressure through pinching the nostrils together for a minimum of 10 minutes. This technique may be utilized alone or in conjunction with a nasal spray containing a vasoconstrictor such as Afrin or Neo-Synephrine.

If this technique fails to stop the bleeding, packing the nasal cavity should be performed. This can be done with a variety of materials including cotton balls, plain gauze, nasal pledgets, Vaseline gauze, commercially available expandable nasal packing such as Merocel or a Rhino Rocket, or an anterior epistaxis balloon. Cotton balls, plain gauze, and pledgets should be soaked in Afrin or Neo-Synephrine. Expandable nasal packing and anterior epistaxis balloons should be coated in Vaseline or antibiotic ointment prior to insertion.

If a specific area of bleeding can be localized on the nasal septum, chemical cautery with silver nitrate may reduce or arrest the bleeding.

Patients with posterior nosebleeds require posterior nasal packing and evacuation for careful monitoring. While facilitating evacuation, posterior nasal packing may be done with a Foley catheter lubricated with Vaseline and inserted through the nasal cavity into the posterior pharynx. The balloon is then inflated with 10–15 cc of saline or clean water and gently pulled back until resistance is met with the inflated balloon resting in the posterior nasopharynx. The catheter may be held in place with tape to the patient's forehead or cheek. The patient with posterior packing in place must be evacuated and continuously monitored for respiratory suppression.

GASTROENTERITIS

Gastroenteritis is a very common complication of international travel associated with many expeditions. Symptoms include abdominal pain, nausea and vomiting, and diarrhea. It may result from simple dietary change, food intolerance, or infection. Infectious gastroenteritis may be viral, bacterial, or parasitic. The majority of gastroenteritis is self-limiting requiring only symptomatic treatment and supportive care; however, blood or pus in the stool or fever indicates more severe disease requiring treatment with antibiotics such as ciprofloxacin.

A potential complication of gastroenteritis is dehydration secondary to fluid and electrolyte losses via the gut. The level of dehydration should be quantified using symptoms of thirst or lethargy and signs including color of the urine, orthostasis, tachycardia, and decreased skin turgor. Rehydration should begin as soon as possible. In the absence of vomiting, oral rehydration should be adequate, even for severely dehydrated patients. A variety of fluids may be used including commercial rehydration solution or homemade solutions based on recommendations by the World Health Organization (WHO). Diarrheal disease is discussed further in Chapter 25.

SKIN AND SOFT TISSUE

Perhaps the most common problems encountered during expeditions are related to skin and soft tissues including contact dermatitis, heat rash, infections, insect bites, and sunburn. The occurrence and severity of many of these problems may be reduced through prevention. This begins with simple hygiene with soap and water daily, or as often as possible. Wearing a hat, long pants, and long sleeves and the use of sunscreen with a high sun protection factor (SPF) and insect repellant containing DEET (N, N-diethyltoluamide) or permethrin will minimize skin exposure and reduce potential mosquito and arthropod illness. Individuals should perform frequent body and clothing checks for ticks and other insects. Light-colored clothing may help deter ticks. There is no additional benefit of DEET concentrations greater than 50%, and in many situations, significantly less concentrated formulations are adequate.

Evaluation of the patient with a skin and soft tissue problem includes obtaining a history focusing on the relationship between the host (the patient), the environment, and potential vectors of disease. This includes obtaining information about exposure to environmental hazards including water, plants and animals, sick contacts, and vectors such as mosquitoes, sand flies, ticks, and other parasites. This is accomplished by detailing a precise travel history asking the patient to recall personal activity in each location such as bathing in a pond or walking on a beach. Additionally, patients should be questioned regarding onset of systemic signs and symptoms such as fever, rash, arthralgias, myalgias, and headache.

Among the most common skin and soft tissue problems encountered during expeditions are bites from arthropods including mosquitoes, fleas, ticks, and flies. They are generally a localized pruritic eruption beginning at the site of the bite within minutes to hours and persisting for days to weeks. Many of these are inflammatory rather than infectious and should be closely followed to determine if and when antibiotics are indicated. Arthropod bites may also transmit infection, and it is important to monitor patients for systemic signs and symptoms.

Infections

Infections from a variety of causes including arthropod bites are common skin and soft tissue problems, and it is essential that expedition medical personnel understand their treatment. This should include an understanding of endemic diseases specific to the area of travel and their vectors and modes of transmission. In addition to optimizing treatment, this may provide opportunities for prevention of illness. A wealth of this information is available on the World Wide Web through the U.S. Department of State (*http://www.travel.state.gov/travel/*), the Centers for Disease Control (*http://www.cdc.gov/travel*), and the World Health Organization (*http://www.who.int/topics/travel/en*).

Many bacterial infections of the skin are caused by group A streptococcus or *Staphylococcus aureus*. Typical initial treatment includes oral beta-lactam antibiotics such as cephalexin or dicloxacillin. Several specific infections are discussed next.

Cellulitis is an infection of the dermis and subcutaneous layers of the skin leading to localized pain, swelling and redness. It is characterized as an erythematous, often raised plaque with indefinite borders. Cellulitis is usually tender to palpation, shiny, and edematous and can be associated with localized lymphadenopathy and fever. The causative agent is typically group A streptococcus or *S. aureus*, and it often develops from a preexisting wound, trauma, laceration, or insect bite.

Uncomplicated cellulitis may be treated with a variety of antibiotics including cephalexin and dicloxacillin. In regions with endemic methicillin-resistant *S. aureus* (MRSA) bactrim or clindamycin may be substituted. Cellulitis with associated fever or unresponsive to oral antibiotics may require intravenous or intramuscular antibiotics such as ceftriaxone or cefazolin.

Cellulitis due to exposure to freshwater may be caused by *Aeromonas* species and ciprofloxacin may be indicated. Cellulitis after exposure to saltwater may be caused by *Vibrio vulnificus* requiring treatment with doxycycline.

Folliculitis is an infection of the hair follicles that may be bacterial, sterile, or fungal. Bacterial folliculitis is usually caused by *S. aureus* ; however, folliculitis associated with spa or hot tub use may be due to *Pseudomonas* species. This variant tends to occur in skin folds under bathing suits. Sterile folliculitis often occurs over the torso and under restrictive clothing, and fungal folliculitis may occur on the lower extremities associated with shaving. Bacterial folliculitis is described as pruritic red papules that progresses to pustules with crusting and surrounding erythema. Folliculitis caused by *S. aureus* can be treated with cephalexin and folliculitis caused by *Pseudomonas* with ciprofloxacin. Fungal folliculitis can be treated with fluconazole. Sterile folliculitis requires no antibiotics but, rather, wearing loose-fitting clothing.

Impetigo is a common superficial bacterial skin infection most commonly found in children caused by group A streptococcus and *S. aureus*. Impetigo has a worldwide distribution and is classified as bullous and nonbullous. Nonbullous lesions are described as "honey-crust" typically found around the mouth and nose. Bullous lesions are commonly found in the intertriginous areas. Treatment includes proper hygiene, cephalexin or dicloxacillin, and mupirocin ointment.

An *abscess* is a fluctuant, erythematous, circumscribed collection of pus within the dermis commonly associated with cellulitis or folliculitis. The etiology is often staphylococcal. Abscesses can occur anywhere on the body and may be treated with incision, drainage, and packing. It may be difficult to determine the extent of an abscess, and in certain cases additional imaging may be necessary.

Acute lymphangitis is an infection involving the subcutaneous lymphatic channels most commonly with group A streptococcus. The infection is often characterized by erythematous linear streaks extending from a wound on the extremity proximally along the lymphatic channels. Cephalexin is a reasonable first-line treatment.

Necrotizing subcutaneous infections are a severe form of cellulitis. The involved area is swollen, erythematous, warm, painful, and tender. Within several days, the skin color becomes purple, bullae develop, and cutaneous gangrene ensues. At this stage, the involved area is no longer tender; it has become numb due to the destruction of the superficial nerves of the subcutaneous tissues. Crepitance is often present. The causative agent can be anaerobic or mixed. The patient should be given intravenous antibiotics such as flagyl and clindamycin and intravenous fluids and transferred immediately for surgical debridement.

Tinea infections, which include infection of the scalp (tinea capitis), the body/trunk (tinea corporis), the feet (tinea pedis or athlete's foot), the nails (tinea unguium), and the inguinal crease (tinea cruris or "jock itch"), are also commonly seen in expedition participants.

The causative agent is *Trichophyton species*. These infections are generally characterized by pruritus and well-circumscribed red rings with central clearing and raised borders. More specifically, tinea pedis presents with scaling and macerated skin between the toes, tinea capitis with hair loss and scaling of the scalp, and tinea unguium with thick, yellow and distorted nail beds. Topical antifungal medications work well for mild infections; however, more extensive infection especially involving the scalp or nails may require oral antifungals including terbinafine or fluconazole.

Pediculosis is an infestation of the scalp or eyelids (pediculus capitis), body (pediculus corporis) and/or pubic area (*Phthirus pubis*) by lice. These small, flat, wingless insects use sharp claws to attach to the human host and feed on blood. They lay eggs or nits on the hair shaft. Transmission is through direct contact. Pediculus capitis and corporis are typically described as small erythematous papules, usually 2–4 mm in diameter. Phthirus pubis is usually described as pinpoint hemorrhagic spots; however, small bluish grey macules can be seen in the suprapubic area. Lice infestation causes intense pruritus and excoriation of the affected area is common. Treatment includes using permethrin rinse/shampoo and a nit removal kit and washing all clothes, bed sheets, and hairbrushes/combs.

Scabies, caused by the mite *Sarcoptes scabiei*, is a common dermatologic infection transmitted directly by skin-to-skin and sexual contact and indirectly through shared clothing or bedding. Skin manifestations include dirty appearing lines or burrows, papules, nodules, blisters, and eczematous or erythematous changes due to excoriation. The most commonly affected areas are the finger web spaces, flexor surfaces of the wrists and elbows, the axillae, the breast and inframammary areas in females, the buttocks and the genitalia. Typically the scalp and face are unaffected. Diagnosis is based on history, clinical exam, and skin scrapings. Lesions are scraped with a sterile scalpel blade that has a drop of mineral oil on it. The scrapings and oil are then placed on a microscope slide with a coverslip, and examined for mites, mite eggs, or mite feces (Freedman et al., 2006). The differential diagnosis includes body lice and atopic dermatitis. Topical scabicides remain the mainstay of treatment, although oral agents are also available. Permethrin cream and lindane are the two most studied topical agents, although the neurotoxic side effects of lindane have resulted in its limited use. A key to treatment is that all close physical contacts are treated and all bedding and clothing laundered at the same time.

Contact Dermatitis

Contact dermatitis is characterized by an inflammatory reaction of the skin to an allergen or irritant that may be a chemical, physical, or biologic agent. Allergic contact dermatitis is a form of delayed hypersensitivity mediated by lymphocytes sensitized by contact of the skin with the allergen. Irritant contact dermatitis results when caustics, industrial solvents, detergents, or similar compounds contact the skin. It may result from brief contact with a potent caustic substance or from repeated or prolonged contact with milder irritants. Clothing, jewelry, soaps, cosmetics, plants, and medications contain allergens that commonly cause allergic contact dermatitis. These include rubber compounds, plants, nickel (often used in jewelry alloys), paraphenylenediamine (an ingredient in hair dyes and industrial chemicals), and ethylenediamine (a stabilizer in topical medications).

Contact dermatitis often has a characteristic distribution, suggesting that the eruption was caused by external stimuli. This can range from vesicles in a linear distribution to generalized erythema and fissuring of the skin seen in irritant dermatitis from continued exposure. Cold compresses may provide some relief in the initial stages. Mild or moderate erythema may respond to topical steroids; however, severe or systemic reaction may require enteral steroids. Diphenhydramine will help to control itching.

Rhus dermatitis, a specific form of contact dermatitis, results from sensitization to the resinous sap material in poison ivy, oak, and sumac. Other plants in this family contain allergens that are identical and may cause crossreactivity when exposure occurs either on the skin or through ingestion.

Contact dermatitis may be reduced through covering exposed skin with appropriate clothing and gloves. Barrier creams and products that contain 5% quaternium-18 such as Ivy-Block may prevent Rhus dermatitis. This compound may also be found in some antiperspirants.

When an exposure is suspected, washing the skin may inactivate the allergen but should be done quickly. After 10 minutes, only 50% of Rhus resin may be removed, and after 60 minutes, none will be removed by washing.

Heat Rash

Miliaria rubra or prickly heat is another frequent skin complaint of individuals traveling in tropical environments especially when wearing tight clothing. It is characterized by pruritic vesicles or papules on an erythematous base and is caused by an obstruction of the sweat glands and maceration of the sweat gland ducts resulting in leakage of sweat around the ducts into the epidermis. The lesions are located in areas where the clothing is tightly bound to the body such as the waist, armpits, flexures, upper back, and chest. The eruption usually spares hair follicles. Treatment includes bathing in cool water and gently applying dry talcum powder or calamine lotion. Wearing loose clothing may aid in prevention.

Sunburn

One of the most common medical problems experienced by expedition participants is sunburn. This may be especially true in individuals traveling to the tropics where the amount of ultraviolet light from the sun is greater than what they are accustomed to. Within the ultraviolet spectrum, ultraviolet A (UVA) and ultraviolet B (UVB) are the most important. UVB (290–320 nm) is the main cause of sunburn, and UVA (320–400 nm) is the main cause of photosensitive diseases such as solar urticaria and drug eruptions.

Prevention of sunburn includes wearing widebrimmed hats, long sleeves, and long pants, sunglasses with UV protective lenses, and appropriate sunscreen especially on uncovered and exposed areas of the body.

The chemicals in sunscreens absorb or scatter ultraviolet light, reducing its penetration into the skin. Sunscreens are described or rated by this ability referred to as the sun protection factor or SPF. It is the ratio of the amount or dose of UV radiation needed to develop minimal sunburn with sunscreen to the amount of dose of UV radiation needed to develop the same minimal sunburn without sunscreen. Typical commercially available sunscreens range in SPF from 2 to 50. The minimum recommended SPF is 15; however, those with fair skin may require significantly higher SPF. Lightweight clothing provides an SPF of approximately 5–7; thus, it may be important to apply sunscreen under clothing in certain circumstances.

The treatment of mild to moderate sunburn includes nonsteroidal antiinflammatory drugs (NSAIDs) and cool compresses. Severe sunburn may be treated with the addition of topical or oral steroids; however, their use is controversial. Topical indomethacin has also been used.

UROLOGICAL EMERGENCIES

In conditions under which medical resources are limited and advanced diagnostic testing is not readily available, general management of urological emergencies may prove challenging. However, expedition medical personnel should be familiar with and able to readily identify and treat a number of common urological emergencies.

Hematuria

Gross hematuria is generally not a life-threatening condition, and significant hematuria would be a highly unusual situation in the field unless renal or possibly lower urinary tract trauma has occurred. Relatively small amounts of gross hematuria can be associated with common urologic conditions such as urinary calculi, lower urinary tract infections, a substantially enlarged prostate, and renal or bladder tumors, but it is also seen in uncommon conditions such as renal papillary necrosis and sickle cell disease. Urinary calculi and infections are often associated with painful symptoms, can certainly be encountered, can develop into a urologic emergency, and must be treated.

However, gross painless hematuria need not be treated in the field and most likely will not require evacuation. The patient needs to be referred for timely urological evaluation because gross painless hematuria can be the first sign of malignancy or urinary calculi.

Renal Colic

Renal calculi, commonly referred to as kidney stones, may be a source of severe pain. Prolonged dehydration, such as occurs in high altitude or dry, hot climates can precipitate stone formation and onset of renal colic. Renal colic usually presents as flank pain, often very intense in nature, which can wax and wane. Radiation to the lower abdomen, testicle, or labial area can occur at the onset or develop as the stone moves. Nausea and vomiting as well as diaphoresis may occur, and patients are often very restless. Gross hematuria may accompany renal colic. Passage of small stone fragments or the entire calculus (if small) may occur.

Calculi 5 mm or smaller will often pass spontaneously but larger stones may become obstructed in the ureter. A low-grade fever may accompany an uncomplicated urinary calculus but high-grade fever or persistence of fever signifies an emergency that requires evacuation and relief of obstruction for impending sepsis.

Other conditions that may mimic renal colic include acute appendicitis, testicular torsion, pyelonephritis, salpingitis, pyelonephritis, or abdominal aortic aneurysm.

The most important early consideration is achieving an adequate level of pain control. Nonsteroidal anti-inflammatory medications may be useful but narcotic medications are often required for analgesia. Other medications such as anti-emetics may be used to control nausea or vomiting symptoms. The use of selective α-1 antiadrenergic antagonist medication such as tamsulosin or alfuzosin is often useful to decrease ureteral smooth muscle spasm and allow passage of smaller calculi. These medications are commonly used for relief of lower urinary tract symptoms in older men and should be used if available concomitantly with pain medication.

Acute Urinary Retention

The hallmark of acute urinary retention is an inability to pass urine accompanied by severe discomfort. Most frequently found in males, patients with acute urinary retention typically may describe prior symptoms of out-flow obstruction and occurrence of obstruction is most often preceded by an exacerbation of these symptoms.

Urinary incontinence due to overflow with obstruction can be the presenting symptom.

Some common causes of urinary retention include enlargement of the prostate known as benign prostatic hyperplasia (BPH), urethral stricture, and urinary tract infection (in males). Urinary retention can also be manifested by neurological disorders, but this is unlikely to be the cause in the setting of an expedition. One of the most common causes of acute urinary retention is the use of antihistamines in men. Often one will elicit a history of some decreased urinary flow and the antihistamine effect on bladder neck smooth muscle can trigger the onset of acute urinary retention.

Acute urinary retention requires relief of obstruction by a catheter. Since this is unlikely to occur in a truly sterile manner in the field, administration of a broad-spectrum antibiotic for the duration of catheterization is advised. If no catheter is available, a straw or other similar diameter tube may be considered for temporary insertion in the bladder, but this should not be undertaken unless in extreme circumstances due to the potential for injury and infection. Cessation of antihistamines, initiation of selective α-1 antiadrenergic antagonist medication such as tamsulosin or alfuzosin if available, and avoidance of opiate analgesics may help relieve obstruction or prevent recurrence until the patient undergoes proper evaluation by a urologist. Inability to relieve urinary retention is an emergency and should precipitate immediate evacuation.

Paraphimosis

Paraphimosis is defined as swelling of the glans penis resulting from trapping of the foreskin behind the corona of the glans. Principle management consists of analgesia followed by steady firm compression of the glans and distal penis to reduce swelling with the goal of pulling the retracted foreskin forward over the glans. Patients with predisposition to infection in this condition, such as diabetics, should be treated with antibiotics. This condition may recur and urological referral is advised upon return to the community.

SUGGESTED READINGS

Auerbach P, ed. *Wilderness Medicine*. 4th ed. St. Louis: Mosby; 2001: 1082–3.

Basnyat B, Cumbo TA, Edelman R. Infections at high altitude. *CID*. 2001;33:1887–91.

Centers for Disease Control and Prevention. *Traveler's Health: Yellow Book Health Information for International Travel, 2005–2006*. Atlanta: U.S. Department of Health and Human Services, Public Health Service; 2005.

Corren J. Allergic rhinitis and asthma: how important is the link? *J Allergy Clin Immunol*. 1997;99:S781–6.

Dawson C, Whitfield H. ABC of Urology: Urological emergencies in general practice. *BMJ*. 1996;312:838–40.

Freedman DO, Weld LH, Kozrarsky PE, et al. Spectrum of disease and relation to place of exposure among ill travelers. *N Engl J Med*. 2006;354:119–30.

Gilbert DN, Moellering RC, Eliopoulos GM, Sande MA. *The Sanford Guide to Antimicrobial Therapy 2006*. 36th ed. Antimicrobial Therapy, March 2006.

Gottlieb T, Atkins BL, Shaw DR. Soft tissue, common and joint infections. *MJA*. 2002;176:609–15.

Habif. Contact dermatitis and patch testing. In: *Clinical Dermatology*. 4th ed. St. Louis: Mosby; 2004.

Harrigan E, Rabinowitz L. Atopic dermatitis. *Immunol Allergy Clin North Am*. 1999;19:383.

Hussmann J, Kucan JO, Russel RC, et al. Electrical injuries morbidity, outcome and treatment rationale. *Burns*. 1995;21:530–5.

International Travel and Health 2005. The World Health Organization.

Joint Task Force on Practice Parameters. The diagnosis and management of urticaria: a practice parameter; part I: acute urticaria/angioedema; part II: chronic urticaria/angioedema. *Ann Allergy Asthma Immunol*. 2000;85:521.

Kain KC. Skin lesions and returned travelers. *Med Clin North Am*. 1999;83:1077–101.

Minevich E, Tackett L. Testicular torsion. eMedicine. Available at: *http://www.emedicine.com/med/topic2780.htm*.

Plaut M, Valentine MD. Allergic rhinitis. *NEJM*. 2005;353:18, 1934–44.

Sampson HA, et al. Second symposium on the definition and management of anaphylaxis: summary report – second national institute of allergy and infectious disease/food allergy and anaphylaxis network symposium. *Ann Emerg Med*. 2006;47(4):373–80.

Sarry J, et al. A systematic review of contact dermatitis treatment and prevention. *J Am Acad Dermatol*. 2005.

Simons FE, Gu X, Simons KJ. Epinephrine absorption in adults: intramuscular versus subcutaneous injection. *J Allergy Clin Immunol*. 2001;108:871–3.

Skoner DP. Allergic rhinitis: definition, epidemiology, pathophysiology, detection and diagnosis. *J Allergy Clin Immunol*. 2001;108:S2–8.

Spies C, Trohman RG. Narrative review: electrocution and life-threatening electrical injuries. *Ann Intern Med*. 2006;145(7):531–7.

Steffan R, DuPont HL, Wilder-Smith A. *Manual of Travel Medicine and Health*. 2nd ed. London: Dekker; 2003.

Swartz MN. Cellulitis. *N Engl J Med*. 2004;350:9.

Valentine MD, Sanico A. Allergy and related conditions. In: Barker LR, Burton JR, Zieve PS, eds. *Principles of Ambulatory Medicine*. 6th ed. Baltimore: Lippincott Williams & Wilkins; 2003: 387–405.

Weldon D. Differential diagnosis of angioedema. *Immunol Allergy Clin North Am*. 2006;26(4).

Worldwide variation in prevalence of symptoms of asthma, allergic rhinoconjunctivitis, and atopic eczema: ISSAC. *Lancet*. 1998;351:1225–32.

25 | The Diarrhea of Travelers

R. Bradley Sack, MS, MD, ScD

INTRODUCTION

International travel, which is increasing at a rapid rate, is a most rewarding way to experience different cultures, wonders of nature and the beauties of human inventiveness, and, of course, the culinary arts. Traveling to the developing world, however, where water and sanitation are less than adequate, becomes a significant obstacle when ingesting the wonderful cuisine of those countries. The traveler then often faces the challenge of dealing with the most common of travelers' diseases, acute diarrhea, or as it is usually referred to, travelers' diarrhea. Over the years, this illness has been given colorful names to describe its symptomatology, based on its location: Montezuma's Revenge, Delhi Belly, and Aztec two-step, to name a few. All of these very appropriate names refer to the same illness: travelers' diarrhea. This illness was first officially recognized and named in the 1950s by Kean (Kean, Waters, 1958) when it commonly occurred among students and vacationers traveling to Mexico and other developing countries. Initial studies for etiologic agents were all negative (using the available techniques at the time), and it was thought perhaps to be due to changes in the mineral concentrations of the drinking water, changes in gut flora, or even jet lag.

Our understanding of the disease changed remarkably in the mid-1970s, when it became clear that most cases of travelers' diarrhea were, indeed, due to infectious agents, the most common being enterotoxigenic E. coli (ETEC). This organism was first identified in 1968 in Calcutta, India (Sack, Gorbach, Banwell, et al., 1971; Qadri, Svemmerholm, Faruque, et al., 2005); where it was found to produce a cholera-like illness in adults and children. Later it was identified as the major cause of diarrhea in travelers to Mexico (Gorbach, Kean, Evans et al., 1975; Merson, Morris, Sack, et al., 1976). Subsequently, it has been identified as the major cause of travelers' diarrhea throughout the developing world.

Because ETEC has been described as the major bacterial cause of diarrhea in young children living in the developing world (Qadri, Svemmerholm, Faruque, et al.,

2005), it became clear that travelers from a developed country behave as a child when entering this environment (i.e., they are both immunologically naïve with respect to these bacterial pathogens). As children age, they develop antibodies to these organisms and thus become relatively resistant. This scenario is also seen in long-term travelers to the developing countries; with time they also develop immunity to these organisms. This immunity is relatively transient, however, once they leave these endemic areas, and probably lasts no longer than 1–2 years.

Adult populations living in the developing world, having acquired immunity as children, are relatively resistant to the development of travelers' diarrhea when they visit another developing country.

It is estimated that during a 3-week trip by travelers from the developed world who visit a developing country, the attack rate is about 30%, making it the most common illness suffered by travelers. Indeed, it is the most common illness in adults in any defined population, with the exception of common source outbreaks due to contaminated water.

Because of the wide interest in this disease, there have been many research and review articles (DuPont, 2006), as well as one book published (Ericsson, DuPont, Steffen, 2003).

THE CLINICAL ILLNESS

Travelers' diarrhea usually occurs within a few days of entering an area where water and sanitation are inadequate, but it may occur anytime during the travel. It not infrequently occurs on the trip home (in the airplane) following a going-away party, or a dietary indiscretion by the traveler who thinks the risk is over. The illness begins acutely, with watery diarrhea, nausea, sometimes vomiting, abdominal cramps, weakness, and rarely a low grade fever. Usually the traveler has from 3–8 watery or loose bowel movements in a 24-hour period, but sometimes it can be much more. Without specific treatment, the illness may last on average of 2–3 days, but sometimes it can continue for up to 10 days. Diarrhea that continues for a longer period of time is usually caused by another group of organisms, particularly protozoa. (See discussion in "Protozoa.")

The illness is usually relatively mild; it rarely is severe enough to require hospitalization. (Hospitalization in some developing countries can be an uncomfortable and even dangerous experience.) The disease usually causes at least an interruption in travel plans such as postponing expeditions in favor of remaining in the hotel where the bathrooms are close. A change in eating habits is also almost inevitably a result of such an experience. There is excellent treatment for the disease (see discussion in "Treatment") and the traveler should be armed with the appropriate medications.

If the diarrheal stool contains blood, and the patient experiences fever, abdominal pain, and tenesmus, an invasive organism (not an enterotoxin-producing organism) is probably responsible for the illness. Adequate antimicrobial therapy is essential for treatment of such diarrhea. (See discussion in "Treatment.")

ETIOLOGIC AGENTS

The presently known causes of travelers' diarrhea are shown in Table 25.1. All are found as relatively frequent causes of diarrhea in children living in the developing world.

Enterotoxigenic *E. coli*

In most studies around the world, this is the most common agent identified. ETEC (Figure 25.1) may be

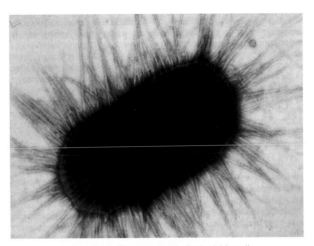

Figure 25.1. Enterotoxigenic *Escherichia coli.*

found in from 20 to 60% of cases, varying with geographical areas.

ETEC produce both enterotoxins and colonization factors which are responsible for the diarrheal illness (Qadri, Svemmerholm, Faruque, 2005). The enterotoxins are LT (heat-labile enterotoxin) or ST (heat-stable enterotoxin). ETEC may produce one or both of these two enterotoxins. LT is a large molecular weight protein that is very similar to cholera toxin, whereas ST is a small molecular weight polypeptide that is not antigenic. These enterotoxins activate adenylate cyclase (LT) or guanylate cyclase (ST), which results in secretion of chloride by the crypt cells of the small intestine and a decrease of neutral sodium chloride absorption by the villus cells, resulting in the diarrheal illness. Colonization factors (of which there are more than 25) allow the ETEC to adhere to the mucosa of the small bowel, and thereby effectively produce the enterotoxins that cause the diarrhea.

These organisms are susceptible to antimicrobial agents and, therefore, can be effectively treated with the appropriate ones. Unfortunately, ETEC are almost impossible to identify in the routine laboratory unless relatively sophisticated techniques are available.

Enteroaggregative *E. coli*

Another *E. coli*, enteroaggregative *E. coli* (EAEC), has been found more recently also to be an important agent in travelers' diarrhea (Matthewson, Johnson, DuPont, et al., 1985). These organisms are also found as a significant cause of diarrhea in children living in the developing world. They were first identified by their aggregation pattern when placed in a Vero cell tissue culture. The exact mechanism of action of these small bowel pathogens is not as well known as ETEC; they are also difficult to identify in a routine laboratory.

Note also that enterohemorrhagic *E. coli* are almost never seen as causes of travelers' diarrhea. These

Table 25.1. Estimates of the most frequent causes of travelers' diarrhea

Etiologic agents	Frequency (%)
Enterotoxigenic *Escherichia coli*	30–50
Enteroaggregative *E. coli*	15–25
Shigella	5
Campylobacter jejuni	5[a]
Salmonella	2
Giardia lamblia	1–2
Entamoeba histolytica	<1
Cyclospora	<1[b]
Cryptosporidium	3
Rotavirus	1
Norovirus	<1[c]
Other agents	1[d]
Unknown agents	20–40

[a] Found more frequently in Thailand.
[b] Found most frequently in Nepal.
[c] Found frequently in passengers on cruise ships.
[d] These include *Vibrio* sp (including *V. cholerae, V. parahemolyticus*), *Aeromonas*, and other diarrheogenic *Escherichia coli*.
Data from Ericsson, DuPont, Steffen (2003); Sack (2005); Taylor, Bourgeois, Ericsson, et al. (2006a)

organisms are seen primarily in processed food, or food that is fecally contaminated with cow's manure. Many studies in tropical areas have failed to identify these organisms as a cause of diarrhea in the local population.

Campylobacter jejuni/coli

For reasons not well understood, *Campylobacter jejuni* and *Campylobacter coli* are a frequent cause of travelers' diarrhea in Thailand and surrounding areas, perhaps because they are frequently found in poultry and meats prepared for sale in the markets. This mildly invasive organism produces a disease similar to *Shigella*. This organism is a microaerophilic organism that requires an atmosphere of reduced oxygen to grow in the laboratory. It is frequently resistant to antimicrobials and has become more resistant in the last few years.

This organism, which is also seen frequently in children of the developing world, is the most common cause of diarrhea among adults living in the United States. This is probably because poultry sold in supermarkets is frequently contaminated with the organism; as much as 50% of fresh chickens sold may harbor these organisms.

Shigella and Salmonella

Shigella and *Salmonella* are infrequently found as causes of travelers' diarrhea. An illness in which stools with blood are found, or fever is present, should suggest the presence of these organisms.

Vibrio cholerae

Cholera is a very rare cause of travelers' diarrhea, but it is clearly the most severe and can be fatal if not treated adequately. The infecting dose of *V. cholerae* (Figure 25.2) is quite large, usually requiring the ingestion of grossly contaminated water or food, which explains why travelers are rarely affected.

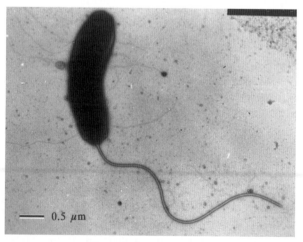

Figure 25.2. *Vibrio cholerae.*

V. cholerae and ETEC are very similar in their mode of action. *V. cholerae* produces a single enterotoxin (often called cholera toxin) that is nearly identical to the LT toxin produced by ETEC; it activates adenyl cyclase as the primary mode of action; it also uses fimbria to facilitate colonization of the small intestine.

Diarrhea produced by *V. cholerae*, however, is usually more severe than that produced by ETEC. Diarrheal stool rates may be as high as one liter per hour, leading to the development of shock that can occur within 12 hours of the onset of symptoms, making this a true medical emergency. If this occurs, intravenous fluids, either normal saline or Ringer's lactate, must be given rapidly until the patient is out of shock; then oral rehydration salts (ORS) can be used to complete the rehydration and to replace continued stool loss. ORS alone is adequate in patients with lesser degrees of dehydration. The addition of antibiotics will shorten the disease to about 36 hours and thus obviate the need for prolonged rehydration. Antibiotics of choice include doxycycline – in areas where the organisms are sensitive – or ciprofloxacin, which will be effective against all *V. cholerae*.

V. cholerae grows well on selective bacteriologic media (thiosulfate citrate bile salts sucrose agar media is the preferred one), but treatment does not depend on the bacteriologic diagnosis. Correcting the dehydration is the most important part of therapy.

Viruses

Viruses, with one exception, are a relatively infrequent cause of travelers' diarrhea. The exception is Norovirus, which may be found as a cause of travelers' diarrhea on cruise ships (Gunn, Terranova, Greenberg, et al., 1980). Such aggregations of persons living in close quarters seem to be an ideal place for this virus to spread and cause disease. This organism characteristically causes vomiting ("winter vomiting disease") as the primary symptom and is self-limited; no specific therapy is needed other than maintaining hydration. The organism is also found as a frequent cause of diarrhea among adults and children in the United States.

Rotavirus is the major cause of severe diarrhea in children living in developing countries, but it is infrequently found in adult travelers. This is probably because all persons experience at least one episode of diarrhea due to Rotavirus early in life, regardless of whether a person lives in a developed or developing country. Therefore most adult travelers will already have some immunity to this organism.

PROTOZOA

Protozoa are infrequent causes of travelers' diarrhea. Diarrhea due to these organisms is usually prolonged rather than acute. The most frequent of these organisms is *Giardia lamblia*. This disease is characterized by a prolonged, mild diarrhea, often with symptoms of excessive belching of foul-smelling gas. Abdominal pain may be present, but rarely is there fever. This organism is ubiquitous, found everywhere where sanitation is less than optimal. In the United States, it is a well-recognized cause of diarrheal disease among hikers and campers who drink out of streams that are contaminated with beaver feces. Fortunately, this organism can be eradicated with appropriate drugs. (See discussion in "Treatment.") *Entamoeba histolytica* is very uncommon in travelers but may present as a serious illness, "amebic dysentery," which needs to be treated aggressively. *Cryptosporidium parvum* is a relatively common cause of acute diarrhea in young children living in the developing world, but it has been only an infrequent cause of travelers' diarrhea (Jokipii, Pohjola, Jokipii, 1985). The organism may cause prolonged severe diarrhea in immunocompromised persons, such as those with HIV/AIDS. *Cyclospora cayetanensis* is a more recently described protozoon that has been found to cause diarrhea in travelers to Nepal, particularly in the spring. It is rarely found in other parts of the world. (Shlim, Hoge, Shlim, et al., 1995). It produces a chronic diarrhea that can last for months, associated with weight loss.

Blastocystis hominis is frequently found in stools of travelers from developing countries. However, no data show this to be a cause of the diarrhea.

ETIOLOGIC DIAGNOSIS

Unfortunately the laboratory is not very helpful in the etiologic diagnosis of travelers' diarrhea. The recognition of ETEC and EAEC is very difficult, and most laboratories will not have these capabilities. Fortunately, laboratory diagnosis is not usually necessary because the treatment is so successful. (See discussion in "Treatment.") Furthermore the traveler is usually moving about, and not staying in a place where a laboratory would be of help. *Shigella* and *Salmonella* can be cultured in most minimally equipped laboratories, and this may be necessary in rare cases. Except for Rotavirus, viruses would not be recognized easily in the laboratory, and it is an infrequent cause of travelers' diarrhea. Norovirus is very difficult to identify and can be done only in special research settings. Etiologic diagnoses of protozoa require stool exams by experienced technicians. *Giardia* and *E. histolytica* are the easiest to recognize, but *Cryptosporidium* and *Cyclospora* may not be recognized by a lab in the developing world.

EPIDEMIOLOGY

As is true for the diarrhea of children living in the developing world, travelers' diarrhea is a product of inadequate potable water and poor sanitation. The measure of the risk for developing the disease is to know how common diarrhea is among the children living in that area.

The clinical syndrome of travelers' diarrhea was described earlier in the chapter. However, when doing epidemiologic studies of diarrhea, it is important to have a definition of the illness that is generally agreed upon, so that the disease can be compared in different geographic areas and seasons. The generally accepted definition is at least 3 loose or watery stools in a 24-hour period with at least one other symptom, such as nausea, vomiting, or abdominal discomfort. One episode is differentiated from another by having at least 2–3 days of normal stools between episodes. Using these definitions, studies have been carried out throughout the developing world, and the risk of developing the illness can best be compared using a map, as shown in Figure 25.3 (Steffen, 2005).

The major risk factors for developing travelers' diarrhea are the destination of travel, the country of origin (developed countries), the age of the traveler, the duration of stay, the season of the year, and the travel style, including compliance with dietary recommendations. Travelers living in the developing world who visit another developing country have a considerably lower incidence of travelers' diarrhea than those from the developed world; if these travelers visit the developed world, they have a very low incidence of diarrhea, estimated at 1–2%, similar to the local population.

In adults, the younger, more adventuresome travelers are at higher risk, probably because they are more likely to eat in less sanitary places and to do more hiking in even less developed areas. In children, the rates are also increased, but fewer studies have been done to define this. Their risk is known to be particularly high when children from the developed world visit their families, particularly grandparents, living in the developing world.

Most cases develop with increasing frequency during the first 3 weeks of the visit. With longer durations, the rates of diarrhea level off, probably as a result of local antibody formation from exposure to the enteric pathogens.

The seasonal incidence of bacterial diarrhea is seen throughout the world. During the warm season, diarrhea rates are increased, whereas they are less frequent during the cool season. This almost certainly relates to the increased growth of bacterial pathogens in food at more elevated temperatures.

Persons traveling frugally are probably more likely to be exposed to contaminated food and water just because of the types of food that they eat. Also, persons doing adventure travel, backpacking, and carrying food are more likely to encounter the organisms. It has also been shown that individuals staying in certain hotels in developing countries have a high risk of developing diarrhea. Clearly, lack of attention to water and sanitation is the most likely explanation.

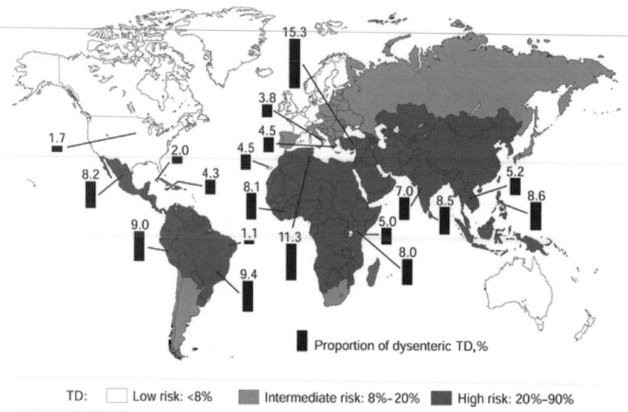

Figure 25.3. Risk of developing travelers' diarrhea (Steffen, 2005).

Traveling on cruises sometimes becomes a risk. All the passengers eat from the same kitchen so the possibility of an outbreak of diarrhea is a real one. That is, of course, if there is a break in the attention to hygiene. Both bacteria (enterotoxigenic *E. coli*) and viruses (Noroviruses) have been known to cause large outbreaks on cruise ships.

Compliance with dietary recommendations, that is carefully observing food and water precautions, is easy to spell out but very difficult to carry out. Scientific studies have given various results, mostly negative, on how protective these actions are. These are difficult studies to carry out, and data are based on the travelers' documentation or recall of foods eaten. However, as few as 2–5% of travelers may actually adhere to these recommendations.

PREVENTION

Prevention guidelines are summarized in Table 25.2.

Water and Food Precautions

As mentioned previously, compliance with strict food and water guidelines is often difficult to adhere to. However, here are several suggestions that will decrease the risk of being exposed to enteric pathogens.

Drinking water must be treated in some way; commercially bottled, filtered, boiled, or chlorinated water are all safe. Travelers should be instructed not to drink tap water, or even brush their teeth with it. Ice should be avoided, unless one is certain that it is being made from safe water. Freezing does not kill these microbes; therefore, iced drinks may not be safe.

The most hazardous food items are fresh vegetable salads (such as lettuce and tomatoes) because these have been handled and washed with water that may not be safe. However, fresh vegetables used for salads can be made safe by soaking in hypochlorite solutions (or other similar solutions depending on the country). Restaurants, even the best ones, usually do not disinfect salads. Milk products that have not been pasteurized are also unsafe. Meat and seafood should be adequately cooked before eating. Fresh fruit that can be peeled, such as bananas, oranges, mangoes, and papayas, are always safe if carefully peeled. However, unpeeled fruit or berries are hazardous and should be avoided. Eating from food vendors on the street is risky, unless the food served is piping hot. Coffee and tea are always safe because they are made using heated water. Breads are usually safe, unless they have been sitting out where flies can land on them.

Medications

Both over-the-counter and prescription medications have been used to prevent travelers' diarrhea.

Table 25.2. Guidelines for prevention and treatment of travelers' diarrhea

Food and water precautions: Riskiest foods are fresh vegetable salads, fruits eaten with peel, and untreated water and ice.

Antimicrobials (optional, see text): Fluoroquinolones can be used OD, beginning 1 day before travel, and continuing to 1 day after travel. This regimen can be used safely for at least 3 weeks. This provides about 80–90% protection against developing travelers' diarrhea.

Other agents: Bismuth subsalicylate, given qid, has been found to prevent about 60% of travelers' diarrhea. It should not be taken with antibiotics. Lactobacillus GG given as capsules has been found to protect up to 45% of travelers.

Treatment of travelers' diarrhea:

Hydration:
Increase intake of fluids such as soups, juices, other fluids containing carbohydrates and salt to prevent/treat dehydration. Packets of ORS can be carried by the travelers, and are ideal for this purpose.
IV replacement of fluids (Ringer's lactate is preferred) may be necessary in severe cases.

Antibiotics: [a]
Ciprofloxacin (or other fluoroquinolones) 500 mg every 12 hours for 1 to 2 days
Or azithromycin (for children or adults) 500 mg daily for 1 to 2 days
Or rifaximin, 200 mg twice a day for 3 days

Symptomatic treatment:
Loperamide: Imodium-like drug that can be used after antibiotic is started to decrease frequency of bowel movements; not recommended to be used alone for treatment.

[a] Doxycycline and trimethoprim-sulfamethoxazol are no longer drugs of choice because of the high degree of bacterial resistance to these antimicrobials.
Adapted from Sack (2005); DuPont (2006); *Medical Letter (2004)*.

Nonantimicrobials

Bismuth subsalicylate (Pepto-Bismol), when taken four times a day, has been shown to give about 60% protection. The specific actions of the medication include some antimicrobial and antisecretory properties, but it is not clear exactly how the drug works in prevention. The amount of salicylate in the preparation is not high enough to cause toxicity (Ericsson, DuPont, Steffen, 2005).

Probiotics are preparations of live organisms (usually lactobacilli) found normally in the intestine that can be ingested to colonize the bowel and thus prevent infection with diarrheogenic organisms. There are many different preparations on the market, some of which have been studied for the prevention of travelers' diarrhea. No studies have conclusively shown any of them to be protective.

Antimicrobials

A number of studies have shown that certain antimicrobials, taken daily during travel are highly effective in preventing travelers' diarrhea. The earliest studies done in late 1970s showed both doxycyline and trimethoprim-sulfamethoxazole to be highly (85%) effective (Sack, 2005). However, due to increasing bacterial resistance, these drugs are no longer used for either prevention or treatment of travelers' diarrhea. Following these early studies in 1985, a consensus conference held at the National Institutes of Health (Gorbach, Edelman, 1986) came to the conclusion that these prophylactic antimicrobials should not be used by travelers. This recommendation applied to the general traveling public.

Since that time, newer agents, such as Ciprofloxacin and other fluoroquinolones have been shown to be as highly (80–90%) protective as prophylaxis (DuPont, 2006). For these studies, medications were taken once a day beginning on the day before travel, continuing during the trip, and stopping on the last day of the trip. They were not used longer than 3 weeks.

In spite of their efficacy, however, use should be limited to specific situations because of the possibility of allergic reactions, the development of resistant enteric strains that could become a problem for the traveler, and the fact that early antimicrobial treatment is very effective. In most developing countries, these antimicrobials are sold over-the-counter and are widely used; therefore, the addition of antimicrobials to the environment by travelers would be relatively insignificant.

Who, then, are good candidates for antimicrobial prophylaxis? Possible recipients could be travelers on a very tightly scheduled trip that does not allow for changes due to illness. This might be a musician who must perform on schedule or a business or academic person with meetings or lectures. Also persons with medical conditions that could be aggravated significantly by an episode of travelers' diarrhea would be candidates for prophylaxis. For most travelers, however, we recommend carrying along a dose of antimicrobials that can be used for treatment if necessary.

There is, however, a new drug on the market that has the potential for providing effective prophylaxis. The drug is rifaxamin (Xifaxan) (*Medical Letter*, 2004). It has been used effectively in studies of both treatment and prophylaxis for travelers' diarrhea in Mexico (DuPont, Jiang, Ericsson, et al., 2001; DuPont, Jiang, Okhuysen, et al., 2005). The drug is poorly absorbed, achieves very high concentrations in the bowel, and has no significant side effects (DuPont, 2006). Though the drug has been shown not to be effective against invasive pathogens, such as *Shigella* or *Campylobacter*, when given prophylactically in treatment studies, it has prevented *Shigella* infections in volunteers, even though it does not provide effective treatment (Taylor, McKenzie, Durbin, et al., 2006b) A clinical study of travelers to Mexico showed that from 1 to 3 tablets (200 mg) taken per day gave significant (up to 70%) protection against travelers' diarrhea (DuPont, Jiang, Okhuysen, et al., 2005).

At present, the drug is marketed only for treatment of travelers' diarrhea, but has the potential for being effectively used for prophylaxis, without the concerns originally expressed by the consensus conference.

Vaccines

At present, there are no vaccines on the market in the United States that are specifically for prevention of travelers' diarrhea. Vaccines are, however, being developed to provide protection against the major causes of travelers' diarrhea, ETEC and *Shigella*. ETEC vaccines contain the most common colonization factors of ETEC in addition to the B subunit of the heat labile toxin, LT. Any effective ETEC vaccine would be useful not only for travelers, but much more importantly for children of the developing world, where this organism is the primary bacterial cause of their diarrheal illnesses.

All travelers' diarrhea vaccines being developed are to be used orally to primarily stimulate the local immune mechanisms of the gut. Both killed and live ETEC vaccines are being studied. For their use by travelers, vaccines would need to be given at least 1–2 weeks before travel and may, ideally, provide protection up to a year or more. In the developing world, ETEC vaccines would be given to children very early in life because this is the time when the disease is most frequent.

Interestingly a cholera vaccine (Dukoral) made from whole cells of *V. cholerae* and its B subunit of cholera toxin is being marketed in Canada and parts of Europe (but not in the United States) as a vaccine to prevent travelers' diarrhea due to ETEC (Hill, Ford, Lallopo, 2006). The rationale for protection is that the antigenic B subunit of the cholera toxin is closely related structurally and immunologically to the LT enterotoxin of ETEC and may thus provide protection. No studies have shown conclusively, however, that Dukoral is useful for the prevention of travelers' diarrhea, and it is not recommended for this purpose.

Vaccines against *Shigella* and *Campylobacter jejuni* are also in progress, but none are yet available for use.

TREATMENT

Treatment consists of two principles: prevent the development of dehydration, and eliminate the source of the infection (Table 25.2).

Rehydration

The prevention of dehydration can be done with the intake of oral fluids and electrolytes during the course of the illness. Increasing normal fluid intake, such as soups and juice, is usually adequate if the diarrhea is mild. ORS can be taken to prevent dehydration when the stool output is large. The traveler can carry these packets or purchase them in the country visited. Ceralyte (available from Cera Products, 9017 Mendenhall Court, Columbia, MD, 21045, or travel stores) is the only packaged ORS sold in the United States. An adequate oral rehydration solution can also be homemade with salt and sugar by adding ½–¾ teaspoon of table salt and 6–8 teaspoons of table sugar to 1 quart of clean water.

ORS was developed initially to be used in patients with cholera, but it was quickly found to be effective in treating and preventing dehydration in acute diarrhea due to any cause, and was particularly useful in small children in the developing world. ORS is now recommended by the World Health Organization (1995) and all public health programs as the mainstay of treatment for use in any type of diarrhea and in any age group, in which the stool volume may be enough to cause dehydration. The fluid contains electrolytes (sodium chloride, potassium, citrate) and some form of carbohydrates (glucose, sucrose, or starch, like rice powder). The combination of the glucose molecule with the sodium molecule results in the increase in absorption of sodium chloride from the small bowel to prevent or treat the dehydration.

In the infrequent but severe cases of diarrhea with large amounts of stool loss, hospitalization and intravenous fluids may be necessary. Either normal saline or Ringer's lactate can be used initially to correct shock, after which ORS can be given to replace ongoing stool losses. Fortunately, ORS, if used adequately, can usually prevent the need for intravenous therapy and a visit to a local medical facility.

Antimicrobials

Following the identification of the major infectious bacterial agents of travelers' diarrhea, studies of the effectiveness of antimicrobials for treatment became imperative. Because ETEC was found as the major cause of travelers' diarrhea, the studies were directed at those organisms. Initial studies were done with doxycyline and trimethoprim-sulfamethoxazole, and both agents were shown to be effective in shortening the course of the illness (Sack, 2005; DuPont, 2006). With time, however, many ETEC were developing resistance to these drugs, and new ones were evaluated. At present, Cipro is the drug most widely used worldwide, although other fluoroquinolones are also effective (DuPont, 2006). Azithromycin has also been found to be highly effective and is often used in Thailand and the surrounding countries because one of the causes of travelers' diarrhea in this part of the world, *Campylobacter jejuni*, has developed resistance to Cipro. Travelers are advised to have the medication with them at the time of travel. They then take the antimicrobial with the first symptoms of diarrhea: Cipro (500 mg tab) is given followed in 12 hours with a second dose. For azithromycin, a 500 mg tablet is taken with a second dose at 24 hours. Thus, only two doses of medication are needed for a full course of treatment. After 24 hours, the diarrhea is usually much improved, or completely cured.

As discussed earlier, a new poorly absorbed antimicrobial agent, refaximin (Xifaxan), has now also been shown to be an effective treatment for travelers' diarrhea and is now available in the United States (Taylor, Bourgeois, Ericsson, et al., 2006a). This drug that has been available in other parts of the world, particularly Europe, for many years for the general treatment of diarrheal disease. In the bowels, it reaches high concentrations, which are more than 200 times higher than the minimum inhibitory concentrations of any of the known bacterial diarrheal pathogens. The drug was first studied extensively in Mexico and later in other parts of the world. In double-blind controlled studies, using a dose of 200 mg tablets taken three times a day, it has an efficacy equivalent to Ciprofloxacin for the treatment of travelers' diarrhea (Taylor, Bourgeois, Ericsson, et al., 2006a). It is not, however, effective in the treatment of invasive agents of travelers' diarrhea (Taylor, McKenzie, Durban, et al., 2006b).

Nonantimicrobial Agents

Antisecretory agents, other than loperamide, have also been studied for treatment of travelers' diarrhea, but none have been found to be effective and are not marketed in the United States.

Loperamide, an antisecretory and antimotility drug is useful, when given in addition to antimicrobials (Ericsson, 2005). The combination therapy results in an even quicker resolution of the diarrhea. It is not recommended that antimotility agents be used alone because they have no antimicrobials properties; thus, the disease may persist in spite of temporary symptomatic improvement.

Some episodes of travelers' diarrhea may persist and last longer than 2 weeks. Treatment of these illnesses requires the specific identification of an additional set of etiologic agents, particularly protozoa. The general recommendation is three stools collected over several days for microscopic examination, and an assay for *Giardia* antigen. Occasionally, the use of a string capsule may be useful in identifying *Giardia* in the upper small intestine. Serology is useful only with infection by E. histolytica. Metronidazole is the drug of choice for treating both *Giardia* and E. histolytica infections. Trimethoprim-sulfamethoxazole is the drug for cyclospora infections (Schlim, Hoge, Schlim, et al., 1995). The only drug that has been shown to be effective against *Cryptosporidium* is nitazoxanide, now available in the United States, but experience with the drug has not yet been extensive (Ochoa, White, 2005).

POSSIBLE SEQUELA TO TRAVELERS' DIARRHEA

In most cases, there are no significant sequela following travelers' diarrhea. However, recently Connor (2005) and DuPont, Jiang, Okhuysen, et al. (2005) have demonstrated that the diagnosis of irritable bowel syndrome may be a sequel to an episode of travelers' diarrhea. This association is currently being extensively evaluated.

In some instances in which the episode of travelers' diarrhea persists, underlying illnesses may be unmasked, such as irritable bowel syndrome and inflammatory bowel disease. These underlying diseases are usually diagnosed after returning from travel, when all other diagnoses for infectious causes are exhausted. Tropical Sprue has also rarely been diagnosed in travelers with persistent diarrhea.

SUMMARY

In spite of the fact that we understand much about travelers' diarrhea – its cause, epidemiology, prevention, and treatment – it appears that travelers' diarrhea will be of importance to travelers to the developing world for a long time to come. Improvements in water and sanitation in the developing countries are the ultimate ways to decrease and eliminate this disease. Because this long-term solution is many years away, the use of newly developed medications for prophylaxis and effective vaccines will provide some much-needed protection.

REFERENCES

Connor BA. Sequelae of traveler's diarrhea: focus on postinfectious irritable bowels syndrome. *Clin Infect Dis.* 2005;41: S577–86.

DuPont HL. New insights and directions in travelers' diarrhea. *Gastroenterology Clinics of North America.* 2006;35:337–53.

DuPont HL, Jiang ZE, Ericsson CD, et al. Rifaximin versus ciprofloxacin for the treatment of travelers' diarrhea: a randomized double-blind clinical trial. *Clin Infect Dis.* 2001;33:1807–15.

DuPont HL, Jiang ZE, Okhuysen PC, et al. A randomized double-blind placebo-controlled trial of rifaximin to prevent travelers' diarrhea. *Ann Intern Med.* 2005;142:805–12.

Ericsson, CD. Nonantimicrobial agents in the prevention and treatment of traveler's diarrhea. *Clin Infec Dis.* 2005;41: S557–63.

Ericsson CD, DuPont HL, Steffen R, eds. *Travelers' Diarrhea.* Hamilton, Ontario: Decker; 2003.

Gorbach SL, Edelman R, eds. Travelers' diarrhea: National Institutes of Health Consensus Development Conference. *Rev Infect Dis.* 1986;8(Suppl 2):S109–S233.

Gorbach SL, Kean BH, Evans DG, et al. Travelers' diarrhea and toxigenic *Escherichia coli. N Engl J Med.* 1975;5;292: 933–6.

Gunn RA, Terranova WA, Greenberg HB, et al. Norwalk virus gastroenteritis aboard a cruise ship: an outbreak on five consecutive cruises. *Am J. Epidemiol.* 1980;112:820–7.

Hill DR, Ford L, Lallopo DG. Oral cholera vaccines: use in clinical practice. *Lancet Infect Dis.* 2006;6:361–73.

Jokipii L, Pohjola S, Jokipii AM. Crpytosporidiosis associated with traveling and giardiasis. *Gastroenterology.* 1985;89: 838–42.

Kean, BH, Waters S. Diarrhea of travelers. I. Incidence in travelers returning to United States from Mexico. *Arch Indust Health*. 1958;18:148–50.

Mathewson H, Johnson, PC, DuPont HL, et al. A newly recognized cause of travelers; diarrhea enteroadherent *Escherichia coli*. *J Infect Dis*. 1985;151:471–5.

Merson MH, Morris GK, Sack DA, Creech WB, Kapikian AZ, Gangarosa EJ. Travelers' diarrhea in Mexico: a prospective study of physicians and family members attending a congress. *N Engl J Med*. 1976;294:1299–305.

Ochoa, TJ, White AC. Nitazoxanide for treatment of intestinal parasites in children. *Pediatric Infec Dis J*. 2005;24: 641–2.

Qadri F, Svemmerholm AM, Faruque ASG, et al. Enterotoxigenic *Escherichia coli* in developing countries: epidemiology, microbiology, clinical features, treatment and prevention. *Clin Microbiol Rev*. 2005;18:465–83.

Rifaximin (Sifaxan) for travelers' diarrhea. *Medical Letter*. 2004;46:74–5.

Sack RB. Prophylactic antimicrobials for the traveler's diarrhea: an early history. *Clin Infect Dis*. 2005;41:S553–6.

Sack RB, Gorbach SL, Banwell JG, et al. Enterotoxigenic *Escherichia coli* isolated from patients with severe cholera-like disease. *J Infect Dis*. 1971;123:378–85.

Sack, DA, Sack, RB, Nair, GB, Siddiue AK. Cholera. *Lancet*. 2004;353:223–33.

Shlim DA, Hoge CW, Shlim DR, et al. Placebo-controlled trial of cotrimaxazole for cyclospora infections among travelers and foreign residents in Nepal. *Lancet*. 1995;345:691–3.

Steffen R. Epidemiology of traveler's diarrhea. *Clin Infect Dis*. 2005;41:S536–40.

Taylor DN, Bourgeois AL, Ericsson CD, et al. A randomized, double-blind, multicenter study of rifaximin compared with placebo and with ciprofloxacin in the treatment of travaelers' diarrhea. *Am J Trop Med Hyg*. 2006a;74:1060–6.

Taylor DN, McKenzie R, Durbin A, et al. Rifaximin, a nonabsorbed oral antibiotic, prevents shigellosis after experimental challenge. *Clin Infect Dis*. 2006b;42:1283–8.

World Health Organization. International study group on reduced-osmolarity ORS solutions: multicentre evaluation of reduced-osmolarity oral rehydration salts solution. *Lancet*. 1995;345:282–5.

26 | Malaria

Diagnosis, Prevention, and Treatment for the Traveler

Christian F. Ockenhouse, MD, PhD

Disclaimer: The views herein are solely those of the author and are not to be construed as official or representing those of the U.S. Army or the Department of Defense.

INTRODUCTION

Throughout the ages, explorers, adventurers, soldiers, and travelers have met a determined foe. The human disease caused by the malaria parasite, the most important parasitic disease of mankind, has extracted a devastating toll on the serious explorer as well as the vacationing traveler resulting not only in failed missions, curtailed voyages and expeditions, but ultimately in death. Nevertheless, the devastating effects of malaria can be countered through diligent preparation before embarking on an adventure. Currently, the World Health Organization (WHO) estimates that over 100 countries frequented by 125 million travelers each year are endemic for malaria (Figure 26.1), resulting in thousands of cases of imported malaria to the United States, Europe, and Australia.[1-4] It is expected that the number of cases of imported malaria will increase due to the rapid spread of drug-resistance, an increase in transmission due to climactic changes and global warming in areas previously at low risk for malaria, and an increase in international travel, adventure voyages, and expeditions. According to WHO estimates, between 350 million and 500 million cases of acute clinical malaria occur each year worldwide with greater than one million deaths primarily in children in sub-Saharan Africa.[5-6] The exact number is unknown due to vast underreporting and incorrectly diagnosed cases. This chapter will summarize the critical and practical steps that health care providers and travelers alike can apply to prevent and minimize the devastating consequences of this disease if encountered on one's journey.

HISTORY

The history of infectious diseases of mankind would not be complete without summarizing the devastation wrought by malaria for adventurers on expedition to Africa, Asia, and Central and South America. Expeditions set out not only for the thrill of adventure, prestige, or the sole pursuit of new knowledge but also to search for the means to discover and extract the curative treatments for the "ague" or malaria fever from the powdered bark of the cinchona tree. Such excursions are thoroughly described in two recent books, which portray the heroic actions of brave men who ventured to the hills of the Peruvian Andes and the jungles of Java to gather the bark from the cinchona tree in order to extract, purify, and formulate the active ingredient into the antimalarial quinine.[7-8] Throughout history, malaria spared neither the famous, including Alexander the Great, Oliver Cromwell, George Washington, Abraham Lincoln, Ulysses S. Grant, Mahatma Gandhi, and Lord Horatio Nelson, nor the infamous Jesse James. Outdoorsmen and explorers such as Davy Crockett, Christopher Columbus, Meriwether Lewis, Henry Morton Stanley, Dr. David Livingstone, and Commodore Oliver Hazard Perry are among those reported to have contracted malaria during their lives. To be sure, military campaigns throughout history were adversely affected by malaria and in some cases accounted for more casualties than enemy fire. Commanders such as Napoleon used malaria to oppose the British in the Walcheren Expedition by flooding the Dutch countryside to allow malaria to flourish. Reportedly, Napoleon stated, "We must oppose the English with nothing but fever, which will soon devour them all".[8] The lessons learned from the conflicts and wars of the United States have been slow and painful. From the Revolutionary War to present-day conflicts, both *Plasmodium falciparum* and *Plasmodium vivax* malaria have accounted for millions of cases and countless avoidable deaths in U.S. military personnel.[9] Not withstanding the illnesses borne by the mighty and powerful, the burden of malaria disease throughout the ages has been borne primarily by those most vulnerable to its devastating consequences, namely infants residing in tropical and subtropical regions of the world. Malaria stills extracts a deadly toll especially in those younger than 5 years old in sub-Saharan Africa where more than one million children die each year primarily due to lack of access to quality health care. Like the malaria-naïve

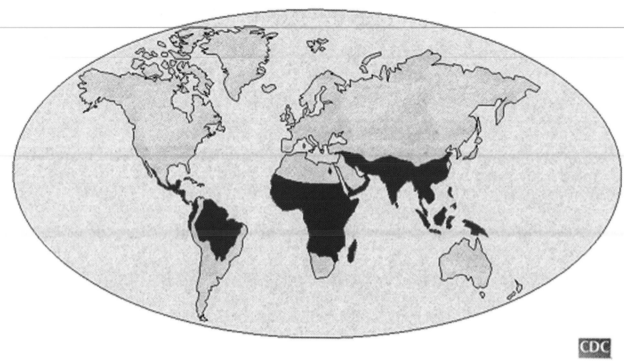

Figure 26.1. Geodistribution of malaria worldwide. Courtesy of the Centers for Disease Control and Prevention at *http://www.cdc.gov*.

child, the healthy nonimmune traveler is equally at risk for acquiring the infection and dying from an untreated and unrecognized infection. However, all too often after returning to their home country, the patient's history of travel and possible exposure to malaria parasites is either ignored or not considered in the formulation of a differential diagnosis of a febrile patient.

GEOGRAPHIC DISTRIBUTION

There are four species of human malaria caused by the protozoan parasite, *Plasmodium* (*Plasmodium falciparum, Plasmodium vivax, Plasmodium ovale*, and *Plasmodium malariae*), and each species has evolved along with its anopheles mosquito vector, environment, and host to uniquely cause disease in man. The primary means to acquire infection is through the bite of an *Anopheles* mosquito. The risk for infection to the traveler differs markedly from continent to continent, from region to region, and in urban versus rural environments and depends upon such factors as intensity of transmission, seasonality, elevation, rainfall, and host genetic differences that account for innate resistance or susceptibility to infection and disease. The choice of antimalarial medications depends also upon drug-resistance patterns that have emerged in practically all regions of the world where malaria is transmitted. Most geographic regions of the world have chloroquine-resistant *P. falciparum* malaria except for focal areas where chloroquine is still indicated for both prophylaxis and treatment. Regions of chloroquine-sensitive *P. falciparum* malaria include Haiti and the Dominican

Republic, Mexico, Central America, and parts of the Middle East. In most parts of the world, *P. vivax* remains sensitive to chloroquine except for isolated areas within Indonesia, Papua New Guinea, and Vanuatu.

PARASITE BIOLOGY AND LIFE CYCLE

The malaria parasite subverts the human host to its own survival advantage by adopting a complex life cycle in both the vertebrate and invertebrate host. Central to its survival is the uncanny ability of the parasite to completely transform itself by changing its antigenic repertoire depending upon the stage of development, enabling the parasite to quickly replicate intracellularly in hepatocytes during the pre-erythrocytic liver stage of development or in red blood cells during the erythrocytic stage. After mosquito inoculation of as few as 10–100 sporozoite-stage organisms into the subcutaneous tissue, the parasite migrates from the subcutaneous tissue to the lymphatics and circulation and continues its journey to the liver (pre-erythrocytic stage) where it invades, develops, and multiplies within the liver hepatocyte for 5–7 days. A single sporozoite can multiply within a hepatocyte to release tens of thousands of merozoite-stage parasites, which enter the peripheral circulation in search of its final destination, the red blood cell. The pre-erythrocytic liver stage of parasite development is completely asymptomatic in the host. Yet during this developmental period within the liver, the parasite undergoes transcriptional activation inducing the expression of a new repertoire of proteins. The appearance of parasite proteins that are expressed only during specific developmental stages of its life cycle protect the pathogen from host immune responses by limiting exposure of antigenic epitopes to antigen-presenting cells prior to entering the erythrocytic blood stage of development. In select cases of *P. vivax* and *P. ovale* infections, some of the parasites may remain dormant or quiescent within the hepatocyte (known as a hypnozoite parasite) for weeks to months. The molecular basis for parasite latency of hypnozoites remains unknown, although it is presumed that host cell processes trigger reactivation of parasite development in the liver culminating in blood-stage parasitemia that initiates a clinical malaria attack. Consequently, the asymptomatic latent liver phase caused by *P. vivax* and *P. ovale* parasites accounts for both delayed onset of malaria and clinical relapses that occur weeks to months after an infectious mosquito bite. Most antimalarial drugs do not preferentially target the parasite while it resides within the hepatocyte; therefore, they would have little to no activity against the hypnozoite forms of *P. vivax* or *P. ovale* malaria. However, a single class of antimalarial compounds, the 8-amino-quinolines, eradicates liver-stage parasites from all human malarias. Primaquine, the most prominent member of this class of compounds is indicated for radical cure for hypnozoite-stage parasites in individuals diagnosed with primary *P. vivax* malaria whose asexual blood-stage parasitemia has been treated, and in addition is a second-line chemoprophylaxis drug that may used to prevent infection.[10]

The merozoite-stage parasites released from ruptured hepatocytes invade erythrocytes and multiply synchronously over 48 hours (*P. falciparum, P. vivax, P. ovale*) or 72 hours (*P. malariae)* before rupturing to release progeny merozoites that perpetuate the life cycle resulting in an exponential rise in the parasite density within the host. The erythrocytic blood-stage infection phase of the parasite life cycle is responsible for the clinical manifestations of the disease. In order for transmission to continue, some asexual-stage parasites are triggered by incompletely understood molecular processes to form sexual-stage gametocytes, which are picked up by uninfected female *Anopheles* mosquitoes during a blood meal. The gametocytes quickly exflagellate within the insect vector, mate to form a zygote, and reproduce within the midgut to form sporozoites, which eventually find their way to the mosquitoes, salivary glands whereupon the life cycle is completed during the next blood meal on its victim.

CLINICAL MALARIA

In a nonimmune traveler, clinical malaria is a medical emergency that must be investigated promptly because if left untreated may result in rapid end-organ damage and death. Infection with *P. falciparum* is responsible for the vast majority of severe and complicated malaria that

may result in coma (cerebral malaria), renal and hepatic failure, pulmonary edema, and death. In *P. falciparum* infections, the malaria-infected erythrocyte sequesters along the endothelium of the postcapillary venules as the parasite matures within the red blood cells.[11–13] The adhesion of large numbers of trophozoite and schizont-infected erythrocytes in the vascular beds of the brain, heart, intestines, kidneys, liver, and spleen is responsible one of the factors responsible for the major manifestations of complicated malaria infection.

Severe malaria anemia is an insidious complication of *P. falciparum* malaria observed principally in young children residing in areas of high malaria transmission. Severe malaria anemia is not generally considered a serious complication in the adult traveler.

There are no specific signs and symptoms that differentiate clinical malaria from a multitude of other infectious diseases; however, malaria does not cause a rash, which distinguishes it from a variety of viral (i.e., dengue fever, hemorrhagic viruses) and rickettsial diseases. Although initial symptoms may be mild, fever is first manifestation in a traveler returning from a malaria-endemic area and is often accompanied by other nonspecific systemic complaints including chills, rigors, headache, gastrointestinal distress including vomiting and diarrhea, myalgias, low back pain, and fatigue. Fever results when the intraerythrocytic parasites burst out of the red blood cells releasing a cascade of proinflammatory mediators such as TNF-α, interleukin 1, and interferon-γ. People experiencing any symptoms consistent with malaria should seek immediate medical care and prompt diagnosis and should inform the health care provider about possible prior exposure to mosquito bites or presence in an area with possible malaria transmission. The health care provider who evaluates a returning traveler with fever must obtain a detailed travel history and perform a physical examination and request immediate thick and thin blood films for malaria diagnosis.[14]

PREVENTION

All nonimmune travelers who journey to regions with malaria transmission and are exposed to mosquitoes between dusk and dawn are at risk for infection. To minimize the risk for infection, specific preventive measures can and should be employed. Presently, there is no approved effective vaccine to prevent malaria. The most important factor that increases the risk for malaria is noncompliance with preventive measures! Travelers should follow the four principles (ABCD rule) of malaria prevention as recommended by the World Health Organization.[15]

A. Situational **A**wareness
B. Avoid mosquito **B**ites
C. Compliance with **C**hemoprophylaxis
D. Seek early **D**iagnosis and treatment for fever

Situational Awareness

Situational awareness is the assessment of the variables that may substantially impact the relative risk of acquiring malaria in one's travels/expedition. It requires sufficient time in pretravel preparation and necessitates good judgment. Important considerations include assessing the malaria risk for transmission in the specific geographic area one is entering as this may impact the extent of preventive measures (i.e., prevention of mosquito bites only or the addition of specific chemoprophylaxis regimens). Additional considerations include length of stay and the type of sleeping accommodations in urban or rural areas. Estimating the risk for malaria infection can be difficult because the epidemiology of transmission often is not known and can change substantially according to geographic region, altitude, and seasonal (rainy versus dry), or yearly variations.

Avoid Mosquito Bites

Avoiding mosquito bites is an effective countermeasure to protect against malaria in an area of very limited transmission. Prevention using mosquito bednets (Figure 26.2) impregnated with Permethrin

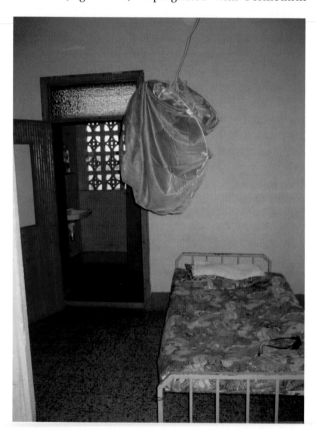

Figure 26.2. An important part of malaria prevention is the prevention of mosquito bites at night through the use of bednets like the one in this hotel room in Sudan. Bednets impregnated with permethrin have been shown to be even more effective than nontreated nets. Photo courtesy of Gregory H. Bledsoe.

has been shown to be particularly effective in preventing malaria.[16–17] Permethrin is also available in a spray or liquid formulation to treat clothing. Importantly, especially during the hours from dusk till dawn, most of the body surface should be covered by loose-fitting clothes. All travelers should be advised to use an effective mosquito repellent such as DEET (N, N-diethyl-3-methyl-benzamide) at concentrations between 30–50%. DEET-containing formulations have been approved for both children and adults.[18–22] The traveler should examine the label of several commercially available insect repellents for the concentration of DEET because lower concentrations (20% or less) provide substantially shorter duration of effectiveness (< 3 hours) compared to higher concentrations of DEET. An alternative to DEET are repellents containing the active ingredient, Picardin.[23] Picardin-containing repellents are odorless and have less skin irritation than DEET-containing formulations and are widely available in the United States, Europe, and Australia. However, the duration of protection using Picardin-formulated repellents varies according to the concentration, and protection may be limited to no more than a couple of hours.

Compliance with Chemoprophylaxis

No antimalarial chemoprophylaxis regimen provides complete protection against infection! However, chemoprophylaxis is an effective and important prevention strategy against malaria when used as directed with full and complete compliance.[24–27] Despite appropriate use of chemoprophylaxis, malaria may still occur in a traveler due to several factors that include poor absorption or inadequate blood levels of the drug. Travel medicine health care providers should consider the travel itinerary, the risk for *P. falciparum* and/or *P. vivax* transmission, and weigh the possible side effects of antimalarials with the convenience of taking their prophylaxis medications either daily versus weekly before making specific recommendations. Clinical malaria due to *P. vivax* or *P. ovale* may occur in travelers (even those compliant with chemoprophylaxis) long after departure from an at-risk area.[28] Due to the latency of the exoerythrocytic-stage hypnozoite parasites within the liver hepatocyte, most chemoprophylaxis regimens are inadequate to prevent relapses. Therefore, the traveler should strongly consider taking terminal prophylaxis using primaquine to eliminate the hypnozoite-stage parasites after leaving an area at risk for *P. vivax* or *P. ovale* malaria transmission.

No specific recommendations for malaria prevention or treatment for the pregnant woman traveler is included here, but excellent sources of information are referenced.[29–30] Women who are pregnant should be advised against traveling to an area with high malaria transmission. Pregnant females who become infected with malaria are at high risk for severe and complicated malaria that may result in premature termination of the pregnancy or low birth weight of the infant. In addition, several of the licensed antimalarials have not been adequately tested in pregnancy.

The following guidelines for recommended chemoprophylaxis regimens should be carefully considered when planning a trip to a malaria zone and are not meant as an endorsement for any particular drug. The nonpregnant traveler should seek advice and guidance from knowledgeable physicians experienced in travel medicine well in advance of scheduled travel not only to plan to protect against possible malaria exposure but also to receive immunizations against other preventable infectious diseases such as typhoid fever and hepatitis A that may be encountered. Table 26.1 describes the available antimalarial chemoprophylaxis regimens recommended for adult travelers, the dosages and frequency of the regimen, and the side effects and contraindications

of each drug. Except where indicated in Table 26.1, all are licensed by the Food and Drug Administration within the United States.

The traveler should be advised when to start and stop a specific regimen because some regimens such as weekly mefloquine or chloroquine require longer times to achieve therapeutic blood levels, whereas alternative regimens such as doxycycline or atovaquone-proguanil (Malarone®) taken daily achieve faster effective blood concentrations. The convenience of weekly chemoprophylaxis (chloroquine or mefloquine) versus daily prophylaxis (doxycycline or atovaquone-proguanil) must be also considered in the context of side effects, drug resistance, protective efficacy, and other additional benefits conferred upon the traveler against forms of travelers' diarrhea provided by doxycycline.

All travelers should be warned of the possible side effects that may be encountered.[31] All antimalarial drugs have some degree of potential side effects that cannot be predicted and that affect some but not all individuals.

Table 26.1. Malaria chemoprophylaxis regimens recommended for adult and pediatric travelers

Antimalarial drug	Dosage	Frequency	Possible side effects	Contraindications
Doxycycline	Adult: One tablet (100 mg) Pediatric: < 5 kg or < 8 yr old – contraindicated 25–35 kg; 50 mg 36–50 kg; 75 mg > 50 kg or age > 14 yr, 100 mg	Daily	Gastrointestinal distress, and esophageal irritation, photosensitivity	Hypersensitivity to tetracyclines
Atovaquone-proguanil (Malarone®)	Adult: One tablet (250 mg atovaquone plus 100 mg proguanil) Pediatric: 11–20 kg; 1 pediatric tablet 21–30 kg 2 pediatric tablets 31–40 kg 3 pediatric tablets (pediatric formulation; one-quarter strength = 62.5 mg atovaquone and 25 mg proguanil)	Daily	Abdominal pain, nausea, vomiting, headache	Hypersensitivity to atovaquone and/or proguanil
Mefloquine (Lariam®)	Adult: One tablet (250 mg) Pediatric: < 15 kg; not recommended 15–19 kg; one-quarter tablet 20–30 kg; one-half tablet 31–45 kg; three-quarters tablet > 45 kg; 1 tablet	Weekly	Neuropsychiatric event, sleep disturbances, vivid dreams, insomnia, dizziness, dysphoria	Hypersensitivity to mefloquine, psychiatric or convulsive disorders, not recommended for pilots
Chloroquine (Aralen®)	Adult: One tablet contains 300 mg of chloroquine phosphate base (equivalent to 500 mg chloroquine salt, USP) Pediatric: 5 mg base/kg (8.3 mg salt/kg) 5–6 kg; 25 mg base 7–10 kg; 50 mg base 11–14 kg; 75 mg base 15–18 kg; 100 mg base 19–24 kg; 125 mg base 25–35 kg; 200 mg base 36–50 kg; 250 mg base >50 kg or > 14 yr old	Weekly	Abdominal pain, diarrhea, blurred vision, tinnitus, skin itch	Hypersensitivity to chloroquine, epilepsy, seizures, may aggravate psoriasis

Consequently, the traveler and his or her physician must weigh the benefits of protection from a potentially deadly infection against the adverse effects that range in intensity from mild to severe. In fact, the two primary reasons often cited for lack of compliance to a prescribed regimen are the side effects of the medication and the total length of time and the frequency that the traveler must take their malaria pills. To mitigate and minimize side effects from antimalarial drugs, the physician should provide clear and explicit directions by instructing the traveler to take the chemoprophylaxis drugs with food and plenty of water.

Because of the widespread distribution of chloroquine–resistant *P. falciparum* malaria worldwide, chloroquine (Aralen®) should NOT be used for chemoprophylaxis except when travel is restricted only to certain specific geographic locales where chloroquine-sensitive malaria is transmitted. Chloroquine may be considered for primary chemoprophylaxis against *P. falciparum* when traveling to areas of Central America, Haiti, parts of the Middle East, and for *P. vivax* malaria when traveling to the Republic of Korea near the demilitarized zone (DMZ), but should never be used for prophylaxis when traveling to Africa. For most regions of the world, *P. vivax* remains sensitive to chloroquine except for isolated areas in Papua New Guinea and Indonesia. However, because both *P. falciparum* and *P. vivax* malaria are frequently found together in the same geographic area of South America, the Pacific Islands, South Asia, Southeast Asia, and Papua New Guinea, it is prudent to avoid using chloroquine for chemoprophylaxis in these areas.

Multidrug-resistant malaria is an emerging threat especially in parts of Southeast Asia along the eastern and western borders of Thailand. In such regions, neither chloroquine nor mefloquine (Lariam®) should be used for prophylaxis due to the high degree of parasite resistance. Mefloquine should be taken weekly starting at least 2 weeks prior to travel to an affected area so that adequate blood levels can be achieved and possible side effects assessed. Alternatively, a loading dose of mefloquine (once daily for 3 days prior to travel) may be taken prior to departure and can be used to gauge tolerability to the drug and assess if any untoward side effects occur. Side effects to mefloquine occur in 25–50% of travelers and include nausea and diarrhea, bizarre dreams, mood changes, and dizziness but most resolve spontaneously.[32–35] Severe psychiatric complications such as psychosis and seizures are quite rare (~1 in 10,000 users), while less severe reactions include depression and anxiety and in such persons mefloquine should be avoided. Tolerability to mefloquine prophylaxis can be assessed within the first few days after taking the loading dose to determine whether compliance may become an issue and permitting sufficient time to identify alternative regimens.

Nevertheless, the vast majority of users (97–98%) tolerated mefloquine chemoprophylaxis without problems. Mefloquine should continue to be taken weekly up to 4 weeks after departing an area at risk for malaria transmission.

Doxycycline taken 1–2 days before travel and continuing daily for the entire length of possible exposure and for 30 days upon leaving an area at risk for malaria is an effective prophylaxis drug against both multidrug resistant *P. falciparum* malaria and *P. vivax* malaria.[36–38] Full compliance with the regimen is required as missing even a single dose is sufficient to permit parasite breakthrough with corresponding onset of clinical malaria. As doxycycline is known to cause gastrointestinal distress, it should always be taken with food and plenty of water. To prevent sun sensitivity that may result from taking daily doxycycline, the traveler should wear protective clothing and use sunscreens to protect against ultraviolet A rays.

Atovaquone-proguanil (Malarone®) available as a fixed-dose tablet containing 250 mg atovaquone and 100 mg proguanil is relatively new to the market and provides excellent protection against malaria.[39–43] The combination of these two drugs is synergistic and has activity against both blood-stage and liver-stage parasites. Like doxycycline, atovaquone-proguanil must be taken 1–2 days before beginning travel and continued daily for up to one week after departing a malaria at-risk area. In addition, the side-effect profile is acceptable to most travelers. In a recent randomized trial comparing four frequently prescribed antimalarial drug regimens for travelers, both doxycycline and atovaquone-proguanil were found to be better tolerated than either mefloquine or the combination of chloroquine-proguanil.[44] The combination of chloroquine-proguanil is not approved in the United States and is not recommended for chemoprophylaxis due to the high number of breakthrough cases of malaria.[45]

Primaquine has been shown to be quite effective for chemoprophylaxis against both *P. falciparum* and *P. vivax* malaria and is considered by the U.S. Centers for Disease Control and Prevention as a second-line chemoprophylaxis agent.[46–49] Primaquine, 8-aminoquinoline, discovered in the 1940s and extensively tested in military personnel returning from the Korean conflict during the 14-day journey back to the Unites States has been shown to kill the hypnozoite forms of the parasites in the liver. Primaquine is the only approved medication to eradicate latent *P. vivax* and *P. ovale* parasites in persons with a documented clinical case of malaria resulting from either one of these two species. Primaquine also has broad activity against liver-stage *P. falciparum* parasites but little to no activity against the asexual blood-stage parasites.[50]

Because of its activity against liver-stage parasites, primaquine (30 mg base) taken daily should be started

1–2 days prior to entering an area at risk for malaria and should be continued for 3–7 days after leaving the at-risk area. Dosing should be prescribed with reference to the base concentration of the drug. A single 26.4 mg tablet of primaquine contains 15 mg of the base; therefore, two tablets daily (30 mg base) are required. The primary FDA-approved indication for primaquine is for the radical cure of P. vivax and P. ovale hypnozoite parasites after a documented clinical attack due to one of these parasites. The dose of primaquine to eradicate latent hypnozoites has recently been recommended to be increased to 30 mg base from the traditional dose of 15 mg base daily for 14 days due to reports of breakthrough parasitemia at the lower 15 mg dose. For patients with clinical malaria due to P. vivax, it is critical that a blood schizont-icide treatment regimen such as chloroquine be used initially to kill the asexual blood-stage parasites prior to commencing radical cure with primaquine.

In persons who may be exposed to P. vivax and/or P. ovale malaria and for whom primaquine is recommended as terminal prophylaxis, or in travelers who choose to use primaquine as chemoprophylaxis, all such individuals must be screened for the glucose 6-phosphate dehydrogenase (G6PD) deficiency by a simple blood test. A normal level of G6PD enzyme level in the blood must be documented before prescribing primaquine. Primaquine is contraindicated in persons with G6PD deficiency as acute hemolysis may result. There are several variants of G6PD deficiency. Individuals such as most Africans and African Americans with enzyme levels that are 20% normal G6PD activity may have mild hemolysis, whereas those with enzyme levels less than 5% normal G6PD activity are associated with severe intravascular hemolysis.

Seek Early Diagnosis and Treatment for Fever

Rapid diagnosis and treatment of malaria in travelers with unexplained fever is essential to prevent the severe complications from malaria as any delay may compli-cate successful treatment. Diagnosis is required for any person who develops a fever one week or more after entering a high-risk malaria area and up to 3 months after departure from an area at risk for P. falciparum or up to 12 months after departure from an area at risk for P. vivax. The diagnosis of malaria still relies primarily on the microscopic examination of both thin and thick malaria blood smears. In many developing countries, malaria smears are not routinely available, and pre-sumptive treatment is given based solely on a clinical suspicion of malaria. Even when available, the interpret-ation of malaria blood films requires experts trained in interpreting malaria blood smears and the reliability of accurate diagnosis cannot always be assured. Unfortu-nately, many laboratory technicians including those in the United States, Europe, and Australia are ill-equipped

and inexperienced to prepare a proper malaria blood smear and even less experienced in evaluating that smear under a microscope. The differences in size and morphology between the different parasite species and stages of parasite development (ring, trophozoite, sch-izont, gametocyte) require both training and experi-ence. Frequently, a thick smear is not prepared resulting in underreporting true malaria prevalence because the level of parasitemia in the peripheral circulation is below the threshold level of detection that is possible when only a thin blood smear is examined by microscopy. The health care provider must request that an unfixed thick blood smear be made where parasite density levels as low as 10–100 parasites per microliter blood can be detected. The improper preparation of the thick smear and the inexperience in distinguishing a parasite from a staining artifact (or platelet), make the correct diag-nosis in many hospital-based clinical laboratories chal-lenging. If no parasites are seen on the initial blood film, then serial blood samples should be collected every 8–12 hours for a total of three sets of thick and thin blood smears.

Because of the difficulties in preparing and exam-ining thick and thin blood smears, new antigen-based malaria diagnostic assays or rapid diagnostic tests have been developed that detect the presence of Plasmodium parasites.[51–53] The World Health Organization's site (ht-tp://www.wpro.who.int/sites/rdt) details the products available for diagnosis of malaria. These tests can pro-vide accurate results in as little as 10 minutes and are available worldwide. We make no recommendations or endorsements of any product but consider FDA licen-sure (for the U.S. market) a required factor in ensuring that any marketed test meets the minimally acceptable standards for diagnostic accuracy and sensitivity, and reproducibility with good quality control in manufac-ture.

TREATMENT

The treatment of malaria is complex and depends upon the species of malaria, the severity of disease, drug-resistance patterns, history of prior antimalarial chemoprophylaxis, and serious adverse events that may occur from the use of particular medications. For these reasons, a traveler with fever in an area of malaria transmission should seek immediate medical attention. There may be however special circumstances when a traveler either is unable to obtain expedient medical care and treatment, refuses to take chemo-prophylaxis, or is in an area of low malaria transmission where emergency standby antimalaria treatment may be appropriate.[54–55] It should be emphasized that such emergency standby treatment is NO substitute for pre-vention of malaria and such treatment may be ineffec-tive if the likelihood of clinical malaria is low or when a

Table 26-2. Treatment regimens recommended for adult and pediatric travelers with uncomplicated malaria

Antimalarial drug	Dosage	Regimen	Possible side effects/contraindications
Artemether/lumefantrine (Coartem®, Riamet®)	Adult:1 tablet (20 mg artemether plus 120 mg lumefantrine) Pediatric: no pediatric formulation – adult tablet used per regimen instructions	Adult: 4 tablets per dose at 0 and 8 hr on day 1 followed by 4 tablets q12 hr on days 2 and 3. Pediatric: 5–14 kg; 1 tab q12 hr × 3 days 15–24 kg; 2 tabs q12 hr × 3 days 25–34 kg; 3 tabs q12 hr × 3 days > 35 kg; adult regimen	Hypersensitivity to artemether or lumefantrine
Atovaquone proguanil (Malarone®)	Adult: 1 adult tablet (250 mg atovaquone plus 100 mg proguanil) Pediatric: 1 pediatric tablet (2.5 mg atovaquone plus 25 mg proguanil)	Adult: 4 tablets per dose daily for three consecutive days Pediatric: 5–8 kg; 2 pediatric tab qd × 3 days 9–10 kg; 3 pediatric tabs qd × 3 days 11–20 kg; 1 adult tab qd × 3 days 21–30 kg; 2 adult tabs qd × 3 days 31–40 kg; 3 adult tabs qd × 3 days > 40 kg; 4 adult tabs qd × 3 days	Hypersensitivity to atovaquone and/or proguanil, abdominal pain, nausea, vomiting, headache, avoid use with creatinine clearance < 30 ml/min
Quinine sulfate/doxycycline	Quinine: 8 mg base/kg (600 mg tablets) doxycycline: 100 mg tablets	Adult: Quinine: 600 mg tablet 3 times daily for 7 days; Doxycycline: 1 tablet q 12 hr on day 1 followed by 1 tablet per day from days 2–7 of treatment regimen Pediatric: quinine sulfate 25 mg/kg/d in 3 divided doses × 7 days plus 2 mg/kg/d up to 100 mg × 7 days (contraindicated for < 8 yr old)	Stomach cramps, diarrhea, blurred vision, lightheadedness, dizziness, unusual bleeding, arrhythmias, tinnitus
Mefloquine (Lariam®)	Adult: 1 tablet (250 mg) Pediatric: 20–25 mg/kg	Adult: 3 tab po at time of diagnosis followed by 2 tabs 8 hr later Pediatric: divided dose taken at time of diagnosis and 8 hr after first dose	Neuropsychiatric event, sleep disturbances, vivid dreams, insomnia, dizziness, dysphoria, contraindicated in persons with depression or history of seizures

fever is due to causes other than malaria. There is also a danger in the under- and overuse of such standby treatment; however, in certain circumstances the treatment may be life-saving if no access to medical care is available. The choice of emergency standby treatment is unfortunately quite limited and should be prescribed cautiously based on clear written instructions to the traveler on how and when to take the medication. As a rule of thumb, malaria treatment regimens should not use the same drugs that may have been used for chemoprophylaxis as resistant parasites may emerge and

side effects may be compounded. Qualified medical care should be sought at the first opportunity.

The treatment of malaria depends upon the severity of disease and dictates whether oral or parenteral treatment is indicated.[56] Antimalarial drugs used for the treatment of malaria are summarized in Table 26.2. Many of the same drugs used for chemoprophylaxis are also used for the treatment of uncomplicated malaria albeit at different dosage regimens. The physician should take a careful travel history in the clinically ill patient with malaria to document which if any antimalarials may have been used previously and to avoid the same drugs for treatment that may have been used for chemoprophylaxis.

Artemisinin-based combination therapy (ACT) is a new class of antimalarials with potent activity resulting in a rapid clearance of parasitemia and is currently the therapy-of-choice for treatment of uncomplicated malaria. Artemisinin is a sesquiterpene lactone extracted from the sweet wormwood plant *Artemisia annua*, and has long been used by the Chinese as an herbal remedy for malaria. It is particularly effective against multidrug-resistant malaria. However, because of its relatively short half-life, it must be combined with a longer acting antimalarial to avoid the induction of drug resistance. A highly efficacious fixed-dose combination of artemether (20 mg) and lumefantrine (120 mg) has been produced for the treatment of the *P. falciparum* malaria and is marketed in endemic countries as Coartem® or in industrialized countries as Riamet® (it is not FDA-cleared for use in the United States).[57] The combination of these two drugs rapidly clears malaria parasites from the blood and prevents recrudescence. Unfortunately, either counterfeit artemisinin-based drugs or artemisinins manufactured under poor quality control with variable or no antimalarial activity are frequently sold in foreign countries and caution is advised when purchasing such medications.

The combination of sulfadoxine and pyrimethamine (Fansidar®) is no longer considered first-line therapy for uncomplicated malaria as resistance to this drug combination has rapidly emerged on several continents. Infrequent but severe cutaneous skin reactions that include Stevens-Johnson syndrome and other adverse reactions such as megaloblastic anemia and severe liver dysfunction have been described. Quinine sulfate (7 days duration) is still a very effective antimalarial for uncomplicated *P. falciparum* malaria especially when it is combined with doxycycline (200 mg daily for 7 days) or in some cases when combined with clindamycin (300 mg base 4 times daily for 5 days). Patients should be cautioned that quinine may induce nausea and vomiting and tinnitus and should be used cautiously in patients on beta-blockers, or other cardiosuppressant medications. Amodiaquine is readily available over-the-counter in many foreign countries although its effectiveness due to emerging drug resistance is variable. It is not generally considered first-line therapy. Halofantrine should not be used unless there are no alternative antimalarial medications available, and it should only be used under medical supervision due to its known risk of fatal cardiotoxicity associated with QTC interval prolongation.

The treatment of severe and complicated *P. falciparum* malaria in a critically ill patient with prostration, impaired consciousness, respiratory distress, shock, or acute renal failure or in a moderately ill patient with high parasitemia in excess of 1% requires intravenous administration to rapidly kill circulating and sequestered parasites.[58–60] Until recently only quinine dihydrochloride or quinidine gluconate were the drugs of choice for severe and complicated *P. falciparum* malaria. Quinine can induce severe hypoglycemia and should be administered slowly after an appropriate loading dose (see Table 26.3) with frequent glucose monitoring. In the United States, intravenous quinine is not available, and limited supplies of quinidine gluconate are available. Quinidine (10 mg salt/kg equivalent to 6.25 mg base/kg) should be infused over 2 hours followed by a continuous infusion of 0.02 mg salt/kg/min (0.0125 mg/kg/min base) until the parasitemia drops and the patient can take quinine sulfate orally (600 mg every 8 hours) to complete the treatment course for 7 days. Continual cardiac telemetry monitoring is essential as both quinidine and quinine may induce life-threatening cardiac arrhythmias. In certain situations, exchange transfusion may be indicated to rapidly lower the peripheral parasitemia and correct the metabolic acidosis; however, its effectiveness has not been proven.

Recent clinical trials have shown that an intravenous formulation of artesunate (an artimisinin derivative) reduced mortality from *P. falciparum* malaria to 15% compared to 22% in patients who received quinine, the drug recommended for the treatment of severe malaria throughout Africa, South America, and most of Asia.[61–62] Intravenous artesunate is currently undergoing clinical trials using a product manufactured under Good-Manufacturing Practices (GMP) to support the licensure application to the U.S. Food and Drug Administration for use in the United States and abroad.

CONCLUSION

A traveler planning an expedition to a remote region where malaria may be transmitted should strongly be encouraged to consult an expert in travel medicine. The objective is to ensure that the voyager remains healthy and fit to engage in the adventure with confidence that he or she has prepared for any encounter with the deadly malaria enemy. There are excellent resources available on the Internet regarding travelers' malaria.

Excellent up-to-date information on geographic risk for malaria, sources for travel medicine clinics, chemoprophylaxis, and treatment recommendations include:

1. U.S. Centers for Disease Control
   Hotline (770) 488–7788 or (770) 488–7100 after hours. Ask to page the malaria person on call.
   http://www.cdc.gov/malaria/index.htm
   http://www.cdc.gov/travel/
2. World Health Organization links to malaria
   http://www.who.int/malaria/home
   http://www.euro.who.int/malaria/about/ 20020611_3

Table 26.3. Treatment regimens for severe and complicated malaria adults and children

Antimalarial drug	Dosage	Possible side effects/contraindications
Quinine dihydrochloride (intravenous)	Rapid loading dose: 7 mg/kg (salt) infused over 30 minutes followed by 10 mg/kg (salt) infused over 4 hr in 5% dextrose solution. Repeat infusion every 8 hr till parasitemia falls below 1% then switch to oral quinine/doxycycline as per instructions in this table.	Hypoglycemia, cardiac arrhythmias, tinnitus. Do not give loading dose if quinine or mefloquine given within previous 24 hr.
Quinine sulfate/doxycycline initiate after parasite density declines to < 1% and able to tolerate oral intake	Quinine (600 mg three times q 8 hr po) and doxycycline (100 mg q 12 hr po) × 7 days).	Stomach cramps, diarrhea, blurred vision, lightheadedness, dizziness, unusual bleeding, arrhythmias, tinnitus. Doxycycline NOT for children younger than 8 yr of age.
Quinidine gluconate	Loading dose: 10 mg/kg (salt) infused over 2 hr followed immediately by continuous infusion of 0.02 mg/kg/min (salt) until parasite density < 1% and patient able to tolerate oral intake. Then continue with oral quinine sulfate /doxycycline per instructions in this table.	Cardiac conduction arrhythmias.
Artesunate (not available in United States 2007)/ doxycycline	Infuse artesunate 2.4 mg/kg × 1 time then 1.2 mg/kg at 12 hr and 24 hr, then 1.2 mg/kg daily until parasites no longer detectable. After parasites clear continue with doxycycline 100 mg q 12 po × 7 days.	Insufficient data available to assess side effects.

http://www.who.int/ith/en/
http://whqlibdoc.who.int/publications/ 2005/9241580 364_chap7.pdf
3. Travex®
http://www.travax.nhs.uk
4. U.K. National Travel Health Network and Centre
http://www.nathnac.org
5. U.K. Health Protection Agency (HPA Malaria Reference Laboratory)
020 7636 3924 weekdays 10:00–15:00 hrs
http://www.malaria-reference.co.uk
http://www.hpa.org.uk/infections/topics_az/malaria
6. Fit for Travel
http://fitfortravel.nhs.uk

REFERENCES

1 Kain KC, Keystone JS. Malaria in travelers: epidemiology, disease, and prevention. *Infect Dis Clin North Am.* 1998;12(2):267–84.
2 Newman RD, Parise ME, Barber AM, Steketee RW. Malaria-related deaths among U.S. travelers, 1963–2001. *Ann Intern Med.* 2004;141(7):547–55.
3 Muentener P, Schlagenhauf P, Steffen R. Imported malaria (1985–95): trends and perspectives. *Bull World Health Organ.* 1999;77(7):560–6.
4 Skarbinski J, James EM, Causer LM, Barber AM, Mali S, Nguyen-Dinh P, Roberts JM, Parise ME, Slutsker L, Newman RD. Malaria surveillance – United States, 2004. *MMWR Surveill Summ.* 2006;55(4):23–37.
5 Guerra CA, Snow RW, Hay SI. Mapping the global extent of malaria in 2005. *Trends Parasitol.* 2006;22(8):353–8.
6 Anon. World malaria situation in 1994. Part I. Population at risk. *Wkly Epidemiol Rec.* 1997;72(36):269–74.
7 Honigsbaum M. *The Fever Trail: In Search of the Cure for Malaria.* New York: Farrar, Straus and Giroux; 2001: 1–307.
8 Rocco F. *The Miraculous Fever-Tree. Malaria and the Quest for a Cure That Changed the World.* New York: HarperCollins; 2003: 1–348.
9 Ockenhouse CF, Magill A, Smith D, Milhous W. History of U.S. military contributions to the study of malaria. *Mil Med.* 2005;170(4 Suppl):12–16.
10 Baird JK, Hoffman SL. Primaquine therapy for malaria. *Clin Infect Dis.* 2004;39(9):1336–45.
11 Beeson JG, Brown GV. Pathogenesis of *Plasmodium falciparum* malaria: the roles of parasite adhesion and antigenic variation. *Cell Mol Life Sci.* 2002;59(2):258–71.

12 Chen Q, Schlichtherle M, Wahlgren M. Molecular aspects of severe malaria. *Clin Microbiol Rev.* 2000l;13(3):439–50.

13 Planche T, Krishna S. The relevance of malaria pathophysiology to strategies of clinical management. *Curr Opin Infect Dis.* 2005;(5):369–75.

14 Lesho EP, George S, Wortmann G. Fever in a returned traveler. *Cleve Clin J Med.* 2005;72(10):921–7.

15 Anon. *International Travel and Health 2005/2006.* WHO publication. *http://www.who.int/ith/en/*; Chapter 7, pp. 132–51.

16 Guyatt HL, Snow RW. The cost of not treating bednets. *Trends Parasitol.* 2002;18(1):12–16.

17 Lengeler C. Insecticide-treated bednets and curtains for preventing malaria. *Cochrane Database Syst Rev.* 2000;(2): CD000363. Update in: *Cochrane Database Syst Rev.* 2004;(2): CD000363.

18 Fradin MS. Mosquitoes and mosquito repellents: a clinician's guide. *Ann Intern Med.* 1998;128(11):931–40.

19 Fradin MS, Day JF. Comparative efficacy of insect repellents against mosquito bites. *N Engl J Med.* 2002;347(1):13–18.

20 Frances SP, Van Dung N, Beebe NW, Debboun M. Field evaluation of repellent formulations against daytime and night-time biting mosquitoes in a tropical rainforest in northern Australia. *J Med Entomol.* 2002;39(3):541–4.

21 Brown M, Hebert AA. Insect repellents: an overview. *J Am Acad Dermatol.* 1997;36(2 Pt 1):243–9.

22 Sudakin DL, Trevathan WR. DEET: a review and update of safety and risk in the general population. *J Toxicol Clin Toxicol.* 2003;41(6):831–9.

23 Anon. Picardin – a new insect repellent. *Med Lett Drugs Ther.* 2005;47(1210):46–7.

24 Franco-Paredes C, Santos-Preciado JI. Problem pathogens: prevention of malaria in travellers. *Lancet Infect Dis.* 2006;6(3):139–49.

25 Petersen E. Malaria chemoprophylaxis: when should we use it and what are the options? *Expert Rev Anti Infect Ther.* 2004;2(1):119–32.

26 Chen LH, Keystone JS. New strategies for the prevention of malaria in travelers. *Infect Dis Clin North Am.* 2005;19(1): 185–210.

27 Shanks GD, Edstein MD. Modern malaria chemoprophylaxis. *Drugs.* 2005;65(15):2091–110.

28 Schwartz E, Parise M, Kozarsky P, Cetron M. Delayed onset of malaria – implications for chemoprophylaxis in travelers. *N Engl J Med.* 2003;349(16):1510–16.

29 Garner P, Brabin B. A review of randomized controlled trials of routine antimalarial drug prophylaxis during pregnancy in endemic malarious areas. *Bull World Health Organ.* 1994;72(1):89–99.

30 Phillips-Howard PA, Wood D. The safety of antimalarial drugs in pregnancy. *Drug Saf.* 1996;14(3):131–45.

31 Croft AM, Whitehouse DP, Cook GC, Beer MD. Safety evaluation of the drugs available to prevent malaria. *Expert Opin Drug Saf.* 2002;1(1):19–27.

32 Lobel HO, Kozarsky PE. Update on prevention of malaria for travelers. *JAMA.* 1997;278:1767–71.

33 Schlagenhauf P. Mefloquine for malaria chemoprophylaxis 1992–1998: a review. *J Travel Med.* 1999; 6:122–33.

34 Croft AMJ, Garner P. Mefloquine to prevent malaria: a systematic review of trials. *BMJ.* 1997;315:1412–16.

35 Steffen R, Fuchs E, Schildknecht J, Naef U, Funk M, Schlagenhauf P, Phillips-Howard P, Nevill C, Sturchler D. Mefloquine compared with other malaria chemoprophylactic regimens in tourists visiting east Africa. *Lancet.* 993;341 (8856):1299–303.

36 Ohrt C, Richie TL, Widjaja H, Shanks GD, Fitriadi J, Fryauff DJ, Handschin J, Tang D, Sandjaja B, Tjitra E, Hadiarso L, Watt G, Wignall FS. Mefloquine compared with doxycycline for the prophylaxis of malaria in Indonesian soldiers. A randomized, double-blind, placebo-controlled trial. *Ann Intern Med.* 1997;126(12):963–72.

37 Shanks GD, Roessler P, Edstein MD, Rieckmann KH. Doxycycline for malaria prophylaxis in Australian soldiers deployed to United Nations missions in Somalia and Cambodia. *Mil Med.* 1995;160(9):443–5.

38 Pang LW, Limsomwong N, Boudreau EF, Singharaj P. Doxycycline prophylaxis for falciparum malaria. *Lancet.* 1987;1(8543):1161–4.

39 Hogh B, Clarke PD, Camus D, Nothdurft HD, Overbosch D, Gunther M, Joubert I, Kain KC, Shaw D, Roskell NS, Chulay JD; Malarone International Study Team. Atovaquone-proguanil versus chloroquine-proguanil for malaria prophylaxis in non-immune travellers: a randomised, double-blind study. Malarone International Study Team. *Lancet.* 2000;356(9245):1888–94.

40 Overbosch D, Schilthuis H, Bienzle U, Behrens RH, Kain KC, Clarke PD, Toovey S, Knobloch J, Nothdurft HD, Shaw D, Roskell NS, Chulay JD; Malarone International Study Team. Atovaquone-proguanil versus mefloquine for malaria prophylaxis in nonimmune travelers: results from a randomized, double-blind study. *Clin Infect Dis.* 2001;33 (7):1015–21.

41 Berman JD, Nielsen R, Chulay JD, Dowler M, Kain KC, Kester KE, Williams J, Whelen AC, Shmuklarsky MJ. Causal prophylactic efficacy of atovaquone-proguanil (Malarone) in a human challenge model. *Trans R Soc Trop Med Hyg.* 95(4):429–32.

42 Shanks GD, Gordon DM, Klotz FW, Aleman GM, Oloo AJ, Sadie D, Scott TR. Efficacy and safety of atovaquone/proguanil as suppressive prophylaxis for *Plasmodium falciparum* malaria. *Clin Infect Dis.* 1998;27(3):494–9.

43 Ling J, Baird JK, Fryauff DJ, Sismadi P, Bangs MJ, Lacy M, Barcus MJ, Gramzinski R, Maguire JD, Kumusumangsih M, Miller GB, Jones TR, Chulay JD, Hoffman SL; Naval Medical Research Unit 2 Clinical Trial Team. Randomized, placebo-controlled trial of atovaquone/proguanil for the prevention of *Plasmodium falciparum* or *Plasmodium vivax* malaria among migrants to Papua, Indonesia. *Clin Infect Dis.* 2002;35(7):825–33.

44 Schlagenhauf P, Tschopp A, Johnson R, Nothdurft HD, Beck B, Schwartz E, Herold M, Krebs B, Veit O, Allwinn R, Steffen R. Tolerability of malaria chemoprophylaxis in non-immune travellers to sub-Saharan Africa: multicentre, randomised, double blind, four arm study. *BMJ.* 2003;327(7423):1078.

45 Baudon D, Martet G, Pascal B, Bernard J, Keundjian A, Laroche R. Efficacy of daily antimalarial chemoprophylaxis in tropical Africa using either doxycycline or chloroquine-proguanil; a study conducted in 1996 in the French Army. *Trans R Soc Trop Med Hyg.* 1999;93(3):302–3.

46 Fryauff DJ, Baird JK, Basri H, Sumawinata I, Purnomo, Richie TL, Ohrt CK, Mouzin E, Church CJ, Richards AL, et al. Randomised placebo-controlled trial of primaquine for prophylaxis of *falciparum* and *vivax* malaria. *Lancet.* 1995;346(8984):1190–3.

47 Baird JK, Fryauff DJ, Basri H, Bangs MJ, Subianto B, Wiady I, Purnomo, Leksana B, Masbar S, Richie TL, et al. Primaquine for prophylaxis against malaria among nonimmune transmigrants in Irian Jaya, Indonesia. *Am J Trop Med Hyg.* 1995;52(6):479–84.

48 Schwartz E, Regev-Yochay G. Primaquine as prophylaxis for malaria for nonimmune travelers: a comparison with mefloquine and doxycycline. *Clin Infect Dis.* 1999;(6):1502–6.

49 Baird JK, Fryauff DJ, Hoffman SL. Primaquine for prevention of malaria in travelers. *Clin Infect Dis.* 2003;37(12):1659–67.

50 Arnold J, Alving AS, Hockwald RS, Clayman CB, Dern RJ, Beutler E, Flanagan CL, Jeffrey GM. The antimalarial action of primaquine against the blood and tissue stages of falciparum malaria (Panama, P-F-6 strain). *J Lab Clin Med.* 1955;46(3):391–7.

51 Whitty CJM, Armstrong M, Behrens RH. Self-testing for *falciparum* malaria with antigen-capture cards by travelers with symptoms of malaria. *Am J Trop Med Hyg.* 2000;63 (5–6):295–7.

52 Murray CK, Bell D, Gasser RA, Wongsrichanalai C. Rapid diagnostic testing for malaria. *Trop Med Int Health.* 2003;8(10):876–83.

53 Moody A. Rapid diagnostic tests for malaria parasites. *Clin Microbiol Rev.* 2002;15(1):66–78.

54 Chen LH, Keystone JS. New strategies for the prevention of malaria in travelers. *Infect Dis Clin North Am.* 2005;19(1): 185–210.

55 Chen LH, Wilson ME, Schlagenhauf P. Prevention of malaria in long-term travelers. *JAMA.* 2006;296(18):2234–44.

56 Lalloo DG, Shingadia D, Pasvol G, Chiodini PL, Whitty CJ, Beeching NJ, Hill DR, Warrell DA, Bannister BA; HPA Advisory Committee on Malaria Prevention in UK Travellers. UK malaria treatment guidelines. *J Infect.* 2007;54(2): 111–21.

57 Wernsdorfer WH. Coartemether (artemether and lumefantrine): an oral antimalarial drug. *Expert Rev Anti Infect Ther.* 2004;2(2):181–96.

58 Pasvol G. The treatment of complicated and severe malaria. *Br Med Bull.* 2006;75–76:29–47.

59 Pasvol G. Management of severe malaria: interventions and controversies. *Infect Dis Clin N Am.* 2005; 211–16.

60 Mishra SK, Mohanty S, Mohanty A, Das BS. Management of severe and complicated malaria. *J Postgrad Med.* 2006;52(4):281–7.

61 Dondorp A, Nosten F, Stepniewska K, Day N, White N; South East Asian Quinine Artesunate Malaria Trial (SEAQUAMAT) group. Artesunate versus quinine for treatment of severe *falciparum* malaria: a randomised trial. *Lancet.* 2005;366(9487):717–25.

62 Jelinek T. Intravenous artesunate recommended for patients with severe malaria: position statement from TropNetEurop. *Euro Surveill.* 2005;10(11):E051124.5.

Jenny R. Hargrove, MD, and Luanne Freer, MD, FACEP, FAWM

Wild animal attacks are a unique subset of injuries. Multiple injuries in any combination occur such as extensive complex lacerations and puncture wounds, crush injuries, evisceration, and blunt trauma. In addition to the challenge of managing these in less than ideal environments, there is often a hysteria that goes along with these types of attacks. Mainstream news headlines such as the mauling and subsequent eating of the "Grizzly Man" Timothy Treadwill and his girlfriend by bears in Alaska; Steve Irwin's unnerving demise after a "freak" accident involving a stingray (AP, 2006); and the tiger attack on Roy of Siegfried and Roy have served to feed into public misunderstanding of wild creatures and their behaviors (Marquez, 2003; Herzog, 2005). In this chapter, we will explore prevention, management, and treatment of bites and injuries inflicted by large and small mammals, herbivores, predators, large birds, reptiles, and hazardous aquatic life.

EPIDEMIOLOGY

In the United States, 2 million to 4.5 million animal bites occur annually. Only 1% of these require hospitalization. The majority of these reported bites are dogs (80–85%) and cats (10%), with other animals (rodents, rabbits, horses, raccoons, bats, skunks, and monkeys) making up the remaining 5–10% (2006).

A study done in the United States estimated 177 animal-related fatalities a year (excluding zoonotic infections and animal–vehicle collisions), and 61% of these fatalities were caused by nonvenomous animals. The majority of these cases were caused by "other specified animal" on chart review. However, it can be inferred from mechanism of injury that the majority of these were likely caused by farm animals. Dogs accounted for the second largest category of fatalities. Males had a two to three times greater risk than females for venomous and nonvenomous fatalities. Fatalities were overall much greater in the southern region of the United States (Langley, 2005). These statistics, however, are largely from domestic animals and cannot be reliably extrapolated to the wild animal population. Children ages 5–9, predominately male, are at greatest risk of injury from dog bites and males have an almost two times greater risk of death from dog bite injury (Spence, 1990; Sinclair and Zhou, 1995; Holmes, 1998). Bites are reportedly underestimated in children; in one survey of children 4–18 years old, the animal bite rate was 36 times greater than the reported bite rate (Beck and Jones, 1985; Beck, 1991).

There are no reliable estimates of annual worldwide animal attacks. In sub-Saharan Africa several thousand people are killed every year by big game animals including man-eating lions (Freer, 2007). A 2002 World Health Organization (WHO) survey conducted in India reported an incidence of major injury from mammal attack to be 5.3 per 1,000 population (2003). It is unclear how many of these were domestic versus wild animal attacks. It is reasonable to assume, however that the frequency of bites as well as morbidity and mortality are much higher in underdeveloped countries due to a greater exposure to wild animal populations and relative paucity of medical care in these regions.

PREVENTION

Rural and country living is on the rise in the United States. It is estimated that 50 million people now live in nonmetropolitan areas within the United States (Cromartie, 2007). Civilization is steadily encroaching on wildlife habitat and this increases the likelihood of encounters with wild animals; preventing dangerous encounters is becoming ever more important.

Travel to wild and exotic locations is becoming increasingly popular. Stepping into the wilderness as humans puts us into an environment and hierarchy of other living creatures. Human encounters with wild animals occasionally provoke aggressive behavior resulting in attack and injury to the human. When one is traveling to a particular region known to be inhabited by dangerous wild animals, it behooves the visitor to educate him/herself about that animal's patterns of behavior, habitats, mannerisms, and perceived provocations. Knowing what to do and what not to do in certain situations may be the difference between life and death.

Individual animal patterns and behaviors and methods for prevention will be discussed within each section.

PREHOSPITAL CARE

Patient assessment and treatment in the field can be challenging, and rescuers should remember that scene safety is the priority. Large cats and other predatory creatures may remain in the vicinity following a recent attack, placing rescuers and bystanders at risk. A watchful, observant eye should be kept for return of the animal while rapid patient evaluation takes place, and, ideally, animal control specialists should attend the scene. Large attacking animals can cause life-threatening injuries such as blunt or penetrating trauma. As per conventional trauma life support protocol, rapid assessment of ABCs (airway–breathing–circulation) should take place. Airway stabilization, spinal immobilization, and control of major blood loss by direct pressure should be initiated immediately while plans for evacuation are made since these injuries will likely require definitive trauma care. Delay in delivery to definitive medical care may result in serious complications, including infection. Most victims of large animal attack should be considered multiply traumatized and transported to a capable medical facility.

If delay in transportation to definitive care is inevitable, wound care should be initiated immediately on scene. Early irrigation and cleansing are effective for prevention of wound infection. Debridement of the wound and pressurized irrigation with a syringe and copious potable water is preferred. If a syringe is not available, a plastic bag punctured by a safety pin can be used to produce pressurized irrigation. Use of 1% povidone-iodine solution provides antibacterial and virucidal properties and even use of hand soap can be effective in killing rabies and other viruses. Use at least a liter of water for irrigation and then cover wounds with clean, dry dressings.

Field closure of bite and claw wounds is generally not recommended. However, with certain wounds (for example, those very deep and open to muscle and deep subcutaneous tissues), loose closure and careful dressing after irrigation and cleansing may prevent further exposure to pathogens.

For those bites at high risk for infections, early antibiotic therapy should be initiated. Oral doses of amoxicillin-clavulanate, azithromycin, or ciprofloxacin should be given within one hour of injury (Goldstein, Citron et al., 1998a; Fleisher, 1999; Goldstein, Citron et al., 2002). If care is delayed for days and the wound is especially infection-prone, packing the wound with honey may be effective at prevention of infection as honey has intrinsic antibacterial properties (Phuapradit and Saropala, 1992; Al-Waili and Saloom, 1999).

Reporting the injury, including its location and a description of the animal and its behavior to animal control authorities is important. Capture of the animal by professionals for quarantine and evaluation for rabies may be required. If the animal was killed during the attack, then attempt to transport the animal to authorities, if possible with refrigeration. Care must be taken when handling the animal; gloves and eye protection should be used to avoid potential exposure to rabies especially when handling the head and mucous membranes.

EVALUATION AND TREATMENT

Trauma life support protocols should guide hospital evaluation and treatment of victims of animal attack; life-threatening injuries should be addressed first (Klein, 1985). Patterns of injury from certain animals can be predicted; penetrating injuries from goring, biting, and clawing as well as blunt trauma caused by kicking, trampling, or falls may be present. In one study of injuries from large animals falls from horses resulted in extensive craniofacial injury, whereas bull and cow injuries from trampling and kicks resulted in a predominance of torso injuries (Norwood, McAuley, et al., 2000). Fractures of the upper extremity had a higher association with torso and craniofacial injuries than did those of the lower extremity (Norwood, McAuley, et al., 2000). In another study of large animal abdominal trauma, the majority of patients had blunt trauma (93%). Of 33 patients, 22 required surgical intervention and 17 of these patients had small bowel or mesenteric injury; 6 suffered liver or spleen injury (Dahl, 1998).

Resuscitation with intravenous fluids and/or blood products may be needed for patients with extensive bleeding and volume loss. Appropriate diagnostic imaging should take into account patterns of injury from different animals. Surgical consultation may be required depending on the injury. Long bone fractures should be immobilized. Prophylactic antibiotics should be used in high-risk wounds or in patients with comorbidities associated with immune compromise. High-risk cases include wounds with open fractures, penetrating torso injuries, severe craniofacial trauma associated with fractures, and deep, extensive, contaminated lacerations and crush injuries among others. Hospital admission may be required for extensive injuries requiring surgery or observation and should be considered for patients with wounds at high risk for infection, or for those in need of pain control.

WOUND CARE

Wounds from animal attacks should be treated with a presumption of polymicrobial contamination.

Bite wounds introduce oral flora, and the bacterial content varies between species. Soil, urine, and feces contamination from claw and scratch injuries should be assumed. Wounded tissue is often crushed and macerated, leading to higher rates of infection. These wounds may not only develop local infection but are also at risk for development of zoonotic infection and systemic disease.

Even after field treatment wound care, hospital treatment should again be directed at aggressive irrigation and debridement of wounds. Debridement is most effective for removing soil, clots, and bacteria (Fleisher, 1999). In one study, high-pressure, low-volume irrigation versus low-pressure, high-volume techniques were found to be equally effective (Pronchik, Barber, et al., 1999). High-pressure irrigation of 15 psi or higher reduces bacterial counts in the wound by approximately 90% (Granick, Tenenhaus, et al., 2007), and a 19-gauge needle attached to a 35cc or 65cc syringe can produce psi of 25–35 (Singer, Hollander, et al., 1994). Tap water appears to be as effective as sterile solutions for irrigation (Valente, Forti, et al., 2003). Iodine in 1% solution has broad antimicrobial and virucidal properties and is safe and nontoxic to wounds in this concentration (Viljanto, 1980; Oberg, 1987). Other solutions such as hydrogen peroxide, alcohols, and higher concentrations of iodine are toxic, inhibit wound healing, and should not be used on open wounds.

When considering wound closure, one must factor risk of infection, functional recovery, and cosmesis. High-risk wounds are those to the hands and feet, deep puncture wounds, crush injuries, bites overlying joints or vital structures or those with risk of cranial, orbit, or sinus penetration. Primate bites (including humans) have an extremely high risk of infection as do bites of cats, swine, crocodiles, and alligators. Any patient who has significant medical comorbidities or who is in an immunocompromised state (patients with diabetes, HIV, on chronic steroid or immunosuppressive therapy, or

with prosthetic heart valves or prosthesis) is at increased risk for infection. Primary wound closure in all high-risk cases should be undertaken only with extreme caution, if at all.

Hand injuries and bites are quite frequent and carry a high risk of infection due to multiple compartments and relatively reduced vascularity (Maimaris and Quinton, 1988). In one study, the infection rate in bites to the hand rose from 18.8 to 25% after suture closure (Aigner, Konig, et al., 1996). However, a recent study has shown similar outcomes in small, uncomplicated bites to the hand that were closed primarily vs treated conservatively (Quinn, Cummings, et al., 2002). Immobilization is an important component of treatment of extremity bites as movement will increase the risk of bacterial spread to different compartment (Bennett, 1988).

Facial and scalp wounds (Figure 27.1) have a much lower rate of infection even after repair and tend to do very well (Aigner, Konig, et al., 1996). Facial injuries carry cosmetic consequences and should, in general, be closed primarily (Wolff, 1998; Stefanopoulos, Karabouta, et al., 2004).

Small, linear, uncomplicated lacerations may be repaired within 12–24 hours. Delayed primary closure is another alternative to consider, and if this option is chosen, wounds must be kept clean and moist with saline dressing until closure. Wounds left open require special care with ongoing debridement, irrigation, wet to dry dressing changes, and close daily monitoring. Please see Chapter 35 for further discussion of specific wound closure techniques. Triple antibiotic ointment therapy may aid healing of abrasions and minor scratches, but it is less useful for deeper, repaired lacerations or punctures (Geronemus, Mertz, et al., 1979; Leyden and Sulzberger, 1981). Clean, nonadhesive absorptive dressings are appropriate for lacerations or abrasions that continue to ooze. Follow-up care and daily wound inspections for high-risk wounds are highly recommended.

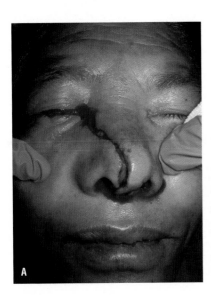
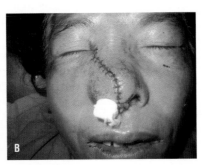

Figure 27.1. Yak goring in Nepal. (A) initial injury (B) repaired. Photo courtesy of Anne Perry.

Wound cultures of fresh wounds provide no useful information and do not guide therapy. Cultures of *infected* wounds, however, should help practitioners choose appropriate antibiotic treatment. Blood cultures should be obtained if patients show signs of systemic infection. Unusual or uncommon pathogens that infect bite wounds may be missed by local lab workers on routine cultures; cultures taken from patients with sepsis and high-risk infections should be sent to both local labs and reference labs or to the CDC as this strategy increases the likelihood of identifying the offending pathogen (Talan, Citron, et al., 1999).

INFECTION

Prophylactic antibiotics for low-risk wounds are no longer routinely recommended if thorough debridement and irrigation techniques are employed expeditiously. Certain species associated with high risk of infection and extensive bites to the hand are scenarios where antibiotic prophylactic therapy is likely appropriate (Wiggins, Akelman, et al., 1994; Fleisher, 1999; Medeiros and Saconato, 2001; Tuncali, Bingul, et al., 2005). If used, prophylaxis should be directed against pathogens known to be associated with the attacking species.

The list of aerobic and anaerobic bacteria that cause infections is extensive. These pathogens may cause infections ranging from cellulitis to abscess formation to bacteremia and sepsis. Patients should be examined daily for wound redness, heat, induration, swelling, fluctuance, and tenderness, as well as for lymphangitic streaks, lymphadenopathy, and fever. Once infection is established, empiric therapy should be initiated. Appropriate empiric therapy recommendations, established on the Emergency Medicine Animal Bite Infection Study Group, includes a beta-lactam antibiotic and a beta-lactamase inhibitor, a second-generation cephalosporin with anaerobic activity, or a combination therapy with penicillin and a first-generation cephalosporin or clindamycin and a fluroquinolone (Talan, Citron, et al., 1999). Azithromycin has also been shown to be effective against certain unusual animal pathogens (Goldstein, Citron, et al., 1998a; 1998b). As with any infection, cultures and sensitivities should guide antibiotic therapy. Gangrene requiring amputation, osteomyelitis, septic joints, endocarditis, meningoencephalitis, pneumonitis, and septic deaths have all been reported in victims of animal attack (Findling, Pohlmann, et al., 1980; Kullberg, Westendorp, et al., 1991; Alberio and Lammle, 1998).

TETANUS

Clostridium tetani spores are ubiquitous, wild animal oral flora included. Tetanus spores take about 7–21 days to incubate. Any victim who has received a full vaccination series and a booster within 5 years is usually sufficiently protected from tetanus. If a patient has had the vaccination series but is not within 5 years of booster administration, then a 0.5 cc intramuscular injection of diphtheria-tetanus toxoid (Td) booster vaccine or tetanus-acellular pertussis-diphtheria toxoid (Tdap) booster vaccine should be prescribed. If the patient has a high-risk wound and there is any question of the vaccination status, then they should receive 250 to 500 units of tetanus human immune globulin (TIG) as well as the vaccine, administered in separate arms. If the patient received his last tetanus booster more than 10 years prior, but has had the vaccination, then TIG administration should be considered because 4 days may be needed to mount an appropriate immune response from a booster dose. Booster doses should be repeated at 30 and 60 days to complete the vaccination series for immunization.

ZOONOSES

Wild animals not only are known to transmit a myriad of systemic diseases and parasites but also are vector carriers. Some transmission occurs through bites and scratches; however, a large number of diseases are transmitted through saliva, nasal secretions, urine, and feces. Examples include rabies, cat-scratch disease, monkeypox virus, simian herpes virus, tularemia, Hantavirus, tetanus, Q fever, and toxoplasmosis.

RABIES

Rabies is a neurotropic rhabdovirus transmitted through saliva of infected animals. It is rapidly progressive with an extremely high mortality rate, and victims typically die within several days. According to the CDC, over 55,000 cases are diagnosed worldwide each year. There is currently no known reservoir host. Only six people have been known to survive rabies, most of these with long-term neurologic sequelae, and all but one received pre- or postexposure prophylaxis (Willoughby, Tieves, et al., 2005).

In the United States and Puerto Rico in 2004, 92% of reported rabies occurred in wildlife. Raccoons, skunks, and bats represented the majority of these cases (Krebs, Mandel, et al., 2005). Most human rabies in the United States is linked to exposure to rabid bats (Noah, Drenzek, et al., 1998). Worldwide the majority of rabies in Africa, India, and Southeast Asia is transmitted by dogs (Sriaroon, Sriaroon, et al., 2006; Sudarshan, Madhusudana, et al., 2007).

Risk of exposure to rabies depends on the type of animal, behavior of the animal, and country/region of exposure. In any developing country, the rate of rabies in dogs is so high that postexposure prophylaxis is almost always warranted (Figure 27.2). Unusual or aggressive behavior in the daylight in a typically docile wild animal should raise suspicion.

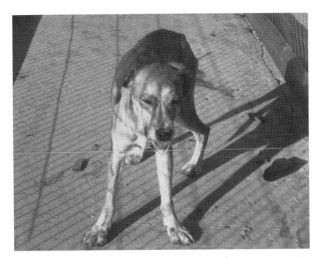

Figure 27.2. Rabid dog. Photo courtesy of Centers for Disease Control and Prevention.

Thorough and prompt cleansing of all wounds with a virucidal agent (povidone-iodine) may substantially decrease viral load (Smith, Fishbein, et al., 1991; Smith, Meadowcroft, et al., 2000). Most soaps have virucidal properties against rabies as well (Larghi, Savy, et al., 1975). Those who frequently travel to rabies endemic regions or those at high risk of exposure through their profession should consider preexposure prophylaxis. Current Centers for Disease Control and Prevention (CDC) guidelines for pre- and postexposure prophylaxis are as follows: preexposure rabies vaccine is administered 1 mL intramuscularly on days 0, 7, 21, and 28. Postexposure prophylaxis for previously unvaccinated persons includes rabies immune globulin 20 IU/kg infiltrated subcutaneously at the wound site (the entire dose if possible) as well as the rabies vaccine administered similar to preexposure schedule except on days 0, 3, 7, 14, and 28. Any expedition participant who has received a significant rabies exposure – including all bat bites and all dog bites in developing countries – should receive prompt wound care and immediate evacuation. Rabies vaccine is discussed in more detail in Chapter 4.

PSYCHIATRIC CONSEQUENCES OF ANIMAL ATTACK

Posttraumatic stress disorder (PTSD) is well documented in adolescents after dog bites. In one study of 22 children bitten by dogs, 12 showed signs and symptoms of PTSD two to nine months after the bite. Violent attacks, multiple or deep bites seemed to have a higher association with symptoms (Peters, Sottiaux, et al., 2004). Panic attacks, flashbacks, and nightmares may afflict the victim and can become disabling. Wild animal attacks have as much potential, if not more to cause PTSD. One case of PTSD was documented in a young girl after a severe cougar mauling (Denholm, 1995). Immediate debriefing after the stressful event, ongoing psychotherapy, and occasional drug therapy

may all be beneficial in treatment for victims of animal attack (Denholm, 1995).

ANIMALS THAT ATTACK

Rodents

Rats, mice, and other small rodents have long had the stigma of transmitting all zoonoses including plague, tularemia, and hantavirus. Rat-bite fever, from infection with *Streptobacillus moniliformis* or *Spirillum minus*, found in oral flora of wild rodents, causes an acute relapsing febrile illness with flu-like symptoms. Wild rat carrier rates may range from 50 to 100% and can be transmitted to other wild or domestic animals. Although few cases have been reported in the United States, rat-bite fever carries a 10% mortality rate and requires high suspicion to enable proper diagnosis and prompt treatment (Shvartsblat, Kochie, et al., 2004; Elliott, 2007).

Transmission of rabies from a rodent bite is rare due to low rates of viral secretion in the saliva and the fact that rodents do not become infected with rabies as readily as other wild animals. Local epidemics do occur, however, and in one epidemic, woodchucks represented the majority of carriers. One rabid woodchuck reportedly attacked an elderly woman knocking her down and biting her multiple times (Ordog, Balasubramanium, et al., 1985; Moro, Horman, et al., 1991).

Prairie-dog transmission of the monkey-pox virus to humans was documented in a 2003 Indiana outbreak in diseased pets, when transmission occurred with direct handling of sick prairie dogs (Kile, Fleischauer, et al., 2005). The virus was initially endemic in imported African rats and squirrels and was subsequently transmitted to prairie dogs (Georges, Matton, et al., 2004). Routes of transmission seem to influence the severity of the disease with bites and scratches producing more severe symptoms than direct contact (Reynolds, Yorita, et al., 2006). Since the small pox vaccine is protective against monkey-pox virus, the CDC recommends those at high risk (pet handlers, veterinarians, lab workers) receive the vaccine. Some experts believe a postexposure vaccine confers protection as well.

Rodent bites represent a small percentage of bites brought to medical attention (Ordog, Balasubramanium, et al., 1985). Laboratory workers, pet owners, and lower socioeconomic groups represent the highest risk groups. Children 5 years and younger are at high risk, and most bites to the hands and face occur during sleep between the hours of midnight and 8 A.M. (Hirschhorn and Hodge, 1999). A survey done in New York correlated risk of bite with degree of rat infestation (Childs, McLafferty, et al., 1998). There have been case reports of globe rupture in an infant, orbital cellulitis, and significant loss of eyelids due to rat bites (Wykes, 1989; Myers and Christmann, 1991; Ouazzani, Dali, et al., 2006). Oral flora is similar to other animal species, and bite infection rates are estimated to be 2–10% even without treatment (Ordog, Balasubramanium, et al., 1985). One case of sporotrichosis was reported in a rat bite victim (Frean, Isaacson, et al., 1991).

Skunks

Skunks represent 27% of rabies carriers in the United States (Krebs, Mandel, et al., 2005). Very few skunk bites are reported; those that do occur are from skunks kept as pets or rabid skunks in the wild. There are no medical reports of infection from skunk bites.

A skunk's main defense mechanism is its well-known spray of a noxious secretion from its anal sac. The animal will often give a warning to offenders by stomping its front feet, then turning and raising the tail in the air, spraying with surprising accuracy to distances up to 12 feet. The spray contains butyl mercaptan, which can cause severe skin irritation, keratoconjunctivis, temporary blindness, nausea and vomiting, excessive salivation, and temporary loss of consciousness. There are no reports of death or serious morbidity in humans from skunk spray. There is one report of methemoglobinemia and Heinz body anemia in a pit bull after being sprayed by a skunk (Wood, Sollers, et al., 2002).

Strong oxidizing agents such as mixture of household bleach (5% hypochlorite solution) diluted 1:5 in water, followed by washing with strong dish soap, followed with another dilute bleach rinse lessen the irritation and odor of skunk spray. Another recipe uses 3% hydrogen peroxide solution (1 quart), ¼ cup of baking soda, and strong liquid dish soap; tomato juice mixed with strong detergent or shampoo may help as well. All methods work by oxidizing the mercaptan and freeing the sulfur to be washed away. It is the authors' opinion after two encounters of this noxious substance with the authors' dog, that nothing works as well as claimed, and that only time is effective at wearing the odor away.

Raccoons

Raccoons are notoriously curious animals that frequent suburban areas raiding trash cans and dump sites. They represent the highest rabies carrier rate, nearly 38%, in the United States (Krebs, Mandel, et al., 2005). The first human death from raccoon variant rabies was reported in 2003 in Virginia although it was unclear how it was contracted as there was no history of bite (Silverstein, et al., 2003). This is significant as epizootic raccoon rabies infections are increasing along the east coast (Wandeler et al., 2000).

Raccoons carry *Baylisascaris procyonis*, a parasite that is known to cause a severe neurologic disorder and ocular disease when acquired by humans. Transmission occurs when raccoon feces laden with infectious eggs are ingested (Gavin, Kazacos, et al., 2005; Shafir, Wise, et al., 2006).

Porcupines

Porcupine attacks injure their victims by impaling them with their quills (Figure 27.3), which are long, barbed, and spongy in the center and can migrate as much as 10 inches under the skin. The quill core will readily absorb bodily fluids and expand, work its way deeper with muscular movement. There are reports of intestinal perforation and intraperitoneal granuloma formation from porcupine quill (McDade and Crandell, 1958; Milrod and Goel, 1958). Dogs have suffered septic arthritis, orbital perforation, and brain penetration secondary to quill migration (Daoust, 1991; Grahn, Szentimrey, et al., 1995; Brisson, Bersenas, et al., 2004).

There are no medical reports of human infections from imbedded quills. This is likely due to quills' mild antiseptic quality as well as prompt removal of the quills in humans. Removal of quills by simple extraction is the best method, but location of the quill, duration of penetration, and surrounding anatomy should be considered before proceeding with extraction. Veterinarian experience with quill extraction guides the techniques used for impaled humans.

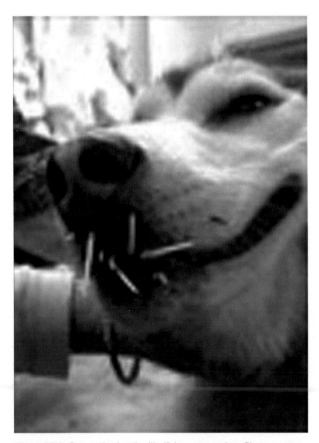

Figure 27.3. Domestic dog "quilled" by a porcupine. Photo courtesy of Luanne Freer.

Bats

The majority of cases of human rabies from exposure to bats in the United States have no definitive history of a bite. This may be due to minimally recognized bite wounds (most likely), nonbite transmission such as aerosol transmission (which has never been clearly documented), or another hypothesis of an intermediate animal that acquires rabies from the bat and then transmits it to humans (less likely) (Gibbons, 2002). Insect-eating bats have very small teeth and therefore produce minimally detectable bites (Noah, Drenzek, et al., 1998). The risk of serious bacterial wound infection from bat bite is low.

Vampire bats found in Central and South America have larger teeth and feed from the blood of animals (including humans) by making a small incision in the skin and drinking the blood meal. In humans, this occurs on any exposed skin surface while they are sleeping at night, but it can be prevented by use of mosquito nets. Blood loss is not significant as one bat feeds a maximum of 1 oz of blood per night.

In July 2004, a rabies outbreak due to bites from vampire bats occurred in a Colombian village resulting in 14 deaths, the largest rabies outbreak in that country to date (Valderrama, Garcia, et al., 2006). In a 2004 survey of rabies in animals in the United States and Puerto Rico, bats represented almost 20% of cases (Krebs, Mandel, et al., 2005). Any history of exposure to a bat should prompt serious consideration of rabies post-exposure prophylaxis. All bat bites should receive wound care and immediate evacuation for rabies prophylaxis.

Swine

Domestic pigs can be aggressive and dangerous, often goring or biting the lower extremities as they attack from behind (Barnham, 1988). Wounds tend to be deep and can carry the usual wide range of bacteria as well as *Pasteurella multicoda* and *Pasteurella aerogenes,* resulting in high rates of infection (Barnham, 1988; Barss and Ennis, 1988; Goldstein, Citron, et al., 1990; Ejlertsen, Gahrn-Hansen, et al., 1996; Lindberg, Frederiksen, et al., 1998). Care must be taken to thoroughly irrigate, explore, and debride these wounds; they are at high risk for infection and prophylactic antibiotics and admission should be considered.

Wild pigs have been known to be even more aggressive than their domestic counterparts. In 2006, a man was gored to death by a wild boar outside of Mangalore, India (Manipady, Menezes, et al., 2006). Feral pigs are quite common in many regions of the world, including Papua New Guinea and can be easily provoked and inflict significant injury (Barss and Ennis, 1988).

Canines

Coyote populations have flourished in recent years and have become an increasing problem in suburbia due to attacks on pets and children. In California alone, there were 41 coyote attacks on humans from 1998 to 2003; the majority of these were on children, and unprovoked and increasingly aggressive behavior in nonrabid coyotes has been observed (Timm, 2004). Rabies has become less problematic in this species due to the success of the oral rabies vaccination of coyote and fox populations (Sidwa, Wilson, et al., 2005; Slate, Rupprecht, et al., 2005).

Wolves are known to be efficient pack hunters and throughout history have represented a threat to humans, particularly in Europe and Asia. "Child lifting" is still reported in India where lone wolves have reportedly picked up children to carry off for a meal. It is presumed wolves resort to human depredation when there is lack of natural prey, close proximity to humans, or lack of fear of humans. In Uttar Pradesh, India, in 1996, over 76 children from villages in the region were preyed on by wolves; over 50 of these children were killed (Jhala, 1997). In North America, where wolves are typically shy and stay well away from man, there have been very few wolf attacks, and the majority of those were reportedly rabid. In 2006, a student hiking alone in northern Saskatchewan was eaten by animals; there continues to be speculation about the actual cause of death, but some believe this case was the first recent-day North American fatality caused by wolves (George, 2006).

Coyote and wolf bites should be treated using the same guidelines as with domestic dogs in terms of closure and antibiotics. Canine bites are often associated with crushed, macerated tissue; lacerations require very thorough debridement.

Most coyotes are shy and can be easily chased away, discouraging attack. Wolves however, can be provoked by a direct stare. With either species, a human at a run may provoke a predatory instinct to chase and attack.

Foxes are shy and rarely attack. Those that do are usually rabid. Rabies is on the decline in this population as well, due to oral vaccination programs (Sidwa, Wilson, et al., 2005). Foxes induce more puncture wounds than other canines; therefore, the bite may be more prone to infection.

Hyenas are notorious for attacking humans, especially children in Africa. They have very powerful jaws and have been known to behead young children and amputate limbs (Loro, Franceschi, et al., 1994). Some develop a taste for human flesh after scavenging on dead or dying human bodies and can rival lions as "man-eaters." Those who survive a hyena attack are frequently quite disfigured.

Dingos are disappearing at an alarming rate in Australia (Johnson, Isaac, et al., 2007). Even though they are one of the top predators of Australia, they pose very little human threat. However, reports of a handful of attacks make these animals potentially dangerous, especially around children (Cameron, 1984).

PRIMATES

Primate bites are infamous for their infectious potential in both human and nonhuman victims. Those at risk for NHP (nonhuman primate) bites are laboratory workers, zookeepers, and pet owners in developed countries. In underdeveloped countries, there are many incidences of aggressive monkey and baboon attacks on humans. Monkeys notoriously populate temples within some Asian cities, where they eat food offerings and come into close contact with locals and tourists and exhibit little if any fear of humans. Bands of monkeys have been known to attack villages in Africa and steal food out of homes and stores when their own source is scarce (Francisco, 2004). Monkeys in India have reportedly developed a taste for ceremonial brew and have been known to become inebriated and attack villagers outside of their homes (Agrawal, 2005). Baboons can be especially aggressive and have been known to kill humans (Figure 27. 4).

Monkey bites tend to be directed at the extremities, and finger amputations are common (Figure 27.5). Bites commonly result in infection rates despite use of prophylactic antibiotics (Goldstein, Pryor, et al., 1995) *Staphylococcus epidermidids, Enterobacteriaceaea enterococci,*

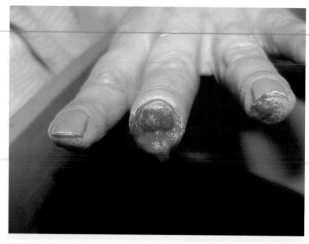

Figure 27.5. Distal finger amputation from gorilla bite. Photo courtesy of Gregory H. Bledsoe.

Beta-hemolytic streptococci, Bacteroides, Fusobacterium, and *Eikenella corrodens* have all been isolated from NHP bites (Goldstein, Pryor, et al., 1995). These bites should be treated with broad spectrum prophylactic antibiotics and close follow-up.

The simian herpes virus (B-virus) infection is an emerging problem; although transmission rate to humans is low, it carries a mortality rate of 80%. The *Macaca* genus is most commonly infected and the adult captive infection rate is 73–100%. These types of monkeys represent the majority of those used in research, which places laboratory workers at high risk. Infected monkeys are typically asymptomatic. Free-ranging feral macaque populations have been found in parts of Texas and Florida (Ostrowski, 1998). Whole bands of rhesus monkeys found to have simian herpes virus have been humanely eradicated in Africa due to their close proximity to villages or safari camps (Identification of Simian Herpes Virus B, 2000). Immediate wound care requires use of virucidal agents such as povidone-iodine solution and cetrimide. Out of 61 persons bitten by infected monkeys and cleaned with these viricidal solutions, none became infected (Tribe and Noren, 1983). Some experts recommend prophylactic use of antiviral medications such as Valacyclovir in the event of monkey bite (Cohen, 2002).

Reclusive and shy, gorillas routinely avoid humans. When confronted they may attack in defense but often will bite once and flee. They usually can be dissuaded from further attack and are very seldom responsible for serious injury. Male chimpanzees are very territorial and occasionally will attack humans. There have been reports of a few cases of chimps killing and eating humans. There are multiple reports of baboon attacks, frequently from visitors in South Africa. Most of these episodes involve baboons searching for food (Yeld, 2004).

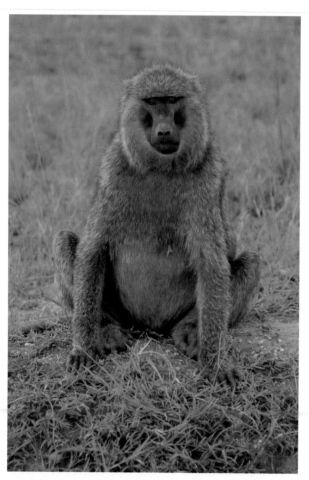

Figure 27.4. Baboon. Photo courtesy of Jenny Hargrove.

HERBIVORES

Deer and Elk

Motor vehicle collisions with deer and elk (Figure 27.6) account for most of the animal-related injuries and fatalities in the United States (Conn, 2004). Most deer–auto collisions occur 1 hour after sunset, so prevention includes slowing down and remaining alert during dusk and night driving, or avoiding driving during these hours in densely deer-populated areas (Haikonen and Summala, 2001). Prevention methods such as the use of deer whistles and road side reflectors have proven useless. Long-term, well-designed, well-maintained fencing combined with herd over- or underpasses are effective collision prevention methods (Hedlund, Curtis, et al., 2004).

Deer are a host for ticks carrying Lyme disease as well as other tick-related illnesses. The increasing deer population in New England directly correlates with the rise in incidence of Lyme disease (Barbour, 1998).

A 73-year-old man died of antler injuries to his face when attacked by a deer outside in his garden. Male deer may become more aggressive during mating season (Kasindorf, 2005), and with diminishing natural habitat and increasing population, injuries can result from goring, kicking, stomping, or rarely biting (Figure 27.7). Bull elk occasionally attack during rutting season and cows will sometimes butt or stomp when protecting their young (Figure 27.8).

Most deer and other ungulates can be easily intimidated and scared away by aggressive behavior (yelling, waving of hands, and even pretending to charge the animal).

Moose

Moose are responsible for a large number of motor vehicle collisions in New England and Sweden (Bjornstig,

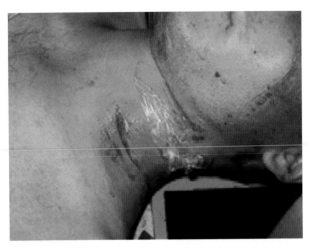

Figure 27.7. Goring from an ungulate horn. Photo courtesy of Luanne Freer.

Eriksson, et al., 1986; Farrell, Sutton, et al., 1996). Moose–vehicle collisions produce a rear and downward deformity of the roof of the car resulting in more head, face, and spine injuries to human occupants (Farrell, Sutton, et al., 1996; Bashir and Abu-Zidan, 2006).

Bull moose in rutting season and cows in calving season can be particularly aggressive. These large animals are capable of inflicting significant injury by stomping, butting, and goring (Figure 27.9). Moose may show signs of raised rump hairs, laid back ears, or licking of lips prior to charging. To avoid attack, a person should seek shelter behind a solid object, climb a tree, or at last resort roll into a ball protecting the head with arms and hands until the moose leaves the scene (Alaska Department of Fish and Game, 1997).

American Bison

Bison reside mainly in and around Yellowstone National Park (Figure 27.10) where the last remaining North

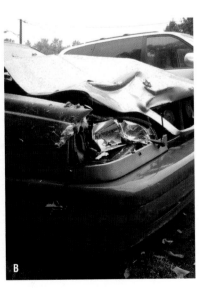

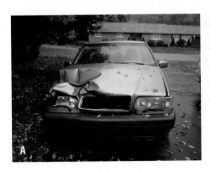

Figure 27.6. Extensive damage to car after high-speed collision with a deer at night. Photo courtesy of Gregory H. Bledsoe.

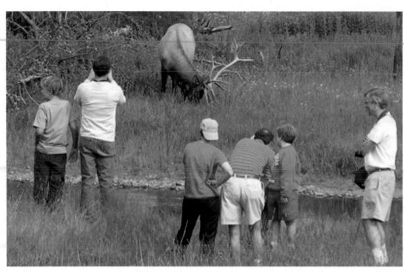

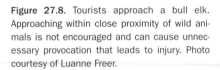

Figure 27.8. Tourists approach a bull elk. Approaching within close proximity of wild animals is not encouraged and can cause unnecessary provocation that leads to injury. Photo courtesy of Luanne Freer.

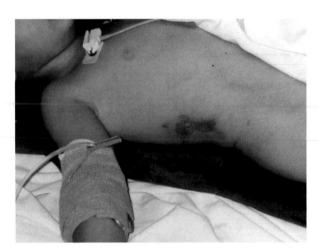

Figure 27.9. Patient stomped by moose. Injuries included fractured ribs and hemopneumothorax. Photo courtesy of Luanne Freer.

American wild herd was brought back from near extinction in the latter half of the twentieth century. From 1975 to 1993, 56 injuries and 3 deaths were reported (Conrad, 1994). When provoked, the bison's massive head and powerful chest are capable of inflicting significant blunt trauma by butting or tossing victims into the air. Gorings with significant penetrating injury and even evisceration have been reported (Conrad, 1994).

Buffalo

One of African's top five big game animals, Cape buffalo (Figure 27.11) are notorious for the severity of their attacks, as they kill more big game hunters than any of the other big game animals. Unprovoked, the buffalo will not generally attack, but if injured, it can turn into a cunning predator, and they are known to double back on the trail

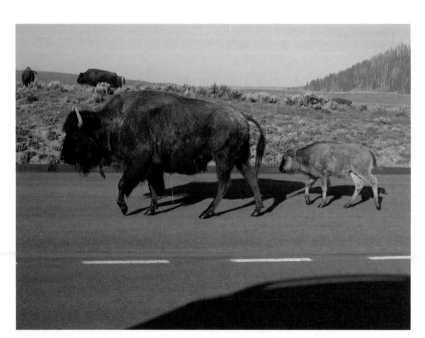

Figure 27.10. American bison in Yellowstone. Photo courtesy of Jenny Hargrove.

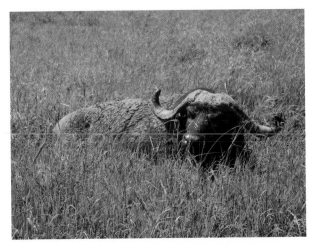

Figure 27.11. Cape buffalo. Photo courtesy of Jenny Hargrove.

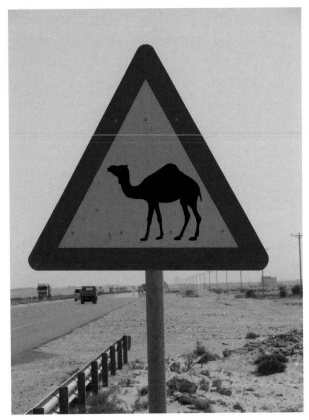

Figure 27.13. Motor vehicle crashes involving camels are a serious concern in certain countries. Photo courtesy of Gregory H. Bledsoe.

to surprise a hunter from behind. Old solitary bulls that are sick or injured may be dangerously aggressive without the safety of the herd. Buffalo can toss their victims up to 10 feet in the air, trample, gore, and disembowel by whipping the head and horns side to side; they kill from 20 to 100 people per year in Africa (Shattock, 1968).

Water buffalo, found on the Indian subcontinent and Southeast Asia, are largely domesticated, and very few if any are left in the wild. They are docile for the most part, but occasionally, if provoked, are capable of attack.

Camels

Largely domesticated, the camel functions as a pack and transportation animal in areas of the Middle East, Africa, and Asia; however, feral populations exist throughout those regions as well as in western Australia. The camel is a temperamental creature capable of spitting, biting, and kicking. Multiple case reports cite significant facial trauma with open fractures and lacerations as a result of camel attack (Singh, Gulati, et al., 1994; Ogunbodede

and Arotiba, 1997; Suess, Magerkurth, et al., 2004; Nawaz, Matta, et al., 2005). Camel jaws are powerful, and their bites are unpredictable (Figure 27.12); open fractures and crushing injuries of shoulders and extremities have been reported (Janjua, 1993; Janjua and van den Berg, 1994).

Camels are also associated with significant motor vehicle collision and injuries (Figure 27.13) because, when struck, the camel usually falls on the roof of the car producing head and cervical spine injury to the occupants inside (Ansari and Ashraf Ali, 1998a; 1998b; Bashir and Abu-Zidan, 2006).

Tapirs

Various species of tapirs reside in Central and South America and Southeast Asia. Almost all species are considered endangered, and they tend to be docile and avoid confrontation. A Brazilian man was attacked in his corn field by a tapir after provoking and attempting to injure it. The farmer was bitten and sustained lacerations to the neck and thighs; he died from exsanguination (Haddad, Assuncao, et al., 2005).

Rhinoceros

Rhinos are large mammals weighing 1–2 tons and are capable of speeds of up to 50 mph (Figure 27.14). They

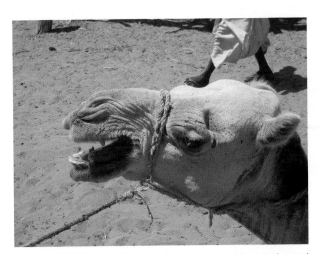

Figure 27.12. The powerful jaws of the often temperamental camel contain large canine teeth. Photo courtesy of Gregory H. Bledsoe.

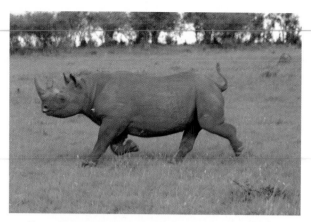

Figure 27.14. Rhinoceros. Photo courtesy of Jenny Hargrove.

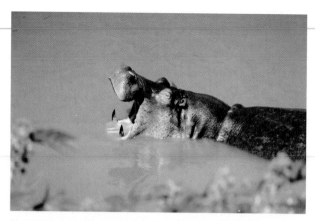

Figure 27.16. The large canine teeth of the hippopotamus are capable of causing significant damage. Photo courtesy of Libby Beatty.

are verily easily provoked and have been known to charge motor vehicles, even trains. Owing to their poor eyesight, they tend to charge at any small sound, movement, or smell. If charged, a victim may attempt to side step. Those who have fallen during pursuit may be given a sniff or two then ignored. If the victim is in the line of charge, however, there is high risk of significant trauma from blunt force at high velocity. At the end of his charge, the rhino will typically hook its horn right or left tossing its victim several feet in the air. Every year a handful of victims are killed by black rhinos in Africa (Durrheim and Leggat, 1999). White rhinos are typically docile and not as aggressive.

Hippopotamus

The hippopotamus (Figure 27.15) is one of the most dangerous land mammals in Africa. If a person is trapped between the hippo and water, or if someone is

in its direct line of travel, the hippopotamus will almost always attack. The males can weigh in excess of 3 tons and can reach speeds of up to 45 miles an hour. Once in motion, they rarely change course. On land there is little chance of surviving a charging hippo if the victim cannot get out of the way. In the water, it is also easily provoked and aggressive. The cows will diligently protect their young. Hippos have gaping jaws with huge canines (Figure 27.16) and can easily chop boats and people in half. Survivors of a hippo attack are rare; injuries tend to be extensive with internal organ injuries, long bone fractures, and other crush injuries (Pickles, 1987; Lin and Hulsey, 1993; Durrheim and Leggat, 1999).

Elephants

Most reported elephant attacks in Africa are from injured, hunted elephants or occur when humans approach too closely. In these two scenarios attacks

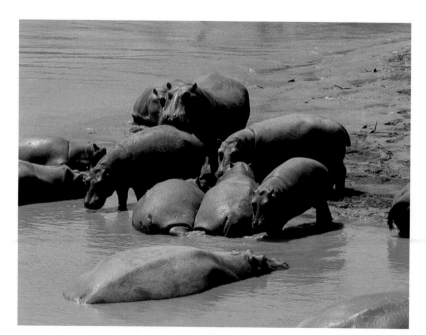

Figure 27.15. Hippopotamus. Photo courtesy of Jenny Hargrove.

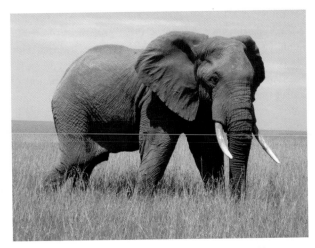

Figure 27.17. African elephant. Photo courtesy of Jenny Hargrove.

are provoked. Occasionally a rogue elephant that is injured or intoxicated from eating fermented marula berries may seek out and kill humans for unknown reasons. In one instance, a rogue elephant was captured and found to have a bad tooth that likely caused foul temperament. Each year a few hundred tourists, hunters, and locals are killed in Africa by elephants (Figure 27.17) (Durrheim and Leggat, 1999; Albrecht, Breitmeier, et al., 2003).

After losing land and food sources to deforestation, bands of rogue elephants in Assam, India, caused significant damage to property and crops and killed 22 people in 2004. Reportedly, the rogues repeatedly stampeded the area, eating crops and trampling homes. Loss of habitat and vegetation are thought to be the main reason why over 600 people have been killed by elephants in this region within the last 15 years. Elephants in the area also developed a taste for rice beer and frequented village barrels in search of the beverage (Associated Press, 2004).

Elephants can kill by a variety of methods, goring with their trunks, crushing by stepping on the victim, throwing the victim up in the air, strangulating them with their trunk, or using a weapon such as a tree branch to club them. Once the victim has fallen, elephants tend to kneel on and crush their victims (Begoian, 1979; Durrheim and Leggat, 1999; Albrecht, Breitmeier, et al., 2003).

BIG CATS

Patterns of big cat injuries differ from those of canines. The cat's incisors are narrower and sharper, can penetrate more easily, and contain proprioreceptors that allow them to detect when they have hit bone. The upper and lower teeth fit together in an overbite that allows for locking on prey. The majority of big cat bites and attacks are to the head and neck, especially the base of the skull and cervical spine (Cohle, Harlan, et al., 1990; Matter and Sentinella, 1998). The cat will shake its head violently sided to side damaging the spinal cord and immobilizing their prey. They may also bite directly into the spine severing the spinal cord (Cohle, Harlan, et al., 1990; Rollins and Spencer, 1995). Cheetahs (Figure 27.18), lions, and leopards will also attack the frontal neck, strangling and asphyxiating their prey by crushing the larynx (Loefler, 1997). Injury to the phrenic nerve, carotid artery laceration, spinal cord injury, and deep head and neck lacerations have been reported in cougar attacks on children (Kadesky, Manarey, et al., 1998). Big cats also scratch their victims with long claws, which can produce significant lacerations and bleeding. Reports of exsanguination have occurred (Rollins and Spencer, 1995).

After encountering a big cat in the wild, humans should stand their ground and make themselves appear as large and threatening as possible, making loud noises and shouting. Running will provoke a predatory instinct

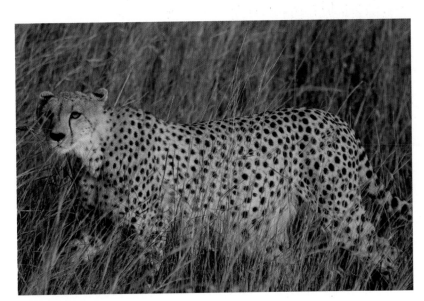

Figure 27.18. Cheetah. Photo courtesy of Jenny Hargrove.

to chase on the part of the cat. Humans should never turn their backs or crouch down in the presence of a big cat. Aggressive behavior (fighting back) once an attack has begun may cause a cat to terminate his attack (Chester, 2006).

Big cats carry similar flora to their smaller domestic counterparts; infection from *Pasteurella* species has been reported in lion, cougar, and tiger bites (Kizer, 1989; Garcia, 1997; Kadesky, Manarey, et al., 1998).

Cat-scratch disease (CSD) resulting from a scratch and inoculation of *Bartonella henselae* is well documented in domestic cats. CSD is a real possibility from big cat scratches; this gram-negative rod has been also isolated from puma and bobcats in North, Central, and South America (Chomel, Kikuchi, et al., 2004; Chomel, Kasten, et al., 2006). The resulting illness occurs 3–5 days after exposure and results in regional lymphadenopathy, fever, and systemic symptoms. CSD is usually treated symptomatically, and antibiotics are reserved for systemic cases. Prognosis is good.

Tigers

Royal Bengal tiger habitat is rapidly being deforested in India and Southeast Asia. These cats have long been known as man-eaters and are the number one cause of death by mammals in these regions, posing a significant risk to people. Bengal tigers prey on children and women when natural prey is lacking, and as with most big cats, they prey on unsuspecting persons and strike without forewarning. Their bite is extremely powerful, and their massive paws can kill in a single swipe. Extremity amputation and spinal cord transection have occurred after one bite (Steinbok, Flodmark, et al., 1985; Clark,

Sandusky, et al., 1991; Associated Press, 2007) Carotid artery laceration, spinal fractures, and multiple other facial, intracranial, as well as internal organ injuries have been reported (Prasad, Madan, et al., 1991; Wiens and Harrison, 1996). Tigers have the dubious distinction of being the animal kingdoms' worldwide reigning "man-eater" consuming approximately 80 people per year in India alone. In a 20-year time span from 1972–1992, 800 people were killed by tigers within India and Bangladesh (AP, 1992).

Pasteurella infection, including meningitis and infection from a new *Pasteurella* subset, *Neisseria weaveri*, have complicated tiger bites (Burdge, Scheifele, et al., 1985; Steinbok, Flodmark, et al., 1985; Capitini, Herrero, et al., 2002).

Lions

Lions (Figure 27.19) are strong, powerful hunters though not as efficient as tigers. Wounded lions are extremely likely to attack hunters. Lionesses protecting their cubs may be provoked more easily. Lion attacks tend to occur during harvest time and in times when prey is scarce (Packer, Ikanda, et al., 2005). Man-eating lions are probably created when they scavenge on human corpses disposed of in the bush following famine and epidemics and develop a taste for human flesh. Recently, in war-torn countries, illegal immigrants or victims of war fled at night through lion territory, which resulted in an increase in lion-associated fatalities and injuries; lions kill and eat about 300–500 people a year in Africa (Treves and Naughton-Treves, 1999). The same patterns of injury and infection rates apply for lion attacks as for other big cats. They frequently kill in one swipe or one bite.

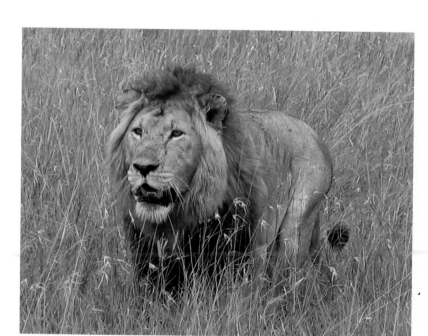

Figure 27.19. Lion. Photo courtesy of Jenny Hargrove.

Leopards

Leopards are shy and reclusive, live in trees, and show much more fear of humans than other big cats. They need much more provocation to attack and tend to attack when trapped or cornered by a dog. Leopards tend to claw and bite more than other cats, but they also inflict head and neck injury (Bahram, Burke, et al., 2004). They are scared away more easily, and the probability of surviving a leopard attack is greater than that of the tiger or lion. There are reports of man-eating leopards, but they are rare.

Cougars

Also known as mountain lions, catamounts, or pumas, cougars are smaller than other big cats, and their hunting behavior is similar to domestic cats. They are found throughout the Americas and are increasingly encroaching on populated areas in the Western United States. Cougars reside in suburban Colorado and Southern California where they have been seen crouched in trees outside of day cares, homes, and parks and trails in close proximity to people (Chester, 2006).

From 1991 to 2003 there were 73 attacks and 10 deaths from mountain lion attacks in Canada and the United States (Chester, 2006). Two attacks on the same day in 2004 occurred in Southern California – one fatal, the other with critical injuries to the neck and face. Both victims were riding mountain bikes at the time (Chester, 2006). The vast majority of attacks are on children, but cougars also attack hikers, trail runners, and mountain bikers (Chester, 2006). This is presumably a predatory attack, and the cougar perceives a moving person as fleeing prey. Cougar attacks on children are more likely to be fatal than attacks on adults.

Patterns of injury resemble other big cat attacks with injury mainly to the head and neck (Grant, 1979; Kadesky, Manarey, et al., 1998; McKee, 2003). Cougars usually consume their human victims but prefer natural prey. Infection after injury from cougar attack follows patterns described with other big cats (Kizer, 1989).

BEARS

Bears are as variable as their worldwide distribution. They occupy a variety of habitats and display different behaviors and body habitus. Bear maulings are sensationalized and have led to a misunderstanding of the animal. As their wild territory diminishes, however, encounters will become more frequent (Dieter, Dieter, et al., 2001).

Humans can prevent most bear attacks from ever occurring if they are properly educated before entering bear habitat. Techniques for avoiding contact with bears differ for the species of bear encountered. Almost all bears will avoid human contact if given advance warning of an approaching human. When hiking in bear country, humans should make a steady medium volume noise, with conversation, whistling, or singing. ("Bear bells" sold in many campground stores are probably not loud enough.) Visitors should stay alert while in bear country and while around feeding grounds, such as rivers with fish and berry patches, and should avoid approaching a carcass (scavenger birds may herald a carcass and a feeding bear). Watch for signs of tree scratchings, bear droppings (which can contain a lot of seeds), or breaking of branches and heavy underbrush indicating a large animal has passed (Floyd, 1999).

During a sudden (provoked) encounter with a brown bear, the human should appear nonthreatening. Stand still, avoid making sudden movements, and avoid direct eye contact. Talking to the bear in a soft voice may help them identify you as human; running may ellicit a predatory response. A provoked encounter with a black bear is more likely to end in their fleeing the scene, and a human should behave more aggressively. If charged by any type of bear, hold your ground, resisting the urge to run. If attacked, "play dead" by rolling face down, covering head and neck with arms and hands, and remain stationary. Hopefully the bear will presume there is no threat and will retreat (Floyd, 1999). Use of pepper spray (5–10% capsicum oleoresin) when discharged within 20–30 feet of an approaching bear is an effective deterrent. Improper use of pepper spray on tents and clothing to act as a deterrent may actually attract bears (Haecker, 1998; Temte, 1998). Storage of food well away from camp in impenetrable canisters or high in trees, cooking away from the campsite, and keeping any fragrant products (lotions, gum, flavored lip balm) out of the campsite will help deter bears (Smith, 1997; Floyd, 1999). There is no evidence to support bear attraction to menstrual odors, but unscented feminine products should be used in bear country and used products should be disposed of properly.

An unprovoked or predatory attack by any type of bear is unusual but occasionally reported. Humans should act aggressively and fight back if being pursued by a predatory bear.

Brown Bears

Grizzly, Kodiak, and Mexican brown bears are all part of the brown bear family; they are large and powerful with tremendous strength and can run up to 45 mph. Brown bears have huge heads, strong jaws, large canine teeth, and claws as long as fingers attached to massive paws (List of Fatal Bear Attacks, 2007). Most encounters with brown bears that end in attack are provoked, with bears perceiving humans as threats to their food source, their cubs, or their habitat (e.g., sudden surprise encounters). Sows typically aggressively defend their young and account for the majority of brown bear attacks on

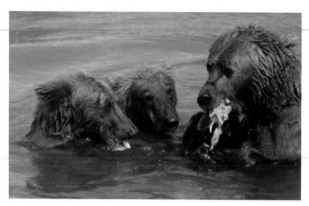

Figure 27.20. Grizzly bear sow with cubs. Photo courtesy of Luanne Freer.

humans (Figure 27.20). In the Yukon, a young man at a flagging job was killed by a female grizzly when he unknowingly came within 15 feet of the den containing two cubs (Dube, 2006). Typically attacks are brief; the bear often loses interest fast and leaves the area. An exception to this is an injured or shot bear whose attacks are more lengthy and extended and resulting injuries more extensive (Dieter, Dieter, et al., 2001). Bears habituated to human food are much more likely to incite bear–human conflict and are also more likely to consume their human kill (Tough and Butt, 1993; Gunther and Mark, 2004). Injuries include extensive tearing, ripping, and crushing, with deep lacerations from their teeth and claws affecting primarily head and neck, chest, and abdomen (Budrin Iu, Khitrov, et al., 1976; Rose, 1982; Ullah, Tahir, et al., 2005). Penetrating head injuries from bear claws have been reported (Gunther and Mark, 2004; Raveenthiran, 2004). There have been at least 50 recorded deaths from brown bears in North America from 1900–2003 (List of Fatal Bear Attacks, 2007).

Grizzly bear bite wounds (Figure 27.21) can develop significant infections, and deep wound culture pathogens include *Serratia fonticola, Serratia marcescens, Aeromonas hydrophila, Bacillus cereus,* and *Enterococcus durans* (Kunimoto, Rennie, et al., 2004).

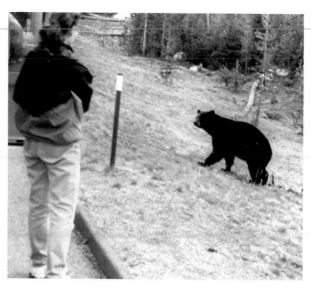

Figure 27.22. Tourists approach a black bear. Bears seen in the wild should not be approached in this manner as their behavior could become aggressive if provoked or threatened. Photo courtesy of Luanne Freer.

Black Bears

Black bear territory in North America is extensive, and their population is much greater than their brown bear counterparts (Figure 27.22). As a result there are far more documented encounters with humans. Attacks resulted in a similar number of fatalities from 1900 to 2003 with 52 deaths recorded, but overall black bear attacks result in more minor injuries, with higher survival rates (Floyd, 1999; List of Fatal Bear Attacks, 2007). Attacks tend to be more predatory than defensive, as was the case in 2002 in New York State when an infant was dragged from her stroller and into the woods and killed (Floyd 1999; Associated Press, 2002). Improper food storage and development of a taste for human food has led to significant bear management problems in national parks (Townes, Laughlin, et al., 2000). Female black bears are less likely to become aggressive in defense of their cubs and will often retreat into a tree with their cubs (Floyd, 1999).

Polar Bears

Despite the large size and rumored aggressive behavior, polar bears are statistically less likely to attack than a grizzly. However, the number of both humans and bears in polar bear habitat is substantially lower so conflicts are much less likely to occur. Only 5 reported deaths occurred in North America from polar bear attack from 1900 to 2003 (List of Fatal Bear Attacks, 2007). The majority of attacks is predatory or associated with an attractant and likely involves habituated bears (Floyd, 1999). Fishing villages near the Arctic Circle are notoriously frequented. Injuries from attacks might be higher; however, most people carry firearms for protection in these regions.

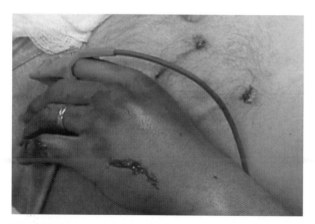

Figure 27.21. Wounds from a grizzly bear attack. Photo courtesy of Luanne Freer.

In Norway, from 1971 to 1975 of the 10 people seriously or fatally injured, none carried an appropriate firearm (Risholt, Persen, et al., 1998). The occasional killing of polar bears in this region for protection does not impose an immediate threat on the population. The pattern of injury in polar bear attack is similar to other bear species (Risholt, Persen, et al., 1998).

Other Bears

Brown bears in Asia and Europe have similar aggressive patterns to their North American brothers. The sloth bear in Europe and Asia is reported to be quite aggressive, and there are a few reported deaths each year, likely from perceived threat as this animal is mainly an insectivore. Panda bears are herbivores, shy, and pose little threat if any to humans.

MARSUPIALS

Kangaroos account for a substantial number of motor vehicle collisions in Australia every year. Injuries from these collisions are more minor compared with that of larger animals (Abu-Zidan, Parmar, et al., 2002; Bashir and Abu-Zidan, 2006). Kangaroo interactions have increased in Australia likely due to loss of habitat and human feeding (Peatling, 2005). They have powerful hind legs and can inflict serious injury when kicking. The toenail on the hind leg is capable of disemboweling a human. Their forepaws are functionally versatile, and they can grapple and box with them. Kangaroo are capable of inflicting serious lacerations and puncture wounds as in the case of an attack on Brisbane woman picking flowers in her garden (Viellaris, 2004).

Opossums are North Americas' only marsupial. Although nocturnal, quiet, and shy, when backed into a corner they can become very aggressive. Bites have been documented in captivity. Often, in extreme danger, an opossum will play dead (Figure 27.23) and can remain in

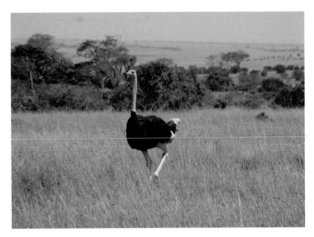

Figure 27.24. Ostrich. Photo courtesy of Jenny Hargrove.

comatose state with drooling, stiff body, and very shallow respirations for up to 4 hours. Cultures from seven opossum's mouths grew out streptococci, coagulase-positive and coagulase-negative staphylococci, *Aeromonas* species, *Citrobacter freundii*, *Eikenella corrodens*, and *Escherichia coli* (Howell and Dalsey, 1990).

LARGE BIRDS

Ostriches (Figure 27.24) can inflict injury with their powerful kicks and sharp toenails. One to two deaths a year occur due to ostrich attack. These giant birds can run up to 45 mph; if being chased, a human should lie prone to protect the abdomen, covering the neck with hands and arms. Ostriches may peck at the victim until interest is lost. Disembowelment, globe and orbit perforations, and even esophageal perforation have been documented after ostrich attack (Chaudhry, Al-Sharif, et al., 2003; Mostafa and Galiwango, 2004; Khan and Olumide, 2006).

The New Guinea cassowary, which is similar in appearance to the ostrich, also produces patterns of injury and attack that are similar in style to the ostrich.

Emus, mostly domesticated farm animals, are native to Australia. These usually shy birds, if provoked or cornered, may kick producing injury as well.

As with many birds, ostriches and emus are fascinated by shiny objects. Care should be taken not to wear shiny buttons, jewelry, or other such objects when in close proximity to these creatures as these items may be attractants.

VENOMOUS MAMMALS

The platypus, a furry, duck-billed creature native to parts of Australia is usually shy but, when provoked, may inject venom from a hollow spur located in its hind leg. The venom has been characterized as a C-peptide that is a potent activator of nocioreceptors resulting in severe

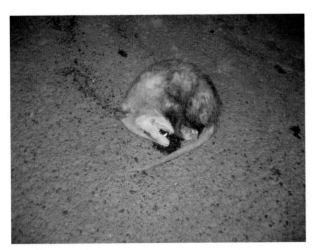

Figure 27.23. Opossum playing dead. Photo courtesy of Jenny Hargrove.

pain (Kourie, 1999; de Plater, Milburn, et al., 2001). Although the venom is not lethal, it produces local swelling, lymphadenopathy, and pain in the envenomated limb that may be unresponsive to narcotics and may last for days to weeks. Immobilization and regional nerve blocks have been shown to be effective (Fenner, Williamson, et al., 1992).

The short-tailed shrew resides in the northeastern United States and contains a potentially lethal toxin, which has been identified as blarina toxin (Kita, Nakamura, et al., 2004; Kita, Okumura, et al., 2005). The venom, injected from the salivary glands through lower incisors can produce severe burning pain and swelling that may persist for several weeks. Envenomation was first described in the late 1800s; however, there have been no reported cases since the early 1900s (Dufton, 1992).

HAZARDOUS AQUATIC LIFE

Alligators and Crocodiles

Alligators (Figure 27.25) live in southern U.S. coastal states and are opportunistic feeders. The number of alligator attacks has grown recently, likely due to the expansion of suburbia into their natural habitat; from 1948 to August 1, 2004, 376 injuries and 15 deaths were reported (Langley, 2005). Alligators have large steel trap-like jaws with which they seize their prey, causing substantial crushing injuries. After locking onto their prey, alligators drag them into the water in an attempt to drown the victim. Death occurs from the massive crush injuries to the torso, dismemberment with resulting exsanguination, or drowning (Harding and Wolf, 2006). Alligator oral flora includes gram-negative species, most notably *Aeromonas hydrophila* and anaerobic species including *Clostridium*. Overwhelming infection from bite wounds and death secondary to sepsis have been reported (Harding and Wolf, 2006). It is best not to walk, swim, or boat (especially with children or dogs) near water in alligator territory in the evening.

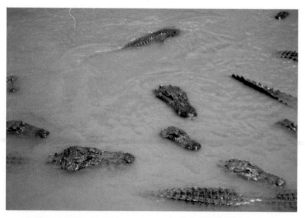

Figure 27.25. Alligators. Photo courtesy of Howard Backer.

Alligator eyes reflect green with light and may be distinguished at night by this feature.

Nile crocodiles are one of the leading causes of death in Africa each year, and humans are routinely regarded as prey. Most attacks occur along riverbanks, where the attacking crocodile locks its jaws around the victim, dragging its prey back to the water where it twirls round and round in an attempt to drown and dismember its victims. Their bites are powerful and can decapitate and transect human torsos (Mekisic and Wardill, 1992). Salt water crocodiles in Australia are responsible for multiple deaths each year as well. In one study of 16 attacks, most occurred at night while swimming or wading in shallow water, and alcohol was involved in 50% (Mekisic and Wardill, 1992). Wound infections are frequently caused by *Aeromonas hydrophilia*, *Clostridium*, *Pseudomonas*, *Vibrio*, *Proteus*, *Entercoccus*, and *Bacteroides*. Death from sepsis has occurred (Vanwersch, 1998), and when victims do survive, they frequently suffer severe deformity (Vanwersch, 1998).

AMAZONIAN SPECIES

Candirú

The candirú, sometimes referred to as the toothpick fish, is a small parasitic catfish found in the Amazon; they are thin, translucent, and range from ½ to 6 inches long. They have evolved to occupy a singular niche in the food chain by swimming into the gills of other fish and then extending their gill covers that have a spinous process to hold themselves in place. The rasp-like teeth around their circular mouth allow the candirú to feed on the host's blood. This adaptation for attraction to the egress of fluid from the gills of fish may be either to the force of the flow itself or perhaps a chemical attractant. These fish are seemingly able to swim up the human urethra and lodge themselves with their umbrella-like spinous process leading to urinary obstruction. While there are various descriptive reports of this occurrence from natives, explorers, and missionaries to the area, there are no well-documented cases of this event in recent medical literature. Interestingly, there are no reports of this occurring in any other animal species. There are even claims of penile amputation in the native population after obstruction with candirú; however, these also have not been documented. Urethral invasion by the candirú remains yet to be well described in medical literature and is likely a rare event. The locals report that the green fruit of the jugua tree (*Genipa americana L.*), the buitach apple, will dissolve the spines because of its high citric acid content. High-dose vitamin C may also work. Natives wear pudendal shields when urinating in bodies of fresh water (Herman, 1973; Breault, 1991) in attempts to prevent possible urethral penetration by this fish.

Piranhas

Piranhas are found ubiquitously in South American rivers and lakes. These small, carnivorous fish with razor sharp teeth hunt in schools and are attracted to blood or dead fish or carcasses in the water. Piranhas are ferocious hunters capable of reducing a horse to its skeleton within a matter of minutes. In spite of their reputation, there are few reports of piranhas attacking and eating humans. Almost all known cases of human consumption are of humans who had already died of another cause such as drowning. The vast majority of reported attacks are of a single bite to the feet or hands. Piranha bites are circular, crater-shaped lacerations, with missing tissue. Bites are increasing in frequency in river areas that have been dammed, where piranha populations are increased; bites are likely caused by defensive protective of breeding grounds rather than predatory intent. Bite injuries tend to heal well, but there are a few reports of toe amputations and extensive bleeding (Haddad and Sazima, 2003). There is one reported case of a severe infection from *Aeromonas hydrophila* secondary to a piranha bite; however, the patient had a preexisting history of neutropenia (Revord, Goldfarb, et al., 1988). To prevent piranha bites, avoid swimming or wading in dammed areas with underbrush along the shore, or blood, dead fish, food, or carcasses in the water. Splashing or flailing movement in the water will also attract piranha and may explain why children are at a higher risk of being bitten (Haddad and Sazima, 2003; Mol, 2006). There are two reports of epileptic victims having sustained severe lacerations from piranha bites after they were attacked following a seizure in the water (Mol, 2006).

Electric Eels

Electric eels are a type of knifefish indigenous to Central and South America. They are capable of producing up to 650-V shock, which is enough to paralyze a human and cause drowning. Humans report a tingling sensation when in the vicinity of electric eels. A human is capable of being shocked by touching the skin of the eel up to 9 hours after its death (Valasco, 2003).

Anaconda

Anacondas are an aquatic constrictor native to South American jungles; they kill prey by looping their coils around and constricting and suffocating their prey. They also have teeth and powerful jaws that can latch on to prey, pulling it underwater to drown; they then swallow their prey whole, headfirst. There are reports of anacondas preying upon humans; the most recent report was of an 8-year-old boy attacked by an anaconda while playing in a creek bed on a farm outside of Sao Paulo. The boy's grandfather ran to the rescue and was nearly caught in the snake's coils as well, but fought it off with stones and a machete. The boy survived but required 21 sutures on his chest due to a laceration from the bite of the snake (Reuters, 2007).

SUMMARY

Remote and wilderness areas provide amazing opportunities to see wildlife in their natural habitat. The risk associated with encountering a potentially dangerous animal can be dramatically reduced by taking appropriate precautions when entering the animal's natural domain. When traveling to a remote region, it is important to learn about the local animal life and know both how to prevent attack and how to deal with an attack if it does occur.

REFERENCES

Abu-Zidan F M, Parmar KA, et al. Kangaroo-related motor vehicle collisions. *J Trauma*. 2002;53(2):360–3.

Agrawal, Premenra. Drunk monkeys attack humans. *Times of India*. Available at: *http://timesofindia.indiatimes.com/articleshow/1080182.cms*. 2005.

Aigner N, Konig S, et al. [Bite wounds and their characteristic position in trauma surgery management]. *Unfallchirurg*. 1996;99(5):346–50.

Al-Waili NS, Saloom KY. Effects of topical honey on post-operative wound infections due to gram positive and gram negative bacteria following caesarean sections and hysterectomies. *Eur J Med Res*. 1999;4(3):126–30.

Alaska Department of Fish and Game. (1997). What to Do about Aggressive Moose? Available at: *http://www.wildlife.alaska.gov/index.cfm?adfg=aawildlife.agmoose*.

Alberio L, Lammle B. Images in clinical medicine. *Capnocytophaga canimorsus* sepsis. *N Engl J Med*. 1998;339(25):1827.

Albrecht K, Breitmeier D. [Fatalities after injuries by wild animals]. *Arch Kriminol*. 2003;212(3–4):96–103.

Ansari S, Ashraf Ali KS. Camel collision as a major cause of low cervical spinal cord injury. *Spinal Cord*. 1998a;36(6):415–17.

Ansari S, Ashraff Ali KS. Camel collision as a major cause of low cervical spinal cord injury. *Spinal Cord*. 1998b; 36:415–417. *Spinal Cord*. 1998:36(11): 804.

Associated Press. Bear Mauls and Kills Infant in New York State. *http://news.bbc.co.uk/2/hi/americas/2204256.stm*. 2002.

Associated Press (AP). "Crocodile Hunter" Steve Irwin Dead. CNN.com. September 4, 2006.

Associated Press (AP). Elephants Rampage through Villages in India. Available at: *http://www.foxnews.com/story/0,2933,138495,00.html*. 2004.

Associated Press (AP). Heavy death toll to tigers in Bangladesh. *Cat News*. 1992;16:6.

Associated Press (AP). Tiger Bites Off Woman's Arm at Zoo in Montenegro. Available at: *http://www.foxnews.com/story/0,2933,258543,00.html*. 2007.

Azar-Cavanagh M, Chan, T. Simian Exposure (Herpes B & SIV). UCSD Department of Emergency Medicine, San Diego, Calif. Available at: *http://health.ucsd.edu/ClinicalResources/simian21.pdf*. 2005.

Bahram R, Burke JE, et al. Head and neck injury from a leopard attack: case report and review of the literature. *J Oral Maxillofac Surg*. 2004;62(2):247–9.

Barbour AG. Fall and rise of Lyme disease and other Ixodes tick-borne infections in North America and Europe. *Br Med Bull.* 1998;54(3):647–58.

Barnham M. Pig bite injuries and infection: report of seven human cases. *Epidemiol Infect.* 1988;101(3):641–5.

Barss P, Ennis S. Injuries caused by pigs in Papua New Guinea. *Med J Aust.* 1988;149(11–12):649–56.

Bashir MO, Abu-Zidan FM. Motor vehicle collisions with large animals. *Saudi Med J.* 2006;27(8):1116–20.

Beck AM. The epidemiology and prevention of animal bites. *Semin Vet Med Surg (Small Anim).* 1991;6(3):186–91.

Beck AM, Jones BA. Unreported dog bites in children. *Public Health Rep.* 1985;100(3):315–21.

Begoian AG. [Death from compression of the neck by an elephant's trunk]. *Sud Med Ekspert.* 1979;22(2):56–7.

Bennett JB. Repairing cuts and lacerations of the hand. *Postgrad Med.* 1988;83(8):157–61.

Bjornstig U, Eriksson A, et al. Collisions with passenger cars and moose, Sweden. *Am J Public Health.* 1986;76(4):460–2.

Breault J. Candirú: Amazonian parasitic catfish. *J Wilderness Med.* 1991;2(4):304–12.

Brisson BA, Bersenas A, et al. Ultrasonographic diagnosis of septic arthritis secondary to porcupine quill migration in a dog. *J Am Vet Med Assoc.* 2004;224(9):1467–70, 1453–4.

Budrin Iu P, Khitrov LN, et al. [Injuries by the claws and teeth of a bear]. *Sud Med Ekspert.* 1976;19(1):49–50.

Burdge DR, Scheifele D, et al. Serious *Pasteurella multocida* infections from lion and tiger bites. *JAMA.* 1985;253(22):3296–7.

Cameron JM. The Dingo murder in retrospect. *Med Leg J.* 1984; 52(3):164–79.

Capitini CM, Herrero IA, et al. Wound infection with *Neisseria weaveri* and a novel subspecies of *Pasteurella multocida* in a child who sustained a tiger bite. *Clin Infect Dis.* 2002;34(12): E74–6.

Chaudhry IA, Al-Sharif AM, et al. Severe ocular and periocular injuries caused by an ostrich. *Ophthal Plast Reconstr Surg.* 2003;19(3):246–7.

Chester T. Mountain Lion Attacks on People in the U.S. and Canada. Available at: *http://tchester.org/sgm/lists/lion_attacks. html.* 2006.

Childs JE, McLafferty SL, et al. Epidemiology of rodent bites and prediction of rat infestation in New York City. *Am J Epidemiol.* 1998;148(1):78–87.

Chomel BB, Kasten RW, et al. Bartonella infection in domestic cats and wild felids. *Ann NY Acad Sci.* 2006;1078:410–5.

Chomel BB, Kikuchi Y, et al. Seroprevalence of Bartonella infection in American free-ranging and captive pumas (*Felis concolor*) and bobcats (*Lynx rufus*). *Vet Res.* 2004;35(2): 233–41.

Clark MA, Sandusky GE, et al. Fatal and near-fatal animal bite injuries. *J Forensic Sci.* 1991;36(4):1256–61.

Cohen J, David D. Recommendations for prevention of and therapy for exposure to B virus (Cercopithecine Herpesvirus 1). *CID.* 2002;35:1191–1203.

Cohle SD, Harlan CW, et al. Fatal big cat attacks. *Am J Forensic Med Pathol.* 1990;11(3):208–12.

Conn, JM, et al. Nonfatal motor-vehicle animal crash-related injuries – United States, 2001–2002. *MMWR Morb Mortal Wkly Rep.* 2004;53(30):675–8.

Conrad LB, Balison J. Bison goring injuries: penetrating and blunt trauma. *J Wild Med.* 1994;5(4):371–381.

Cromartie, John. Rural Population and Migration. U.S. Department of Agriculture. *http://www.ers.usda.gov/Briefing/Population/.* 2007.

Dahl E. [Animal bites at the casualty department of the Oslo City Council]. *Tidsskr Nor Laegeforen.* 1998;118(17):2614–17.

Daoust PY. Porcupine quill in the brain of a dog. *Vet Rec.* 1991;128(18):436.

de Plater GM, Milburn PJ, et al. Venom from the platypus, *Ornithorhynchus anatinus*, induces a calcium-dependent current in cultured dorsal root ganglion cells. *J Neurophysiol.* 2001;85(3):1340–5.

Denholm CJ. Survival from a wild animal attack: a case study analysis of adolescent coping. *Matern Child Nurs J.* 1995;23(1):26–34.

Dieter RA. Jr, Dieter DL, et al. Bear mauling: a descriptive review. *Int J Circumpolar Health.* 2001;60(4):696–704.

Dube, Jonathan. Grizzly Bear Kills Man in Yukon. Available at: *http://www.cbc.ca/canada/story/2006/05/01/grizzly-yukon060401.html.* 2006.

Dufton MJ. Venomous mammals. *Pharmacol Ther.* 1992;53(2): 199–215.

Durrheim DN, Leggat PA. Risk to tourists posed by wild mammals in South Africa. *J Travel Med.* 1999;6(3):172–9.

Ejlertsen T, Gahrn-Hansen B, et al. *Pasteurella aerogenes* isolated from ulcers or wounds in humans with occupational exposure to pigs: a report of 7 Danish cases. *Scand J Infect Dis.* 1996;28(6):567–70.

Elliott SP. Rat bite fever and *Streptobacillus moniliformis. Clin Microbiol Rev.* 2007;20(1):13–22.

Farrell TM, Sutton JE, et al. Moose-motor vehicle collisions: an increasing hazard in northern New England. *Arch Surg.* 1996;131(4):377–81.

Fenner PJ, Williamson JA, et al. Platypus envenomation – a painful learning experience. *Med J Aust.* 1992;157(11–12): 829–32.

Findling JW, Pohlmann GP, et al. Fulminant gram-negative bacillemia (DF-2) following a dog bite in an asplenic woman. *Am J Med.* 1980;68(1):154–6.

Fleisher GR. The management of bite wounds. *N Engl J Med.* 1999;340(2):138–40.

Floyd T. Bear-inflicted human injury and fatality. *Wilderness Environ Med.* 1999;10(2):75–87.

Francisco. Monkey's Attack Women and Children; Kassala, Sudan Aug 19, 2004. Available at: *http://lists.ibiblio.org/pipermail/monkeywire/2004-August/000665.html.* 2004.

Frean JA, Isaacson M, et al. Sporotrichosis following a rodent bite: a case report. *Mycopathologia.* 1991;116(1):5–8.

Freer L. Bites and injuries by wild and domestic animals in Auerboch PS. *Wilderness Medicine.* 5th ed. CU Mosby, St. Louis, 2007; pp. 1133–1155.

Garcia VF. Animal bites and *Pasturella* infections. *Pediatr Rev.* 1997;18(4):127–30.

Gavin PJ, Kazacos KR, et al. Baylisascariasis. *Clin Microbiol Rev.* 2005;18(4):703–18.

George J. Death of a student hiking in remote northern Saskatchewan. *San Francisco Chronicle.* January 14, 2006;F-1.

Georges AJ, Matton T, et al. [Monkey-pox, a model of emergent then reemergent disease]. *Med Mal Infect.* 2004;34(1):12–19.

Geronemus RG, Mertz PM, et al. Wound healing. The effects of topical antimicrobial agents. *Arch Dermatol.* 1979;115(11):1311–14.

Gibbons RV. Cryptogenic rabies, bats, and the question of aerosol transmission. *Ann Emerg Med.* 2002;39(5):528–36.

Goldstein EJ, Citron DM, et al. Trovafloxacin compared with levofloxacin, ofloxacin, ciprofloxacin, azithromycin and clarithromycin against unusual aerobic and anaerobic human and animal bite-wound pathogens. *J Antimicrob Chemother.* 1998a ;41(3):391–6.

Goldstein EJ, Citron DM, et al. Activities of HMR 3004 (RU 64004) and HMR 3647 (RU 66647) compared to those of erythromycin, azithromycin, clarithromycin, roxithromycin, and eight other antimicrobial agents against unusual aerobic and anaerobic human and animal bite pathogens isolated from skin and soft tissue infections in humans. *Antimicrob Agents Chemother.* 1998b;42(5):1127–32.

Goldstein EJ, Citron DM, et al. Recovery of an unusual Flavobacterium group IIb-like isolate from a hand infection following pig bite. *J Clin Microbiol.* 1990;28(5):1079–81.

Goldstein EJ, Citron DM, et al. In vitro activities of the desfluoro(6) Quinolone BMS-284756 against aerobic and anaerobic pathogens isolated from skin and soft tissue animal and human bite wound infections. *Antimicrob Agents Chemother.* 2002;46(3): 866–70.

Goldstein EJ, Pryor EP 3rd, et al. Simian bites and bacterial infection. *Clin Infect Dis.* 1995;20(6):1551–2.

Grahn BH, Szentimrey D, et al. Ocular and orbital porcupine quills in the dog: a review and case series. *Can Vet J.* 1995;36(8):488–93.

Granick MS, Tenenhaus M, et al. Comparison of wound irrigation and tangential hydrodissection in bacterial clearance of contaminated wounds: results of a randomized, controlled clinical study. *Ostomy Wound Manage.* 2007;53(4):64–72.

Grant DF. Massive trauma to the head and face, attack by a cougar: report of case. *ASDC J Dent Child.* 1979;46(3):226–9.

Gunther KAH, Mark A. Grizzly bear–human conflicts in the Greater Yellowstone ecosystem, 1992–2000. *BioOne.* 2004;15(1):10–22.

Haddad V Jr, Assuncao MC, et al. A fatal attack caused by a lowland tapir (*Tapirus terrestris*) in southeastern Brazil. *Wilderness Environ Med.* 2005;16(2):97–100.

Haddad V Jr, Sazima IO. Piranha attacks on humans in southeast Brazil: epidemiology, natural history, and clinical treatment, with description of a bite outbreak. *Wilderness Environ Med.* 2003;14(4):249–54.

Haecker C, Tom S. *USGS Cautions Proper Use of Pepper Spray to Avoid Bear Attacks.* Anchorage: U.S. Geological Society Alaska Science Center; 1998.

Haikonen H, Summala H. Deer-vehicle crashes: extensive peak at 1 hour after sunset. *Am J Prev Med.* 2001;21(3):209–13.

Harding BE. Wolf BC. Alligator attacks in southwest Florida. *J Forensic Sci.* 2006;51(3):674–7.

Hedlund JH, Curtis PD, et al. Methods to reduce traffic crashes involving deer: what works and what does not. *Traffic Inj Prev.* 2004;5(2):122–31.

Herman JR. Candiru: urinophilic catfish: its gift to urology. *Urology.* 1973;1(3):265–7.

Herzog W. *Grizzly Man.* Documentary Film. 2005.

Hirschhorn RB, Hodge RR. Identification of risk factors in rat bite incidents involving humans. *Pediatrics.* 1999;104(3):e35.

Holmes J, ed. *United States Population: A Profile of America's Diversity – The View from the Census Bureau.* The World Almanac and Book of Facts 1999. Mahwah, NJ: Primedia References; 1998.

Howell JM, Dalsey WC. Aerobic bacteria cultured from the mouth of the American opossum (*Didelphis virginiana*) with reference to bacteria associated with bite infections. *J Clin Microbiol.* 1990;28(10):2360–1.

Identification of Simian Herpes Virus B in a Colony of 215 Rhesus Monkeys at Woburn Safari Park Lead to Their Humane Destruction Because of the Potential Health Risk to Humans. *http://www.provet.co.uk/health/diseases/simianb.htm.* 2000.

Janjua KJ. Camel bite injury: an unusual report of left shoulder mutilation with major vascular and bony injuries. *Injury.* 1993;24(10):686–8.

Janjua KJ, van den Berg AA. Animal injuries presenting to Riyadh Armed Forces Hospital: a survey. *Trop Doct.* 1994;24(2):84.

Jhala DSV. Childlifting by wolves in eastern Uttar Pradesh, India. *J Wildlife Res.* 1997;2(2):94–101.

Johnson CN, Isaac JL, et al. Rarity of a top predator triggers continent-wide collapse of mammal prey: dingoes and marsupials in Australia. *Proc Biol Sci.* 2007;274(1608):341–6.

Kadesky KM, Manarey C, et al. Cougar attacks on children: injury patterns and treatment. *J Pediatr Surg.* 1998;33(6):863–5.

Kasindorf M. Deer attacks: nature, civilization lock horns. *USA Today.* December 1, 2005.

Khan MA. Olumide AA. Head injury caused by an ostrich: A rare entity. *Pediatr Neurosurg.* 2006;42(5):308–10.

Kile JC, Fleischauer AT, et al. Transmission of monkeypox among persons exposed to infected prairie dogs in Indiana in 2003. *Arch Pediatr Adolesc Med.* 2005;159(11):1022–5.

Kita M, Nakamura Y, et al. Blarina toxin, a mammalian lethal venom from the short-tailed shrew Blarina brevicauda: isolation and characterization. *Proc Natl Acad Sci USA.* 2005;101(20):7542–7.

Kita M, Okumura Y, et al. Purification and characterisation of blarinasin, a new tissue kallikrein-like protease from the short-tailed shrew *Blarina brevicauda*: comparative studies with blarina toxin. *Biol Chem.* 2004;386(2):177–82.

Kizer KW. Pasteurella multocida infection from a cougar bite: a review of cougar attacks. *West J Med.* 1989;150(1):87–90.

Klein M. Nondomestic mammalian bites. *Am Fam Physician.* 1985;32(5):137–41.

Kourie JI. Characterization of a C-type natriuretic peptide (CNP-39)-formed cation-selective channel from platypus (*Ornithorhynchus anatinus*) venom. *J Physiol.* 1999;518(2): 359–69.

Krebs JW, Mandel EJ, et al. Rabies surveillance in the United States during 2004. *J Am Vet Med Assoc.* 2005;227(12):1912–25.

Kullberg BJ, Westendorp RG, et al. Purpura fulminans and symmetrical peripheral gangrene caused by Capnocytophaga canimorsus (formerly DF-2) septicemia – a complication of dog bite. *Medicine (Baltimore).* 1991;70(5):287–92.

Kunimoto D, Rennie R, et al. Bacteriology of a bear bite wound to a human: case report. *J Clin Microbiol.* 2004;42(7):3374–6.

Langley RL. Alligator attacks on humans in the United States. *Wilderness Environ Med.* 2005;16(3):119–24.

Langley RL. Animal-related fatalities in the United States - an update. *Wilderness Environ Med.* 2005;16(2):67–74.

Larghi OP, Savy VL, et al. [Inactivation of rabies virus by chemical agents]. *Rev Assoc Argent Microbiol.* 1975;7(3):86–90.

Leyden JJ, Sulzberger MB. Topical antibiotics and minor skin trauma. *Am Fam Physician.* 1981;23(1):121–5.

Lin HH, Hulsey RE. Open femur fracture secondary to hippopotamus bite. *J Orthop Trauma.* 1993;7(4):384–7.

Lindberg J, Frederiksen W, et al. Problems of identification in clinical microbiology exemplified by pig bite wound infections. *Zentralbl Bakteriol.* 1998;288(4):491–9.

List of Fatal Bear Attacks in North America by Decade. Available at: *http://en.wikipedia.org/wiki/List_of_fatal_bear_attacks_in_North_America_by_decade.* 2007.

Loefler IJ. Big cats attack at the nape of the neck. *J Trauma.* 1997;43(3):560.

Loro A, Franceschi F, et al. The reasons for amputations in children (0–18 years) in a developing country. *Trop Doct.* 1994;24(3):99–102.

Maimaris C, Quinton DN. Dog-bite lacerations: a controlled trial of primary wound closure. *Arch Emerg Med.* 1988;5(3):156–61.

Manipady S, Menezes RG, et al. Death by attack from a wild boar. *J Clin Forensic Med.* 2006;13(2):89–91.

Marquez M. Roy of Siegfried and Roy Critical after Mauling. Available at: *http://www.cnn.com/2003/SHOWBIZ/10/04/roy.attacked/.* 2003.

Matter HC, Sentinella A. The epidemiology of bite and scratch injuries by vertebrate animals in Switzerland. *Eur J Epidemiol.* 1998;14(5):483–90.

McDade HC, Crandell WB. Perforation of the gastrointestinal tract by an unusual foreign body; a porcupine quill; report of two cases. *N Engl J Med.* 1958;258(15):746–7.

McKee, D. Cougar attacks on humans: a case report. *Wilderness Environ Med.* 2003;14(3):169–73.

Medeiros I, Saconato H. Antibiotic prophylaxis for mammalian bites. *Cochrane Database Syst Rev.* 2001;(2): DOI: 10.1002/14651858.CD001738.

Mekisic AP, Wardill JR. Crocodile attacks in the Northern Territory of Australia. *Med J Aust.* 1992;157(11–12):751–4.

Milrod S, Goel DP. Intraperitoneal foreign body granuloma caused by a porcupine quill. *Med Serv J Can.* 1958;14(7):504–7.

Mol J. Attacks on humans by the piranha *Serrasalmus rhombeus* in Suriname. *Stud Neotrop Fauna Environment.* 2006;41(3):189–95.

Moro MH, Horman JT, et al. The epidemiology of rodent and lagomorph rabies in Maryland, 1981 to 1986. *J Wildl Dis.* 1991;27(3):452–6.

Mostafa MB, Galiwango B. Traumatic oesophageal perforation in a male ostrich (*Struthio camelus australis*). *Vet Rec.* 2004;154(21):669.

Myers CB, Christmann LM. Rat bite – an unusual cause of direct trauma to the globe. *J Pediatr Ophthalmol Strabismus.* 1991;28(6):356–8.

Nawaz A, Matta H, et al. Camel-related injuries in the pediatric age group. *J Pediatr Surg.* 2005;40(8):1248–51.

Noah DL, Drenzek CL, et al. Epidemiology of human rabies in the United States, 1980 to 1996. *Ann Intern Med.* 1998;128(11):922–30.

Norwood S, McAuley C, et al. Mechanisms and patterns of injuries related to large animals. *J Trauma.* 2000;48(4):740–4.

Oberg MS. Povidone-iodine solutions in traumatic wound preparation. *Am J Emerg Med.* 1987;5(6):4553–5.

Ogunbodede EO, Arotiba JT. Camel bite injuries of the orofacial region: report of a case. *J Oral Maxillofac Surg.* 1997;55(10):1174–6.

Ordog GJ, Balasubramanium S, et al. Rat bites: fifty cases. *Ann Emerg Med.* 1985;14(2):126–30.

Ostrowski SRL, Mira J. B-virus from pet macaque monkeys: an emerging threat in the United States? *Emerg Infect Dis.* 1998;4(1):117–121.

Ouazzani BT, Dali H, et al. [Rat bite: an unusual cause of orbital cellulitis]. *J Fr Ophtalmol.* 2006;29(6):e14.

Packer C, Ikanda D, et al. Conservation biology: lion attacks on humans in Tanzania. *Nature.* 2005;436(7053):927–8.

Peatling, Stephanie. Kangaroo Attacks in Australia Spotlight Growing Turf War. Available at: *http://news.nationalgeographic.com/news/2005/05/0506_050506_kangaroos.html.* 2005.

Peters V, Sottiaux M, et al. Posttraumatic stress disorder after dog bites in children. *J Pediatr.* 2004;144(1):121–2.

Phuapradit W, Saropala N. Topical application of honey in treatment of abdominal wound disruption. *Aust N Z J Obstet Gynaecol.* 1992;32(4):381–4.

Pickles G. Injuries by wild animals in the African bush. *J R Army Med Corps.* 1987;133(3):159–60.

Prasad A, Madan VS, et al. Tiger assault: an unusual mode of head injury. *Clin Neurol Neurosurg.* 1991;93(2):171.

Pronchik D, Barber C, et al. Low- versus high-pressure irrigation techniques in *Staphylococcus aureus*-inoculated wounds. *Am J Emerg Med.* 1999;17(2):121–4.

Quinn J, Cummings S, et al. Suturing versus conservative management of lacerations of the hand: randomised controlled trial. *BMJ.* 2002;325(7359):299.

Raveenthiran V. Comment on "Penetrating head injury caused by bear claws: case report." *J Trauma.* 2004;57(5):1141.

Reuters. Brazilian pries grandson from anaconda's death grip. ABC News Online. Available at: *http://www.abc.net.au/news/newsitems/200702/s1844688.htm.* 2007.

Revord ME, Goldfarb J, et al. Aeromonas hydrophila wound infection in a patient with cyclic neutropenia following a piranha bite. *Pediatr Infect Dis J.* 1988;7(1):70–1.

Reynolds MG, Yorita KL, et al. Clinical manifestations of human monkeypox influenced by route of infection. *J Infect Dis.* 2006;194(6):773–80.

Risholt T, Persen E, et al. Man and polar bear in Svalbard: a solvable ecological conflict? *Int J Circumpolar Health.* 1998;57(Suppl 1):532–4.

Rollins CE, Spencer DE. A fatality and the American mountain lion: bite mark analysis and profile of the offending lion. *J Forensic Sci.* 1995;40(3):486–9.

Rose SC. Bear maulings in Alaska. *Alaska Med.* 1982;24(3):29–32.

Shafir SC, Wise ME, et al. Central nervous system and eye manifestations of infection with *Baylisascaris procyonis. Curr Infect Dis Rep.* 2006;8(4):307–13.

Shattock FM. Injuries caused by wild animals. *Lancet.* 1968;1(7539):412–15.

Shvartsblat S, Kochie M, et al. Fatal rat bite fever in a pet shop employee. *Am J Ind Med.* 2004;5(4):357–60.

Sidwa TJ, Wilson PJ, et al. Evaluation of oral rabies vaccination programs for control of rabies epizootics in coyotes and gray foxes: 1995–2003. *J Am Vet Med Assoc.* 2005;227(5):785–92.

Silverstein MA, et al. First human death associated with raccoon rabies – Virginia, 2003. *MMWR Morb Mortal Wkly Rep.* 2003;52(45):1102–3.

Sinclair CL, Zhou C. Descriptive epidemiology of animal bites in Indiana, 1990–92 – a rationale for intervention. *Public Health Rep.* 1995;110(1):64–7.

Singer AJ, Hollander JE, et al. Pressure dynamics of various irrigation techniques commonly used in the emergency department. *Ann Emerg Med.* 1994;24(1):36–40.

Singh A, Gulati SK, et al. Multiple fractures following camel bite of the face (a case report). *Acta Chir Plast.* 1994;36(3):85–8.

Slate D, Rupprecht CE, et al. Status of oral rabies vaccination in wild carnivores in the United States. *Virus Res.* 2005;111(1):68–76.

Smith D. *Backcountry Bear Basics: The Definitive Guide to Avoiding Unpleasant Encounters.* Seattle: The Mountaineers; 1997.

Smith JS, Fishbein DB, et al. Unexplained rabies in three immigrants in the United States: a virologic investigation. *N Engl J Med.* 1991;324(4):205–11.

Smith PF, Meadowcroft AM, et al. Treating mammalian bite wounds. *J Clin Pharm Ther.* 2000;25(2):85–99.

Spence G. A review of animal bites in Delaware – 1989 to 1990. *Del Med J.* 1990;62(12):1425–33.

Sriaroon C, Sriaroon P, et al. Retrospective: animal attacks and rabies exposures in Thai children. *Travel Med Infect Dis.* 2006;4(5):270–4.

Stefanopoulos P, Karabouta Z, et al. Animal and human bites: evaluation and management. *Acta Orthop Belg.* 2004;70(1):1–10.

Steinbok P, Flodmark O, et al. Animal bites causing central nervous system injury in children: a report of three cases. *Pediatr Neurosci.* 1985;12(2):96–100.

Sudarshan MK, Madhusudana SN, et al. Assessing the burden of human rabies in India: results of a national multi-center epidemiological survey. *Int J Infect Dis.* 2007;11(1): 29–35.

Suess O, Magerkurth O, et al. Camel bite: an unusual type of head injury in an infant. *J Pediatr Surg.* 2004;39(10):e11–13.

Talan DA, Citron DM, et al. Bacteriologic analysis of infected dog and cat bites: Emergency Medicine Animal Bite Infection Study Group. *N Engl J Med.* 1999;340(2):85–92.

Temte JL. Grizzly bear and pepper spray: a word of caution. *Wilderness Environ Med.* 1998;9(4):262.

Timm RM, Genoways HH. The Florida bonneted bat, *Eumops floridanus* (Chiroptera: Molossidae): systematics, distribution, geographic variation, and ecology. *J Mammal.* 2004; 85(6):51.

Tough SC, Butt JC. A review of fatal bear maulings in Alberta, Canada. *Am J Forensic Med Pathol.* 1993;14(1):22–7.

Townes DA, Laughlin MK, et al. The black bears of Yosemite National Park: bear-induced injuries – the role of improper food storage. *Wilderness Environ Med.* 2000;11(1):67–8.

Treves A, Naughton-Treves L. Risk and opportunity for humans coexisting with large carnivores. *J Hum Evol.* 1999;36(3): 275–82.

Tribe GW, Noren E. Incidence of bites from cynomolgus monkeys in attending animal staff – 1975–80. *Lab Anim.* 1983;17(2):110.

Tuncali D, Bingul F, et al. Animal bites. *Saudi Med J.* 2005;26(5):772–6.

Ullah F, Tahir M, et al. Mammalian bite injuries to the head and neck region. *J Coll Physicians Surg Pak.* 2005;15(8):485–8.

Valasco T. *Electrophorus electricus.* Animal Diversity Web. Available at: *http://animaldiversity.ummz.umich.edu/site/ accounts/information/Electrophorus_electricus.html.* 2003.

Valderrama J, Garcia I, et al. [Outbreaks of human rabies transmitted by vampire bats in Alto Baudo and Bajo Baudo municipalities, department of choco, Colombia, 2004–2005]. *Biomedica.* 2006;26(3):387–96.

Valente JH, Forti RJ, et al. Wound irrigation in children: saline solution or tap water? *Ann Emerg Med.* 2003;41(5): 609–16.

Vanwersch K. Crocodile bite injury in southern Malawi. *Trop Doct.* 1998;28(4):221–2.

Viellaris, R. AR-News (AU): Ferocious Kangaroo Attacks Woman. Available at: *http://lists.envirolink.org/pipermail/ar-news/ Week-of-Mon-20040315/021653.html.* 2004.

Viljanto J. Disinfection of surgical wounds without inhibition of normal wound healing. *Arch Surg.* 1980;115(3):253–6.

Wandeler AL, et al. Update: raccoon rabies epizootic – United States and Canada, 1999. *MMWR Morb Mortal Wkly Rep.* 2000;49(2):31–5.

Wiens MB, Harrison PB. Big cat attack: a case study. *J Trauma.* 1996;40(5):829–31.

Wiggins ME, Akelman E, et al. The management of dog bites and dog bite infections to the hand. *Orthopedics.* 1994;17(7): 617–23.

Willoughby RE, Tieves KS, Hoffman GM, Ghanayem NS, Amlie-Lefond CM, Schwabe MJ, Chusid MJ, Rupprecht CE. Survival after treatment of rabies with induction of coma. *N Engl J Med.* 2005;352(24):2508–14.

Wolff KD. Management of animal bite injuries of the face: experience with 94 patients. *J Oral Maxillofac Surg.* 1998;56(7): 838–43; discussion 843–4.

Wood WF, Sollers BG, et al. Volatile components in defensive spray of the hooded skunk, *Mephitis macroura.* *J Chem Ecol.* 2002;28(9):1865–70.

World Health Organization. WHO Project No: ICP DPR 00. New Delhi, India. 2003.

Wykes WN. Rat bite injury to the eyelids in a 3-month-old child. *Br J Ophthalmol.* 1989;73(3):202–4.

Yeld J. Baboon attacks Cape Point visitor. Available at: *http:// www.capeargus.co.za/index.php?fSectionId=49&fArticleId=21 94506.* 2004.

28 | Snake and Arthropod Envenoming

Michael V. Callahan, MD, DTM&H, MSPH, and Marie Thomas

Note: *If this chapter is being consulted for a medical emergency please turn immediately to Table 28.4 on page 406.*

INTRODUCTION

Few topics in backcountry medicine have proved as controversial as the field management of venomous injuries from wild animals and arthropods. One reason for the controversy is that recommendations for stabilizing and treating venomous or "envenoming" injuries in the resource-constrained settings are often in conflict, require capabilities beyond those available in the wilderness, or endorse interventions later found to be injurious to the victim.[1,2] For expedition medical personnel and others providing care in austere environs, adapting front-country medical protocols for the management of venomous injuries to the backcountry can prove a daunting challenge. The need for evidence-based recommendations for the prevention and treatment of envenoming injuries has increased in recent years, along with the number of international sojourners and military personnel who are injured by venomous exotic fauna. As international travel and ease of access to previously denied regions continues to improve, increased numbers of untrained travelers will continue to come in contact with a large number of medically significant venomous animals. A compiled list of medically significant venomous terrestrial animals is provided in Table 28.1. The problem has been complicated further by the emergence of new high-risk adventure activities, which increases the risk of encounters with several types of venomous animals. For example, four expatriate envenoming cases seen by one western air medevac service over a 3-year period resulted from "extreme adventure" tour operators who intentionally created close encounters between venomous snakes and paying customers.[3] When encounters result in envenoming mishaps, the injured traveler may receive first-aid from well-intentioned but inexperienced bystanders, which could prove dangerous to life and limb. Upon repatriation to developed countries, victims of envenoming routinely require continued medical care from physicians who may lack experience managing venomous bites caused by exotic species. This chapter will address principles for the prevention, stabilization, and management of venomous injuries caused by terrestrial animals based on recent clinical experiences and prospective studies. The chapter will focus on field-viable technologies, practices, and methodologies appropriate for the expedition and delayed-care environment. Principles for the prevention and treatment of envenoming injuries are divided into two sections: medically significant arthropods including arachnids and venomous insects, and a separate discussion of venomous snakes. A discussion of venomous marine animals is found in Chapter 29. Each section includes recommendations for preventing venomous bites and stings during wilderness activities, followed by principles for stabilization and management in austere environments and follow-on care in the hospital. Since a growing number of expeditions have on-hand medical expertise and satellite communication, and may even be equipped with small, cartridge-based serum chemistry and complete blood count assays, a discussion of laboratory criteria for monitoring injured patients is included. The primary communication objective in each section is that *predeployment education* of team members will play a major role in preventing these injuries during expeditions to virtually every destination.

APPROACH TO THE ENVENOMED PATIENT

Human injuries caused by envenomation, the process by which an animal injects venom, are invariably the result of defensive actions of threatened animals (Figure 28.1). Venom may be delivered through a caudal stinger, as in the case of scorpions and the hymenoptera (bees and wasps); fangs, or grooved teeth, as with the reptiles and spiders; or through specialized spines as in certain caterpillars. One mammal capable of envenoming is the male duck billed platypus,[4] an aquatic oddity that lives in Australia's eastern regions. When defending itself, the male can deliver venom by forcibly driving caudal spurs into the hand of the unwary handler. In the majority of cases, venomous injury will vary significantly with the

Table 28.1. Representative venomous animals by region

Type	Name	Region
Spiders	Widow spiders (*Latrodectus*)	Worldwide
	Violin spiders (*Loxosceles*)	Western hemisphere
	Banana spiders (*Phoneutria*)	Tropical Americas
	Wolf spiders (*Lycosidae*)	Worldwide
	Funnel web spiders (*Atrax*)	Australia
	Hobo spiders (*Tegeneria*)	Europe, Asia, Northwest United States
Scorpions	Amazon yellow (*Tityus*)	South America
	African scorpions (*Leiurus*)	North Africa
	African scorpions (*Buthus*)	North Africa, Spain
	Indian scorpions (*Buthotus*)	India, Sri Lanka, Bangladesh
	American bark scorpions (*Centruroides*)	Southern United States to Colombia
Venomous snakes		
Vipers	Daboia (*Daboia russelli*)	Asia, Australia
	European asp (*Vipera berus*)	Europe
	Forest vipers (*Atheris*)	Africa
	Gaboon viper/puff adder (*Bitis*)	Africa
	Sand vipers (*Cerastes*)	Asia, Australia
	Saw-scale vipers (*Echis*)	Asia, Australia
Ground viper	Stiletto snakes/burrowing asps (*Atractaspis*)	Africa
Elapsids	Australian elapids (*Notechis, Oxyuranus, Pseudechis*)	Asia, Australia
	Mambas (*Dendroaspis*)	Africa
	Asian coral snakes (*Maticora/ Caliophus*)	Asia, Australia
	Cobra (*Naja, Walterinnesia*)	Africa, Asia, Australia
	Coral snakes (*Micrurus*)	Americas
	Kraits (*Bungarus*)	Asia, Australia
	Sea snakes (*Enhydrina*)	Asia, Australia
	African coral snakes (*Aspidelaps*)	Africa
Rear-fanged colubrids	Boomslang (*Dispholidus*)	Africa
Pit vipers	Central/Southern pit vipers (*Bothrops*)	Americas
	Cottonmouth/copperhead (*Agkistrodon*)	Americas
	Green tree viper group (*Trimeresurus*)	Asia, Australia
	Malayan pit viper (*Calloselasma*)	Asia, Australia
	Rattlesnakes (*Crotalus*)	Americas
Mammals	Solenodons (*Atopogale cubana*)	Caribbean Islands
	Platypus (*Ornithorhyncus*)	Australia
	Shrews (*Blarina*)	North and Central America
	Loris (*Nycticebus*)	Tropical Asia and Africa

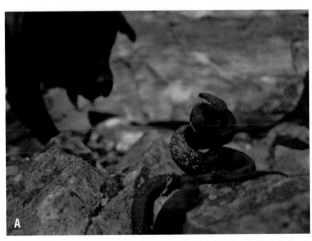
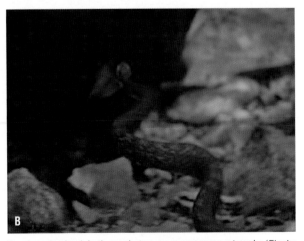

Figure 28.1. A snakebite is usually the result of defensive actions taken by a threatened animal. In these photos, a nonvenomous rat snake (*Elaphe obsoleta*) displays the defensive posture (A) and striking kinematics (B) common to many venomous snakes. Photo courtesy Michael Callahan.

offending species, the amount of venom, its toxicity, the location where the venom was injected, and the body mass and sensitivity of the patient. In the case of bites by the more dangerous snake and spider species, definitive treatment is only possible using specific antivenin. In situations where the expedition member is envenomed in a remote settings, antivenin is often unavailable at local clinics, of dubious quality when present, and prone to dangerous side effects when administered by inexperienced care providers (see Treatment section).

The physician treating a patient on the trail, or directing care from a distant location, will need to provide comfort and assurances to the patient while simultaneously attempting to obtain an accurate description of the offending animal and identify factors relevant to characterizing the gravity of the incident. Critical information includes a description of the offending animal's size, color, behavior, and location; initial description of symptoms; and presence of any well-intentioned but injurious first-aid measures such as tourniquets, cryotherapy, scarification, and electrical shock treatment. Details obtained from the history and physical must be compared with medically significant species native to the region. If envenoming is likely, the patient must receive care at local health facilities as specific antivenin – and expertise – is more likely to be available *in the country where the bite occurred* than in the traveler's home country. A critical point underscored by recent tragedies is that international air medical evacuation flight teams may lack expertise managing the critically envenomed patient; as such, medevac may actually extricate the patient from clinicians with expertise managing complications unique to certain species. In the majority of cases, air medical evacuation should be deferred until after local experienced clinicians have seen the patient and appropriate immunotherapy for local species has been initiated.

Successful assessment and treatment requires that the clinician be familiar with the range, habitat, and behavior of native venomous animals and can make judgments on the quality of local medical resources and the availability of appropriate antivenin. The point is stressed that a physician with expertise treating the bite of a rattlesnake (*Crotalus*) in Texas may be hard-pressed to accurately assess and manage the bite of a saw-scaled viper (*Echis*) in a remote African clinic. An understanding of the natural history and initial effects of a given species' venom can play an important role in identifying the offending species when the animal itself is not available. Examples of this information at work include the purely clinical diagnosis of scorpion sting and the differentiation of necrotic from neurotoxic spider bites, the use of potentially life-saving compression wraps for krait bites but not viper bites, and witholding immunotherapy for the frequent "dry" non-envenoming bites of many venomous snakes.

PRETRAVEL

The expedition clinician preparing in advance for the possibility of venomous injuries during an exotic adventure is likely to be overwhelmed by the diversity of venomous creatures in the destination region. Under these circumstances it is helpful to separate principles of prevention, early field care, and definitive management according to the most consistently available data point: *the identity of the offending species.* Therefore, in the following sections, treatment will be addressed under the premise that the general identity of the offending animal is known (e.g., spider vs. snake). Special emphasis will be given to the most dangerous venomous animals: terrestrial venomous snakes, in particular the old world elapids (cobras, kraits, and coral snakes) and vipers. Because definitive treatment requires specific immunotherapy, a listing of current international antivenins with proven efficacy is provided for reference (Table 28.9). This list will need to be updated annually as products are frequently discontinued or changed without warning.

Prior to departure, the expedition physician will need to identify itineraries and activities likely to increase the risk of encounter with venomous species. Intransigent thrill seekers and others prone to taking unnecessary risks need to be identified as they pose a threat to others and should be excluded from the expedition. For extreme expeditions and circumstances where the consequences of backcountry envenoming are especially dire, the expedition leader should insist that everyone sign a safety contract that requires all team members to abide by guidelines that reduce unnecessary risk, in this case resulting from encounters with venomous species. For example, a recent expedition to India's Kashmir required team members to sign a safety contract warning them against participating in the "cobra handling" workshops in the Lucknow region, which have resulted in bites to participants. A list of risk reduction behaviors for reducing encounters with venomous animals is provided in Table 28.2.

For expeditions traveling without a qualified clinician, pretravel safety education should include a review of the emergency evacuation plan and principals for "first aid" for venomous injuries. Those traveling in regions without medical facilities should receive quality wilderness-specific medical training such as that provided through the Wilderness Medical Society (*http:// www.wms.org*). This training assists the front-country practitioner to adapt their knowledge and experience to the management of patients in the backcountry. When appropriate, at-risk groups should also be provisioned with medical equipment to stabilize a bitten extremity and assess for coagulopathy in the field and be provided with antibiotics to prophylax high-risk bites. In rare cases, research teams working intimately with venomous species may choose to add intravenous fluids, neurotropic

Table 28-2. Prevention of venomous injuries in the backcountry

	Venomous arthropods	
	Bees and wasps (Hymenoptera)	Do not wear brightly colored clothing.
		Avoid perfumes and aromatic cosmetics.
		Avoid trash cans, flowers, unprotected meat, and rotting fruit.
		Keep meat and high-sugar foods and drinks covered.
	Stinging caterpillars	Look before grabbing shrubbery, vines, and branches.
	Centipedes (*Scolopendra*)	Keep bed sheets off floor.
		Wear footwear at night.
		Shake out shoes before wearing.
	Venomous arachnids	
Spiders	Widow spiders (*Latrodectus*)	Avoid webs.
	Banana leaf spiders (*Phoneutria*)	Keep bed sheets from touching floor.
	Violin spiders (*Loxosceles*)	Use insecticide to reduce prey species.
	Web spiders (all)	Inspect privies before sitting (widow spiders).
	Funnel web spiders (*Atrax*)	Watch for burrows; do not play with adults.
Scorpions	*Tityus, Buthus, Centruroides*	Check tub before entering.
		Use UV light wands at night.
	Venomous snakes	
Cobras (Naja), mambas		Do not attract rodents (which attract snakes).
		Do not play with "de-venomed" cobras in Asia.
Elapids		Do not handle unknown species – even if "dead."
		Do not handle docile species of kraits (bites occur suddenly).
		Use a flashlight and walking stick after dark.
		Shake out boots and clothing.
		Avoid sleeping on the ground (especially for kraits).
	Venomous lizards	
Heterodon lizards		Do not handle Gila monsters or beaded lizards even if they are "tame." Bites occur suddenly.

pharmaceuticals, sedatives, analgesics, and antivenin to the field medical kit. However, in the authors' experience, the highest yield investment is to prioritize training of team members to avoid encounters with dangerous species rather than to invest in advanced, cumbersome, and resource-intensive medical therapeutics. One notable exception is an expedition that must work in close contact with venomous species for purposes of medical, zoologic, or ecological research.

VENOMOUS ARTHROPODS

Throughout history, humans have experienced the misfortune of defensive stings and bites of venomous arthropods belonging to either the insects (e.g., bees, wasps) or the arachnids (e.g., spiders, scorpions, and ticks). The spectrum of arthropod envenoming ranges from mild discomfort to life-threatening anaphylactic reactions, tissue destruction, paralysis, and death.[5,6] Hematophagous arthropods seek human contact for purposes of a blood meal, but venomous species have little to gain from an encounter with humans; therefore, injuries are usually the result of the spider or wasp being slapped or stepped upon. It is no surprise then that injuries resulting from the defensive actions of scorpions, spiders, and bees may be prevented by field behaviors

that increase vigilance, or that decrease encounters. For example, avoiding use of fragrant cosmetics, and floral print clothing, and cleaning up leftover food around the campsite all help to reduce attractants for stinging hymenoptera. Established methods for preventing encounters with venomous arthropods are listed in Table 28.2.

Hymenoptera: Bees, Wasps, and Stinging Ants

In terms of the *number* of injuries, the most medically significant venomous arthropods are the Hymenoptera, which include bees, wasps, and stinging ants. Hymenoptera stings cause considerable morbidity through the sting injuries, and by inducing Type I hypersensitivity (anaphylactic) reactions.[7] Hymenoptera venom can however be significant. One insect species, the Central American bullet ant (*Paraponera clavata*), causes such significantly painful stings that they have been compared to a gunshot wound by individuals unfortunate enough to be able to compare the two injuries.[8] The venom of Hymenoptera contains varying concentrations of serotonin, histamine, and acetylcholine, as well as simple enzymes and small peptides. Patients stung by large numbers of bees, wasps, or ants may exhibit signs and complain of symptoms caused by bioactive amines. In the majority of cases however, sting injuries produce immediate pain, which typically abates over a 30- to 120-min period. The infamous "killer bees," a name denoting an Africanized strain of honeybee, have venom that is comparable to that of the common honeybee (*Apidae*). This species' reputation is derived from its spirited defense of the hive, often after minimal provocation. Local reactions to Hymenoptera stings result in a raised papule, usually with a central blanched region, surrounded by blanching erythema, and mild edema at the bite site.

Unlike the predatory wasps, which sting and paralyze prey to feed to their larvae (Figure 28.2), members of the honeybee family have a barbed stinger that cannot be retrieved from the wound. After stinging the offender, the bee eviscerates itself as it flies off, leaving the stinger and the venom gland behind. In these circumstances, the stinger-gland should be quickly removed as the gland will continue to contract, driving more venom into the wound. In contrast with reports to the contrary, grasping the gland between the thumb and fingers during removal has not been shown to increase the amount of venom delivered to the wound.[9] After ensuring the patient is not exhibiting symptoms of hypersensitivity, the wound should be inspected for a retained stinger and cleaned with mild soap and water. The tetanus vaccine status of the team member should always be verified, and the patient should be counseled to look for signs of secondary infection. Oral H1 antihistamines such as diphenhydramine are effective at reducing itching, which can persist for hours following the sting injury. Topical antiinflammatory creams (ketorolac) or oral nonsteroidal antiinflammatory agents (NSAIDs) are also effective in reducing discomfort. Cold compresses help to reduce pain associated with Hymenoptera stings, but they should *never* be used to treat venom injuries that cause tissue destruction, such as those seen with snake and spider bites.

In the backcountry, anaphylactic reactions can prove more difficult to treat than in the emergency department. Suspected hypersensitivity reactions associated with sting injury should be treated promptly before the onset of more severe symptoms. The most reliable therapy is an intramuscular injection with 1:1,000 epinephrine hydrochloride (0.25–0.5 mL IM). Although easy to use, portable single- and double-dose epinephrine injectors (e.g., EpiPen™) are less preferable in the expedition environment as patients with severe reactions may need repeated injections. Also, many field medics report that commercially available epinephrine injectors do not withstand the rigors of backcountry travel. In the authors' experience, expedition kits equipped with multidose epinephrine vials may be kept protected in plastic sleeves allowing for the use of repeat treatment of recalcitrant hypersensitivity reactions. Following injection of epinephrine, the skin should be rigorously massaged to speed drug delivery. Hymenoptera sting injuries to the foot and ankle have a high risk of becoming infected with gram-positive skin flora; consequently, the team member is cautioned to look for erythema, edema, tenderness, and warmth and to treat empirically with appropriate antibiotics.

Centipedes

Centipedes are multisegmented arthropods consisting of over 3,300 species of which the majority of medically significant species live in the tropics. Of these, approximately 100 species belonging to the genus *Scolopendra* are both the largest – with one species growing up to 38 cm and capable of catching and killing small rodents and bats – and the most medically significant (Figure 28.3). Throughout the tropical Americas and

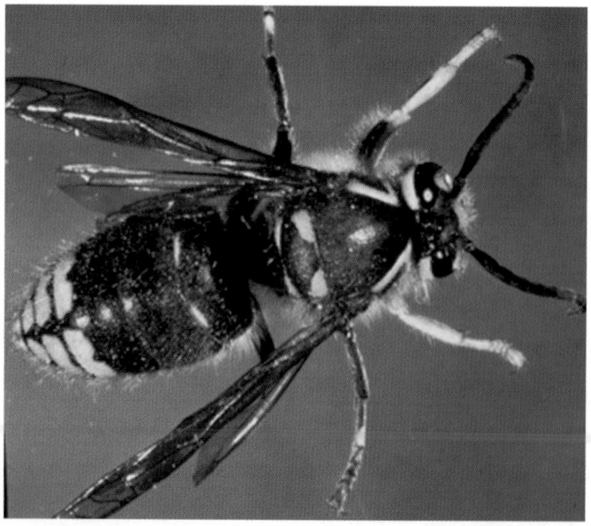

Figure 28.2. Hymenoptera include bees, wasps, and stinging ants. This bald-faced hornet (*Dolichovespula maculata*) is quick to attack and possesses a painful sting. Photo courtesy Michael Callahan.

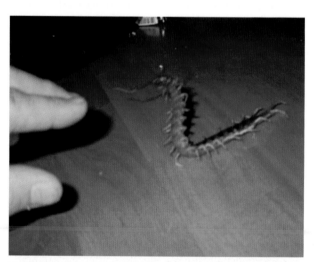

Figure 28.3. Tropical centipedes can cause venomous bites with local and systemic symptoms. This Asian centipede (*Scolopendra*) is acting defensively, having just missed biting the handler. Photo courtesy Michael Callahan.

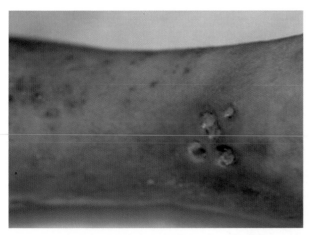

Figure 28.4. Bites from tropical centipedes such as *Scolopendra* can cause necrotic, slow-healing injuries and systemic reactions. The patient in this photo was bitten during a Laotian jungle trek when he put on his socks. Expedition team members should always store clothes in sealed bags or backpacks. Photo courtesy Michael Callahan.

Asia, several species of *Scolopendra* are increasingly recognized as capable of significant envenoming characterized by local tissue destruction (Figure 28.4), and systemic effects ranging from rhabdomyolysis to nephrotoxicity and myocardiotoxicity. Rarely, deaths are reported usually involving small children in rural Asia and Amazonia. The stinging bites by centipedes are delivered through horizontally opposed fangs and result in injuries that are both traumatic and venomous. Management of these injuries is supportive as no antivenin exists. There are anecdotal reports from the zoological community that laboratory-acquired bites are extremely painful and slow to heal. At this time, there is one known prospective clinical trial in Brazil that may result in an evidence-based comparison of management protocols for large centipede envenoming injuries. At this time, management recommendations are supportive and should be based on the clinician's judgment.

Caterpillars

Stinging caterpillars are specialized larvae (the "worm" forms) of butterflies and moths. Worldwide, an estimated 1000 species are capable of causing stinging injuries to humans. All species of stinging caterpillars have a distinct head and a body composed of between 13 and 15 segments. The dorsal surface of the body is adorned with specialized urticaceous or venomous setae (spines). The setae are hollow and contain simple toxins produced in cutaneous venom glands. Stinging is a defensive response to predators and requires direct contact with the setae. When the offending animal comes in contact with setae, the spines penetrate the epidermis and fracture off, releasing venom. Local reactions range from mild itching to moderate pain and may cause dermatitis or pustules. Systemic symptoms

include malaise, fever, and nausea. Management of cutaneous envenoming is supportive and includes local and systemic antihistamines and monitoring of the injury for evidence of secondary infection.

VENOMOUS ARACHNIDS: SPIDERS, SCORPIONS, AND TICKS

Spiders

Medically significant arachnids cause injuries ranging from benign, self-limiting bites to dermatonecrotic injuries, systemic paralysis, and death. With the exception of ticks, which envenomate as a consequence of blood feeding, injuries caused by the arachnids are defensive in nature; therefore, adopting safety practices will help reduce the chance of a harmful encounter. Arachnid venoms vary widely with species and cause symptoms ranging from intense local pain to system reactions, including severe systemic neurotoxemia. Among the arachnids, only the spiders use their venom to initiate digestion of prey, which helps justify the observation that dermatonecrosis is common in spider bite but rare for scorpion stings and noninfectious tick bite. In both the eastern and western hemispheres, the venom from several species of spiders can lead to significant tissue destruction. The species most commonly implicated in necrotic arachnidism are running spiders (Figure 28.5) belonging to the violin spider group (violin or recluse spiders; genus *Loxosceles*); hobo spiders (*Tageneria*), jumping spiders (*Phidippidus*), Mediterranean sac spiders (*Chiracanthium*), and wolf spiders (*Lycosa*). The bites from several members of the *Loxosceles* spiders, in particular the South American species *L. laeta*, can cause catastrophic necrosis and destruction of underlying structures resulting in severe cosmetic disfigurement and death (Figure 28.6).[10,11] Although there is a simple polyspecific *Loxosceles* antivenin produced in Brazil,

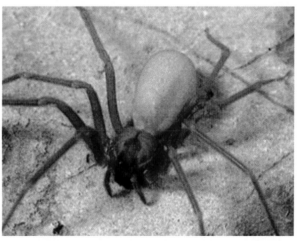

Figure 28.5. Running spiders of the genus *Loxosceles* (violin spiders) are responsible for thousands of necrotizing bites in the Americas each year. Photo courtesy M. Pitts.

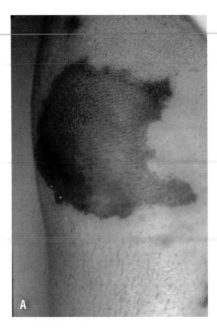

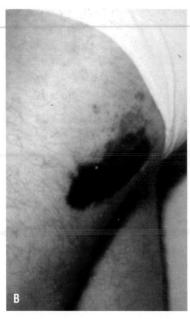

Figure 28.6. Necrotic spider bites can cause significant injury. The victim in this photo was bitten by *Loxosceles laeta* while traveling in the Andes. The bite was photographed at 12 hr (A) and 60 hr (B). Photo courtesy Michael Callahan.

there is a decades-long debate about its value,[12] and there are no FDA-approved indications for its use.

Widow spiders (*Latrodectus*) (Figure 28.7) epitomized by the American black widow (*L. hesperens, L. mactans*) and Australian brown widow and red-back spider (*L. hasseltii*) are dangerous web-bound spiders, which are found throughout the world. All widow spiders possess potent neurotoxic venom, which induces painful muscle cramps and spasms. The larger female spiders, which are responsible for most bites, build chaotic, untidy webs near sources that attract insects, such as pit privies and trash dumps. When working with this spider (*L. mactans*) in the laboratory, the authors observe these species are reluctant to bite; however, under natural circumstances, patients occasionally report being bitten

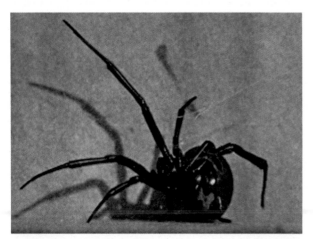

Figure 28.7. Widow spiders (*Latrodectus*) are significantly venomous and have a worldwide distribution. Bites occur when humans intrude on webs or when spiders are trapped against human skin. Local symptoms are mild, but if left untreated, bites can be fatal. Photo courtesy Michael Callahan.

after minimal disturbance of the webs. Patients with confirmed widow spider bites present with inconsequential local symptoms, typically mild redness and pain at the bite site. Initial descriptions of a mild sting, are quickly replaced by escalating aching and numbness. Within minutes of the bite, optimism that symptoms will be mild vanishes with the onset of proximal muscular aches and spasms. Systemic envenoming is heralded by severe abdominal cramping, hypertension, and diaphoresis. In severe bites, cramping affects large muscle groups of the abdomen, back, and shoulders. Small children are at increased risk of severe envenoming and may present with the combined constellation of findings of abdominal rigidity, mild fever, and catecholamine-induced leukocytosis, which together may suggest an acute abdomen. Several times each year a *Latrodectus* envenoming in a noncommunicative patient is misdiagnosed as an appendicitis, resulting in a trip to the operating theater. Fortunately, a number of antivenins are produced against *Latrodectus* spiders many of which have demonstrated efficacy against bites by other members of the genus. At the time of this writing, quality *Lactodectus* antivenins are produced by manufactures in Australia, South Africa, South America and the United States.

Over the last several years, the tropical and travel medicine community has come to respect an overlooked but impressively venomous New World species of spider that is responsible for considerable morbidity and occasionally, fatalities in Central and South America. This genus, known commonly as the wandering or banana spiders (genus: *Phoneutria*), were only recently recognized for the potency of their venom. One Brazilian species (*P. nigriventer*) is large, is persnickety, and possesses a neurotoxic venom implicated in a number of fatal bites.[13] The foraging behaviors of the American wandering spiders frequently bring them into contact with humans, particularly in rustic settings where trekkers are sleeping on the floor. In the two cases known to the authors, the victims were handling shrubbery at night resulting in bites to the hands. The observation was made that the *Phoneutria* spiders confused the hand movement of the victim with that of the spiders' prey species, large insects, or small birds, bats, or mice. There is a Brazilian antivenin developed against *Phoneutria*, which appears active against species in other South American countries.[14]

The distinction of "most dangerous" neurotoxic spider belongs to the funnel web spiders (*Atrax*) of Australia and the Indonesian islands. These formidable, aggressive spiders are robust in build, possess highly neurotoxic venom strong enough to kill humans, and have powerful fangs that allow them to bite through clothing and footwear. An effective updated antivenin against funnel web spiders is produced in Australia by Commonwealth Serum Laboratories (see *http://www.toxinology.com/generic_static_files/cslavh_antivenom_funweb.html*).

Scorpions

Scorpions (Figure 28.8) are responsible for a significant number of fatalities in the Middle East, Africa, and the neotropical Americas. The most dangerous species are the African and Middle Asian *Leiurius* and *Tityus*, the Asian *Buthus*, and members of the *Centruroides* scorpions in the western hemisphere. Most fatalities involve stings to small children and the elderly. Scorpions are thigmotropic and nocturnal in habitat, prompting them to take cover in any suitable haven during daytime. Expedition members are most frequently envenomed when they don footwear that was left on the ground or when they enter the shower stall without first checking

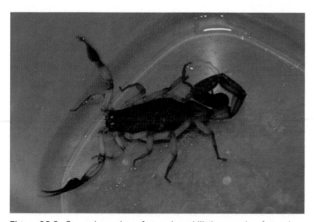

Figure 28.8. Several species of scorpions kill thousands of people a year. Travelers are frequently stung by large tropical species, such as this *Hadurus* specimen, when they step barefoot into shower stalls without looking. Photo courtesy Michael Callahan.

for the presence of trapped scorpions. In all cases of stings by dangerous species, the priority is expeditious administration of appropriate antivenin and control of severe pain. In the backcountry, first-aid measures that are likely to improve outcome include centripetal application of a compression dressing as for *neurotoxic* snake envenoming (see Snakebite section). Scorpion antivenins are produced worldwide by numerous manufacturers but are often unavailable in rural health clinics where they are needed most.

Ticks

Several species of hard ticks are capable of envenoming, which is clinically manifest as an unusual symmetric ascending flaccid paralysis known as "tick paralysis." The most frequently implicated species are female members of the wood ticks (genus *Dermacenter*, especially *D. andersonii* and *D. variabilis*), found throughout the Americas and Europe, and the deer ticks (*Ixodes*, especially *I. holocyclis*), which have a worldwide distribution.

The ticks produce a postsynaptic venom in their salivary glands and deliver it to the patient during a phlebotamine meal. The 48- to 60-kDa venom antigen responsible for symptoms is extremely labile in mammals, perhaps explaining why prompt removal of the tick results in resolution of symptoms in 1–24 hr.

Tick paralysis most commonly affects children. In the authors' experience with cases from the southeastern United States, small children from rural regions who have long hair (which obscures the attached ticks), seem to be the most frequently affected. For clinicians who have seen tick paralysis, symptoms are pathopnuemonic for the syndrome and are unlikely to be missed. Patients typically report that initial symptoms are progressive onset of weakness of large muscle groups of the lower extremities.

Patients with early tick paralysis may complain only of fatigue or exhibit ataxia. Affected children with tick paralysis will often attempt to rise from a sitting position by using their arms to extend their knees, a finding known as Gower's sign. Progression of symptoms progresses centripedally, from lower to upper extremities and torso. Bulbar muscle function tends to be preserved until late, and death is due to respiratory failure.

Unlike other cases of life-threatening neurotoxic envenoming, tick paralysis can be reversed without definitive therapy other than tick removal. The labile protein is rapidly degraded after the tick is removed resulting in quick return of function. The syndrome is prevented by implementation of tick-deterrent behaviors such as trap cuffs on legwear, "tick checks," the use of permethrin-impregnated clothing, and application of extended formulation DEET (N, N- diethyl-m-toluaminde).

VENOMOUS MAMMALS

There are four groups of venomous mammals worldwide, and all belong to different taxonomic groups. Venomous mammals deliver venom through either modified teeth – as in the case of the solenodons and shrews – or through caudal spurs, as in the case of the platypus. Mammalian venom tends to be simple, consisting of several small kD peptides and rarely, bioactive amines. Fatalities from mammalian envenoming are rare, and cases that have undergone retrospective review indicate that the victim had significant medical comorbidities or that death was due to other causes.

Solenodons are primitive mammals that resemble extremely large shrews with body weights of 0.5–3 kg and that are restricted to the central Caribbean islands. Two species are capable of an envenoming bite. Venom is produced in mandibular acinar glands located in the buccal mucosa and is delivered into wounds created by canaliculated incisors. The larger Cuban solenodon (*Atopogale cubana*) is both more dangerous and more frequently implicated in human envenoming. The Haitian solenodon (*Solenodon paradoxus*), which is also found in the Dominican Republic, is infrequently implicated in human cases. Symptoms include pain and erythema at the bite site.

Shrews (*Blarina*) are small, hypermetabolic mammals that are capable of delivering venomous saliva through bites. Patients bitten by shrews, usually as a consequence of research activities, report sharp stinging pain followed by a persistent achy sensation that can last several days. Species reported to deliver the strongest bite include the North American northern short-tailed shrew (*Blarina brevicauda*), southern short-tailed shrew (*Blarina carolinensis*), and Elliot's short-tailed shrew (*Blarina hylophaga*). It is likely that shrews from other regions are also venomous.

The platypus (*Omithorhyncus anatinus*) is an aquatic oddity of 40–60 cm and 1–3 kg size that is found in select parts of Australia. The male platypus is able to deliver venom through a spur modified from the calcaneus on the hind leg.

Lorises (genus *Nycticebus*), slow moving arboreal primates found in Old World jungles, produce a simple venomous secretion in modified axillary glands located proximal to the animal's elbow. Lorises distribute the venom to the fur of offspring to protect them from predators. There is evidence that an adult loris can also transfer venom to its mouth to allow the animal to deliver a venom-laden bite.

VENOMOUS SNAKES

After man, venomous reptiles are the vertebrates that pose the greatest threat to human lives, accounting for between 100,000 and 120,000 fatalities each year. Ven-

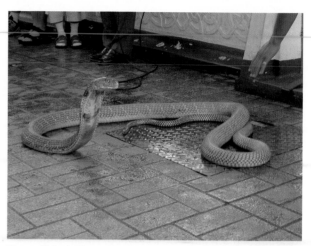

Figure 28.9. A king cobra (*Ophiophagus hannah*) is handled at a snake farm in Bangkok, Thailand. Travelers should be wary of viewing venomous snakes in uncontrolled environments, especially if the handler is a street amateur and not a trained professional. Photo courtesy Christian Tomaszewski.

omous snakes are a primary concern for the international traveler because these adventurers are likely to be exposed to the same level of risk as the local population but lack experience in how to recognize and avoid dangerous species. Familiarity with methods for avoiding dangerous species, or "snake sense," helps to prevent bites in developing tropical countries where snakes and humans live in intense contact with each other. This point is illustrated by the higher incidence of snake envenoming among expatriate and backcountry travelers compared to local field workers and others with regular contact with dangerous species. Principle factors associated with snake envenoming *among travelers* include the following:

1. In many cases, the snake was purposely disturbed, and the bite was defensive.
2. The handler was often "familiar" with snakes from his or her home country but unfamiliar with local species.
3. Photo opportunities (Figure 28.9) are routinely implicated in promoting unwise behaviors.
4. Bites are likely to occur in rural areas, and are often inflicted upon individuals lacking resources, resulting in delayed, complex, and costly medical evacuations.
5. Ambiguity in effective first-aid measures result in procedures that aggravate injury to limb and that may threaten the life of the patient.

Kinematics of Snake Envenoming

Venomous snakes possess specialized grooved or canaliculated fangs in the maxilla of the upper jaw that are connected to venom glands. Venoms are produced in specialized salivary glands and delivered to fixed fangs in the case of elapids (*Elapidae*) and erectile fangs in

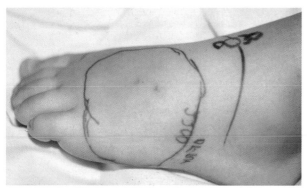

Figure 28.10. Fang marks of a copperhead (*Agkistrodon*) bite on the foot of a pediatric patient in North Carolina, USA. Photo courtesy Christian Tomaszewski.

the case of the vipers (*Viperinae*) and pit vipers (*Crotalinae*). The pit vipers, specialized predators of mammals and birds, possess elongated, deeply penetrating fangs (Figure 28.10) and heat-sensitive pits located between the eye and the nostril, which together help the vipers to target and envenom warm-blooded prey. Several species of rear-fanged colubrids such as the Asian keelbacked snakes (*Rhobdophis*) are significantly venomous,

possessing a procoagulant that quickly defibrinates the blood of envenomed patients. The most dangerous rear-fanged species are found in Southeast Asia. A list of venomous snakes and geographic ranges is provided in Table 28.3.

Assessment of Snake Envenoming

Venomous snakebite is a medical emergency until clinical assessment by an experienced physician proves otherwise. In contrast with many wilderness medical problems, snake envenoming is one condition that if untreated is virtually guaranteed to have an unfortunate outcome in the backcountry. Table 28.4 lists general first-aid principles for wilderness settings. One contributing factor to bad outcomes in the tropics is the lack of uniform criteria for assessing, triaging, and managing the bites of over 300 venomous species. The risk to life and limb (Figure 28.11), and the permanent disfigurement that complicates the bites of many species underscore the value of educating wilderness travelers about venomous snakes. Expedition physicians and team leaders should implement strategies for avoiding snake encounters and review priorities in assessing and managing

Table 28-3. Representative genus and species of venomous snakes

Type	Family	Genus and species	Common name	Range
Vipers	Crotalidae	C. adamantus	Eastern diamondback rattlesnake	Southeastern United States
	Agkistrodon	A contortrix	Copperheads and moccasins	North and Central America
	Bothrops	B. atrops	Fer de Lance	Central and South America
	Lachesis	L mutis spp.	Bushmaster	Central and South America
	Azmiops	A. feae	Fea's viper	Southeast Asia (rare)
	Trimeresurus	T. stejnegeri	Chinese bamboo pit viper	Southern China
	Tropidolaemus	T. wagleri	Wagler's temple viper	Indonesia
Elapidae	Bungarus	B. fasciatus	Banded krait	India, Laos
		B. caeruleus	Indian krait	Western India, Nepal Sri Lanka
	Calliophis	C. bibroni	Bibron's coral snake	India, Thailand
	Micrurus	M. fulvius	Eastern coral snake	Southeastern coastal United States
	Micruroides	M. euryxanthus	Western coral snake	Texas, Mississippi, New Mexico
	Maticora	M. bivirgata	Blue long-glanded coral snake	Malaysia, Indonesia
	Naja	N. nivia	African Cape cobra	China, northern Laos, Vietnam
		N. naja	Indian cobra	Pakistan, Nepal, Sri Lanka
		N. kaouthia	Monocellate cobra	India, Thailand
		N. oxiana	Central Asian cobra	Northern India, Nepal
		N. sumatrana	Malay spitting cobra	Sumatra, Malaysia
		N. philippinensis	Mindora/Philippine cobra	Philippines
	Ophiophagus	O. hannah (only)	King cobra	India, Philippines
	Oxyuranus	O. microlepidotus	Inland taipan	Australia (Northern territory to Queensland)
	Walterinnesia	W.aegyptia (only)	Desert cobra	Middle East, Northern Africa
Colubridae	Ahaetulla	A. nasuta	Long-nosed vine snake	India, Southeast Asia
	Balanophis	B. ceylonicus	Sri Lankan keel-backed	Sri Lanka
	Boiga	B. dendrophilia	Mangrove snake	Thailand, Singapore, Sulawesi
	Cerebrus	C. rhynchops	Dog-faced watersnake	India, Southeast Asia, Philippines
	Coluber	C. ravergieri	Steppe racer	Northwest India, Xinjiiang province
	Enhydris	E. enhydris	Rainbow watersnake	Southern India, southern China
	Rhobdophis	R. subminiatus	Red-necked keel-backed	Southeast Asia

Table 28.4. First-aid for snake envenoming

ABCs: Place patient in the lateral recumbent position. If non-breathing, insert an oral airway or pull tongue forward. In unconscious patients, tongue may be perforated with pin and externally fixed. Perform rescue breathing if needed. If hypotensive, use IV fluids if available; otherwise, place in shock position, raise extremities, and protect airway with recumbent positioning.

Do no harm.

Initiate evacuation plan immediately.

If patient is alert, place patient at rest and provide reassurance.

Wash bite wound to remove unabsorbed venom.

Immobilize the bitten extremity in a functional position at or below heart level.

Remove rings, watches, and other potentially constrictive items.

Delay the spread of venom (see compression bandages for neurotoxic species – see text and Table 28.7).

If patient is alert, without nausea, and evacuation is prolonged, provide fluids (po). Avoid alcohol.

Painkillers, especially narcotic analgesia and NSAIDs[a], should not be used early, except at the recommendation of a physician familiar with snake envenoming.

---

[a] NSAIDs, nonsteroidal antiinflammatory drugs.

Table 28.5. Patient history

All Cases

Name, age, weight of victim

Size, color, shape, and distinctive feature of the snake

Geographic location where bite occurred (country, region, swamp, forest, zoo)

Anatomic location of bites and number of bites received

Initial symptoms

Type of first aid or traditional therapy received

Past medical history (e.g., asthma, COPD)

Medication (especially warfarin, β-blockers, recreational drugs, alcohol)

Prior history of antivenom or animal product immune therapy

Change in symptoms during transport

Presence of priority symptoms: nausea, vomiting, blurred vision, dizziness, dyspnea, syncope, weakness, chest pain, urinary retention, bleeding from rectum or gums, dark-colored urine, melena, hematochezia

Tetanus immunization status

For viper and *Rhabdophis* Bites

Blood type

Recent surgery

History of cardiac disease, anemia, or hemoglobinopathy

For cobra, krait, mamba, taipan, and coral snake bites

Time of last meal

History of prior intubation

History of bronchospasm or arrhythmias

Edrophonium hypersensitivity

Location of responsible support personnel (to assist in care of paralyzed patients)

Advanced directive

---

the bites by the species that may be encountered. Many teams traveling en-route to a backcountry objective are likely to be called upon to treat bites to the rural poor. It should be noted that two New World lizards, the Gila monster and the Mexican beaded lizard (*Heloderma*), are also venomous. These species possess mandibular venom glands, which secrete moderately toxic venom into the wounds made by grooved teeth. The clinical presentation resulting from successful envenoming includes local pain, erythema, edema, nausea, vomiting, and diaphoresis. Deaths from lizard envenoming are rare; bites are occasionally reported when hobbyists are bitten by "pet" lizards.[15] No antivenin is available for bites by Heloderma lizards.

Following successful envenoming, the clinical features of snake venom may cause remarkable variations in clinical presentation. Interpretation of symptoms in the backcountry may be difficult to reconcile with clinical observations and the patient's history (see Table 28.5). For this reason, management of acute snake envenoming

in resource poor settings benefits from a basic division of clinical assessment into the following broad categories: (1) local effects restricted to the bitten extremity; (2) hematotoxic effects upon coagulation, vascular beds, and red cells; (3) myonecrotic effects to muscle and dermis; (4) local and systemic neurologic effects such as paralysis; (5) cardiotoxicity; (6) nephrotoxicity; and (7) endocrinopathies resulting from delayed and indirect toxicities.

A number of spectacular cases have emphasized limitations of applying experience gained from treating snakebite from local species to bites from foreign snakes. In general, physicians experienced in treating snakebite in the tropics agree that although vipers account for the greatest number of bites (Figure 28.12), it is likely that

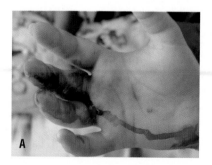
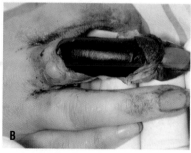

Figure 28.11. Injury from the bite of an African puff adder (*Bitis arietans*). Injury to finger at 6 hr postbite (A) and 36 hr postbite (B). This injured middle finger was eventually amputated. Photo courtesy Christian Tomaszewski.

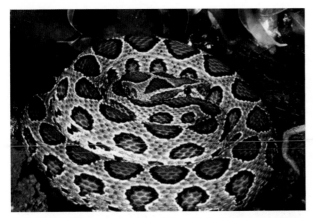

Figure 28.12. Vipers, such as this Asian daboia (*Daboia russelli*), are commonly implicated in human and have venom capable of causing devastating tissue damage and systemic coagulopathy. Photo courtesy Beat Akeret.

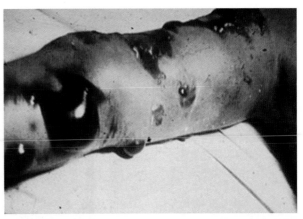

Figure 28.14. Viper and many cobra venoms possess enzymes that cause significant local tissue injury as well as systemic defibrination and direct toxicity to end organs and vascular beds. This patient was bitten by a New World rattlesnake resulting in extensive hemorrhagic blebs, hemolysis, and hypotension. Photo courtesy Michael Callahan.

the elapids, such as the kraits and cobras (Figure 28.13), account for the greatest number of deaths. The venom of the vipers is, however, likely to cause death through near-term or delayed mechanisms. Viper venom contains a large number of complex enzymes that can cause tremendous local pain, swelling, clotting abnormalities, and tissue destruction (Figure 28.14 and 28.15). The venom of many Old and New World vipers induces defibrination, either through procoagulant activity or the indirect activation and consumption of specific clotting factors. The clinical result of the activity of many viper venoms is sustained coagulation dyscrasias (Figure 28.16) that can cause thrombi and infarction damage to the adrenals, kidneys, and pituitary gland.[16] Venom from many Asian and African cobra species is capable of causing either devastating tissue injury, or pure neurotoxic reactions including respiratory failure; however, in most cases of cobra bite, patients present with a mixture of signs and symptoms rather than isolated evidence of neurotoxicity.

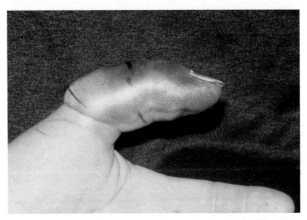

Figure 28.-15. Local tissue destruction secondary to the bite of an eastern diamondback rattlesnake (*Crotalus adamanteus*) at 12 hr postbite. Photo courtesy Christian Tomaszewski.

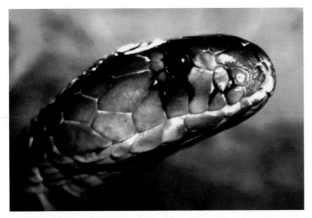

Figure 28.13. In tropical Asia, elapids such as this cobra (*Naja naja siamensis*) are likely responsible for the greatest number of snakebite fatalities in areas without antivenin. Photo courtesy Beat Akeret.

The prognosis of the snake-envenomed patient who is far from medical care and antivenin ranges from inconsequential to hopeless. In the case of viper bites, tissue damage and end-organ damage may unfold over days; however, in the case of intravenous bites, death may occur within minutes. Death between 12 hours and 5 days is likely associated with uncorrected coagulopathies complicated by hypovolemic, metabolic, and hemorrhagic shock, and rarely endocrine crises secondary to infarction of pituitary or adrenal glands. Bites by extremely neurotoxic species, in particular the kraits, mambas (Figures 28.17 and 28.18), and Philippines cobra, can cause death within hours (Figure 28.19). In the expedition environment, where rescuer breathing is the usual source of positive pressure ventilation, victims are likely to die from failure of patient ventilation due to fatigue among the rescuers and improper airway management rather than the delayed complication of shock, renal failure, or secondary wound infection.

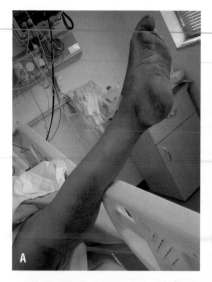

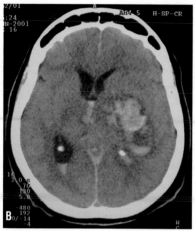

Figure 28.16. Viper bites can cause sustained coagulopathies in addition to local tissue destruction. This patient was bitten by a saw-scaled viper (*Echis carinatus*) while on coumadin. The patient suffered local tissue destruction at less than 24 hr postbite (A) and then intracranial bleeding causing death at 48 hr postbite (B). Photo courtesy Christian Tomaszewski.

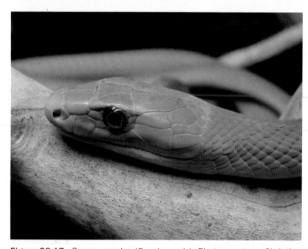

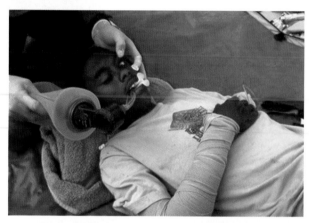

Figure 28.19. Individuals bitten by certain neurotoxic snakes such as the kraits, coral snakes, mambas, and several cobras may display virtually no local symptoms but proceed to have severe systemic reactions. This patient bitten by a mamba was quickly paralyzed. Note the bulbar palsy and the use of compression wrap. Photo courtesy of Michael Callahan.

Figure 28.17. Green mamba (*Dendroaspis*). Photo courtesy Christian Tomaszewski.

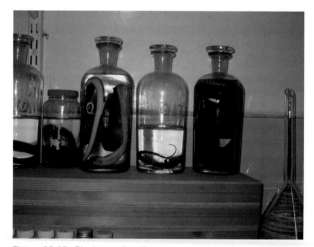

Figure 28.18. Black mamba (*Dendroaspis polylepis*) preserved in a specimen jar in a hospital lab in Tanzania (third jar from left). Black mambas are named for the color of their deeply pigmented mouth interiors, not their body color, which is usually a shade of gray. Photo courtesy Gregory H. Bledsoe.

Accurate assessment of snakebite is improved through an understanding of the snakes themselves. For example, the observation that between 25 and 40% of venomous snakebites do *not* result in envenoming helps in the evaluation of seemingly asymptomatic bites by vipers, which typically cause local pain and swelling within minutes of striking. Assessment of bites caused by neurotoxic species is more complicated as symptoms heralding envenoming may be delayed in excess of 15 hours.

Clinical assessment of bites may be complicated by symptoms that may be the result of venom or the patient's terror from the snakebite itself. The treating physician will need to determine that hyperventilation and associated symptoms of perioral anesthesias and carpopedal flexion, as well as tachycardia, diaphoresis, and faintness are due to anxiety and do not indicate systemic envenoming. In austere environments, differentiating envenoming from dry bites inflicted by purely neurotoxic species such as the kraits (*Bungarus*), mambas (*Dendroaspis*), coral snakes (*Maticora, Caliopsus, Micrurus*), and several Australian species (*Oxyuranus*) is challenging as local findings are often minimal and the onset of systemic symptoms may be delayed many hours.[17] It should be stressed that snakebite fatalities have occurred on expeditions when bites by neurotoxic species were initially determined to be "dry" due to the absence of local symptoms.[18] Indeed, cryptic envenoming by many elapids is often unrecognized until early neurotoxic symptoms such as bulbar paralysis is obvious. In the authors' experience with early assessment of envenoming by two highly neurotoxic species, the banded krait (*B. fasciatus; n* = 7) and West African mambas (*Dendroaspis; n* = 4), the first symptoms to present were mild, nonspecific muscle discomfort or weakness and/or tingling at the bite site. In contrast, the majority of envenoming by cobras and virtually all vipers result in *severe* local pain, swelling, and erythema. Coagulopathy, as evidenced by persistent bleeding from fang marks, venipuncture site, gingiva, or gastrointestinal track or a failed whole blood clotting test, or WBCT, (see discussion in Treatment section) is commonly associated with bites by the vipers (*Crotalids, Bitis, Bothrops, Echis, Daboia*, etc.), boomslangs (*Dyspholidus*), or members of the Asian keel-backed snakes (*Rhabdophis*). The venom of one African colubrid, the Natal green snake (*Philothamnus*), has a potent procoagulant that could induce thrombosis or infarction of small and mid-sized vessels.

Common findings following viper envenoming include local pain, swelling, and echymosis. Systemic coagulopathy may occur within 20–30 min following the bites of certain vipers. In the case of patients bitten by African and Asian cobras, these symptoms may also include neurotoxic findings. In southern India, Sri Lanka, and Bangladesh, envenoming by members of the Russell viper complex, now named daboia (*Daboia russelli russelli/D. r. pulchella*), may cause pain, swelling, myolysis, disseminated intravascular coagulation (DIC), and severe neurotoxic symptoms.[19] Physicians treating snakebite by unfamiliar species may have misplaced confidence in the quality and specificity of foreign-produced antivenins. For example, several Asian manufacturers produce antivenin using the venom of snakes that are easily procured from nearby sources and fail to include venom from specimens found in more distant parts of the species' range. For this reason and when choices are available, snakebite should be treated with antivenin produced using the snakes *from the same region* as where the bite occurred. In other regions, notably West Africa and Asia, our team has recently discovered antivenins that were counterfeit, possessing no neutralizing immunoglobins

at all.[20] The specter and consequences of administering a faux therapeutic of dubious and uncertain composition into the central venous circulation of an envenomed patient is potentially a new concern for the wilderness physicians.

TREATMENT

A generalized protocol for the treatment of snakebite is provided in Table 28.6. All cases of snake envenoming require immediate attention to the ABCs (airway–breathing–circulation) and other near-term threats to life, an accurate history from the patient and bystanders, rapid implementation of measures proven to delay the spread of venom, and immediate activation of the evacuation plan. Evacuation from the backcountry should not be delayed by the availability of advanced on-scene medical care, except in the unlikely case where antivenin is both present and can be administered safely. The emphasis on rapid transport to more advanced medical care is based on unfortunate cases where envenomed patients who were seemingly stable would suddenly succumb to catastrophic internal hemorrhage, endocrine crises, myocardial infarction, cardiac dysrthymias, or other complication that are neigh impossible to manage in resource-constrained settings. Most cases of envenoming are immediately obvious; however, cryptic neurotoxic envenoming cannot be ruled out until the patient has remained symptom-free for 18–24 hours. Early assessment may be complicated by differentiating symptoms resulting from the venom from those caused by the patient's emotional state. The consequences of unfamiliar or dubious first-aid practices and traditional remedies should be closely monitored. Injurious first-aid practices such as cold treatment, tourniquets, electrical shock treatment, scarification, alcohol ingestion, and cutaneous burns should be documented and addressed as permitted by time, resources, and expertise. There is no first-aid measure that in itself is therapeutic, and none of these measures is a substitute for antivenin treatment. Definitive treatment of snakebite requires an understanding of local species, appropriate methods to delay spread of venom, and expedited access to obtain species specific or polyvalent antivenin.

Initial care in the wilderness and in the medical clinic includes immediate attention to the ABCs and rapid assessment of cranial nerve findings. After ensuring ABCs are intact, the care provider should obtain a quick history to determine the circumstances surrounding the bite and a description of the offending animal. In the first minutes of medical care, all potentially constrictive items such as rings, watches, and decorative body piercings should be removed and the locations splinted in a functional position at or slightly below heart level. Bitten extremities should be splinted using a padded rigid

Table 28.6. Emergency management of snake venom poisoning

1. Complete primary assessment (airway–breathing–circulation) and obtain quality vital signs. If stable, go to number 4.
2. Ventilation: If patient is in respiratory distress, increase FiO_2 (if available) using simple mask[a] or ambu bag (BVM) supplemented with portable field O_2 concentrator or micro tank. For venom-paralyzed patients, consider immediate anticholinesterase inhibitor therapy. Patients should be pretreated with atropine, 0.6–1.0 mg/L (children: <20 µg/kg) and tested for edrophonium sensitivity (1 mg IV). Patients without contraindications are treated with edrophonium 8 mg IV (0.15 mg/kg for children) and evaluated clinically for improvement. Patients who show improvement within 3–10 minutes should be treated either with edrophonium or neostigmine (0.5– 1.0 mg IM or over 4 min IV) and atropine every 2–3 hr. Note: anticholinesterase inhibitors have little value after complete paralysis is present.
3. Hemodynamics: determine BP at bilateral locations and compare between bitten and unbitten extremity. Initiate whole blood clotting test using blood obtained from a peripheral site (see text). If necessary and resources exist, correct hypotension with 300–500 ml infusion every 5 min (children 20ml/kg) until normal pressure is restored. Use of vasopressors should be reserved for cases that do not respond to IV hydration and that do not have hemorrhage. Location of cryptic bleeds should be identified using focused clinical exam and stool guaiac studies. Initiate trial CPR for any pulseless patient but be prepared to terminate if heart rate does not spontaneously return. Cardiac arrest in the envenomated patient has an extremely grim prognosis.
4. Assign tasks to team members: delegate someone to identify the snake, to initiate medical evacuation plan, and to collect compression bandage and the team medical kit; deploy two trail runners to nearest medical facility; designate satellite/cell phone operator to notify health care assets of inbound snake bite (e.g., start search for antivenin, identify in-country ALS and helicopter availability).
5. Local Care: fang marks should be closely inspected and retained fangs removed with forceps. The bite site should be irrigated and blotted with gauze to wash away excess venom, which is frequently sprayed onto skin. Do not otherwise manipulate the bite site. Suction device may be considered if applied within 1–3 minutes of the bite but are otherwise useless and should be removed (see text). Consider pressure bandages for suspected neurotoxic bites (see discussion). If a tourniquet was erroneously applied, consider removal based on situation, circumstance, and clinical judgment. If tourniquet requires removal, first place BP cuff proximal to TK and inflate to 100–120 mmHg. Control reperfusion with diligent monitoring. Obtain circumferential measurements and compare to unbitten extremity and repeat Q 15 min. Remove potentially constrictive items such as rings, watches, body piercings and elastic bands. Keep bitten extremity immobilized at or below heart level using SAM® splint or equivalent. Monitor extremity for pain and complications resulting from edema.
6. Antivenin: If envenoming is confirmed, give appropriate antivenin as soon as available. Mitigate against hypersensitivity reactions by oral antihistamine pretreatment and placing epinephrine (0. 5 mL of 1:10,000 dilution) at side of litter. Do not skin test if there is a chance antivenin will *not* be used. Stop antivenin to treat for anaphylactic reactions and then resume at a slower rate. For moderate envenomings, administer antivenin at 1 vial Q 5 min in 250 ml appropriate diluent; control rate using micro-drip adjustment. Generally, monovalent antivenins are administered in 1–2 vial aliquots and polyvalent antivenins at 2–3 vial aliquots. If patient is deteriorating quickly, give antivenin IV push. If patient is alert, inquire about change in symptoms and compare with clinical exam (e.g., circumferential measurements). Administer additional aliquots as determined by patient symptoms and clinical judgment. Note: hyper-immune serums ("wet antivenin") tend to be weaker than lyophilized preparations.
7. Extended evacuation: nasogastric tubes can reduce airway disasters in spontaneously breathing patients who are being evacuated over difficult terrain. If skill and resources permit, cricothyrotomy should be considered for paralyzed patients as bag-mask and bystander mouth-to-mouth ventilation is near impossible to maintain during ground evacuation. Enteral fluids should be considered for conscious patients if there is no IV support. The team physician should not turn the patient over to personnel with lower levels of medical experience, and others unfamiliar with modern wilderness medical devices, technologies, and treatment protocols.

[a] The best of the simple masks for extended field ventilation is the SealEasy™ mask produced by Respironics, Inc.

material. On rare occasions when the victim is bitten on the torso, the bite site should be kept superior providing this does not impede evacuation. If a neurotoxic species is suspected, a compression dressing (pressure bandages) should be applied proximal to the bite and extended beyond the fang marks (Figure 28.19). Compression dressings, which were originally developed in Australia for use in neurotoxic snakebite,[21] have had apparent success against the bites of many species.[22,23] One caveat to the use of compressive bandages is with regard to bites by vipers and cobras possessing venom that causes tissue destruction: the application of compression bandages to bites by these species may exacerbate local injury as swelling tissue is restrained by the dressing. In the authors' experience managing bites by the Asian cobra *Naja kouthia*, which possesses potent myonecrotic venom, compression bandages increased tissue destruction only in the distribution of the area covered by the dressing. The point is reiterated that compression dressings are intended for bites by snakes with neurotoxic venoms and *not* for snakes possessing venom known to cause tissue destruction. Patients treated with compression dressings require close supervision because, as consequence of increasing pain, the unsupervised patient is likely to release the dressing allowing sequestered venom and by-products of tissue injury to be suddenly released into the systemic circulation. General guidelines for the use of compression bandages are provided in

Table 28.7. Contraindications to pressure bandages

Bite by unknown species with local evidence of tissue damage

Any bite with pain, swelling, and bleeding from fang marks

Bites associated with severe coagulopathy

Bites >24 hr, without symptoms

Bites by colubrids (e.g., *Boiga, Rhabdophis*)

Bite by any Asian viper or pit viper (possible exception: *Daboia r. russelli* in southern India and Sri Lanka)

Any cobra bite with local pain, swelling, or significant discoloration

Comment: pressure-immobilization bandages seem beneficial for envenoming by kraits, coral snakes (*Calliopus, Maticora*), king cobra (*Ophiophagus hannah*), and Philippine cobra (*Naja philippinensis*) (see text).

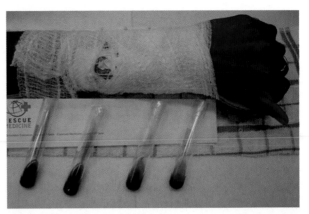

Figure 28.20. WBCT can help assess for coagulopathy and guide antivenin use. The patient in this photo was bitten by an *Echis* viper. Early WBCT demonstrates incoagulable blood (left two tubes). Following antivenin therapy, the WBCT became positive as indicated by a clot and clearing serum (right two tubes). Note persistent bleeding from fang marks in forearm and the use of SAM® splint. Photo courtesy Michael Callahan.

Table 28.7. Venom extraction devices, cauterization, stun guns and native remedies common in the backcountry of Asia (e.g., bamboo cupping), Africa (e.g., hot stones and palauces), and the Americas (e.g., whiskey, gasoline) should be strictly avoided as none have been shown to be of clinical value.

In the backcountry, the presence of venom-induced coagulopathy can be determined at trailside by improvising a WBCT from available materials. In this test, whole blood is obtained from a safe peripheral site and allowed to clot on a non-silica-coated glass surface such as the cover of a compass or a microscope slide. Note that the glass lenses of sports sunglasses, which are coated, are ineffective as they do not reliably catalyze coagulation. On arrival at a local clinic, coagulopathy may be assessed using the traditional WBCT. In this case, 5–8 cm of freshly drawn blood is placed in a clean (red top) vacutainer or test tube and allowed to remain undisturbed at ambient temperature for 20–30 minutes (Figure 28.20). If no clot is noted, the tube should be decanted and inspected for the presence of small thrombi. Incoagulable blood suggests that the offending species was likely a viper, boomslang (*D. typhus*), Asian keel-backed snake (*Rhabdophis*), or other species possessing defibrinating venom. In clinical settings where serial measurement of prothrombin and partial thromboplastin is not possible, the WBCT can be adapted to monitor for the effectiveness of antivenin therapy by placing several drops of blood (100 µl) on a clean glass microscope slide and monitoring for return of clot formation. Protocols for determination of clotting disorders in the wilderness are provided in Table 28.8.

Critical Envenoming: patients bitten by a neurotoxic species require close monitoring for at least 15 hours. Early symptoms of elapid neurotoxins include anxiety, diplopia, ptosis, and other evidence of bulbar palsy. Neurologic abnormalities that can not be attributed to other causes (i.e., hyperventilation, narcotic analgesia) are an indication for immediate treatment using antivenin directed against local neurotoxic species. Polyvalent antivenins, developed to protect against the venom of neurotoxic species, are commonly used in sub-Saharan Africa, Asia, and the tropical Americas. The majority of these antivenins will be unfamiliar to Western physicians (Figure 28.21) and none are approved for use by the U.S. Food and Drug Administration (FDA). Antivenin supplies in rural hospitals throughout the tropics are often in short supply, have expired, have been stored without refrigeration, and may even be counterfeit. If the patient is critically envenomed and no alternatives exist, unrefrigerated and expired antivenin should still be used. In all cases where unfamiliar, foreign, and dubious antivenin is being administered, the clinician should initiate delivery using highly dilute concentrations or at very low rates while monitoring for unusual adverse reactions.

Table 28.8. Field and bedside tests for coagulopathy

Whole-blood clotting test

5 mL of blood is collected in a red-top vacutainer tube or other non–silica-coated test tube and left undisturbed for 20 min at room temperature (>21°C). After 20 min, tube is tipped, allowing unclotted blood to be decanted. Unclotted blood suggests defibrination, which in Asian snakebite cases suggests envenoming by vipers or *Rhabdophis*

Rapid clot test

100 µL of blood is placed carefully on an untreated microscope slide, with one edge resting on top of another slide to form a slight angle. Within 5–8 min, normal blood clots. Defibrination of blood collects at the bottom of the droplet and fails to clot or slowly rolls off the slide. After 10–12 min, slide may be tipped to evaluate further the degree of anticoagulation. The advantage of this technique is that it allows for internally controlled coagulation estimates using simple methods and inexpensive equipment.

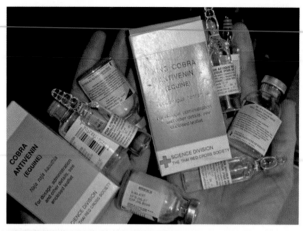

Figure 28.21. Antivenin may be stored as lyophilized powder or hyper-immune serum and may cover one species (monovalent) or many species (polyvalent) in a region. Use of antivenin in austere settings requires familiarity with local species, advanced medical training, and the ability to treat severe hypersensitivity reactions (see discussion). Photo courtesy Michael Callahan.

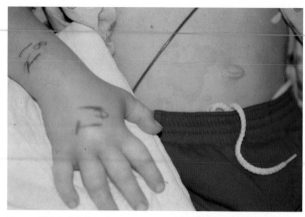

Figure 28.22. Allergic reaction to antivenin. In this patient, the antivenin was temporarily stopped due to evidence of an allergic reaction (note rash on abdomen) and then restarted after symptoms were controlled. The patient developed no further allergy symptoms and responded well to treatment. Photo courtesy Christian Tomaszewski.

Antivenin is produced as either hyper-immune serum or as lyophilized powder, which is kept refrigerated and must be reconstituted and delivered as a dilute intravenous infusion. After removal from the refrigerator, antivenin should be warmed to room temperature while gently swirling the vial to increase solubility of precipitated protein. Attempts to give antivenin by arterial infusion have proven catastrophic in the patient with coagulopathy and are strongly discouraged. Intramuscular injection of antivenin is also not recommended as it squanders supply without achieving appropriate physiologic distribution. Although potency and recommended dosing vary widely among manufacturers, antivenin is generally administered in 1–2 vial aliquots over 5–10 min providing the initial therapy does not cause adverse effects. Use of an IV microdrip at the initiation of antivenin therapy will allow for careful controlled increases in antivenin infusion while monitoring for hypersensitivity reactions. Pain, numbness, muscle fasciculations, and clotting abnormalities will often improve transiently during antivenin treatment; however, prolonged therapy is usually necessary. Antivenin should be interrupted to manage hypersensitivity reactions (Figure 28.22) and may be stopped when no further progression of pain, swelling, or erythema is noted, and when coagulopathies have reversed. If neurotoxicity of bulbar or respiratory muscles is noted, anticholinesterase inhibitors such as neostigmine and edrophonium may be used in an effort to buy time for antivenin to work. In the case of Asian krait envenoming, no pharmaceutical intervention has been shown to reverse the effects of neuroparalysis after it has become clinically apparent. A list of international antivenins is provided in Table 28.9.

Following successful resuscitation and antivenin treatment, patients will still need to be monitored for sequela of envenoming. Common complications include tissue necrosis, renal failure, endocrinopathies, and serum sickness reactions from antivenin. Wound care includes delayed and judicious debridement of necrotic tissues, daily wound care as for burn injuries, and close monitoring for secondary infection. After being stabilized and treated at an in-country hospital, patients injured by myonecrotic venoms should be transported to an appropriate facility for wound evaluation and initiation of physical therapy. Clinical pearls for avoiding pitfalls while treating the bites of international species are listed in Table 28.10.

SUMMARY

It is important for the expedition medical officer to be aware of the local venomous species and have a prepared plan for treating envenomed patients. Medical evacuation service providers should be queried about management of envenoming injuries and strategies for evacuation from remote locations. Prevention of envenomation is the key to maintaining safety while on an expedition and the medical officer should review strategies for bite prevention prior to departure. If an expedition member becomes the victim of an envenomation, systematic steps for evaluating the wound, identifying the species causing the injury, assessing the patient using field viable studies, initiating treatment, and evacuating the patient should be followed. Effective antivenin and clinical expertise is more likely to be present in the country where the team member was envenomed than it is in the country of repatriation. Physical therapy is a key aspect of rehabilitation of destructive envenoming and should not be delayed.

Table 28.9. Snake antivenins

Genus	Species	Subspecies	Range	Antivenin
New World Crotalids	American rattlesnakes, cottonmouths	*Sistrurus*	Neotropical and tropical Americas	Polyvalent Crotalidae: Protherics "CroFAb" (Previously Therapeutic Antibodies) Runcorn; Cheshire WA7 4QX, UK, phone: +44 (0)1928 518000 Fax: +44 (0)1928 518002
South and Central American vipers	Lachesis, Bothrops, Crotalids, Agkistrodon	*Lachesis muta* (*bushmaster*)	Central and South America	Monovalent and polyvalent antivenins: Instituto Butant Av. Vital Brasil 1500 05503–900 – São Paulo – SP Brazil, phone: ++(011) 3726-7222 **Fax:** ++ (011) 3726-1505 **E-mail:** *instituto@ butantan.gov.br*
Agkistrodon-Mamushis group (Gloydius)		*A. blomhoffi blomhoffi*	eastern Japan Japanese Island	(1) Mamushi Antivenin, The Chemo-Serotherapy, Research Institute, Kumamota, Japan, phone: ++ 81963441211 (2) Mamushi Antivenin, Takeda Chemical Industries Ltd., Osaka, Japan, phone: ++ 8162042111
		A. blomhoffi brevicaudus	Southern China to Korea	(3) Mamushi, Shanghai Institute of Biological Products, Ministry of Health, Shanghai, China, phone: ++ 86212513189 Alternative: (1), (2)
		Deinagkistrodon acutus (previously *A. acutus*)	China, Taiwan, North Vietnam, Laos	(4) Monovalent long-nosed pit viper antiserum: Shanghai Institute of Biological Products, Shanghai, China, phone: ++86212513189 (5) *Agkistrodon* antivenom, National Institute of Preventative Medicine, Taipei, Taiwan, phone: ++88627857559
	Hypnale hypnale and *Hypnale nepa*		Southern India, Sri Lanka	No specific antivenom; bivalent antisnake venom may be effective: Serum Institute of India Ltd., Pune-411 028 India, phone: ++91-51-240946/240973/241720
Bungarus	*B. caeruleus*		Eastern Pakistan, southern Nepal to Bangladesh, India, Sri Lanka	(6) Monovalent krait antiserum, Central Research Institute, Kasauli, India, phone: ++9117932060 (7) polyvalent snake antiserum (includes *D. russelli, Naja, E. carinatus*), Central Research Institute, Kasauli, India, phone: ++9117932060 (8) Polyvalent antisnake venom (includes *Naja*, Indian *Daboia*, and *Echis*), Haffkine Biopharmaceutical Co. Ltd., Parel, Bombay, phone: ++9122-412932023/4129224
	B. multicinctus		Eastern Myanmar to Guiyang, China, northern	(9) *B. multicinctus* antivenom (monovalent), Shanghai Institute of Biological Products, Shanghai, People's Republic of China, phone: 86212513189
			Thailand, Laos	(10) *Naja-Bungarus* antivenom (*N. atra*), National Institute of Preventative Medicine, Taipei, Taiwan, phone: ++88627857559 Alternative: (6), (11)
	B. faciatus		Eastern India to southern China, Southeast Asia	(11) Banded Krait Antivenin, Thai Red Cross Society, Bangkok, Thailand, phone: ++ 66225201614

(continued)

Table 28.9. *(continued)*

Genus	Species	Subspecies	Range	Antivenin
Calliophis and Maticora			Asia, Southeast Asia	No antivenom produced; consider antivenom for *Bungarus* (9) or a polyvalent anti-*Micrurus* (e.g., Anti-coral, Instito Clodomiro Picado, Universidade de Costa Rica, San Jose, Costa Rica, phone: ++506-290-344
Calloselasma	*C. rhodostoma*		Southeast Asia: from northern	(12) Malayan pit viper antivenom, Thai Red Cross Society, Bangkok, Thailand, phone: ++66225201614
			Thailand, Vietnam to Sumatra, Java	(13) Anti-Malayan pit viper polyvalent antivenom serum, Serum Bio Farma (Pasteur Institute), Bandung, Indonesia, phone: ++622283755
Daboia	*D. russelli siamensis* (China and Taiwan) (previously *D. r. formosensis*)		Taiwan, southern China (Kunming)	(14) Monovalent Russell viper antivenom, Central Research Institute, Kasauli, India, phone: ++9117932060 Alternative: consider (15) (monovalent) and (8) (polyvalent: includes *Naja*, Indian *Daboia*, and *Echis*)
0	*D. russelli siamensis* (Thailand)		Thailand, Laos, Kampuchea	(15) Russell viper antivenom (monovalent), Thai Red Cross Society, Bangkok, Thailand, phone: ++ 66225201614 (now using venoms isolated from throughout Southeast Asia) Alternative: (14) (monovalent); (16) (monovalent F(ab) 2), (8) (low efficacy)
	D. russelli siamensis (Indonesia) (previously *D. r. limitis*) *D. russelli russelli* (India)		Indonesia, Komodo, Flores, Northern Kanpur to lowlands between the Ghats, Intergrades common	(16) Russell viper antivenom (monovalent), Perum Bio Farma, Bandung, Indonesia, phone: ++ 83755/83756 Alternative: (15), (14) (14), (8), (16)
	D. russelli russelli (Sri Lanka) (previously *D. r. pulchella*)		Sri Lanka	(17) PolongaTab (anti-Daboia F(ab) 2), Protherics PLC, London, EC4V5DR, UK, phone: 44(0)2072469950 Alternative: (15) > (14) > (8)
	D. russelli russelli (Myanmar)		Myanmar, eastern Bangladesh	(18) Monovalent Russell viper antiserum, Industrie & Pharmaceutical Corporation, Rangoon, Myanmar (outdated inventory; no contact number at this time) Alternative: (15), (16), (8)
Echis	*E. carinatus*		Pakistan, northwestern India	(19) Monovalent Echis antisnake, Central Research Institute, Kasauli, India, phone: ++ 9117932060 Alternative: (8) (polyvalent); (20) monovalent Echis antivenom, Haffkine Biopharmaceutical Co. Ltd., Parel, Bombay, phone: ++9122-412932023/4129224 Note: In United States, envenoming by captive Indian *Echis*, EchiTab, an anti-African *Echis* F(ab) 2 antivenom has been used with evidence of efficacy. (Protherics PLC, London, EC4V5DR, UK, phone: 44(0)2072469950)
	E. sochureki		Pakistan, northern India to southern Kashmir	As above

Genus	Species	Subspecies	Range	Antivenin
Naja	*N. atra*		China, Vietnam, northern Laos	(21) Monovalent cobra antiserum, Central Research Institute, Kasauli, India, phone: ++ 9117932060 (22) Cobra antivenin, Thai Red Cross Society, Bangkok, Thailand, phone: ++66225201614 (preparation has included venom from spitting cobras)
	N. kaouthia		Eastern India, Yunnan, China, Malaysia, Vietnam	As above
	N. naja		Nepal, southeastern Pakistan to Sri Lanka	As above
	N. oxiana		Iran, southern Tajikistan, Afghanistan to central Pakistan and northern India	As above
	N. philippinensis		Manila, Mindanao	(23) "Cobra" (monovalent), serum and vaccine Laboratories, Rizal, Philippines
	Spitting cobras			
	N. siamensis		Eastern Myanmar, Thailand, Cambodia, South Vietnam	(21), (22), (24), (25)
	N. sputatrix		Thailand (south of Chang Mai), Cambodia, Laos, South Central Vietnam	(22) (see note) (24) Malayan cobra (monovalent), Perum Bio Farma, Bandung, Indonesia, phone: 83755/83756 (25) Cobra antivenin (monovalent), Twyford Pharmaceuticals, Rhein, Germany, phone: 0621-589-2688
	N. sumatrana		Java, Flores, Bali, Malaysia to Singapore, Sumatra	(22), (24) Alternative: (21), (25)
	N. sumarensis		Philippines	No data or case studies; consider (22)
Ophiophagus	*O. hannah*		India, southern Nepal	(26) King cobra antivenin, Thai Red Cross Society, Bangkok, Thailand, phone: ++66225201614
			China, Southeast Asia, Philippines	Other Asian cobra antivenoms may be used as alter natives; however, efficacy seems to be much less
Rhabdophis	*R. subiminiatus,* *R. tigrinus*		Western India, southern China, all of Southeast Asia, Khabarovsk (southern Russia), Japan, south-central China, Taiwan	(27) Anti-Yamakagshi antivenin, The Japan Snake Institute, Gunma Prefecture 379-23, Japan, phone: ++81277785193 (27)
Trimeresurus	*T. albolabris*		Kashmir, Bhutan, Southeast Asia	(28) Green pit viper antivenin, Thai Red Cross Society, Bangkok, Thailand, phone: ++66225201614; (this antivenom will soon be prepared using an increased number of species)
	T. mucrosquamatus		Western India, southern China, Central Vietnam	(29) Habu antivenom, The Chemo-Serotherapy Research Institute, Kumamoto, Japan, phone: ++81963441211 Alternative: (28); other *Trimeresurus* antivenoms also have neutralizing activity

Table 28.10. Clinical pearls for snake envenoming

Local pain, swelling, and erythema are the hallmarks of viper and *most* cobra envenoming bites.

Non-envenoming "dry" bites by vipers and most cobras (exceptions below) are *likely* if there are *no* local findings or complaints after the first hour. Exception: bites from kraits (*Bungarus*), mambas (*Dendroaspis*), Cape Cobra (*N. nivea*), Philippines cobra (*N. philippinensis*), and coral snakes (*Micrurus*), among others, can cause life-threatening paralysis with minimal local symptoms.

Antivenin should be given urgently to any patient showing neurotoxic effects. For some species (e.g., kraits), neurotoxin binding is not reversed by antivenin treatment. It is common for krait-paralyzed patients to be artificially ventilated for weeks.

Many Asian cobras may possess both myelonecrotic and neurotoxic venoms.

The venoms of several vipers are significantly neurotoxic (*Daboia*; several *Crotalids*).

The venom of most old world vipers cause local tissue injury, and often, systemic coagulopathy.

The venom of several rear-fanged Colubrid snakes cause minimal local reaction but may cause severe coagulopathy (e.g., *Rhabdophis*, Asian keel-backed).

Persistent or recrudescing hemorrhage from fang marks or IV sites (after 10 min) indicates coagulopathy.

Anticholinesterase inhibitors may delay the onset of paralysis and buy time for antivenin to work.

REFERENCES

1 Bush SP, Hegewald KG, Green SM, et al. Effects of a negative pressure venom extraction device (Extractor) on local tissue injury after artificial rattlesnake envenomation in a porcine model. *Wilderness Environ Med.* 2000;11(3):180–8.

2 Holstege CP, Singletary EM. Images in emergency medicine: skin damage following application of suction device for snakebite. *Ann Emerg Med.* 2006;48(1):105, 113.

3 Bailey SE, Callahan MV, Mossessian, CE, et al. *Case Studies in Air Medical Evacuation From Austere Asia and Africa.* Innsbruck, Austria: International Society of Travel Medicine; May 2001.

4 Tonkin MA, Negrine J. Wild platypus attack in the antipodes: a case report. *J Hand Surg [Br].* 1994;19(2):162–4.

5 Smalligan R, Cole J, Brito N, et al. Crotaline snake bite in the Ecuadorian Amazon: randomised double blind comparative trial of three South American polyspecific antivenoms. *BMJ.* 2004;329(7475):1129.

6 Warrell DA, Looareesuwan S, White NJ. Severe neurotoxic envenoming by the Malayan krait *Bungarus candidus* (Linnaeus): response to antivenom and anticholinesterase. *Br Med J (Clin Res Ed).* 1983;286(6366):678–80.

7 Nall TM. Analysis of 677 death certificates and 169 autopsies of stinging insect deaths. *J Allergy Clin Immunol.* 1990;75:185.

8 Schmidt, JO. Hymenopteran venoms: striving toward the ultimate defense against vertebrates. In: Evans DL, Schmidt, eds. *Insect Defenses, Adaptive Mechanisms and Strategies of Prey and Predators.* Albany: State University New York Press; 1990: 387–419.

9 Visscher PK, Camazine S, Vetter RS. Removing bee stings. *Lancet.* 1996;348:301–2.

10 Tambourgi DV, Paixao-Cavalcante D, Goncalves de Andrade RM. Loxosceles sphingomyelinase induces complement-dependent dermonecrosis, neutrophil infiltration, and endogenous gelatinase expression. *J Invest Dermatol.* 2005;124(4):725–31.

11 Ribeiro LA, Von Eickstedt, VR Rbuio GBG, et al. Epidemiologia do Acidente por Aranhas do Gênero *Loxosceles* Heinecken & Lowe no Estado do Paraná (Brasil). *Mem Inst Butantan.* 1993;55:19–26.

12 Pauli I, Puka J, Gubert IC, et al. The efficacy of antivenom in loxoscelism treatment. *Toxicon* [On-line]. 2006;48(2): 123–37.

13 Bucaretchi F, Deus Reinaldo CR, Hyslop S. A clinico-epidemiological study of bites by spiders of the genus *Phoneutria. Rev Inst Med Trop Sao Paulo.* 2000;42(1):17–21.

14 Isbister GK, Graudins A, White J, et al. Antivenom treatment in arachnidism. *J Toxicol Clin Toxicol.* 2003;41(3):291–300.

15 Strimple PD, Tomassoni AJ, Otten EJ. Report on envenomation by a Gila monster (*Heloderma suspectum*) with a discussion of venom apparatus, clinical findings, and treatment. *Wilderness Environ Med.* 1997;8(2):111–16.

16 Tun-Pe, Phillips RE, Warrell DA, et al. Acute and chronic pituitary failure resembling Sheehan's syndrome following bites by Russell's viper in Burma. *Lancet.* 1987;ii:763–7.

17 Callahan, MV. Asian snakes. In: Brent, Wallace, Burkhardt, Phillips, Donovan, eds. *Critical Care Toxicology: Diagnosis and Management of the Critically Poisoned Patient.* St. Louis: Mosby; 2005:1138, 1146.

18 Pe T, et al. Envenoming by the Chinese krait (*Bungarus multicintus*) and banded krait (*B. fasciatus*) in Myanmar. *Trans R Soc Trop Med Hyg.* 1997;91:686–8.

19 Moffat MA. Death by snakebite. *Outside.* March 2002:74–6.

20 Jayanthi GP, Gowda TV. Geographic variation in India in the composition and lethal potency of Russell's viper venom. *Toxicon.* 1988;26:257–64.

21 Callahan MV, Bailey SE, Mossessian CE, Tsarhinghaovih S, et al: Discovery of counterfeit antivenin immunotherapy in hospital inventories in rural Nigeria and Thailand. Presented at: Southeast Asian Conference on Rational Use of Antibiotics; May 29–30, 2006; Bangkok, Thailand.

22 Sutherland SK, Coulter AR, Harris RD. Rationalization of first-aid measures for elapid snakebite. *Lancet.* 1979;I: 183–6.

23 Tun-Pe, Aye-Aye-Myint, Khin-Ei-Han, et al. Local compression pads as a first-aid measure for victims of bites by Russell's viper (*Daboia russelii siamensis*) in Myanmar. *Trans R Soc Trop Med Hyg.* 1995;89(3):293–5.

24 Pe T, Mya S, Myint AA, et al. Field trial of efficacy of local compression immobilization first-aid technique in Russell's viper (*Daboia russelii siamensis*) bite patients in Southeast Asian. *J Trop Med Public Health.* 2000;31(2):346–8.

Craig Cook, MD

INTRODUCTION

Due to the diversity of marine species with their range in physical size and inhabited environments, anyone who ventures into the sea has the potential to come into contact with hazardous marine life, and that encounter may result in an injury. Even though the vast majority of these are accidental and unintentional, close contact with dangerous marine life may be sought as the goal of an expedition for scientific purposes.

As a result, marine life injuries may occur and will have to be treated on-site. Fortunately, the majority of these will be minor and self-limiting if attended to promptly. In the rare instance there is a serious injury, immediate first-aid must be rendered, and evacuation must be arranged to the nearest medical facility.

Avoidance is the most important measure and certainly the easiest if everyone is well educated to the various hazardous species endemic to the area that will be visited. This, then, is the theme of what will follow in this chapter. The higher the level of awareness, the less likely an injury will occur. If a bite or envenomation should occur, those involved will have the knowledge to institute prompt treatment, potentially limiting the symptom duration with a faster recovery.

Marine life dangerous to man can be classified as those that bite and those that cause envenomations. What follows is not a comprehensive list, but rather the most common hazardous marine life that may be encountered

MARINE LIFE THAT BITE

Sharks

There are more than 350 species of sharks distributed throughout the world's oceans. Of these, approximately fewer than 20 species have been involved in attacks on man. Only a handful of species have attacked divers. The majority of attacks involve swimmers or surfers probably as incidents of mistaken identity. If we eliminate the attacks on divers spearfishing as cases of provocation, then we have only a small number of species of sharks and situations where the diver may find himself at risk.

These are still very rare occurrences. The frequently quoted statistics comparing the odds of a shark attack to lightning strikes or fatal bee stings is misleading. Divers can find themselves in a situation analogous to being caught on an open mountaintop during an electrical storm. In this case, the odds of being bitten could become likely unless they recognize their exposure and are able to remove themselves. In an expedition, there may be a high likelihood of shark encounters due to the remoteness of a visited area, large shark populations, and the longer times spent underwater. On the other hand, in some areas, a team may spend hundreds of hours underwater and never even see a shark.

The family Lamnidae contains the great white shark (*Carcharodon carcharias*), which has been responsible for the majority of attacks on divers (Figure 29.1). In most cases, the diver did not see the shark before the attack, which illustrates the suddenness of the attack and that circling behavior is often not observed. Its large size (up to 20 feet) accounts for the massive trauma and frequent fatalities. As soon as a great white has been spotted, diving activities should be suspended, and divers should exit the water. Its close relative the mako (*Isurus oxyrinchus*) is also considered dangerous but, being pelagic, is rarely encountered by divers.

The tiger shark (*Galeocerdo cuvieri*) also grows to a large size (reported to 20 feet) and has attacked divers (Figure 29.2). It is not typically observed by divers preferring deeper depths during the day and approaching shallows during the night. It has a reputation for feeding on virtually anything from horseshoe crabs to sea turtles and even trash has been found in its stomach. Its reaction to divers ranges from a casual curiosity and departure to aggressive interest. Despite its slow moving behavior, it is intelligent and capable of rapid bursts of speed. As with the great white, a large tiger shark should be considered reason for leaving the water.

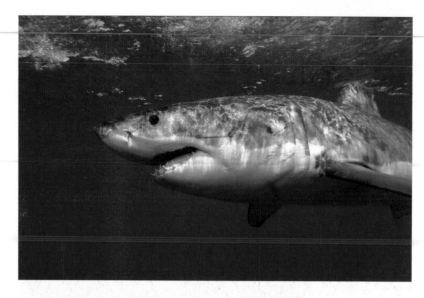

Figure 29.1. The great white shark (*Carcharodon carcharias*). Courtesy of Stephen Frink.

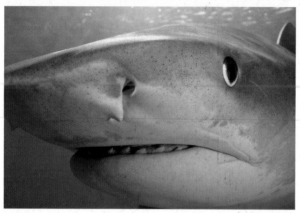

Figure 29.2. The tiger shark (*Galeocerdo cuvieri*). Courtesy of Stephen Frink.

Another potentially dangerous shark is the oceanic white tip (*Carcharhinus longimanus*), which is primarily a pelagic shark but can be occasionally encountered in open water off deep water drop-offs. It has been documented as the main species responsible for many of the attacks in open ocean ship disasters. Its response

to divers is either a single close circling pass and exit or definite interest with increasingly closer approaches. Due to its bold behavior and large size of up to 10 feet, it should be treated with caution.

The bull shark (*Carcharhinus leucas*) is a common and widely distributed shark that has been known to attack divers. Its name reflects its large bulky size of up to 12 feet and bold behavior. When displaying aggression, it has been described as moving its snout in small quick side-to-side movements. It is commonly found in shallow coastal waters and is known to travel considerable distances up freshwater tributaries. The large size, aggressive behavior, and determination need to be considered should this shark appear.

The most commonly encountered shark with the potential for aggression is the pacific grey reef shark (*Carcharhinus amblyrhynchos*) (Figure 29.3). Attacks committed by the larger sharks mentioned previously are probably due to the diver being seen as a potential food source. In the case of the grey reef shark, the attacks are thought to be the result of threat or territorial behaviors. In locations where they are familiar with divers,

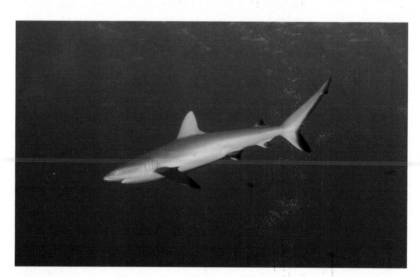

Figure 29.3. Pacific grey reef shark (*Carcharhinus amblyrhynchos*). Courtesy of Craig Cook.

they may be observed but do not seem to be interested or make close passes. In remote areas where contact with humans is infrequent, they can become quite curious, joining divers in small numbers and remaining close by throughout the dive. In some situations, a grey reef shark will exhibit signs of aggression in a display unique to it and perhaps several other species.

This antagonistic display consists of extreme arching of its back, with its snout elevated, pectoral fins dropped and the mouth slightly opened (Figure 29.4).[1] While in this position, the swimming changes to a more exaggerated form of head swinging and tail motion where the head and tail almost seem to meet and the body axis often lies at a slight side tilt (Figures 29.5 and 29.6).

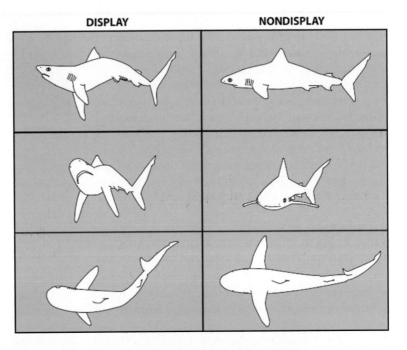

DISPLAY   **NONDISPLAY**

Figure 29.4. The antagonistic swimming display of the grey reef shark. When agitated, the shark lifts its snout, lowers its pectoral fins and arches it back. The swimming motion becomes more exaggerated with greater side-to-side head movements. Courtesy of R. H. Johnson.

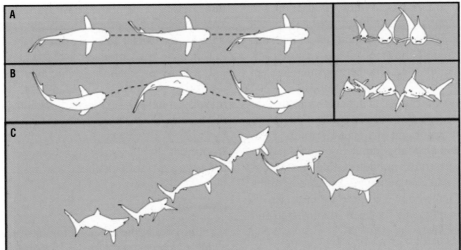

Figure 29.5. The antagonistic swimming display of the grey reef shark. (A) Normal swimming. (B and C) Exaggerated swimming behavior. Courtesy of R. H. Johnson.

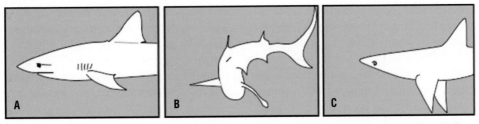

Figure 29.6. The antagonistic swimming display of the grey reef shark. (A) Normal pectoral fin position. (B) Exaggerated tail swimming. (C) Lowered pectoral fin position. Courtesy of R. H. Johnson.

Anyone who has witnessed these displays will immediately notice the difference. Whether these displays are an indication of territoriality, anger, or fear is unknown. What is known is that the possibility of an attack may be imminent and the diver should keep the shark in view and slowly retreat keeping an object (such as a camera) ready to interpose between the charging shark and the diver's body. Should an attack occur, these are typically lightning fast with a quick "defense" bite and not a feeding style of bite. Fortunately, this type of attack is rare, and when one has occurred it was preceded by a threat display that was ignored. All divers should be aware of these display patterns in order to avoid their consequences. It should be noted that all sharks are unpredictable, and their behavior is poorly understood and is mostly based on anecdotal reports.

Other sharks have been involved in attacks on divers, but these are rare. It is important that divers seek out knowledge of species distribution and behavior from local authorities in the area that will be explored.

Treatment

As can be expected, bite wounds exhibit massive tissue injury with deep lacerations, puncture wounds, tissue loss, and crush injury, with the possibility of amputation. Treatment centers on controlling the bleeding with direct pressure, tourniquets, and pressure points and administering intravenous fluid resuscitation. The affected limb should be elevated above the heart level. The diver should not be moved until the bleeding has stopped and is under control. If there appears there will be a long delay in evacuation transport, then oral fluids can be administered if intravenous fluids are not available and the patient is alert. The patient must be kept supine and warm, and signs of shock must be watched for and treated should they occur. If there is going to be a significant delay in transport, the wound should be irrigated with sterile water and any debris (sand or teeth removed) if this can be done without any additional loss of blood. Broad spectrum antibiotics should be administered due to wound contamination. Evacuation to the nearest medical facility should be undertaken as soon as possible after initial first-aid has been administered and the bleeding controlled.

Prevention

Numerous devices can be used for self-defense including the shark billy, Kevlar mail suits, powerheads, and even portable devices that generate electrical fields. All have limitations, especially against large sharks. The best defense is avoidance. If a potentially dangerous large shark is spotted, it should be kept in sight and a slow retreat made back to the boat or shore keeping close to the bottom or reef. All divers should remain close together. In the case of an attack or close pass, defensive blows should be directed against the shark's sensitive areas

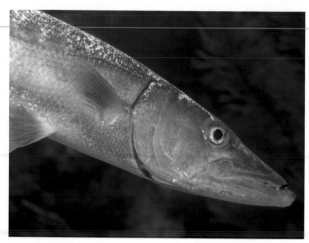

Figure 29.7. The great barracuda. Courtesy of Craig Cook.

such as the snout, eyes, or gills. Rescuers have only rarely attracted the interest of the shark while assisting the victim.

Barracuda

Usually the barracuda follows the shark in most discussion of hazardous marine life, which is undeserved (Figure 29.7). With its large prominent teeth and unnerving, motionless approaches close to divers, it is easy to see how the barracuda has gotten its reputation. However, (there may have been only) one or two known cases of a barracuda actually attacking a diver. The greater danger involves divers who are spearfishing or have tried to spear a barracuda. It is thought that jewelry or small flashy metallic objects worn by a diver can be mistaken for a small fish and lead to a mistaken bite. Wearing jewelry should be avoided for this reason.

Treatment

See treatment for shark bite.

Killer Whales

Without a doubt the top predator in the ocean, the killer whale (*Orcinus orea*) also has an undeserved reputation (Figure 29.8). Until recently, these extremely intelligent and social mammals were considered dangerous despite there not being a single credible report of a killer whale attacking a diver. Now a common sight at many aquariums, there are also specialized adventure tours that have provided hundreds of divers the opportunity to dive alongside them without incident. However, these human–orca interactions are still a relatively new occurrence, and divers encountering orcas need to exercise common sense as in the case of any animals in their own habitat.

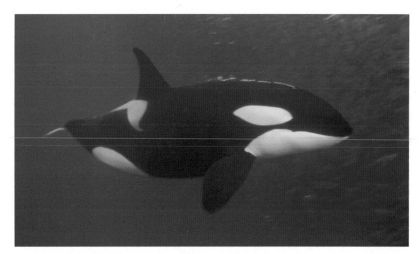

Figure 29.8. The killer whale. Courtesy of Amos Nachoum.

Crocodiles and Alligators

Both alligators and crocodiles are responsible for isolated deaths every year and these numbers can be expected to increase as human habitation and tourism continues to encroach on their natural habitat (Figure 29.9). They are known to be intelligent and territorial and hunt by stalking their prey (including humans). The danger of attack increases in proportion to their size, which can approach 18–20 feet in both the crocodile and alligator. Individuals traveling to areas where these large reptiles make their home should contact locals knowledgeable about their range. In areas where they are present, care should be taken in walking along river tributaries, canoeing, or kayaking. If an attack should occur, treatment is the same as for shark attack with control of bleeding and tissue trauma.

Moray Eels

Bites from a moray eel are usually due to either a misplaced hand or intentional feeding. Unprovoked attacks virtually never occur. They are shy and typically try to remain out of sight in a coral crevice though they can occasionally be encountered free swimming across a reef while feeding (Figure 29.10). At many popular dive sites, a moray eel frequently becomes a common fixture and attraction. These eels become used to the frequent feeding and may become quite bold in approaching divers. Accidents have occurred with serious bites in these circumstances and serve to illustrate that even though things appear safe, risk is still present.

Treatment

A bite usually involves a high degree of tissue trauma and bleeding. The teeth are directed backward and care must be taken not to cause more trauma in removing the eel, which is often slow to release its bite. As in the case of a shark bite, bleeding must be controlled first before transporting the victim to a medical facility. Shock must be watched for and the victim reassured and kept warm. The wounds tend to become infected easily and it is important to thoroughly clean the wound and administer antibiotics and tetanus prophylaxis.

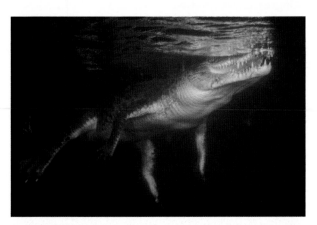

Figure 29.9. The saltwater crocodile in Papua New Guinea. The author swam in the water with this specimen which exhibited no signs of aggression. Courtesy Bob Halstead.

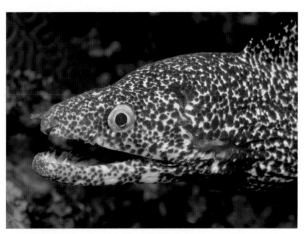

Figure 29.10. Black spotted moray eel. Courtesy of Craig Cook.

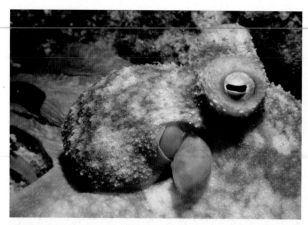

Figure 29.11. The common Caribbean octopus. Courtesy of Craig Cook.

Octopuses

Large octopuses have been the subject of legend and fear since mariners first went to sea (Figure 29.11). In reality, these are probably one of the most intelligent creatures in the ocean. They are unaggressive and curious, often extending a tentacle to probe the hand of a diver who approaches in a slow and gentle manner. Tales of the octopus enveloping a diver in its tentacles in order to drown him are the equivalent of octopus bringing down ships and are simply myth. Their tentacle grip can be quite firm and take a surprising amount of force to free oneself, and there is a danger that a diver could panic causing injury to himself by losing his mouthpiece or mask in such circumstances. The mouth of both the octopus and the squid are composed of a beak-like appendage that can produce puncture-like wound if bitten. There may be a mild venom that does not cause symptoms beyond that of the puncture wound. This is not so in the case of a blue-ringed octopus bite, which will be discussed later.

Squid

Despite the docile behavior of the octopus, large squid can be dangerous to divers. The Humboldt squid (*Dosidicus gigas*) is known to grow to 6 feet in length and weigh more than 100 pounds. It feeds ferociously and will attack other hooked squid. It inhabits the Pacific coasts of Central and South America where it can be found in large numbers at night near the surface of deep waters, where they come to feed. It has been reported that under these conditions, larger squid have attempted unsuccessfully to pull divers that were filming them down into deeper water. Certainly, the real danger posed by contact with these squid is risk of loss of a mask or regulator. Because they are deep-water inhabitants, divers will not normally encounter them. Aside from the incidents mentioned here, there are no reported cases of divers being deliberately attacked.

Treatment

An octopus or squid bite should be treated as a puncture wound by thoroughly washing it with soap and then irrigating it with fresh water. Pain may be treated with hot water immersion if needed (see following discussions of hot water immersion). The major risk is secondary infection by marine organisms.

Needlefish

Though impalement by needlefish or related members of the order Belonidae is rare, several cases have been reported. These fish range in size from 2 to 5 feet and have an elongated pointed jaw with abundant small teeth. They typically hunt small fish near the surface and are generally shy. The injury results from the long beak of the fish penetrating the unfortunate victim. Injuries have been reported in fishermen, divers, windsurfers, and surfers. In a few cases, severe injury – such as traumatic carotid cavernous sinus fistula[2] or ruptured globe[3] – has been reported. Divers and fishermen need to be cautious using lights with needlefish in the vicinity as these creatures seem to be attracted to lights. As with any penetrating injury, first-aid consists of not removing or disturbing any retained bill pieces and immediately evacuating the patient to the nearest medical facility.

MARINE ENVENOMATIONS

Marine life in this category pose a hazard by venom injected by either a bite, puncture from a barb, or contact with stinging cells. The reaction and symptoms depend on the species and can range from mild irritation to life-threatening. Hundreds of species are potentially dangerous to humans, but this section will cover only those that are most likely to be encountered and pose the greatest hazard.

Stingray Envenomation

It has been estimated that these shy and gentle creatures are responsible for over a thousand injuries per year with 18 recorded deaths. Most injuries result from contact with the tail barbs belonging to species from the family Dasyatididae or common stingrays, usually from fishermen who handle them carelessly or swimmers or waders who step on them (Figure 29.12). It is extremely rare for unprovoked injuries to occur in divers, and only a few cases have been documented.

(The serrated barb (Figure 29.13A) is found further distally on the tail than in other ray families and gives the stingray a greater striking force.) The barb itself is covered by a layer of enveloping tissue called the integumentary sheath, which also contains the venom glands. When the barb and sheath penetrate the tissue, the sheath ruptures as the barb punctures it and venom is

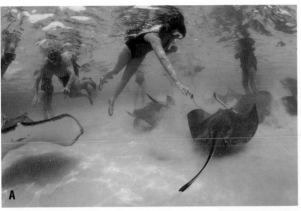

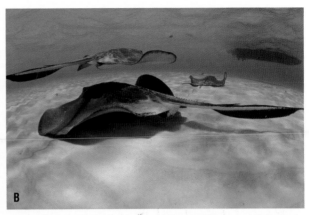

Figure 29.12. (A) Snorkelers enjoying stingrays at Grand Cayman Island. Courtesy of Craig Cook. (B) Southern stingrays. Courtesy of Craig Cook.

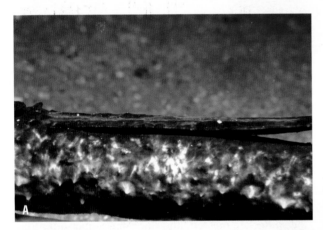

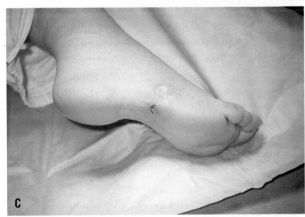

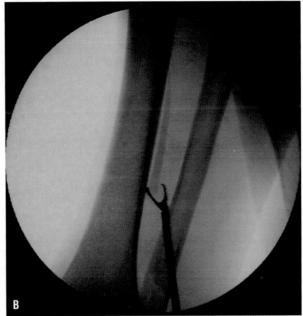

Figure 29.13. (A) Stingray barb. It is not uncommon to find more than one barb on larger rays. Courtesy of Craig Cook. (B) A retained barb parallel to the tibia in the lower leg. The first X-ray missed the barb, which was obscured by the bone. Repositioning the limb slightly showed the barb. The patient required surgery in order to remove it. Courtesy of Craig Cook. (C) Penetrating injury from a stingray barb. Courtesy of Alan Hodgdon.

released into the wound. The venom has been shown to contain a necrosis factor as well as a cardiotoxin. In animal models, the cardiotoxin produces cardiac conduction abnormalities; however, this appears to be rare in human envenomations.[4]

The most common symptom is immediate onset of pain followed by local swelling and paleness with a bluish perimeter. Systemic symptoms are uncommon in mild punctures but may include nausea, vomiting, fever, cramping, and tremors. Intensity of symptoms appears to be dependent on the wound depth and extent, presence of spine fragments, and amount of venom delivered. Bleeding may be present, and the potential of a large vessel being involved must be considered. The spine is quite fragile, and it is not unusual for a large portion of spine to be imbedded in the wound. For this reason, X-rays should always be taken, and any wound that is slow to heal should be carefully reexamined for retained spine fragments or integumentary sheath (Figure 29.13B).

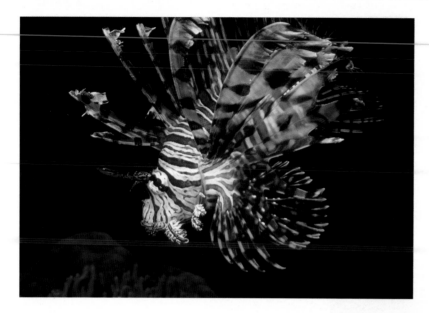

Figure 29.14. Pacific lionfish. Courtesy of Craig Cook.

Treatment

Initial treatment consists of removing any visible remaining barb or organic matter. The wound should be irrigated with fresh water, then cleaned with soap and water and finally reirrigated. Pain may be relieved by immersion in water up to 45°C (110–113°F) for 30- to 60-minute periods as needed and the affected part elevated (another person and not the patient should test the water temperature). Medical attention should be sought and X-rays taken. The wound should be initially left open for delayed closure if needed (Figure 29.13C), antibiotics and tetanus prophylaxes should be administered and the patient observed. As with any marine envenomation, it is essential for the wound to be clean of all debris or contamination in order for rapid and optimal healing to occur.

The special cases of barb penetration into a body cavity, neck, or face are medical emergencies, and the majority of deaths have resulted from this type of injury. It is critical then, to control any hemorrhage and provide cardiorespiratory support until arrival at a medical facility.

Prevention

Waders and swimmers should shuffle their feet while walking on the bottom to avoid stepping on a ray. Divers should be cautioned not to swim directly over a ray or block its escape route. Finally, fishermen who have caught a ray should not attempt to unhook a ray but cut the line to release it.

Venomous Fish

The family Scorpaenidae contains most of the common venomous species that divers would encounter such as the lionfish, scorpionfish, and stonefish. Other species are either rare or deep-water inhabitants and are rarely seen by divers and will not be mentioned. Stonefish envenomation will be covered separately.

Lionfish are well-known to divers due to their spectacularly colored dorsal and pectoral fins which are displayed when threatened (Figure 29.14). They are slow moving and are often encountered close to ledges or coral outcroppings. Their dorsal, pectoral, and anal fins sport spines containing a venom apparatus covered by an integumentary sheath (Figure 29.15). When alarmed, the spines are erected, and the fish assumes a position with the dorsal spines directed toward the threat.

The majority of lionfish envenomations occur in home aquariums, whereas diver envenomations usually occur accidentally due to unawareness of their presence or poor buoyancy control. Symptoms range from a mild stinging to excruciating pain. The wound and surrounding area may become erythematous with varying degrees of swelling. Systemic signs such as nausea, vomiting, and fever may often be present as well. Generally, the presentation depends on the puncture depth, amount of venom injected, and host reaction to the foreign protein.

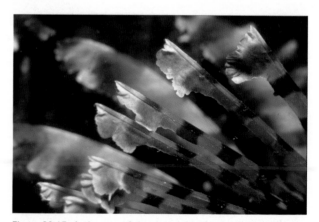

Figure 29.15. A close-up of the dorsal fin of a lionfish showing the spine covered by the integumentary sheath. Courtesy of Craig Cook.

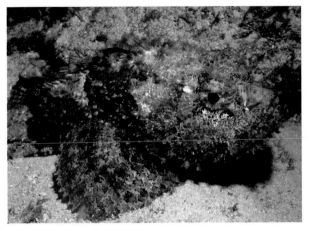

Figure 29.16. Scorpionfish. Courtesy of Craig Cook.

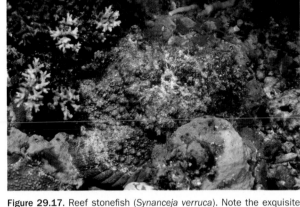

Figure 29.17. Reef stonefish (*Synanceja verruca*). Note the exquisite camouflage rendering it almost invisible. Courtesy of Craig Cook.

Scorpionfish are usually sessile bottom dwellers, partially buried in and/or hidden among coral rubble, and rely on their camouflage for predation and defense (Figure 29.16). They are often first noticed when stepped on or when a diver accidentally places a hand on them for buoyancy support. As with other members of this family, a number of species contain venomous dorsal spines. Symptoms of envenomation are the same as for lionfish and vary among species.

Treatment consists of removal of any retained spine fragments and then immediate immersion of the affected area in hot water no hotter than 45°C (110–113°F).[5] The water should be tested by someone other than the victim first. Recommended immersion times are for 30–90 minutes or until relief. If the wound is in a nonimmersible area, then hot compresses or heat packs can be used. These periodic immersions may be repeated if needed. It is thought that this may detoxify the heat-soluble venom or act to inhibit local pain mediator pathways. With more severe or painful wounds, lidocaine 1% without epinephrine may be injected into the puncture wound for temporary relief. The wound should then be washed with soap and water and thoroughly irrigated with sterile water. A topical antibiotic such as neomycin should be applied and then the area immobilized and elevated. The patient should be observed closely for any signs of an anaphylactic reaction, infection, or shock.

Stonefish Envenomation

The stonefish is also a member of the Scorpaenidae family but requires special mention. It has been described as the most venomous fish in the world and, based on the degree of pain produced, rightly deserves this recognition. There are ten species, but two are common. The estuarine stonefish (*Synanceja horrida*) inhabits shallow estuaries, while the reef stonefish (*Synanceja verruca*) is commonly found on shallow reefs throughout the Indo-Pacific (Figure 29.17). Their extraordinary camouflage makes them virtually indistinguishable from their surroundings and is the primary reason for envenomations. They are extremely hardy and reported to be able to live out of water if kept moist for over 24 hours. Their venom remains toxic for several days in dead specimens.[6]

The venom apparatus consists of 13 dorsal spines, each consisting of a central spine surrounded on the distal ends by paired venom glands and covered by a tough integumentary sheath. The spine punctures its sheath and then the victim's skin, allowing the venom access into the puncture. The venom is a heat-labile protein containing several toxic factors.

After envenomation, there is an abrupt onset of excruciating pain in the affected part, so severe as to cause the victim to writhe in absolute agony. Few descriptions of an envenomation approach that of a stonefish. There is local swelling and discoloration that can spread and affect the entire extremity. Systemic symptoms are minor when compared to the intense pain. Despite the impressive nature of pain elicited, there are surprisingly few fatalities reported, and these may possibly have been due to anaphylactic reactions or underlying cardiovascular disease.

Treatment

Treatment centers on pain relief and hot water immersion described earlier. In addition, stonefish antivenom should be administered if available. Narcotics and analgesics are often insufficient to control the pain, and the large doses required often approach respiratory depression. Optimal pain relief can often only be achieved by regional anesthetic blocks. Antivenom also appears to reduce the recovery period.

Prevention

In shallow waters, thick-soled shoes or boots should be worn (thin-soled shoes have been punctured) and attention should be directed to foot placement. Divers need to be aware of hand or finger placement on reefs or bottom rubble and exercise good buoyancy control.

Blue-Ringed Octopuses

This small octopus, *Hapalochlaena lunulata,* is named for its colorful pattern of blue rings that appear on its body and tentacles when disturbed or frightened (Figure 29.18). It is found in the western Indo-Pacific and normally inhabits shallow bottom close to shore where it may be encountered inhabiting shells or other debris. Deaths have resulted from bites while handling this shy creature. Usually the bite is painless and not remembered.[7] There may be small puncture marks or blood blister present at the bite site, but this is often overlooked.

Envenomation may quickly lead to paralysis and death unless prompt resuscitation and ventilatory support is given. The toxin is a tetrodotoxin-like compound that acts to inhibit neuronal transmission resulting in weakness, paralysis of the respiratory muscles, smooth muscle relaxation, decreased blood pressure, and other autonomic manifestations.[8] Early signs of mild envenomation include circumoral numbness, double vision or other ocular symptoms, difficulty in swallowing or speech, and weakness, all representing nervous system impairment. The envenomation by a blue-ringed octopus is unique in that there is no pain component.

Treatment

The patient must be closely watched for signs of respiratory arrest so that ventilatory support can be given. The toxin itself is not fatal, and the bite is survivable with appropriate and rapid treatment. It should be noted that in severe cases the patient may be paralyzed but completely alert and support must be given recognizing this potential.

During institution of the initial assessment and support measures, the bite site should be irrigated and immobilized quickly with a pressure bandage (see following discussion of pressure bandages) to slow the systemic spread of the toxin. Prompt evacuation is critical to what should be a survivable episode.

Sea Snake Envenomation

Sea snakes are endemic to Indo-Pacific tropical waters above 20°C with the number of species decreasing moving east across the Pacific (Figure 29.19). There are no species inhabiting the Atlantic Ocean. They are known to possess some of the most toxic venom on the planet and deserve the respect of those who come in contact with them. The majority of the species are bottom feeders occasionally surfacing for air. Members of the family Hydrophiidae, or true sea snakes, spend all of their life in the water, whereas those in the family Laticaudidae emerge to breed and rest on dry land (Figure 29.20). Almost all cases of sea snake bites occur in fishermen or waders inadvertently making contact with them. Most are nonaggressive and must be provoked to bite. In one study, among 19 species, only 4 species were considered aggressive, and even these would seldom attack if unprovoked.[9] The majority of deaths have resulted from one species (*Enhydrina schistosa*); however, there are no reports of any deaths occurring in divers. This species is found in muddy estuarine waters and would not usually be encountered.

Despite their toxic venom, sea snakes have small fangs of less than 4 mm, which are barely long enough to penetrate a wet suit. In addition, they do not inject a venom dose in more than half of the bites. However, should envenomation occur, the symptoms are severe and life-threatening. The venom has been shown to consist of a neurotoxin that inhibits release of acetylcholine and results in muscle paralysis in addition to a myotoxin that destroys skeletal muscle. Early signs are weakness, eyelid drooping, double vision, and difficulty with speech, swallowing, and breathing, which can progress to complete paralysis within minutes to hours.

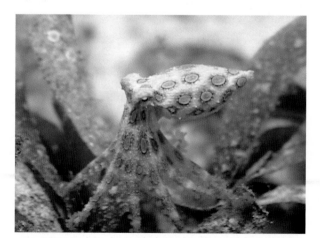

Figure 29.18. Blue-ringed octopus (*Hapalochlaena lunulata*). The blue rings become visible when threatened. Courtesy of Mike Schnetzer.

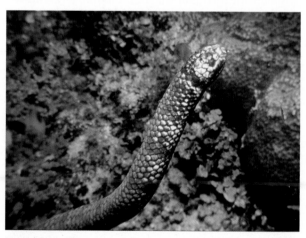

Figure 29.19. Olive sea snake (*Aipysurus laevis*), Marion reef coral sea. Courtesy of Craig Cook.

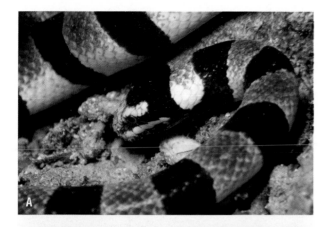

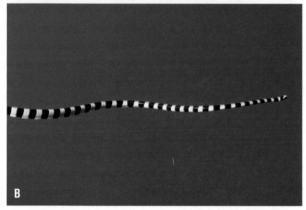

Figure 29.20. Black-and-white sea krait (*Laticauda colubrine*). Courtesy of Craig Cook.

The myotoxin often produces muscle aches and pain that become severe with movement and myoglobinuria (dark urine) may be present along with elevation of creatine kinase.

Treatment

If a bite occurs or is suspected, the area should be wrapped with a compression bandage and immobilized in order to keep the venom localized until a medical facility with full resuscitative resources and antivenom can be reached. For a bite on a toe, this would involve wrapping the limb up to the knee with enough pressure to feel snug but not uncomfortable. Pulses should remain present and the skin should remain pink; otherwise, the bandage may be too tight. The bandaging should begin over the bite and then cover up or down the limb. A splint should be applied to further immobilize the limb and prevent muscle contractions from spreading the venom. Incision and suction over the puncture site is not recommended and may be harmful.

The victim needs to be monitored for any respiratory impairment, and prompt resuscitation should be instituted if needed. If available, sea snake antivenom should be administered in serious cases. The venom is from the *Enhydrina schistosa* species but is effective for most other sea snakes. If sea snake venom is unavailable, then

tiger snake venom is also effective but may need to be given in larger quantities. There is always the potential for allergic reaction, which must be considered; however, antivenom should not be withheld if the condition warrants its use.

Cone Shell Envenomation

Of the more than 300 species of cone shell, several dozen can produce severe envenomation including death. These are usually found buried under ruble or sand during the day; at night they emerge to hunt other mollusks, crustaceans, or small fish. They employ a harpoon-like dart, which pierces and then envenomates their prey. The danger to humans is being stung while handling a live specimen. The shell has an opening running the length from the larger to small end. It was once thought that the shell could be safely handled by picking it up by the large end, but it is now known that almost all areas of the shell can be reached by the stinging apparatus. A number of toxins have been identified with the most important being the alpha conotoxin, which blocks acetylcholine at the neuromuscular junction causing a flaccid paralysis.[10]

Symptom of envenomation include pain, numbness, swelling, and, in severe cases, weakness and paralysis leading to respiratory arrest. Many of the dozen or so deaths reported could probably have been saved with respiratory support.

Treatment

Treatment is the same as in sea snake or blue-ringed octopus envenomation with pressure immobilization and ventilatory support if required. Currently, there is no antivenom available.

Jellyfish Envenomations

Although most jellyfish stings experienced by divers usually are minor, several families and species can deliver life-threatening stings. The true jellyfish from the class Scyphozoa are encountered most commonly, but they only rarely cause serious stings. The class Hydrozoa, in addition to the stinging corals and hydroids, contains *Physalia physalis* or the Portuguese Man-of-War, which can cause severe stings that have resulted in several deaths (Figure 29.21). The class Cuboza contains the box jellyfish, which deserve separate discussion.

Box Jellyfish

The cubozoans are comprised of two subclasses, the chirodropids and carybdeids. The distinction is made by multiple versus single tentacles at each end of the four corners of the bell of the jellyfish.[11] Among the chirodropids, *Chironex fleckeri* is responsible for the majority

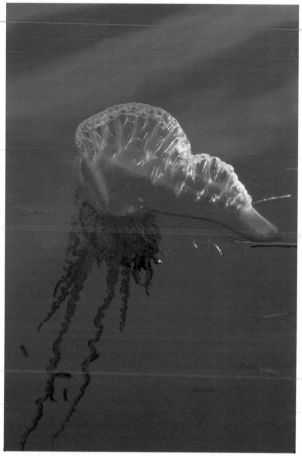

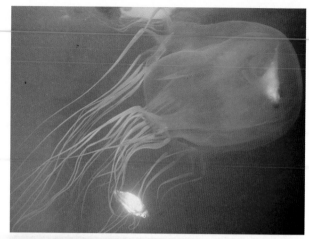

Figure 29.22. The feared box jellyfish (*Chironex fleckeri*). Courtesy of Jamie Seymour, James Cook University.

Figure 29.21. Portuguese man-of-war (*Physalia physalia*). Courtesy of Stephen Frink.

of the envenomations from this group (Figure 29.22). It is probably the most venomous creature known today causing 63 deaths in Australia alone and is speculated to cause dozens of deaths each year in other locations. It inhabits shallow coastal waters in the western Indo-Pacific primarily the northeastern Australian coasts but has been reported to be found in the Philippines. It is usually observed swimming close to the surface, trailing tentacles that can extend up to 3 meters in length in search of small fish or shrimp. It has been shown to exhibit a primitive from of intelligence and appears to have a rudimentary form of eyesight that allows it to avoid objects (including humans).

The venom system consists of six distinct types of stinging cells (nematocysts) present on their tentacles that discharge on contact. One type acts as a grappling hook to bring (the tentacle) in closer so other nematocysts can fire. The tentacle is often in a partially contracted state preventing contact with other nematocysts, and it is important to prevent these from discharging while removing adherent tentacles. The toxin is composed of a skin toxin that produces the dramatic erythematous wheal and two poorly characterized lethal factors. The lethal factors seem to work clinically by either a respiratory or cardiac mechanism thought to be associated with interference with the sodium or calcium channel conduction in these tissues.

Symptoms of an envenomation are dramatic, with agonizing pain and the victim attempting to remove the usually adherent tentacles. Unfortunately, these efforts only serve to cause the remaining undischarged nematocysts to discharge, worsening the envenomation. The lesion rapidly forms a distinct erythematous wheal following the location of the tentacle. These will darken and may eventually scar from effects of the skin toxin. Systemic manifestations in severe cases consist of a rapid deterioration with either respiratory or cardiac arrest.

Treatment

Immediate treatment consists of keeping the victim calm and lying down as movement will increase the venom absorption. Undischarged nematocyts should be deactivated by pouring vinegar over any adherent tentacles for at least 30 seconds. The tentacles can then be removed using tweezers but reportedly they can be removed by using the fingertips due to protection from the thickened finger pads.[12] If they are removed by this manner, care must be taken not to touch any exposed areas, and the hands must be washed to remove any undischarged nematocyst present.

Ice pack compression has been shown to decrease the pain, but it will not completely relieve it.[13] It must be noted that although vinegar is effective at preventing nematocyst discharge, it is ineffective at relieving pain or inactivating venom. Chironex antivenom is available for administration and should be administered in all cases but the mildest envenomation. It is the only effective treatment for pain relief, and there is some evidence that it may decrease scarring.[14] Every effort should be made to get the victim to a medical facility as soon as possible, and preparations should be made to support and treat the victim should cardiovascular deterioration appear.

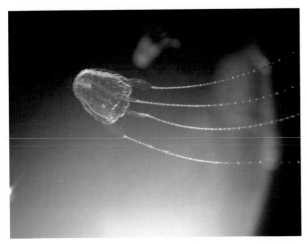

Figure 29.23. The box jellyfish (*Carukia barnesi*) producing the Irukandji syndrome. Courtesy of Jamie Seymour, James Cook University.

Irukandji Syndrome

Some members of the carybdeids contain venom that produces systemic symptoms unlike other jellyfish envenomations (Figure 29.23). First described in the species *Carukia barnesi* by its discoverer who deliberately envenomated himself, the Irukandji syndrome consists of local pain, muscle and lower back or thoracic pain, sweating, nausea, and vomiting.[15] Many of the signs and symptoms appear to be a result of catecholamine excess due to the venom's action on presynaptic neurons. Malignant hypertension in the range of 300/160 has been reported with deaths from intracerebral bleeding, heart failure, or pulmonary edema.[16] In severe cases, the outcome depends on the degree of envenomation and health state of the victim. There appears to be species-specific range of venom toxicity, but this is not completely understood.

Treatment

Treatment is the same as for chironex envenomation except that antivenom is not available. Emphasis will need to be placed on treatment of hypertension or other cardiac manifestations. Irukandji syndrome can be misidentified as decompression illness, but a careful history and physical exam can usually differentiate between the two.

Coral Cuts and Stings

Contact with coral results in either superficial cuts, lacerations, or abrasions. The extent of the injury and recovery is dependent on other factors such as wound contamination or local allergic factors. Coral is composed of a calcium framework supporting the organic coral polyp, and the sharp edges can easily produce a cut or scrape. Inevitably, some amount of this organic proteinacous material gets into the wound causing a contact dermatitis (Figure 29.24). Usually, this results in

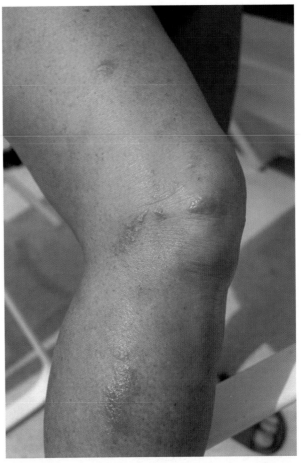

Figure 29.24. An example of coral cuts showing a contact dermatitis presentation. Courtesy of Craig Cook.

an itchy, erythematous papule or wheal that may eventually evolve into vesicles with surface crusting. These lesions resolve in several days to a week but may last longer in humid environments or if there is secondary infection. Though all corals have nematocysts present, there is no sting or envenomation with the exception of fire coral (*Millepora*).

Fire coral is not a true coral but is a member of the class Hydrozoa and differs in the type of nematocysts present. These are able to deliver a potent sting on light contact. It is widely distributed throughout tropical waters and is identifiable by its growth patterns and smooth outside surfaces (Figures 29.25 and 29.26). Another member of the class Hydrozoa that is able to deliver a contact sting is the hydroids. These soft branching structures attach themselves to areas of reef or rubble in shallow depths. Because they are small, ranging from, a few cementers to 20 cm, and tend to blend in which other parts of the environment, they are easy to come in contact with (Figure 29.27). The appearance of these hydrozoan stings present as distinct erythematous papules or wheals with varying degrees of localized swelling. The course is generally benign with resolution within several days.

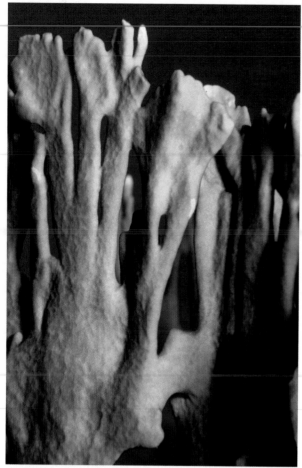

Figure 29.25. Fire coral (*Millepora*). Courtesy of Craig Cook.

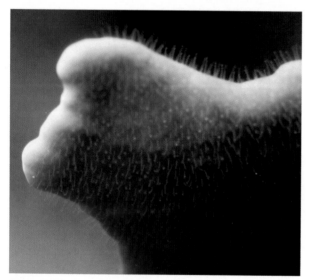

Figure 29.26. Fire coral close-up showing stinging cells. Courtesy of Craig Cook.

Treatment

Coral cuts or abrasions that are quickly cleaned will result in a more rapid recovery than those that were neglected. The wound needs to be scrubbed using a soft brush and fresh water containing a soapy detergent in order to rid the wound of any debris from the polyps or coral. The

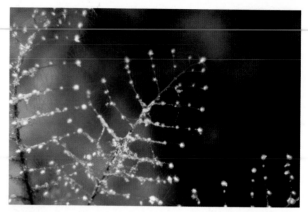

Figure 29.27. Hydroids. Courtesy of Craig Cook.

quicker this is done, the less chance that a more severe dermatitis will result with faster resolution. The wound should be covered and observed for infection. Deep lacerations will require medical attention and tetanus prophylaxis.

Fire coral and hydroid stings can be treated with vinegar irrigation though the efficacy has not been shown to be consistent across all species. Cold ice pack to the sting sites have been shown to be effective for some stings.

Sea Urchins

Sea urchin spine punctures are commonly encountered due to their wide distribution and seemingly uncanny ability to be in exactly the wrong place much to the dismay of those who make contact with them. Some species may have venom contained in the organic coverings of their spines; however, the majority do not and result in localized puncture wounds (Figure 29.28). The spines typically break off and remain in the dermis until they are either reabsorbed or expressed to the surface. In some instances, neither will occur, and the spine will need to be excised.

In addition to their spines, some species contain shorter appendages called pedicellariae, which are containing a terminal spinous jaw-like structure that

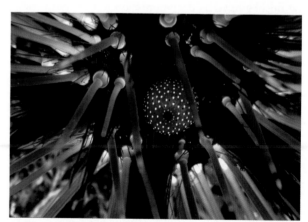

Figure 29.28. Long spined sea urchin common in tropical and semitropical waters. Courtesy of Craig Cook.

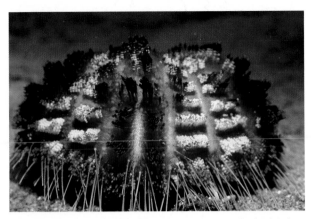

Figure 29.29. Fire urchin from Papua New Guinea showing both spines and pedicellariae. Courtesy of Craig Cook.

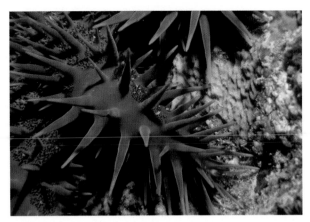

Figure 29.31. Close-up of magnesium calcite spine of a crown of thorns. Courtesy of Craig Cook.

contains venom (Figure 29.29). Punctures by these spines result in severe pain and swelling.

Treatment

Treatment consists of hot water immersion as described earlier. Large spines should be removed carefully with tweezers with smaller buried fragments left to be re-absorbed. Excision or exploration should be avoided unless there is joint involvement or infection. The often described breaking up of spine fragments into smaller pieces by object impact is not effective and is not recommended.

Crown of Thorns

Injuries from the crown of thorns are uncommon due to its distribution. This is indeed fortunate from the perspective of the coral reef due to the destruction that these sea stars cause. Feeding on coral polyps, they can destroy entire segments of reef during outbreaks and rank as one of the great risks to the health of coral reefs. A crown of thorns can reach up to 60 cm across, though it is typically less than this (Figure 29.30). The body, with its 18–24 arms, is covered with sharp magnesium calcite spines 2–6 cm in length enveloped with several tissue layers

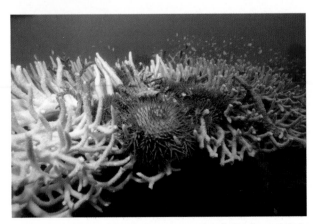

Figure 29.30. Crown of thorns (*Acanthaster planci*). Courtesy of Craig Cook.

containing glandular structures (Figure 29.31). These contain venomous compounds that probably account for the symptoms experienced after a puncture. The body also contains defensive steroid-like compounds called saponins. The spines are brittle and break easily after contact usually after an unintentional encounter.

Symptoms are usually described as pain out of proportion to the injury. The area immediately around the puncture appears inflamed and swollen. Limb and lymph node swelling are usually not seen unless there has been extensive contact with multiple punctures. Pain often resolves in mild cases after several hours. In severe cases, there may be systemic symptoms with nausea and vomiting more likely due to pain than to a systemic toxin. As with any marine puncture, a local contact dermatitis may ensue from foreign organic material entering the wound. The wound should be carefully washed after removal of any spines. Greater than expected bleeding from the puncture site may be noticed, probably due to the presence of a local anticoagulant.

The wound should be closely examined by medical personnel for retained spines or foreign material and, if present, carefully removed. Any retained spines that cannot be easily removed will need to be examined at a medical facility with capability for radiographic detection. Pain may be relieved by hot water immersion (no greater than 45°C) for 30–90 minutes and may be repeated. Cold packs have also been reported as being helpful in certain cases. A local anesthetic injection such as xylocaine may give some relief, and tetanus toxoid may be administered if required.

Bristle Worms

This common worm is found throughout tropical and semitropical waters. It may reach 15 cm in length and is covered with fine setae or bristles that break off when touched (Figures 29.32 and 29.33). When threatened these bristles are splayed apart offering a greater surface area for contact. These setae remain intradermally causing swelling, erythema, and pain that may last for

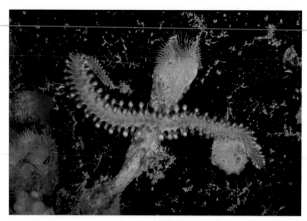

Figure 29.32. Bristle worm or fire worm. The fine bristles break off and become embedded in the skin causing a severe reaction. Courtesy of Craig Cook.

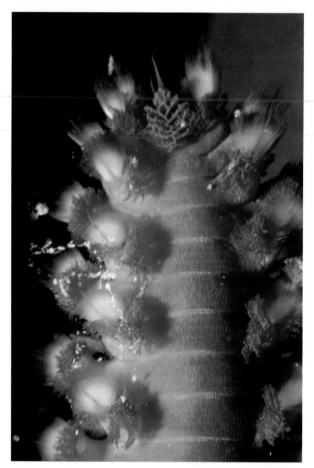

Figure 29.33. Bristle worm close-up showing fine bristles. Courtesy of Craig Cook.

days. No venom presence has ever been reported, and it is presumably the setae that cause the symptoms, however out of proportion these may be.

Treatment

Removal of bristles by using tape may be useful followed by cleaning with soap and water. Topical lidocaine,

steroids, and antihistamines have been used with varying degrees of relief.

Sea Bather's Eruption

Also referred to as sea lice, this aptly named description refers to the itchy, erythematous papular rash that is produced by contact with the various small larval forms of coelenterates. The most common offender, at least in the Caribbean, is *Linuche unguiculata* or the thimble jellyfish. Serum immunoglobins against *unguiculata* have been identified in some individuals.[17] Other larva ranging from anemones to crab larvae have also been implicated. Cases are often seasonal and are worldwide in distribution. Symptoms are usually described as a burning or itchy type of papular rash, lasting for up to 5 to 7 days. The distribution often corresponds to the elastic pressure from bathing suits or wet suits such as at the wrist, neck or waist (Figure 29.34). A low grade fever is not uncommon especially in repeat cases.

Treatment

Topical steroids and antihistamines may provide some relief from symptoms; however, this is highly variable.

Marine Seafood Poisonings

A minor sting or envenomation from any of the previously described marine life could be expected to cause only a small inconvenience, whereas a major envenomation could result in the incapacitation of an individual. In contrast, marine poisonings tend to infect more than one individual and have often affected the entire crew. History has recorded more than one incident where entire military campaigns and expeditions have been changed due to seafood poisonings. The theme of the remainder of this chapter centers again on recognition and avoidance, which remains central to the following discussion on marine poisonings. The expedition that

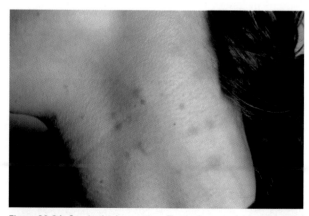

Figure 29.34. Sea bather's eruption. The lesions are typically located under tight fitting clothing such as the collar of this woman's wetsuit. Courtesy of Craig Cook.

has meticulously planned for every contingency cannot afford to place itself in jeopardy for something as simple as the wrong seafood choice at a single meal. It is important to note that all of these toxins are not deactivated by heat or refrigeration and give off no disagreeable taste or appearance. The following discussion is not all encompassing but covers some of the most common marine poisonings or those that could be life-threatening.

Ciguatera Poisoning

The most common marine poisoning reported in tropical and semitropical areas is ciguatera poisoning. This syndrome differs from other cases of gastrointestinal illness due to the neurologic symptoms frequently present and the course length. It results from ingestion of large carnivorous fish whose flesh is toxic from ingestion of other similarly infected fish lower in the food chain.

The toxic organism is a bottom dwelling dinoflagellate (*Gambierdiscus toxicus*), which is fed on by herbivorous fish that are eaten by larger carnivorous fish. This results in the toxin being concentrated in fish and then converted to ciguatoxins. There are at least three different forms of these toxins, the most serious of which is the action on sodium conduction channels, particularly in nerve cells.[18] It is speculated that this mechanism may result in the long-term neurologic symptoms often seen.

Ciguatera poisoning is unique in that there are endemic regions where certain species are known to be infected, followed by other regions where there are sporadic outbreaks. Fish species affected tend to be those at the top of the predator chain, such as barracuda, red snapper, grouper, Spanish mackerel, and coral trout among others. Pelagic or deep-water fish are rarely affected. Unfortunately, these species vary from region to region, and it is usually impossible to know for sure which are infected. In some areas of Australia, certain species are prohibited for sale, but this is no help to individuals in more remote regions. Often, the local population is knowledgeable as to which fish may be toxic, but it borders on recklessness to rest the operational success of an expedition on such sources. Similarly, local "tests" such as feeding portions of fish to cats or observing whether or not flies land on it, have no basis on which to be relied on. Recently, a commercial testing kit has become available for individual use.

The symptoms of ciguatera poisoning comprise varying degrees of gastrointestinal and neurologic signs and symptoms.[19] Onset is anywhere from less than one hour after ingestion to greater than 24 hours and dependent on the amount of toxin ingested. Gastrointestinal symptoms include diarrhea, vomiting, and abdominal pain. The abdominal pain can become chronic and last for months. Common neurologic symptoms are described are paresthesias, myalgias, and hot-cold

sensation reversal.[20] In cases where GI symptoms are minor with prominent neurologic symptoms, and the patient has dived in the preceding 24 hours, there could be confusion with decompression sickness. These cases should be able to be properly differentiated according to clinical presentation however. Finally, nonspecific symptoms such as fatigue and weakness are experienced by the majority of those infected. The distribution of gastrointestinal to neurologic symptoms varies from case to case. Duration seems to be related to severity and can last for months and be incapacitating in severe cases.

Treatment

Treatment has generally been supportive, including rehydration with fluid and electrolytes. Vomiting may be induced if it has been several hours or less since the fish was consumed. Tricyclic antidepressants such as amitryptyline have shown to be of benefit in some patients in relieving some long-term neurologic symptoms. Diphenhydramine (Benadryl) may be useful for symptoms of itching. Recently, mannitol in doses of 1g/kg of a 20% solution has been advocated in acute cases with dramatic improvements being reported in some individuals.[21] It is speculated that the intravascular osmotic changes may lessen the degree of myelin swelling and damage from the toxin. This effect seems to be of most benefit early in the course as later administration shows decreasing efficacy.

A number of postinfection complaints, perhaps immune in nature, have been described. Certain nontoxic fish species when eaten have produced symptoms along with shellfish, pork, and chicken or nuts. It is recommended that patients refrain from eating seafood for this reason. Alcohol has been well documented to also reproduce or exacerbate symptoms particularly in the acute phase and should also be avoided.

Pufferfish Poisoning

Pufferfish poisoning probably ranks as the most serious of all marine poisonings. Its toxin, tetrodotoxin, found in its ovaries, liver, intestines, and skin is extremely lethal causing dozens of deaths each year and even more morbidity requiring hospitalization. Fortunately, the fish is very easy to identify and cases result from the extremes of either complete ignorance or deliberate ingestion as a prepared delicacy.

The pufferfish and its relatives the sunfish and porcupinefish, all have a distinctive appearance and behavior. Their scales have been replaced with small spines and they are able to enlarge their bodies by ingesting water in order to avoid being swallowed (Figure 29.35). As a result, the potential for misidentification is low. However, in Japan it is prepared as "fugu" by specialized licensed chiefs who carefully remove the toxic organs leaving the fins and flesh for the discriminating diner. Enough toxin

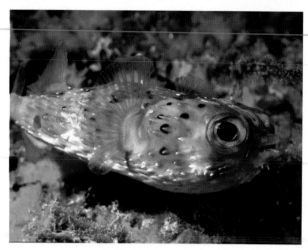

Figure 29.35. Pufferfish.

still remains to impart a slight tingling in the palate further enhancing its gastronomic appeal.

The toxin, which has been very well researched and described, works by inhibiting sodium channels in nerve cells. This produces muscular weakness eventually progressing to paralysis and death in severe cases. Clinically, symptoms appear rapidly ranging from minutes to several hours. There is often circumoral numbness of the lips, tongue, and face which may extend to involve the extremities and rest of the body.[22] The small and rapidly fatiguing motor nerves of the eyes may be involved resulting in diplopia (double vision) along with the pharyngeal muscles resulting in difficulty in swallowing. Any patient showing these symptoms with a history of possible pufferfish ingestion will need immediate transport to a medical facility capable of ventilator support.

Continued progression will manifest itself as further muscular weakness finally cumulating as respiratory paralysis and death. As in the case of blue-ringed octopus and cone shell envenomation, it must be emphasized that cardiopulmonary resuscitation and support are life-saving.[23] These cases should be survivable with the proper treatment as these toxins have no permanent damaging effects. Tetrodotoxin has no effect on nerve cells in the brain, and mentation and awareness remain unaffected. A patient may be paralyzed but is able to hear and understand what is happening around them, a situation that can be terrifying to many individuals. Every effort should be made to thoroughly explain what is occurring and then sedative and amnestic medications administered.

Scombroid Poisoning

Specific species of poorly prepared and refrigerated fish can produce a poisoning syndrome with symptoms similar to an allergic reaction. Fish from the Scombridae family such as tuna, albacore, bonitos, mackerel, and other game fish were traditionally described as the primary culprits of this syndrome. Now, other fish such as

dolphin (mahi-mahi), amberjack, and bluefish have also been implicated.

Fish that are allowed to remain at room temperature undergo a chemical reaction where histadine is converted into histamine and saurine.[24] Histamine is one of the primary mediators responsible for allergic reactions, and when ingested these substances produce similar symptoms. The fish itself appears normal and gives off no abnormal odor. The taste has often been described as bitter or peppery, but not disagreeable. Cooking does not deactivate the toxins. Symptoms appear fairly rapidly often within minutes and usually under an hour. An erythematous rash with urticaria (hives) and pruritus is common along with diarrhea, vomiting, and abdominal cramps. Systemic symptoms such as flushing, hypotension, tachycardia, dizziness, and throbbing headache are also common.[25] Bronchospasm has also been described and asthmatics would be at higher risk for these symptoms.

Treatment is symptomatic with intravenous (IV) hydration, histamine (H2 and H1) blockers such as cimetidine and diphenhydramine, IV hydrocortisone, or inhaled bronchodilators if needed.[26] The symptoms usually subside within 6–12 hours. Prompt and careful attention to refrigeration of these fish is completely effective in preventing scombroid poisoning.

Shellfish Poisoning

Shellfish poisoning encompasses at least four syndromes, each produced by a specific toxin.[27] All result from eating toxic shellfish such as mussels, clams, oysters, and other bivalves. The toxins are either dinoflagellates or polyethers that are filtered and then concentrated in the shellfish. Most poisonings are due to personal harvesting and consumption with numbers being usually small. Many localities monitor for shellfish toxins further keeping infection low. Symptoms are of gastrointestinal or neurologic nature and, with the exception of amnesic shellfish poisoning, can present within minutes, usually within 2 hours.

Paralytic Shellfish Poisoning

By far the most serious of all shellfish poisonings, paralytic shellfish poisoning (PSP) results from saxitoxin produced by a number of dinoflagellates. This neurotoxin acts similarly to tetrodotoxin by blocking sodium channel transmission in nerves. Cooking does not deactivate the toxin. Symptom onset is rapid and described as circumoral numbness or tingling in the mouth or tongue, extremity weakness, difficulty talking, double vision along with gastrointestinal symptoms.[28] In severe cases, the weakness continues to progress to paralysis, and death results. In some cases, a dysphoria described as a floating sensation has been experienced. As in the case of all marine poisoning, there is no antidote, and treatment is supportive. Induced vomiting or gastric lavage and use of activated charcoal are helpful if administered early in the first few hours. The patient must be monitored for any sign of respiratory compromise. There are no lasting side effects for those affected.

Neurotoxic Shellfish Poisoning

Symptoms of neurotoxic shellfish poisoning (NSP) are generally similar but milder than PSP.[29] In this case, the dinoflagellate-produced toxin is a polyether called brevetoxin that is often associated with red tides. (It has been described as potentially infectious as an aerosol form under these conditions.) As in PSP, both neurologic and gastrointestinal symptoms may be present with progression to paralysis and death (though rare). Treatment is the same as for PSP.

Amnesic Shellfish Poisoning

Another form of shellfish poisoning is caused by domoic acid formed by specific species of diatoms.[30] In addition to the gastrointestinal symptoms, the neurologic presentation has included mental confusion and short-term memory loss, hence its name. The memory loss may be permanent and is most severe in the elderly where it may present as dementia-type syndrome.

Diarrhea Shellfish Poisoning

Gastrointestinal symptoms are predominant in this form of shellfish poisoning, but neurologic manifestations are absent.[31] Okadaic acid is the demonstrated toxin that increases the permeability of the intestinal cells to fluid passage and produces a secretory diarrhea. Hydration and symptomatic treatment are usually all that is required with complete recovery within 1 or 2 days.

SUMMARY

Marine environments offer a considerable range of hazardous animals that could threaten expedition participants. The expedition medical officer needs to be aware of potential threats as well as the best means of diagnosing and treating these various injuries and exposures.

REFERENCES

1 Johnson, RH, Nelson DR. Agonistic display in the grey reef shark *Carcharhinus menisorrah* and its relationship to attacks on man. *Copeia*. 1:76–84.

2 McCabe MJ, Hammon WM, Halstead BW, Newton TH. A fatal brain injury caused by a needlefish. *Neuroradiol*. 1978;15(3):137–9.

3 Thakker MM, Usha KR. Orbital foreign body and ruptured globe from needlefish impalement. *Arch Ophthalmol*. 2006;124(2):284.

4 Williamson J, Fenner P, Burnett J, eds. *Venomous and Poisonous Marine Animals: A Medical and Biological Handbook*. Sydney, Australia: NSW University Press; 1996.

5 Williamson J, Fenner P, Burnett J, eds. *Venomous and Poisonous Marine Animals: A Medical and Biological Handbook*. Sydney, Australia: NSW University Press; 1996: 112–13.

6 Maretic Z. Fish venoms. In: Tu AT, ed. *Handbook of Natural Toxins, Vol 3, Marine Toxins and Venoms*. New York: Marcel Dekker: 445–78.

7 Flecker H, Cotton BC. Fatal bite from octopus. *Med J Aust*. 2:329–32.

8 Williamson J. The blue-ringed octopus bite and envenomation syndrome. *Aquatic Dermatology. Clin Dermatol*. 1987;5(3):127–33.

9 Heatwolfe H. *Sea Snakes*. Malabar, Fla: University of New South Wales Press and Krieger Publishing Company; 1999: 121–2.

10 Kurigan J. Snail toxins yield fast-paced advances in drug research. *J NIH Res*. 1995;7:30–2.

11 Fenner PJ. Venomous jellyfish of the world. *SPUMS J*. 2005;35:131.

12 Fenner PJ. Dangerous Australian box jellyfish. *SPUMS J*. 2005;35:78–9.

13 Exton DR, Fenner PJ, Williamson JA. Cold packs: an effective topical analgesia in the treatment of painful stings by *Physalia* and other jellyfish stings. *Med J Aust*. 1989;151: 625–6.

14 King PF. Acute analgesia and cosmetic benefits of box-jellyfish antivenom. *Med J Aust*. 1991;154:365–6.

15 Flecker H. "Irukandji" stings to North Queensland bathers without production of wheals but with severe general symptoms. *Med J Aust*. 1952;1:89–91.

16 Fenner PJ. Dangerous Australian box jellyfish. *SPUMS J*. 2005;35:81.

17 Wong DE, Meinking TL, Rosen LB, et al. Seabather's eruption: clinical, histological, and immunological features. *J Am Acad Derm*. 1994;30:99–406.

18 Bidhard JM, Vijverberg HP, Frenlin C, et al. Ciguatoxin is a novel type of Na+ channel toxin. *J Bio Chem*. 1984;259:8353–7.

19 Morris JG, Lewin P, Hargrett NT, et al. Clinical features of ciguatera poisoning. *Arc Intern Med*. 1982;142:1090–2.

20 Bagnis R, Kuberski T, Laugier S. Clinical observations on 3,009 cases of ciguatera (fish poisoning) in the South Pacific. *Am J Trop Med Hyg*. 1979;28:1067–73.

21 Palafox A, Jain LG, Pinano AZ, et al. Successful treatment of ciguatera fish poisoning with intravenous mannitol. *JAMA*. 1988;259:2740–2.

22 Cook J. *The Three Voyages of Captain James Cook Around the World*. Vol. IV. London; Longman, Hurst, Rees, Orme and Brown; 1821:103.

23 Sun K, Wat J, So P. Puffer fish poisoning. *Anaesth Intens Care*. 1994;22:307–8.

24 Morrow JD, Margolies GR, Rowland J, et al. Evidence that histamine is the causative toxin of scombroid-fish poisoning. *N Engl J Med*. 1991;324(11):716–20.

25 Kim R. Flushing syndrome due to mahimahi (scombroid fish) poisoning. *Arch Dermatol*. 1979;115(8):963–5.

26 Blakesley ML. Scombroid poisoning: prompt resolution of symptoms with cimetidine. *Ann Emerg Med*. 1983;12(2): 104–6.

27 Eastaugh J, Shepherd S. Infectious and toxic syndromes from fish and shellfish consumption: a review. *Arch Intern Med*. 1989;149(8):1735–40.

28 Sobel J, Painter J. Illnesses caused by marine toxins. *Clin Infect Dis*. 2005;41(9):1290–6.

29 Lehane L. Paralytic shellfish poisoning: a potential public health problem. *Med J Aust*. 2001;175(1):29–3.

30 Jeffery B, Barlow T, Moizer K, et al. Amnesic shellfish poison. *Food Chem Toxicol*. 2004;42(4):545–57.

31 Isbister GK, Kiernan GC. Neurotoxic marine poisoning. *Lancet Neurol*. 2005;4(4):219–28.

30 | Expedition Toxicology

Timothy B. Erickson, MD, and Janet Y. Lin, MD, MPH

INTRODUCTION

In the international wilderness and expedition setting, familiarization with commonly prescribed and abused drugs available to a specific region or group of people is important. Expanded urbanization and worldwide travel has increased illegal drug trafficking exponentially. Awareness of prescription medications any expedition team members may be taking is essential. Additionally, the expedition health care provider should be familiar with the poisonous plants, mushrooms, natural toxins, herbal products, and venomous creatures indigenous to the area of exploration and travel.

The poisoned victim may present with a variety of clinical symptoms including dermatologic changes, gastroenteritis, altered mental status, seizures, cardiac dysrhythmias, and respiratory distress. In many cases, during the initial management, the offending agent is unknown. To complicate matters, a large percentage of overdoses involve multiple drugs, making the diagnosis of the primary causal agent more challenging. Accidental environmental exposures and natural toxins may add to or complicate the presentation of a poisoned victim.

In developing countries and in the remote wilderness, access to medicinal agents is limited. Advanced treatment modalities commonly available in industrialized nations (antidotes, ventilators, dialysis equipment, intensive care units) are usually unavailable in underdeveloped countries or in the expedition environment. Therefore, the provider must be resourceful and, at times, creative. Fortunately, the majority of poisonings can be treated by removing the patient form the source of exposure, taking general decontamination measures, and offering supportive care. In adverse weather conditions, providing shelter away from the elements also represents an essential aspect of supportive care.[1]

CRITICAL ACTIONS

As with any acutely ill patient, attention to the ABCDs is critical when evaluating the acutely poisoned patient.

Airway	If the patient is obtunded or having a seizure, assess that the oral cavity is clear of debris, such as food or vomitus.
Breathing	Make sure the patient is breathing spontaneously and without difficulty. Provide oxygen if the patient is acutely short of breath, either by mask or nasal cannula.
Circulation	Check the blood pressure and pulse. If there are signs of shock, establish an IV line and hydrate.
Decontamination	Dermatological exposures should be decontaminated with clothing removal and copious irrigation with water or saline solution.

After addressing the ABCDs, it is important to look for signs and symptoms of serious poisonings and life-threatening conditions, which may be associated with a toxic exposure.

Coma and Decreased Level of Consciousness: Alcohols, sedatives such as benzodiazepines, opioids (heroin), carbon monoxide exposure, cyanide, and antidepressants

Shortness of Breath: Insecticides/organophosphates, hydrocarbon aspiration, herbicides (paraquat), salicylates, and chemical pneumonitis

Severe Vomiting and Diarrhea: Acetaminophen, salicylates, iron, lead, organophosphates, caustics, digitalis, plants, and mushrooms

Status Epilepticus and Tetany: Cocaine, antidepressants, insecticides, carbon monoxide, lead, isoniazid, salicylates, water hemlock, and *Giromitra* mushrooms

Cardiac Dysrhythmias: Antidepressants, antimalarials, digitalis, cocaine, amphetamines, volatile substance abuse

HISTORY AND PHYSICAL EXAM

In the expedition setting, resources are limited and the health care provider needs to rely more on a thorough history and physical exam. However, in adverse weather conditions or a remote setting, a thorough history may not be prudent, and evacuation of the patient represents a more important action. Historical questions include: the time of exposure, the route of exposure (oral, intravenous, dermal, inhalation), reason for the poisoning (accidental, suicidal), amount of drug ingested, whether the patient has vomited, the patient's significant past medical history, and whether other victims in the expedition team or surrounding area were affected (vital information particularly with environmental toxins).

Certain classes of drugs present with specific symptoms or characteristic physical findings. These clinical presentations are termed toxic syndromes or toxidromes. Some of the more common toxidromes and agents that cause them follow:[2,3]

Cholinergic (mnemonic "DUMBELS")

Diarrhea, defecation

Urination

Miosis

Bronchosecretions, bradycardia

Emesis

Lacrimination

Salivation

Agents: Organophsphate/carbamate insecticides, betel nut (chewed worldwide, common in India), *Inocybe* and *Clitocybe* mushrooms

Anticholinergic

Dry as a bone (dry skin)

Blind as a bat (dilated pupils)

Hot as hell (hyperthermic)

Red as a beet (flushed skin)

Mad as a hatter (delirium)

Agents: Antihistamines (diphenhydramine), atropine, tricyclic antidepressants, jimson weed, mandrake, henbane, nightshade

Opioid

Miosis

Coma

Respiratory depression

Decreased bowel sounds

Bradycardia

Hypothermia

Agents: Heroin, codeine, morphine, poppies, methadone, fentanyl

Sympathomimetic

Tachycardia

Hyperthermia

Dilated pupils

Hypertension

Seizures

Tachypnea

Agitation

Agents: Cocaine, amphetamines, PCP, nicotine, caffeine, khat

In the international expedition setting, laboratory facilities are often limited, if available at all. As a result, qualitative urine toxicology screens or quantitative blood levels for specific toxins may not be practical for diagnostic purposes. If available, baseline labs can be obtained and used to narrow the differential diagnosis. Random diagnostic studies or "shot gunning" laboratory data with scarce resources is greatly discouraged.

The anion gap equation, which is calculated by taking the patient's serum sodium minus the sum of the chloride and bicarbonate. $Na - (Cl + HCO_3)$ Normal = 8–12, may be valuable.

Several toxins cause an elevated anion gap metabolic acidosis in the overdose setting. (The mnemonic is: METAL ACID GAP).[4]

Methanol, metformin, massive exposures to any toxin

Ethylene glycol

Toluene

ASA

Lactic acidosis

Aminogycosides (uremia-inducing agents)

Carbon monoxide, cyanide

INH, iron

DKA

Generalized seizures (toxin induced)

Alcohol ketoacidosis

Paraldehyde

When cardiotoxic agents are suspected the patient should be placed on a cardiac monitor, and a 12-lead ECG should be obtained if available. If the medical facility has radiographic capabilities, a chest radiograph should be obtained on patients with respiratory compromise or acute dyspnea. Additionally, an abdominal radiograph may be diagnostic with certain radioopaque toxins such as the heavy metals (iron, lead, mercury, arsenic) or in "body packers" smuggling illegal contraband across international borders.

Decontamination Measures

If the patient presents with a recent toxic ingestion, gastric decontamination is usually warranted. The most efficacious decontamination method with the fewest side effects is oral-activated charcoal. In powdered form, it can easily be transported and should be part of any expedition medical kit (Table 30.1). Activated charcoal (AC) possesses a high surface area, which will absorb the majority of toxic agents when given in doses of 1–2 g/kg prepared in a slurry of water. If the amount of toxin ingested is known, providing charcoal in a 10:1 ratio (10 g of AC to every 1 g of toxin) makes more pharmacologic

Table 30-1. Expedition medical kit for toxicological emergencies	
Product	Indication
Powdered activated charcoal	Gastric decontamination
Powdered PEG solution	Gastric decontamination
Gastric lavage tube	Gastric decontamination
Naloxone (Narcan)	Opioid overdose
MARK II, autoinjectors (Atropine 2-PAM)	Organophosphates, nerve agents
Diazepam	Seizures, sympathomimetics
Pyridoxine, vitamin B_6	INH, false morel mushrooms
Diphenhydraine	Dystonic reactions, allergic reactions
EpiPen	Anaphylaxis allergic reactions
Oxygen tank/mask	CO poisoning, hypoxia
N-actetylcysteine	Acetaminophen poisoning
Succimer (DMSA)	Lead, mercury, arsenic poisoning
Peptol-Bismol, ciprofloxacin	Food poisoning
Sodium bicarbonate	Metabolic acidosis, TCA toxicity, salicylates
Antimalarials	Malaria, mosquito-borne diseases
DEET insecticide	Arthropod, tick, mosquito deterrent
CroFab	Pit viper envenomation
Bottle of whiskey	Ethylene glycol, methanol poisoning
Normal saline IV tubing – angiocaths	Hydration, irrigation
Cyanide antidote kit*	Cyanide toxicity from fire exposure
Digibind*	If expedition member on Digoxin
Glucagon*	If expedition member on beta-blockers
Calcium*	HF burns, calcium channel blockers
*Optional	

sense.[3] For several drugs, such as aspirin, theophylline, phenobarbital, digitoxin, and carbamazepine, multiple dosing of activated charcoal (every 2–4 hours) may enhance elimination due to enterohepatic or enteroenteric recirculation of the drug. Activated charcoal is relatively ineffective against pesticides, hydrocarbons, caustic agents, alcohols, and small ionic metals such as iron and lithium. In some Asian countries and Australia, where activated charcoal is less available, a similar clay-like substance called Fuller's Earth is commonly used. In some charcoal preparations, cathartics (e.g., magnesium citrate and sorbitol) are added in order to induce diarrhea. Administration of a cathartic with the first dose of charcoal in older children and adults is often recommended. However, overzealous use of cathartics can result in patient dehydration and electrolyte imbalance if not used cautiously.

The emetic agent, syrup of ipecac, is harvested from the *Cephaelis ipecacuanha* plant in Brazil and Central America. In the average patient, it will induce vomiting within 20 minutes after oral administration. It is contraindicated in patients with active seizures and depressed mental status due to its aspiration potential. It is also contraindicated following caustic and hydrocarbon ingestions due to reintroduction of the agent to the esophagus and lung, respectively. Additionally, when effective, syrup of ipecac may delay administration of activated charcoal. Ipecac may have a limited role in victims who have recently ingested plants, berries, and mushrooms or agents not well absorbed by charcoal. Although no longer recommended in the hospital or home setting, in the expedition and remote wilderness environment, syrup of ipecac may be the only decontamination modality accessible. In this scenario however, oral activated charcoal would be a preferred method, if available.

Gastric lavage is indicated in patients who present within 1 hour after ingestion of a potentially lethal poison. The procedure uses a large bore orogastric tube. The patient's stomach is irrigated and suctioned with several liters of water or normal saline until the gastric effluent is clear of pill fragments or gastric debris. Like ipecac, it is contraindicated in caustic and hydrocarbon ingestions. If the patient is lethargic, comatose, or experiencing airway difficulties, oral intubation should be performed prior to lavage in order to protect the airway from aspiration.[2]

Whole bowel irrigation with high molecular weight polyethylene glycol (PEG) solution (commonly used for presurgical bowel preparations and radiologic procedures) is osmotically and electrolyte safe. This Go-Lytely solution can be used following ingestions of iron, lead by international drug smugglers (intestinal body packers of cocaine and heroin). The typical dose is 1–2 liters per hour administered via a nasogastric tube. Premixed, PEG solution comes in a small powdered packet making it a practical addition to an expedition medical kit (Table 30.1).

Enhanced Elimination

Urinary alkalinization with bicarbonate may be efficacious in promoting renal excretion following overdoses of weak acids (e.g., salicylates and phenobarbital). The goal is to maintain a urinary pH of 7.0–8.0. In this intervention, maintenance of potassium is essential for effective renal excretion. Urinary acidification is never clinically indicated and may exacerbate toxin-induced rhabdomyolysis.

If the poisoned victim can be transported to a higher-level medical care facility, hemodialysis may be indicated following life-threatening doses of agents with low molecular weights, low volumes of distribution, and water-soluble properties.[4]

U	Uremia-inducing agents
N	Not responsive to conventional therapy
S	Salicylates
T	Theophylline
A	Alcohols (methanol, isopropanol)
B	Barbiturates
L	Lithium
E	Ethylene glycol

Table 30.2. Common toxins and their antidotes

Toxin	Antidote
Acetaminophen/paracetamol	N-acetylcysteine
Carbon monoxide	Oxygen, HBO
Cyanide	Cyanide antidote kit (hydroxycobalamin)
Arsenic	BAL, succimer
Lead	BAL, CaEDTA, succimer
TCAs	Sodium bicarbonate
Opiates	Naloxone
Anticholinergics	Physostigmine
Organophosphates	Atropine, pralidoxime (2-PAM)
Digibind, FAB fragments	Digitalis, digoxin
Beta-blockers, calcium channel blockers	Glucagon
Calcium channel blockers, hydrofluoric acid	Calcium
Iron	Deferoxamine
Methemoglobinemia	Methylene blue
Isoniazid (INH)	Pyridoxime
Methanol/ethylene glycol	Ethanol/4-methylpyrazole (4-MP)
Benzodiazepines	Flumazenil
Calcium channel blockers/ beta-blockers	Glucose/insulin
Oral hypoglycemic agents	Octreotide
Pit viper envenomations	Cro-Fab

Antidotes

A small number of poisons have a direct antagonist or antidote to counteract its toxic properties. However, in regions of exploration and expedition, these tend to be undersupplied and overly expensive to stock. Common toxins and their specific antidotes are listed in Table 30.2.

SPECIFIC TOXINS

Acetaminophen (Paracetamol)

Introduction

Acetaminophen or paracetamol is available worldwide as a pain reliever and fever reducer and is found in many over-the-counter cold and flu preparations. In an overdose setting, large doses of acetaminophen deplete glutathione stores in the liver, resulting in the accumulation of toxic metabolites (such as NAPQI) via the cytochrome P450 pathway. Acute doses of 7–8 g of acetaminophen in an adult or 200 mg/kg in children are considered toxic. Chronic ingestion of alcohol or other drugs which are metabolized through the liver P450 system (e.g., INH) may exacerbate acetaminophen's hepatotoxicity at lesser doses. (See Figure 30.1.)

Clinical Features

Patients with acetaminophen toxicity typically present with nausea, vomiting, and abdominal pain during the first 24 hours after ingestion. At 36–48 hours, the patient usually experiences resolution of GI symptoms or enters a "quiescent phase." From 72–96 hours postingestion, the patient suffers renewed nausea, vomiting, RUQ pain along with jaundice, bleeding, and mental status changes consistent with hepatic encephalopathy.

Diagnosis

The diagnosis is made based on the history of ingestion along with laboratory data consistent with liver damage. If possible, SGOT (AST), SGPT (ALT), bilirubin, and protime (PT) levels should be assessed and followed in a serial manner. However, liver function tests may not be abnormal until 48–72 hours after ingestion. In the first 4–24 hours following an acute ingestion, if available, a serum acetaminophen level can be measured and plotted on the Rumack nomogram (Figure 30.2). Optimally, the level is drawn at 4 hours postingestion and plotted on the nomogram.[5] If the level falls within the potential hepatotoxic range, antidote therapy is indicated as discussed later. Serum BUN and creatinine should also be measured because the severely poisoned patient may suffer hepatorenal failure. If mental status changes occur, ammonia levels can be followed.

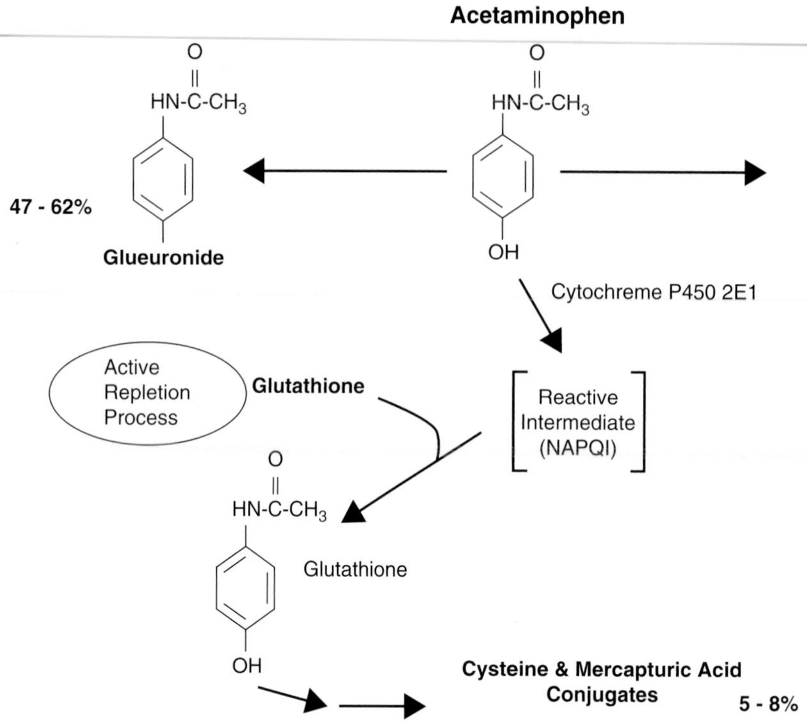

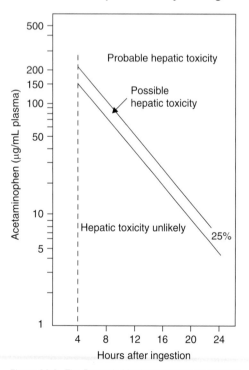

Acetaminophen

Figure 30.1. Metabolism of acetaminophen (*http://www.fda.gov*).

Acetaminophen Toxicity Nomogram

Figure 30.2. The Rumack–Matthew nomogram, relating expected severity of liver toxicity to serum acetaminophen concentrations. From Smilkstein MJ, Bronstein AC, Linden C, et al. Acetaminophen overdose: a 48-hour intravenous N-acetylcysteine treatment protocol. *Ann Emerg Med* 1991;20(10):1058, with permission.

Treatment

Initial treatment consists of gastric decontamination with gastric lavage following a large overdose if the patient presents within one hour of ingestion and has not already vomited. Activated charcoal can also be administered orally to adsorb excess drug in the gut. The mainstay of therapy is the antidote N-acetylcysteine (NAC), which acts to replenish depleted glutathione stores in the liver.[6] Indications for use include 4- to 24-hour hepatoxic acetaminophen level as plotted on the nomogram, single acute ingestion of 7–8 g in the adult and 200 mg/kg in the child, or late presentation of a patient already demonstrating liver toxicity. The antidote is administered orally (140 mg/kg single loading dose, followed by 70 mg/kg maintenance dose, every 4 hours × 17 doses). In patients with vomiting unresponsive to antiemetics, the antidote can also be given intravenously. Recently, this IV form of the antidote (Acetadote) has been approved by the Food and Drug Administration (FDA) for use in the United States. If levels are unavailable in the international setting, and a significant overdose is suspected, it is best to administer the full course of antidote as the benefits greatly outweigh the risks. If the patient has advanced irreversible liver damage, hepatic encephalopathy, hepatorenal syndrome, or severe coagulopathy, a liver transplant, if available, may be ultimately indicated.

Prevention

Prevention includes keeping acetaminophen products away from children or suicidal adults as well as public education as to the potential danger of this seemingly "benign" medication with misuse. Be aware that many international over-the-counter products contain acetaminophen or paracetamol.

Acetazolamide (Diamox)

Introduction

Acetazolamide is a carbonic anhydrase inhibitor that is widely used by mountaineers to prevent or treat high-altitude disorders. The medication works to increase excretion of bicarbonate, thus establishing a metabolic acidotic state. This in turn increases ventilation, which subsequently increases arterial oxygen concentrations in a few hours. This physiologic change mimics acclimatization.[7] Controversy exists as to the adequate dose and how and when it is administered (range from 125 to 750 mg a day).

Clinical Features

Acetazolamide toxicity generally occurs in those with impaired renal function or in those who take the medication for chronic conditions (e.g., glaucoma). These people will present with severe metabolic acidosis, oftentimes with altered mental status. At altitude, patients suffering from high-altitude sickness may present with headache, dizziness, nausea, vomiting, weakness, insomnia, and progress to confusion and difficulty breathing. In an expedition setting, it may be important to differentiate acute high-altitude sickness that may progress to high-altitude cerebral edema or high-altitude pulmonary edema from a possible overdose of acetazolamide, although the incidence of toxicity in a normal person is rare.

More common are adverse effects associated with acetazolamide intake. Because it is a diuretic, people will experience increased urination and must watch for dehydration. Other common side effects are paresthesias of the hands and feet and altered taste, especially of carbonated drinks (makes beer taste flat). Some people complain of blurred vision while taking the medication. All these side effects resolve with cessation of the medication.[8]

Treatment

At altitude, the first step in treatment of a possible toxicity should be descent. If there is no improvement after this maneuver, the patient will require more intensive treatment and support which will be dictated by what is available. If laboratory capabilities are available, blood work to rule out other causes of metabolic acidosis are important.

Prevention

A prolonged acclimatization plan will help to reduce the incidence of altitude sickness and thus potentiate the need for pharmacological treatment or prophylaxis. However, if this is impossible, judicious use of Diamox or other agents will prevent any misuse.

Alcohols

Introduction

The toxic alcohols include methanol (windshield washer fluid, gasohol, moonshine), ethylene glycol (antifreeze, coolant), and isopropanol (rubbing alcohol). Globally, homemade "brews" of hard liquor products can potentially contain toxic alcohol additives. In 2006, a methanol epidemic in Nicaragua resulted from contaminated "guaro" cane alcohol causing over 500 poisonings and 40 deaths. Internationally, epidemics of ethylene glycol poisoning have been described in Russia and Scandinavia and methanol poisoning in India and Europe when used as an ethanol substitute. With each toxin, it is not the parent compound, but rather the resultant metabolites formed by the enzymatic pathway via alcohol dehydrogenase, that are poisonous. The toxic metabolites of methanol are formaldehyde and formic acid; ethylene glycol: glycolic and oxalic acid; and isopropanol: acetone.

Clinical Features

Patients poisoned by the toxic alcohols, whether intentionally or accidentally, will typically present inebriated with a depressed mental status and respiratory drive. All three compounds will cause some form of GI distress. Significant methanol toxicity will eventually result in ocular damage and blindness. Ethylene glycol poisoning results in renal failure and cardiopulmonary edema. Isopropanol can cause gastric bleeding.

Diagnosis

Diagnosis is based on the history of ingestion and clinical features. Additionally, unlike ethanol and isopropanol toxicity, methanol and ethylene glycol will result in a metabolic acidosis with elevated anion gap: Anion gap = $Na - (Cl + HCO_3)$ normal 8–12.

Methanol, ethylene glycol, and isopropanol all exhibit an elevated osmolal gap calculated by the equation: $2(Na) + Glucose/18 + BUN/2.8 + ETOH/4.6$. The osmol gap is the measured osmol minus the calculated osmol (normal < 10).

If available, serum methanol, ethylene glycol, and isopropanol can be measured. However, the turnaround time for lab results is often too long to withhold therapy. In the expedition setting, laboratory measurement will be virtually impossible. Since fluorescein is present in antifreeze products, fluorescence of the patient's urine or gastric contents under a wood's lamp (black light)

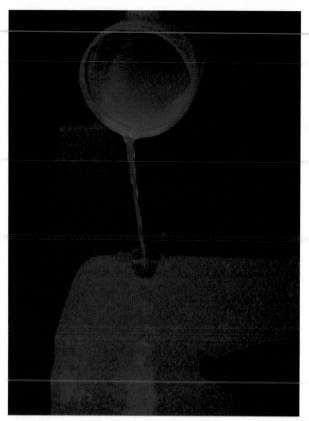

Figure 30.3. Urine fluorescing under a black light in a patient who ingested ethylene glycol. Photo courtesy of Gregory H. Bledsoe.

may be another diagnostic clue (Figure 30.3). However, the absence of this finding in the urine does not rule out ethylene glycol toxicity.

Treatment

Toxic alcohol poisoning, particularly with ethylene glycol and methanol is life-threatening. Therefore, management should never be withheld while awaiting definitive laboratory results.

Gastric lavage and activated charcoal is rarely efficacious as the alcohols are rapidly absorbed through the gastric mucosa. Ipecac should not be used because of the patient's lethargic state and aspiration potential.

Ethanol therapy is inexpensive, is readily available worldwide, and can competitively inhibit the alcohol dehydrogenase enzyme-induced pathway described previously. It can be administrated intravenously as a drip, or given orally. Four "shots" of whiskey, four glasses of wine, or six beers should be enough to induce a level of 100–150 mg%, necessary to inhibit the formation of the toxic metabolites. However, this level of inebriation needs to be maintained until the toxic alcohol is excreted through the kidneys. Because of its wide availability and low cost, ethanol represents the best method of detoxification in the remote expedition setting.

If the patient is severely poisoned, acidotic, has elevated serum level and/or evidence of end-organ damage,

if available, therapy with hemodialysis should be instituted. In the United States and Europe, the new antidote 4-methylpyrazole (4-MP) has been approved for the management of ethylene glycol and methanol poisoning.[9,10] It directly inhibits alcohol dehydrogenase and obviates the need for ethanol therapy. However, in most countries, it is too expensive to be adequately stocked.

Prevention

Prevention of toxic alcohol poisoning includes proper storage and labeling to keep these agents away from children, animals, and suicidal adults. The development of less toxic additives to engine coolants such as propylene glycol and the addition of bittering agents to make the sweet taste of these toxic alcohols less palatable, are other preventative measures. Even though foreign homemade alcohol concoctions are offered as a form of hospitality and may certainly be tempting, members of an expedition team should avoid drinking them.

Amphetamines

Introduction

Amphetamines or "speed" once commonly abused in the 1960s have regained popularity with newer "designer" forms. Drugs like Ecstacy, Adam, Eve, Ice, Crystal Meth, and Crank are abused worldwide and easier to manufacture and distribute than cocaine or heroin. Recently, in Europe, Ecstacy overtook heroin as the most commonly abused drug. In Yemen, Ethiopia, and Eastern Africa, a plant with amphetamine-like properties called khat is commonly chewed and abused. In the rural United States, a crystal methamphetamine epidemic has been well documented over the past decade.[11] As with cocaine, amphetamines are sympathomimetic agents with powerful alpha and beta receptor stimulation. Amphetamines can be abused orally, nasally, and intravenously.[12]

Clinical Features

Patients with amphetamine toxicity typically present with tachycardia, tachypnea, anxiousness, and dilated pupils. Severely intoxicated individuals will suffer chest pain, seizures, hyperthermia, and intracranial bleeds. Chronic users of crystal methamphetamine may have skin ulcerations and poor dental hygiene with advanced gingival disease.

Diagnosis

In any patient with access to drugs and presenting with the preceding sympathomimetic signs and symptoms, amphetamine abuse should be considered. Urinary toxicology screens can quantitatively screen for amphetamines if used within 72 hours of sampling. However, several of the newer designer drugs will test negative on typical amphetamine screens. If the patient experiences chest pains, an ECG should be obtained. If seizures occur, a CT scan of the head should be ordered, if available.

Treatment

Management of patients intoxicated on amphetamines includes supportive care and immediate attention to abnormal vital signs. If hyperthermic, the patient should be aggressively cooled with mist/sprays, fans, and strategic ice packs. If evidence of rhabdomyolysis or myoglobinuria exists, the patient should be given fluids, alkalinization, and mannitol to force diuresis. If hyperactive, anxious, tachycardic, and tachypnic, as with cocaine, liberal doses of benzodiazepine can be administered. Seizure activity can also be treated with benzodiazepines. If the amphetamine was recently ingested, standard doses of activated charcoal can be given.

Prevention

Similar to cocaine and heroin abuse, stricter drug laws may lessen abuse of amphetamines. Public education as to the potential dangers of these drugs is also essential.

Antibiotics

Introduction

In many parts of the world, medications that require a prescription in the United States are available to be purchased by any consumer without restriction. There are also medications for treatment of certain conditions that are available in other parts of the world that are not available in the United States or are no longer commonly used in the United States. Antibiotics are a good example. Available antibiotics may be those that one is less familiar with its indications or side effect profile. Two more commonly encountered antibiotics globally are chloramphenicol and tinidazole.

Clinical Features

Chloramphenicol is used extensively in less-developed areas of the world because of efficacy and expense. It is not used in the United States primarily because of its toxicity profile. It is important to be aware of its potential toxicity if one travels into a less-developed country. Toxicity is dose-related and primarily affects children, those with liver impairment, or those on medications that could alter serum concentrations of chloramphenicol. The known toxicities are aplastic anemia (rare), which can occur through oral or intravenous administration at any age, and Gray Baby Syndrome, a phenomenon affecting neonates because they lack the liver enzymes to metabolize the drug. Babies will present with hypotension, cyanosis, and death.[13]

Another common medication available worldwide that one may encounter is tinidazole (trade names Tindamax, Fasigyn). It is a second-generation synthetic imidazole in the same family as metronidazole and is not yet widely available in the United States. Indications for use are the same as for metronidazole: giardiasis, amebiasis, trichomonas. As with metronidazole, this medication should not be taken with alcohol because it can precipitate a disulfiram reaction.

Antidepressants

Introduction

Antidepressants are prescribed worldwide. The most common agents are cyclic antidepressants (e.g., tricyclic antidepressants or TCAs, amytriptyline, doxepine), and the SSRIs or serotonin reuptake inhibitors (e.g., fluoxetine, sertraline, St. Johns Wort). Regarding toxic potential, the cyclic antidepressants are more severe and will be focused on here. TCAs have anticholinergic properties and powerful alpha blockade (resulting in hypotension) along with sodium channel interaction at the myocardial cell channels causing cardiotoxicity.

Clinical Features

Following TCA overdose, the patient can present with an anticholinergic toxidrome (hyperthermic, dry, flushed skin, dilated pupils, and mental status changes or delirium). In addition, they are tachycardic and hypotensive. In severe overdoses, lethargy, coma, and generalized seizure activity can result.

Diagnosis

Diagnosis is based on the history of ingestion or history of depression and access to antidepressants. In addition, a patient with depressed mental status, seizures, and anticholinergic properties is a TCA overdose until proven otherwise. If available, an ECG often demonstrates a QRS widening (> 100ms) along with tachydysrhythmias, and ventricular tachycardia/fibrillation.

Urine and blood toxicology screens to detect TCAs are available but are often inaccurate with poor clinical correlation. With a moderate to severely poisoned patient, baseline labs including an arterial blood gas should be determined.

Treatment

Management of the patient with TCA overdose includes rapid control of the airway since patients will develop acute mental status changes within the first 2 hours of ingestion. Cardiac dysrhythmias and widening of the QRS are best controlled with administration of sodium bicarbonate (1–2 amps IVP) to stabilize the sodium channels in the myocardium and to alkalinize the serum, thereby enhancing TCA protein binding.[14] The goal is to maintain a serum pH of 7.45–7.55. In addition to IV fluids, alpha agonists such as Levophed may be required for refractory hypotension. Gastric lavage followed by activated charcoal administration is indicated in recent ingestions after the patient's airway is protected with intubation. Generalized seizure activity is best controlled with liberal doses of benzodiazepines. The antidote physostigmine, although indicated with severe poisonings of pure anticholinergic agents such as diphenhydramine and atropine, is *contraindicated* in TCA overdoses.

Poisoning with SSRI agents is less severe than TCAs and generally does well with supportive care alone along with gastric decontamination.

Prevention

Prevention of TCA poisoning includes keeping these medications away from children and suicidal adults. Unfortunately, many depressed patients on TCAs have suicidal ideations; hence, safer agents with fewer side effects such as SSRIs may be more appropriate.

Antihistamines

Introduction

Antihistamines (such as diphenhydramine) are common over–the-counter medications for allergic reactions and cold symptoms, and they are often used as sleep aids in adults. Diphenhydramine has anticholinergic, sedative, antiemetic, antivertigo, antidyskinetic, and local anesthetic properties. It is a common agent ingested in suicide attempts, and toxicity is well documented. Toxicity is reported in acute doses greater than 5 mg/kg and potentially lethal doses greater than 10mg/kg.

Clinical Features

Patients that present with a diphenhydramine overdose usually present with anticholinergic findings: hyperthermia, dry, flushed skin, dilated pupils, and mental status changes or delirium. Patients may present with or without tachycardia. Dysrhythmias are common. In a severe overdose, lethargy, seizures, or coma may be present. Respiratory depression may also be present. Because of the easy access to antihistamines and common combination OTC meds containing antihistamines, it is important to keep in mind that that there may be other toxidromes or symptoms present as well that can confuse the presentation.

Diagnosis

Diagnosis is based on the history of ingestion. An ECG may reveal QRS widening (> 100 ms) along with tachydysrhythmias.[15] In the moderate to severely poisoned patient, baseline labs including an arterial blood gas should be determined, as well as other toxicological assays to rule out concomitant ingestions.

Treatment

Management of the patient with a diphenhydramine overdose includes rapid control of the airway if patients present with severe respiratory depression. Cardiac dysrhythmias and widening of the QRS may be controlled with administration of sodium bicarbonate (1–2 amps IVP) in order to stabilize the sodium channels in the myocardium, similar to TCA overdose treatment. Gastric lavage, followed by activated charcoal administration is indicated in recent ingestions after the patient's airway is protected with intubation. Generalized seizure activity is best controlled with liberal doses of benzodiazepines. The use of the antidote physostigmine is indicated in severe poisonings especially if seizures, cardiac dysrhythmias, or hyperthermic reactions, are refractory to conventional therapy.

Prevention

Because many antihistamines are readily available over-the-counter, increased attention to ensuring that medication bottles are not accessible to children is imperative.

Antimalarials

Introduction

Malaria is caused by infection of the *Plasmodium* parasite, transmitted by the female mosquito.

Antimalarial agents are commonly prescribed in tropic and equatorial regions for prophylaxis against, and treatment of malaria. Agents include chloroquine (developed during World War II), quinine (obtained from the bark of the cinchoma tree), and mefloquine. These drugs have arrhythmic properties and therefore, potential cardiotoxicity. Large overdoses of chloroquine can cause myocardial depression, vasodilation and hypotension. The automaticity and conductivity of the heart are also decreased. With quinine overuse or poisoning, a clinical syndrome called *Cinchonism* may result, producing vision loss, tinnitus, palpitations, and mental status changes.[16]

Clinical Features

If the patient has malaria, they may already present with chills, diaphoresis, high fever, headache, and mental status changes (cerebral malaria). Onset of action in an overdose setting with the more common antimalarials is rapid (within 2 hours). Initially the patient may have abdominal pain, nausea, and vomiting due to the irritation of the esophageal and gastric mucosa. Mildly toxic patients often complain of palpitations, drowsiness, headache, tinnitus, vision changes, and "irregular heart beats." If the overdose has been chronic from misuse of the medication, the patient can also report insomnia and nightmares.

Diagnosis

Diagnosis is based on the history of ingestion or IV administration along with the preceding clinical features. If malaria is suspected in the patient, a malaria smear can confirm this. In critically ill patients, baseline labs (if available) can be sent for CBC, electrolytes, and

BUN/creatinine. Serum drug levels are not available in the majority of hospital settings and are not clinically applicable to the patient's presentation or management. The electrocardiogram can demonstrate sinus bradycardia, widened QRS, T wave changes, ST segment depression, prolonged QT intervals, complete heart block and ventricular tachycardia and fibrillation.

Treatment

Treatment is largely supportive. Be prepared to treat cardiorespiratory arrest in cases of large overdose. Hypotension can be managed with IV fluids and pressor agents. Because the patient may become rapidly unstable, syrup of ipecac should be avoided. With recent potentially life-threatening ingestions, gastric lavage may be efficacious. Activated charcoal should be administered. Extensive clinical experience in Africa has demonstrated successful use of early mechanical ventilation, high-dose benzodiazepines, and epinephrine in severe poisoning cases of chloroquine.[17]

Prevention

Prevention includes keeping these agents out of the reach of children as well as public education regarding their potential toxicity. Other measures to prevent malaria may also be recommended including mosquito netting, insecticides, as well as antimalarials with fewer side effects such as tetracycline and atremisinin.

Newer Antimalarial Agents

The most important newer antimalarial agents to enter the market are the atremisinin-based medications. Although they are not readily available in the United States, they are now considered WHO's first-line combination therapy in areas where there is monotherapy resistence of *P. falciparum*. The active ingredient is derived from a shrub, *Artemisia annua*. Traditional Chinese herbal medicine practitioners have used this for thousands of years; however, its antimalarial properties were only discovered in 1972. Atremisinin is also known as qinghaosu. The mechanism of action is not well understood, but it seems to affect all cycles of the malaria life cycle.[18]

While its use has increased, interest in determining potential toxicity has also increased. So far, it has shown a very high safety profile. The most common adverse reaction reported is gastrointestinal upset. With respect to neurotoxicity, seizures and altered brainstem function have been reported, but only in animal models with extremely high doses.

Arsenic

Introduction

Arsenic is most widely recognized for its potentially harmful capabilities as a suicidal or homicidal agent. Tasteless, odorless, and sugar-like in appearance, arsenic can cause chronic as well as acute intoxication, and can be lethal. Pope Pius III and Napoleon Bonaparte are both theorized to have died as a result of arsenic exposure. Arsenic has also played a role as a component of certain chemical warfare agents, including adamsite and lewisite. Arsenic has been responsible for several civilian mass poisonings, primarily due to contamination events.

Arsenic exists in both organic and inorganic forms. Organic sources for arsenic are primarily the Earth's crust, seawater, and seafood, which contain arsenobetaine and arsenocholine. The inorganic arsenic compounds are more potentially harmful than are the organic forms.[20]

Clinical Features

Acute toxicity. The onset of symptoms after an acute ingestion is usually rapid, within 30–60 minutes, but it may be delayed if ingested with food. Patients may initially complain of garlicky breath or stool, a metallic taste, fever, dry mouth, and dysphagia. Gastrointestinal symptoms are common, and patients usually have nausea, vomiting, abdominal pain, and profuse watery diarrhea or rice water (cholera-like) stools. Hematemesis or hematochezia can occur. Cardiovascular collapse may occur due to capillary leakage, plasma transudation, and extravascular fluid loss.[19] Patients may develop ventricular arrhythmias, prolonged QT, ST depression, torsade de pointes, cardiomyopathy, and acute respiratory failure. Acute neurological symptoms can include changes in mental status, seizures, delirium, and encephalopathy. Bone marrow failure can occur leading to pancytopenia and hemolytic anemia. Renal failure can occur with vasodilation and may lead to acute tubular necrosis. Other symptoms may include skin flushing, toxic erythroderma, and exfoliative dermatitis. Arsine gas can cause immediate death when present in very high concentrations. In lower concentrations, exposure to arsine may lead to gastrointestinal and neurological symptoms, as well as renal failure and hemolysis.

Chronic toxicity. The onset of chronic arsenic poisoning is insidious. Patients may develop jaundice, liver dysfunction, and hepatomegaly with portal hypertension. Diabetes and pancreatitis can occur. Axonal degeneration with peripheral neuropathies can develop, as can an ascending paralysis similar to Guillain Barre Syndrome. Patients can under certain circumstances develop headaches and cranial nerve palsies. Other patients present with a dry cough, hemoptysis, and patchy lung infiltrates. Hematologic abnormalities similar to those seen in acute toxicity can also develop. Chronic arsenic toxicity has a variety of dermatologic manifestations, including hyperpigmentation, brawny desquamation, dermatitis, and hyperkeratosis. Some patients may develop Aldrich-Mee's lines, transverse white bands in the nail beds that occur approximately 30–40 days after initial exposure. Another chronic development largely seen in Taiwan is known as blackfoot disease, or gangrene of the feet.[20]

Treatment

If recent seafood ingestion has been excluded as a confounding variable to an elevated arsenic level, the management of acute arsenic poisoning involves the basic principles of decontamination, supportive care, and chelation therapy. If ingestion is recent, gastric lavage should be considered. This can be followed by orally administered activated charcoal with a mixed ingestion. However, since charcoal does not efficiently adsorb arsenic, the use of activated charcoal is of limited value. Consideration should be given to the use of whole bowel irrigation (WBI) with polyethylene glycol in cases of acute ingestion, particularly with radiographic evidence, as with iron and lead poisoning.

The definitive treatment for acute arsenic poisoning involves the administration of chelation therapy. British Anti Lewisite (BAL) or 2,3-dimercaptopropanol is the chelating agent of choice in cases of acute arsenic intoxication. Contraindications to BAL include pregnancy, G6PD deficiency, and peanut allergy since the drug is suspended in peanut oil. In the setting of renal failure, BAL may need to be supplemented with hemodialysis. Oral analogues of BAL include meso-2,3-dimercaptosuccinic acid (DMSA, succimer), and 2,3-dimercaptopropanesulphonate sodium (DMPS), which are both water-soluble agents.

Benzodiazepines/Sedative Hypnotics

Introduction

Benzodiazepines are widely prescribed all over the world. They are used for anxiolytic and sedative properties as well as for muscle relaxation. Of great concern are their addictive properties in the chronic setting. Benzodiazepines such as diazepam (Valium) and lorazepam (Ativan) are first-line medications for seizure control via their interaction with GABA receptors.

Clinical Features

Like other sedative hypnotics (e.g., barbiturates) patients who overdose on benzodiazepines typically present with respiratory depression and bradycardia along with lethargy or coma. Rarely do they suffer from cardiovascular collapse. The popular sedative hypnotic agent GHB (gamma hydroxy butyrate) is widely abused in Europe and North America. Toxicity can result in coma, respiratory depression, and seizures.[21]

Diagnosis

Diagnosis of benzodiazepine overdose is based on the history of ingestion or chronic use, along with the clinical features described previously. If available, baseline lab data can be sent including a pulse oxymetry or ABG to assess the patient's respiratory status. Specific serum benzodiazepine levels are usually unavailable and have poor clinical correlation.

Treatment

Treatment is mainly supportive, targeted at airway control. Because these patients present with central nervous system (CNS) and respiratory depression, intubation and mechanical ventilation is often required with larger overdoses. Pressor agents are rarely indicated with typical scenarios. Once the airway is controlled, if the ingestion is recent (within one hour), the patient may be lavaged or given activated charcoal via an orogastric tube. The benzodiazepine antagonist flumazenil will rapidly reverse the sedative effects of benzodiazepines. It can be given intravenously in dose of 0.5–1.0 mg (0.01–0.02 mg/kg in children). It should be reserved for acute, isolated benzodiazepine overdoses with airway complications. Mixed ingestions and reversal of patients who are chronically on benzodiazepines may result in withdrawal seizures after administration of flumazenil.[22]

Botulism

Introduction

Botulism is a neuroparalytic disease caused by certain toxigenic *Clostridia* species. Spores from three genetic variants have been reported to cause botulism: *C. botulinum*, *C. butyricum*, and *C. barati*. These spores are ubiquitous in soil and dust and are highly resistant to heat. In contrast, the toxins they liberate are heat labile and are destroyed by temperatures greater than 80°C. Although eight distinct toxins exist, toxins A, B, or E cause most disease in humans.

The toxin binds irreversibly to presynaptic receptors and prevents acetylcholine release.[23]

Nerve endings in the peripheral nervous system and at neuromuscular junctions are affected, which manifests as a symmetric descending paralysis. Recovery requires regeneration of receptors, which may take weeks to months.

Four syndromes of botulism exist. The most commonly reported type is infant botulism, which accounts for the majority of botulism cases reported to the Centers for Disease Control and Prevention (CDC). The source of spores is often not found, although many reports have implicated the use of raw honey as a sweetening agent for infant food. Food-borne botulism is the second most common type, followed by wound botulism. Therapeutic botulism is a recently reported phenomenon resulting from the use of botulinum antitoxin for cosmetic and medicinal purposes. A few cases of this form have been reported.[24]

Clinical Features

Food-borne botulism results from ingestion of preformed botulinum toxin in putrefied food. Approximately 25 cases per year are reported in the United States and are usually sporadic in nature. Canned fruits and vegetables are the most commonly identified source. As a result, this is an important potential source of toxicity in the expedition setting. The incubation period of botulism averages 12–36 hours, after which mild gastrointestinal symptoms occur. As the illness progresses, patients develop malaise, fatigue, and small muscle incoordination. This classically manifests as diplopia, dysarthria, or dysphagia. As the descending motor weakness progresses, respiratory compromise occurs, which may require emergent ventilatory support.

Diagnosis

The diagnosis of acute botulism toxicity is based primarily on a history of exposure and characteristic clinical findings. Within the first 3 days of illness, toxin may be isolated from stool or blood; after this time, identification generally requires stool culture.

Treatment

Recent advances in the management of respiratory failure have had the greatest impact on improving mortality in botulism. Trivalent (A,B,E) equine antitoxin may be useful in food-borne botulism. Studies have demonstrated improved mortality and shortened hospital stay. One 10 cc vial contains an amount of antitoxin that is 100-fold greater than that needed to neutralize the largest amount of toxin ever measured at the CDC.[23] Only toxins not yet bound to nerve endings can be neutralized; thus, antitoxin can prevent but not reverse existing paralysis. Hypersensitivity is a potential adverse side effect, and the clinician should be prepared to manage possible anaphylaxis. Antitoxin has been administered to both children and pregnant women without complications. With early recognition and appropriate supportive care, death is rare (5–10%) and usually results from complications of mechanical ventilation. Recovery occurs over weeks to months; residual weakness may persist for years.

Caffeine

Introduction

Caffeine is ubiquitous. It is a potent stimulant that crosses many cultures. Persons on expeditions may also utilize caffeine supplementation for increased energy or alertness, especially on strenuous treks or endurance activities. The most common sources of caffeine are coffee, teas, sodas, chocolate, or cocoa-containing foods (Table 30.3). In addition, caffeine is an added ingredient in many energy bars or supplements that cater to athletes. More than 60 species of plants contain caffeine. Several caffeine-containing plants people may encounter internationally are cocoa pods, kola nuts, mate leaves, guarana seeds, and yoco bark. Some authorities consider caffeine a drug of dependence. Normal intake of moderate amounts of caffeine is considered safe (i.e., 250–500 mg/day). The U.S. Food & Drug Administration allows a maximum of 72 mg of caffeine per 12-oz serving (6 mg/oz) (Tables 30.4, 30.5).

Clinical Features

Caffeine toxicity, also referred to as caffeinism, generally presents as hyperstimulation of the nervous system. Symptoms of anxiety, tremulousness, tachycardia, restlessness, excitement, insomnia, gastrointestinal upset, rambling flow of thought and speech, diuresis, muscle

Table 30.3. Caffeine content of beverages[25,26]

Beverage	Caffeine content
Coffee	
Regular drip	106–164 mg/5 oz
Regular percolated	93–134 mg/5 oz
Regular Instant	7–68 mg/5 oz
Decaffeinated	2–5 mg/5 oz
Tea	
1 minute brew	21–33 mg/5 oz
3 minute brew	35–46 mg/5 oz
5 minute brew	39–50 mg/5 oz
Canned iced tea	22–36 mg/5 oz
Cocoa and chocolate	
Cocoa beverage (mix)	2–8 mg/6 oz
Milk chocolate	6 mg/oz
Sweet chocolate	20 mg/oz
Baking chocolate	35 mg/oz
Hot cocoa	14 mg
Chocolate milk	2–7 mg/8 oz

Table 30.4. Caffeine content in soft drinks

Soft drink	Average caffeine content (mg)	Soft drink	Average caffeine content (mg)
Krank20 (bottled water)	71 mg/12 oz	Sugar-free Mr. Pibb	58
Surge	53	Mountain Dew	55
Water Joe	45 mg/12 oz	Mello-Yello	53
Kick	58	Coca-Cola Classic	47
Red Bull (8.3 oz)	80	Diet Coke	47
Jolt	72	Dr. Pepper	40
Josta	58	Sunkist Orange	40
RC Edge	70	Pepsi Cola	38
XTC Power Drink	70	Canada Dry Jamaica Cola	30
Battery Energy Drink	46	Shasta Cherry Cola	44
KMX	53	Tab	47

Table 30.5. Over-the-counter and prescription medications	
Medication	Caffeine content
Stimulants	
No-doz	100
Vivarin	200
Pain relievers	
Anacin	32
Excedrin	65
Excedrin P.M.	0
Midol (for cramps)	32
Midol (P.M.S.)	0
Vanquish	33
Dexatrim	200
Prescription	
Cafergot	100
Darvon compound-65	32.4
Fioricet / Fiorinol	40
Migralam	100

twitching, periods of inexhaustibility, and psychomotor agitation occur. The dose of caffeine causing these symptoms is variable, depending on tolerance and sensitivity of an individual, but generally is dependent on at least a 250-mg caffeine intake.

Withdrawal symptoms also occur in those habituated to caffeine. They are not life-threatening. The most common symptoms of acute caffeine withdrawal are headache, fatigue, drowsiness, decreased concentration, and irritability. Usually, onset of symptoms occurs between 12 and 24 hours after last consumption with a peak at 20 to 48 hours postconsumption. Symptoms may last from 1 day to 1 week.[25–27] This is an important consideration because many expedition health team members will experience caffeine withdrawal headaches when not drinking their normally daily intake, which can be confused with other disease entities such as high-altitude sickness.

Diagnosis

Diagnosis of caffeine toxicity is clinical along with historical information of caffeine intake. There are no tests specific to caffeine. If tachycardia is present and electrocardiography is available, consider getting an electrocardiogram to rule out an arrhythmia. Also, consider other stimulant ingestions as a cause.

Treatment

Acute caffeine toxicity symptoms are usually short lived. The half-life of caffeine is 4–6 hours. No long-term consequences of acute caffeine toxicity are usually present. Hence supportive therapy or no therapy may be needed. In caffeine withdrawal, even small amounts of caffeine can thwart symptoms. Abrupt cessation of caffeine intake in a habituated person should not be done.[26]

Carbon Monoxide

Introduction

Carbon monoxide (CO) is the leading cause of poisoning deaths in industrialized nations. It is an odorless, tasteless, invisible gas that binds to hemoglobin 240× more readily than oxygen, thus resulting in cellular hypoxia. Sources of CO poisoning include automotive exhaust, heavy cigar/cigarette smoking, industrial furnaces with poor ventilation systems, faulty camping methane and propane heaters, as well as open household fires, whether ignited accidentally or used purposefully for cooking and heating. The latter is extremely common, and an underestimated source of CO poisoning in rural, underdeveloped countries, and colder expedition environments.

Clinical Features

Patients exposed to carbon monoxide will present with a wide variety of nonspecific symptoms including flu-like symptoms, headache, dizziness, vomiting, ataxia, syncope, dyspnea, chest pain, seizures, and coma. The classic "cherry red" skin is a rare finding and is only seen in severe, fatal cases (Figure 30.4).

Diagnosis

The diagnosis is made on clinical suspicion in a patient presenting with any of the aforementioned signs and symptoms. In countries with cold seasons, CO poisoning epidemics result when furnaces are fired up for the first time. Additionally, CO poisoning typically affects an entire household making it imperative that health care providers inquire about exposure to other members of the expedition team.

If available, a carbon monoxide level can be measured using the same co-oximetry laboratory equipment that analyzes arterial blood gases. Additionally, a venous blood sample can be measured for CO. Although levels do not correlate well with the degree of toxicity and clinical signs, patients are generally symptomatic with levels over 35–40%, and severely poisoned at levels over 60%.

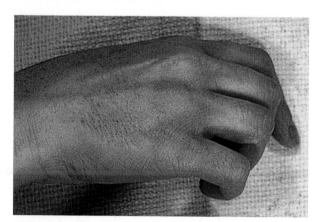

Figure 30.4. The cherry red skin findings associated with fatal carbon monoxide poisonings. From *http://www.forensicindia.com/copoisoning.*

Pregnant patients with CO poisoning are a great concern since the fetal hemoglobin has a much higher affinity for CO and therefore, lower threshold for toxicity.

Treatment

Treatment of CO poisoning includes removing the victim from the source of exposure into the open air and ventilating the enclosed area. If the patient is symptomatic, the antidote for CO is high-flow oxygen therapy. The half-life of carbon monoxide is approximately 5 hours in room air and drops to 90 minutes with 100% O_2 mask delivery. The patient should be given oxygen therapy until asymptomatic, or, if blood can be measured, when the CO level drops below 10%. The exception to this rule is if the patient is pregnant.[28] In this scenario, the mother should be given oxygen therapy for an additional 5× the length of time it took for her to be completely symptom-free or for her CO level to drop to zero. In this way, the fetal hemoglobin can be adequately cleared of CO poisoning.

If available, hyperbaric oxygen (HBO) is indicated in patients with CO levels over 40% (if pregnant, levels over 15%) or those patients with significant CNS symptoms (i.e., syncope, seizures, coma).[29,30] With severe CO exposure resulting in altered mental status or seizures (even if a CO level cannot be obtained), the patient should be transported out of the expedition environment for a higher level of care. When HBO is unavailable, high-flow oxygen or the use of a high altitude Gamow Bag represent the best treatment modalities[31] and can be immediately administered in remote wilderness and high-altitude settings.

Prevention

Prevention includes education regarding the dangers of CO poisoning and advice on proper heating and cooking systems as well as improved regulation of potential CO sources.

Caustics

Introduction

Caustic agents are compounds that cause tissue destruction on contact. They are generally categorized as either acids or alkali (basic). Common acids include sulfuric and hydrochloric acid and are found in car batteries and toilet bowl cleaners. Upon ingestion, acids generally cause a coagulation necrosis within the gastric mucosa. Alkalis such as sodium hydroxide are found in drain cleaners and lye products. Ingested alkalis generally cause liquefaction necrosis causing deep penetrating damage predominantly to esophageal tissue.

Clinical Features

Patients who ingest caustics typically present with oropharyngeal blisters, dysphagia, drooling, throat pain, stomach pain, and vomiting. Patients with dermal or ocular exposure complain of severe skin with evidence of irritation, burns, or ulceration.

Diagnosis

Diagnosis of caustic burns is based on a history of exposure along with the clinical features described previously. There are no practical laboratory tests that measure specific acid or base levels.

An arterial blood gas can be analyzed if systemic toxicity is suspected, although the damage is typically limited to a localized area thus not affecting total body pH. If ingested, an upright chest and abdominal radiograph should be obtained to rule out perforation as demonstrated by free air.

Regardless of the specific agent, if the patient is symptomatic, when available, an endoscopic examination should be performed to assess the degree of caustic damage to the GI mucosa.

Treatment

If the ingestion is acute, vomiting should not be induced. Immediate field dilution with small aliquots of milk or water may lessen the degree of tissue damage. A base should never be used in an attempt to neutralize an acid or vice versa. With dermal or ocular exposure, the skin or eyes should be irrigated with copious amounts of normal saline or tap water on site, prior to transportation to the health care facility. In the outdoor expedition setting with no hospital facility available, copious irrigation with any natural or man-made source of water is the most important intervention. Once at the medical facility, syrup of ipecac or gastric lavage is generally contraindicated with caustic ingestions as the procedure may reintroduce the esophagus to the offending agent. If endoscopic examination of the GI tract demonstrates first-degree burns, no treatment is necessary. If a second or circumferential burn results, treatment with corticosteroids and antibiotics are recommended. If third-degree burns or perforation has occurred, steroids are contraindicated as they will exacerbate the resultant mediastinitis or peritonitis.[32]

Hydrofluoric Acid

Hydrofluoric acid deserves special consideration. Although a weak acid, it behaves like a strong base causing liquefaction and deep tissue damage on contact. It is a common compound used in cleaning masonry and etching glass products. Typically, the patient's degree of pain is out of proportion to the appearance of the burn on physical exam. Treatment of dermal burns includes copious irrigation and application of calcium gluconate gel or IM injections around the circumference of the burn.[33]

Prevention

Proper storage and labeling of acids and alkali are essential to prevent accidental ingestion, particularly in children. Improved occupational safety measures will lessen severity of dermal and ocular burns in the industrial setting.

Cocaine

Introduction

Cocaine is a highly addictive sympathomimetic drug that stimulates both alpha and beta receptors. It is abused and smuggled across international borders worldwide, but it is primarily harvested in South American countries such as Colombia and Bolivia. Cocaine powder is typically "snorted" nasally, but is commonly smoked in a "rock" or "crack" form. Historically, Robert Louis Stevenson (the author of *Treasure Island*) was suspected to have been addicted to cocaine during his tuberculosis therapy. Legend has it he authored the entire novel of *Dr. Jekyll and Mr. Hyde* in a 3-day period while under the influence of cocaine.

Clinical Features

Patients under the influence of cocaine experience a euphoric high that is short lived and highly addictive. Patients typically present with tachycardia, tachypnea, diaphoresis, anxiety, and dilated pupils (mydriasis). If severely intoxicated, the patient can suffer chest pain from cardiac ischemia, seizures, profound hyperthermia, rhabdomyolysis, cerebral vascular accidents, intracranial bleeds, and death.

Diagnosis

The diagnosis of acute cocaine toxicity is based on a history of abuse or access to the drug. If the history is unobtainable, a patient presenting with the preceding sympathomimetic signs and symptoms is cocaine intoxication until proven otherwise. Urine toxicology screens can quantitatively test positive for cocaine metabolites if the drug was abused within the 72 hours of sampling. If the patient presents with chest pain, serial ECGs and cardiac enzymes should be followed, if available. If the patient suffers seizure activity, a CT scan of the head should be ordered if the health care facility has radiologic capabilities. An abdominal radiograph or KUB of an alleged cocaine smuggler may be diagnostic if the patient has ingested several latex-wrapped packets.

Treatment

Management of the patient with cocaine toxicity includes supportive care and immediate attention to abnormal vital signs. If the patient is hyperthermic, rapid cooling measures with spray/mist, circulating fans, and strategic ice packs should be applied. If evidence of myoglobinuria and rhabdomyolysis, the patient should be given fluids, alkalinized, and given mannitol. If the patient is tachycardic, anxious, hyperactive, and experiencing chest pains, benzodiazepines in liberal doses are required. If the chest pain is truly ischemic in nature, nitroglycerin can be administered. However, beta-blockers are discouraged since the patient may suffer from the resultant effects of unopposed alpha receptor stimulation. Seizure can also be managed with high doses of benzodiazepines. If the patient is a body packer, the GI tract can be flushed with high molecular weight polyethylene glycol solution (PEG) at 1–2 liters per hour along with activated charcoal administration to adsorb leaking cocaine.[61]

Prevention

Prevention of cocaine trafficking includes stricter international laws against drug smuggling and abuse. Detoxification programs are also necessary to treat those individuals highly addicted to this drug.

Cyanide

Introduction

In fires, hydrogen cyanide gas is formed as a combustion product of wool, silk, synthetic fabrics, and building materials. Additional sources include ignited polyurethane and polyester materials commonly found in tent camping material and outdoor wear. Cyanide exposure by this route is now recognized as a major cause of toxicity among fire victims previously thought to be poisoned by carbon monoxide. Historically used as a diabolical homicidal agent, poisoning has also occurred from accidental ingestion of cyanide-containing metal cleaning solutions imported from Southeast Asia. Amygdalin and other cyanogenic glycosides, found in the seeds and pits of certain plants such as apples, apricots, and peaches, are hydrolyzed in the gut to cyanide.[34]

If masticated, fruit pit ingestion has led to outbreaks of cyanide poisoning in children in Turkey and Gaza. Cassava food products also contain cyanogenic glycosides and have been frequently implicated in accidental cyanide poisoning in developing countries. Examples of these products are the fufu of Ghana, dumbot of Liberia, atiéké of Ivory Coast, and bami in other regions.

The primary mechanism of toxicity in cyanide poisoning is disruption of the cytochrome oxidase system, which results in cellular hypoxia. Cyanide binding at cytochrome aa3 in the Krebs cycle disrupts oxygen utilization in ATP production. As a result, cells shift to anaerobic metabolism, and severe lactic acidosis occurs. The critical targets of cyanide are those organs most dependent on oxidative phosphorylation, namely the brain and heart.[35]

Clinical Features

The clinical presentation depends on the route and dose of exposure. Inhalation of cyanide gas causes loss of consciousness within seconds, whereas symptoms from an oral exposure develop anywhere from 30 minutes to several hours from the time of ingestion. Since cyanide poisoning results in profound cellular hypoxia, the central nervous system and the cardiovascular system are the most rapidly affected. Initial symptoms in victims not experiencing rapid loss of consciousness include headache, anxiety, confusion, blurred vision, palpitations, nausea, and vomiting.[36]

Diagnosis

In industrialized nations, whole blood cyanide levels may be obtained, but results are not available emergently. Levels less than 0.5 mg/L are considered nontoxic. Blood gas analysis and serum chemistries may be helpful in the acute setting. Arterial blood gases will typically show a marked metabolic acidosis. Obtaining a venous blood gas analysis for comparison may demonstrate a diminished arterial–venous O_2 difference (bright red venous blood) because tissue extraction of oxygen from the blood is severely impaired. The AO_2–VO_2 may approach zero. Serum chemistries will demonstrate an elevated anion gap due to the presence of a lactic acidosis.

Treatment

The management of cyanide poisoning requires immediate supportive care as well as specific antidotal therapy. Oxygen therapy and rapid sequence intubation may be necessary. Mouth-to-mouth resuscitation is avoided in primary rescuers because of the theoretical risk of secondary cyanide exposure. Fluid resuscitation is initiated in patients with hypotension. Sodium bicarbonate should be considered in profound acidosis. Contaminated clothing should be removed, and skin and eyes should be copiously irrigated. Standard decontamination procedures should be followed in order to limit any further absorption by the patient. Gastric decontamination with activated charcoal may be considered only in a patient who arrives with minimal symptoms soon after an oral exposure.

Although some victims of cyanide poisoning have survived with supportive care alone, antidotal therapy clearly improves survival and shortens the recovery period. The only antidote currently approved for use in the United States is the Taylor Cyanide Antidote Kit (Figure 30.5), which contains amyl nitrite perles, sodium nitrite solution, and sodium thiosulfate. Nitrites produce methemoglobin, which has a higher affinity for cyanide than does cytochrome oxidase. This combination of methemoglobin and cyanide forms the relatively nontoxic cyanmethemoglobin. Cyanmethemoglobin production displaces cyanide from cytochrome aa3 and allows resumption of oxidative phosphorylation and aerobic metabolism.[35,36] A new antidote recently approved by the FDA is hydroxocobalamin (vitamin B-12a).[37] Cyanide couples with the cobalt component of hydroxocobalamin, producing cyanocobalamin, which is nontoxic.

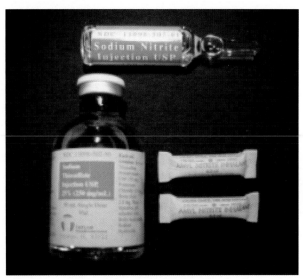

Figure 30-5. The Cyanide Antidote Kit.

DEET

Introduction

N, N-diethyl-3-methylbenzamide (DEET) is the most common insect repellent used on the market today to prevent vector-borne diseases, especially in the international setting. It is effective against mosquitoes, ticks, biting flies, chiggers, and fleas. It was developed in 1946 by the U.S. Department of Agriculture and registered for public use in 1957. It is estimated that 38% of the U.S. population and more than 200 million people worldwide use DEET each year. Many formulations and concentrations are available to the consumer. In general, the higher the concentration of DEET, the longer the effectiveness of the product. The lowest effective dose is generally believed to be 30%; however, it is lower for extended-release formulas. The repellent is applied topically, so most potential toxic exposures occur dermally. However, accidental exposures, such as ingestions of liquid formulations, are possible especially by young children.[38]

Clinical Features

Given the millions of people who have used DEET worldwide in over 40 years, DEET has an extremely high safety profile. Studies have failed to reveal significant and sustained toxicity. The most commonly reported reactions to DEET are related to either accidental inhalational or ocular exposures. DEET can be a self-limited eye irritant. Other reactions that may occur are local skin reactions, urticaria, or contact dermatitis. More serious reactions have been reported in two case reports: one case of psychosis induced by topical exposure and another with cardiovascular toxicity that presented as hypotension and bradycardia. Perhaps the most concerning adverse reaction reported is encephalopathy presenting as seizures in children. However, there have been only 12 cases documented, and further studies have failed to substantiate the direct correlation between DEET and encephalopathy. The adverse reactions are generally not thought to be related to the concentration of the substance.[38,39]

Diagnosis

Diagnosis of DEET toxicity will most likely be made by historical use of the insect repellent and the preceding clinical features. Most toxicity cases are thought to be related to improper or excessive application of the repellent. There are no available laboratory tests that will help in the immediate clinical situation.

Treatment

Most exposures require only local removal of the agent. A very small amount of topical repellent is actually absorbed by the skin (an estimated 8%), and it is rapidly excreted in the urine. In severe cases requiring hospitalization, supportive therapy is the mainstay of treatment. Seizure activity is generally self-limited and responsive to benzodiazepines.

Prevention

Even though there is no direct correlation between the concentration of DEET and its adverse effects, using the lowest effective dose of repellent for a given type of activity or setting is encouraged. Careful application of DEET on children will also help to minimize unnecessary toxicity.

Dietary Supplements

Although not recommended, these products may be misused by expedition team members with the intent of increasing strength, stamina, and endurance.

Dehydroepiandrosterone

A naturally occurring adrenal precursor to testosterone, dehydroepiandrosterone (DHEA), is converted to androstenedione and ultimately testosterone. It is commonly used to increase strength and athletic performance. Banned from prescription sale by the FDA, it is now marketed as a dietary supplement. Administration of dehydroepiandrosterone and androstenedione is associated with increased serum concentrations of testosterone precursors, testosterone and estradiol. An overall sense of well-being, which occurs with chronic administration of anabolic steroids, is commonly reported. Most reported toxicity from chronic use of these agents consists of androgenic side effects such as acne, increased body hair, and chronic muscle, tendon, and ligamentous injuries. Treatment should start with discontinuation of product use. Supportive care is the mainstay of therapy.[76]

Creatine

Athletes wishing to boost their performance ability commonly use creatine-containing preparations. Creatine, in the form of creatine phosphate, is an amino acid that is utilized by the muscle cell to maintain the availability of adenosine triphosphate (ATP) during times of extreme muscular activity. These preparations frequently include carbohydrates since the combination appears to increase skeletal muscle creatine stores more than creatine alone.

The popularity of these agents and overall lack of reported complications suggest that toxicity is limited. However, there are few systematic studies of the toxicity of creatine. Weight gain, water retention, diarrhea, and muscle cramping are among the more commonly reported side effects. There are rare reports of renal complications that were associated with creatine product use, although these most likely resulted from exertional rhabdomyolysis. Treatment is cessation of product use and supportive care.

Metals

Some cultures believe in the medicinal value of metals to prevent and treat certain diseases. As a result, various metals are commonly added to traditional healing preparations. Some of the more common metals implicated in toxicity from topical exposure, as well as products for ingestion, include lead, mercury, silver, cadmium, arsenic, and chromium. Lead-containing preparations are among the most commonly reported contaminants among herbal products from around the world. Lead oxide preparations are commonly used in the Mexican–Hispanic culture as digestive tonics (azarcon). Lead may also be found in multiple cosmetic preparations used in India (surma), the Middle East, and Africa. Arsenic and mercury contamination from hand-rolled mixtures of herbs and honey produced in China has occurred in the United States. Other metals implicated in toxicity include colloidal silver products advertised as antimicrobials and antiinflammatory agents.[77]

Digitalis

Introduction

Digitalis (Europe) or digoxin (United States) is a common cardiac glycoside that is used worldwide for the treatment of atrial fibrillation and congestive heart failure. It has positive inotropic properties. Digitalis toxicity results in the poisoning of the sodium potassium ATPase pump of the myocardial cell resulting in hyperkalemia, as manifested by brady- and tachydysrhythmias. Without aggressive therapy, digitalis poisoning carries a high mortality rate.

Clinical Features

Patients presenting with a digitalis overdose initially experience nausea and vomiting. The patient may also describe dizziness, vertigo, and altered color perception. Classically, the patient suffers hypotension and bradydysrhythmias, secondary to AV nodal blocks. The patient can also present with any type of atrial and ventricular tachydysrhythmia. With severe poisoning, the patient may also experience CNS toxicity ranging from subtle mental status changes to seizures and coma.

Diagnosis

Diagnosis of digitalis poisoning is based on a history of ingestion or access to cardiac drugs in a patient presenting with the preceding clinical features. In addition, cardiac monitoring and ECGs can demonstrate dysrhythmias consistent with digitalis poisoning. Potassium levels with acute poisoning are usually elevated. With chronic poisoning, the patient may be eukalemic or hypokalemic depending on whether they are concomitantly on a diuretic. If available, serum digoxin or digitalis levels can be obtained. Therapeutic digoxin levels range between 0.8 and 1.8ng/ml. In general, acute toxicity levels over 5.0 ng/ml denote moderate poisoning; levels over 10.0 ng/ml, severe poisoning.

Treatment

Management of acute digitalis overdose consists of gastric decontamination with activated charcoal if following a recent ingestion. Bradycardia and hypotension can be treated with atropine and pressors, although they are usually refractory. The mainstay of digitalis poisoning consists of administration of the intravenous FAB fragment antidote Digibind. Indications include any patient with digitalis or digoxin poisoning and a potentially unstable dysrhythmia, potassium levels over 5.5, and digoxin levels over 10.0 ng/ml. In the setting of hyperkalemia associated with digitalis toxicity, calcium administration is contraindicated. Dosing is 10 vials IV if the digoxin level is unknown and the patient is too unstable to await levels. Otherwise, the number of vials can be calculated using the specific formula available in the FAB package insert.[40] Unfortunately, Digibind is expensive and rarely available in developing countries.

Prevention

Prevention includes proper education of cardiac patients taking digitalis or digoxin. In addition, this dangerous medication should be kept out of the reach of children. Expedition team members should be aware of cardioglycoside-containing plants such as foxglove, oleander, and lily of the valley as potential sources of digitalis poisoning. (See Plant section.)

Hallucinogenics

Introduction

Hallucinogenic agents include many drugs such as LSD, marijuana, PCP, peyote, mescaline, anticholinergic plants, morning glory seeds, nutmeg, and mushrooms. Hallucinogenic agents alter one's perception and reality through visual and auditory changes. These drugs are commonly abused worldwide. In some parts of the world, many of these agents are legal for use in religious and heritage ceremonies.

Clinical Features

Patients under the mild influence of a hallucinogenic agent typically present with "mellowing" and loss of inhibitions. Patient with moderate toxicity may present with altered mental status, tachycardia, tachypnea, and mydriasis. Patients with severe intoxication can present with violent behavior, traumatic injuries (PCP), profound hyperthermia, and evidence of rhabdomyolysis.

Diagnosis

Diagnosis includes a history of use and access to drugs. In addition, patients who present with altered mental status and visual and auditory hallucinations should be considered under the influence of any of these agents. Urine toxicology screens do exist for drugs like marijuana, but if positive, they may not indicate recent use since this drug is fat-soluble and remains in the system for several weeks with heavy, chronic use. PCP may also test positive if abused within 72 hours of sampling. LSD levels are usually not available in the clinical setting.

Treatment

Management of the majority of patients under the influence of hallucinogenic drugs includes providing supportive care, offering reassurance, and placing them in an environment with minimal external stimulus until the effect of the drug wears off. Patients with severe intoxication and violent behavior (high dose LSD and PCP) often need physical restraints and chemical sedation with either benzodiazepines or haloperidol. In addition, they need to be rapidly cooled if hyperthermic and alkalinized with bicarbonate along with mannitol diuresis if in rhabdomyolysis.[42]

Prevention

Prevention of severe intoxication with hallucinogenic agents includes public education as to the potential dangers of these mood-altering drugs. In the international setting, many hallucinogenic agents are legal, but expedition team members should abstain from these drugs in order to avoid unexpected side effects.

Herbicides (Paraquat)

Introduction

Paraquat is an herbicide that has widespread use in Cental America, Australia, Asia, and the Orient. In these countries, it is also a common suicidal agent with an extremely high mortality rate (up the 50%) if a significant exposure is left unrecognized or untreated.

Clinical Features

The patient typically presents with oropharyngeal burns that resemble those of a caustic ingestion. Additionally, several hours after ingestion, the patient develops a pulmonary fibrotic syndrome as paraquat causes lipid peroxidation and pulmonic cell damage. As a result, the patient will exhibit tachypnea, respiratory distress, and hypoxia. Within 48–72 hours, the patient can develop oliguria, anuria, and renal failure.

Diagnosis

Diagnosis of paraquat poisoning is made by history of ingestion or exposure. Additionally, the clinical syndrome of oral caustic-appearing burns, respiratory distress, and renal failure should cause the health care provider to suspect paraquat poisoning. Blood paraquat levels can be obtained and plotted on a nomogram to predict mortality, but they are rarely available emergently in industrialized countries and never available in more remote international settings.

Treatment

Treatment includes airway protection with intubation, and decontamination with gastric lavage followed by administration of activated charcoal or Fuller's Earth. High-flow oxygen is contraindicated with paraquat poisoning because it will actually exacerbate the patient's pulmonary fibrotic state. The renal failure is best treated with emergent hemodialysis, if available. Unfortunately, the mortality rate of paraquat poisoning is very high, particularly in suicidal victims who ingest significant quantities.[43]

Hydrocarbons

Definition

Hydrocarbon-containing agents are widespread internationally and available in almost every household whether used as a heating or light source, fuel, or lubricant. As a result, these compounds are commonly ingested accidentally by children and are accessible to those adults with suicidal intent. Several classes exist including aliphatic, straight-chained, chlorinated, and aromatic hydrocarbons. The toxicity of hydrocarbons is based on the particular compound's aspiration potential. The lower the viscosity and higher the volatility, the greater the aspiration risk.[44]

Clinical Features

Patients who ingest hydrocarbons typically present with gastrointestinal distress, including vomiting and diarrhea. A characteristic gasoline-like odor will be noted on the breath. When aspirated, patients may exhibit coughing, gagging, tachypnea, respiratory distress, fever, and hypoxia. With significant overdoses, the patient may present with CNS depression.

Diagnosis

Hydrocarbon toxicity should be suspected in any pediatric patient with coughing or respiratory distress with access to these household agents. A chest radiograph may exhibit signs of aspiration pneumonitis if taken within 6–24 hours postingestion. An arterial blood gas or pulse oximetry will usually demonstrate signs of hypoxia. There are no blood levels diagnostic of hydrocarbon poisoning in the typical clinical setting.

Treatment

With the majority of hydrocarbon ingestions, administration of ipecac or gastric lavage is contraindicated due to the fact it will reintroduce the agent to the trachea thereby potentiating aspiration. However, if the patient has ingested greater than 5 cc/kg or the hydrocarbon contains a dangerous additive such as an organophosphate, heavy metal (leaded gasoline), or aromatic hydrocarbon (benzene, toluene), gastric lavage may be indicated, as long as the patient's airway is protected. If there are clinical or radiographic signs of aspiration pneumonitis, the patient should be given oxygen therapy and possible antibiotics. Corticosteroid administration is not recommended.

Prevention

Prevention of hydrocarbon poisoning includes patient education, proper storage, and regulation of the more dangerous additives accessible to the public. Additionally, safer fuel and heating sources will decrease the need for more potentially dangerous compounds.

Iodine

Introduction

Iodine and other products containing iodine are widely used by travelers for water purification in areas where drinkable water is not readily available. The portability and effectiveness of purifying contaminated water with iodine have perpetuated its use, despite advancements in water filtration systems. In addition, some filters available on the market are also iodine-based. Also in some areas of the world, higher concentrations of iodine are found in the local cuisine, such as seaweed in Asia. In general, the benefits of water filtration outweigh the risks of iodine toxicity.[45]

Clinical Features

The main features of iodine toxicity relate to thyroid disorders: thyroiditis, development of a goiter, and hypothyroid or hyperthyroid states. Symptoms may also include tachycardia, palpitations, and GI distress. These findings develop after significant and prolonged exposure to iodine-containing products. Other potential health effects are hypersensitivity reactions. Patients with predisposed thyroid disorders or autoimmune diseases may be more susceptible to iodine toxicity (i.e., unmasking a previously undiagnosed disorder). Generally, the health effects of intoxication are not long term. They resolve after the source of iodine exposure is eliminated. The maximum recommended dietary dose is 2 mg/day for no longer than 3 weeks' duration; however, these limits are controversial, as there exists variability in individual sensitivity to iodine.[46]

Diagnosis

Diagnosis of iodine toxicity may occur with the detection of a goiter or clinical signs of hypothyroid or hyperthyroid along with a history eliciting substantial iodine use. Thyroid hormone panel testing, such as TSH levels, are useful in definitively diagnosing a thyroid disorder, but often the panel is not available in less-developed countries or remote settings.

Treatment

As mentioned previously, most cases of thyroid dysfunction due to excess iodine intake or exposure resolve on their own once removed from the agent. No medical intervention is usually required. However, thyroid replacement therapy may be required if one were persistently hypothyroid.

Prevention

The benefits of water filtration through iodine-containing products outweigh the risks of iodine toxicity. Judicious use of iodine as a water filtration strategy is effective and safe. If prolonged water purification means are required, one can consider alternating filtration systems.

Inhalants/Volatile Substances

Introduction

Inhalants or volatile substances deserve special mention because they are rapidly becoming some of the more commonly abused drugs by children and adolescents in industrialized and developing countries worldwide.[11,47,48] These agents have become popular because they are easy to access and inexpensive, have addictive properties, and, in general, are not considered illegal substances. Commonly abused agents include model glue, spray paints, Scotch-gard, typewriter correction fluid, gasoline, butyl ethers, and cleaning solvents. Routes of administration include direct sniffing, huffing (rag saturated, then inhaled), and bagging (product sprayed into a plastic bag then inhaled). Chronic use of these agents can have profound effects on the cardiac, renal, and central nervous systems.

Clinical Features

Adolescents under the influence of volatiles may have mental status changes, behavior abnormalities,

tachycardia, tachypnea, and a characteristic hydrocarbon odor on the breath or skin. Profound intoxication can result in pulmonary aspiration, seizures, cardiac dysrhythmias, and death.[47,48]

Diagnosis

Diagnosis is based on the patient's history of exposure, access to these products, and presentation with the previously described clinical features. There are no standard tests to detect these individual agents. If severely intoxicated, baseline labs, chest radiograph, and electrocardiogram should be obtained, if available.

Treatment

Management of the majority of patients under the influence of an inhalant includes supportive care and reassurance, alone. If in respiratory distress, the patient's oxygen status should be assessed and the airway protected because these agents have high aspiration potential. Due to the fact many of the volatile substances can sensitize or irritate the myocardium, the patient should be monitored for cardiac dysrhythmias and treated appropriately. Liberal use of epinephrine is discouraged because it may overstimulate the already sensitized myocardium. Beta-blockers and lidocaine may be indicated if the patient suffers tachydysrhythmias.

Prevention

Prevention of volatile substance abuse includes widespread public awareness as to the high prevalence and dangers of these substances. Also, parents and community leaders need to be made aware and take an active part in curtailing access of these products to children and adolescents.

Insecticides (Organophosphates)

Introduction

Pesticide overuse, poisoning, and improper storage are worldwide concerns. Additionally, chemical warfare agents commonly contain insecticide-type nerve agents (e.g., Sarin, Tabin VX).[49] The most commonly used insecticides include organophosphates, carbamates, and pyrethrums. Some organochlorine agents such as DDT, although prohibited in the United States and other industrial nations, may still be used in many developing countries where federal and environmental regulation is lacking.

Organophosphate and carbamate insecticides exert their toxicity by linking with and inactivating acetylcholinesterase. This leads to accumulation of acetylcholine at cholinergic receptor sites and paralyzes cholinergic transmission at parasympathetic, certain sympathetic nerve endings, and neuromuscular junctions while penetrating the central nervous system.

Clinical Features

Due to cholinergic excess, initial signs and symptoms of organophosphate and carbamate toxicity is muscarinic in nature. These are best remembered by the mnemonic "DUMBELS"

D   Diarrhea, defecation, diaphoresis

U   Urination

M   Miosis

B   Bronchosecretion, bradycardia

E   Emesis

L   Lacrimation

S   Salivation

Unlike carbamates, organophosphates also affect nicotinic receptors, causing fasciculations, twitching, weakness, tachycardia, and areflexia. CNS effects of organophosphates include confusion, seizures, coma, and respiratory depression.

Diagnosis

In acute poisonings, no specific tests can identify organophosphate toxicity; therefore, the initial diagnosis is based on the history of exposure and clinical features. Organophosphates cause depression of RBC and plasma cholinesterase. The test is a measurement of cholinesterase enzyme activity; therefore, the lower the value is, the worse the scenario will be. Depression of the enzyme by 50% denotes mild to moderate toxicity, while depression by more than 90% is consistent with severe toxicity. In reality, most health care facilities worldwide do not have access to this test. Other laboratory data may include electrolyte measurement if the patient has severe diarrhea, an arterial blood gas or percutaneous oxygen saturation (pulse oximetry) to assess for hypoxia, and a chest radiograph if bronchosecretions and pulmonary edema are present.

Treatment

The patient should be removed or evacuated from the source of insecticide exposure. If dermal exposure has occurred, the patient's clothing should be removed and skin irrigated with copious amounts of water. The health care provider must use caution in this setting to wear protective gowns and gloves since insecticides can be rapidly absorbed dermally causing systemic toxicity.

Once in the health care facility, the patient's airway must be assessed. Often, with severe organophosphate poisoning, the patient is suffering from copious bronchosecretions thereby requiring intubation and frequent suctioning. Once the airway is protected, the patient should be lavaged if a significant amount of insecticide was recently ingested. If the patient is exhibiting muscarinic signs and symptoms of poisoning, atropine at dose of 2–4 mg every 15 min should be administered

IV (or via the ET tube if IV access is unobtainable). This inexpensive antidote is usually available in most countries worldwide. The endpoint of therapy is the drying of secretions. Historically, grams of atropine have been required. The antidote pralidoxime or 2-PAM is indicated if the patient is exhibiting nicotinic toxicity or if the patient requires multiple doses of atropine. The dose is 1–2 g IVPB in adults and 25–50 mg/kg in children.[49] Unfortunately, 2-PAM is unavailable in most underdeveloped countries where the incidence of insecticide exposure is highest. However, military autoinjectors containing vials of both atropine and 2-PAM are now readily available due to the increasing worldwide threat of nerve agent exposure.

Prevention

Prevention of insecticide poisoning includes public health education, proper storage, and use of safer agents with less human toxicity (e.g., pyrethroid agents). Additionally, international federal and environmental regulatory agencies are required to control the overuse of the more dangerous pesticides.

Iron

Introduction

Iron is commonly found in prenatal and multivitamins and prescribed for patients with iron deficiency anemia. It is a common overdose among pregnant patients because of prenatal accessibility and in children because of the sweet-tasting outer coating. In fact, in the United States, it has recently been responsible for nearly one-third of all pediatric pharmaceutical poisoning deaths. Iron is a direct mucosal irritant causing GI bleeding. In the overdose setting, it can also cause metabolic acidosis and hepatic failure.

Clinical Features

In the overdose setting, patients typically present with vomiting and abdominal pain along with hematemesis and hematochezia. Like acetaminophen toxicity, the initial GI phase is followed by a quiescent phase 12–24 hours after ingestion. Within 24–48 hours, the patient suffers liver damage and may present with jaundice and bleeding abnormalities. With severe poisoning the patient may develop hepatic encephalopathy.

Diagnosis

The diagnosis of iron poisoning is based on the history of ingestion and accessibility to iron-containing products. Patients typically develop hyperglycemia, a leukocytosis, metabolic acidosis with elevated anion gap, and elevated liver function tests. In addition, if available, an abdominal radiograph will demonstrate radioopaque iron tabs if the ingestion was recent. A serum iron level can also be followed. Serum iron levels over 350 mg/dl denote moderate toxicity, and levels over 500 mg/dl are consistent with severe or potentially life-threatening poisoning.

Treatment

Management of patients with iron poisoning consists of gastric lavage if the ingestion is within one hour and the patient has not already vomited. Activated charcoal does not bind iron well due to its small ionic size. If the abdominal radiograph is positive for pill fragments, therapy with whole bowel irrigation (polyethylene glycol solution) is indicated at 1–2 L/hr (25 cc/kg in children) until the radiograph is clear of radioopaque fragments. If no radiographic equipment is available, it is reasonable to start whole bowel irrigation empirically following a potentially toxic overdose.

If available, chelation therapy with the antidote deferoxamine is indicated (15 mg/kg/hr IVPB, not to exceed 6–8 g in the first 24 hours).[50] If administered too rapidly, hypotension can ensue. If the IV access cannot be established, deferoxamine can be given IM; however, the absorption is more erratic. Following chelation therapy, if body iron-binding sites are saturated (as in the overdose setting), the patient's urine will change to a "vin rose" color. However, this color change may be subtle; therefore, the decision to chelate should not be based solely on this criterion.[51]

Prevention

Prevention includes keeping these products in safety capped containers and blister packaging to deter pediatric access.

Isoniazid

Introduction

Isoniazid (INH) is widely prescribed for antituberculosis therapy. With incidence of tuberculosis (TB) increasing exponentially worldwide, many patients are on INH. Because of the sweet-tasting elixir preparation used for children, it is a very common pediatric poisoning in Asian countries. INH causes a severe metabolic acidosis and generalized seizure activity refractory to most conventional therapies. Patients who are slow acetylators (African American, American Caucasian) are more prone to toxicity. Fast acetylators include Japanese, Thais, Koreans, Chinese, and Inuit populations.

Clinical Features

Patients with INH poisoning may present with a history of ingestion or history of being treated for TB. Clinically they may have nausea, vomiting, altered mental status, and generalized seizure activity.

Diagnosis

Diagnosis of INH poisoning is based on the history of ingestion or TB therapy. Also, the combination of severe metabolic acidosis and elevated anion gap with refractory seizures is INH toxicity until proven otherwise. The patient may also have radiographic evidence of TB (cavitary lesions) on chest radiograph. Patients chronically on INH may have signs of hepatic damage on liver function testing. In industrialized countries, serum INH levels can be measured, but the turnaround is too long to have an impact on clinical management.

Treatment

Management consists of supportive care and gastric decontamination with lavage and charcoal administration if the ingestion was recent. Ipecac is contraindicated because of potential seizure activity. Severe acidosis should be corrected with sodium bicarbonate administration. Seizure activity is often refractory to benzodiazepines, barbiturates, and phenytoin. The antidote of choice for INH poisoning is pyridoxine (vitamin B-6). It interacts with the GABA receptors counteracting seizure activity. The dose is 1 g of B-6 for every gram of INH ingested. If the amount of INH ingested is unknown, a starting dose of 5–10 g is recommended.[52] If the IV pyridoxine is unavailable, B-6 tabs can be crushed up and mixed into a slurry and administered via an NG tube. Oral B-6 is readily available as an over-the-counter product in most drug and health food stores.

Prevention

Prevention of INH poisoning includes keeping these preparations away from children and suicidal adults as well as the concomitant administration of pyridoxine on a daily basis. Also, newer generation anti-TB drugs may have fewer side effects in the overdose setting.

Ketamine

Introduction

Ketamine has been used as an agent for consciousness sedation since the 1960s. It is widely available in hospital settings internationally. It is a potent dissociative anesthetic that typically does not produce the cardiorespiratory depressant effects of other anesthetics. Even though an emergence phenomenon has led to a decrease in use of ketamine in developed countries as a general anesthetic agent, its use is widespread in developing countries, battlefield settings, and veterinary medicine. This is due to a relative decrease in the necessity to monitor patients who are administered the drug, the multiple routes of administration (oral, intravenous, intramuscular, topical, inhaled), a relatively high safety profile, and low cost. Because of its hallucinatory side effects and safety profile, ketamine has also infiltrated the recreational drug market, used commonly at raves parties and other social gatherings. Common street names include vitamin K, Special K, Kit-Kat, and Ket.

Clinical Features

Ketamine overdoses usually present with prolonged sedation. Other symptoms of an overdose may be hypertension, tachycardia, increased tonic clonic movements that may resemble seizure activity, tremors, and vocalization. Severe overdoses may present with seizures and respiratory depression. Cardiac dysrhythmias are rare. Common side effects associated with ketamine administration are increased tracheobronchia, secretions, emergence phenomena, visual hallucinations, vivid dreams, and nystagmus.[53]

Diagnosis

Diagnosis of ketamine overdose is based on the history of ingestion or treatment with the anesthetic. Serum levels of the drug are not generally useful in the acute clinical setting.

Treatment

Treatment is primarily supportive. Early attention and protection of the airway is imperative, especially with the hypersecretion state associated with ketamine. Laryngospasm can occur but is rare. The increased secretions can be treated with an anticholinergic agent, such as atropine or glycopyrolate. If ketamine was recently ingested, gastric decontamination can be performed. Because ketamine is lipid-soluble and has a large volume of distribution, there is no effective means of enhanced elimination.

Lead

Introduction

Lead poisoning or "plumbism" has been long recorded historically, including theories that it may have contributed to the fall of the Roman Empire as the aqueducts delivering fresh water to the political leaders were lined with lead. Present day, it remains as a significant environmental problem in industrialized nations, and its impact is vastly underestimated in developing countries. Sources of lead poisoning include old paint chips accidentally ingested by children, aerosolized lead dust in urban settings, house and building renovations, and leaded gasoline (still readily available in many countries). Other sources include lead-lined ceramics used in cooking and drinking, retained lead bullets in war-torn regions, occupational exposures (e.g., bridge painters), and lead-containing cosmetic products (popular in the Middle East and India). Lead poisoning inhibits heme synthesis in the bone marrow resulting in hematologic and central nervous system toxicity.

Clinical Features

In the acute setting, lead poisoning presents with colicky abdominal pain and vomiting, weakness, and dizziness. Chronically it can result in microcytic, iron deficiency anemia. With severe poisoning, the patient can present with mental status changes, cognitive dysfunction, motor abnormalities, and encephalopathy.

Diagnosis

The diagnosis of lead poisoning can be made on clinical suspicion with a history of exposure along with presenting signs and symptoms. If available, blood lead levels can be analyzed. Although levels do not always correlate clinically, generally, levels over 40 µg/dl are considered consistent with mild toxicity (weakness, abdominal complaints, anemia), whereas levels over 70 µg/dl can result in CNS toxicity and encephalopathy. A hemoglobin or complete blood count should be followed. Abdominal radiographs may detect radioopaque lead paint chips in children with pica. Also, radiographic skeletal lead lines can be detected in children chronically poisoned with lead representing growth plate arrest.

Treatment

Management of lead poisoning begins with recognition and removal of the patient from the source of exposure. If a child has ingested multiple lead paint chips as demonstrated on abdominal radiograph, whole bowel irrigation with polyethylene glycol solution can be instituted. If lead poisoning has resulted from retained lead bullets or shrapnel, surgical removal is indicated. If elevated lead levels are documented and the patient is symptomatic, chelation therapy is recommended. With mild to moderate toxicity, oral chelation with succimer (DMSA) has been proven efficacious.[54] Because this is a newly approved antidote, it may not be available in most international settings. If the patient is demonstrating severe toxicity with CNS dysfunction, chelation with intravenous calcium EDTA and intramuscular BAL is recommended.

Prevention

Prevention of lead poisoning begins with public awareness as worldwide urbanization is increasing exponentially. Once recognized, the most important preventive therapy is the removal of the patient from the source of exposure coupled with environmental lead abatement. Members of an expedition team should avoid cooking and drinking from utensils potentially glazed or soldered with lead products.

Mercury

Introduction

Mercury is a concerning environmental toxin internationally. This metallic element may present with three forms of varying toxicity: elemental, inorganic, and organic.[19]

Clinical Features

Elemental mercury. The gastrointestinal absorption of elemental mercury is of negligible clinical significance and is considered essentially nontoxic. Caregivers should be reassured that the main concern of a broken mercury thermometer in the mouth is the potential injury from glass.

Inhalation of large amounts of elemental mercury vapor results in an acute, severe illness that may include respiratory distress and noncardiac pulmonary edema. Erosive dermatitis and a characteristic neurologic syndrome called erethism may ensue following an acute inhalational exposure. Patients with erethism often complain of mood swings and exhibit social withdrawal.

Inorganic mercury. The acute ingestion of mercury salts is rare, but it is seen on occasion following accidental or suicidal ingestion of pesticides containing mercuric chloride. The patient presents with vomiting, abdominal cramps, and diarrhea; volume loss and third-spacing may lead to cardiovascular collapse. Nephrotoxicity manifesting as acute tubular necrosis and glomerulonephritis have also been reported.

Organic mercury. Symptoms following acute exposures to organic mercurials are often delayed several days. Examples of environmental organic mercurials include methyl mercury, ethylmercury, and phenylmercury. Personality changes, visual field constriction, cerebellar dysfunction, and coma characterize the progressive neurologic deterioration. Organic mercury is a well-known teratogen and may be contained in freshwater fish and seafood.

Treatment

In a significant exposure to elemental mercury when elevated urinary concentrations are documented, chelation therapy may be initiated after the patient is removed from the source of exposure. Dimercaprol (BAL) was the mercury chelator of choice for years. Currently, it is reserved for severe mercury poisoning but is not recommended for organic mercury toxicity because of the potential of increasing CNS mercury concentrations secondary to postchelation redistribution. In more recent years, less toxic, water-soluble congeners of dimercaprol (DMSA and DMPS) have become available. The dosing of DMSA (succimer) is 10 mg/kg/dose, TID for 5 days; then BID for 14 days. A 2-week hiatus or drug holiday is recommended for repeat cycles of therapy. The end point of therapy is guided by clinical symptoms and if measurable, declining mercury levels in the urine.[55]

Prevention

Significant symptoms require exposure to amounts of mercury in vapor form much greater than those found after a typical household or small mercury spill. Minimizing vaporization after a spill is the most important intervention. Protocols for spill management include visualizing mercury droplets with a bright light, scraping together all visible mercury using an adsorbent product and avoiding dispersion or vaporization by such methods as sweeping or vacuuming.

Methemoglobinemia

Introduction

Methemoglobin is a form of hemoglobin in which the deoxygenated heme moiety has been oxidized from the ferrous (Fe^{2+}) to the ferric (Fe^{3+}) state. Deoxygenated hemoglobin must be maintained in the ferrous state to perform the physiologic role of oxygen transport properly. Therefore, methemoglobinemia, which is the accumulation of methemoglobin within the blood, causes decreased efficiency of oxygen delivery to tissues.

Sources of methemoglobinemia include nitrates, nitrites, inorganic contaminated well water, meat preservatives (as found in beef jerky, a favorite staple of expedition diets), dapsone, amyl nitrite, benzocaine sprays and gels, and antimalarials (chloroquine, primaquine).

Clinical Features and Diagnosis

Cyanosis unresponsive to oxygen, despite normal arterial oxygen tension, is the hallmark of methemoglobinemia.[56] Cyanosis is typically most notable in the skin, lips, and nail beds. Rapid accumulation of methemoglobin will be clinically more severe than a similar degree of methemoglobinemia that develops gradually. The arterial blood of patients with methemoglobinemia is classically described as "chocolate brown." Comparison of suspect blood to control blood on a white paper towel or filter paper highlights this distinction. In contrast to deoxygenated blood from patients with cardiopulmonary disease, methemoglobin-darkened blood does not redden upon exposure to room air. In general, the nonanemic patient tolerates the acute accumulation of less than 30% methemoglobin. As with carbon monoxide, methemoglobin levels can be measured using a standard hospital CO-oximeter.

Treatment

Antidotal therapy with intravenous methylene blue should be considered for patients with overt signs of tissue hypoxia, central nervous system depression, or cardiovascular instability.[57] If no contraindications exist (such as G6PD deficiency), methylene blue therapy is otherwise generally recommended for methemoglobin levels in excess of 30%, or when comorbid conditions limit a patient's tolerance for decreases in oxygen delivery.[56,57]

Table 30.6. Mushrooms

Major toxicity of mushrooms

Mushroom	Major toxic effect
Group I Cyclopeptide (*Amanita phalloides*)	Hepatotoxicity[a]
Group II Monomethylhydrazine (*Gyromitra*)	Hepatotoxicity, seizures[a]
Group III Muscarine (*Clitocybe* spp.)	Cholinergic excess
Group IV Antabuse (*Coprinus* spp.)	Antabuse reaction
Group V Ibotenic/Muscimol (*Amanita muscaria*)	CNS excitation or depression
Group VI Hallucinogenic (*Psilocibin* spp.)	Hallucinations
Group VII Gastrointestinal irritants (*Chlorophyllum*)	Gastrointestinal irritation
Group VIII Orellanine (*Cortinarius* spp.)	Renal failure[a]
Group VIII Allenic norleucine (*Amanita smithiana*)	Renal failure[a]
Group IX *Tricholoma equestre*	Rhabdomyolysis[a]

[a] Potentially life-threatening

Mushrooms

Mushroom collection and ingestion is extremely popular worldwide, particularly in Europe, North America, and Asia. Each mushroom group varies from region to region and should be considered poisonous until proven otherwise. (See Table 30.6.)

Mushroom Groups/Pathophysiology/ Clinical Findings

Mushroom poisonings can be categorized into nine distinct clinical syndromes. Cyclopeptide (Group I) and monomethylhydrazine (Group II) containing mushrooms tend to have delayed onset of symptoms, which can lead to fulminant hepatic failure and neurotoxicity, respectively. Groups III through VII, can cause significant toxicity, but are generally not life-threatening. Mushrooms from these groups tend to have an early onset of clinical symptoms. Group VIII, primarily certain species of *Cortinarius* and *Amanita smithiana*, tend to cause a syndrome of delayed-onset renal failure. *Amanita smithiana*, unlike the other life-threatening mushroom ingestions, can cause gastrointestinal symptoms early after ingestion. Group IX are newly described mushrooms that may induce rhabdomyolysis.[78]

Although most mushroom poisonings will fall into one of these nine groups, other non-life-threatening illnesses from mushroom ingestion are possible. Examples include gastroenteritis from bacterial contamination, absorption by the mushroom of pesticides or other environmental chemical contaminants, ingestion of raw or undercooked mushrooms, individual sensitivity, or ingestion of large quantities. It is also possible for more than one toxic species to be ingested, which can confuse the clinical picture. In these cases, identification of each involved mushroom species becomes more important.

Group I: Cyclopeptide-Containing Mushrooms

This is one of the major groups of mushrooms that can lead to life-threatening toxicity. Some examples of mushrooms in this group include *Amanita phalloides* (Figure 30.6), *Amanita verna, Amanita virosa, Conocybe filaris,* and certain species of *Galerina* and *Lepiota* spp. These mushrooms contain amatoxins, phallatoxins, and virotoxins. Only the amatoxins are considered significant in human poisoning. They are felt to cause toxicity by interfering with RNA polymerase reactions.[79]

Initial toxic effects, which consist primarily of nausea, vomiting, and abdominal pain, are usually delayed 6–24 hours postingestion. This is an important clinical distinction from the very large group of GI irritants (Group VII), which tend to produce gastrointestinal symptoms much sooner after ingestion. Other clinical effects include fluid and electrolyte imbalance, hypotension, CNS depression, fulminant hepatic failure, coagulopathy, and, rarely, seizures. After the period of initial GI distress, the patient may seem to improve clinically while having a subclinical deterioration in hepatic status. Fulminant hepatic failure is the most important consequence of cyclopeptide toxicity and is seen approximately 3 days postingestion.

Treatment generally centers on supportive care and replacement of fluid and electrolytes. Activated charcoal is generally recommended early in the course. A number of interventions have been attempted for cyclopeptide poisoning, including hemoperfusion, high-dose penicillin, high-dose cimetidine, N-acetylcysteine, silibinin, and thioctic acid. None of these therapies have been subjected to controlled studies in humans, and the data regarding their effectiveness is variable. Liver transplant

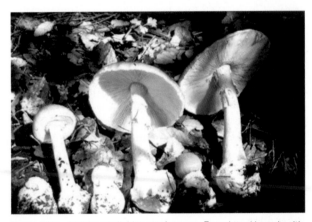

Figure 30.6. *Aminita phalloides* mushrooms. From *http://www.health. act.gov.au/gfx/pubs.*

has been used successfully in cases of cyclopeptide-induced fulminant hepatic failure. Extracorporeal liver assistance methods have been used successfully to avoid transplant in cases of *Amanita phalloides* poisoning.

Group II: Monomethylhydrazine-Containing Mushrooms

The monomethylhydrazine containing group can also lead to life-threatening neurotoxicity. Like the Group I mushrooms, there can be a delay in onset of symptoms for 6–12 hours postingestion. This group contains the "false morels." The true morel or *Morchella* species is a choice edible mushroom found throughout North America. The *Gyromitra* species of mushrooms can be confused with this delicacy, hence the term "false morel." (See Figures 30.7 and 30.8.) Representative examples of these mushrooms are: *Gyromitra ambigua, Gyromitra esculenta,* other *Gyromitra* sp., and *Helvella* sp. These mushrooms contain the toxin gyromitrin which is converted to monomethylhydrazine (MMH), and N-methyl-N-formylhydrazine (MFH). Hydrazines are also used as rocket fuels. The hydrazines act by reacting with pyridoxine and inhibiting pyridoxal phosphate-related enzyme reactions. MFH is also felt to deplete hepatic cytochrome P450.

Nausea, vomiting, diarrhea, and abdominal cramps are commonly seen 6–12 hours after the mushroom is ingested. As with Group I mushrooms, hepatic failure can occur. Important hematologic effects include hemolysis and methemoglobin production. The mechanism of toxicity of the hydrazine-containing mushrooms is similar to that of isoniazide, which is well known to cause seizures in overdose. Likewise, delirium, altered mental status, and metabolic acidosis can be seen after ingestion.

Treatment is primarily focused on supportive care, with replacement of fluid and electrolytes. Like INH toxicity, seizures can be managed with vitamin B-6

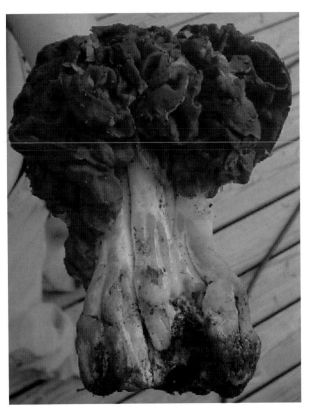

Figure 30.8. False morels. From *http://www.thegreatmorel.com/ images/falsemorel2s.jpg.*

(pyridoxine). In adults, a dose of 5 g can be administered. Benzodiazepines can be used synergistically with vitamin B-6 for seizures. For methemoglobinemia, methylene blue can be utilized for the symptomatic patient.

Group III: Muscarine-Containing Mushrooms

The muscarine-containing mushrooms cause a cholinergic toxidrome. The onset of symptoms is early after ingestion, usually between 30 minutes and 2 hours. A useful mnemonic to recall the clinical effect of muscarinic poisoning is DUMBELS:

Diarrhea, defecation

Urination

Miosis

Bronchosecretions, bradycardia

Emesis

Lacrimination

Salivation

Some muscarine-containing species include *Clitocybe dealbata,* certain other species of *Clitocybe,* and numerous species of *Inocybe.* Treatment is generally supportive, and usually no specific antidotes need to be administered. Atropine may be administered for excessive muscarinic effects. Atropine can be given with a

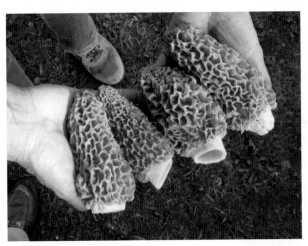

Figure 30.7. True morels. From *http://www.doorbell.net/lukes/ a061204a.jpg.*

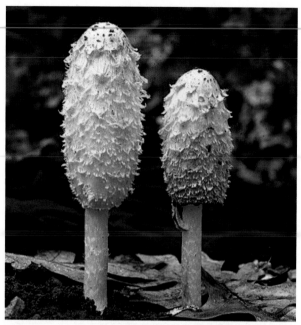

Figure 30.9. Inky caps. From *http://www.botit.botany.wisc.edu/toms_fungi/images/copr1.jpg.*

test dose of 1 mg IV. The dose can be doubled every 5–10 minutes until there is clearing of tracheobronchial secretions.

Group IV: *Coprinus* species (Antabuse)

Several species of *Coprinus* contain the toxins coprine and 1-aminocyclopropanol. The representative mushroom is *Coprinus atramentarius* is also know as the "alcohol inky cap" as it turns into a puddle of inky-like liquid as it decomposes (Figure 30.9). The toxin acts as an inhibitor of aldehyde dehydrogenase and can therefore lead to an antabuse-like reaction when consumed with alcohol.

Clinically the onset of symptoms is between 30 minutes and 2 hours postingestion. The duration of effects is typically 6–8 hours, but enzyme inhibition may last several days, during which patients should not consume alcohol. Typical symptoms include flushing, nausea,

vomiting, abdominal cramps, and diarrhea. Dizziness, headache, and rarely seizures can be seen. Hypotension and cardiovascular compromise can occur.

Treatment of toxicity is essentially supportive. Hydration with crystalloids may be necessary. If a pressor agent is needed for disulfiram-induced hypotension, norepinephrine is theoretically the pressor of choice. Dopamine beta hydroxylase may be inhibited, which may impair dopamine's efficacy.

Group V: Ibotenic Acid/Muscimol

This category of mushrooms has previously been felt to cause anticholinergic effects (80). However, more recent information shows that effects are predominantly due to GABA and glutamate effects. These mushrooms are commonly ingested for their dissociative and hallucinogenic effects.

Some representative species of this group include *Amanita gemmata, Amanita muscarina,* (Figure 30.10), and *Amanita pantherina.* The specific mechanism of toxicity is related to ibotenic acid, which is structurally similar to glutamic acid, and muscimol, which is related to GABA. Effects of glutamate agonism include central nervous system (CNS) excitation, whereas GABA agonist effects include CNS depression. Symptoms of overdose begin as early as 30 minutes and up to 3 hours after ingestion. The patient may exhibit ataxia, hallucinations, hysteria or hyperkinetic behavior, CNS depression myoclonic jerking, and seizures. Unlike other toxic mushroom ingestions, vomiting is rare.

Treatment of this mushroom group is focused on supportive care. Benzodiazepines and phenobarbital have been used successfully for hallucinations and CNS excitation symptoms.

Physostigmine, once thought to be the antidote of choice, is not indicated.

Group VI: Hallucinogenic Mushrooms

Clinicians may encounter this group of mushrooms due to recreational use by adolescents. Young adults involved

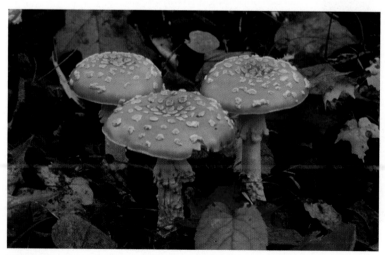

Figure 30.10. *Amanita muscaria* mushrooms. From *http://www.gdccc.org.*

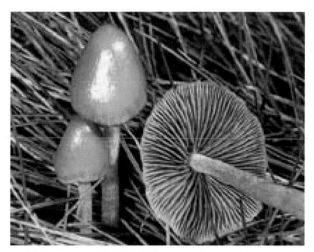

Figure 30.11. *Psilocybe semilanceata.* From *http://www.enteogenos. com/images/plantas/semi_stm.jpg.*

in expedition and exploration of the remote wilderness may ingest these for euphoric effects. Hallucinogenic mushrooms may be found either in the wild or purchased in the form of kits and cultivated at home.

Some representative examples of these mushrooms include certain species of *Conocybe, Gymnopilus, Panaeolus,* and *Psilocybe* (Figure 30.11). The toxins are indole alkaloids such as psilocybin and psilocin. These substances have LSD-like effects and possibly cause some serotonin agonism.

Clinically patients can present with delirium, visual hallucinations, psychosis, or erratic and agitated behavior. On physical examination, the patient may have mydriasis, tachycardia, flushing, vomiting, tremors, and rare seizures.

Treatment is supportive. Keeping a patient in a darkened environment with minimal stimuli will help as the effects abate. Benzodiazepines are indicated for very agitated patients. There may be a role for antipsychotic agents (such as haloperidol) for severe agitation or psychotic symptoms.

Group VII: Gastrointestinal Irritants

This comprises the largest group of toxic mushrooms. As stated earlier, most of these mushrooms will cause symptoms within 3 hours after ingestion. This property can help distinguish them from mushrooms in Groups I, II, and VIII. It is also possible that a specimen of a Group I, II, or VIII mushroom could be ingested along with a gastrointestinal irritant. This would mask the characteristic delay of onset of symptoms from the potentially deadly toxins. Therefore, it is important to obtain identifications of all of the mushrooms consumed if more than one species was potentially ingested.

There is a diverse range of species included in this group. *Chlorophyllum molybdites* and *Omphalotus olearius* are two common examples. Other Group VII mushrooms include certain species of *Agaricus,*

Boletus, Gomphus, Hebeloma, Lactarius, and *Lepiota tricholoma.*

These mushrooms contain a wide variety of irritant chemicals that will lead to nausea, vomiting, and diarrhea. Hypovolemic shock, attributed to severe hydration, has been reported after ingesting *Chlorphyllum molybdites.* The cornerstone of management is distinguishing this category from the more serious forms of mushroom ingestion. Therapy includes adequate hydration and maintaining fluid and electrolyte balance.

Groups VIII: Renal Toxins

Two groups of mushrooms that are potentially renal toxic include the *Cortinarius orellanus* group and the newly described *Amanita smithiana* (Figure 30.12).[81] The *Cortinarius* species include *Cortinarius gentiles, Cortinarius orellanus,* and *Cortinarius rainierensis.*[82] These mushrooms contain the toxins orellanine and orelline, which lead to renal toxicity. Like the Group I and II mushrooms, Group VIII species typically cause delayed symptoms and can lead to life-threatening toxicity. Renal failure is estimated to occur in 30–45% of these cases. The symptoms from these mushrooms can be delayed 24 hours to 2 weeks after ingestion. Some of these species are found in the United States, but the cases of poisoning have mainly occurred in Europe. No deaths due

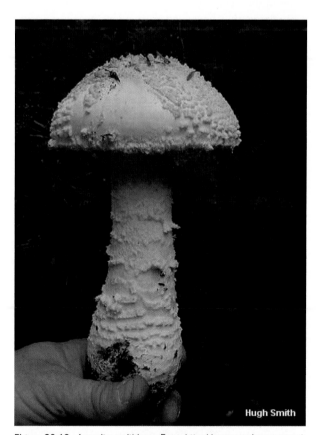

Hugh Smith

Figure 30.12. *Amanita smithiana.* From *http://www.mushroomexpert. com/images/smith/smith_amanita.*

to ingestion of these mushrooms have been reported in North America.

The nephrotoxic mushroom *Amanita smithiana* is found in the Pacific Northwest of the United States. The toxins in this mushroom include allenic norleucine (aminohexadienoic acid) and chlorocrotylglycine. These toxins specifically lead to renal toxicity. In one series, the time to onset of symptoms ranged from 20 minutes to 12 hours. Therefore, this species is an exception to the general rule of mushroom poisoning in that it can cause serious toxicity with an early onset of symptoms. The treatment for both of these mushroom groups is supportive. Hemodialysis should be instituted for patients developing worsened renal failure.

Group IX: Rhabdomyolysis-Inducing Mushrooms

A newly reported mushroom that can cause clinically significant toxicity is *Tricholoma equestre*. This mushroom has been implicated in cases of delayed rhabdomyolysis in France.[83] The mushroom is found throughout the world, and is know as "Man on Horse mushroom." The North American representative called *Tricholoma equestre* has been considered as an excellent edible, and there are no reports of toxicity in the United States. It is possible that the North American mushroom is a different species than the mushroom of the same name in Europe, or the different populations of the fungus may differ in their chemical composition. Currently, it is recommended that health care providers treat ingestions of this mushroom as potentially serious. The toxic constituent has yet to be identified. In the French series, 12 patients became ill and 3 died. Patients reported fatigue, muscle weakness, and myalgias, primarily in the lower extremities, 24–72 hours after consuming three consecutive meals containing *Tricholoma equestre*. All of these patients had clinically significant rhabdomyolysis. Treatment for this mushroom ingestion would focus on IV hydration along with management of rhabdomyolysis and its complications.

Nonsteroidal Antiinflammatory Agents

Introduction

Many nonsteroidal antiinflammatory agents (NSAIDs) are currently available, with several more awaiting approval. Both ibuprofen and naproxen are available without prescription. A second generation of NSAIDs known as the COX-2 inhibitors, or coxibs, was introduced in the late 1990s. These were touted to cause less gastrointestinal and renal toxicity with chronic use, as well as have platelet-sparing effects when compared to the traditional NSAIDs. Recently, several of these products have been associated with cardiovascular disease in certain higher risk patients. Traditional NSAIDs act by inhibiting both cyclooxygenase 1 and 2, and thus inhibiting synthesis of prostaglandins from arachidonic

acid. Toxicities associated with prostaglandin synthesis involve two major organs, the gut and kidney. Gastric irritation and bleeding occur when synthesis of the cytoprotective prostaglandins I_2 and E_2 is inhibited. These prostaglandins are also involved in maintaining fluid and electrolye balance, renin release leading to aldosterone regulation, potassium loss, blood pressure control, and renal blood flow, especially in states when renal perfusion is decreased.

Celecoxib, rofecoxib, and valdecoxib are the coxibs that are currently available in the United States. By specifically blocking cyclooxygenase-2 (COX-2) these agents have reduced gastrointestinal toxicity and bleeding that are complications of traditional NSAIDs. They are generally well tolerated by younger adult patients who are well hydrated and who have normal renal function. These agents should be avoided in older patients with preexisting renal impairment or cardiovascular disease.

Clinical Features

Patients who ingest NSAIDs typically exhibit gastrointestinal toxicity, including nausea, vomiting, and epigastric pain. Ulceration and bleeding are associated with chronic use.[58] Patients may exhibit central nervous system toxicity with large overdoses. Symptoms include drowsiness, dizziness, and lethargy. Rarely, patients may develop hypotension and tachycardia, usually as a result of hypovolemia.

The traditional NSAIDs have been associated with renal failure from both acute and chronic use, especially in high-risk individuals such as diabetics and patients with hypertension. Acute interstitial nephritis/proteinuria may develop at any time, but it typically develops after months to years of NSAID therapy and is reversible upon discontinuation of therapy. NSAID-induced papillary necrosis is the least common renal toxicity and is irreversible. An anion gap metabolic acidosis is associated with NSAID toxicity, usually from massive suicidal ingestions of more than 25 g.[59]

Diagnosis

Laboratory tests that should be performed in symptomatic patients include serum electrolytes, a complete blood count, serum blood urea nitrogen, and creatinine. Assays for determining ibuprofen levels are available in industrialized nations, although there is no clinical correlation between levels and toxicity. Arterial blood gases should be obtained if acidosis is suspected. Serum salicylate and acetaminophen levels should be obtained to rule out analgesic coingestants, particularly in patients who have deliberately overdosed.

Treatment

Patients are managed with supportive care. Gastric decontamination with activated charcoal is indicated in recent ingestions. There are no antidotes for the NSAIDs. Extracorporeal methods and multiple doses of activated charcoal are ineffective for NSAID removal because of their high degree of plasma protein binding and short half-lives. Enhanced elimination techniques have not been studied in the NSAIDs with prolonged half-lives.

Prevention

Avoid NSAIDs with a history of gastrointestinal complications, renal insufficiency or in the case of COX-2 inhibitors, cardiovascular disease. Also, in individuals who are dehydrated, fatigued, and overheated (common in expedition settings), liberal NSAID use should be discouraged.

Opioids

Introduction

Heroin is an opioid narcotic harvested from poppy seeds. Although it has traditionally been smuggled across international borders from regions surrounding Southeast Asia, Nigeria, and Afghanistan, most recently, Colombian cocaine cartels have dramatically increased trafficking of heroin throughout North America. Adulterated heroin is usually abused intravenously (mainlining), but a more pure form is snorted, much like cocaine. Because heroin is highly addictive, infiltration of narcotics into a country can have a grave impact on the economy, crime rate, and health status. In North America, a recent highly fatal fentanyl epidemic has emerged.

Clinical Features

Patients presenting following an opioid overdose will have central nervous system and respiratory depression, along with miotic or pinpoint pupils. An exception is meperidine (Demerol) toxicity, which may result in dilated pupils or mydriasis. Opioids will also produce hypothermia and bradycardia. In addition, if abused intravenously, the patient may have needle track marks on examination of the extremities.

Diagnosis

Diagnosis of an opioid overdose is based on a history of abuse or a patient presenting with the classic triad of miotic pupils, coma, and respiratory depression. If available, urine toxicology screens will quantitatively test positive for opiates if the agent has been abused within the last 72 hours. It should be noted that standard urine toxicology screens may not detect methadone or the potent opioid, fentanyl. A dramatic response to IV administration of the pure opioid antagonist naloxone also confirms the diagnosis. Diagnosis of heroin body packers may be established by noting several radioopaque densities on an abdominal radiograph.

Treatment

The mainstay of treatment is recognition and administration of the antidote naloxone.[60]

The patient should be placed in restraints prior to administration because it will precipitate acute withdrawal in chronic abusers. An initial dose of 0.4–2 mg can be given IV. If no response, up to 10 mg can be given. Because the effect of heroin lasts up to 4 hours, and the response to naloxone is no more than 1 hour, repeated doses may be necessary. If naloxone administration does not resuscitate the patient, the airway should be protected with intubation, and the other etiologies for altered mental status should be considered. Treatment of body packers, who smuggle heroin by ingesting many (up to 100) packets of latex-wrapped, pure heroin, includes whole bowel irrigation, activated charcoal administration, and if ineffective, emergent surgical removal.[61]

Prevention

Prevention includes stricter drug trafficking laws and control at international borders as well as improved narcotic detoxification programs to cure addicted individuals.

Plant-Derived Dietary Supplements

See Table 30.7.

Introduction

The term "dietary supplement" generally refers to any particular ingredient, usually a vitamin, mineral, herb, amino acid, or other product. Although new dietary supplements are introduced on a continuous basis, those ingredients classified as "supplements" are not subject to the same oversight by the FDA. Supplement manufacturers, marketers, and sellers currently receive little prospective governmental regulation. Until pharmaceutical drugs, there was no need for the manufacturer to submit evidence of either efficacy or safety prior to marketing a new dietary supplement formulation. The removal of these products from the market by the FDA now occurs only after the product is proven unsafe. The terminology used in classification of these agents can also be confusing, since the terms "alternative," "complementary," and "homeopathic" are often used interchangeably.

Dietary supplement ingredients may differ in both actual content and amount from that indicated on the product label. Contamination of these products may occur during harvesting, manufacturing, or processing. Patient beliefs about the efficacy of alternative medicines may delay presentation for medical evaluation and treatment. Recently, the United States Pharmacopeia's (USP) Dietary Supplement Verification Program has been established to help better regulate the distribution

Table 30.7. Herbal medications[72,73]

Ginkgo	Used to treat peripheral vascular disease, free radical scavenger, increase cerebral circulation
St. John's Wort	Used to treat depression and sleep disorders; better than placebo, similar to standard SSRI antidepressants (6 week onset); "herbal Prozac"
Ephedra (Chinese Ma Huang)	Marketed as an alternative to Ecstasy, weight reducer, increase stamina (initially product claimed euphoria/ hallucinogenic effect with "no health risks"); deaths reported
Feverfew	European antipyretic, for migraines, contains parthenolide (serotonin antagonist)
Ginseng	Used for centuries in China as an aphrodisiac; builds up general viability, increased physical capacity (most products don't contain enough to make a difference)
Ginger (Chinese rhizome)	For motion sickness and indigestion
Pennyroyal (Hispanic)	Used to treat colic in adults and infants; also used as an abortifacient; can cause hepatotoxity and liver failure
Echinacea (Native American)	Acts as an immunostimulant; increases phagocytosis; promotes activity of lymphocytes; used to prevent the common cold
Saw palmetto (Native American)	Used to treat Benign Prostatic Hypertrophy (BPH); increases urinary flow; reduces conversion of testosterone to dihydrotestosterone (DHT)
Kava	Root of the tropical black pepper; South Pacific psychoactive drug; sleep aid; relaxant; benzodiazepine-like effect; made into a tea
Yohimbine	Bark of the West African yohimbe tree; alpha 2 antagonist; aphrodisiac properties; priapism

and content of newer herbal and dietary supplement products.[73,77]

St. Johns Wort (*Hypericum perforatum*)

This flowering plant is commonly used as an herbal antidepressant.[72] Most preparations are standardized by their hypericum (naphthodianthrones) content, which until recently was thought to be the major active ingredient. Subsequent research suggests that hyperforin (phloroglucinols) significantly inhibits reuptake of serotonin, norepinephrine, and dopamine in nanomolar concentrations and is more likely to be responsible for the herb's antidepressant effects.

Toxicity is uncommon, but it may include mild gastrointestinal and neurologic symptoms such as fatigue and dizziness. *H. perforatum*'s ability to inhibit biogenic amine reuptake, possibly in conjunction with weak monamine oxidase inhibition, may predispose it to the development of the serotonin syndrome when used in conjunction with other serotonergic agonists. Signs and symptoms include altered mental status, autonomic instability, and hyperthermia.[74]

Echinacea

Plants from the genus *Echinacea* are commonly used for the prevention and treatment of viral upper respiratory infections. Efficacy is weakly supported by animal models in which *Echinacea* increases circulating white blood cells, cytokine production, and phagocytosis. Most clinical trials looking at outcomes of therapy are methodologically flawed and inconclusive. There is little reported toxicity associated with *Echinacea*, although rare events include hepatitis, nausea, asthma, and anaphylaxis. Management consists primarily of supportive care.

Ephedra

A common component of many over-the-counter central nervous system stimulant and weight loss formulations; ephedra alkaloids are extracted from plants of the *Ephedra* genus.[75] They are known in traditional Chinese medicine as Ma Huang. The ephedra alkaloids include ephedrine, pseudoephedrine, and methylephedrine. Ephedrine is an indirect-acting sympathomimetic alkaloid that affects α-1, β-1, and β-2 adrenergic receptors. This causes vasoconstriction, increased chronotropy, hypertension, mydriasis, headache, and nervousness.

The toxicity of ephedra is similar to other sympathomimetic agents. Among the more commonly reported adverse effects are myocardial ischemia and infarction, stroke, seizures, hyperthermia, and rhabdomyolysis. The general treatment of ephedrine-induced complications consists of supportive care. Benzodiazepines may be used to control psychomotor agitation. Management of cardiovascular or central nervous system ischemia includes the use of direct-acting vasodilating agents or alpha-adrenergic receptor-blocking agents, such as phentolamine. In most states in the United States, ephedra-containing products have been banned.

Ginseng

Ginseng preparations are used for an extremely wide variety of reasons; its reputation as a medicinal panacea accounts for the name of its genus, *Panax*. Ginseng is commonly used to improve stamina and concentration, relieve stress, and augment general well-being.[72] Historically, ginseng has also been used as an aphrodisiac, an antidepressant, and a diuretic. The most likely pharmacologically active components in ginseng are the gingenosides, which have a variety of clinical effects. They may cause changes in serum glucose concentration, serum cholesterol levels, hemoglobin production, blood pressure, and heart rate and may also induce central nervous system stimulation.

The most recognized complication of long-term use includes hypertension, nervousness, sleeplessness, and morning diarrhea known as the Ginseng Abuse Syndrome.[72,77] Other infrequently reported complications include central nervous system overstimulation, insomnia, headache, epistaxis, and vomiting. Management of side effects associated with ginseng use should begin with the cessation of use. Supportive and symptom focused therapy are recommended.

Cardioactive Glycosides

Digoxin-like compounds that share the pharmacologic profile of digoxin are present in numerous preparations marketed as aphrodisiacs (Rock Hard, Love Stone, and Black Stone), herbal remedies for congestive heart failure (Ch'an Su), and contaminants in dietary supplements. The aphrodisiacs are topical preparations used for their local anesthetic effects but are not safe to ingest. Ingestion of any cardioactive steroid in a sufficient dose can result in life-threatening digoxin-like toxicity. Digoxin levels are generally either undetectable or slightly elevated, depending on the particular assay and the cross-reactivity between the cardioactive glycosides and digoxin. As a result, poisoning may occur with a negative or only mildly elevated digoxin level. Treatment of symptomatic or potentially severe cardioactive steroid poisoning should include administration of digoxin-specific antibody fragments, regardless of the level measured.[77]

Radiation Exposure

Introduction

Radiation exposure is an environmental concern worldwide. Catastrophes such as Hiroshima, Japan, in 1945, Three Mile Island, Pennsylvania, in 1979, and Chernobyl, Ukraine, in 1986 are well-known examples. Recent international concerns have risen over potential clear terrorist attacks and "dirty bomb" detonations. Profound radiation exposure can result in bone marrow depression, sterility, leukemias, cancers, and death if not recognized and patients not rapidly evacuated. Radiation waves include alpha, beta, gamma, and neutron particles with gamma and neutron rays having the greatest clinical impact.

Clinical Features

Patients exposed to radiation may present with little physical findings unless they suffered a skin burn or traumatic injury, following an explosion. Within 6 hours, the patient experiences fatigue, nausea, and vomiting. Within 24–72 hours, depending on the proximity and amount of exposure, the patient may show signs of bone marrow depression (anemia, pancytopenia) and fever secondary to their immunocompromised state. With massive doses of radiation, death can ensue within 1–4 days.

Diagnosis

Diagnosis is based on a history of exposure whether through an environmental disaster or occupational mishap. Baseline lab tests should be sent including a complete blood cell count with platelets and differential. If available, the absolute lymphocyte count should be monitored at baseline and 48 hours postexposure to predict a patient's clinical outcome. An absolute lymphocyte count below 200 mm at 48 hours reflects a very poor prognosis for survivability (Figure 30.13).[62] The amount of radiation exposure may be measured in rads using special equipment (Geiger counter and dosimeters)

Treatment

Management includes rapid evacuation of patients from the site of exposure, removing clothing, decontaminating skin and eyes with copious irrigation, showering, cleansing with soap, and properly disposing of all contaminated clothing and body fluids. A scrub brush may be used but not to abrade the skin. The patient's vitals should be stabilized and wounds treated appropriately.

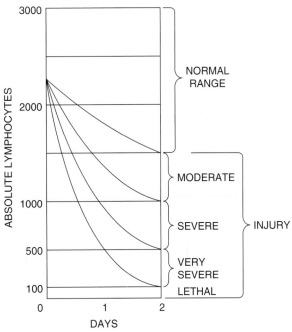

Figure 30.13. Andrews lymphocyte nomogram

Following severe exposure resulting in leukemia and pancytopenia, transfusion with blood products and bone marrow transplants have been described. Early treatment with potassium iodine (KI) may help prevent subsequent thyroid cancer.

Prevention

Prevention includes stricter industrial regulation of facilities using nuclear power as an energy source, disarmament of nuclear war weapons, and heightened security against potential nuclear attacks.

Rodenticides

Introduction

Older rodenticides contained highly toxic additives such as arsenic and strychnine; however, most current rodenticide exposures and ingestions involve anticoagulants. Initially, warfarin was found in rodenticide bait in concentrations of 25–50 mg/100 g of product. Two problems arose with warfarin: Several feedings of bait over a number of days by the target animal were required to reach a lethal dose; and a genetic selection process led to the emergence of warfarin-resistant rats. These problems were overcome by the development and introduction of the "super warfarin," or long-acting anticoagulant products, which are approximately 100 times more potent than warfarin and kill the target animal with a single feeding.

Clinical Features

With significant ingestion of anticoagulant rodenticides by humans, bleeding abnormalities may occur. These range from easy bruising, epistaxis and hemoptysis, to life-threatening GI bleeding and intracranial hemorrhage.

Treatment

For the patient with a reliable history of an accidental "taste" amount of anticoagulant rodenticide bait, referral to a health care facility, home GI decontamination, and outpatient coagulation studies are not necessary. Caregivers should be advised to observe for signs of bleeding or easy bruising for several days and report any unusual symptoms.[63]

For the patient suspected of ingesting large amounts of anticoagulant bait, GI decontamination with activated charcoal may be considered, followed by a 48-hr outpatient PT/PTT or INR monitoring. Initiate vitamin K_1 therapy as indicated. For any symptomatic patient who is actively bleeding, admit to a critical care unit for definitive care with FFP and vitamin K_1.

Prevention

Ingestions of any amount of foreign, outdated, illegal, or unapproved products for indoor use should be considered extremely serious as these products may contain arsenic, cyanide, strychnine, sodium monofluoroacetate, thallium, white phosphorus, aldicarb, or other highly toxic chemicals.

Salicylates (Aspirin)

Introduction

Like acetaminophen, aspirin is available worldwide and is used as a pain reliever, fever reducer, and prophylaxis against cardiac disease. Salicylates are contained in bismuth subsalicylate (Peptol-Bismol) and in herbal willow bark products. It is also contained in high concentrations in balms or rubefacients containing oil of wintergreen. Acetylsalicylate acid (ASA) uncouples oxidative pathways in the Krebs cycle resulting in anaerobic metabolism and acidosis. It also directly stimulates respiratory centers causing tachypnea and respiratory alkalosis. Aspirin overdose can result in significant morbidity and mortality if not recognized and managed aggressively.

Clinical Features

Patients typically present with nausea, vomiting, tinnitus, and abdominal distress. Because of the irritating effect of ASA on the gastric mucosa, the patient may also present with melanotic stools. Patients are usually tachypnic, tachycardic, and hyperthermic. In severe overdoses, the patient may suffer generalized seizure activity and noncardiogenic pulmonary edema.

Diagnosis

Diagnosis is based on the history of acute ingestion or the fact the patient is chronically taking aspirin on a daily basis. A complete blood count, serum electrolytes, glucose, BUN/Cr, and arterial blood gas should be determined. If available, serum ASA levels should be followed in a serial fashion to ensure a declining level. Levels above 100 mg/dl in an acute setting are considered severe and life-threatening. Patients chronically on ASA are severely poisoned at lower levels (over 70 mg/dl) because of the resultant long-term CNS exposure. Like acetaminophen, there does exist a salicylate nomogram, however, it has little practical use and does not correlate well clinically.

Treatment

Management of acute aspirin poisoning consists of gastric decontamination with lavage, if recent postingestion, followed by oral activated charcoal administration. Because aspirin has a propensity to form concretions in the gut, multiple doses of activated charcoal may be indicated with larger ingestions. Since ASA is a weak base, elimination can be enhanced by urinary alkalinization with sodium bicarbonate. In order to cause the proper ionic exchange at the renal tubules, the patient's potassium level needs to remain in the normal range and should be monitored closely. If the patient's ASA level is in the severe range (over 100 mg/dl), remains acidotic despite alkalinization, has generalized seizures, or is exhibiting pulmonary edema, emergent hemodialysis is indicated.[64]

Prevention

Prevention includes keeping aspirin products away from children and suicidal adults. Also, public education as to the dangers of this commonly ingested drug in an overdose setting is necessary. Herbal products containing large amounts of willow bark or oil of wintergreen should be avoided.

Sleep Aids

Introduction

Many different sleep aids are available either over-the-counter or by prescription. These are widely used by travelers because of sleep deprivation, poor sleep environments, or jet lag. Two of the more common sleep aids on the market today are zolpidem (Ambien) and melatonin.[65]

Clinical Features

Zolpidem is a short-acting non-benzodiazepine sedative hypnotic that has shown alleviation of jet lag severity when used for short periods of time. Even though it is not devoid of any abuse potential, the risk of dependence is markedly less than that of benzodiazepines. The drug is believed to act on central benzodiazepine receptors. One known side effect of zolpidem intake is sleep walking, which may be occur with normal therapeutic doses. An overdose will present similar to a benzodiazepine overdose. Most common symptoms will be drowsiness, short-lasting coma, and respiratory failure. Miosis is common. Cardiac abnormalities are rare.

Diagnosis

Diagnosis is usually made in conjunction with historical information of ingestion of zolpidem and the previously mentioned clinical features. It may be difficult to differentiate zolpidem poisoning from a benzodiazepine poisoning or other sedative hypnotic medication. If available, baseline lab data can be sent including a pulse oximetry or ABG to assess the patient's respiratory status. Specific serum levels are usually unavailable and do not often affect treatment or outcome.

Treatment

Treatment of zolpidem overdose is largely supportive, similar to that of benzodiazepine treatment. In addition, there are reports that flumazenil, the benzodiazepine antagonist, can rapidly reverse the toxic effects of zolpidem overdose. Naloxone has not been shown to have any effect.[66,67]

Clinical Features

Melatonin is another popular sleep aid that may be used with or without zolpidem (or other sedative hypnotic) often in the attempt to alleviate jet lag symptoms. It is considered a "chronobiotic" that acts on circadian phase regulation. Because it is an endogenous substance produced in the pineal gland, exogenous formulations are believed to be relatively safe. However, the typical therapeutic amounts are much greater than the physiologic amounts. Because melatonin is considered a nutritional/herbal supplement, there are very limited data on its toxicity profile. Treatment doses widely vary from 0.5 mg to greater than 50 mg; the typical dose is 5 mg for jet lag. Possible overdose patients present with drowsiness or disorientation, and rarely seizures.

Diagnosis

It is important to exclude concomitant ingestion of other potentially more dangerous medications or drugs with melatonin, such as opiates and sedative hypnotics because these could be more detrimental to the clinical outcome of the patient. Serum levels are usually unavailable and do not correlate clinically because these levels often vary, even following a fixed dose.

Treatment

Treatment is largely supportive and reports document generally uneventful outcomes. Melatonin taken in the recommended doses is considered safe.

Specific Toxic Plants

Introduction

Evaluation of a patient with a plant exposure presents several challenges to the expedition health care provider. Significant geographical variation in plant species exists. (See Table 30.8.) Historical information regarding the species of plant as well as the amount ingested is often lacking. The degree of toxicity expected may depend on the particular part of the plant structure ingested (e.g., seeds, fruit, stem, root). Plants vary in toxicity during different stages of their growth cycle. Mechanical preparation of the plant material may also affect the overall toxicity. Furthermore, there is considerable overlap in the clinical manifestations of toxicity of many plants. Although the vast majority of plants are nontoxic, a small number are mildly toxic and a few can be deadly with even a small exposure.[84]

Historical information to be elicited includes whether the plant is an indoor or outdoor variety, and a description of the plant's flower, stem, leaves, height, location, and, if possible, name. It is useful to consider certain plants according to the predominant and most serious manifestations of toxicity.

Table 30.8. Plants

Castor bean *Ricinus*: Brown/white speckled seeds; Clinical: mimics septic shock, leukocytosis, hypotension, dehydration; Treatment: Supportive care, fluids, activated charcoal

Foxglove *Digitalis*: Ornamental, tubular pink, purple, white flowers; Clinical: gastritis, cardiac conduction disturbances; Treatment: supportive, AC, Digibind

Hemlock *Water Cicuta Poison Conium*: Fernlike leaves white umbrella-like flowers; Clinical: salivation, vomiting, seizures, bradycardia, hypotension, death; Treatment: supportive, AC, atropine, intubation, control seizures.

Holly *Ilex*: Green leaves with barbs bright red berries; Clinical: gastritis; Treatment: supportive

Jimsonweed *Datura*: Funnel shaped white or purple lower many seeds in star-shaped fruit; Clinical: anticholinergic effect: dry skin, tachycardia, dilated pupils, delirium, flushed skin; Treatment: supportive, AC, physostigmine if severe toxicity

Lily of the Valley *Convallaria*: Long green leaves, white bell shaped flowers; Clinical: gastritis cardiac disturbances; Treatment: supportive, AC, Digibind

Mandrake *Mandraora*: Green leaves resemble lettuce; Clinical: anticholinergic; Treatment: supportive, AC, physostigmine

Mistletoe *Phroradendron*: Green leaves with white berries; Clinical: gastroenteritis, potential cardiotoxicity; Treatment: supportive care, AC

Nightshades *Solanum* sp.: Potato shrub-like, small flowers (yellow purple, white) with red or black berries; Clinical: nausea, vomiting, abdominal pain, hallucinations; Treatment: supportive care, AC

Oleander *Nerium*: Ornamental shrub, flowers, white, pink, yellow in clusters Clinical: gastroenteritis, conduction disturbances; Treatment: supportive, AC, Digibind

Pitted fruits: Apricots. Peach, cherry, apple (amygdalin, cyanide-like) Clinical: dyspnea, cyanosis, seizure, vomiting cardiovascular collapse; Treatment: supportive, AC, Cyanide antidote kit

Pokeweed *Phytolacca*: Shrub like clusters of dark purple berries, made into poke salad when properly cooked; Clinical: abdominal cramping, nausea, vomiting, may cause convulsions with large ingestions; Treatment: supportive, AC

Rhubarb: Large green leaves with edible reddish/pink stalks, calcium oxalate crystals; Clinical: oral burns gastritis, renal compromise; Treatment: AC, oral calcium gluconate

Rosary or jequirity pea *Abrus*; Popular with beaded jewelry, bright scarlet seed with black hilum; Clinical: severe gastritis, bloody diarrhea; Treatment: supportive, fluids, AC

Tobacco *Nicotinia*: Yellow, white tubular flowers; Clinical: salivation, GI distress, confusion, convulsions, tachycardia, hypertension; Treatment: supportive, AC

Yew *Taxus* sp. (Chinese, Japanese, and Western): Evergreen tree, seed waxy red with open end Clinical: nausea, vomiting, abdominal pain, with severe overdose may cause convulsions and cardiac conduction disturbances; Treatment: supportive, AC, monitor cardiac activity

Mucosal Irritants

When ingested, a wide variety of plant species cause mucous membrane irritation due to microscopic needle-shaped bundles of calcium oxalate (raphides) present throughout the plant structures. Plants containing calcium oxalate include philodendron, dumbcane (dieffenbachia), pothos (*Epipremnum aureum*) caladium, calla lily (*Zantedeschia*), peace lily (*Spathiphyllum* sp.), Jack-in-the-pulpit (*Arisaema atrorubens*), elephant ear (*Colocasia esculenta*), and skunk cabbage (*Symplocarpus foetidus*).

When masticated, the raphides release the calcium oxalate crystals, which penetrate mucous membranes, and in conjunction with proteolytic enzymes cause immediate burning and inflammation. Symptoms may persist for a week or more. Of the species listed, philodendron and dieffenbachia account for the highest percentage of exposures. Most exposures do not produce toxicity. Oral irritation was the most common complaint, followed by dermal pain, and vomiting. In the majority of cases, airway obstruction is not a significant concern. Treatment is symptomatic, with demulcents such as milk, popsicles, and cool drinks.

Analgesics may be required; pruritus may respond to antihistamines.

Chili pepper or jalapeno (*Capsicum annuum*) is one of the most common plant exposure reported. Exposure often occurs by handling or ingesting the pepper, with subsequent mucous membrane contact. Additionally, the toxin responsible for causing symptoms, capsaicin, is the active ingredient in many self-defense sprays. Capsaicin causes release of Substance P from sensory nerve endings and its potency is measured in Scoville units. Clinical effects consist of intense burning pain, irritation, and erythema. Profuse lacrimation may occur with ocular exposure. Vesication is typically not seen. Eating too many capsaicin-containing peppers can also produce intense rectal pain commonly known as jaloproctitis. Symptoms can persist for hours to days depending on the duration of exposure. A number of remedies have been suggested in the medical literature, including water, vinegar, isopropyl alcohol, antacids, vegetable oil, and lidocaine gel. Immersion or flushing of the exposed area with cool water may bring temporary relief. Washing the affected area with soap and warm water may help to remove some of the residual capsaicin. Exposure does not result in any long-term injury.

Gastrointestinal Irritants

Mistletoe (*Phoradendron* sp.). Reports of significant toxicity from mistletoe involve *Viscum album*, the European variety, which contains a toxin known to cause cardiotoxicity in animals. There are a few reports of death due to this variety, but the toxic effects are not well studied. The common variety found in the United States contains an alkaloid that may cause gastroenteritis. In general, the overall incidence of ingestions causing symptoms is low in this variety.

Poinsettia (*Euphorbia pulcherrima*). The poinsettia was first introduced to the United States in the 1800s. The plant's reputation for toxicity in the early half of 1900s was based on a single unconfirmed report of death in a 2-year-old child. Despite no further reports, many published sources and the general public continue to regard this plant as seriously toxic. Most exposures result in no symptoms and can be managed without a health care referral. No confirmed fatalities have been reported. Management of these exposures requires no more than supportive care; gastric decontamination is not necessary with small ingestions.[85]

Holly (*Ilex* sp.). There are 300 to 350 species of holly, but *Ilex aquifolium* or Christmas holly is most frequently implicated in plant exposures. The plant produces green berries that mature into red berries; they highlight the foliage and are used in holiday decorations. Both the leaves and berries contain irritants that may produce gastroenteritis, which is usually not severe.

Pokeweed (*Phytolacca americana*). The alkaloid phytolaccine is found in pokeweed. It primarily causes irritation of the skin, mucous membranes, and gastrointestinal tract. The plant also contains a mitogen that causes mitosis of lymphoid cells and lymphocytosis. Careful boiling can inactivate the toxin. In fact, pokeweed has been prepared as "poke salad" in the southern United States. As the green berries ripen to purple their toxic content also diminishes (Figure 30.14). Gastrointestinal symptoms after ingestion of the raw plant or unripe berries can become severe, and admission may be required for supportive care and hydration.

Systemic Toxins

Plants containing anticholinergic substances. Jimsonweed (*Datura stramonium, Datura meteloides*), deadly nightshade (*Atropa belladonna*), black henbane (*Hyoscyamus niger*), and mandrake contain anticholinergic substances. Jimsonweed, also called Jamestown weed (described by early seventeenth-century New World colonists), locoweed, and devil's trumpet, is a tall plant

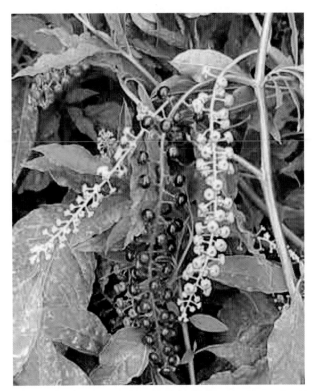

Figure 30.14. Pokeweed. From *http://www.kaweahoaks.com/html/poke_berry_clusters.jpg.*

with a musty odor and spiny seedpods. The plant grows wild throughout the United States, making it a common plant exposure. Patients may intentionally make a Jimsonweed-laced tea for euphoric reasons. Jimsonweed and other plants that cause anticholinergic poisoning contain belladona alkaloids, including atropine, hyoscyamine, and scopolamine. Patients with significant ingestion will manifest an anticholinergic toxidrome with tachycardia, fever, mydriasis, dry mucous membranes, GI hypomotility, and urinary retention. Central anticholinergic syndrome results in altered mental status, ranging from somnolence to severe agitation. Hallucinations are common. Decontamination with activated charcoal may be considered in the cooperative patient; however, its use in the symptomatic patient is of questionable value. Agitation should be initially treated with benzodiazepines. The use of the antidote physostigmine is reserved for patients with seizures, severe agitation, or arrhythmias. The dose for adolescents and adults is 1–2 mg administered slowly IV over several minutes. Because of the short half-life, it may need to be readministered after 30–40 minutes. The majority of patients may be adequately managed with supportive care alone. Symptoms of toxicity usually resolve within 24 hours.

Plants containing solanine. Plants containing solanaceous alkaloids grow throughout the United States, and include common nightshade (*Solanum* sp.), tomato (*Lycopersicon esculentum*), nettle (*Solanum* sp.), and

Jerusalem cherry (*Solanum tuberosum*). This does not include deadly nightshade (*Atropa belladonna*). Even though all parts of the plant are poisonous, many nightshades also produce berries that are most toxic when green or unripe. Ingestion of "green potatoes" may also cause illness due to solanine poisoning, as may ingestion of the sprouts that grow from potato eyes. However, toxicity is unlikely to occur unless the ingestions are significant. Small ingestions of these plants generally result in no more than self-limited gastrointestinal effects. Severe intoxications manifest with CNS and respiratory depression, as well as heart rate abnormalities, but fatalities are rare.

Plants containing cardiac glycosides. Foxglove (*Digitalis purpurea*), lily-of-the-valley (*Convallaria majalis*), common oleander (*Nerium oleander*), yellow oleander (*Thevetia peruviana*) all contain digitalis-like glycosides. (See Figures 30.15 and 30.16.) Of all varieties of oleander, yellow oleander has been responsible for the greatest

number of fatal poisonings worldwide. Yellow oleander is a common ornamental shrub found primarily in warmer climates, but it is not common in the United States. All parts of the plant contain several cardiac glycosides and can produce a syndrome similar to digoxin poisoning when ingested. The patient may manifest abdominal pain, nausea, vomiting, and diarrhea, as well as weakness, bradycardia, and AV block. Because some of the plant glycosides are structurally similar but not identical to digoxin, a serum digoxin level may not be accurate. Treatment with digoxin-immune Fab fragments is safe and effective for significant cardiac arrhythmias.[86] It has been shown to restore sinus rhythm and to correct bradycardia and hyperkalemia. The exact dose required is unknown, but recent investigations suggest that much higher doses may be needed than those used to treat digoxin overdose. Patients with symptomatic ingestions from these plants should be transferred to a hospital for cardiac monitoring.

The yew (*Taxus* species) (Figure 30.17) is a short evergreen bush commonly used in landscaping design. Seeds and leaves of the plant contain the toxins taxine A and B. Reported ingestions peak in late summer, probably due to the appearance of the fleshy red aril surrounding the seed. The aril, while attractive to children, is relatively nontoxic. While deaths have been reported in the medical literature, significant toxicity requires a large ingestion. Most exposures result in no symptoms. The most frequently encountered symptoms are gastrointestinal upset and dermal irritation. Hypotension, arrhythmias, and seizures rarely occur. Treatment is supportive.[87]

Tobacco (*Nicotiana* sp.). Most deaths from tobacco exposure reported in the literature result from occupational exposure to green tobacco or ingestion/inhalation of highly concentrated nicotine preparations such as chewing tobacco or cigars. Clinical response to nicotine intoxication follows a biphasic course. Initially there is a stimulatory effect at cholinergic receptors in the parasympathetic and sympathetic ganglia, as well as at the neuromuscular junction. Tachycardia, mydriasis, diaphoreis, tremor, and seizures may be seen. The stimulatory phase is then followed by autonomic and neuromuscular blockade from persistent stimulation, resulting in fasciculations and skeletal muscle paralysis. Death is usually due to respiratory arrest or cardiovascular collapse. Treatment is supportive, and most patients may require only a brief period of observation. Patients without spontaneous vomiting in the first hour are unlikely to have ingested a toxic amount.

Poison hemlock (*Conium maculatum*). *Conium* can be found throughout the United States. The plant can be identified by the "mousy" odor that it emits. *Conium* contains coniine, which is structurally similar to nicotine. The concentration of coniine is highly variable and depends

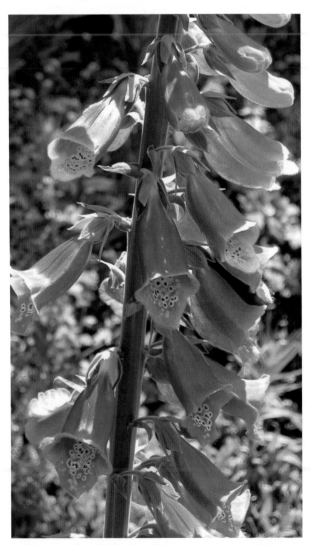

Figure 30.15. Foxglove. From *http://www.huntingtonbotanical.org*.

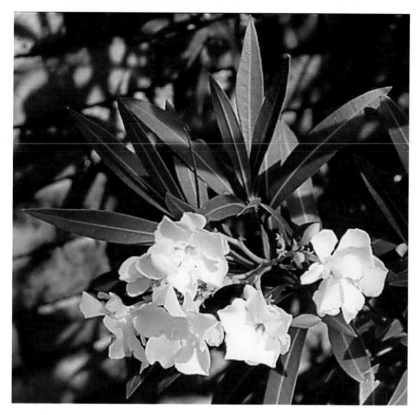

Figure 30.16. Oleander. From *http://www. museums.org.za/bio/images/enb6/enb06271x. jpg.*

on the age of the plant, geographical location, and time of year. Manifestation of toxicity is also similar to that seen with nicotine, with an initial stimulatory phase that may include tachycardia, diaphoresis, tremor, and seizures, followed by a depressant phase that may involve bradycardia, muscular paralysis, and coma. Gastrointestinal symptoms are also prominent. Death occurs rarely (the poison allegedly killed Greek philosopher Socrates) and

usually results from respiratory arrest. Ingestion of poison hemlock is a potentially significant exposure, and close observation is highly recommended. Supportive care is the mainstay of treatment.

Water hemlock (*Cicuta douglasitis*). Water hemlock (Figure 30.18) is easily confused with the wild carrot or water parsnip and may be mistaken for edible tubers

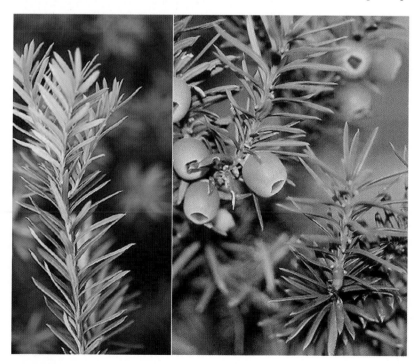

Figure 30.17. Yew (*Taxus* sp.). From *http:// oregonstate.edu/dept/ldplants/tamehic4.htm.*

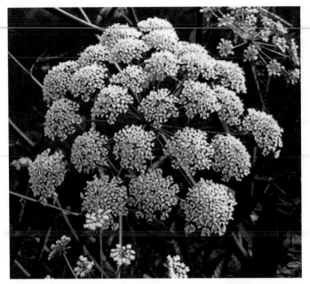

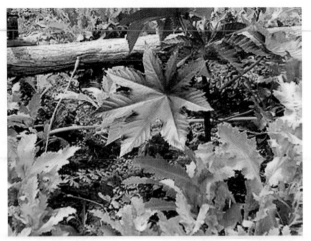

Figure 30.19. Caster beans. From *http://www.summerville-novascotia. com/.../CasterBean-c.jpg*.

Figure 30.18. Common water hemlock. From *http://www.biosurvey. ou.edu/okwild/images/comhem*.

by inexperienced outdoorsmen. The flowering portion of the plant also mimics that of Queen Anne's lace. The plant is often found growing along the borders of freshwater lakes and streams. The plant contains cicutoxin, a potent neurotoxin that is present in highest concentration in the root. These exposures have a higher documented case fatality rate than any other plant ingestions. Patients may rapidly progress to status epilepticus, respiratory distress, and death.[88] Because there is no available antidote, treatment consists of aggressive supportive care. All patients who ingest water hemlock should be transported and monitored in an intensive care setting.[89]

Monkshood (*Aconitum napellus*). There are nearly 100 species of monkshood in the United States. Fatality from ingestion of this herbaceous perennial has been reported and is due to the toxin aconite. Symptom onset is generally rapid with cardiovascular symptoms predominating. Bradycardia or AV block may develop and be responsive to atropine, suggesting a parasympathetic effect. Ectopy manifests as ventricular dysrhythmias. Antiarrhythmics or cardiac pacing may be needed as part of intensive care support. Respiratory paralysis may ensue, requiring ventilatory support. No antidote exists.

Plants containing grayanotoxins. Grayanotoxins are the principal toxins produced by azaleas, rhododendrons (*Rhododendron* sp.), and mountain laurel (*Kalmia latifolia*). They bind to and activate voltage-dependent sodium channels in cell membranes. Not all *Rhododendron* species produce grayanotoxins. Symptoms following ingestion may include salivation, emesis, and perioral paresthesias. Although poisoning in humans is rare, hypotension, cardiac conduction disturbances, and muscle weakness have also been reported. With

adequate supportive care, symptoms generally resolve within 24 hours.

Plants containing toxalbumins. This plant group includes castor bean (*Ricinus communis*) (Figure 30.19) and rosary pea or jequirity bean (*Abrus precatorius*). The toxalbumins of the castor bean (ricin) and the rosary pea (abrin) are some of the most toxic substances known. The bright scarlet and black seed of the rosary pea is used for jewelry and in the making of rattles and maracas in the tropics. Castor beans are used in the production of castor oil and are cultivated commercially throughout the United States. The seeds have a thick waxy shell and must be thoroughly chewed to liberate the toxin. Seeds swallowed whole will likely pass the GI tract without harm. Both toxins inhibit cellular synthesis, affecting cells with rapid turnover such as GI mucosal cells. Additionally, the toxins can cause red blood cell agglutination. Symptoms are commonly delayed and may include severe vomiting, diarrhea, and life-threatening hemorrhage. Historically, ricin has been used in isolated cases of espionage-related homicide. While theoretically beneficial, use of whole bowel irrigation to expedite expulsion of seeds has been studied and not found to be beneficial.[84]

Plants containing colchicines. Poisonings from these members of the Lily family – autumn crocus (*Colchicum autumnale*) and glory lily (*Gloriosa superba*) – are rare but serious and potentially fatal. All parts of the plant contain colchicine, an antimitotic agent used therapeutically in the treatment of gout.[90] Acute nausea, vomiting, and abdominal pain may result. In more severe intoxications, delayed effects may be seen, including hematologic derangements, liver injury, gastrointestinal hemorrhage, and disseminated intravascular coagulation (DIC). Worldwide, deaths have been reported, and generally occur several days after exposure. Treatment is supportive. Research involving colchicine-immune Fab therapy is encouraging, but not commercially available.

Rhubarb (*Rheum rhaponticum*). The stalk of the rhubarb is edible, but the leaves contain high concentrations of soluble oxalate. Once concentrated in the kidneys, theoretically the oxalate could precipitate with calcium and cause renal injury; however, this is unlikely with episodic exposures. Symptoms may be delayed up to 24 hours. Because of the precipitation of calcium, patients could develop hypocalcemia, although this has not been commonly reported. Manifestations of hypocalcemia include electrocardiographic changes, paresthesias, tetany, hyperreflexia, muscle twitches, muscle cramps, and seizures. As with most plants, gastrointestinal symptoms predominate. Serum calcium should be monitored and supplemented with calcium gluconate as needed. Typically, sufficient quantities of leaf material to produce toxicity are not ingested by children. Rhubarb leaf ingestion presents a more significant potential problem for farm animals such as cattle.

Ackee (*Blighia sapida*). Named after Captain Bligh and introduced to Jamaica from West Africa, well-ripened ackee fruit is a component of many Caribbean diets. The unripe fruit contains a potent toxin, hypoglycin, which inhibits metabolic pathways and can cause profound hypoglycemia. The illness, which also manifests with severe gastrointestinal distress and CNS derangements, is also known as Jamaican vomiting sickness. The onset of symptoms may be delayed several hours. The clinical impression appears similar to that of Reye's syndrome, with liver injury resulting in identical pathological changes. Fatalities from this exposure are more common in children, possibly due to lower liver glycogen stores and a greater tendency to hypoglycemia. Treatment requires hospital admission, with careful attention to blood glucose levels as well as hydration status.[91]

Psychoactive Plants
LSD congeners. Seeds from morning glory (*Ipomea violacea*), Hawaiian baby woodrose (*Argyreia nervosa*), and Hawaiian woodrose (*Merremia tuberosa*) contain amides of lysergic acid and cause effects similar to LSD. Generally several hundred morning glory seeds must be chewed in order to achieve a psychogenic effect. In addition to sensory distortion and hallucinations, gastrointestinal upset may occur. Commercial preparations of the seeds are often sprayed with a noxious chemical, which may increase the likelihood of emesis. While not life-threatening, intoxication may cause hallucinations and anxiety. Patients should receive supportive treatment in a quiet, nonthreatening environment.[92] Sedation with benzodiazepines may be required.

Peyote (*Lopophora williamsii*). Featured in many Native American ceremonies, peyote is a small, fleshy, rounded cactus that grows throughout the southwestern United States and northern Mexico. The tops of the cactus are generally sliced off and dried, forming brown "buttons" that have a high content of the hallucinogen, mescaline. A second toxin, lophophorine, is believed to have weak strychnine-like activity and may account for some of the cactus' gastrointestinal effects. Shortly after ingestion, peyote produces nausea, vomiting, headache, and abdominal pain, as well as distortion of awareness. Visual hallucinations are common. Symptoms generally subside after a few hours, although the patient may experience disturbing flashbacks and loss of reality for the next several days.

Vitamins

Introduction
A variety of vitamin products account for exposures, including multiple vitamins in pediatric and adult formulations, products with or without iron and/or fluoride, tablet and liquid preparations, and single ingredient formulations. The most important factor leading to overdose is the accessibility of multiple vitamin preparations. Given the wide use of vitamins, the lack of reported adverse effects suggests that these products as a group are fairly safe. Ingestion of vitamin products that do not contain iron or fluoride is unlikely to cause acute toxicity, but the chronic use of vitamins A and D certainly may cause morbidity.

Vitamin A
No expedition text would be complete without a reference to vitamin A toxicity, classically described in artic exploration from consumption of polar bear liver. Artic explorers in the 1800s knew of the poisonous qualities of polar bear liver and described acute illness following ingestion. The first documented death due to vitamin A poisoning was Xavier Mertz, a Swiss scientist who died in January 1913 on an Artic expedition. Just 0.3 g of the liver of the polar bear contains the upper intake level. If eaten in one meal, 30–90 g is enough to cause serious toxicity in a human. The toxic substance in polar bear liver was not identified as vitamin A until 1942.[68]

Vitamin A is a fat-soluble vitamin that when absorbed is transported by retinol-binding protein to its primary hepatic storage site. Hypervitaminosis A occurs when the retinal-binding protein carrying system and the liver become saturated from excessive intake of vitamin A. The free Vitamin A in plasma binds with lipoprotein membranes, causing increased permeability and decreased stability, and is responsible for dermatologic abnormalities and bone malformations. Excessive deposition of vitamin A in liver cells leads to hepatoxicity.[70]

Acute exposure may produce significant increases in intracranial pressure. This may result in anorexia, vomiting, irritability, lethargy, and, in infants, bulging fontanelles.[69] With chronic use of vitamin A, it is common to see alopecia, skin desquamation and erythema, fissuring at lip corners, pruritus, photophobia, headache, hepatomegaly, joint pain, bone pain, and tenderness and premature epiphyseal closure.

Exposure to the vitamin A preparation should be discontinued. There are no specific antidotes for vitamin toxicity. Gastric decontamination is generally unnecessary except with acute vitamin A exposures exceeding 300,000 IU.[70] Fluid loss caused by gastroenteritis should be treated with oral or intravenous fluids. Antiemetics or antidiarrheals are helpful for prolonged or severe vomiting and diarrhea. Increased intracranial pressure from acute and chronic hypervitaminosis A commonly improves upon discontinuation of vitamin A. Rarely, more aggressive therapy with mannitol, steroids, and hyperventilation may be necessary.

Vitamin B-6

Vitamin B-6, or pyridoxine, described previously as the antidote for INH toxicity, is a water-soluble vitamin that, when taken, manifests no toxic effects. Chronic low-dose therapy can produce a sensory neuropathy in some individuals. Muscular incoordination, decreased or absent deep tendon reflexes, and decreased sensation to touch, pain, and temperature in a "stocking-glove" distribution is common. Muscle strength is preserved. With time most patients recover fully, although permanent deficits can result.

Vitamin C

Vitamin C, or ascorbic acid, is a water-soluble vitamin that is metabolized to oxalic acid. A lack of vitamin C is classically described in exploration accounts in the form of scurvy.[71] Excessive doses may increase oxalate excretion and produce nephrolithiasis. Self-limited gastrointestinal symptoms such as nausea and vomiting are common with overdose. Acute renal failure, hemolysis, anemia, and hemoglobinuria can rarely occur.

Vitamin D

Vitamin D is a fat-soluble vitamin synthesized in the skin from a combination of cholesterol and exposure to sunlight. Toxic effects are usually due to oversupplementation; acute ingestion rarely causes toxicity. Chronic ingestion of more than 2,000 IU/day from supplements or fortified dairy products causes an increase in calcium levels by facilitating calcium absorption and mobilizing calcium from bone. A lack of vitamin D affects boney development causing osteomalacia and rickets.

Symptoms seen with chronic excessive intake of vitamin D are similar to those of hypercalcemia: gastrointestinal upset, headache, irritability, weakness, hypertension, renal tubular injury, and occasionally cardiac arrhythmias. Patients with hypercalcemia from vitamin D toxicity should be placed on a low-calcium diet. In severe cases, hydration, loop diuretics, steroids,

calcitonin, sodium EDTA, or mitramycin may be considered.

Niacin

Niacin, or vitamin B-3, is a water-soluble vitamin that commonly produces an acute vasodilatory syndrome that is prostaglandin-mediated. Acute ingestion of regular release formulations of niacin commonly causes transient cutaneous flushing, vasodilation, headache, and pruritus. Niacin-induced hepatoxicity is uncommon, but when it occurs, it is generally dose related and associated with sustained-release products.

REFERENCES

1 Erickson T. Toxicology. In: VanRooyen M, Kirsch T, Clem K, Hollimen J, eds. *Field Medicine: Emergency Medicine for International Health Workers.* 1st ed. New York: McGraw-Hill; 2002.

2 Erickson T, Aks S, Gussow L. Diagnosis and management of the overdosed patient: a rational approach to the toxic patient. *EM Practice.* August 2001: 1–25.

3 Erickson T, Ahrens W, Aks S, Baum C, Ling L. *Pediatric Toxicology: Diagnosis and Management of the Poisoned Child.* 1st ed. New York: McGraw-Hill; 2005.

4 Erickson T, Thompson T, Lu J. Approach to the patient with an unknown overdose. *Emerg Clin North Amer.* In press.

5 Smilksein MT, Bronstein AC, Linden C, et al. Acetaminophen overdose: a 48 hour IV N-AC treatment protocol. *Ann Emerg Med.* 1997;20(10):1058.

6 Rumack BH. Acetaminophen hepatotoxicity: the first 35 years. *Clin Toxicol.* 2002;40:3.

7 Hillenbrand P, Pahari AK, Soon Y, et al. Prevention of acute mountain sickness by acetazolamide in Nepali porters: a double-blind controlled trial. *Wilderness Environ Med.* 2006;17(2):87–93.

8 Dumont L, Mardirosoff C, Tramer MR. Efficacy and harm of pharmacological prevention of acute mountain sickness: quantitative systematic review. *BMJ.* 2000;321(7256):267–72.

9 Brent J, McMartin K, Phillips S, et al. Fomepizole for the treatment of ethylene glycol poisoning. *N Engl J Med.* 1999;340:832–8.

10 Brent J, McMartin K, Phillips S, et al. Fomepizole for the treatment of methanol poisoning. *N Engl J Med.* 2001;344: 424–9.

11 Johnston LD, O'Malley PM, Bachman JG. Monitoring the Future national survey results on adolescent drug use: overview of key findings, 2002. NIH Publication No. 03–5374. Bethesda, MD: National Institute on Drug Abuse, 2003.

12 Albertson TE, Derlet RW, Van Hoozen BE. Methamphetamine and the expanding complications of amphetamines. *West J Med.* 1999;170:214–9.

13 Sutherland JM. Fatal cardiovascular collapse in an infant receiving large amounts of choramphenicol. *Am J Dis Child.* 1969;97:761.

14 Glauser J. Tricyclic antidepressant poisoning. *Clev Clinic J Med.* 2000;67(10):704–19.

15 Clark RF, Vance MV. Massive diphenhydramine poisoning resulting in a wide-complex tachycardia: successful treatment with sodium bicarbonate. *Ann Emerg Med.* 1992;21:318–21.

16 Wolf LR, Otten EJ, Spadafora MP. Cinchonism: two case reports and review of acute quinine toxicity and treatment. *J Emerg Med.* 1992;10:295–301.

17 Riou B, Barriot P, Rimailho A, et al. Treatment of severe chloroquine poisoning. *N Engl J Med.* 1988;318:1–6.

18 Gordi T, Lepist EI. Artemisinin derivatives: toxic for laboratory animals, safe for humans? *Toxicol Lett.* 2004;147(2): 99–107.

19 Graeme KA, Pollack CV. Heavy metal toxicity, part I: arsenic and mercury. *J Emerg Med.* 1998;16:45–56.

20 Haroz R, Greenberg M. Arsenic poisoning. In: Erickson T, Ahrens W, Aks S, et al., eds. *Pediatric Toxicology: Diagnosis and Management of the Poisoned Child.* 1st ed. New York: McGraw-Hill; 2005: 445–9.

21 Mason PE, Kern WP. Gamma hydroxybuteris acid: GHB intoxication. *Academ Emerg Med.* 2002;9(7):730–9.

22 Gueye PN, Hoffman JR, Talboulet P, et al. Empiric use of flumazenil in coma patients: limited applicability of criteria to define low risk. *Ann Emerg Med.* 1996;266:24.

23 Carlson A. Food poisoning and botulism. In: Erickson T, Ahrens W, Aks S, et al., eds. *Pediatric Toxicology: Diagnosis and Management of the Poisoned Child.* 1st ed. New York: McGraw-Hill; 2005: 515–23.

24 Shapiro RL, Hatheway C, Swerdlow DL. Botulism in the United States: a clinical and epidemiologic review. *Ann Intern Med.* 1998;129:221–7.

25 Harris C. Caffeine. In: Erickson T, Ahrens W, Aks S, et al., eds. *Pediatric Toxicology: Diagnosis and Management of the Poisoned Child.* 1st ed. New York: McGraw-Hill; 2005: 231–5.

26 Cheesebrow D. Caffeine. In: Harris CR, ed. *Emergency Management of Selected Drugs of Abuse.* Dallas: ACEP Publishing; 2000.

27 Nawrot P, Jordan S, Eastwood J, et al. Effects of caffeine on human health. *Food Addit Contam.* 2003;20(1):1–30.

28 Caravati EM, Adams CJ, Joyce SM. Fetal toxicity associated with maternal carbon monoxide poisoning. *Teratology.* 1984;30:253–7.

29 Snook C. Carbon monoxide poisoning. In: Erickson T, Ahrens W, Aks S, et al., eds. *Pediatric Toxicology: Diagnosis and Management of the Poisoned Child.* 1st ed. New York: McGraw-Hill; 2005; 533–40.

30 Weaver LK, Hopkins RO, Chan KJ, et al. Hyperbaric oxygen for acute carbon monoxide poisoning. *New Engl J Med.* 2002;347:1057–67.

31 Scheinkestel CD, Bailey M, Myles PS, et al. Hyperbaric or normobaric oxygen for acute carbon monoxide poisoning: a randomised controlled clinical trial. *Med J Aust.* 1999;170:203–10.

32 Lamireau T, Rebouissoux L, Denis D, et al. Accidental caustic ingestion in children: is endoscopy always mandatory? *J Pediatr Gastroenterol Nutr.* 2001;33:81–4.

33 Cadello D, Hertig F. Acids and alkali. In: Erickson T, Ahrens W, Aks S, et al., eds. *Pediatric Toxicology: Diagnosis and Management of the Poisoned Child.* 1st ed. New York: McGraw-Hill; 2005: 331–40.

34 Suchard JR, Wallace KL, Gerkin RD. Acute cyanide toxicity caused by apricot kernel ingestion. *Ann Emerg Med.* 1998;32:742–4.

35 Mycyk M, Kranz A. Cyanide poisoning. In: Erickson T, Ahrens W, Aks S, et al., eds. *Pediatric Toxicology: Diagnosis and Management of the Poisoned Child.* 1st ed. New York: McGraw-Hill; 2005: 486–91.

36 Ruangkanchanasetr S, Wananukul V, Suwanjutha S. Cyanide poisoning, 2 case report and treatment review. *J Med Assoc Thai.* 1992;82:S162–7.

37 Mannaioni G, Vannacci A, Marzocca C, et al. Acute cyanide intoxication treated with a combination of hydroxycobalamin, sodium nitrite, and sodium thiosulfate. *J Toxicol Clin Toxicol.* 40: 181–183, 2002.

38 Sudakin DL, Trevathan WR. DEET: a review and update of safety and risk in the general population. *J Toxicol Clin Toxicol.* 2003;41(6):831–9.

39 Goodyer L, Behrens RH. Short report: the safety and toxicity of insect repellents. *Am J Trop Med Hyg.* 1998;59(2):323–4.

40 Jeger A, Bilbault P, Meziana F, et al. Digoxin antibodies, when, how much. *J Toxicol Clin Toxicol.* 2003;414; 424–5.

41 Miller PL, Gay GR, Ferris KC, et al. Treatment of acute, adverse psychedelic reactions: "I've tripped and I can't get down." *J Psycho Drug.* 1992;24:277–9.

42 Gussow L. LSD and other hallucinogens. In: Erickson T, Ahrens W, Aks S, et al., eds. *Pediatric Toxicology: Diagnosis and Management of the Poisoned Child.* 1st ed. New York: McGraw-Hill; 2005: 398–402.

43 Erickson T, Brown K, Wigder H. A case of paraquat fatality in a suburban ED. *J Emerg Med.* 1997;15(5).

44 Machado B, Cross K, Snodgrass WR. Accidental hydrocarbon ingestion cases telephoned to a regional poison center. *Ann Emerg Med.* 1988;17:804.

45 Goodyer L, Behrens RH. Safety of iodine based water sterilization for travelers. *J Travel Med.* 2000;7(1):38.

46 Pearce EN, Gerber AR, Gootnick DB, et al. Effects of chronic iodine excess in a cohort of long-term American workers in West Africa. *J Clin Endocrinol Metab.* 2002;87(12): 5499–502.

47 Beauvais F, Wayman JC, Jumper-Thurman P, et al. Inhalant abuse among American Indian, Mexican American, and non-Latino white adolescents. *Am J Drug Alcohol Abuse.* 2002;28:171.

48 Kurtzman TL, Otsuka KN, Wahl RA. Inhalant abuse by adolescents. *J Adolesc Health.* 2001;28:170.

49 Holstege CP, Kirk M, et al. Chemical warfare: nerve agent poisoning. *Crit Care Clin.* 1997;13(4):923–42.

50 Tennenbein M. Benefits of parenteral deferoxamine for acute iron poisoning. *J Toxicol Clin Toxicol.* 1996;34:485–9.

51 Aks S, Tennenbein M. Iron poisoning. In: Erickson T, Ahrens W, Aks S, et al., eds. *Pediatric Toxicology: Diagnosis and Management of the Poisoned Child.* 1st ed. New York: McGraw-Hill; 2005: 455–60.

52 Henry GC, Haynes S. Isoniazid and other antituberculosis drugs: isoniazid. In: Ford MD, Delaney KA, Ling LJ, Erickson T, eds. *Clinical Toxicology.* Philadelphia: W. B. Saunders; 2001: 440–4.

53 Hayase T, Yamamoto Y, Yamamoto K. Behavioral effects of ketamine and toxic interactions with psychostimulants. *BMC Neurosci.* 2006;16(7):25.

54 Rogan J, Dietrich KN, Ware JH, et al. The effect of chelation therapy with succimer on neuropsychological development in children exposed to lead. *N Engl J Med.* 2001;344:1421–6.

55 McKay C, Perez A, Goldstein R. Mercury poisoning. In: Erickson T, Ahrens W, Aks S, et al., eds. *Pediatric toxicology: Diagnosis and management of the poisoned child.* 1st ed. New York: McGraw-Hill; 2005, 468–75.

56 Wright RO, Lewander WJ, Woolf AD. Methemoglobinemia: etiology, pharmacology, and clinical management. *Ann Emerg Med.* 1999;34:646–56.

57 Osterhoudt KC. Methemoglobinema. In: Erickson T, Ahrens W, Aks S, et al., eds. *Pediatric Toxicology: Diagnosis and Management of the Poisoned Child.* 1st ed. New York: McGraw-Hill; 2005, 492–500.

58 Hall AH, Smolinske SC, Conrad FL, et al. Ibuprofen overdose: 126 cases. *Ann Emerg Med.* 1986;15:1308.

59 Zell Kanter M. Nonsteroidal anti-inflammatory drugs. In: Erickson T, Ahrens W, Aks S, et al., eds. *Pediatric Toxicology: Diagnosis and Management of the Poisoned Child.* 1st ed. New York: McGraw-Hill; 2005: 228–30.

60 Sporer KA. Acute heroin overdose. *Ann Intern Med.* 1999;130:584–90.

61 Traub SJ, Hoffman RS, Nelson LS. Body packing – the internal concealment of illicit drugs. *N Engl J Med.* 2003;349(26): 2519–26.

62 Andrews GA, Auxier JA, Lushbaugh CC. The importance of dosimetry to the medical management of persons exposed to high levels of radiation. In: *Personal Dosimetry for Radiation Accidents.* Vienna: International Atomic Energy Agency; 1965.

63 Sheperd G, Klein-Schwartz W, Anderson B. Acute, unintentional pediatric brodifacoum ingestions. *Ped Emerg Care.* 2002;18(3):174–8.

64 Yip L, Dart RC, Gabow PA. Concepts and controversies in salicylate toxicity. *Emerg Med Clin North Am.* 1994;12: 351–63.

65 Suhner A, Schlagenhauf P, Hofer I, et al. Effectiveness and tolerability of melatonin and zolpidem for the alleviation of jet lag. *Aviat Space Environ Med.* 2001;72(7):638–46.

66 Gock SB, Wong SH, Nuwayhid N, Venuti SE, Kelley PD, Teggatz JR, Jentzen JM. Acute zolpidem overdose – report of two cases. *J Anal Toxicol.* 1999;23(6):559–62.

67 Garnier R, Guerault E, Muzard D, et al. Acute zolpidem poisoning – analysis of 344 cases. *J Toxicol Clin Toxicol.* 1994;32(4):391–404.

68 Russel FE. Vitamin A content of polar bear liver. *Toxicon.* 1966;5:61–2.

69 Fishman RA. Polar bear liver, vitamin A, aquaporins, and pseudotumor cerebri. *Ann Neurol.* 2002;52(5):531–3.

70 Hathcock JN, Hattan DG, Jenkins MY, et al. Evaluation of vitamin A toxicity. *Am J Clin Nutr.* 1990;52:183–202.

71 Olmedo JM, Yiannias JA, Windgassen EB, Gornet MK. Scurvy: a disease almost forgotten. *Int J Dermatol.* 2006 Aug;45(8):909–13.

72 Ernst E. The risk-benefit profile of commonly used herbal therapies: ginkgo, St. John's wort, ginseng, echinacea, saw palmetto, and kava. *Ann Intern Med.* 2002;136:42–53.

73 O'Hara MA, Kiefer D, Farrell K, et al., A review of 12 commonly used medicinal herbs. *Arch Fam Med.* 1998;7: 523–36.

74 Greeson JM, Sanford B, Monti D. St. John's wort (*Hypericum perforatum*): a review of the current pharmacological, toxicological, and clinical literature. *Psychopharmacology.* 2001;153: 402–14.

75 Haller CA, Benowitz NL. Adverse cardiovascular and central nervous system events associated with dietary supplements containing ephedra alkaloids. *N Engl J Med.* 2000;343: 1833–8.

76 Leder BZ, Longcope C, Catlin DH, et al. Oral androstenedione administration and serum testosterone concentrations in young men. *JAMA.* 2000;283:779–82.

77 Schier J, Nelson L. Herbal products. In: Erickson T, Ahrens W, Aks S, et al., eds. *Pediatric Toxicology: Diagnosis and Management of the Poisoned Child.* New York: McGraw-Hill; 2005: 508–14.

78 Fischbein C, Aks S, Mueller R. Mushroom poisoning. In Erickson, T, Ahrens W, Aks, S, et al., eds. *Pediatric Toxicology: Diagnosis and Management of the Poisoned Child.* 1st ed. New York: McGraw-Hill; 2005: 533–40.

79 Satora L, Pach D, Butryn B. Mushrooms, amatoxins and the liver. *J Hepatol.* 2005;42(2):166–9.

80 Satora L, Pach D, Ciszowski K, Winnik L. Fly agaric (*Amanita muscaria*) poisoning, case report and review. *Toxicon.* 2005;45(7):941–3.

81 Warden CR, Benjamin DR. Acute renal failure associated with suspected *Amanita smithiana* mushroom ingestions: a case series. *Acad Emerg Med.* 1998;8:808–12.

82 Leathem AM, Purssell RA, Chan VR, et al. Renal failure caused by mushroom poisoning. *J Toxicol Clin Toxicol.* 1997;35: 67–75.

83 Bedry R, Baudrimont I, Deffieux G, et al. Wild-mushroom intoxication as a cause of Rhabdomyolysis. *N Engl J Med.* 2001;345:798–802.

84 Carlson A, Krenzelak E. Poisonous plants. In: Erickson T, Ahrens W, Aks S, et al., eds. *Pediatric toxicology: Diagnosis and management of the poisoned child.* 1st ed. New York: McGraw-Hill; 2005, 541–7.

85 Krenzelok EP, Jacobsen TD, Aronis J. Poinsettia exposures have good outcomes . . . just as we thought. *Am J Emerg Med.* 1996;14:671–4.

86 Eddleston M, Rajapakse S, Rajakanthan, et al. Anti-digoxin Fab fragments in cardiotoxicity induced by ingestion of yellow oleander: a randomized controlled trial. *Lancet.* 2000;355:967–72.

87 Krenzelok EP, Jacobsen TD, Aronis J. Is the yew really poisonous to you? *Clin Toxicol.* 1998;36:219–23.

88 Krenzelok EP, Jacobsen TD, Aronis J. Hemlock ingestions: the most deadly plant exposures. Abstract. *J Toxicol Clin Toxicol.* 1996;601–2.

89 Biberci E, Altunas Y, Cobanoglu A, et al. Acute respiratory arrest following hemlock (*Conium maculatum*) intoxication. *J Toxicol Clin Toxicol.* 2002;40:517–18.

90 Danel VC, Wiart JF, Hardy GA, et al. Self-poisoning with *Colchicum autumnale* L. flowers. *J Toxicol Clin Toxicol.* 2001;39:409–11.

91 Meda HA, Diallo B, Buchet J, et al. Epidemic of fatal encephalopathy in preschool children in Burkina Faso and consumption of unripe ackee (*Blighia sapida*) fruit. *Lancet.* 1999;353:536–40.

92 Schultes RE. Hallucinogens of plant origin. *Science.* 1969;163:245–54.

Environmental Injuries

Kenneth Kamler, MD

Human beings can survive weeks without food, days without water, but only hours without heat. Humans must, at all costs, preserve and protect their internal temperature, for it holds the key to all their life functions. The human body is a mass of billions of exquisitely sequenced chemical reactions all of which are temperature-sensitive. Individual changes in the cadence of those reactions will quickly lead to internal chaos, like a symphony orchestra with each member playing at a different tempo. The timing, and thus the temperature, of these reactions is so critical that if body temperature varies by more than 4°F from 98.6°F, systems begin to malfunction, and the body's formidable defenses will start to crumble. A variation of 10–15°F, unless quickly reversed, will generally be fatal. This is a frightening thought when you consider that we live on a planet where, depending on location and season, we can be assaulted by temperature variations of 100°F or more.

THERMAL REGULATION

In temperate climates, air temperature is generally lower than body temperature, and, as a result, body heat is constantly being given off into the space around it. The rate of heat loss depends upon the temperature differential between the environment and the body. When the air is 16°F cooler than the body, the rate of heat production is exactly offset by the rate of heat loss.[1] This means that a resting human body will be in optimum heat balance when the outside temperature is 82°F. That is the average temperature on the African plains, one piece of evidence that human life evolved there.

But it didn't stay there. Humans have migrated nearly everywhere and explored everywhere else. Years ago, when adaptation to temperature extremes was first being examined from a scientific point of view, it was assumed, reasonably enough, that people living at the poles would have lower body temperature than those living at the equator. In fact, regardless of where we are on this planet, whether we've just begun exploring or lived

there for generations, all people guard the same internal temperature. We are indeed able to survive extreme environments, but we do it by fiercely defending that temperature through adjustments in our body systems and in our behavior.

Methods of Heat Transfer

Conduction
When there is direct contact between two objects, heat will flow from the warmer one to the colder one. Conductive heat transfers are generally not significant unless you are sitting in snow or on a hot rock, or sleeping on the ground without adequate insulation. It becomes very significant, though, if you're wet. Water has 25 times the conductivity of air[2] and will literally suck the life out of you. All of the survivors of the *Titanic* disaster were dry. None of those immersed in the sea survived though the water was warmer than the air.

Convection
Convection is a kind of facilitated conduction that occurs when air or fluid circulates over one of the contact surfaces, transferring the heat faster. The driving force can be external (the wind) or internal (blood flow). This is why a heater with a fan will make a room warmer much faster than an oven with its door open. Conversely, wind will rapidly blow away body heat – not in linear proportion to its velocity, but much faster as the square of its velocity.[3] So compared to a one-mile-per-hour wind, a ten-mile-per-hour wind will extract heat one hundred times faster. Wind chill tables were developed in recognition that moderately cold air combined with high winds can be life-threatening. Clothing that traps air against the skin will greatly reduce this type of heat loss, which is otherwise the major cause of wilderness hypothermia.[4]

Radiation
Every object in our world contains heat in the form of vibrating molecules that radiate energy completely independent of contact. During the day, the sun releases vast amounts of energy in the form of waves that radiate

through space until they collide with something, such as one of us. This speeds up the molecular vibrations within our bodies, which we sense as "getting hotter." On a cool night, we're hotter than the air and the energy flow reverses. We emit energy in the infrared spectrum, making us and other animals detectable by night sensors. Infrared emissions are not affected by clothing or skin color. The sun's energy, however, is mostly in the visible spectrum, so its absorption will be increased by darker clothes or darker skin.

Evaporation

The body is constantly losing water, as perspiration that collects on the skin and as vapor in exhaled air. Sweating may be obvious in the heat, but there is "insensible" perspiration even in cold climates. Respiratory water loss will be augmented by dry air and deep and rapid mouth breathing. As water evaporates, it draws energy, and therefore heat, from the body making sweating a fine-tuned way to cool off. If the sweat gets trapped under impermeable clothes, it will collect as water and cool the body too rapidly by conduction instead of by evaporation.

PHYSIOLOGIC CONTROL

Sensors

Our body's margin of survival is precariously thin. It must continually balance the laws of thermodynamics to maintain a constant body temperature despite the thermal onslaught from without and within that can vary by 100°F or more. To mount an effective defense, the body must first gauge the outside temperature so that it can begin to respond long before its core temperature becomes affected. The entire outer surface of the body is supplied with nerve endings called thermoreceptors – thermometers sensitive either to hot or to cold.[5] The receptors are not evenly distributed; there are more on the forehead and upper torso than in the arms and legs. This makes sense for survival because the brain and other internal organs are more critical to maintain body function, and it explains why it's easier to immerse your arms and legs into cold water than your head and chest. There are more cold receptors than warm receptors. This also makes survival sense. The body was designed in a warm climate, so it is more threatened by cold.

Thermoreceptors have overlapping ranges, but heat receptors fire more frequently as temperature rises, while cold receptors fire more when temperature falls.[6] When the change is sudden, the firing rate increases dramatically, like alarm bells going off. And when the temperature reaches either extreme of the range, a separate set of receptors is activated; they add the element of pain – an effective way to motivate you to do something about the situation.

Signals from thermoreceptors are transmitted to the hypothalamus, the brain's maintenance center, located at the base of the skull.[7] The front of the hypothalamus contains the body's thermostat, which actively monitors internal body temperature while also remaining exquisitely sensitive to skin temperature – its vital early-warning system. At 98.6°F, the warm and cold receptor inputs are balanced. When the hypothalamus receives increased input from either set of its "front line" receptors, it sends modulating signals to its internal organs that facilitate heating or cooling, and it sends an arousal signal to the conscious brain, warning it that it needs to reduce thermal stress. Without the alarm set off at the skin surface, the hypothalamus would be unable to react to an increase in body temperature until after it occurred. This would be highly dangerous given that a 4°F differential is enough to disrupt the body's functions.[8] Should the thermostat in the hypothalamus itself become disrupted, the entire thermoregulatory system would rapidly spin out of control.

Effectors

As critically important as temperature regulation is for all humans, we have no systems designed specifically to heat or cool our bodies, other than sweat glands, which are actually highly modified hair follicles. Thermostatic control depends on organs and tissues borrowed from other systems. The body recruits blood vessels, skin, fat, muscles, and most important of all, because of its ability to modify behavior, the conscious brain.

The most energy-efficient way, and the body's immediate response to regulate temperature, is by fine-tuning the vascular system.[9] Blood flow through arteries and arterioles is regulated by smooth muscles that respond to nervous and hormonal signals. The muscles ring the blood vessels and act as control valves. As they dilate or contract, they correspondingly increase or decrease flow rates and can preferentially divert blood to the skin surface for cooling, or below the subcutaneous fat layer for insulation and countercurrent warming. Blood can be directed away from body parts that have high surface areas and lose heat extravagantly, such as ears, noses, and toes, and toward organs more critical for survival, such as the heart, lungs, and brain.

Vascular control is rapid and elegant, but when core temperature begins to drift outside the narrow safe range, the body has two powerful techniques to bring it back – shivering and sweating. Shivering is the rhythmic contraction of skeletal muscle that serves no purpose other than to generate heat. Sweating is the extrusion of water onto the skin surface to promote evaporative cooling. Additionally, the body will release varying amounts of epinephrine and thyroid hormone – regulators of metabolism and therefore heat production – to restore thermal balance.[10]

But by far the most effective way for a human to maintain body temperature is through behavior. Our thermal receptors make us aware of temperature changes and can stimulate the hypothalamus to create a sense of discomfort in our consciousness. If we don't take effective action, the pain receptors at the temperature end-ranges will fire, adding additional motivation to make some change – like putting on a hat or taking off a sweater, moving into the shade or building a snow cave.

Body Temperature

There is no one specific location within the body that emits the core temperature.[11] Because no biochemical reactions are 100% efficient, all organs give off heat as a by-product. The busiest organs, the brain, heart, lungs, liver, and muscles, generate the most heat. Organs and tissues that are at the surface or excrete water or waste, like the skin, respiratory lining, bladder, and rectum, lose the most heat. Nevertheless, because of the efficiency with which heat is transferred to the blood (by conduction) and then circulated around the body (convection), temperature throughout the body remains remarkably constant.

Given that body heat is so uniformly distributed, decisions on where and how to measure it can be based on practical considerations. The underside of the tongue is easily accessible and well perfused. A probe placed there will rapidly reflect changes in core temperature – faster than a probe in the rectum, which is also quite a bit more uncomfortable. Axillary measurements, tympanic membrane infrared probes, and liquid crystal bubbles taped on the forehead are noninvasive, but there is some question as to their accuracy in reflecting core temperature.[12] Electronic thermometers have an equilibration time of one minute or less, digital displays as fine as a tenth of a degree, and the probe placed in the oral cavity is easy to tolerate. Mercury thermometers have longer equilibration times, can be misread and are more fragile, but are useful as backups. So the best combination of speed, accuracy, and minimal invasiveness is probably an electronic thermometer in the mouth.

Core temperature, although uniform throughout the body, does undergo normal physiologic variations.[13] The most obvious is fever, a generally beneficial response to infection that stimulates the immune system. Body temperature is affected by circadian rhythm. It will fall perhaps 1° in the early morning and rise 1° in the late afternoon. Women in the luteal phase of their menstrual cycle (between ovulation and menses) may have up to a 1.5° rise in body temperature. It can temporarily increase up to 2° after vigorous exercise. Although fitness has no direct effect on body temperature, an exercise program carried out in either a cold or warm environment will lower the temperature at which sweating begins and, therefore, reduce the rise in core temperature that would otherwise occur. The primary benefit of exercise, however, is that a fitter person can better sustain intense physical activity and, therefore, generate more heat for a longer time.

Thermal regulation will also be affected by other factors over which we have no control: age and gender. Temperature adjustment is dependent, in part, on blood vessels and muscles – tissues that tend to deteriorate as we age and are often affected by chronic illnesses.[14] Individuals older than 60 will have less responsive blood flow, less sweating, and less shivering. Women will generally be more susceptible to outside temperature because even though they have a greater relative amount of subcutaneous fat, they have a smaller blood volume and a higher proportion of surface area compared to body mass.[15] However, given that the most decisive factor in tolerating temperature changes is behavior, women or elderly adults – if they're smart, knowledgeable, and prepared – are far more likely to survive than clueless young males.

HYPOTHERMIA

Human bodies were designed in and for the tropics. Although we have adapted certain body systems to fend off cold, we are woefully inadequate physiologically to deal with extreme cold. Our first adjustment is to redirect blood flow from along the skin surface, which dissipates heat like a car radiator, to below our insulated layer of subcutaneous fat. The effect is like tucking your toes inside a blanket. Next, we begin shivering starting in the trunk, arms, and legs. When the contractions spread to the jaw muscles, we start chattering. Shivering produces only about as much heat as walking. Vigorous motion of the large muscles of the arms and legs is a far more effective way of combating the cold, especially if the movements are coordinated to transport you out of danger.

When heat production can no longer fend off the cold, the body conserves its warmth by shutting down blood flow to the areas that leak the most heat.[16] Hands and feet, noses and ears, become pale and cold. The head and neck is another highly exposed area, but the body plays favorites. Despite the heat loss, flow to the head remains high in order to ensure an adequate supply of blood to the brain. Scientists have only recently discovered the prioritizing of body parts; mothers, who insist their children wear hats and scarves on the coldest days, have long known it.

The only other protective response humans have against cold is goose bumps – which occur when the tiny muscles attached to hair follicles contract to straighten out our body hairs, creating loft to trap warm air against the skin. It works well for the feathers of high-flying birds and the fur of arctic foxes, but for humans with their relative paucity of hair, the mechanism seems almost pathetic. When the body starts to lose the battle, core temperature drops. Since a drop of 4°F (to about 95°F) will begin to affect biochemical reactions, it is generally considered to be the start of hypothermia.[17]

Below 95°F, there is a steady drop in cerebral metabolism that affects cortical function.[18] The mind becomes apathetic. Thinking is sluggish, and fine motor dexterity is lost, critically affecting our ability to get out of the very situation that is causing the problem. More primitive systems such as brainstem pacing of pulse and respiration, and hypothalamic thermostatic regulation aren't affected until the temperature drops another 20°F (to about 77°F) because blood flow will be disproportionately shunted to these areas so critical for survival.

The cold response of vasoconstriction and increased flow rate will at first increase blood pressure and cardiac load. As temperature drops below 90°F, nerve conduction velocity slows, and cardiac muscle begins to stiffen, leading to various types of cardiac arrhythmias.

Respiratory rate, although initially stimulated by cold, will progressively decline as temperature drops. Stiffening diaphragm and rib muscles make it harder and harder to drive lungs which are losing elasticity and filling with increasingly viscous secretions.

Peripheral vasoconstriction redirects fluids centrally where volume receptors interpret it as fluid overload and stimulate a diuretic response from the kidneys.

Diagnosis

What's going on inside the body is directly reflected by what we see on the outside – the symptoms of hypothermia.[19] They begin as body temperature drops the first 4°. With mild hypothermia, the victim will feel cold, then painfully cold, though exposed skin may be numb. Shivering will begin and become progressively stronger. Pulse and respiration will be increased. There may be difficulty with fine hand coordination. Though this will not be noticeable to an observer, it can be critical to a lone victim unable to close a zipper or tie a hood.

As temperature drops another 5° (to about 90°F), the incoordination becomes obvious. The victim will lag behind and stumble. Speech and thought will be slow, and the victim will be apathetic to his or her own condition. Pulse and respiration begin to slow. Reflexes are hyperactive. Uncontrolled urination may occur.

Below 90°F comes severe hypothermia, generally marked by the cessation of shivering. The victim will be unable to walk. Reflexes are diminished, and cardiac arrhythmias develop. The victim will be irritable and confused. With the steady decrease in temperature, consciousness progressively decreases as well. At around 85°F, the bizarre phenomenon of paradoxical undressing may occur:[20] Hypothalamic control is lost, blood flushes back to the skin creating a sensation of warmth, and a confused lone victim will remove his or her clothing. Cases where a female removes her clothing often initially lead to suspicion of rape.

At a core temperature of 80°F or below, voluntary motion will stop. There will be no reflexes and no response to pain. At about 70°F the heart will stop but until then heartbeat and breathing will be extremely slow and shallow – barely perceptible and easy to miss. That's why no hypothermia victim should be declared cold and dead until he or she has been warm and dead.[21]

It doesn't take extreme weather to cause hypothermia. Moderate cold and wind combined with sweaty clothes and open zippers on hikers who are thirsty, hungry, and tired is enough to do it. But those conditions are commonplace on many cold weather expeditions, so it is important for members to observe each other carefully and keep a high index of suspicion. Severe hypothermia is so hard to treat that early diagnosis of mild hypothermia will likely make the difference between life and death.

Treatment

Treating mild hypothermia is simple – restrict heat loss and promote heat production. Block the wind and remove the wet clothes. Add extra warming and wind-resistant layers and close the zippers and sleeves. If you have no dry clothes, at least wring out the wet ones before putting them back on. Take a drink and eat something, preferably carbohydrates. Get up off the ice or cold rocks and get moving to generate heat; even better if the movement gets you out of the hostile environment.

Treating severe hypothermia is much more problematic because the individual cannot take care of him- or herself and cannot generate adequate internal heat to rewarm his or her body. A core temperature of 90°F is not physiologically incompatible with life but, as a practical matter, it is fatal for someone who doesn't get outside help. At that temperature, the severe incoordination and confusion make self-rescue impossible.

Once shivering has stopped and metabolism has slowed, core temperature will fall precipitously until it equilibrates with ambient temperature. External heat must be provided. The situation is urgent and critical, but every step must be done very gently since a chilled heart has irritable hair-trigger muscles ready to set off arrhythmias at the slightest disturbance – or with no disturbance at all.[22] The victim should not move under his or her own power, but rather should be carefully carried away from any heat-dissipating elements – wind, water, ice, and snow – to a shelter if possible. A tent will block the wind, but a snow cave is warmer. The shelter must have an insulated bottom. A closed cell foam pad is better than an inflatable thermorest pad because foam traps the air within rather than allowing it to circulate. If pads are lacking, use clothes, backpacks or leafy tree branches. Lay the victim out horizontally. Check for any wet clothes including, and especially, the underwear. Remove them, or cut them away if necessary to minimize manipulation of the extremities. Loosen tight clothing, particularly boots, but boots should not be removed. The feet are likely to swell and the boots may be impossible to put back on.

After heat loss is minimized, adding heat is essential. Boil water to warm and humidify the shelter or start a fire if you're still outside. Use the hot water to fill water bottles and to create hot packs out of clothes or blankets wrapped in plastic bags. Place the bottles and packs in areas that will transmit heat most rapidly – the neck, axillae, and groin, anatomical regions that have thin skin and high rates of subcutaneous blood flow.

If appropriate equipment is available, other methods can be used to warm the victim: Inhalation devices that deliver heated, humidified air through a face mask transfer some heat by condensation but their effectiveness lies more in preventing respiratory heat loss. Heat can be transferred by gastric lavage – a tube is inserted through the nose, down the esophagus and into the stomach. Warm fluids are repeatedly instilled via syringe and then withdrawn once they've cooled. Warm water bladder irrigation is attempted through much the same way using a Foley catheter to infuse warm liquids into the urinary bladder of a patient. Warm peritoneal dialysis has also been recommended as a possible means of rewarming a hypothermic victim, but it requires significant skill and specific equipment to be attempted in the field. Femoral–femoral bypass and extra-corporeal membrane oxygenation are extremely invasive and require significant hospital support and, because of this, are not covered in this chapter.

One final method sometimes used to transfer heat is to place the victim naked in a sleeping bag and have someone, also naked, get in the bag with him or her. All this takes is a willing volunteer. These transfers through the lungs, the stomach, the bladder, and the skin can all be tried, but none of them seem capable of transferring more than a very modest amount of heat.[23]

In a cold, dehydrated victim, warmed intravenous fluids can be administered if sweet hot liquids cannot be taken orally, but with constricted blood vessels, starting an IV is extremely difficult. If it can be started, the fluid of choice would be 5% dextrose in normal saline. Since the IV is exposed to the ambient temperature, there's the real risk that the infusion will cause further body cooling. Treating hypothermia victims in below zero temperatures on Everest, the author has managed, with some success, to avoid this problem by taping chemical hand warmers around the IV bags and frequently alternating the hanging bag with one that was floating in warm water.

Cardiopulmonary resuscitation should not be administered unless 3 minutes have elapsed with no detectable pulse either on portable EKG or by palpation. If there is even a faint heartbeat, the shock of CPR will probably cause an arrhythmia. If it is elected to start CPR, the rate should be half that normally given because less oxygen is needed to support the lower metabolism, circulation is slow, and the stiff heart needs more time to complete a cycle.[24]

Severe hypothermia in the wilderness is a desperate situation. The best way out is immediate evacuation by helicopter. Overland evacuation will most likely provoke an arrhythmia and CPR cannot be done on a moving stretcher. If an air lift is not going to happen and the other members of the expedition are safe, on-site rewarming should be tried, bearing in mind that the process may take many hours, even a day or more to be successful.

Prevention

The best way to deal with hypothermia is to not get it at all. For the most part, humans can perform safely in extreme cold, but the prevention of cold injury requires preparation, knowledge, and intellect. Humans must know how to dress, eat, and shelter themselves. Our brain is by far the most powerful tool we have for cold weather survival.

Clothing

A cold wind poses a great risk of hypothermia because of the geometric rise in the potential convective heat loss. A barrier is needed to prevent body-heated air adjacent to the skin from being blown away. This barrier is clothing. At the same time, the barrier must be able to disperse water vapor that collects on the skin but not allow water droplets to penetrate from the outside, since skin contact with water will greatly accelerate heat loss by conduction. Cold weather clothing must, therefore, remove water, trap air, and block wind and rain. The three different functions are best performed with three different layers, with the added advantages that multiple layers, worn loosely, trap air between them and can be added and subtracted to adapt to changes in heat load.

Inner layer – underwear to remove water: Polypropylene and polyester fabrics will wick perspiration away from the skin to eliminate the conductive heat loss and evaporative cooling of water.

Middle layer – insulation to trap air: Shirts and pants should generally be made of pile or fleece (light synthetic fabrics that retain heat well) or wool (a somewhat heavier but warmer fabric that is able to retain heat even when wet). The most effective insulating material per weight is goose down, which, although it loses heat when wet, would be the best choice for big mountains or anywhere else where the snow is dry.

Outer layer – a shell to block wind and rain: Parkas and wind pants should be made of a synthetic fabric woven tightly enough to resist penetration by wind and water, yet not so tight that skin vapor cannot pass through.

Heat loss from the head and neck must be prevented if the core temperature is to be maintained. A body under cold stress will not constrict blood flow to the head as it will to hands and feet because it prioritizes the brain, the organ we need most for survival. A bare head can account for 50% of the heat loss in an individual wearing winter clothing.[25] Wool hats or balaclavas are essential – hoods alone won't do. Adding a scarf or gaiter is a very effective way to warm blood as it flows through the neck.

Blood flow to the feet and hands will be the first to be sacrificed if core temperature is under attack; it is impossible to keep them warm if your body is not warm. Feet can otherwise be well protected with the right combination of socks and boots. Wearing a polypropylene liner and one or two pairs of wool socks inside a double boot – an inner layer of felt or foam with an outer layer of hard plastic – is like walking in a thermos.

Gloves remain an unsolved problem in cold weather gear. Fingers have a large surface area and therefore a high rate of radiant heat loss. Mittens greatly reduce surface area and so are much warmer than gloves, but also much clumsier. One compromise solution is to wear a thin synthetic glove inside a wool or fleece glove inside a windproof, water-resistant mitten. The mitten should be removed only when fine dexterity is required but it is often too tempting to take it off, and no mitten will work if it isn't worn. The author has treated many more frost-bitten fingers than frostbitten toes.

Food

Food is transported through the blood in the form of a sugar called glucose, a simple carbohydrate that enters cells easily and burns rapidly, like paper. This is why eating sugar gives you a quick burst of energy. Blood resupplies its load of glucose constantly by tapping into the liver and muscles for their stores of glycogen, a slightly more complex carbohydrate that burns slower, like wood, and provides a more sustained energy release. Carbohydrates are pure fuel; they have no function in the body other than to provide heat and power. If their resupply is not adequate, the body will burn its own fat and protein to provide fuel.

Hiking with a heavy pack through deep snow on a cold day will more than double your body's energy requirement. Although a human can last weeks without food, when energy supplies fall short of demand, the ability to sustain exercise and generate heat will be compromised. The best way to maintain fuel reserves, and thereby avoid hypothermia, is to carbohydrate-load to maximize glycogen stores and then to eat carbohydrate-rich foods at regular meals and frequently as supplemental snacks.

Water

Dehydration is common in cold environments. Heavy exercise and open-mouth breathing of dry air increases respiratory water loss. Peripheral vasoconstriction increases central fluid load that the body responds to by increasing diuresis. Also, as skin temperature falls, the thirst sensation is blunted. Although dehydration does not impair vasoconstriction or shivering, it can degrade performance. Hydration should be monitored by checking urine volume (a pee bottle kept inside the tent should be filled by morning) and urine color (snow flowers should be yellow, not orange).

With heavy exertion, at least four quarts of liquid a day may be necessary. It's a good idea to consume water or energy drinks at every meal and to sip them frequently in between. It is not a good idea to eat snow. It doesn't provide an adequate volume of water and it drains body heat.

Shelter

Cold weather survival depends more on protecting yourself from the environment than adapting to it. In that regard, shelters are an extension of clothing. A good shelter will trap air, eliminate moisture, and block wind to contain body heat. Additionally, shelters have the potential to generate external heat. Look for natural shelters and then try to improve them. Caves and alcoves under rock overhangs are obvious choices. Hillsides are generally warmer than valleys since warm air rises. Standing trees will act as barriers to the wind and may have sunken ground or snow-wells at their bases. Large fallen trees often have depressions behind them.

Improve the shelter by adding a wall of rocks or snow or leafy tree branches. Dig the hole deeper into the ground or snow. Snow is an excellent insulator provided direct contact is avoided. Cover the floor with a foam pad or leaves. Cover the top with a tarp or branches. If you have a shovel, or something you can use as a shovel, you can dig into a snow drift to make a cave. Keep it small to retain body heat unless you are able to put a fire inside, in which case there must be a ventilation hole. Of course if it is not too cold, a tent or even a bivouac sack is a lot easier (Figure 31.1).

FROSTBITE

Frostbite occurs when body parts freeze. Since the water in cells contains electrolytes and is heated from within, ambient temperature has to be below 21°F before skin will freeze.[26] Less of a temperature drop and less time of exposure is required if heat loss is facilitated by wind or moisture. Frostbite can come on very rapidly when skin comes in contact with cold metal, and instantaneously when in contact with cold gasoline or alcohol, which remain liquid at –40°F.

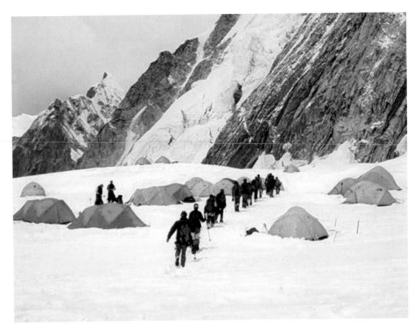

Figure 31.1. Proper shelter is imperative in an extremely cold environment like Everest Camp One. Photo courtesy Naurang Sherpa.

Body parts that have high ratios of surface area to volume – ears, noses, fingers, and toes – are often left exposed and are the most at risk for freezing because the body will quickly shut down blood flow to these areas to conserve heat (Figure 31.2). Ice crystals will form within the cells and between them. When the cooling takes place over hours, the ice is primarily extracellular and less disruptive than the intracellular crystals that form when cooling is more rapid. Formation of ice crystals is not necessarily fatal for cells. They can survive freezing and return to health once they are thawed. What destroys frozen body parts is the damage the cold inflicts on the endothelial lining of their blood vessels. Plasma leaks through the vessel walls and the loss of liquid causes the blood to sludge, further reducing the flow through the already constricted vessels. As thawing occurs, warmed blood encounters injured endothelial linings forming clots that can completely obstruct circulation. Without blood flow, the tissues necrose.

A resting human is in heat balance when skin temperature is 82°F. Below this level, we begin to feel cool. By 70°F, we feel cold, then painfully cold. At about 60°F, blood vessels are maximally constricted and skin is maximally pale. Once skin temperature reaches 50°F, the "hunting response" or cold-induced vasodilation (CIVD) occurs.[27] This is a curious phenomenon more developed in people indigenous to the Arctic. Vessels begin to alternately dilate and constrict in 5- to 10-minute cycles, thus intermittently replenishing blood flow to the cold stressed part. In measured doses, the body is sacrificing heat to try to maintain functioning extremities.

Below a skin temperature of 50°F, cutaneous sensation is lost and the feeling of painful cold is replaced by numbness. This is the first warning sign of impending frostbite. With no circulation, skin temperature can drop precipitously. Below 25°F, ice crystals begin to form, blood vessels leak, and blood coagulates. Tissues become hard and purple.

The best treatment for frostbite is rapid and steady rewarming of the body part in a water bath maintained between 100°F and 108°F.[28] Unfortunately, field logistics often make this impossible and an unsuccessful attempt will leave the victim worse off. Resist the temptation to immediately thaw the part until you've realistically assessed your situation. Partially thawed tissue or thawed tissue that refreezes will sustain additional damage. The unavoidable plasma leakage and clot formation that occur with the recommencement of blood flow is a cycle you don't want repeated more than once.

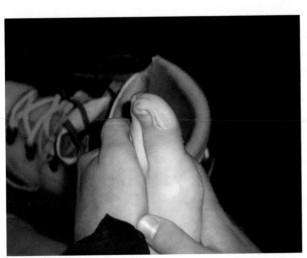

Figure 31.2. Mild frostbite. Photo courtesy Howard Donner.

You will need enough fuel and water to allow for full thawing, which may take half an hour or more. You will need a thermometer to control the temperature within a narrow range. After thawing, the extremity must be kept warm through the entire evacuation and cannot be traumatized. Thawed hands can be used for balancing but cannot do heavy gripping, and thawed feet can't be walked on. If the victim is hypothermic as well, his or her body temperature must first be brought above 93°F before thawing or the cold blood suddenly released from the extremity may shock stiff heart muscles into an arrhythmia. It may well be better to leave the part frozen and opt for quick evacuation, especially since longer freezing time doesn't necessarily mean more severe permanent damage.

Field rewarming (Figure 31.3) is not easy to do when the air temperature is below zero and the body part is a block of ice. Hot water may need to be added and cold water drawn off, almost continuously. The larger the tub, the easier it will be to maintain a stable temperature. Gentle active motion is helpful to stimulate blood flow and, at the same time, it stirs the water to keep the temperature uniform. Don't massage the part; massage will only traumatize the fragile tissues. Too cool a bath will be ineffective. Too warm a bath will cause further thermal injury, the first sign of which in an insensate hand or foot may be the victim smelling his own flesh burning. It is important not to use dry heat (such as a fire or an oven) to rewarm frostbitten tissue as this dry heat can further desiccate and damage the tissue.

Rewarming should be continued until the hard waxy skin has become soft and pliable, indicating essentially that the ice has melted and the direct cellular injury has been reversed. The part will turn red as blood flow returns. Nerves are reactivated bringing on severe pain. Strong analgesics may be necessary. Nonsteroidal anti-inflammatory medications (NSAIDs) such as ibuprofen have the added advantage of reducing both inflammation and clot formation.

If the redness and swelling subside within a few days, leaving no permanent damage, the condition is often referred to as frostnip. If blisters appear after thawing, the injury is more severe, and the prognosis is guarded. Clear blisters that extend to the tip of the digit indicate superficial damage with a likelihood of full recovery. Blood-filled blisters that stop short of the tips carry a much worse prognosis. Blister formation requires active nervous and vascular input. If the end of the digit (the portion most severely exposed to the cold) is unable to generate a blister, nerves and blood vessels have been destroyed and recovery is unlikely. In general, blisters should not be debrided unless they are likely to break anyway and become infected.

The part should be sterilely, or at least cleanly, wrapped with pads between the digits, and then elevated.

The goal in the field is to prevent infection and protect from contact until evacuation. Dressings should be changed daily if supplies allow. Antibiotics can be given, tetanus toxoid if necessary. A hand or foot may need to be placed in a frame at night to avoid pressure from a blanket or sleeping bag. No matter how ugly the part looks, unless it is infected, no amputations should be done. The degree to which tissues can revascularize is sometimes amazing, though it may take weeks. The vasculature, however, is permanently compromised. Frostbite often leaves behind dystrophic nail growth and less responsive blood vessels, making recovered tissues cold-sensitive for years or forever. Tissues that can't recover will eventually demarcate and fall off.

First and foremost, prevent frostbite by preventing hypothermia. If body temperature is not threatened, peripheral vessels won't need to constrict and start the cooling process. Maintain heat production with food and exercise. Maintain insulation by eliminating moisture

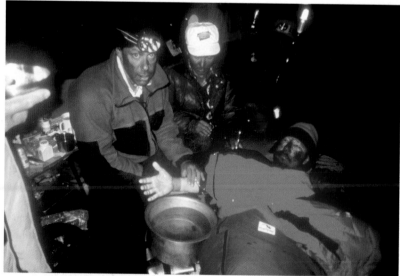

Figure 31.3. The author rewarming a severely frostbitten patient in a tent on Everest. Photo courtesy Kenneth Kamler.

and wearing adequate layers of nonconstrictive clothing. While in Antarctica, the author saw a dramatic example of how critical clothing can be. The author and his climbing partner had the same socks and boots on during a 36-hour climb, except his partner's wool sock had a hole in it over the big toe where his nail had cut through. When they got back to the tent, his partner's first three toes were purple. It took 5 days to evacuate him, and he eventually lost all three toes (though he is back climbing again).

NONFREEZING COLD INJURIES

Although frostbite will not occur in air above freezing, body parts are vulnerable to other injuries as temperature drops. When feet are wet and cold, they are at risk of developing chilblain, pernio, and trenchfoot – progressively more severe conditions related to increased time of exposure. Together they form a continuum of injury descriptively known as "river rot." In temperatures below 60°F, it can take as little as 3 hours for a wet foot (or wet hand or face) to develop chilblain – a condition of swollen, itchy, aching skin. Exposure for a day or so will lead to pernio – the skin becomes more painful and small red vesicles appear. Both chilblain and pernio resolve with drying and rewarming and lead to no permanent damage.

Trenchfoot is a far more serious condition that develops after feet have been left for several days in cold wet socks and boots. The feet turn white, cold, and numb. After drying and rewarming, they become red, hot, and painful. Over the next days and weeks, pain intensifies, and skin becomes hypersensitive and may necrose, much like frostbite. Pain, weakness, and loss of motor control may become permanent disabilities. To avoid the condition, feet must be kept dry. Allow boots to dry out thoroughly. Vapor barrier boots that do not allow sweat to evaporate are especially risky. Change socks twice a day, and spray the feet with an antiperspirant each time.

In some people, contact with cold air induces itching, redness, and swelling of the skin – a condition known as cold urticaria. Onset is from 2 minutes to 2 days after exposure. Resolution generally occurs 2 hours to 2 days later. Antihistamines are the standard treatment for most urticaria, with EpiPen injection being used for refractory or systemic reactions. Avoidance of cold would seem to be the easy preventative, though it seems to be the rate of skin cooling rather than the absolute temperature that provokes the symptoms.

Cold dry air and intense exercise can combine to cause cold-induced bronchoconstriction. Narrowing of the upper airways seems to be due to a reflex response generating a high amount of inflammation. It is far more common in people with underlying asthma, but pulmonary congestion can be seen in anyone. Cold air increases respiratory secretions and decreases ciliary clearance, degrading respiration function in all of us.

HYPERTHERMIA

Humans are designed to endure heat far better than cold. They survive in external temperatures that surpass 120°F and can perform vigorous exercise capable of raising internal temperature to 140°F in one hour.[11] Human protein, especially nerve tissue, will congeal at temperatures above 112°F. So, why aren't our brains cooked like hard-boiled eggs? We are protected from the onslaught of heat from without and within by our thermal regulatory system. If it breaks down, we'd be no different from pieces of meat roasting in an oven.

Even at rest in a temperate climate, our basal metabolism generates enough heat to raise body temperature 2.5°F per hour. Strenuous activity can increase that rate 15 times.[29] Humans lose most of their heat through the skin, which acts like a car radiator. (Significant heat loss through the lungs occurs only in cold climates.) Blood, our liquid coolant, passes through all our organs, picking up heat and carrying it to the skin surface where it is cooled by proximity to the outside temperature. As the heat load increases, more blood is shunted to the skin by arterial control, and veins dilate to prolong surface contact time. This process, heat loss by radiation, depends on ambient temperature being significantly lower than skin temperature, 95°F. A higher ambient temperature will actually heat the blood.

There are two environments on our planet where air temperature routinely exceeds body temperature – the desert and the jungle. To survive in either one, or to do vigorous exercise in any environment, a human being needs an additional system to dissipate heat. When blood vessels alone are not getting the job done and the skin is heating up, the body turns on its sprinkler system.

Sweating may be inelegant, but it works. Sweat glands spread a layer of water onto the surface of the skin. As the water evaporates – an energy absorbent process – it draws heat from the body, vaporizing it into the air. High temperatures speed up evaporation and actually improve cooling efficiency, which would otherwise steadily diminish and then reverse as the outside temperature rose. Sweating can dissipate heat more than 20 times faster than radiative cooling,[30] but for the system to work, the body needs a steady input of water and a steady output of vapor. The threat of the desert is too little water: The body can't make sweat. The threat of the jungle is too much water: Fully saturated air has little capacity to add more moisture so sweat simply sits on the skin or drips off, unable to evaporate.

About three million sweat glands are distributed unevenly on the skin.[1] Most are located on the forehead, face and neck, chest, and back (areas that need priority cooling to protect the brain, heart, and lungs) and in the armpits and groin (efficient sites for cooling because of the large volume of blood circulating just beneath thin skin). The number of sweat glands activated and the range at which sweat flows are adjusted by the hypothalamus as it monitors both skin and core temperature. Sweating may be a profligate use of water in the dry desert or a worthless waste of water in the humid jungle, but when the body is fighting to maintain its temperature, it knows no limits.

Two-thirds of the human body is water. The average person contains about 50 liters of fluid and loses a minimum of 2 liters in daily maintenance.[32] The kidneys use water to flush out waste as urine; the lungs use it to moisturize inhaled air so that it won't irritate the sensitive pulmonary linings. Some water also seeps out passively through the skin – the body's not-quite-watertight container. At rest on a hot day, with sweat glands turned on, the body can easily use up 5 liters of water. Hiking can cost an additional liter or more per hour, and increased sweating is an autonomic response to nervous tension. In the desert or jungle where heat, exercise, and anxiety are a common combination, water losses can mount rapidly. When the body is down even 1 liter, its function becomes impaired. Once it is down 5 liters, fatigue and dizziness set in. A loss of 10 liters disturbs vision and hearing and sets off convulsions. A deficit of 15–20 liters, roughly a third of the body's total water, is fatal.[32]

If the water is not replaced or if it can't evaporate, core temperature will rise. To stay alive, the body must dissipate its heat load, continue oxygen intake, and develop a survival strategy. Therefore, it will shunt more blood to the skin, the lungs, and the brain, at the expense of other less immediately essential organs, such as the stomach, intestines, liver, and muscles. Faced with the need to supply more blood to the network of heat-dissipating vessels that have opened up under the skin, while still maintaining flow to the brain and lungs, the heart pumps harder and faster. The chest pounds, and the pulse rises. To aggravate matters, the drier blood is thicker and, therefore, harder to propel through the vessels. Increased work generates more body heat, which requires even more blood flow to the skin, creating a vicious cycle. A core temperature rise of 2°F will increase the speed of metabolic reactions 15%. When the temperature climbs to 102°F, blood flow won't be able to keep up, and the body will show signs of heat exhaustion. Above 104°F, metabolic speed will be about 50% above normal and blood supply to even the most vital organs will fall short, with the brain affected first.[32] The victim will lose consciousness and collapse into heat stroke.

Increasingly severe signs of hyperthermia, from heat exhaustion to heat stroke, reflect the body's progressive breakdown as it fails to adequately offset its heat load. Symptoms of heat exhaustion are nonspecific and gradual in onset – fatigue, weakness, nausea, dizziness, headache, muscle cramps. Sweating may or may not be present. Skin may be pale and have goose bumps. The heart rate will be rapid. Decreased blood flow to the brain may cause the victim to swoon or to momentarily faint (syncope). If the heat load continues to mount, the onset of heat stroke is typically sudden and severe. Since the brain is the most oxygen-sensitive organ, the first indications are often confusion and incoordination, followed by unconsciousness.

Because the early signs are of gradual onset and occur commonly in the field for many other reasons, it is important to recognize risk factors in the environment and in team members and then to maintain a high index of suspicion. The ultimate outdoor setting to induce hyperthermia would be a performance of sustained vigorous activity under stressful conditions in an environment of high temperature and humidity, with no easy access to water. The ultimate team-member-at-risk would be someone with high body fat or mass and low fitness, who is inadequately acclimatized, behind on fluids, and highly motivated to get the job done no matter what. Certain medications, like antihistamines, diuretics, amphetamines, and antipsychotic drugs, will further reduce heat tolerance. Women may be more heat-sensitive during the luteal phase of their menstrual cycle.[15]

Interestingly, a person's risk of developing heat illness on any given day significantly increases if he or she had to deal with adverse environmental or personal health conditions the day before.[11] Heat stroke in these people often occurs during the early part of the day, suggesting that their thermal regulatory systems were already compromised by the stress of the previous day. An afternoon of high heat and humidity, or a member with a fever, a gastrointestinal problem, or even a muscle injury, should make you especially vigilant the following day.

Early recognition and treatment of heat illness can literally mean the difference between life and death. In a high-risk setting, weakness, nausea, cramps, or profuse sweating should be considered a warning signal. The person should be immediately stopped from the activity, though this is not always easy to do when motivation or ego get in the way. Move him or her to the shade, loosen clothing, and apply wet towels. Encourage fluid consumption – either water or electrolyte drinks. Enforce an appropriate rest period, from a few hours to overnight. If the signs are caught early, that should do it. The victim will be able to very quickly return to productive activity. If the condition is ignored, blood will be relentlessly drawn to the periphery for cooling and to the muscles for work. The supply to the brain will come up short, and the victim may faint – a syncopal attack.

The author was alerted to one such episode while on an expedition in the Amazon. One of our Cofan Indian guides came to fetch me when the zoologist he was escorting suddenly collapsed while chasing monkeys. By the time I arrived on the scene, however, she had recovered. The collapse put an abrupt end to her exertion and, since in an upright position 70% of blood volume is below heart level, the horizontal position greatly eased the stress on her heart, which no longer had to work against gravity. She was in the shade, lying on cool ground, and smiling. Her body temperature was back to normal.

When signs are ignored, and victims don't cure themselves by fainting in the shade, heat exhaustion will progress to heat stroke. Confusion and incoordination are signs of imminent collapse. This is not fainting. The victim who collapses will not come around readily. He or she will likely still be sweating profusely. The idea that the skin will be dry is a fallacy, based on the delayed observation of desert victims whose sweat had quickly evaporated or who were severely dehydrated in the first place. The diagnosis can be confirmed by measuring body temperature, which will be above 104°F if it is taken immediately. Usually, there is some delay, and although the collapse and unconsciousness will persist, the dramatic reduction in muscle activity will quickly allow the body temperature to drop. A reading below 104°F doesn't mean it wasn't above that number at the time of collapse. In a heat-stressed environment, anyone who collapses and does not rapidly regain consciousness must be treated for heat stroke immediately. The longer the body remains hot, the worse the outcome will be. Heat stroke is a medical emergency.

Survival depends on rapidity of cooling. Move the victim to the shade and remove any constrictive clothing. Apply cold water or ice water in large quantities – total body immersion if possible, or at least a spray or wet sheets. Fan the victim to accelerate evaporation. Do not sponge with alcohol. Skin absorption may lead to poisoning. If available, start an IV of normal saline or Ringer's lactate. Carefully monitor vital signs: At the start, pulse will be high, and blood pressure and urine output will be low. Give 1–2 liters of fluid in the first hour then titrate accordingly. For seizures or convulsions, administer 5–10 mg of diazepam to prevent body temperature from rising due to muscle activity. Do not give antipyretics – the body set point for thermal regulation is not elevated – this is not a fever. Serially monitor rectal temperature and discontinue active cooling once core temperature falls to 102°F. Evacuate the victim as soon as possible.

About 90% of heat stroke victims survive.[33] Some neurological deficits may last a year or more, but they eventually clear up. After there has been a full recovery, there is no increased risk for that individual to reenter a heat-stressed environment – and perhaps even a lesser risk because he or she will have a higher than average motivation to prevent a recurrence.

Heat stroke is a preventable disease – so much so that in the Israeli army, contracting heat illness is punishable by court-martial.[34] It is prevented by acclimatizing to the environment, drinking adequate fluids, and matching the activity to the risk of heat overload.

Acclimatization is what we commonly call "getting used to the heat." Several adaptive body processes get underway as soon as we are exposed to the heat. The process is the same whether the source of that heat is external (desert or jungle) or internal (sustained exercise). The exposure must be sufficiently stressful to elevate body temperature and provoke profuse sweating. Exercising in a temperate climate or resting in a tropical one will improve performance in the heat, but the gains will be modest compared to those obtained by training in a hot environment. The minimum daily workout should be 2 hours (can be two 1-hour sessions) of cardiovascular endurance exercises, with duration and intensity increased daily. Optimal adaptation to the climate can be achieved after 7–10 days. Acclimatization can be induced by working out in a "simulated" hot environment indoors, but fluid deprivation will not facilitate the process and can quickly lead to heat stroke.

Acclimatization increases heat tolerance physiologically by expanding blood volume and by improving sweating efficiency. Fluid is added to the plasma; red blood cell mass is maintained, but the blood becomes more liquid. The heart expends less effort to pump the blood, and there's an easier flow into the peripheral skin circulation where heat is dissipated. The volume of sweat also increases. To conserve water, the body begins periodic activation of the sweat glands within each patch of skin. Sweating becomes cyclical.[31] Three million sweat glands, all with their valves wide open at the same time, would cause the skin's surface to flood, and water that drips off the body before it evaporates is a complete waste. To give each released droplet the time and space to evaporate, adjacent valves open and close sequentially so that the body obtains maximum cooling from each drop of water it sacrifices. To prevent wholesale loss of salt and other electrolytes, they are withdrawn from the sweat so efficiently that sweat no longer stains or even smells bad, having become nearly pure water. Sweating also becomes easier, beginning sooner after starting exercise and occurring at a lower outside temperature; this serves to keep the body's engine cool before it even starts to overheat.

Signs that the body has achieved acclimatization are a lower heart rate, lower body temperature, and increased sweating during exercise. The effect can be quite dramatic, with team members able to easily complete tasks that were difficult or impossible a week earlier, but acclimatization is transient. Without continued heat–exercise exposure, it will be retained for about 1 week and then gradually decline, with most of it being lost after 3 weeks.[35]

Besides the physiological changes, heat stress generates changes at the molecular level. Repeated heating of body tissues leads to the development of an acquired thermal tolerance by the creation of "heat shock proteins"[36] – proteins that are synthesized in response to stress of any kind including heat, but also exercise and even anxiety. Heat shock proteins stabilize normal proteins against thermal injury and can even refold proteins that have been denatured by heat. They can add a protective advantage against a 3–4°F rise in body temperature. The proteins form within an hour of the stress and can remain active for a week or more. This temporary protection is not acclimatization, but the processes are complementary. Acclimatization reduces the absorbed heat load, while thermal tolerance increases the body's ability to withstand it.

Dehydration by more than 1% of body weight will degrade both physical and mental performance.[30] Minimum body maintenance extracts 2% daily; hard work in the heat can drain that much in an hour. A body that reaches 7% water deficit will be exhausted and on the brink of collapse. Yet humans don't even begin to feel thirsty until their water deficit reaches 3% and even then will only voluntarily drink enough to replace two-thirds of their water loss. What these numbers add up to is that dehydration is insidious and dangerous, and that humans in hot climates need to be "forced" to drink.

Two percent body dehydration is equivalent to the loss of about 1 liter of water. Ideally, restoration of fluid volume should be immediate and ongoing, but this is impractical and unappealing to highly motivated individuals who have a job to get done. The best way to maintain fluid balance is to get a head start by preloading, and then to keep the deficit to a minimum by frequent reloading. At least ½ liter of fluid should be drunk before starting exercise – if possible, about 2 hours before since it takes time for the kidneys to regulate the proper volume (urinate out the excess). During exercise, there should be water breaks every half hour or so during which everyone drinks to quench thirst and then some. It is possible, however, to be too conscientious in drinking. If plasma salt concentration becomes too diluted, osmotic flow into the brain and lungs can result in cerebral and pulmonary edema. Urine color is the most reliable indicator of hydration state and should be monitored regularly. Relying on thirst will not prevent dehydration.

The best opportunity for fluid intake comes during meals. Fluid should be readily available and drinking should be encouraged at that time and immediately afterward. The composition of the drink is unimportant if balanced meals are being consumed regularly.[30] Sports drinks can be valuable to replace salt, minerals, and carbohydrates if dietary intake is inadequate. In sustained exercise, a drink containing glucose or carbohydrates will improve performance. The primary benefit of sports drinks, however, is that the taste will encourage voluntary fluid consumption. Proteins should perhaps be reduced at mealtime because more water is required to digest them. We realize this instinctively in hot climates where we generally lose our taste for meat and prefer fruits and vegetables.

Finally, to prevent heat illness, dress for the conditions, and behave yourself. Wear loose-fitting, light-weight, light-colored, moisture-wicking clothing. In the sun, all skin, especially the head, should be covered or shaded – use a wide brim hat with a neck drape or bandanna. In the shade, expose the maximum amount of skin to air flow. Schedule vigorous physical activity for the mornings or evenings, but bear in mind that humidity is usually highest in the early morning.

To survive in the heat, take a lesson from Saharan nomads. On caravans, they travel in flowing robes, rest in the afternoon, trap animals rather than chase them, and ensure their water supply by caching water-filled ostrich eggs along the route. Maybe we can't follow that behavior exactly, but you get the idea.

REFERENCES

1. Gagge AP, Gonzales RR. Mechanisms of heat exchange: biophysics and physiology. In: Fregly ML, Blatteis CM, eds. *Handbook of Physiology*, vol. 1. Bethesda, Md: Oxford University Press; 1996.
2. Toner MM, Mcardle WD. Human thermoregulatory responses to acute cold stress with special reference to water immersion. In: Fregly, ML, Blatteis CM, eds. *Handbook of Physiology, Section 4: Environmental Physiology*. New York: Oxford University; 1996: 379–418.
3. Wilkerson, J. *Medicine for Mountaineering*. 5th ed. Seattle: Mountaineers Books; 2001.
4. Department of the Army. *Prevention and Management of Cold Weather Injuries*. Washington, DC: Department of the Army, Technical Bulletin Medicine; 2005.
5. Hensel H. Cutaneous thermoreceptors. In: Iggo A, ed. *Handbook of Sensory Physiology*, vol. 2. Berlin: Springer-Verlag; 1973.
6. Crawshaw LI, et al. Body temperature regulation in vertebrates: comparative aspects and neuronal elements. In: Schonbaum E, Lomax P, eds. *Thermoregulation: Physiology and Biochemistry*. New York: Pergamon Press; 1990.
7. Bruck K, Hinckel P. Thermoafferent networks and their adaptive modifications. In: Schonbaum E, Lomax P, eds. *Thermoregulation: Physiology and Biochemistry*. New York: Pergamon Press; 1990.
8. Crawshaw LI, et al. Thermoregulation. In: Auerbach P, ed. *Wilderness Medicine*. 4th ed. St. Louis, Mosby; 2001: 120.
9. Kenney WL. Control of skin vasodilation: mechanisms and influences. In: Johannsen BN, Nielsen R, eds. *Thermal Physiology*. Copenhagen: August Krogh Institute; 1997.
10. Radomski MW, Cross M, Buguet A. Exercise-induced hyperthermia and hormonal responses to exercise. *Can J Physiol Pharmacol*. 1998;76:547–52.
11. Sawka M, Young A. Physiological systems and their responses to conditions of heat and cold. In: *American College of Sports Medicine's Advanced Exercise Physiology*. Philadelphia: Lippincott; 2006.
12. Young CC, Sladen RN. Temperature monitoring. *Int Anesthesiol Clin*. 1996;34:149.
13. Reinberg A, Smolensky M. Chronobiology and thermoregulation. In: Schonbaum E, Lomax P, eds. *Thermoregulation: Physiology and Biochemistry*. New York: Pergamon Press; 1990.
14. Khan F, Spence VA, Belch JJF. Cutaneous vascular responses and thermoregulation in relation to age. *Clin Sci*. 1992; 82:521.

15 Mitchell JH, et al. Acute response and chronic adaptation to exercise in women. *Med Sci Sports Exer.* 1992;24(suppl. 6): S258.

16 Danzl DF, Pozos RS, Hamlet MP. Accidental hypothermia. In: Auerbach PS, ed. *Management of Wilderness and Environmental Emergencies.* 3rd ed. St. Louis: Mosby; 1995.

17 Pozos RS, Danzl DF. Human physiological responses to cold, stress and hypothermia. In: Pandolf KB, Burr, eds. *Textbooks of Military Medicine: Medical Aspects of Harsh Environments,* vol. 1. Falls Church, Va: Office of the Surgeon General, U.S. Army; 2002: 351–82.

18 Ginsberg MD, et al. Temperature modulation of ischemic brain injury – a synthesis of recent advances. *Prog Brain Res.* 1993;96:13.

19 Wilkerson J. *Medicine for mountaineering.* 5th ed. Seattle: Mountaineers Books; 2001: 266–8.

20 Kinzinger R, Risse M, Puschel K. Irrational behavior in exposure to cold: paradoxical undressing in hypothermia. *Arch Kriminol.* 1991;187:47.

21 Auerbach PS. Some people are dead when they're cold and dead. *JAMA.* 1990;264:1856.

22 Bjornstad H, Tande PM, Refsum H. Cardiac electrophysiology during hypothermia: implications for medical treatment. *Arctic Med Res.* 1991;50:71.

23 Sterba JA. Efficacy and safety of prehospital rewarming techniques to treat accidental hypothermia. *Ann Emerg Med.* 1991;20:896.

24 Stoneham MD, Squires SJ. Prolonged resuscitation in acute deep hypothermia. *Anaesthesia.* 1992;47:784.

25 Gonzalez RR. Biophysics of heat exchange and clothing: applications to sports physiology. *Med Exer Nutr Health.* 1995;4.

26 Position stand. American College of Sports Medicine: prevention of cold injuries during exercise. *Med Sci Sports Exer.* 2006.

27 Daanen H, et al. The effect of body temperature on the hunting response of the middle finger skin temperature. *Eur J Appl Physiol.* 1997;76:538–43.

28 Kamler K. *Surviving the Extremes.* New York: St. Martins Press; 2004.

29 Sawka MN, Young AJ. Physical exercise in hot and cold climates. In: Garrett WE, Kirkendall DT, eds. *Exercise and Sport Science.* Philadelphia: Lippincott, Williams & Wilkins; 2000: 385–400.

30 Position stand. American College of Sports Medicine: exercise and fluid replacement. *Med Sci Sports Exer.* 1996; 28(1).

31 Sato K. The mechanism of eccrine sweat secretion. In: Gisolf C, et al., eds. *Exercise, Heat and Thermoregulation.* Dubuque, Iowa: Brown & Benchmark; 1993: 85–117.

32 Gaffin SL, Moran DS. Pathophysiology of heat-related illnesses. In: Auerbach P, ed. *Wilderness Medicine.* 4th ed. St. Louis: Mosby; 2001.

33 Dematte JE, et al. Near-fatal heatstroke during the 1995 heat wave in Chicago. *Ann Intern Med.* 1998;129:173.

34 Wilkerson J. *Medicine for Mountaineering.* 5th ed. Seattle: Mountaineers Books; 2001: 279–80.

35 Wenger CB. Human heat acclimatization. In: Pandolf KB, Sawka MN, Gonzalez RR, eds. *Human Performance Physiology and Environmental Medicine at Terrestrial Extremes.* Indianapolis: Benchmark; 1988: 153–97.

36 Sonna L, Sawka M, Lilly C. Exertional heat illness and human gene expression. In: Sharma H, ed. *Progress in Brain Research,* vol. 162. New York: Elsevier Press; 2007.

COL Ian S. Wedmore, MD, FACEP, FAWM, and LTC John G. McManus, MD, MCR, FACEP

INTRODUCTION

In the twenty-first century, it is an unfortunate fact that individuals on an expedition could become victims of penetrating and/or explosive trauma, whether as a result of being accidentally shot from hunting occurring nearby, becoming inadvertently shot while being caught up in political turmoil, or being involved in an explosive event that is not uncommon in many parts of the world. The medical provider treating penetrating and explosive trauma in the austere environment is faced with multiple challenges including a lack of medical supplies, prolonged evacuation time, and distance and lack of sophisticated care that is the standard for trauma care in the urban environment. This chapter will cover the evaluation and treatment of penetrating and explosive injuries in the austere environment.

PHYSICS AND EPIDEMIOLOGY

Ballistics

The energy available for a missile to inflict upon the body is dependent on the equation $E = \frac{1}{2}MV^2$, where M is the mass of the bullet (larger bullets impart more energy) and V is the velocity of the bullet as it hits the tissue. Thus, in most cases, the potential damage is greatest with a high velocity round such as that seen with modern assault rifles and high-velocity hunting weapons.

For missile injuries, there are two areas of projectile–tissue interaction.

The first is a permanent cavity, which is a localized area of necrotic tissue and clot, proportional to the size of the projectile as it passes through. The second is a temporary cavity (cavitation) caused by the displacement of tissue away from the passage of the projectile. This temporary cavity results in an area of contusion and concussion some distance from the actual path of the bullet. The amount of damage done to tissue depends on the amount of energy transferred to the tissue as well as the elastic properties of the tissue itself. Elastic tissues, such as skeletal muscle, blood vessels, and skin, may be displaced significantly due to cavitation but then rebound with minimal permanent injury. Inelastic tissue, such as bone, brain, or liver, handles cavitation poorly and tends to fracture resulting in significant damage. There is also a shock (sonic) wave that passes through the tissue; this shock wave does not cause any appreciable clinical effect.[1,2]

Despite the fact that the energy that can be imparted to a tissue is potentially most dependent on V^2, the commonly held belief that high-velocity rounds always cause increased tissue damage is incorrect. Velocity is one factor in wounding. An increase in velocity does not de facto increase the amount of tissue damage. High-velocity rounds, if they do not impact bone or relatively inelastic tissues such as brain or solid organs (liver), shatter or yaw in the tissue they impact may pass through imparting little destructive energy.[3]

For example, the amount of tissue damage in the first 12 cm of an M-16A1 bullet wound has relatively little soft tissue disruption, similar to that of a .22 long rifle bullet, which has less than half the velocity (Figure 32.1).[4] The human thigh is approximately 12 cm wide in the average individual, so a high-velocity round may pass through the body before it imparts any significant energy outside of the bullet path.

It has been suggested that high-velocity bullets will yaw in the tissue, which can create irregular wounds increasing tissue damage. Projectiles actually do yaw minimally in flight; however, unless a projectile hits an intermediate target, the amount of yaw in flight is insignificant from a wounding or wound care perspective. Yaw in tissue is in fact also seldom a consideration as the bullets will not yaw until they penetrate deeply into the body. The AK-47 (7.62mm) bullet, for example, does not yaw until it has penetrated 25 cm into tissue (thus, in most cases, the bullet has already passed through the body before it has reached a depth sufficient to yaw) (Figures 32.2 and 32.3).[5] The AK-74 (5.45mm) assault rifle round, however, does yaw relatively early (after about 7 cm of penetration), which may cause increased tissue damage.

Fragmentation of a bullet will also lead to increased tissue damage. The bullet fragments deviate out of the original bullet path in a multitude of directions and velocities causing damage to all the tissue they pass through. Full metal-jacketed military rounds – in accordance with the Hague agreement of 1899 – are designed to remain intact in the body though many will, in fact, fragment after a certain distance in tissue. For example, the M-193 bullet of the M-16A1 rifle reliably fragments after traversing about 15 cm of soft tissue (see Figure 32.1).[6] Thus again, the bullet may have passed through the body before it fragments, or if it enters tissue greater than

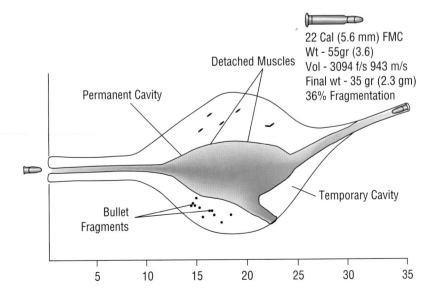

22 Cal (5.6 mm) FMC
Wt - 55gr (3.6)
Vol - 3094 f/s 943 m/s
Final wt - 35 gr (2.3 gm)
36% Fragmentation

Figure 32.1. M16 5.56mm round. The temporary cavity does not occur until the round is more than 12 cm into the tissue. The greatest damage from this round occurs because of its fragmentation at about 15 cm of depth. If the tissue is only 12 cm in diameter (such as the human thigh) and no bone is hit, the round would pass through without causing a huge amount of trauma. Source: U.S. Department of Defense.

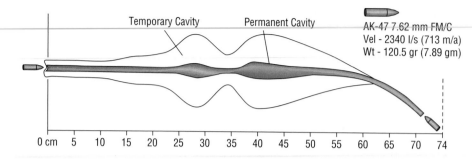

Temporary Cavity   Permanent Cavity

AK-47 7.62 mm FM/C
Vel - 2340 l/s (713 m/a)
Wt - 120.5 gr (7.89 gm)

0 cm 5 10 15 20 25 30 35 40 45 50 55 60 65 70 74

Figure 32.2. AK47 round. The bullet does not yaw until it is 25 cm into tissue, which in almost all cases means it would have passed through a tissue before it yawed. This can, however, occur if the bullet strikes along the length of the body (see Figure 32.3). Source: U.S. Department of Defense.

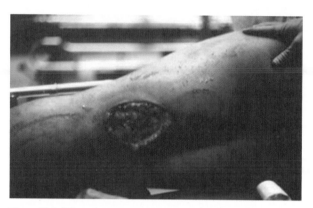

Figure 32.3. Effect of yaw and cavitation from an AKM round. The round entered in the distal calf and traversed along the length of the leg exiting the proximal thigh. This wound was along the path of the projectile at approximately 30 cm where the bullet would have been expected to yaw and create a larger permanent cavity as well as a large amount of cavitation. Photo courtesy of Ian Wedmore.

almost instantaneous transformation of the physical space occupied by original solid or liquid material into gases, filling the same volume within a few microseconds and therefore being under extremely high pressure. The highly pressurized gasses expand rapidly and compress the surrounding environment, generating a pressure pulse that is propagated as a blast wave. As a blast wave passes through the body, it causes damage by several different mechanisms. Patients injured from explosions usually suffer from a combination of blast, blunt, penetrating, and burn injuries (Table 32.1).

Firearm Types

Firearms may be categorized along several lines when evaluating their lethality and probable wounding pattern. When discussing firearm basics it is easiest to

12 cm in depth, it causes significant damage due to multiple fragments formed. Military rounds and assault rifles are in fact designed to wound (though often severely) rather than kill, as wounded individuals require greater resources to evacuate and care for than those killed outright.[7]

Here is one last thought about bullet wounding: It has been often stated that exit wounds are always greater than entrance wounds. This has been shown to be frequently not the case and has no bearing on care, which is always in response to the wound regardless of whether it is an entrance or exit wound.[8]

Explosive

An explosion is caused by the rapid chemical conversion of a liquid or solid material into a gas with a resultant energy release. Low explosives (gunpowder) release energy slowly, by a process called deflagration. In contrast, high-explosive detonation involves the

Table 32.1. Categories of explosive injuries

Category	Mechanism	Injury type
Primary	A form of barotrauma, unique to explosions, which causes damage to air-filled organs	• Blast lung • Tympanic membrane rupture and middle ear damage • Abdominal hemorrhage and perforation • Globe (eye) rupture • Concussion
Secondary	Penetrating trauma caused by the acceleration of shrapnel and other debris by the blast	• Penetrating ballistic (fragmentation) • Blunt injuries • Eye penetration
Tertiary	Casualty becomes a missile and is propelled through the air, with typical patterns of blunt trauma	• Fracture and traumatic amputation • Blunt chest and abdominal trauma • Impalement • Closed and open brain injury
Quaternary	All other explosion-related injuries, illnesses, or diseases which are not due to primary, secondary, or tertiary mechanisms	• Burns (flash, partial, and full thickness) • Crush injuries • Exacerbation of underlying conditions (i.e., asthma, COPD, angina) • Inhalation injury

consider them as handguns, long guns (rifles, assault rifles), submachine guns, and shotguns. When considering the wounding patterns it is easiest to break weapons down into low-velocity versus high-velocity weapons.

Handguns

Handguns are one of the most common causes of penetrating trauma in the United States and are also ubiquitous throughout the world. Handguns are all low-velocity weapons with a short effective range of less than 50 meters, and in the authors' experience typically less than 20 meters for all but well-trained combat marksmen. The importance of this is that if faced by a handgun your chance of not being hit increases significantly as you get beyond 20 meters or more from the assailant and exponentially greater as you get beyond 50 meters. Handguns are the weapon of choice for many police forces and criminals worldwide because they are easy to carry concealed or otherwise and can be utilized in close quarters. Because of these factors, handguns are utilized for close combat and self-defense rather than as a primary military weapon. Examples include the Beretta M9 (the standard US military pistol, see Figure 32.4), Glock pistols, the Colt 45 revolvers, Makarav pistols and, of course, "Dirty Harry's" 44 magnum.

Long Guns

Rifles, carbines, and assault rifles all comprise the long gun group. These are the predominant military and hunting weapons encountered in the world today. They predominantly are very high-velocity weapons with effective ranges of several hundred meters (up to 500 m or longer, but typically the effective range is around 200 m). The AK-47 (AKM), M-16, M-4 carbine, AK-74, German G-3, hunting rifles, and all sniper rifles are part of this class. These guns cannot typically be outrun or outdistanced unless you are already far away from the person shooting at you. They are most effective and accurate when fired on semi-automatic (single

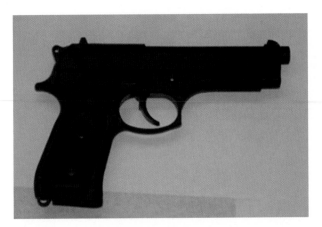

Figure 32.4. M9 Berretta 9mm handgun, the standard pistol of the U.S. military. Photo courtesy of Ian Wedmore.

controlled shots) as they recoil off target easily when fired on full automatic. To quote Robert Young Pelton in his book, *The Worlds Most Dangerous Places*: "If a soldier is careful when squeezing off single shots, he is probably trying to kill you. If soldiers are using full automatic it means you have scared the daylights out of them or they are attacking".[9] The M-16A2 will not fire on full automatic (it is limited to a maximum three-round burst) specifically to reduce the waste of ammunition. Unless you are behind solid cover when threatened with or being fired upon by a long gun within several hundred meters, your chances of being severely wounded are extremely high. Assault rifles are the most common military rifle in the world today and are simply a selective fire (capable of firing single shots or semi- or fully automatic) rifle or carbine.

Submachine Guns

Submachine guns can fire on full automatic but utilize a pistol cartridge for a bullet. They therefore are designed for close combat and self-defense at closer ranges but are lower-velocity weapons than long guns. Examples include the Uzi submachine gun and the MP5.

WEAPON VELOCITY

Low-velocity weapons (less than 2,000 ft/sec and typically less than 1,100 ft/sec) do not as a general rule cause significant tissue cavitation. They also have less propensity to cause significant soft tissue damage. Almost all civilian handguns are prime examples – these cause the majority of urban penetrating injuries.

High-velocity weapons (greater than 2,000 ft/sec) have the potential to cause significant soft tissue damage due to cavitation. Examples include the M-16, M-4 carbine, AK-47(M), and the AK-74 assault rifles. High-velocity civilian hunting rifles have a propensity to cause the most significant tissue damage. They fire large bullets at high velocity, and the bullets are not metal jacketed so they fragment and yaw quickly. These bullets are designed specifically to impart massive tissue damage early.[10] In fact, unjacketed bullets can cause a wound cavity up to 40 times the size of a jacketed bullet.[11]

Commonly Encountered Assault Weapons

The AK-47 rifle is probably the most common weapon seen throughout the world. Originally designed by Russian engineer Mikhail Kalashnikov, it is cheap, easy to use and mass produce, easy to field strip and fix, and easy to utilize by minimally trained individuals. The actual rifle name is the AKM (essentially "modernized" Automated Kalashnikov, Figure 32.5), which replaced the original 1947 AK design in 1959. Yet AK-47 remains the commonly used term to describe most AK rifles. The AK rifle series has an effective range of around

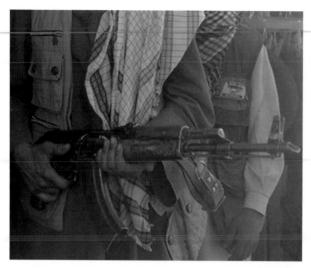

Figure 32.5. Afghan local with AKM rifle. Photo courtesy of Ian Wedmore.

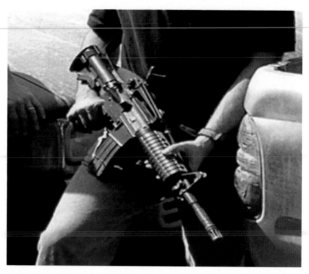

Figure 32.6. M4 carbine. Photo courtesy of Ian Wedmore.

200–300 meters. When firing the standard full metal-jacketed bullet, there is a 25-cm path of relatively minimal tissue disruption before the projectile begins to yaw. This is why relatively minimal tissue disruption may be seen with some wounds.

The AKM was replaced as the standard Soviet infantry assault rifle in 1974 by the AK-74. The AK-74 rifle utilizes a smaller 5.45mm round compared to the AK-47. As previously mentioned, the AK-74 round tends to yaw early at 7 cm; thus, it is more likely to cause increased tissue damage.

The M-16A1 and M-4 carbine (Figure 32.6) fire a 55-grain full metal-jacketed bullet (M-193) at approximately 950 meters/second. The full metal-jacketed bullet (Figure 32.7) penetrates about 12 cm, before it yaws to about 90 degrees, flattens, and then breaks at the cannalure.[4]

There are many types of bullets now used in weapons: incendiary rounds, designed to set fire to whatever they hit; hollow point or "dum dum" bullets designed to flatten when they hit tissue and thus increase tissue damage

earlier upon striking the target and not penetrate objects; armor-piercing rounds designed to penetrate the light armor of vehicles. Clinically this myriad of rounds will cause lesser or greater tissue damage and there is nothing relevant for wound care based solely on what type of round was fired, it is the wound you are looking at and treating rather than what caused it that's important.[12]

In sum, the most important determinant of tissue damage is the amount of energy transferred to the tissue rather than whether the wound is caused by a high- or low-velocity injury. A high-velocity projectile may pass through the body imparting little energy to the tissues and thus only result in a wound similar to a low-energy transfer wound. The depth to which a bullet penetrates can affect wounding – wounds that penetrate to great depth without exiting the body will yaw and fragment, imparting significant damage to the tissues – as well as whether the bullet or fragment hits bone (both cause significant tissue damage due to the fragmentation or in the case of hitting bone the creation of secondary missiles and trauma). Each wound must be approached

Figure 32.7. Standard full metal jacket military rounds found commonly throughout the world. Photo courtesy of Ian Wedmore.

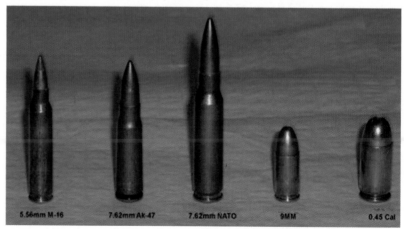

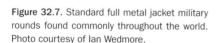

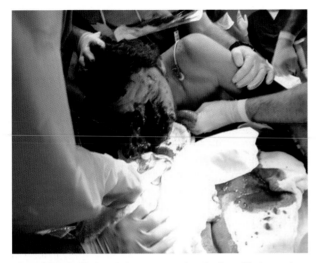

Figure 32.8. Self-induced shotgun wound to the face. Photo courtesy of Ian Wedmore.

individually with those that cause massive tissue injury requiring more extensive debridement than those with minimal tissue damage regardless of being caused by high-or low-velocity projectiles. In other words, treat the wound you are seeing and don't worry about some hidden deep "silent trauma."

Shotgun Wounds

Shotguns at close range are among the most destructive of all weapons as they disperse all of their energy into the affected tissue within a short distance. Shotgun wounds sustained at short ranges (< 3 meters) can be particularly devastating with massive tissue destruction, and the shotgun wadding also penetrates the wound leading to soft tissue contamination and bacterial proliferation (Figure 32.8).[13] In contrast, however, shotguns wounds sustained at a distance may cause minimal injury.[14]

Short-range shotgun wounds will usually require extensive debridement and wound care best carried out in an operating room.[15,16] Field care will be as for all wounds: control of bleeding and if possible removal of necrotic tissue and copious irrigation of the wound.

Grenades and RPGs

Grenades are explosive antipersonnel charges designed to be thrown by hand (hand grenades) or fired from a rifle (rifle grenades) to kill, maim, and otherwise incapacitate an enemy (Figure 32.9). Hand grenades may be subdivided into offensive and defensive grenades. All types of grenade have a high-explosive core, which gives them a blast effect. Offensive grenades are designed to have a limited blast effect (casualty radius), which is smaller than the throwing distance of the grenade so that an assaulter in the open will not be injured by the grenade he has just thrown. Offensive grenades therefore either only utilize the base high-explosive charge core without any shrapnel producing cover or utilize a small charge to limit the diameter of the shrapnel to less than the distance the grenade can be thrown. Defensive grenades have a shrapnel-producing cover over the explosive core. This cover may be made of notched wire, ball bearing, or other metal designed to fragment. They are designated defensive grenades as the fragments can travel farther than the distance the grenade can be thrown and thus must be utilized from cover to prevent the thrower from becoming injured. Many grenades can be converted from offensive to defensive by sliding a fragmentation sheath over the core. Grenades therefore cause injury through their blast effect, the shrapnel they produce, or both.

The rocket-propelled grenade (RPG) is a shoulder fired antitank weapon that has been around in its most recent form, the RPG7, since the 1960s (Figures 32.10 and 32.11). It was derived from antitank weapons of World

Figure 32.9. An M61 grenade from the Vietnam era and an MK II grenade, a common U.S. grenade from World War II. Photo courtesy of Ian Wedmore.

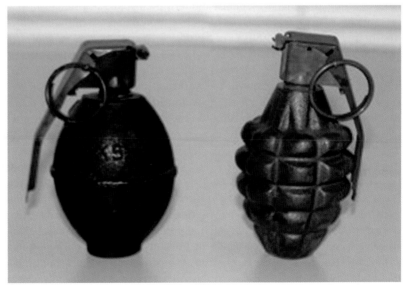

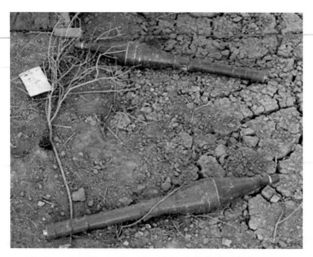

Figure 32.10. RPG7 warheads. Photo courtesy of Ian Wedmore.

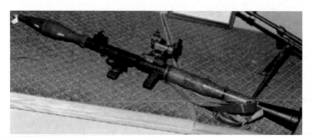

Figure 32.11. RPG7. Photo courtesy of U.S. Department of Defense, Nellis Air Force Base.

War II, most prominently the German Panzerfaust. The RPG7 is the most common form seen worldwide and is used by armies, terrorists, and insurgents throughout the world. If you encounter an RPG in your travels, it will most likely be an RPG7. The RPG7 is very common in both the third world and conflict zones worldwide, where it can be purchased cheaply. (One could be purchased for $50 in Iraq in early 2007.) Although the RPG7 is not particularly effective against modern main battle tanks, it is very effective against lightly armored and unarmored vehicles, buildings, and bunkers. An antipersonnel warhead is available for the RPG7, but it is very uncommon. Most RPG injuries result from the blast effect or shrapnel from whatever the warhead hits. The standard effective range of most RPG warheads is several hundred meters with a maximum range of up to a kilometer.

EXPLOSIVE DEVICES

Because of the current increased terrorist threat and occurrence in many countries, many different explosive devices can be purposefully or accidentally encountered by adventure seekers even outside of previous "war" zones. Most accidental explosive injuries occur from handling or encountering mines, improvised explosive devices (IEDs), or unexploded ordnance (UXO) such as grenades and ammunition. In Afghanistan alone, the death and injury rate was 150–300 per month from accidental UXO even before the current war.

An IED is frequently difficult to detect because it is often uses common items and can be made up of almost any type of material and initiator. It is a "homemade" device that causes injury or death by using explosives alone or in combination with toxic chemicals, biological toxins, or radiological material. IEDs can utilize commercial or military explosives, homemade explosives, or military ordnance and can be found in varying sizes, functioning methods, containers, and delivery methods.

Landmines

Landmines have been sown by the millions around the world, and travel through war-torn or formerly war-torn areas can unfortunately lead to injury from landmines. In fact, a landmine injury reportedly occurs worldwide every 20 minutes.[17] As of 1998, the most heavily mined countries in the world are Egypt (primarily in the Sinai), Iran, Angola, Afghanistan, Iraq, Cambodia, Bosnia, Croatia, and Mozambique with over 85 million mines found in these combined countries.[18] In 2000–1 Afghanistan had the highest number of landmine casualties in the world.[19] Landmines militarily are used primarily as a defensive measure; to protect an area, or as an area denial weapon (to keep individuals out of a piece of terrain, to prevent them from attacking it, or to prevent their travel through it). In recent conflicts, landmines have been used much more indiscriminately to deny individuals their places of work and living, for instance, or solely to cause maiming and death. Landmines can be found anywhere, but they are predominately located around military installations, on specific roads and paths to prevent their use, in fields to prevent their use, in villages to prevent people from living in them, and then unfortunately just about anywhere else as an indiscriminant cause of death and disability. The best source of dangerous versus non-dangerous areas will be the locals in that area. Minefield maps, even if made by those who placed them, are at best unreliable. In highly mined areas, stay on concrete or metaled roads (avoid potholes and recently filled areas) or solid rock. In areas in Afghanistan where significant mine clearing has been performed, risk areas will be marked by red markers with cleared areas marked by white markers. These areas, however, are not traveled without risk. While minefields are theoretically laid according to set patterns, these patterns are so unreliable they are not worth learning.

The Ottawa Convention of 1997 is a UN-sponsored international effort to ban the use of antipersonnel landmines worldwide. As of 2007, it has 155 signatories and 153 countries that have ratified it. Forty countries, however, have not signed or ratified it including the United States, China, North Korea, and Iran among others, nor have any terrorist or insurgent groups agreed to abide by the convention. Despite this, the convention has provided the impetuous for demining to occur in those countries affected the most by heavy mining.

Removing mines requires a lot of time, personnel, and effort. Therefore, even in areas free from conflict, it would not be unusual for the third-world traveler to encounter those involved in demining operations. Despite their training, these individuals are at risk from mines and may end up being patients you have to treat. Demining is done utilizing demining vehicles, metal detectors, and mine dogs that detect mines by the scent given off by the explosive. There are numerous demining organizations worldwide including for-profit agencies and many non-profit and government-supported demining operations; the UN alone has 11 departments or agencies involved in demining.

Landmines are explosive devices that discharge when stepped on or otherwise triggered and are of several types. The two largest categories are antipersonnel and antitank mines. Antipersonnel mines include blast and bounding types. Blast mines are typically pressure-activated and explode when stepped on (Figure 32.12); they thus usually only injure the person who stepped on it. Bounding mines on the other hand are designed to cause multiple injured patients and/or casualties. When "tripped" either by being stepped upon or by activating a trip wire, these bounding mines leap into the air to about chest level and explode, spray-

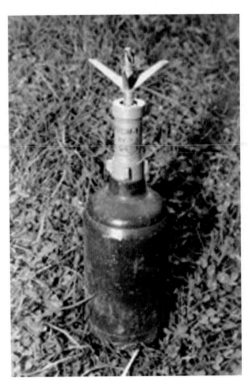

Figure 32.13. Prom-1 Yugoslavian bounding mine. *Source:* U.S. Department of Defense.

ing metal fragments in all directions for many meters (Figures 32.13 and 32.14).

Antitank mines are usually pressure-activated and contain a large amount of explosive since they are designed to immobilize and destroy armored vehicles (Figures 32.15 and 32.16). While antitank mines usually require significant pressure to activate (usually 350 lb of pressure or more) and should therefore be "safe" if stepped on by an individual this should never be assumed. They are often co-placed or booby-trapped with antipersonnel mines to prevent their removal. Many mines also contain anti-tampering devices, which will cause them to detonate when handled.

Landmines cause injuries by their blast effect as well as shrapnel effect. Antipersonnel blast mines are designed primarily to incapacitate and maim when stepped upon. The blast shreds the lower extremity and imbeds dirt and other foreign material into the extremity along the tissue planes (Figures 32.17 and 32.18). It may also cause injuries to the genitals and lower abdomen as the blast travels upward into the standing individual. At the least, the injured individual will require extensive debridement and amputation of the affected extremity. Immediate care of this injury consists of controlling bleeding, providing pain control, cleaning the wound, and evacuating the individual to definitive surgical care as soon as possible.

Bounding mines, on the other hand, cause multiple penetrating wounds to the entire body, particularly the

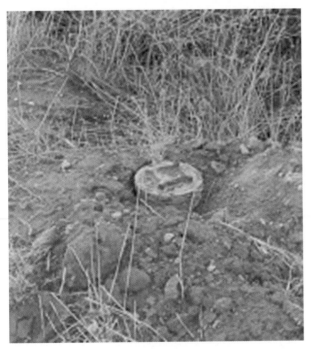

Figure 32.12. Antipersonnel landmine. Photo courtesy of Ian Wedmore.

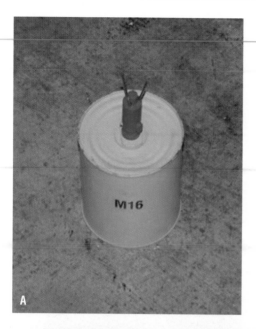

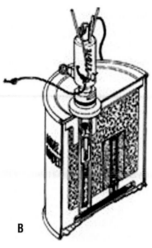

Figure 32.14 (A) M16 U.S. dummy bounding mine. When activated, the M16 leaps to a height of 1.5 meters and explodes, sending fragments to a 30-meter radius. Photo courtesy Ian Wedmore. (B) Cutaway of M16 bounding mine. Courtesy of U.S. Department of Defense.

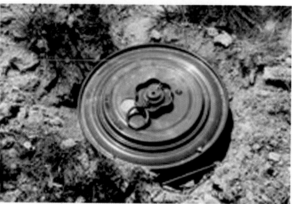

Figure 32.15. TM46 Soviet antitank mine. Photo courtesy of U.S. Department of Defense.

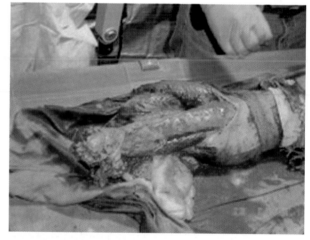

Figure 32.17. Lower extremity injury from antipersonnel landmine. Photo courtesy of T. Gerlinger.

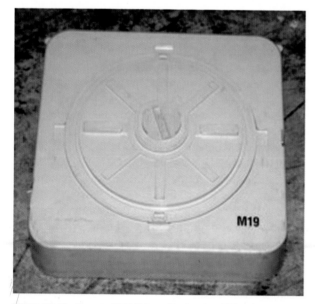

Figure 32.16. Dummy M19 U.S. antitank mine. This mine requires 100–200 kg of pressure to activate. Photo courtesy of Ian Wedmore.

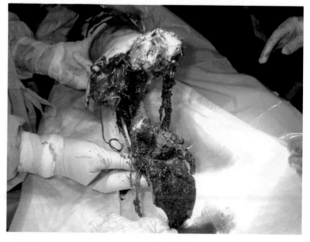

Figure 32.18. Lower extremity injury from landmine. The extensive dirt and contaminated material blown into the wound can be seen. Photo courtesy of T. Gerlinger.

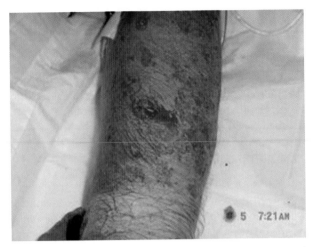

Figure 32.19. Multiple small fragment wounds from antipersonnel mine. Photo courtesy of T. Gerlinger.

chest and lower abdomen, as this is the typical level they "bound" to before exploding. Those close to the mine are hit by large high-velocity fragments; those farther away are at risk of being hit by smaller, slower fragments (Figure 32.19).

Body Armor

One method commonly employed to reduce injury from penetrating projectiles is to use body armor. Body armor or "bullet-proof vests" are commonly used by the military and law enforcement as well as now by terrorist groups. These bullet-proof vests have been shown to be effective in saving lives. According to the U.S. Department of Justice, as of 2005 over 2,700 law enforcement deaths have been prevented by body armor in the United States alone (20). Body armor provides varying degrees of protection from penetrating and blast injury depending on the type and protection factor. The mainstay of body armor is a high-tech mesh. Originally constructed from Kevlar (thus the common name "Kevlar vest"), they are now made from several types of ballistic cloth such as Dyneema, Spectra, and Twaron in addition to Kevlar. This tightly woven ballistic cloth is designed to "net" a projectile slowing it and dispersing its force. Ballistic vests will stop most low-velocity rounds, but they are not effective against high-velocity rounds. To prevent the penetration of high-velocity rounds, a ceramic or metal plate capable of preventing penetration must be added to the ballistic vest. The U.S. National Institute of Justice (USNIJ) has developed standards for the level of protection provided by body armor (Table 32.2).

Most law enforcement vests worn under clothing are Type II and IIA, which will stop most low-velocity bullets, and thus are very effective against handguns but not against high-velocity rifle rounds. Vests must typically be IIIA or better to resist submachine gun rounds. IIIA

Table 32.2. USNIJ classification standards for ballistic resistance of personal body armor[22]

Type I (22 LR; 380 ACP)
This armor protects against. 22 caliber Long Rifle Lead Round Nose (LR LRN) bullets, with nominal masses of 2.6 g (40 gr) impacting at a minimum velocity of 320 m/s (1050 ft/s) or less, and 380 ACP Full Metal-Jacketed Round Nose (FMJ RN) bullets, with nominal masses of 6.2 g (95 gr) impacting at a minimum velocity of 312 m/s (1025 ft/s) or less.

Type IIA (9mm; 40 S&W)
This armor protects against 9mm Full Metal-Jacketed Round Nose (FMJ RN) bullets, with nominal masses of 8.0 g (124 gr) impacting at a minimum velocity of 332 m/s (1090 ft/s) or less, and Smith & Wesson (S&W) 40 caliber Full Metal-Jacketed (FMJ) bullets, with nominal masses of 11.7 g (180 gr) impacting at a minimum velocity of 312 m/s (1025 ft/s) or less.

Type II (9 mm; 357 Magnum)
This armor protects against 9mm Full Metal-Jacketed Round Nose (FMJ RN) bullets, with nominal masses of 8.0 g (124 gr) impacting at a minimum velocity of 358 m/s (1175 ft/s) or less, and 357 Magnum Jacketed Soft Point (JSP) bullets, with nominal masses of 10.2 g (158 gr) impacting at a minimum velocity of 427 m/s (1400 ft/s) or less.

Type IIIA (High-velocity 9mm; 44 Magnum)
This armor protects against 9mm Full Metal-Jacketed Round Nose (FMJ RN) bullets, with nominal masses of 8.0 g (124 gr) impacting at a minimum velocity of 427 m/s (1400 ft/s) or less, and 44 Magnum Semi Jacketed Hollow Point (SJHP) bullets, with nominal masses of 15.6 g (240 gr) impacting at a minimum velocity of 427 m/s (1400 ft/s) or less.

Type III (Rifles)
This armor protects against 7.62mm Full Metal-Jacketed (FMJ) bullets (U.S. Military designation M80), with nominal masses of 9.6 g (148 gr) impacting at a minimum velocity of 838 m/s (2750 ft/s) or less.

Type IV (Armor-Piercing Rifle)
This armor protects against .30 caliber armor-piercing bullets (U.S. Military designation M2 AP), with nominal masses of 10.8 g (166 gr) impacting at a minimum velocity of 869 m/s (2850 ft/s) or less.

armor is also the highest level that is "soft armor" and typically available to wear as concealed armor. To resist high-velocity rifle rounds, armor must be type III or IV. This requires the use of ceramic or metal plates in addition to the ballistic cloth. This level of protection is seen in armor worn by SWAT teams and the military. To prevent penetration by high-velocity rounds, the present U.S. military interceptor body armor utilizes a ceramic SAPI (small arms penetration insert) plate, which is designed to prevent the penetration of three hits from 7.62mm high-velocity rounds fired from 10 meters (Figures 32.20 and 32.21). All body armor is also effective at preventing the penetration of low-velocity fragments from grenades and explosives. High-velocity

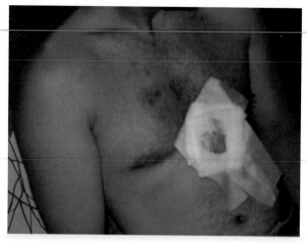

Figure 32.20. Injury from a close range (< 5 meter) hit in the SAPI plate of body armor from an AKM assault rifle. Without body armor this would have been fatal; in this case, it resulted only in a chest wall contusion. Photo courtesy of Ian Wedmore.

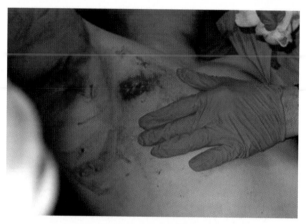

Figure 32.21. Soft Tissue wound to chest wall from AKM rifle. This will need irrigation and dressing only. Photo courtesy of Ian Wedmore.

fragments may penetrate depending on the level of armor and velocity and mass of the fragment. While not a care issue per se, when providing medical oversight to military and law enforcement, it is crucial to reinforce their wearing of body armor as this can do more to prevent injury than anything you can do after the fact. One potential risk from body armor use is that wearing soft armor may be enough to slow a high-velocity bullet to a point at which it will yaw or fragment in the tissues rather than passing "cleanly" through if it hadn't hit the body armor first. In the few studies available, it appears that lower levels of body armor did not affect the velocity of penetrating high-velocity rounds, but as the body armor became thicker, it tended to induce some bullet instability.[21] However, yet again, this does not matter as far as the wound care is concerned, if a bullet does yaw more, it will cause a large wound that will be obvious when it is examined and treated.

WOUND MANAGEMENT

Soft Tissue Wounds

Military wounds and other penetrating wounds sustained in the austere environment are all considered to be contaminated wounds. Treatment should therefore proceed based on this assumption.

Non-Life-Threatening Wounds

Non-life-threatening wounds will typically involve an extremity. These will most often be penetrating wounds, which penetrate through the tissue and exit the body, or grazing wounds, which do not penetrate deeply into body. Several standard principles apply to the treatment of all penetrating wounds. These principles include (1) adequate wound excision; (2) adequate wound drainage; (3) immobilization until the soft tissues are healed; (4) antibiotic therapy; and (5) secondary closure or coverage.[23] All wounds will require that these principles be applied to some extent.

The wound should be debrided minimally of any obviously dead tissue at the entrance and exit. Conservative debridement of only obviously necrotic tissue is preferred to overexuberant debridement of tissue that may be potentially salvageable.[24] The excision of necrotic tissue should remove enough skin from the entrance and exit wounds to allow for adequate wound drainage.

The wound must then be adequately irrigated. This requires the wound to be irrigated with a pressure of at least 7 psi at the wound surface.[25,26] By using a 30–60 cc syringe with an 18-gauge needle or catheter on it, 7 psi can be generated. The quantity of fluid utilized is enough to make the wound appear "clean" though as a general rule at least 250 cc fluid should be used per wound at a minimum. Larger volumes are better than smaller, and there really is no such thing as "too much wound irrigation."

Even though sterile saline or water is the hospital standard for wound irrigation, tap water has been shown to be just as effective without any increased risk of wound infection.[27–30] In the austere environment, since neither sterile saline, sterile water, nor tap water is usually available, any potable water source may be utilized. If water is drinkable, it will be effective. Hydrogen peroxide, bleach solutions, antibiotic solutions, and iodine solutions are no more effective than water for wound cleansing and may actually be deleterious as many of these solutions are tissue toxic.

The wound after irrigation is loosely packed with gauze to allow for free drainage. After the wound is dressed, it can be left covered and dressed until definitive care is reached (up to 72 hours). The dressing need only be removed, evaluated, or changed if there is increased drainage, or pain or fever develops. The injured extremity should be splinted to prevent further soft tissue damage. Penetrating extremity wounds should be treated with antibiotics as soon as possible. This will be covered later in the antibiotic section of this chapter.

Penetrating wounds from projectiles should never be closed primarily. This will lead to an increased risk of infection.[31–33] These wounds, if required, can be closed secondarily 3–6 days after the initial injury. This delay allows the body's host defenses to reduce the wound bacterial counts back down to zero at which time closure can be carried out with a minimal effect on cosmetic outcome. The exception to this is areas with significant vascularity where primary closure is associated with a minimal infection risk such as the face and scalp. These areas may be closed primarily after wound irrigation.

Individuals with penetrating wounds of the extremities are not required to be NPO during their evacuation. They can be given oral liquids for rehydration, take oral medications, and eat normally if evacuation will be prolonged.

Debridement Considerations

In the past it has been considered dogma that all high-velocity projectile tracts must be fully excised and explored, due to the effects of the temporary cavitation. Past literature has suggested that cavitation caused significant injury requiring extensive debridement, up to 30–40 times the diameter of the round.[34] This dogma has since been demonstrated to be untrue (the 30–40 times number occurs only rarely and is probably based on high-velocity hunting rounds). As previously discussed, temporary cavitation may not occur in many high-velocity wounds due to their passing through tissue before obtaining the depth at which cavitation occurs. Elastic soft tissue (skeletal muscle, blood vessels, and nerves) generally heals uneventfully and does not require excision, provided the blood supply remains intact. Temporary cavity effects are analogous to blunt trauma. Animal studies have shown that extensive debridement is not required in most high-velocity wounds.[35,36] These most recent studies on high-velocity wounds found the administration of antibiotics rather than extensive debridement was the most important factor in decreasing the wound infection rate.

Bullet Removal

Despite what most Hollywood movies would suggest, the removal of a bullet from a gunshot wound is not required in most cases. While bullets are in fact not "sterilized" by firing[37] the majority of the contamination from a penetrating round comes from the skin surface and any clothing or surface debris carried into the wound by the projectile or "sucked" into the wound by the vacuum effect of the collapse of the temporary cavitation.[38] This contamination is treated by conservative debridement and irrigation. Lead or copper poisoning does not occur from bullets unless they penetrate and reside in a synovial or cerebral spinal fluid–filled space. Bullet removal therefore is required only in cases of penetration and lodgment in the synovial spaces of the body or cerebral spinal fluid–filled neural structures. Bullets in soft tissue are quickly covered by avascular fibrous scar tissue, which prevents uptake of the metal.[39]

Shrapnel/Fragment Wounds

Shrapnel or fragment wounds are now the most common cause of civilian injuries in third-world conflicts.[40] This unfortunately also means that individuals venturing into austere regions for expeditions are more likely to be injured by fragments rather than bullets. Shrapnel and fragment wounds are managed according to the degree of tissue damaged, though in general small fragments are similar to low-energy-transfer projectiles such as handgun wounds. Large fragments (Figure 32.22) may cause wounds similar to high- or low-velocity projectiles.

Hand grenade fragments tend to cause limited soft tissue injury only as the fragments do not penetrate deeply. They also do not typically result in comminuted fractures.[41] They can often be treated by conservative debridement of only obviously dead tissue, irrigation of the wound, and dressing.[42,43] Similar to bullets, fragments in soft tissue do not require removal.[44] Doing so may lead to excessive morbidity from the probing and incisions used to retrieve the fragments. In general, if the fragments are superficial and easily removed

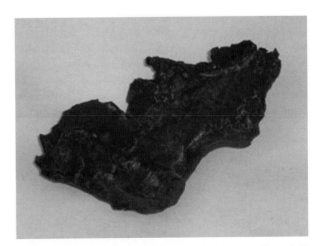

Figure 32.22. Large shrapnel piece. This is from an artillery shell. Photo courtesy of Ian Wedmore.

> High-velocity round wounds do not require aggressive or extensive debridement based *solely* on their velocity. Treat the wound not the weapon velocity.

Small (< 1 cm) fragment wounds without associated hematoma or vital structure involvement can be managed conservatively with minimal debridement and irrigation. The fragments do not need to be removed.

without complication, this can be done; if they are deeper and require substantial removal effort, they should be left in place unless infection develops at the site or as discussed previously in the bullet removal section. The International Committee of the Red Cross, based on experience gained in multiple austere theaters, recommends that soft tissue fragment wounds of less than 1 cm in size that do not have an associated hematoma or vital structure involvement should be managed conservatively.[45] This practice was successfully used by a deployed British Field Hospital during the recent Iraq conflict.[46] Large fragment wounds are treated with debridement and excision as required based on the wound.

Fractures

Fractures from penetrating ordnance and explosives are splinted and stabilized as are fractures from any traumatic cause. However, fractures from high-velocity weaponry tend to have a greater comminution rate[47] and thus are less likely to be well stabilized without surgical intervention. Fractures from low-velocity, low-energy gunshots tend to behave similarly to closed fractures and have a low incidence of infection.[23] Antibiotic prophylaxis is recommended for all fractures associated with high-velocity wounds.[48] In the urban setting, antibiotics may not be required for low-energy transfer wounds, though they are recommended for use in contaminated wounds with associated fractures. Because all austere penetrating wounds are considered "contaminated," all penetrating wounds in the austere environment with or without fractures should receive prophylactic antibiotics.

Pelvic fractures will typically be stable fractures. If unstable, however, stabilization should be undertaken as soon as possible to minimize pelvic bleeding.[49] In the austere environment, this is best carried out by use of some type of pelvic binder. The most easily performed method is to "sheet" the pelvis: a sheet is folded to the width of the pelvis, placed under it and tied across the anterior pelvis. This is a very effective method of temporarily stabilization.[50]

Airway

Civilian prehospital training often requires the placement of the victim in a supine position for evaluation and treatment. In the case of facial and airway wounds, this

may in fact be the completely wrong approach because the airway may be maintained only with the victim sitting in an upright position. In all cases in which an airway is being maintained by an individual in a certain position, the individual should be maintained in that position for evaluation and treatment. The most frequently encountered case again is the facial wound in which the airway remains patent provided the individual is maintained in a sitting–leaning forward position.

Most airway problems can be treated by simple measures such as positioning (the standard jaw-thrust or chin-lift positions) or the placement of a nasopharyngeal airway, which is tolerated by individuals in any state of consciousness. Oropharyngeal airways have little utility in the austere environment as they are poorly tolerated by all but the most deeply obtunded and offer no advantage over nasopharyngeal airways.[51] Numerous airway adjuncts are now available for prehospital use (such as the laryngeal mask airway, Combitube, and King-LT). These adjuncts are easier to effectively place[52–54] and do provide some airway protection,[55,56] though they are not effective in the case of an expanding hematoma compressing the airway or an airway compromised by direct facial trauma.

The greatest risk from penetrating wounds involving the airway is a facial wound causing tissue damage and bleeding that compromises the airway. In these cases, the treatment of choice is a cricothyroidotomy.[57] Although there is morbidity even in the emergency department associated with the procedure, the benefit in penetrating facial trauma and airway compromise typically outweighs these risks.[58]

Endotracheal intubation to provide an airway in penetrating trauma is rarely required; an exception would be a wound to the neck with expanding hematoma. In this case, the early use of intubation prior to the compression of the airway is appropriate. Intubation, however, is problematic due to the equipment required. A cricothyroidotomy kit in contrast is small and light.

With regards to explosive injuries, a high suspicion for occult explosive lung injury should be maintained, and evidence of exposure to overpressure should be determined. The treatment of pulmonary barotrauma is to support gas exchange. Casualties with immediate and severe respiratory distress or massive hemoptysis have less chance of survival, and a definitive airway should be created. In those with mild to moderate respiratory distress, placement of a simple oral or nasal airway may suffice. Oxygenation should be supported by a facemask or non-rebreather mask. Any activity should be minimized;

Simple airway maneuvers such as proper positioning and portable devices will manage most airways compromised by penetrating trauma.

exertion after a blast has been shown to increase the severity of barotraumas. Patients who deteriorate after positive pressure ventilation following explosive injury may have an arterial gas embolism (AGE). AGE is likely to be the cause of rapid death.

Torso/Chest Wounds

Superficial wounds of the chest can be treated as soft tissue wounds as previously described. Penetrating wounds of the chest will most often require tube thoracostomy for definitive treatment; the main goal until evacuation to a medical facility however is to relieve and prevent the life threat of a tension pneumothorax.[59] A needle decompression does this very effectively, and if all that is available is a large-gauge catheter (14 gauge or larger is the standard), needle decompression may be both lifesaving and effective during evacuation.

In animal models, a 14-gauge needle decompression has been shown to effectively decompress a tension pneumothorax, to maintain the decompression for the 4-hour duration of the study and to be as effective as a 32F chest tube during the same 4-hour period.[60] Human experience with needle decompression has also shown it to be as effective as tube thoracostomy in the treatment of tension pneumothorax by prehospital aeromedical providers.[61] A 14-gauge angiocath is placed in the second intercostal space, midclavicular line. The needle is removed. A rush of air will indicate that a pneumothorax has been decompressed. A one-way flutter valve should be utilized if available. This can be made by placing the angiocath through the cut-off finger of a rubber glove prior to its placement in the chest. Should the catheter kink or bend or otherwise obstruct it is left in place and another can be placed. In individuals with large pectoral muscles there may be difficulty in reaching the chest if long catheters (3.5 in.) are not used.[62] It has also been suggested that the site of needle decompression be the fifth intercostal space, midaxillary line in the case of large-chested individuals as well as a site with potentially decreased morbidity.

Open chest wounds should be sealed. This can be done by petroleum gauze and tape, plastic wrap and tape, premade chest seals, hydrogel material, or any other airtight barrier. The authors' preference at the present time is adhesive hydrogel. The standard requirement to leave one side of a closure open is no longer universally recommended. The Present Tactical Combat Casualty Care guidelines[63] do not require this as it is nearly impossible to keep one side of an occlusive dressing open in the combat – and probably also any other austere – setting. If completely sealing a chest wound, one must continue to monitor the patient for the development of a tension pneumothorax. A further rationale is that if the chest is going to be decompressed with a needle anyway then even with a "sucking chest wound," the dressing can be

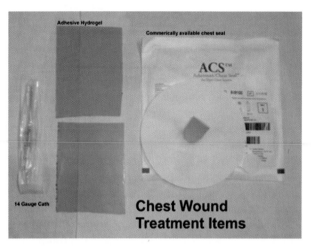

Figure 32.23. Medical items for treatment of penetrating chest trauma. Photo courtesy of Ian Wedmore.

completely sealed. Furthermore, when adhesive sheets such as hydrogel are used to seal a chest wound, it is nearly impossible to leave one side of the chest dressing open. The chest should be dried of blood and sweat as best as possible prior to dressing application because it is difficult to make any dressing stick effectively to the chest. In the authors' experience, hydrogel has the best ability to stick to a chest wound, though several companies are working on premade chest seals with stronger adhesives than are presently available (Figure 32.23).

Abdominal and Pelvic Wounds

The urban standard is that penetrating wounds of the abdomen require surgical exploration and repair in nearly all cases.[64,65] Literature from the last 10 years has shown a role for nonoperative management of selected penetrating wounds of the abdomen;[66–68] however, these cases were evaluated with multiple radiographic studies and observed in the hospital. None of these studies on selective management can be applied to penetrating abdominal wounds in the austere environment. The goal in the austere environment is therefore stabilization of the patient as effectively as possible and rapid transport. Fortunately, even with penetrating abdominal trauma and long delays in evacuation, most individuals will survive. Experience from the factional conflict of the 1980s and 1990s in Afghanistan found that of penetrating abdominal wounds presenting to an ICRC hospital, 25% took 6 hours to arrive and 75% took 6–24 hours to arrive. Nonetheless, the mortality even with delayed laparotomy (due to the patients, delayed presentation) was only between 7 and 20%, respectively.[69]

> The cause of death in penetrating chest wounds is tension pneumothorax. Although not definitive, needle decompression is the rapid treatment of choice.

The austere environment mimics the military environment in that medical supplies will often be limited and evacuation times, prolonged. The use of hypotensive resuscitation has become the standard in the military for frontline treatment of penetrating wounds that cause noncompressible hemorrhage (penetrating wounds of the abdomen or chest). Hypotensive resuscitation will be discussed later.

Penetrating wounds of the abdomen should have a dressing applied to the wound and resuscitation carried out while evacuation is underway. Individuals with penetrating wounds of the abdomen should not be given liquids or medications by mouth. Individuals with penetrating abdominal wounds will all require antibiotic prophylaxis by intravenous or intramuscular route.

Gas-containing abdominal structures are injured in a similar manner and at similar overpressures as the lung. Gastrointestinal (GI) injuries may be as common as pulmonary explosive injuries, but they are often overshadowed by the more immediately life-threatening injuries to airway and breathing. A GI explosive injury tends to affect the colon with injury ranging from edema to hemorrhage to frank rupture. Rupture of the colon, although possible acutely, is generally occult and delayed, occurring after stretching and ischemia lead to bowel wall weakening. Shear forces caused by the explosion may occasionally tear the mesentery, but nonbowel or solid organ injuries after explosions are more likely due to conventional blunt or penetrating mechanisms. Signs and symptoms are often nonspecific and include abdominal pain, nausea, vomiting, diarrhea, tenesmus, decreased bowel sounds, rebound tenderness, guarding, or rectal bleeding.

Hypotensive Resuscitation

The standard Advanced Trauma Life Support (ATLS) teaching for penetrating wounds has in the past been the initiation of two large-bore IVs and the administration of crystalloid solutions to maintain a normal blood pressure. This idea became challenged in the 1990s when it was felt that administration of IV fluids led to increased mortality with wounds causing noncompressible hemorrhage, particularly if evacuation time to definitive surgical care was prolonged. Numerous animal studies[70-73] and case series from World War I and II[74,75] suggested that IV fluid resuscitation in these cases led to a temporary rise in blood pressure, which would "pop the clot" of wounds that had ceased bleeding and lead to further hemorrhage. The administration of crystalloids would further lead to a dilution of the blood and clotting factors leading to further rebleeding and coagulopathy.

The animal studies referenced strongly support hypotensive resuscitation. The largest human study to utilize hypotensive resuscitation in humans, a study by Bickell et al. out of the Houston Ben-Taub trauma center, showed a decrease in mortality with the use of low-volume (hypotensive) resuscitation,[76] and, although criticized, it more importantly showed no decrease in survival due to the use of hypotensive resuscitation. The Cochrane Library of evidence-based medicine also looked at the volume of fluid appropriate for resuscitation and found no advantage to the use of early or large-volume fluid resuscitation.[77] Hypotensive resuscitation has become the standard for frontline combat care in the military. It is just as appropriate for utilization by expeditions or penetrating wounds in any austere environment due to the similar prolonged evacuation times to definitive medical care.

The goal of hypotensive resuscitation is to provide adequate resuscitation to delay irreversible shock in the wounded individual, while also minimizing any over-aggressive rise in blood pressure that standard resuscitation causes that leads to "popping off" the clot and dilutional coagulopathy. Studies have shown that above a systolic blood pressure of 90–95 mm is the point at which rebleeding occurs.[78] The goal of the provider therefore is to resuscitate the individual to this blood pressure but not higher. In the austere setting, this equates to resuscitating an individual with IV fluids until a palpable radial pulse is felt and a normal mental status is noted. A palpable radial pulse has been shown to be an effective field method of determining a systolic blood pressure of at least 80 mm.[79] If the pressure drops below this (radial pulse is weakly or not palpable or mental status is decreased) then small boluses of fluid (250–500 cc over 15–30 minutes) as available are given until these two criteria are met again at which time the resuscitation is stopped. In reality, this means that over a prolonged period of time several boluses may be required depending on the duration of the evacuation. Once in surgery where the bleeding can be controlled, the individual can be fully resuscitated to a normal blood pressure. In the austere environment, there is a further factor involved in the use of hypotensive resuscitation, namely the lack of medical supplies and availability of crystalloid solution.

Austere Resuscitation Fluid Choice

Medical care in the austere environment is similar to frontline military casualty care where availability of medical supplies is limited by the "weight and cube" of the

> A penetrating wound with noncompressible hemorrhage with a systolic blood pressure less than 80 (absence of a radial pulse) or an altered mental status in the absence of head injury should be given IV fluids until a radial pulse is palpated and mental status is normal, at which time resuscitation should be stopped. IV fluids are given again whenever the blood pressure drops and a radial pulse cannot be felt or mental status deteriorates (in the absence of head injury).

supplies to be carried. Controversy abounds in regard to the superiority of crystalloid versus colloids as the ideal fluid for resuscitation. At the present time, there is no definitive evidence to support the use of colloid versus crystalloid.

For austere and military use, colloids do offer a different significant advantage, the ability of a given volume of fluid to increase intravascular volume. Administration of 1,000 cc of normal saline or lactated Ringer's (LR) solution will result in only 200–250 cc of fluid ending up in the intravascular space, whereas only 150–200 cc of colloid solution will result in the same increase in intravascular volume. The entire infused volume of the colloid solution ends up in the vascular space in addition to other fluid that is pulled from the extravascular space into the vasculature by the osmotic pull of the colloid.

Colloids therefore offer the best volume expansion for a given weight and cube. Hetastarch 500 cc provides the volume expansion of 3,000 cc of LR; this makes hetastarch six times more effective in weight and cube as compared to LR. The expert consensus for frontline fluid use in the military, where evacuation times to definitive care may be 6–8 hours or longer, is low-volume colloid for U.S. forces (hetastarch-based fluids: Hespan or Hextend) and hypertonic saline dextran (HSD) for NATO forces. (HSD is not FDA approved and is therefore not available for use by U.S. forces.) HSD also offers the advantage of being antiinflammatory to the injured.[80]

All crystalloids and artificial colloids such as hetastarch induce a systemic inflammatory response in the traumatized primarily through neutrophil activation, a process that can lead to later multisystem organ failure. Hypertonic saline does not induce this response nor does the HSD.[81,82] The use of colloids is limited to 1500 cc (> 20 cc/kg) total infusion; platelet function begins to be negatively affected by hetastarch at greater volumes.[83] After this first 1500 cc (> 20 cc/kg) of colloid, if more fluid is required, crystalloid should be utilized. Hetastarch mixed in a balanced electrolyte solution, a lactate buffer, and physiological levels of glucose (Hextend) has been shown in at least one phase III trial to be superior to hetastarch in saline (Hespan).[84] Hetastarch and dextran both have a risk of anaphylaxis, the risk being approximately 0.08% for hetastarch and 0.5% for dextran.[85]

Hemorrhage Control

In the austere environment, bleeding must be controlled as quickly as possible. The teaching of direct pressure and then the use of pressure points has for

> Colloids provide the best vascular expansion for a weight and volume of fluid carried; however, no more than 1,500 cc of colloids should be given to an individual casualty.

years been the standard. This remains the mainstay for mild to moderate bleeding in the austere environment. For severe bleeding, with long transport to care times, this approach will not always work effectively. Particularly in the case of penetrating trauma and the often high associated incidence of significant venous or arterial bleeding, this approach may not be appropriate. In the combat setting, tourniquets have returned to the forefront of care for the control of major bleeding; they have the same utility for use on expeditions in austere environments.

The use of tourniquets does remain unquestionably controversial, and tourniquets have little utility in the urban setting with rapid transport times to definitive care. Conversely, in the hands of knowledgeable medical providers, tourniquets can prevent morbidity and save the life of a wounded individual in the austere setting. Modern tourniquets are light, fast, and effective and with proper use lead to rapid control of bleeding and the saving of lives with no increase in morbidity. In the Vietnam War, 10% of those who died of penetrating wounds died from compressible hemorrhage (i.e., bleeding that could have been controlled with the use of the tourniquet).[86]

In the combat setting, the tourniquet is utilized in two ways: (1) for immediate control of bleeding for a casualty while still under enemy fire (where direct pressure may not be able to be effectively applied initially); and (2) for control of bleeding when direct pressure and pressure points are not effective. Another advantage of modern tourniquets is that they can be applied and control bleeding more quickly than direct pressure and use of pressure points, thus preventing blood loss until adequate dressings can be applied to control the bleeding and the tourniquet then removed. This is particularly important if there is only one person available to render aid and bleeding control. The placement of the tourniquet allows the provider to treat more severe injuries initially and then address the bleeding when more immediate life threats are controlled. Even if there are no other life threats, rapidly placing a tourniquet allows the provider to utilize both hands to place an effective pressure dressing. It is unlikely but not impossible that you would be under fire on an expedition; however, these other reasons for the use of tourniquets provide their greatest utility for austere use.

Why are tourniquets not used routinely? Tourniquets have lost favor for civilian use due to the morbidity associated with prolonged or inappropriate use. Recent military studies have found that tourniquets both save lives and have little associated morbidity even if placed for inappropriate reasons provided they were removed within several hours.[87,88] The tourniquets now used by the military are quick and effective. The use of ad hoc tourniquets is much less likely to be effective and is much more likely to lead to severe morbidity when used. The tourniquets of choice for the U.S. Army are the CAT® (Combat Application Tourniquet) and the SOFFT tourniquet. In a comparative study of commercially available tourniquets, the CAT was found to be the best combination of compactness, lightweightness, and comfort in addition to effectively stopping arterial blood flow as measured by Doppler.[89]

A tourniquet can be applied and left in place for up to 2 hours with minimal morbidity to the effected extremity (this is the maximum duration tourniquets are left in place during orthopedic surgery without morbidity). A 2006 study on tourniquet use in orthopedic surgery (tourniquet duration less than 2 hours) found the risk of complications to be 1 in 2,442 uses and permanent injury risk to be 1 in 31,742 uses.[90] Tourniquets left on for 6 hours or more typically require the limb to be amputated distal to the tourniquet. Between 2 and 6 hours, morbidity is unclear and depends on a multitude of factors, but the longer a tourniquet is left in place the higher the likelihood of limb loss is.

A tourniquet is properly applied by applying it 1–2 inches proximal to the bleeding (Figures 32.24 and 32.25). After a tourniquet is in place and bleeding is controlled, then the wound may have further dressings, a pressure bandage, and or advanced hemostatic dressings applied. The tourniquet can then be loosened to see if bleeding is controlled. If it is, the tourniquet should be left in

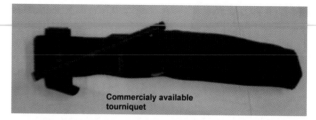

Figure 32.25. The commercially available CAT Tourniquet (Combat Application Tourniquet).

> Tourniquet use can be life-saving in penetrating trauma. The goal of tourniquet use in penetrating trauma in the austere setting is to place it quickly to save loss of blood and then to remove the tourniquet as soon as possible when bleeding is otherwise controlled.

place, but not tightened during evacuation; if bleeding restarts, the tourniquet can be retightened to control the bleeding.

Advanced Hemostatic Agents

Recent advances in hemorrhage control include the development and fielding of modern hemostatic agents. The two most commonly utilized are zeolite powder (Quickclot®) and Chitosan dressing (Hemcon® bandage or Chitoflex® bandage). Both have been shown in animal models to control severe venous and arterial hemorrhage.[91,92] Both have seen significant use in the Afghanistan and Iraqi conflicts. Chitosan (Hemcon) has been shown in an observational case series to be effective in controlling the bleeding of many penetrating wounds without significant side effects.[93] These dressings are most appropriate and effective when utilized where tourniquets cannot be utilized (e.g., neck, buttock, axilla, or groin) (Figure 32.26). They can also be

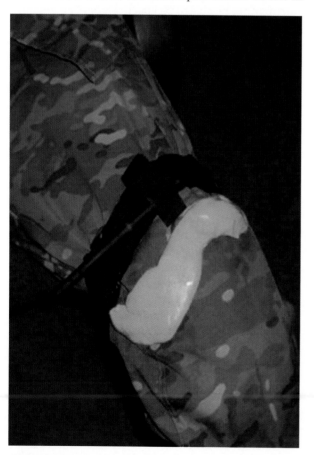

Figure 32.24. CAT tourniquet applied to leg "wound." Photo courtesy of Ian Wedmore.

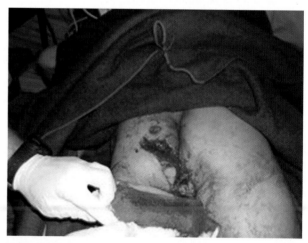

Figure 32.26. A shrapnel wound from an IED. Bleeding could not be controlled with gauze dressings and pressure. A Hemcon bandage was applied with excellent control of bleeding. The patient survived after extensive reconstructive surgery. Photo courtesy of Al Fink.

applied after a tourniquet has been placed to control the bleeding. If effective in their placement (bleeding controlled), the tourniquet can be removed. Both agents are FDA approved for external use.

In the event of a penetrating groin or axillary wound with severe bleeding that cannot be controlled with a tourniquet, the best option available at this time would be the application of an advanced dressing and direct pressure. The authors' first choice would be to stuff Chitoflex or pieces of Hemcon dressing into the wound and then place a pressure dressing. Pressure would then be manually maintained as best as possible and hypotensive resuscitation utilized to limit bleeding and allow clotting to occur in the wound.

Antibiotics

The use of prophylactic antibiotics in penetrating wounds in the literature is based on type of wound (high versus low velocity) and contamination. The literature universally supports the use of prophylactic antibiotics in high-velocity wounds.[94,96] Shotgun wounds are treated like high-velocity wounds due to the massive tissue destruction they inflict.

The use of prophylactic antibiotics in low-velocity wounds is much less clear. In low-velocity wounds in the urban setting, provided there was little wound contamination, good wound care and irrigation was undertaken, there was no advantage found to the use of prophylactic antibiotics.[97,99] In the literature on low-velocity wounds, however, antibiotics are recommended for wounds with any contamination. Penetrating wounds in the austere environment are by definition considered contaminated and should be treated with prophylactic antibiotics. This is also true for fractures that accompany penetrating wounds. In the past, for minimally contaminated wounds, a cephalosporin has been the recommended first-line prophylaxis. If the wound is heavily contaminated, penicillin was recommended to be added to prevent clostridial infection. If a heavily contaminated wound also involves a fracture, then gentamycin should be added. These recommendations were all based on the ideal: IV antibiotic use in a hospital setting. In ideal circumstances, IV antibiotics would be given immediately after wounding; this however is impractical for the austere setting because IV antibiotics require significant supplies and effort to administer. Fortunately, some very effective oral antibiotics with excellent oral bioavailability can be given at the time of wounding with near equivalent efficacy to IV antibiotics.

Its limited side effect profile[100] ability to be used by penicillin- and sulfa-allergic individuals, and once daily dosing recommends the fourth generation fluoroquinolones as the oral agent of choice for penetrating wounds in the austere environment.[101] The fluoroquinolones gatifloxacin or levofloxacin are nearly 99% orally bioavailable and cover the bacteria typically involved in penetrating wounds. Of these two agents, gatifloxacin has the best coverage of Gram-positive, Gram-negative, and anaerobic bacteria to include clostridium.[102] They can be given by mouth to those with extremity wounds shortly after wounding to decrease the risk of wound infections. If levofloxacin is utilized, then better coverage of anaerobes will have to be added. Clindamycin or metronidazole can be utilized.[103] These antibiotics are also effective for penetrating torso injuries.

Penetrating abdominal and pelvis wounds will require IV or IM antibiotics because the individual cannot be given oral medications. A second-generation cephalosporin with anaerobic coverage has previously been recommended for single-agent coverage of penetrating abdominal wounds.[104] A 2000 metaanalysis of antibiotic use in penetrating abdominal trauma recommends the following antibiotics or combinations: cefoxitin, gentamycin with clindamycin, tobramycin with clindamycin, cefotetan, cefamandole, aztreonam, and gentamycin alone.[105] Regardless of which antibiotic regimen is chosen, if an IV is not available, then giving antibiotics via the IM route is a reasonable option.

Hypothermia Prevention and Patient Packaging

Penetrating trauma patients who become hypothermic have a poor prognosis. Hypothermic patients become coagulopathic, which greatly hinders hemostasis.[106] This will worsen and complicate any hypovolemic shock that would otherwise occur. It was recognized in World War I that patients with penetrating injuries must be kept warm to decrease mortality. In the austere setting, this requires packaging the patient in multiple layers of insulation for transport. The patient can be laid on a "space blanket" and then wrapped in blankets and sleeping bags in several layers, dependent on available materials. The use of chemical heat packs between layers has been found to be effective in preventing heat loss.[107]

CPR and Penetrating Wounds

There is no reason to utilize CPR in victims of penetrating trauma in the austere environment. Well-done studies have shown no recovery in trauma patients who required CPR even in the urban civilian setting with its short transport time to medical facilities.[108] It is also

> All penetrating wounds in the austere environment are considered contaminated and therefore should be given prophylactic antibiotics at the time of wounding. Fourth-generation fluoroquinolones make an excellent oral antibiotic choice for extremity and torso wounds.

not recommended for pulseless patients in the austere setting.[109]

Approach to Resuscitation of Penetrating Wounds

A: airway. The airway is usually controllable by positioning and simple airway use. If positioning is effective then placement of a nasopharyngeal airway will typically be effective in maintaining airway patency for transport. In the event of penetrating trauma to the face, cricothyroidotomy may be the airway of choice if those trained to perform the procedure are present.

B: breathing. Eighty-five percent of chest wounds require only tube thoracostomy for definitive treatment.[110] The cause of death from penetrating chest injuries is tension pneumothorax; as such, needle decompression is a life-saving measure. Provided the decompression needle remains patent, the victim will have a pneumothorax, but this in and of itself is not life-threatening in most individuals.

C: circulation. Bleeding control is of paramount importance. While previously not recommended, tourniquets have come back into favor for use in combat wounds for initial control of severe bleeding. Modern tourniquets can be placed in seconds with effective control of bleeding. They also can be removed once placed and do not have to be left in place until definitive care is obtained, provided bleeding can be otherwise controlled. Modern hemostatic bandages can be utilized to control bleeding in areas not amenable to tourniquets. If available, an IV would be placed, and if compressible bleeding has been controlled, the patient would be given IV colloid or crystalloid sufficient to normalize the pulse. If noncompressible bleeding exists such as in penetrating abdomen, pelvis, or torso wounds, then hypotensive resuscitation will be utilized until the patient can be transported to definitive care.

C: c-spine. Numerous studies have shown that high-velocity penetrating wounds do not result in occult spinal injury. If there is no clinical sign of spinal injury at the time of the initial insult, then c-spine precautions do not need to be maintained.[111]

D: disability. Penetrating wounds of the brain require resuscitation to levels that preserve cerebral blood flow. Mental status cannot be used as a guide; a systolic pressure of 90–95 should be the goal.

E: exposure. Any penetrating wound should be *locally* exposed for evaluation. A casualty's clothes do not need to be completely cut off; instead, they can be cut sufficient only to expose the wound. Leaving much of the clothing intact will help prevent hypothermia.

Secondary Survey and Treatment

All wounds should be cleaned with irrigation, minimal debridement carried out as required, and clean dressings placed such that they will remain in place during transport and evacuation. Antibiotics if available should be given as appropriate for the type of wound. The patient should be packaged for transport in multiple layers to prevent hypothermia.

Medical Items/First-Aid Kits

Items for the care of penetrating trauma are extensive and what is taken will be based on how much can be carried. A comprehensive list includes:

IV fluids (colloid and or crystalloid): for fluid resuscitation in the United States, colloids are Hextend and Hespan. Lactated Ringer's and normal saline are standard crystalloid choices.

Irrigation fluid: for cleaning of wounds. If prepackaged solutions are not carried, then any potable water can be used. Water-purifying materials (e.g., filter pumps or iodine solutions) will likely be the most efficient way of providing large volumes of irrigating solutions.

Gauze and fluff or curlex dressings.

Elastic dressings. These are placed over the gauze dressings to provide pressure and hold in place for transport.

Local anesthetics: lidocaine, bupivicaine, marcaine, used to anesthetize wound for debridement and irrigation.

IV and PO antibiotics: oral fourth-generation fluoroquinolone, IV cephalosporins with anaerobic coverage for abdominal wounds.

Minor surgical set: for debridement of wounds.

Catheters for IVs and needle decompression: 18–21 gauge for fluid resuscitation. 14 gauge or larger for needle decompression. IV tubing for resuscitation.

Airway items: nasal trumpets, cricothyroidectomy kit, endotracheal tubes, and intubation equipment. (drugs for rapid sequence intubation if ETT equipment is carried).

Tourniquets: premade tourniquets.

Pain control medication.

Compact Trauma Kit

A small compact kit (Figure 32.27) for emergency treatment of penetrating trauma would include items for treating the most life-threatening conditions. An example utilized by the authors contains:

Tourniquet (1 CAT)

Elastic dressing (1 of the Ace wrap type)

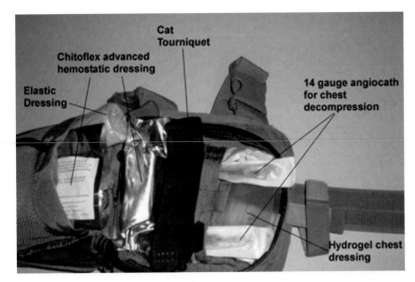

Figure 32.27. Compact kit for care of penetrating trauma. Photo courtesy of Ian Wedmore.

Advanced hemostatic dressings (1 Hemcon, 2 Chitoflex)

1 nasal trumpet

Chest dressing (3 hydrogel)

14-gauge catheters for chest decompression

Trauma shears

1 pair gloves

SUMMARY

Penetrating and explosive injuries in the austere environment present a significant challenge for the medical provider. Basic ATLS principles must be modified to adapt to the prolonged evacuation times to definitive medical care as well as the limited availability of medical supplies. However, the basics remain unchanged with airway control, restoration of effective breathing, and hemorrhage control being the highest priorities. Once the secondary survey is completed, wound care can be undertaken with minimal debridement, copious irrigation, and early administration of antibiotics to decrease morbidity and mortality.

REFERENCES

1. Harvey EN, Korr IM, Oster G, McMillin JH. Secondary damage in wounding due to the pressure changes that accompany the passage of high-velocity missiles. *Surgery.* 1946;21: 218–39.
2. Fackler ML. Wound ballistics: a review of common misconceptions. *JAMA.* 1988;259:2730–6.
3. Santucci RA, Chang Y-J. Ballistics for physicians: myths about wound ballistics and gunshot injuries. *J Urol.* 2004;171:1408–14.
4. *NATO War Surgery Handbook.* 3rd ed. Washington, DC: Government Printing Office; 2004.
5. Barach E, Tomlanovich M, Nowak R. Ballistics: a pathophysiologic examination of the wounding mechanisms of firearms: part I. *J Trauma.* 1986;26:225.
6. Fackler ML. Wounding patterns of military rifle bullets. *Int Defense Rev.* 1989;1:59.
7. Ordog GJ, Wasserberger J, Balasubramanium S. Wound ballistics: theory and practice. *Ann Emerg Med.* 1984;13:1113.
8. Hollerman JJ, Fackler ML. Gunshot wounds: radiology and wound ballistics. *Emerg Radiol.* 1995;2:171–92.
9. Pelton RY. *The World's Most Dangerous Places.* 5th ed. New York: Collins; 2003.
10. Barach E, Tomlanovich M, Nowak R. Ballistics: a pathophysiologic examination of the wounding mechanisms of firearms: part I. *J Trauma.* 1986;26:225.
11. DeMuth WE Jr. Bullet velocity and design as determinants of wounding capability: an experimental study. *J Trauma.* 1966;6:222.
12. Silvia AJ. Mechanism of injury in gunshot wounds: myths and reality [Confronting Forensic Issues]. *Critical Care Nursing Quarterly.* 1999;22(1):69–74.
13. Ordog GJ, Wasserberger J, Balasubramanium S. Shotgun wound ballistics. *J Trauma.* 1988;28:624–31.
14. Ordog GJ, Wasserberger J, Balasubramanium S, Shoemaker W. Civilian gunshot wounds: outpatient management. *J Trauma.* 1994;36:106–11.
15. DeMuth WE. The mechanism of shotgun wounds. *J Trauma.* 1971;11:219–29.
16. Sherman RT, Parrish RA. The management of shotgun injuries: a review of 152 cases. *J Trauma.* 1963;3:76–86.
17. Day W. Removing landmines: one limb at a time? *J Public Health Pol.* 1998;19:261–6.
18. Landmine Database, Department of Humanitarian Affairs, United Nations and Hidden Killers: The Global Landmine Crisis, United States Department of State
19. International Campaign to Ban Landmines. Landmine Monitor Report 2002. Washington DC: Human Rights Watch; 2002.
20. U.S. Department of Justice, Office of Justice Programs, National Institutes of Justice (NIJ).
21. Knudsen PJ, Sorensen OH. The destabilizing effect of body armour on military rifle bullets. *Intl J Legal Med.* 1997;110(2):82–7.

22 National Institute of Justice Ballistic Resistance of Personal Body Armor. NIJ Standard – 0101.04. Revision A. Washington, DC: Office of Science and Technology; June 2001.

23 Bartlett CS. Clinical update: gunshot wound ballistics. *Clin Orthop Rel Res*. 408:28–57.

24 Fackler ML. Ballistic injury. *Ann Emerg Med*. 1986;15: 1451–5.

25 Rodeheaver GT, Pettry D, Thacker JG, Edgerton MT, Edlich RF. Wound cleansing by high pressure irrigation. *Surg, Gyn & Obst*. 1975;141(3):357–62.

26 Pronchik D, Barber C, Rittenhouse S. Low- versus high-pressure irrigation techniques in *Staphylococcus aureus*-inoculated wounds. *Amer J Emerg Med*. 1999;17(2):121–4.

27 Valente JH, Forti RJ, Freundlich LF, Zandieh SO, Crain EF. Wound irrigation in children: saline solution or tap water? *Ann Emerg Med*. 2003;41(5):609–16.

28 Bansal BC, Wiebe RA, Perkins SD, Abramo TJ. Tap water for irrigation of lacerations. *Amer J Emerg Med*. 2002;20(5):469–72.

29 Griffiths RD, Fernandez RS, Ussia CA. Is tap water a safe alternative to normal saline for wound irrigation in the community setting? *J Wound Care*. 2001;10(10):407–11.

30 Moscati R, Mayrose J, Fincher L, Jehle D. Comparison of normal saline with tap water for wound irrigation. *Amer J Emerg Med*. 1998;16(4):379–81.

31 Edlich RF, Rogers W, Kasper G, Kaufman D, Tsung MS, Wangensteen OH. Studies in the management of the contaminated wound. I. optimal time for closure of contaminated open wounds. II. comparison of the resistance to infection of open and closed wounds during healing. *Am J Surg*. 1969;117:323–9.

32 Bowyer GW, Ryan JM, Kaufmann CR, Ochsner MG. General principles of wound management. In: Ryan JM, Rich NM, Dale RF, Morgans BT, Cooper CJ, eds. *Ballistic Trauma*. London: Edward Arnold; 1997.

33 Coupland RM, Howell PR. An experience of war surgery and wounds presenting after 3 days on the border of Afghanistan. *Injury*. 1988;19(4):259–62.

34 Rybeck B. Missile wounding and hemodynamic effects of energy absorption. *Acta Chir Scand*. 1974;450(Suppl):1.

35 Fackler ML, Breteau JP, Courbil LJ, Taxit R, Glas J, Fievet JP. Open wound drainage versus wound excision in treating the modern assault rifle wound. *Surgery*. 1989;105:576.

36 Mellor SG, Cooper GJ. Bowyer GW. Efficacy of delayed administration of benzylpenicillin in the control of infection in penetrating soft tissue injuries in war. *J Trauma*. 1982;40: S128.

37 Adams DB. Wound ballistics: a review. *Mil Med*. 1982; 147: 831.

38 Thoresby FP, Darlow HM. The mechanism of primary infection of bullet wounds. *Br J Surg*. 1967;54:359–61.

39 Berlin R, Gelin LE, Janzon B, et al. Local effects of assault rifle bullets in live tissues. *Acta Chir Scand*. 1976;459(Suppl):1–84.

40 Coupland RM, Samnegaard HO. Effect of type and transfer of conventional weapons on civilian injuries: retrospective analysis of prospective data from Red Cross hospitals. *BMJ*. 1999;319:410–12.

41 Coupland R. Hand grenade injuries among civilians. *JAMA*. 1993;270:624.

42 Gray R. *War Wounds: Basic Surgical Management*. International Committee of the Red Cross; 1994.

43 Bowyer GW. Management of small fragment wounds in modern warfare: a return to Hunterian principles. *Ann R Coll Surg Engl*. 1997;79:175–82.

44 Bowyer GW. Management of small fragment wounds: experience from the Afghan border. *J Trauma*. 1996;40: 170–2.

45 Coupland RM, Korver A. Injuries from antipersonnel mines: the experience of the International Committee of the Red Cross. *BMJ*. 1991;303:1509–12

46 Hinsley DE, Rosell PAE, Rowlands TK, Clasper JC. Penetrating missile injuries during asymmetric warfare in the 2003 Gulf conflict. *Brit J Surg*, 2005;92:637–42.

47 Robens W, Kusswetter W. Fracture typing to human bone by assault missile trauma. *Acta Chir Scand*. 1982; 508(Suppl):223–7.

48 Dahlgren B, Almskog BA, Berlin R, et al. Local effects of antibacterial therapy (benzyl-penicillin) on missile wound infection rate and tissue devitalization when debridement is delayed for twelve hours. *Acta Chir Scand*. 1982;508(Suppl):271–9.

49 Zura RD, Bosse MJ. Current treatment of gunshot wounds to the hip and pelvis. *Clin Orthop Related Res*. 408:110–14.

50 Routt ML Jr, Falicov A, Woodhouse E, Schildhauer TA. Circumferential pelvic antishock sheeting: a temporary resuscitation aid. *J Orthopaedic Trauma*. 2006;20 (1 Suppl):S3–6.

51 Alexander RH, Proctor HJ. *Advanced Trauma Life Support 1993 Student Manual*. Chicago: American College of Surgeons; 1993.

52 Calkins MD, Robinson TD. Combat trauma airway management: endotracheal intubation versus laryngeal mask airway versus combitube use by Navy SEAL and Reconnaissance combat corpsmen. *J Trauma*. 1999;46(5):927–32.

53 Martin SE, Ochsner MG, Jarman RH, Agudelo WE, Davis FE. Use of the laryngeal mask airway in air transport when intubation fails. *J Trauma*. 1999;47(2):352–7.

54 Hagberg C, Bogomolny Y, Gilmore C, Gibson V, Kaitner M, Khurana S. An evaluation of the insertion and function of a new supraglottic airway device, the King LT, during spontaneous ventilation. *Anesthesia & Analgesia*. 2006;102 (2):621–5.

55 Atherton GL, Johnson JC. Ability of paramedics to use the Combitube in prehospital cardiac arrest. *Ann Emerg Med*. 1993;22(8):1263–8.

56 van Zundert A, Al-Shaikh B, Brimacombe J, Koster J, Koning D, Mortier EP. Comparison of three disposable extraglottic airway devices in spontaneously breathing adults: the LMA-Unique, the Soft Seal laryngeal mask, and the Cobra perilaryngeal airway. *Anesthesiology*. 2006;104(6):1165–9.

57 Salvino CK, Dries D, Gamelli R, et al. Emergency cricothyroidotomy in trauma victims. *J Trauma*. 1993;34 503–5.

58 Erlandson MJ, Clinton JE, Ruiz E, et al. Cricothyroidotomy in the emergency department revisited. *J Emerg Med*. 1989;7:115–18.

59 McPherson JJ, Feigi DS, Bellam RF. Prevalence of tension pneumothorax in fatally wounded combat casualties. *J Trauma*. 2006;60:573–8.

60 Holcomb JB, Pusateri AE, Kerr SM, Macaitis JM, Cardenas L, Harris RA. Initial efficacy and function of needle thoracentesis versus tube thoracostomy in a swine model of traumatic tension pneumothorax. *J Trauma*. Accepted for publication.

61 Barton ED, Epperson M, Hoyt DB, Fortlage D, Rosen P. Prehospital needle aspiration and tube thoracostomy in

trauma victims: a six-year experience with aeromedical crews. *J Emerg Med.* 1995;13(2):155–63.

[62] Britten S, Palmer SH, Snow TM. Needle thoracocentesis in tension pneumothorax: insufficient cannula length and potential failure. *Injury.* 1996; 27(10): 758.

[63] Committee on Tactical Combat Casualty Care. *Prehospital Care in the Tactical Environment.* Washington, DC: Government Printing Office; 2003: 9.

[64] Lowe RJ, Saletta JD, Read DR, Radhakrishnan J, Moss GS. Should laparotomy be mandatory or selective in gunshot wounds of the abdomen? *J Trauma.* 1977; 17:903–7.

[65] Fiedler MD, Jones LM, Miller SF, Finley RK. A correlation of response time and results of abdominal gunshot wounds. *Arch Surg.* 1986;121:902–4.

[66] Muckart DJJ, Abdool-Carrim ATO, King B. Selective conservative management of abdominal gunshot wounds: a prospective study. *Br J Surg.* 1990;77:652–5.

[67] Demetriades D, Velmahos G, Cornwell E III, Berne TV, Cober S, Bhasin PS, et al. Selective nonoperative management of gunshot wounds of the anterior abdomen. *Arch Surg.* 1997;132:178–83.

[68] Saadia R, Degiannis E. Non-operative treatment of abdominal gunshot injuries. *Brit J Surg.* 2000;87(4):393–7.

[69] Coupland R. Abdominal wounds in war. *Brit J Surg.* 1996;83(11):1505–11.

[70] Sakles JC. Effect of immediate fluid resuscitation on the rate, volume, and duration of pulmonary vascular hemorrhage in a sheep model of penetrating thoracic trauma. *Ann Emerg Med.* 1997;29(3):392–9.

[71] Bickell WH. The detrimental effect of intravenous crystalloid after aortotomy in swine. *Surgery.* 1991;110(3):529–36.

[72] Riddez L. Central and regional hemodynamics during crystalloid fluid therapy after uncontrolled intra-abdominal bleeding. *J Trauma.* 1998;44(3):433–9.

[73] Owens TM, et al. Limiting initial resuscitation of uncontrolled hemorrhage reduces internal bleeding and subsequent volume requirements. *J Trauma.* 1995;39(2):200–9.

[74] Cannon WB, Fraser J, Cowell EM. The preventive treatment of wound shock. *JAMA.* 1918; 70:618–21.

[75] Beecher HK. Preparation of battle casualties for surgery. *Ann Surg.* 1945:121(6):769–91.

[76] Bickell WH, et al. Immediate versus delayed fluid resuscitation for hypotensive patients with penetrating torso injuries. *NEJM.* 1994;331(17):1105–9.

[77] Kwan I, Bunn F, Roberts I, on behalf of WHO Pre-hospital Trauma Care Steering Committee. Timing and volume of fluid administration for patients with bleeding following trauma. *The Cochrane Library.* 2001;(2).

[78] Sondeen JL, Coppes VG, Holcomb JB. Blood pressure at which rebleeding occurs after resuscitation in swine with aortic injury. *J Trauma.* 2003;54:S110–17.

[79] Deakin CD, Low JL. Accuracy of the advance trauma life support guidelines for predicting systolic blood pressure using carotid, femoral, and radial pulses: observational study. *BMJ.* 2000;321:673–4.

[80] Champion HR. Combat fluid resuscitation: introduction and overview of conferences. *J Trauma.* 2003;54:S7–S12.

[81] Rhee P, Koustova E, Alam H. Searching for the optimal resuscitation method: recommendations for the initial fluid resuscitation of combat casualties. *J Trauma.* 2003;S52–S62.

[82] Coimbra R, Hoyt DB, Junger WG, et al. Hypertonic saline resuscitation decreases susceptibility to sepsis after hemorrhagic shock. *J Trauma.* 1997;42:602–6.

[83] Strauss RG. Review of the effects of hydroxyethyl starch on the blood coagulation system. *Transfusion.* 1981;21: 299–302.

[84] Gran TJ, Bennett-Guerrero E, Phillips-Bute B, et al. Hextend, a physiologically balanced plasma expander for large volume use in major surgery: a randomized phase III clinical trial – Hextend Study Group. *Anesth Analg.* 1999; 88:992–8.

[85] Mishler JM. Synthetic plasma volume expanders – their pharmacology, safety and clinical efficacy. *Clin Haematol.* 1984;13:75–92.

[86] Maughon JS. An inquiry into the nature of wounds resulting in killed in action in Vietnam. *Mil Med.* 1970;135:8–13.

[87] Mabry RL, Holcomb JB, Baker A, Uhorchak J, Cloonan C, Canfield AJ, Perkins D, Hagmann J. U.S. Army Rangers in Somalia: an analysis of combat casualties on an urban battlefield. *J Trauma.* 2000;49:515–29.

[88] Lakstein D, Blumenfeld A, Sokolov T, Lin G, Bssorai R, Lynn M, Ben Abraham R. Tourniquets for hemorrhage control in the battlefield – a four year accumulated experience. *J Trauma.* Accepted for publication.

[89] Walters T. Testing of battlefield tourniquets. Presented at: Advanced Technology Applications for Combat Casualty Care 2004 (ATACCC) Conference; August 16–18, 2004; St. Petersburg, Fla.

[90] Odinsson A, Finsen V. Tourniquet use and its complications in Norway. *J Bone & Joint Surg – British Volume.* 2006;88(8):090–2.

[91] Sondeen JL, Pusateri AE, Coppes VD, Gaddy CE, Holcomb JB. Comparison of 10 different hemostatic dressings in an aortic injury. *J Trauma.* 2003;54:280–5.

[92] Acheson EM, Kheirabadi BS, Deguzman R, Edward J, Dick EJ, Holcomb JB. Comparison of hemorrhage control agents applied to lethal extremity arterial hemorrhages in swine. *J Trauma.* 2005;59:865–75.

[93] Wedmore IS, McManus JG, Pusateri A, Holcomb JB. A special report on the chitosan-based hemostatic dressing: experience in current combat operations. *J Trauma.* 2006 60(3):655–8.

[94] Howland WS, Ritchey SJ. Gunshot fractures in civilian practice. *J Bone Joint Surg.* 1971;53A:47–55.

[95] Patzakis MJ, Harvey JP, Ivler D. The role of antibiotics in the management of open fractures. *J Bone Joint Surg.* 1974;56A:532–41.

[96] Bowyer GW, Rossiter ND. Management of gunshot wounds of the limbs. *J Bone Joint Surg.* 1997;79B:1031–6.

[97] Simpson BM, Wilson RH, Grant RE. Antibiotic therapy in gunshot wound injuries. *Clin Orthop.* 2003;408: 82–5.

[98] Marcus NA, Blair WF, Shuck JM, Omer GE. Low velocity gunshot wounds to the extremities. *J Trauma.* 1980;12:1061–4.

[99] Dickey RL, Barnes BC, Kearns RJ, Tullos HS. Efficacy of antibiotics in low-velocity gunshot fractures. *J Orthop Trauma.* 1989;3:6–10.

[100] Walker RC. The fluoroquinolones. *Mayo Clin Proc.* 1999;74:1030–7.

[101] Mather R, Karenchak LM, Romanowski EG, Kowalski RP. Fourth generation fluoroquinolones: new weapons in the arsenal of ophthalmic antibiotics. *Am J Ophthalmol.* 2002;133:463–6.

[102] Ackerman G, Schaumann R, Pless B, Claros MC, Goldstein EJ, Rodloff. Comparative activity of moxifloxacin in vitro against obligately anaerobic bacteria. *Eur J Clin Microbiol Infect Dis.* 2000;19 228–32.

103 Brooks GF, Butel JS, Morse SA. Infections caused by anaerobic bacteria. In: *Medical Microbiology.* New York: Lange
Medical Books; 2001: 268–9.

104 Osmon DR. Antimicrobial prophylaxis in adults. *Mayo Clinic
Proc.* 2000;75:98–109.

105 Luchette FA, Borzotta AP, Croce MA, et al. Practice management guidelines for prophylactic antibiotic use in
penetrating abdominal trauma: the EAST practice management guidelines work group. *J Trauma.* 2000;48:508–18.

106 Holcomb JB, Pusateri A, Harris RA, Reid TJ, Beall LD,
Hess JR, MacPhee MJ. Dry fibrin sealant dressings reduce
blood loss, resuscitation volume, and improve survival in
hypothermic coagulopathic swine with Grade V liver injuries. *J Trauma.* 1999;47:233–42.

107 Hamilton RS, Paton BC. The diagnosis and treatment of
hypothermia by mountain rescue teams: a survey (abs).
Wild Environ Med. 7(1):28–37.

108 Branney SW, Moore EE, Feldhaus KM, et al. Critical analysis of two decades of experience with postinjury emergency
department thoracotomy in a regional trauma center.
J Trauma. 1988;45:87.

109 Battistella FD, Nugent W, Owings JT, Anderson JT. Field
triage of the pulseless trauma patient. *Arch Surg.* 1999;134:
742–6.

110 Swan KG, Reiner DS, Blackwood JM. Missile injuries:
wound ballistics and principles of management. *Milit Med.*
1987;152:29–34.

111 Arishita GI, Vayer JS, Bellamy RF. Cervical spine immobilization of penetrating neck wounds in a hostile environment. *J Trauma.* 1989;29:332–7.

33 | Drowning and Submersion Injury

Bradford D. Winters, PhD, MD

Drowning and submersion injury are environmental threats that may plague just about any expedition. Environments where this type of injury is a ubiquitous threat include kayaking, sailing, white-water rafting, scuba diving, and, of course, swimming. The threat, however, exists in many places where submersion would seem unlikely such as the desert where flash thunderstorms can rapidly turn dry narrow canyons into raging torrents or alpine environments where a thin snowpack may overlie a glacial runoff river. Urban/suburban environments also offer ample opportunity for drowning and submersion injury. Culverts, drainage canals and ponds, and backyard swimming pools of all sizes pose a threat to young and old alike.

INJURY PREVENTION

Prevention is the central issue in drowning and submersion injury. As will be discussed, treatment of these injuries after the fact has variable effectiveness, which is greatly exceeded in its success by close attention to preparation and safety measures prior to embarking on a trip or going anywhere near the water. Up to 80% of all drowning events are thought to be preventable.[1]

Anyone planning on going into or near an aquatic environment should have adequate swimming skills and be physically fit. A basic knowledge of self-rescue techniques including improvisation of personal flotation devices (PFD) and cardiopulmonary resuscitation (CPR) is imperative. Courses in both are available through several organizations, especially the American Red Cross. Anyone who lacks adequate swimming skills should either reconsider the activity or certainly wear a U.S. Coast Guard–approved PFD during the entire time he or she is on or near the water. Many states do not require adults to wear such devices while on watercraft (though all require that PFDs be present on the craft for all occupants), but it would be wise for all adults to don them regardless of their swimming skills. Accidents may happen at any time and in the event one is knocked unconscious, a PFD may be the only thing that prevents you from drowning. One should be familiar with the safety features, availability of life rafts, and escape routes of any boat you venture upon whether it is a 20-foot outboard or a luxury cruise ship.

Children must wear approved PFDs by law in every state when on a watercraft. When children are swimming, close supervision is critical to the prevention of drowning. Even children who are deemed "good swimmers" need to be watched closely. Rescue equipment should be kept readily available and preferably, one adult should be familiar with rescue techniques and CPR. Children whose swimming skills are suspect should wear a PFD. Have a communication system available so you can call for help. This may be a mobile phone or a marine radio. Access to the water by children should be restricted when adequate adult supervision is unavailable.

Pools and other such bodies of water should be encircled with a fence and gates or doors should self-close and the opening mechanism should be inaccessible to children. Local statutes should be consulted for rules about fence height and other regulations that pertain to pools. Small portable "wading" pools should be emptied as soon as they are no longer being used. A small child can easily drown in a few inches of water, and numerous reports exist describing toddlers drowning in vessels such as mop buckets and toilets because they lack the ability to extract themselves.[2,3]

Prevention in nonaquatic environments that still carry the hazard of drowning should focus on awareness of the threat and caution. You are not going to take a PFD on a mountain climbing trip nor are you going to carry one in the desert when exploring dry canyons. Awareness of the weather, the local conditions, and terrain should be the focus of preparation so that the threat is recognized quickly and hopefully avoided.

As mentioned previously, those going in or near the water should be in good physical shape. People who have certain conditions but who otherwise are in good shape need to take additional precautions. Examples would include those with seizure disorders and those with diabetes who would be advised to always enter the aquatic environment with a partner and to be sure they have taken their medications properly prior to entering.

Finally, the avoidance of alcohol and/or drugs is essential. Like automobile accidents, drowning and submersion injuries are often associated with intoxicated individuals.[4,5] It is estimated that up to 50% of drowning events associated with aquatic recreational activities involve alcohol as a causative factor.[5] Even small amounts of alcohol may impair judgment leading to injury or inadequate response to an emergency situation. Extreme environments of all types are no place for mind-altering substances.

DEFINITIONS

Drowning

Drowning is defined as the process of experiencing respiratory impairment from submersion/immersion in a liquid. The term "drowned" usually implies death as a result of this insult. Some liquids that can support oxygenation such as perflubrons when they fill the lungs, but most liquids and particularly water do not provide a medium that is conducive to gas exchange. Oxygen has a very low solubility in water. Fish exist in the aqueous world through very efficient oxygen extraction using gills. Marine mammals can alter their metabolism and have special adaptations such that many can dive for extended periods of time but they, like we terrestrial animals, must eventually come up for air. Those adapted to terrestrial life however, have extremely limited ability to go without access to air and as such quickly become hypoxic when submerged.

Submersion Injury versus "Near-Drowning"

"Near-drowning" is a common term introduced in the early 1970s[6] to describe those who had been submerged but survived the incident for at least some period of time. This definition is considered imprecise given current resuscitation capabilities. Additionally, definitions that have "drowning" as anyone who dies within 24 hours of a submersion event and all others as "near-drowning"[7] (regardless of if and when they die) cannot take into account subsequent pathological processes that the submersion victim may experience after rescue. More complex classifications have been developed including one that takes into account organ system failures, physiological abnormalities, and use of a scoring system to describe the injury.[8] These have not been widely used and without data to support their prognostic value in terms of outcomes, they unfortunately add little to the state of care.

Most now advocate using the term "submersion injury" to denote that the individual has experienced an injury secondary to submersion that may or may not ultimately lead to death. We will use the term "submersion injury" to broadly describe this situation throughout this text and use the term "drowning" to specifically describe those who are declared dead upon removal from the water.

Wet versus Dry Drowning

Reports of submersion victims (10–15%) who had no water in their lungs led to the development of the concept of "dry" versus "wet" drowning. Various explanations were given for this phenomenon, most notably laryngospasm secondary to the mechanical stimulus of the water.[6,9] Serious doubt has been cast that dry drowning actually occurs.[10] In the cases where "dry" lungs are reported, osmotic forces may have led to absorption of enough water that the lungs only appear dry. Many of these cases may be related to victims who may have had a lethal event such as a myocardial infarction or arrhythmia and enter the water already dead and hence did not take in water. Additionally, laryngospasm as an explanation seems unlikely as once hypoxia progresses sufficiently, muscle relaxation occurs, and the vocal cord spasm ceases allowing ventilatory movements to pull in water. One case series that examined 67 submersion incidents found only one chest film that demonstrated no evidence of water aspiration.[11] In terms of initial management, however, whether this phenomenon is real or not is immaterial, the primary pathological problem in submersion injury is the hypoxia and anoxia that occurs regardless of whether water is found in the lungs at time of rescue.

Other Terms

Some other terms that may be encountered include "immersion syndrome" and the "diving reflex." Immersion syndrome is thought to result from a vagally mediated process upon exposure to very cold water leading to severe bradycardia and asystole.[12,13] This may be an extreme form of the mammalian diving reflex that is known to occur in a variety of marine mammals and thought to be present in humans to a varying degree. This reflex leads to a longer breath-holding ability as peripheral use of oxygen is diminished and blood flow is shunted to the coronary and cerebral circulation.[14] The extent to which this reflex may help humans survive is unclear.

Another common term is "secondary drowning," which often is used to refer to the scenario where a submersion victim is rescued only to succumb later to another complication such as heart failure or Adult Respiratory Distress Syndrome (ARDS).[15,16] This is also sometimes referred to as the "postimmersion syndrome" and is nonspecific to submersion injury. This term should be avoided.

Incidence of Drowning and Submersion Injury

The actual incidence of drowning deaths worldwide is unknown, and accurate estimates are hampered by poor reporting systems, poor definitions, complex coding, and the fact that many drownings occur in poor and rural areas and are vastly underreported.[17,18] The incidence of submersion injury is even more difficult to ascertain though it has been estimated to be at least twice that of fatal drowning.[18,19] With these caveats in mind, the World Health Organization (WHO) reported nearly 450,000 drowning deaths in the year 2000. This places drowning second only behind traffic accidents in terms of unintentional mortality worldwide.[20,21] WHO estimated that in that year 1.3 million disability adjusted life-years were lost as a result of death and disability secondary to submersion injury.

This burden falls disproportionately on the poor and middle-income countries of the world (80%),[1] particularly Southeast Asia (38%), though Africa has the highest mortality rate from drowning (13.1/100,000).[21] Mortality is especially high among the young. Drowning mortality ranks eleventh among 0–4-year-olds, fourth among the 15 leading causes of death for 5–14-year-olds (first among boys and fifth among girls) and tenth in the 15–44 age cohort.

Clearly, drowning and submersion injury are an underappreciated health threat. In 2002, the Society to Prevent People from Drowning, organized a World Congress on drowning to push for progress in drowning and submersion injury prevention, rescue, and treatment. This society has old roots having been established in 1767 with the original goal of promoting bystander rescue and resuscitation.[22,23] This Congress produced a body of expert opinion and recommendations that is available on the Internet.[23] Even though the overall incidence of drowning and submersion injury in most countries is dropping[24,25] it still extracts a heavy toll and much needs to be done to further reduce the threat.

Epidemiology and Risk Factors

As previously described, drowning and submersion injury is experienced across the globe, affecting poor- and middle-income areas the most and disproportionately falling upon the young. It is also a fairly gender-specific problem with males being more prone to drowning mortality than females across all age groups and in all regions of the globe. In the United States, the peak drowning incidence for both genders peaks around age 2 years and then drops until reaching the age of approximately 10 years, and then skyrockets to a second peak at age 18 years. For females, the incidence peaks around age 1 and then steadily falls off never to rise again.[26,27] Drowning is one of the top three causes of accidental death in the 1- to 4- and 15- to 19-year-old cohorts in most countries and is the second most common cause of accidental death in the 1- to 14-year-old age group in the United States.[28]

Despite this, the underlying cause of drowning varies widely from country to country. In countries such as Denmark, the Netherlands, and Japan,[18,19,29] most drowning deaths are the result of suicide. Japan also reports a large number of elderly people die from drowning in home bathtubs.[29] In the United States, New Zealand, and Australia, many drowning deaths are a result of recreational activities, such as boating,[2,30,31] whereas suicide-associated drowning deaths are rare in these countries.[32,33] The Netherlands and New Zealand report that a common cause of drowning involves automobiles being submerged as a result of a roadway mishap.[19,30] In poor countries such as Bangladesh, more children ages 1–4 die from drowning than from respiratory infection or diarrheal diseases.

As one would expect, communities with increased aquatic activities such as recreation water sports or a greater prevalence of swimming pools tend to have a higher incidence of drowning. Interestingly, even though drowning incidences are higher in coastal communities, much of this occurs in fresh water rather than salt water. Some places like Alaska, Nova Scotia, Maine, New Zealand, and the North Sea are notable exceptions to this rule with saltwater rates of drowning deaths reported as high as 415 per 100,000 commercial fisherman per year.[34]

Ethnicity also seems to be a risk factor particularly in children in the United States where as many as three times the number of African American boys drown as compared to Caucasian boys.[35] Overall, African Americans are at higher risk of drowning than Caucasians.[36] Socioeconomic factors also likely play a role here as African American children are also more likely to drown in bodies of water such as canals, flooded quarries, or lakes, whereas white children are more likely to drown in backyard swimming pools.[37]

Even though it is recommended that people have adequate swimming skills when venturing onto or into the water, it is unclear whether swimming ability actually correlates with rates of drowning.[35,37] Reports of swimming ability are often fraught with bias; hence, conclusions are difficult to draw. As mentioned in the section on prevention, alcohol and other intoxicating substances are likely a major risk factor in drowning.[24,31,38] An early Australian report showed that over 60% of males who drowned had measurable blood alcohol levels, and over 50% of those over the age of 26 had levels that would have qualified as driving while intoxicated had they been stopped as a motorist at the time of the event (0.1%).[39] Current definitions of driving intoxicated have been lowered to 0.08% blood alcohol level, and this usually applies to driving a boat as well. The magnitude of other ingested substances both illegal and legal is unknown but certainly not negligible.

Underlying disease such as seizure disorder and cardiac or respiratory disease does not preclude participation in activities that may involve the risk of drowning but can be a contributor to the problem. Cervical spine (c-spine) injury is often thought to be a major problem in submersion victims, and although it should always be suspected, a retrospective study in 2001 suggested that submersion victims with no clinical signs of trauma and no history of diving were at virtually no risk of having sustained a c-spine injury and that cervical immobilization based solely on the history of submersion may be unwarranted. These results do suggest that without the signs or history of trauma, a c-spine injury (i.e., acute paralysis) is not likely the cause of the person's submersion event.[40]

Hyperventilation is an unusual factor that has also been identified as a risk factor for drowning. Hyperventilation is often used just prior to underwater swimming particularly if the distance is long. This lowers the $PaCO_2$ removing the drive to breathe, but if this drive is removed sufficiently to allow the oxygen stores in the muscle and functional residual capacity of the lungs to be used up, the PaO_2 may drop to the point of hypoxia and unconsciousness. The respiratory drive is much more sensitive to CO_2 than O_2, and oxygen levels must become quite low to stimulate breathing. Since the CO_2 doesn't rise to levels where the drive to breathe forces the swimmer to the surface, the person may drown.[41]

Most unfortunately, drowning or submersion injury may be the result of child abuse. A minority of childhood submersion injuries and drowning deaths are never investigated to determine if they result from abuse.[42] Although this oversight may result from health care providers' concern over introducing this issue into an already tragic event, laws regarding the reporting of injuries that may have resulted from abuse are clear. Health care providers including physicians, nurses, and first responders such as EMTs should be familiar with these laws and have a heightened index of suspicion for child abuse in any drowning or submersion incident.[43]

PATHOPHYSIOLOGY

Type of Water: Seawater versus Freshwater

Drowning in other liquids besides water is possible (such as fuel), but they are quite rare. When they occur, they are often not reported as a drowning. Additionally, they are extremely unlikely to occur in terms of expedition medicine, and thus we will restrict this discussion to submersion in water.

Water is usually divided into three categories: fresh, salt, and brackish. Freshwater is hypotonic compared to plasma, and saltwater has three to four times the osmolarity of plasma. This is variable since the salinity of saltwater bodies differs across the world with the

Dead Sea and the Great Salt Lake in Utah having the highest salinities of any major bodies of salt water. Brackish water is also variable in its salinity because it is a mixture of salt and fresh water. This salinity may vary over time with location and tide as well, but is generally hyper-osmolar to plasma whose salinity is equivalent to 0.9% NaCl. Most submersion injuries occur in some type of water, but the water may contain variable amounts of particulates such as sand and algae. The submersion medium may be contaminated with raw sewage or consist entirely of raw sewage. These "contaminants" have implications that will be discussed later.

In terms of management of drowning or submersion injury, the salinity of the water really doesn't matter nearly as much as the volume of water taken into the lungs.[44–48] The primary injury in drowning and submersion injury is from the anoxia that results from the impaired gas exchange that occurs when the alveoli are filled with water. The salinity of the aspirated water may lead to specific biochemical changes in the patient's lungs and blood and hence may be of importance in the interpretation of certain lab values and the forensic analysis of a drowning victim by a pathologist, but all degrees of salinity will induce similar degrees of hypoxia and anoxia if taken in equal volumes.

Abnormalities that may be seen in freshwater submersion injury result from the fact that because water is hypotonic, the concentration gradient is such that water leaves the lungs and passes across the alveoli into the circulation. At least theoretically, blood volume may increase if sufficient water crosses (11 cc/kg), and this may be able to produce enough hypotonicity in the blood that red blood cell hemolysis occurs if more than 22 cc/kg is aspirated. This amounts to 1.5 liters for a 70-kg person.[44,45,49] Experimental models suggest that this is well in excess of that volume normally aspirated by submersion victims.[5] Though it is theoretically possible, it is unusual for submersion victims to aspirate much more than 3–4 cc/kg of body weight.[50] Theoretically, all of this free water may dilute serum electrolytes including sodium, calcium, and magnesium but not potassium since the hemolysis will release significant amounts of potassium from intracellular stores leading to hyperkalemia. This hyperkalemia is exacerbated by the anoxia-induced acidosis as potassium shifts extracellularly from all tissue beds. Animal studies have in fact been able to demonstrate these pathological changes, but they require large volumes (44 cc/kg) of fresh water to do so. These blood volume and electrolyte changes tend to be self-limiting and rarely need specific treatment.[44,51–53]

Seawater will theoretically cause fluid to shift from the intravascular compartment into the alveolar spaces creating pulmonary edema.[46,54] This movement of water out of the plasma along with movement of salts including sodium, magnesium, and potassium from the seawater into the plasma can potentially cause hyper-osmolarity in the plasma. These changes however are unlikely given the typical volume of aspirated seawater in submersion victims, and if they did occur, like those of fresh water, they tend to be self-correcting and rarely need direct intervention. Extreme salinity environments such as the Dead Sea and the Great Salt Lake are thought to be more likely to induce these electrolyte changes.[55] Also some very unusual submersion events such as one reported industrial accident involving a diver working in an offshore oil rig, where high concentrations of calcium salts are often used as part of the drilling process, have been complicated by severe electrolyte disorders such as hypercalcemia.[56] The increase in this and other electrolytes occasionally seen in seawater and other hyper-osmolar environments is thought to be due to absorption from swallowed water rather than inhaled water.[57] Interestingly, the pathological derangements that hypertonic seawater and hypotonic fresh water may cause have been mostly described in victims who have died, whereas they are uncommonly seen in victims who survive to at least arrive in an Emergency Department (ED).[44,45,49]

Aspirated water (fresh and salt water) has a washing-out effect on the alveoli that removes surfactant, which is necessary to maintain open alveoli at the end of expiration. Without surfactant, the alveoli collapse creating atelectasis, and the blood going to those alveoli does not get oxygenated leading to pulmonary shunting. Lung compliance drops, and ventilation becomes more difficult. Adult Respiratory Distress Syndrome (ARDS) may develop. While replacing surfactant in ARDS is undergoing examination, its role in submersion injury and ARDS in general remains unclear.[58–60] We refer readers to other texts for more complete discussion on the specific management of ARDS.

Water Contaminants

Lung injury is often exacerbated by chemicals or contaminants in the aspirated water. Particulates such as sand can be very irritating to the airways and even lead to airway obstruction. Chemicals that may be in the water such as petroleum products, chemical wastes, and heavy metals can all have a deleterious effect on subsequent lung function. Swallowed water that is now rendered acidic from mixing with gastric contents may be regurgitated and aspirated leading to chemical burns in the lung. All of these insults may lead to the development of ARDS. Most aquatic environments contain microbiological organisms including chlorinated swimming pools. These organisms, if aspirated in sufficient quantity, can lead to postsubmersion infections. Aerobic Gram-negative organisms are common, especially *Pseudomonas*, *Aeromonas*, and *Burkholderia pseudomallei*, the latter of which is endemic in South-

east Asia. *Legionella* species are also a common inhabitant of freshwater ecosystems. These infections may develop rapidly and fulminate appearing similar to ARDS (61), which may also occur in and of itself. The infection may progress to sepsis, severe sepsis, and septic shock with multisystem organ failure. Gram-positive organisms particularly the streptococci and staphylococci may also cause infection in postsubmersion injury patients, though the source is usually from aspirated oropharyngeal contents. Anaerobes are unusual,[1] but certain fungi have been reported with a reasonable frequency, particularly *Pseudoallescheria boydii*. This organism's infection may take weeks to become apparent and may progress to a generalized state. It is often resistant to amphotericin B but is usually susceptible to miconazole.[1] Delayed infection may also have a nosocomial source and be unrelated to the original submersion event. This is particularly true for *Pseudomonas*, *Aeromonas*, *Streptococcus*, and *Staphylococcus* and local sensitivity patterns need to be considered when deciding on appropriate antibiotic treatment. Prophylactic treatment directed toward infection in submersion injury is not indicated unless the aspirated water clearly was contaminated with raw sewage. Even with raw sewage aspiration, the data in support of treatment is not overwhelming.

Water Temperature

The temperature of the water can have a significant impact on submersion injury. Immersion syndrome where severe bradycardia and asystole are thought to occur secondary to vagal responses to very cold water can immediately lead to death. In absence of these phenomena, cold water has other serious deleterious effects that may hasten drowning.

Water has a very high thermoconductivity and as such can lead to very rapid conductive heat loss, which may be exacerbated by convective losses in moving water. This is particularly true in children who generally have less subcutaneous body fat and a much higher surface-to-body-volume ratio and in very lean adults. Swallowing and aspiration of very cold water also leads to further heat loss. Hypothermia exerts several deleterious effects on the body that facilitate the process of drowning and submersion injury. As the core body temperature drops and peripheral vasoconstriction occurs, peripheral sensation begins to diminish. Mental status deteriorates, and the sensorium becomes clouded. Paranoia and hallucinations may develop. Thought processes become disorganized. Muscles become weaker and uncoordinated as the core temperature drops below 35°C making it more difficult to tread water or swim, and the victim may develop trouble protecting his or her airway from aspiration. Finally, unconsciousness usually occurs as the core temperature falls below 30°C leading to the inability to stay on top of the water. Atrial fibrillation may then occur and as the core temperature falls below 28°C ventricular fibrillation often occurs with loss of circulation.

The degree to which any one individual loses heat to the environment is quite variable, even with similar body habitus and clothing. Keeping this variability in mind, estimates of survival time suggest that few people will survive for longer than 1 hour in 0°C water and not longer than 6 hours in 15°C water.[62] Strategies to reduce heat loss would seem beneficial. Protective clothing that insulates and reduces conductive losses can significantly prolong survival in cold water. Wet suits, dry suits, and special "survival suits" (Figure 33.1) clearly improve insulation and tolerance to very cold water, but even the more standard clothing such as parkas, polypropylene layers, and wool can have benefit. Using any potentially insulating material at hand such as blankets or extra life preservers may buy that extra time necessary to survive. Based on studies in the 1970s, behavioral methods of conserving body heat have been advocated. These include trying to minimize movement; assuming postures that reduce surface exposure (bringing the knees up to the chest and wrapping the arms around them, which is only practical if using a PFD), and if there is more than one person in the water; and huddling together with children, if present, placed in the middle of the huddle.[62] Even in the absence of submersion, people who are trapped in or on an aquatic environment can easily die of hypothermia alone since even though they may be able to keep their airway above water, they are still wet and may be losing heat rapidly.

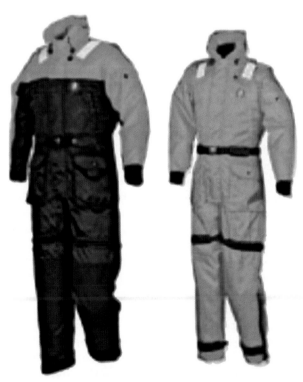

Figure 33.1. Immersion survival suit.

A significant amount of interest has developed in trying to ascertain whether submersion in cold water leads to improved outcomes as compared to warm water. This was spurred by reports of survival, primarily of children, after prolonged periods in very cold water when compared historically to submersions in more temperate water. The mechanism for this benefit is thought to be secondary to cerebral cooling prior to cardiac arrest,[63] and this is most likely to occur in very cold water, particularly when the victim has a high surface-to-volume ratio (such as children) and aspirates the cold water.[64] These reports – plus recent evidence that shows a statistically significant improvement in neurological outcome in patients resuscitated from sudden cardiac death when the patient undergoes deliberate mild hypothermia (32–34°C)[65,66] – have led to renewed interest in the issue of cold water submersion and the use of hypothermia to treat submersion injury of all kinds. Whether the global cerebral ischemia that occurs in submersion victims responds similarly to the global ischemia associated with sudden cardiac death out of the water is not yet clear. There are no randomized controlled trials yet examining this strategy in this patient population. However, this has not dissuaded health care professionals from advocating that submersion victims be treated in a similar fashion. The 2002 World Congress on Drowning published a consensus agreement stating that submersion injury victims, who have return of spontaneous circulation yet remain comatose, should have their core body temperatures maintained between 32–34°C for 12–24 hours followed by re-warming.[5]

The problem in implementing this strategy in the field is that submersion injury may occur far from a hospital and control of body temperature in the expedition environment is likely to be difficult. In the cardiac arrest studies, the patients were rapidly transported to an ED for their care. This may not be available in a wilderness environment. Additionally, in these studies, accurate body temperature measurements were made using invasive devices such as bladder catheters and intravascular catheters. Such accuracy in determining and controlling core body temperature is not possible in the wilderness. Uncontrolled hypothermia can lead to ventricular arrhythmias, coagulapathy with bleeding, and weakness of the ventilatory musculature requiring artificial ventilation. If rescue and evacuation is imminent, initiating cooling or foregoing rewarming in the case of a moderately hypothermic victim may be considered. In situations where evacuation is likely to be delayed, the benefit of this strategy may be outweighed by the risks. Because severe hypothermia carries significant risks, patients whose core temperatures are determined to be below 32°C should probably be warmed until higher-level care can be provided.

On another note, the diving reflex has also been suggested as a potential protective mechanism in submersion victims, and some have suggested the anecdotal reports of survival and good outcome in long-submerged children is secondary to this reflex being sustained in childhood.[67–69] This reflex is rather potent in diving mammals such as seals where their heart rate slows dramatically and blood is preferentially shunted to the brain. In humans, it is much weaker and only discernable in about 10–15% of the population. It is unclear whether this subset of the population accounts for the occasional reports of survival and good outcome after prolonged immersion, with some studies suggesting that its impact is not significant.[70]

Pathogenesis

Animal studies of drowning demonstrate a consistent pattern of events. The first event is struggling sometimes with inhalation. This is followed by lack of movement, some exhalation and a lot of swallowing. The process then becomes one of violent struggle for a variable period of time followed by convulsions, exhalation, and open-mouthed spastic inspiratory efforts. Reflexes diminish and become absent, and death occurs.[71] Similar descriptions of human drownings have been reported, particularly death after a violent struggle, but others have reported no struggle.[72] Humans have been observed to initially struggle, but secondary to exhaustion, panic, or the inability to maintain buoyancy, experience intermittent submersions with breathholding. Water is swallowed and can then cause vomiting. Aspiration is thought to then occur, which may or may not lead to laryngospasm.[73] Whether laryngospasm occurs or frank aspiration of the fluid occurs first, progressive hypoxia occurs. Laryngospasm, if it occurs, eventually relaxes with progressive hypoxia at which point further water aspiration occurs. Eventually the victim becomes unconscious and breathing attempts stop (Figure 33.2). It has been suggested that the "no struggle" scenario may represent initial death from another cause followed by submersion.[5] Other causes of death may be heart attack, seizure, hypoglycemia, trauma, intoxication, or cardiac arrhythmias (especially long QT syndrome, which seems more likely to be triggered by swimming in people who carry this autosomal dominant gene).[5]

The process of drowning centers on a progressive drop in arterial oxygen saturation. The initial response is tachycardia and hypertension but as hypoxia progresses, cardiac output drops, and the heart rate falls progressing to bradycardia and hypotension and eventually pulseless electrical activity and finally asystole. Primary ventricular fibrillation is rare and is usually seen in the setting of extreme hypothermia during resuscitation. Drowning victims usually have no palpable pulse, and their skin is cold, often with a white or purple-bluish color to it.[1] Witnesses may incorrectly judge the victim to be dead

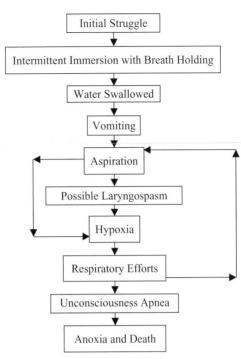

Figure 33.2. Sequence of drowning.

based on this presentation and forego or forestall necessary resuscitation efforts.

Once submersion has occurred, the clock is ticking in terms of outcome. Up to 27% of submersion victims may sustain neurological injury. The incidence of this injury appears to be increasing over the last few years presumably secondary to improved rescue and resuscitation techniques in the field and the ED.[74] Hypoxia and anoxia occur primarily due to the aspiration of the water and the severe shunting that occurs, but if the situation progresses to cardiac arrest or a pulseless arrhythmia, lack of blood flow exacerbates the hypoxia and anoxia.[75] Hypoxia and anoxia rapidly lead to tissue injury and death most notably in the brain. Unfortunately, there is little science examining anoxia and hypoxia specifically in submersion injury. Most of the data are extrapolated from studies of other anoxic/hypoxic insults such as cardiac arrest and stroke.[1] While hypothermia may reduce oxygen demand by the brain and other organs, struggling and shivering may increase oxygen utilization. The human body has extremely limited stores of oxygen in the functional residual capacity of the lungs and in muscle myoglobin. Within minutes, cerebral anoxia begins to occur and injury mounts. If sufficient time goes by without restoration of adequate tissue oxygenation, brain death occurs. Even with rescue and resuscitation, ischemic/reperfusion injury may further worsen neurological outcome. This occurs secondary to a host of inflammatory mediators that are released when ischemic tissue has its oxygen supply restored. Cerebral edema develops and may lead to increased intracranial pressure,[75] which reduces cerebral perfusion pressure. This in turn may lead to the redevelopment of either focal or global cerebral ischemia. Increasing intracranial pressure may eventually lead to a Cushing reflex with hypertension and bradycardia and finally to herniation and death.

Even though brain anoxia and death are the final result of drowning, the primary insult occurs in the lungs. Aspiration of water leads to hypoxia and pulmonary hypertension secondary to pulmonary vascular vasoconstriction.[76] Washout and/or destruction of surfactant occurs,[9] and alveolar collapse and atelectasis results. The combination of atelectasis and alveoli filled with fluid (either aspirated water or exudated fluid) leads to severe pulmonary shunting. It has been estimated that the shunt may be as high as 75%.[77,78] Pulmonary shunting of this magnitude rapidly leads to hypoxia with alveolar to arterial oxygen gradients rising to as high as 600 torr.[79] As the lungs collapse and/or fill with fluid, pulmonary compliance drops. As ventilation-perfusion mismatch worsens, the lungs fail. As hypoxia and anoxia progress, the body switches from aerobic metabolism to anaerobic metabolism leading to lactic acidosis. Additionally, the lack of ventilation leads to severe respiratory acidosis as carbon dioxide cannot be eliminated. This combined respiratory and metabolic acidosis may become quite severe impairing other organ systems such as the brain and cardiovascular system. Hyperkalemia may result from this acidosis and contribute to cardiac dysrhythmias.

Victims of submersion injury who are resuscitated may be plagued with persistent ventilation-perfusion mismatching and with a host of subsequent pulmonary problems that have been touched upon previously including parenchymal injury from particulates and other contaminants in the aspirated water, development of ARDS, and pulmonary infection.

The cardiovascular system is also severely affected by the submersion event though indirectly. The submersion event leads to a massive sympathetic discharge with an outpouring of catecholamines. This occurs even in the face of vagally mediated reflexes such as pulmonary vasoconstriction. Recent evidence has suggested that such massive exposures to catecholamines can lead to myocardial dysfunction in what is referred to a "broken heart syndrome." This phenomenon has been demonstrated in animal models[80] and was suggested in drowning pathology nearly two decades ago.[81] This sympathetic discharge is likely partially driven by the initial panic response and struggle often described in submersion victims, but it primarily results from the hypoxia and acidosis caused by failure of the pulmonary system.

Other organ systems such as the kidney and liver are usually injured secondary to the hypoxia, and when resuscitation occurs, they may manifest their injury as acute tubular necrosis, acute renal failure, and shock liver. We refer readers to other texts for the specifics regarding these two entities.

MANAGEMENT

In the Field

Immediate cardiopulmonary resuscitation is the single most crucial factor influencing survival in submersion injury.[75] The ABCs of airway, breathing, and circulation are the essential principles, and no other treatment or modality matters as much as reestablishing adequate airway, ventilation, oxygenation, and blood flow. It is estimated that CPR is started in submersion victims only about 40–60% of the time. This is unfortunate because it has been reported that only victims who have immediate resuscitation efforts in the field survive. Fifty to eighty percent of submersion victims who receive CPR in the field survive to hospital discharge. When resuscitation efforts were not initiated until emergency medical services (EMS) or the equivalent arrived, no victims survived.[1] It is clear that immediate resuscitation efforts are crucial to survival.

Even though c-spine injuries are unlikely in submersion victims without risk factors or evidence of trauma, if a c-spine injury is suspected, the ABCs must be performed with precautions such as immobilization in mind to stabilize the cervical spine so as to avoid spinal cord injury. If no injury is suspected, immobilization should not be performed. It may increase the risk of aspiration if the victim vomits.[75] It is estimated that almost three-quarters of submersion victims vomit.[57]

Establishment of an effective airway must occur immediately after the victim is brought to the surface. Many have advocated that this be performed in the water if necessary along with mouth-to-mouth or other assisted ventilation. It is unclear whether this has an advantage over getting the victim out of the water onto a stable surface. Additionally the risk to the rescuer must be taken into account. In very cold or rough water, these maneuvers may not only be very difficult but also expose the rescuer to excessive risk and result in more than one person drowning or being injured. Good judgment should prevail based on the conditions and the resources at hand.

If supplemental oxygen is available, it should be applied even to spontaneously breathing victims because of the potential for worsening of their pulmonary status. One hundred percent inspired oxygen is ideal, but it is not likely to be available in the field until EMTs or paramedics arrive for evacuation. Any apneic victim or victim who is judged to have inadequate ventilation should receive assisted ventilation. Bag mask systems are not available in most situations until EMTs arrive, but a rescue mask with a one-way valve is small enough that it should be part of any expedition medical kit. This allows for "mouth-to-mouth" breathing while protecting the rescue breather from the victim's oral secretions and vomitus. There have been reports that CPR in hypothermic submersion victims may precipitate ventricular fibrillation, but there is no contraindication to airway manipulation and rescue ventilation.[75]

Any victim who has lost his or her pulse should receive immediate CPR. In the field without an EKG machine, there will be no way of knowing why the victim is pulseless. It may be secondary to asystole or ventricular fibrillation or even pulseless electrical activity secondary to severe acidosis. As described in CPR, the presence of pulses should be frequently assessed throughout any resuscitation effort.

Pharmacologic therapy for submersion victims is extremely limited, and in the field routes of administration are often few. Intravenous equipment such as a catheter, IV tubing, syringes, and needles are rarely available. The oral route is usually unsatisfactory because of mental status abnormalities that make ingestion of the medication difficult and increase the risk of aspiration of the medication. Additionally, many victims vomit – particularly if their stomachs are full of water – so the medication never gets into their system. If IV equipment is available, it may be prudent to attempt to place an intravenous catheter if someone is present who is capable of doing so. This will facilitate administration of resuscitation drugs when higher-level help arrives. Generally speaking, there is little role for pharmacological therapy in the field for submersion victims. If the victim is thought to be diabetic and is possibly hypoglycemic, dextrose may be administered through an IV or orally if the victim is judged to be able to protect his or her airway. Additional pharmacological therapy will be discussed later.

Submersion victims who are resuscitated will often exhibit shortness of breath, air hunger, rhonchi, or wheezing. Even though some patients may initially look well after being pulled from the water, their pulmonary status can deteriorate rapidly, presumably as proteinaceous fluid fills the alveoli and as alveolar collapse occurs secondary to the washout of surfactant and the leaky capillary membrane effects of hypoxia and acidosis.[74]

Other than the Heimlich maneuver to dislodge aspirated foreign bodies, there is no good evidence to support any of the commonly performed maneuvers to promote drainage of fluid from the lungs. The Heimlich or other similar maneuvers should not be performed to expel water from the lungs. There is no good evidence to support its efficacy in this regard. These attempts only can promote the loss of the airway, exacerbate cervical spine injury if present, and interrupt crucial artificial ventilation and cardiopulmonary resuscitation efforts. Also, in extremely hypothermic victims, the heart is extremely irritable, and there is concern that the Heimlich maneuver could precipitate a ventricular arrhythmia.[82] These maneuvers should be avoided.

Given the cardiac instability and irritability that occurs in extremely hypothermic submersion victims, it has been suggested that rescue from the water needs to be smooth and preferably in the horizontal plane. Vertical rescue may be associated with a greater risk of cardiac instability[1] but clearly is necessary in many situations. Special equipment is available to aid extraction from the water and reduce the risk of death during transfer into boats and helicopters, but it will only likely be available after EMTs or paramedics arrive.[75]

The issue of whether to keep a hypothermic submersion victim cold or attempt to warm them has been the subject of much debate, and different opinions have been expressed in the literature. As mentioned previously, there is very good evidence that global cerebral ischemia from sudden cardiac arrest benefits from induced hypothermia,[65,66] but evidence regarding hypothermia in submersion victim resuscitation specifically has not been conclusive.

When EMS Arrives/In the ED/Hospital

When evacuation rescuers arrive (EMTs, paramedics, etc.), additional resources can be brought to bear. All patients should have 100% oxygen applied and at least one large bore (16-gauge or larger) peripheral IV placed with isotonic crystalloid running. If the patient is apneic or judged to have inadequate ventilatory efforts, artificial ventilation with a bag mask unit should be continued or initiated. Depending on local policies and laws, the EMTs may elect to attempt to intubate the patient for more definitive control of the airway. Other devices such as laryngeal mask airways or esophageal obturator airways may also be used depending on local practices to secure ventilation. Once in the hospital where expertise in advanced airway control techniques is available, a patient with apnea or inadequate ventilation should be intubated. Other indicators for proceeding to intubation include anyone with a Glasgow Coma Scale (GCS) of 8 or less or if the patient fails to maintain a PaO_2 over 60 torr despite a non-rebreather face mask. This latter abnormality is a clear indicator that a pathological process is occurring and runs a very high probability of deteriorating further even if the patient is awake and alert. Endotracheal intubation also facilitates delivering 100% inspired oxygen which non-rebreathers are not able to achieve under the best circumstances.

Another major advantage of endotracheal intubation is that it allows for delivery of Positive End-Expiratory Pressure (PEEP) in a consistent manner. PEEP has several beneficial effects especially in submersion injury.[75] It recruits atelectatic alveoli, helps to prevent alveolar collapse at end-expiration, displaces lung water, improves ventilation/perfusion matching, and decreases shunting. These all lead to improvements in PaO_2. While non-invasive positive airway pressure ventilation (NIPPV) using devices such as Bipap (bi-level positive airway pressure) and CPAP (continuous positive airway pressure) masks can help create PEEP, leaks and intermittent discontinuation of the mask cause the loss of the PEEP benefit. PEEP takes a long time (hours) to achieve its full benefit but only minutes to lose it. PEEP does have its problems. Its use can be associated with pulmonary barotrauma, decreased venous returning with decreased cardiac compliance, and increased afterload all causing hypotension, and high levels of PEEP can diminish venous return from the head leading to increased intracranial pressure (ICP) in patients already at risk for cerebral edema. If the submersion victim appears to be developing ARDS, low tidal volume/high PEEP strategy should be initiated as it has been shown to improve outcome.[83] However, while permissive hypercapnia is acceptable in ARDS without neurological injury, hypercapnia will worsen intracranial pressure and should be avoided in submersion victims with ARDS. This may make it difficult to fully realize the low tidal volume/high PEEP strategy.

Prone positioning has been shown to improve oxygenation in several studies, but it has not been shown to improve survival in lung-injured patients[84] and as such should not be recommended. Wheezing should be managed with beta-2 specific agonists if it is thought to be secondary to bronchospasm from irritants. It is important to differentiate so-called cardiogenic asthma, which is secondary to fluid overload and pulmonary edema.

Restoration of perfusion is crucial. Despite being submersed in water, most victims need close attention to volume resuscitation especially when they are hypothermic.

Bradycardia, asystole, and pulseless electrical activity (PEA) are managed according to ACLS guidelines with chest compression and appropriate administration of epinephrine and/or atropine. When ventricular fibrillation does occur, it is usually very difficult to defibrillate because the primary cause in these patients is extreme hypothermia and cardiac irritability.[1]

After the ABCs are managed and the victim is stable enough from a respiratory and cardiovascular point of view, the secondary survey needs to be performed. Chest X-rays may appear normal or demonstrate obvious pulmonary edema. Cervical and other spine injuries need to be assessed. Head injury may need to be ruled out with a head CT. Other internal and external injuries need to be addressed. Despite the very small possibility that a submersion victim may have aspirated enough fresh water to lead to hemodilution and hemolysis, any drop in hemoglobin or hematocrit should be a red flag that there is either internal or external bleeding. Submersion will not in and of itself cause hypovolemic/hemorrhagic shock. Do not ascribe hemodilution in a submersion patient to the mostly theoretical phenomenon of freshwater absorption. Patients with low hemoglobins or hematocrits should be assessed for internal bleeding. CT scans of the chest, abdomen, and

pelvis may be in order. Focused Abdominal Sonography (FAST) is now a commonly used modality to screen for intraabdominal hemorrhage.

Along with measurements of the hemoglobin and hematocrit, other important laboratory values to obtain include white blood cell count, platelet count, an arterial blood gas, serum electrolyte panel (sodium, potassium, calcium, chloride, bicarbonate), blood urea nitrogen, creatinine, glucose, and creatine phosphokinase.[75] Blood gases may need to be followed serially. Electrolyte disorders, if found, rarely need to be directly managed except possibly in the rare occurrence of submersion in unusual environments like the Dead Sea or certain industrial environments. Serum glucose levels should be tightly controlled. Hypoglycemia and hyperglycemia can have an impact on neurological outcome, and tight glucose control has been shown to improve outcome.[1]

Pharmacologic Therapy

As mentioned previously, pharmacologic therapy for submersion injury is extremely limited. Medications as appropriate for advanced cardiopulmonary resuscitation such as atropine and epinephrine should be administered as dictated by those protocols. In terms of medications specifically for the submersion injury, corticosteroids have often been advocated to treat the pulmonary injury and the cerebral edema associated with ischemia reperfusion injury. However, steroids have been shown to have no benefit in terms of outcomes for conditions such as ARDS (except possibly the late fibrosis stage) or anoxic/hypoxic brain injury from sudden cardiac arrest. Likewise, despite some early studies suggesting benefit from the use of these drugs in submersion victims,[85] currently there is very little evidence to support their use in submersion injury.[57] A Best Evidence Topic Report in 2001 found that most reports of steroid use in submersion victims were anecdotal case reports. The only available prospective study had only ten patients, and the retrospective studies were all reviews of case series. The anecdotal case reports and the very small prospective report generally show favorable results, but the retrospective analyses show no benefit.[86] Until a prospective randomized trial is performed showing statistically significant improvement in a defined outcome, the use of corticosteroids in the treatment of submersion injury should be avoided. Other medications that have been studied in anoxic/hypoxic injuries include nimodipine, lidoflazine, and magnesium. These also have shown no improvement in outcomes.[1] Currently, we have no evidence to support the use of antioxidants and free radical scavengers in submersion victims.[1]

Antibiotics

The use of prophylactic antibiotics has little support in the literature for victims of submersion injury.[75] They should be used only when a documented pulmonary infection has occurred or is highly suspected. Initial coverage should be broad-spectrum and include the likely pathogens described earlier as well as likely ventilator associated pneumonia (VAP) etiologies if the patient is on a ventilator. In the case of submersion injury in raw sewage or waters highly contaminated by raw sewage, many practitioners have elected to prophylactically cover likely pathogens especially the Enterobacteraceae family, though again little evidence exists to support this practice. An infectious disease consult may be appropriate if one is unsure.

Besides death, permanent neurological injury is perhaps the greatest feared complication of submersion injury and much attention has been focused on its management in hopes of improving outcome. Deliberate hypothermia has been the primary modality examined along with the use of barbiturate-induced coma. Very early data[87] suggested benefit of induced hypothermia and barbiturate coma, in terms of mortality and neurological outcome, but subsequent studies suggested that this is not the case[74,88] and that there were increases in sepsis in these patients when it was done. The current thinking, however, has come full circle with the recommendations of the 2002 World Congress on Drowning that all submersion victims be deliberately cooled to a core body temperature of between 32 and 34°C for a period of 12–24 hours followed by rewarming over the next 24 hours. Victims who are below this core body temperature should be rewarmed to within this target range because there is no evidence to support keeping the body temperature below this value.

Warming or rewarming may be done by several methods. Passive internal warming relies on the victim's own thermogenesis and is appropriate for cardiovascularly stable patients. Active external warming involves the use of warm air blankets[1] and is very effective. When victims are in cardiac arrest or cardiovascular failure, active internal warming is the method of choice. Femoral-femoral bypass or extra-corporeal membrane oxygenation is the easiest and most practical method and tends to have fewer complications than atrial cannulation through a sternotomy. Alternatively, the atrial technique achieves higher blood flows. Other internal techniques include bladder irrigation, warm peritoneal dialysis, warm gastric lavage, and hemofiltration.

As the patient warms, regardless of the technique, vasodilation may occur with subsequent hypotension, and this needs to be appropriately resuscitated with volume. Hypothermic patients also tend to develop a cold-induced diuresis that can exacerbate hypovolemia. Hypothermia has certain other deleterious effects including myocardial depression, increased risk of decubitus ulcers and ileus with increased risk of toxic megacolon. It has also been implicated in causing immunosuppression and increased infection rates. The previously discussed studies that suggested hypothermia had no benefit in

submersion victims also suggested a higher incidence of sepsis in the hypothermic groups;[75] however, the very recent studies on sudden cardiac arrest victim found no higher incidence of sepsis in their moderate induced hypothermia group.[65,66]

At one time, some of the principles already addressed were incorporated into a treatment strategy called HYPER. This strategy consisted of treating the victim's *hyper*-hydration with diuretics, *hyper*-ventilating the victim to a $PaCO_2$ of 30 to reduce intracranial pressure, treating *hyper*-pyrexia with cooling to 30°C, treating *hyper*-excitability with high-dose barbiturate coma, and treating *hyper*-rigidity with muscle relaxants. Initial reports in favor of this strategy were published, but subsequent studies by the original researchers and others[89] failed to demonstrate improvement over aggressive supportive care. Diuresis in face of hypothermia is likely to be harmful given the previous discussion. Routine hyperventilating to control ICP is not recommended and should be reserved for immediate use when marked elevations in ICP are identified. Hyperpyrexia should be controlled, and moderate hypothermia for a specified period is now the recommended modality, but cooling to 30°C is well below the target range and carries significant risk. Hyper-rigidity may be treated with muscle relaxants if it interferes with ventilation, but it carries the downside of obscuring the neurological exam. Barbiturate coma, unlike hypothermia, has no beneficial role in treating submersion victims. Thus, few practitioners favor this strategy any longer.

Aggressive supportive care remains the mainstay of treatment. Hemodynamic and respiratory support is central. Seizure activity, if present, should be immediately suppressed. If necessary, continuous EEG monitoring may be warranted. Infection should be vigorously treated. The patient should be placed on deep vein thrombosis prophylaxis. Sudden changes in oxygen or hemodynamics (blood pressure, tachycardia, EKG changes) should prompt an evaluation for pulmonary embolus.

PROGNOSIS

Despite many attempts to delineate prognostic criteria for submersion victims, no satisfactory schema exists to date. No one has been able to identify factors that clearly predict survival or neurological outcome to a satisfactory predictive value. One early attempt at a triage-based classification system relied on a neurological assessment within 1–2 hours after successful CPR and admission to the hospital where victims were categorized into three main groups with group A being awake (alert and conscious), group B being blunted (depressed mental status but arousable with spontaneous respiratory effort), and group C being comatose (nonarousable with abnormal breathing and lack of response or inappropriate response to pain).[75] Some like to subcategorize group C into C1–C3 as was done in Conn's original paper[90] where C is comatose, C1 is decorticate, C2 is decerebrate, and C3 is flaccid. A large retrospective analysis by these same authors suggested a 90% likelihood of survival if the victim was in category A or B. A separate analysis suggested that a GCS of 5 or greater in the ED or ICU was highly predictive of a good neurological outcome.[75] Nearly 20% of submersion victims who still require ongoing resuscitation on arrival in the ED are reported to have functional recovery. Even extreme physiological abnormalities that would otherwise be considered to be predictive of death have been identified in submersion survivors. Some of these include documented submersion time of 66 minutes in a child, core body temperature of 13.7°C, and a pH of 6.29. On the other hand, very low GCS score and Pediatric Risk Mortality scores and a combined scenario of apnea with coma in the ED, need for continued resuscitation in the ED, and pH of less than 7.00 are statistically predictive of death or severe neurological outcome.[1] Another series found that among 24 children who experienced submersion injury and arrived in the ICU with a GCS of 4 or 5, 50% survived with a normal neurological recovery.[57]

Given the variability in these studies, the ever-present uncertainty of submersion time, the potential improved outcomes that might result from submersion in cold versus warm water, the issue of whether cerebral cooling occurred prior to loss of spontaneous circulation, and the effectiveness of CPR and other factors, the prognostic criteria should not be used to determine if a submersion victim should be resuscitated. Every victim, within reason, should receive full and aggressive treatment in the field and at hospital admission.

After the victim is resuscitated, how long to continue care remains controversial. Given the current recommendations for induced moderate hypothermia, care should be continued for at least 48 hours since the cooling period is for 12–24 hours followed by a period of rewarming that generally requires 24 hours. After that point, neurological and general assessment along with attention to the patient's and family's wishes as dictated by living wills, health care proxies, and so on should guide further continuance of care.

Modalities that may aid in prognostication after this initial 48-hour period include EEG, somatosensory evoked potentials, and metabolic MRI. A large meta-analysis[1] showed that when pupillary light reflexes or motor responses were absent on day 3 and there was an absence of SSEP cortical responses within the first week, the outcome was death or severe neurological injury. Neurohumoral markers in serum or CSF have been insufficiently studied to warrant use in submersion victims for the purpose of prognostication.

SUMMARY

Submersion is a ubiquitous threat in both the urban/suburban environment and the more extreme environments including the ocean and the wilderness. Prevention is of primary importance in preventing injury and death. When submersion injury occurs despite taking preventative measures, the most important factor in determining survival is immediate institution of cardiopulmonary resuscitation with the goal of reestablishing perfusion and oxygenation of the tissues. This is amenable to deployment in the field. Many of the other treatment strategies are more complex and require evacuation to a medical center, but the most impact can be realized by those at the scene of the injury. Everyone venturing into the wilderness or an aquatic environment should be familiar with cardiopulmonary resuscitation and be prepared to react in the case of a submersion injury.

REFERENCES

1. Bierens JJ, Knape JTA, Gelissen HP. Drowning. *Curr Opin Crit Care.* 2002; 8:578.
2. Mackie IJ. Patterns of drowning in Australia 1992–1997. *Med J Aust.* 1999; 171:587.
3. Joseph MM, King WD. Epidemiology of hospitalization for near-drowning. *South Med. J.* 1998; 91:253.
4. Roberts SE. Hazardous occupations in Great Britain. *Lancet.* 2002; 360:543.
5. Moon RE, Long RJ. Drowning and near-drowning. *Emerg Med.* 2002;14:377–86.
6. Modell JH. Pathophysiology and treatment of drowning and near-drowning Springfield, IL: Charles C Thomas; 1971.
7. Schuman SH, et al. Risk of drowning: an iceberg phenomena. *J Am Coll Emerg Phys.* 1977; 6:139.
8. Hoff BH. Drowning and near-drowning (letter) *Crit Care Med.* 1980; 8:530.
9. Giammona ST. Drowning: pathophysiology and management. *Curr Problems Pediatrics.* 1971; 3:3.
10. Modell JH, Belefleur M, Davis JH. Drowning without aspiration: is this an appropriate diagnosis? *J Forensic Sci.* 1999; 44:1119.
11. Szpilman D, Elmann J, Cruz Filho FES. Dry-drowning – fact or myth? In: *World Congress on Drowning.* Amsterdam; Springer: 2002.
12. Goode RC, Duffin J, Miller R. Sudden cold water immersion. *Respir Physiol.* 197;23:301.
13. Keatinge WR, Haywar MG. Sudden death in cold water and ventricular arrhythmia. *J Forensic Sci.* 1981;26:459.
14. Daly M deB, Angell-James JE, Elsner R. Role of carotid body chemoreceptors and their reflex interactions in bradycardia and cardiac arrest. *Lancet.* 1979;1:767.
15. Dick AE, Potgeiter PD. Secondary drowning in the Cape Peninsula. *S Afr Med J.* 62:803.
16. Fuller RH. Drowning and post-immersion syndrome: a clinico-pathologic study. *Milit Med.* 1963;128:22.
17. Langley JD, Chalmers DJ. Coding the circumstances of injury: ICD-10 a step forward or backwards? *Inj Prev.* 1999;5:247.
18. Lindholm P, Steensberg J. Epidemiology of unintentional drowning and near-drowning in Denmark in 1995. *Inj Prev.* 2000;6:29.

19 Bierens JJLM. 2944 Submersion victims: an analysis of external causes, concomitant risk factors, complications and prognosis. In: *Drowning in the Netherlands. Pathophysiology, Epidemiology and Clinical Studies*. Utrecht, the Netherlands: University of Utrecht; 1996: 82.

20 Williamson JP, Rowland I, Gertler P, Braude S. Near-drowning treated with therapeutic hypothermia. *MJA*. 2004;9:500.

21 Peden MM, McGee K. The epidemiology of drowning worldwide. *Inj Control Saf Promot*. 2003;10:195.

22 Sternbach GL, Varon J, Fromm R, Baskett PJF. The Humane Societies. *Resuscitation*. 2000;45:71.

23 Drowning Web Site. Available at: *http://www.drowning.nl*. Accessed October 2006.

24 Cummings P, Quan L. Trends in unintentional drowning. *JAMA*. 1999;281:2198.

25 Sibert JR, Lyons RA, Smith BA, et al. Preventing death by drowning in children in the U.K.: have we made progress in 10 years? Population based incidence study. *BMJ*. 2000; 324:1070.

26 Baker SP, O'Neill B, Karpf RD. *The Injury Fact Book*. Lexington, MA: D. C. Health; 1984.

27 Ellis AA, Trent RB. Hospitalization for near-drowning in California: incidence and costs. *Am J Public Health*. 1995;85:1115.

28 Hoyert DL, Kochanek KD, Murphy SL. Deaths: Final data for 1997. *Natl Vital Stat Rep*. 1999;47:1.

29 Tochihara Y. Bathing in Japan: a review. *J Human Environ Syst*. 1999;3:27–34.

30 Langley JD, Warner M, Smith GS, et al. Drowning related deaths in New Zealand 1980–94. *Aust N Z J Public Health*. 2001;25:451.

31 Kohn M, Duthu R, Flood H, et al. Drowning – Louisiana 1998. *JAMA*. 2001;286:913.

32 Byard RW, Houldsworth G, James RA, et al. Characteristic features of suicidal drownings, a 20-year study. *Am J Forensic Med Pathol*. 2001;22:134.

33 Wirthwein, DP, Barnard JJ, Prahlow JA. Suicide by drowning: a 20-year review. *J Forensic Sci*. 2002;47:131.

34 Norrish AE, Cryer PC. Work related injury in New Zealand commercial fishermen. *Br J Ind Med*. 1990; 47:726.

35 Schuman SH, et al. The iceberg phenomena of near-drowning. *Crit Care Med*. 1976;4:127.

36 Centers for Disease Control and Prevention. National Center for Injury Prevention and Control. WISQARS; 2002.

37 Rowe MI, Arango A, Allington G. Profile of pediatric drowning victims in a water-oriented society. *J Trauma*. 1977;17:587.

38 Wintemute GJ, Kraus JF, Teret SP, Wright MA. The epidemiology of drowning in adulthood: implications for prevention. *Am J Prev Med*. 1988;4:343.

39 Plueckahn VD. Drowning: community aspects. *Med J Aust*. 1979;2:226.

40 Watson RS, Cummings P, Quan L Bratton S, Weiss NS. Cervical spine injuries among submersion victims. *J Trauma*. 2001;51:658.

41 Craig AB. Causes of loss of consciousness during underwater swimming. *J Appl Phys*. 1961;10:583.

42 Feldman KW, Monasterasky C, Feldman GK. When is childhood drowning neglect? *Child Abuse Negl*. 1993;17:329.

43 Gillerwater J, Quan L, Feldman K. Inflicted submersion in childhood. *Arch Pediatr Adolesc Med*. 1996;150:298.

44 Modell JH, Graves SA, Ketover A. Clinical course of 91 consecutive near-drowning victims. *Chest*. 1976;10:231.

45 Modell JH, May F. Effects of volume of aspirated fluid during chlorinated fresh water drowning. *Anesthesiol*. 1966;27:663.

46 Modell JH, et al. The effects of fluid volume in seawater drowning. *Ann Int Med*. 1967; 67:68.

47 Orlowski JP, Abulleil MM, Philips JM. Effects of tonicities of saline solutions on pulmonary injury in drowning. *Crit Care Med*. 1987;15:126.

48 Orlowski JP, et al. The hemodynamic and cardiovascular effects of near-drowning in hypotonic, isotonic or hypertonic solutions. *Ann Emerg Med*. 1989;18:1044.

49 Modell JH, Davis JH. Electrolyte changes in human drowning victims. *Anesthesiol*. 1969;30:414.

50 Harries MG. Drowning in man. *Crit Care Med*. 1981;9:407.

51 Modell JH. Near drowning. In: Callaham ML, ed. *Current Therapy in Emergency Medicine*. St. Louis: Mosby; 1986.

52 Rumbak MJ. The etiology of pulmonary edema in fresh water near drowning. *Am J Emerg Med*. 1996;14:176.

53 Fuller RH. The clinical pathology of human near-drowning. *Proc R Soc Med*. 1963;56:33.

54 Cohen DS, et al. Pulmonary edema associated with salt water near drownings: new insights. *Am Rev Respir Dis*. 1992;146:794.

55 Yagil Y, et al. Near-drowning in the Dead Sea: electrolyte imbalance and therapeutic implications. *Arch Intern Med*. 1985;145:50.

56 Fromm RE. Hypercalcemia complicating an industrial near-drowning. *Ann Emerg Med*. 1991;20:669.

57 Denicola LK, Falk JL, Swanson ME, Gayle MO, Kissoon N. Submersion injuries in children and adults: common issues in pediatric and adult critical care. 1997;13:477.

58 Suzuki H, et al. Surfactant therapy for respiratory failure due to near-drowning. *Eur J Pedatr*. 1996;155:383.

59 Straudinger T, et al. Exogenous surfactant therapy in a patient with ARDS after near-drowning. *Resuscitation*. 1997;35:179.

60 Anzueto A, et al. Aerosolized surfactant in adults with sepsis induced ARDS. Exosurf. Acute Respiratory Distress Syndrome Sepsis Study Group. *NEJM*. 1996;334:1417.

61 Ender PT, et al. Near-drowning associated Aeromonas pneumonia. *J Emerg Med*. 1996;14:737.

62 Collis ML. Survival behavior in cold water immersion. Proceeding of the Cold Water Symposium; Royal Life Saving Society of Canada; Toronto; 1976.

63 Golden F. Mechanisms of body cooling in submerged victims. *Resuscitation*. 1997;35:107.

64 Xu X, Tikuisis P, Giesbrecht G. A mathematical model for human brain cooling during cold water near-drowning. *J Appl Physiol*. 1999;86:265.

65 Mild therapeutic hypothermia to improve the neurologic outcome after cardiac arrest. NEJM 2002; 346:549.

66 Bernard SA, et al. Treatment of comatose survivors of out-of-hospital cardiac arrest with induced hypothermia. *NEJM*. 2002;346:557.

67 Conn AW. Near-drowning and hypothermia. *Can Med Assoc J*. 1979;120:397.

68 Gooden BA. Drowning and the diving reflex in man. *Med J Aust*. 1972;2:583.

69 Martin TG. Near-drowning and cold water immersion. *Ann Emerg Med*. 1984;13:263.

70 Ramey CA, Ramey DN, Hayward JS. The dive response of children in relation to cold water near-drowning. *J Appl Physiol*. 1987;63:665.

71 Karpovich PV. Water in the lungs of drowned animals. *Arch Path Lab Med*. 1933;15:828.

72 Modell JH. Current concepts: drowning. *NEJM*. 1993; 328: 253.

73 Boffard KD, et al. The management of near-drowning. *J Roy Army Med Corps.* 2001;147:135.

74 Bohn DJ, et al. Influence of hypothermia, barbiturate therapy, and intracranial pressure monitoring on morbidity and mortality after near drowning. *Crit Care Med.* 1986;14:529.

75 Olshaker JS. Submersion. *Emerg Med Clin N Am.* 2004; 22:357.

76 Colebatch HJH, Halmagyi DJP. Effect of vagotomy and vagal stimulation on lung mechanics and circulation. *J Appl Physiol.* 1963;18:881.

77 Berquist RE, et al. Comparison of ventilatory patterns in the treatment of fresh water near-drowning in dogs. *Anesthesiol.* 1908;52:142.

78 Modell JH, et al. Effects of ventilatory patterns on arterial oxygenation after near-drowning in sea water. *Anesthesiol.* 1974;40:376.

79 Hoff BH. Multisystem failure: a review with special reference to drowning. *Crit Care Med.* 1979;7:310.

80 Eliot RS, et al. Pathophysiology of catecholamine mediated myocardial damage. *J SC Med Assoc.* 1979;75:513.

81 Karch SB. Pathology of the heart in near-drowning. *Arch Pathol Lab Med.* 1985;109:176.

82 Rosen P, et al. The use of the Heimlich maneuver in near drowning: Institute of Medicine Report. *J Emerg Med.* 1995;13:397.

83 The Acute Respiratory Distress Syndrome Network. Ventilation with lower tidal volumes as compared with traditional tidal volumes for ALI and ARDS. *NEJM.* 2000; 342:1301.

84 Gattononi L, et al. Effect of prone positioning on the survival of patients with acute respiratory failure. *NEJM.* 2001; 345:568.

85 Sladen A, Zauder HK. Methylprednisolone therapy for pulmonary edema following near drowning. *JAMA.* 1971;215:1793.

86 Foex BA. Corticosteroids in the management of near-drowning. *Emerg Med J.* 2001;18:465.

87 Conn AW, et al. Cerebral resuscitation in near-drowning. *Pedatr Clin N Am.* 1979;20:691.

88 Nussbaum E, Maggi JC. Pentobarbital therapy does not improve neurological outcome in nearly drowned, flaccid comatose children. *Pediatrics.* 1988;81:630.

89 Modell JH. Treatment of near-drowning: Is there a role of H.Y.P.E.R. therapy? *Crit Care Med* .1986;14:583.

90 Conn A, Montes J, Barker GA. Cerebral Salvage in near-drowning following neurological classification by triage. *Can J Aneasth.* 1980;27:201.

34 | Evaluation and Acute Resuscitation of the Trauma Patient

Elliott R. Haut, MD, FACS, and Rajan Gupta, MD, FACS, FCCP

INTRODUCTION

Trauma is a common disease worldwide. Injuries account for over five million deaths per year across the world.[1] Trauma is the leading cause of death in patients aged 1–44 in the United States. All patients require immediate evaluation and resuscitation to prevent mortality and morbidity after trauma. Trauma centers dedicated to the care of these injured patients are promoted as models to improve care overall and have been documented to have done so in developed nations.[2–6] However, basic initial management has the potential to save more lives globally than the advanced care at specialized centers.

The Advanced Trauma Life Support (ATLS) course sponsored by the American College of Surgeons[7] is the gold standard for teaching initial trauma management and evaluation. The course began in the 1970s in the United States and has since spread around the globe. It clearly emphasizes the importance of the initial resuscitation. ATLS is taught based on the premise that the student may be the only physician treating an injured patient in a small rural hospital.[7] Although not initially designed to do so, this major premise is easily extrapolated to trauma in remote and extreme environments. Although not all diagnostic tools and therapeutic options will be available, the same emphasis on the primary and secondary surveys, therapeutic adjuncts, and a plan for transfer (or evacuation) apply to austere environments. Improvisation and thinking on one's feet are clearly important tools for management of trauma in a non-hospital setting.

The most important first step in trauma evaluation no matter what setting is rapid performance of a primary survey. During the primary survey, definitive diagnosis is less important than identifying diagnoses requiring immediate treatment and performing adjunctive maneuvers. The primary survey sequence is easily remembered with the ABCDE mnemonic. It includes evaluation of the Airway (with cervical spine immobilization), Breathing (and ventilation), Circulation (with adjuncts for hemorrhage control), Disability (evaluation for neurologic defects), and both Exposure and Environmental control.[7]

Decisions and interventions made during this primary survey are crucial. Early trauma deaths may be prevented with appropriate airway, breathing, and circulation management. Strict adherence to the systematic performance of the primary survey is crucial to ensure excellent patient outcomes within trauma centers. In more austere environments, the same algorithm should be followed and standard protocols are equally effective.

Evaluation and management of injuries identified in the primary survey ensure that life-threatening injuries are treated first. Although patients may clearly have other injuries that may look more severe (i.e., complex open extremity injuries), they are usually not immediately life-threatening. The primary survey is done in a stepwise fashion, and if an injury or finding is noted, the primary survey stops and an intervention for that must be undertaken before moving on to the next step. Only after completion of the primary survey can the practitioner move on to the secondary survey. This secondary survey is a rapid, systematic, complete physical examination looking for other potential injuries.

In large urban trauma centers, the trauma team is often comprised of many providers (physicians, nurses, respiratory therapists, etc.) and has the luxury of many practitioners being available to evaluate and manage the patients simultaneously. In the wilderness, there may be only one trained medical person who must prioritize his or her duties (based on ATLS teaching). Interventions associated with the primary survey include control of the airway including by orotracheal, nasotracheal, or surgical airway management. Venous access is also crucial if this modality is available. Other key maneuvers include tube thoracostomy (chest tube placement) or decompression of tension pneumothorax, either by needle decompression or tube thoracostomy. Obtaining venous access often falls under the circulation heading as it enables fluid resuscitation and treatment of hypovolemic shock. Also under circulation would be direct control of hemorrhage. This may be through the use of direct pressure or the use of tourniquets. Pelvic binders prevent ongoing pelvic bleeding after pelvic facture. Gastric and urinary decompression are mentioned within the ATLS course as during the primary survey, although in reality, these often wait until the secondary survey is complete and are almost never used outside of hospital settings.

PRIMARY SURVEY

Airway

Assessing and securing an airway is the first step in the evaluation of the trauma victim. Rapidly establishing a patent proximal or upper airway will facilitate the flow of oxygen and carbon dioxide during breathing. An extremely important underlying principle one must consider at all times during the management of the airway is maintaining in-line cervical spine stabilization. A second underlying principle that should always be considered is weighing the risk/benefit ratio of establishing a definitive airway versus the potential delay in evacuating the patient to an appropriate health care facility.

Assessment of the airway begins with simply asking the patient to speak. If he or she can phonate normally without distress, then the airway is likely secure for the moment, and the primary survey should proceed to the next step – breathing. It is important to note that the trauma victim's status can change rapidly, and constant reevaluation is necessary. However, if the victim is unable to phonate, or there is unexpected hoarseness or stridor, then the airway is potentially compromised and must be evaluated further. Initially, any potential obstructions must be cleared. Visual inspection may identify foreign bodies (e.g., pieces of food) or broken teeth in the oropharynx, which may be removed simply with a finger. If suction is available, this will aid in the removal of fluids such as blood or vomitus.

In the semicomatose or comatose patient, the airway is often occluded secondary to the tongue falling back against the posterior pharyngeal wall. The initial management begins with some basic maneuvers that do not require any special expertise or equipment. This type of occlusion can often be relieved by a jaw thrust or chin lift, simply displacing the mandible forward, thereby lifting the tongue off the posterior wall. To perform a jaw thrust, the rescuer places his or her thumbs on the victim's zygoma and index and long fingers on the angle of the mandible bilaterally and pushes forward (Figure 34.1). To perform the chin lift, the rescuer grasps the victim's chin and lower incisors lifting forward (Figure 34.2), without tilting the head back so as to avoid manipulating the cervical spine. These simple maneuvers should open the proximal airway enough to allow the flow of air to and from the lungs. If no other equipment is available, then one person may need to be dedicated to continuously performing one of these maneuvers to maintain a patent

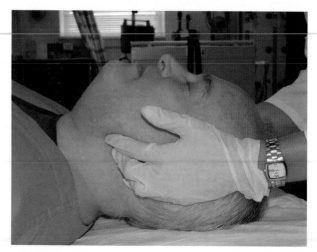

Figure 34.1. Jaw thrust maneuver. Photo courtesy of Gregory H. Bledsoe.

airway in the obtunded patient. However, if either an oropharyngeal or a nasopharyngeal airway is available, then one of these devices can be used to maintain the airway and free the rescuer to proceed with the remainder of the primary survey. The oropharyngeal airway is the most commonly used artificial airway but stimulates the gag reflex in semiconscious patients. The oropharyngeal airway has few applications in the field and the nasopharyngeal airway is preferred. A nasopharyngeal airway is better tolerated by the semiconscious patient, and this airway is simply inserted through one of the nares and directed posteriorly along the floor of the nasopharynx until it is seated. These devices are simple to use and should be carried on any expedition to an austere environment.

A more secure airway can be achieved if more advanced equipment and expertise are available. Placement of a dual lumen airway requires minimal training, and this device has been successfully used in the

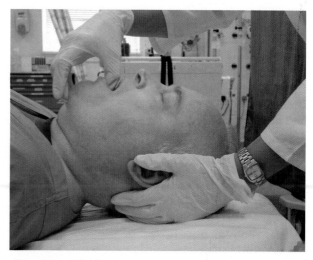

Figure 34.2. Chin lift maneuver. Photo courtesy Gregory H. Bledsoe.

prehospital setting in the civilian experience.[8] As with the oropharyngeal airway, this airway is contraindicated in conscious or semiconscious patients. Additionally, its use is usually limited to patients who are 16 years of age or older and are at least 5 feet tall.[7] To place the dual lumen airway, all previously placed airway adjuncts should be removed, and the chin lift maneuver is performed. The device is advanced through the mouth until the markers on the tube are in line with the victim's teeth. The pharyngeal balloon is then inflated with 100 cc of air, and the distal balloon is subsequently inflated with 15 cc of air. Ventilation is then attempted sequentially through the two lumens (lumen #1 first) until breath sounds are confirmed in the chest, and there is no gastric distension in the abdomen. Once again, every attempt should be made to maintain in-line cervical spine stabilization. The most definitive airway is endotracheal intubation, and this can be achieved via nasotracheal or orotracheal approaches. The nasotracheal approach may be useful in an obtunded patient who has spontaneous respirations. The endotracheal tube (ETT) is introduced through one of the nares and is advanced through the posterior pharynx, using the presence of breath sounds through the tube to guide its placement in the trachea. The orotracheal approach requires sophisticated equipment (e.g., laryngoscope) as well as expertise in direct laryngoscopy. Except for the completely obtunded patient, this approach also often requires sedatives and neuromuscular blocking agents to facilitate the intubation. Thus, availability of these medications as well as knowledge of doses and potential complications is essential.

If all these maneuvers are unsuccessful, or cannot be attempted due to lack of equipment or expertise, then a surgical airway may be another option. This requires making an incision in the anterior neck just below the larynx. A vertical skin incision allows for a greater margin for error in regards to locating the cricothyroid membrane, and avoids lacerating adjacent anterior jugular veins. A horizontal incision in the cricothyroid membrane allows for the passage of a tracheal tube distally into the trachea. If a tracheal tube is not available, any stiff, large-diameter tubing cut to an appropriate length may be used. This technique can be complicated by many potential pitfalls including difficulty visualizing the anatomy in large or obese patients as well as significant bleeding in any traumatic victim (Figure 34.3).

Breathing

After the airway is assessed and secured, the primary survey of the trauma victim proceeds to evaluation of breathing. The two primary components of breathing are oxygenation and ventilation. If available, supplemental oxygen should be applied to all trauma victims. If the patient has absent or inadequate respiratory effort, then ventilation must be assisted.

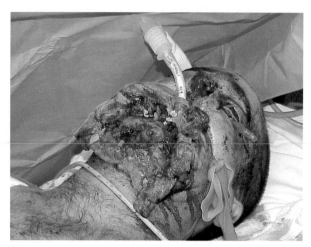

Figure 34.3. Obtaining an airway can be challenging in a patient with significant facial trauma. This patient was orally intubated in spite of severe trauma from a self-inflicted shotgun wound. Had oral attempts failed, a surgical airway would have been necessary. Photo courtesy of Gregory H. Bledsoe.

Assessment of breathing requires auscultation of the chest cavity. If breath sounds are present and equal bilaterally, it can be assumed for the moment that breathing is adequate, and evaluation should proceed to the next step in the primary survey – circulation. Once again, the patient's status can change abruptly, and constant reevaluation is necessary. If breath sounds are absent or diminished, further assessment is necessary. In an intubated patient, diminished breath sounds– especially on the left side of the chest – can indicate that the endotracheal tube may have been advanced too far into the right mainstem bronchus. The trachea should be examined and confirmed to be in the midline. If it is midline, then absent or diminished breath sounds are most commonly secondary to a simple pneumothorax or hemothorax. These require decompression and drainage via a tube thoracostomy; however, such an intervention requires appropriate instruments and expertise. One must consider the necessity versus the risks of this intervention in the austere environment: If the patient is not requiring assistance with ventilation, is oxygenating adequately, and is not in circulatory shock, perhaps the procedure could be delayed for a few hours if the patient can be evacuated expeditiously to a health care facility. If the trachea is deviated away from the side on which the breath sounds are absent or diminished, then the patient may be suffering from a tension pneumothorax, which is a life-threatening entity and requires emergent decompression. This is most expeditiously achieved by inserting a large-bore needle or intravenous catheter into the anterior chest just below the clavicle at the midclavicular line, in approximately the second intercostal space. A tube thoracostomy should subsequently be performed as soon as resources permit.

Circulation

The primary goals during the evaluation of the circulatory state are initiating volume resuscitation and controlling hemorrhage. Ideally, peripheral large-bore intravenous catheters are the preferred access for volume infusion; however, relative hypovolemia can render this technique difficult. If the equipment and expertise are available, central venous access via the subclavian, femoral, or internal jugular veins is a viable option. In a state of shock where femoral and carotid pulses may be weak or absent, the subclavian vein may be the best option since the clavicle is easy to palpate and serves as a good landmark despite blood pressure. A femoral vein, however, can often be cannulated during an aggressive resuscitation even when others are working around the head of the patient and serves as a safe way to obtain intravenous access. An alternative to central venous access, especially in children, is intraosseous access. An intraosseous line may be placed in the anterior tibia approximately one centimeter inferior to the tibial tuberosity, or it may be placed in the sternum.[9–12]

Assessment of circulation begins with an assessment of the mental status of the victim. Confusion, agitation, and lethargy can all be signs of compromised circulation. However, these signs are not necessarily specific because other entities such as head injury and high-altitude cerebral edema can manifest these symptoms as well. If the victim's skin is pale, cold or clammy, or diaphoretic, circulation may also be compromised. Evaluation should include feeling carotid, femoral, and radial pulses. The presence and characteristics of the pulses can be helpful in assessing the circulatory state. Rapid, thready, weak pulses all suggest hypovolemia, and in trauma this is assumed to be from hemorrhage until proven otherwise. A blood pressure should be obtained if appropriate equipment is available. Volume resuscitation with isotonic crystalloid solutions (lactated Ringer's or normal saline) should be initiated. The use of colloids or hypertonic saline for the initial trauma resuscitation has not been proven to improve outcomes, but it has been advocated in the austere environment by some experts due to their reduced weight per resuscitation volume. For persistent hypotension following 2–3 liters of crystalloid, blood products should be infused when available. Placing the patient in a head down position may optimize blood flow to the brain; however, this is contraindicated in the patient with possible head injury. In the austere environment where access catheters or fluids are unavailable, judicious administration of oral fluids may be considered. However, any evidence of abdominal injury is a contraindication for oral intake.

Hypotensive resuscitation is an often-debated management strategy for the prehospital resuscitation plan for patients with hypotension from hemorrhagic shock after trauma. The theory behind this approach is that patients with uncontrollable sources of bleeding such as solid organ injury (i.e., liver, spleen) or other internal bleeding vessels may "pop the clot" that has been formed if the blood pressure is raised too rapidly before surgical hemorrhage control has been obtained. The data on this approach are somewhat conflicting. The first large prospective study on this topic showed that for "hypotensive patients with penetrating torso injuries, delay of aggressive fluid resuscitation until operative intervention improves the outcome".[23] However, a more recent randomized study did not show any benefit for patients treated with the hypotensive resuscitation approach.[24] The variation in practice patterns has also been established in a survey of practicing trauma surgeons about their opinions regarding prehospital care of trauma. Approximately one-third of respondents would suggest IV fluid replacement aimed at normotension (systolic blood pressure 100–120 mmHg), whereas two-thirds of those surveyed would suggest maintaining relative hypotension (systolic blood pressure 70–80 mmHg).[25] ATLS still currently recommends IV fluid administration for most patients, but does state that "rapid restoration of normal blood pressure with a vigorous fluid bolus should be avoided" in austere or hostile environments.[7] Current military medical teaching suggests the hypotensive resuscitation strategy, basing fluid administration on mental status and radial artery pulse examination alone. The Israeli Defense Force guidelines for cases of uncontrolled hemorrhagic shock suggest withholding IV fluids until one of the three parameters is documented: altered sensorium, radial pulse cannot be palpated, or systolic blood pressure below 80 mmHg.[26]

As resuscitation is initiated, evaluation for sites of hemorrhage must be concurrently performed. Life-threatening exsanguination usually occurs in the chest, abdomen, retroperitoneum, pelvis, proximal lower extremities (i.e., femur fractures), or through external wounds. The torso can be difficult to evaluate unless advanced imaging techniques are available. Ultrasound may be used to detect fluid in the pleural spaces, pericardium, and abdomen, but it is unreliable in detecting retroperitoneal bleeds (See Box 34.1.) Portable ultrasound devices are readily available and should be considered for all major expeditions. Fractures of the pelvis and extremities should be reduced and stabilized as soon as possible to reduce bleeding and pain. The pelvis can be stabilized with commercially available devices or by wrapping a sheet around the pelvis and tightening it securely with a knot. Femur fractures should be reduced to length and placed in traction as soon as possible. All external bleeding should be immediately controlled with direct pressure. Several types of hemostatic dressings are currently available to apply to external wounds. External bleeding from extremities can be managed with direct pressure or with the use of a properly applied and managed tourniquet.

Box 34.1. Trauma ultrasound in remote environments
Bret P. Nelson, MD, RDMS, Edward Melnick, MD, and James Li, MD

Background

Rapid triage and diagnosis of seriously injured patients is critical in field medical operations. A wide variety of imaging modalities are utilized in hospital settings, but significant bulk and cost constraints have prohibited their use in the field. Thus, medical providers in out-of-hospital settings have relied almost solely on physical exam and history. Recently, improvements in ultrasound (US) technology have led to lightweight, portable, less expensive machines that may have the capacity to improve diagnostic accuracy in the field.

Modern portable US machines are lightweight (typically less than 6 pounds), provide high image quality, and are built to withstand abusive environmental conditions. These field machines have demonstrated good accuracy when compared to CT scans or radiology department US in the evaluation of hemoperitoneum and pericardial effusion[1-3] as well as pneumothorax.[4,5]

Bedside US has been widely used in U.S. trauma centers since the mid-1990s. In 2001, the American College of Emergency Physicians established guidelines for routine bedside US use in emergency departments.[6] The 1997 Advanced Trauma Life Support (ATLS) guidelines describe the use of US in clinical decision making, and the Focused Assessment with Sonography in Trauma (FAST) exam was formally incorporated into the ATLS guidelines in 2005.[7] Physicians, military medics, and emergency medical services (EMS) personnel have used portable US machines successfully in the field to diagnose traumatic conditions such as hemoperitoneum, hemo- and pneumothorax, and hemopericardium.[8-10]

It is important that any equipment carried to a remote area be lightweight and rugged. In a study of US use during helicopter transport, no mechanical problems were encountered during a one-year study period with one hundred patients assessed.[11] When used in military operations in Iraq, US was used over a 2-month period in conditions of high ambient light and temperature. Fourteen negative cases and one positive case of intraperitoneal fluid were detected.[12] The authors noted the importance of small size, maneuverability, and the option for battery power in the space constraints of a mobile field hospital. Some degradation in expected battery life was attributed to storage in high temperatures during summer months.

When deployed on a medical expedition to remote Amazon jungle settlements, portable US improved diagnostic capacity beyond physical exam alone.[13] In one month, 25 ultrasounds were performed for suspected hemoperitoneum, abdominal aortic aneurysm, and other indications. Disposition was altered because of the scans in seven cases. Batteries were the only means of power for the device due to lack of electricity. The device was used at altitudes up to 5,182 meters as well as sea level.

Thus, there is now extensive experience with nonradiologists using US, and a wide range of experience in deploying portable devices to the point of care in remote environments.

Indications

FAST Exam

Severe torso trauma is a rare but life- and expedition-threatening event. By definition, remote arenas lack the resources to effectively deal with significant injury, and diagnostic modalities are limited. Thus, there is a need to make rapid diagnostic and evacuation decisions.

The FAST exam has been demonstrated in many studies to be accurate in diagnosing hemoperitoneum at the bedside.[14-17] Use of the FAST exam has been shown to decrease time to needed operation and decrease treatment costs.[18] A study of combat deaths in 210 U.S. Marines defined early diagnostic US use as one factor that could decrease overall traumatic mortality.[19]

Preliminary studies in air medical transport have demonstrated that FAST exams are feasible when performed by EMS personnel in confined quarters while moving at high speeds. An initial prospective study of 71 patients transported by helicopter found a complete set of adequate images could be obtained in only 52% of cases, mainly due to time constraints.[9] Another prospective study of one hundred patients transported via helicopter demonstrated adequate image capture of the right upper quadrant view in 90% of cases, with a sensitivity of 60% and specificity of 93% for that single view.[11] In these studies, exams were only performed during retrieval and transport. It is feasible that additional time could have improved the proportion of cases in which studies could be completed.

Physicians deployed on ground transport have used sonography to improve the accuracy of their physical exam, altering trauma management at the scene in one-third of cases.[20] In this study, the average FAST exam was completed in less than 3 minutes. The prehospital US was 93% sensitive and 99% specific compared with diagnoses made in the emergency department. When used by physicians in a French ambulance service, trauma and cardiac US was found to improve diagnostic accuracy in 67% of cases.[8] Ultrasound has been useful in diagnosing hemoperitoneum in forward military operations, as described previously.[12]

An early study of US deployment in a multicasualty environment (after the Armenian earthquake of 1988) demonstrated the potential for sonographic evaluation of a large number of patients in an overwhelmed medical system. Over 400 traumatic casualties were assessed with US in a 72-hour period following the earthquake.[21] Traumatic abdominal pathology was found in 13% of patients assessed, with no false positives and 1% false negatives. Sixteen patients underwent operative intervention based solely upon clinical evaluation and US findings.

Only one study has attempted to asses the value of incorporating US evaluation into a mass-casualty triage system.[22]

(continued)

Box 34.1. *(continued)*

Chart data from 359 patients was used to retrospectively allocate patients within Simple Triage and Rapid Treatment (START) categories of Red (immediate), Yellow (delayed), and Black (expectant). Cases where the management of the delayed (Yellow) patients would have been changed by the results of the FAST exam were assessed. Portable US resulted in 12.9% false negatives and 22.2% false positives, which would have over- or undertriaged many cases. Inconclusive FAST exams were documented in 5.2% patients. The retrospective design of this study makes hard conclusions difficult, but these outcome metrics are important to consider in future prospective design studies.

Intracranial Pressure Assessment
In the setting of closed head injury, rapid diagnosis and management of significant intracranial injury is essential to survival. Early detection of elevated intracranial pressure (ICP) is important, as it may indicate treatable brain disorders such as intracranial hemorrhage, mass effect, or impending herniation. Unfortunately, physical examination is limited in the diagnosis of elevated ICP. Papilledema is an insensitive, nonspecific marker, and one that may take days to develop in the setting of elevated ICP.[23]

The optic nerve sheath diameter (ONSD) can be measured using US and used as a marker for elevated ICP. The optic nerve sheath communicates pressure from the cerebrospinal fluid and is readily visible on US. In a study of 35 patients, ONSD greater than 5 mm correlated with ICP elevations.[24] This bedside test was 100% sensitive and 95% specific when compared to CT scan. A more recent study of 59 head injury patients with suspected elevations in ICP found a sensitivity of 100% and specificity of 63% in detecting elevated ICP.[25] Thus, patients with the ONSD marker for elevated ICP can be identified much more accurately and rapidly than would be possible with serial neurologic exams or other physical exam findings.

Pneumothorax
The ease and accuracy of detecting a pneumothorax with US make it an attractive alternative to plain radiography, which is usually not available in austere settings. A study of 676 thoracic trauma patients found the sensitivity of auscultation in detecting hemopneumothorax was 100% for blunt, but only 50% for penetrating trauma patients.[26] Thus in some settings, physical examination is unreliable for pneumothorax diagnosis. This is often further hampered by uncontrolled environmental factors such as the ambient noise of adverse weather or machinery. In contrast, visualization of the pleura by US is straightforward, and the appearance of lung sliding and comet tail artifacts rules out pneumothorax with a negative predictive value exceeding 99%.[4,5,27]

This technique has been applied at a forward military health service support station to exclude pneumothorax in the setting of deep thoracic shrapnel wounds.[10] Without US, many soldiers would have had to undergo mandated pleural decompression in this setting. The technique has been successfully used in high altitude, where a portable US machine excluded pneumothorax in a patient with blunt chest trauma, hemoptysis, but stable vital signs at 4,000 feet above sea level.[28]

Conclusion
Modern ultrasound is a technology that is ideally suited for field use. It is portable, uses batteries (and can be recharged with a solar panel), can take thousands of images without requiring chemicals or film, and, in most field environments, allows the rapid visualization of tissue and organs that previously could only be visualized by surgical exploration. As the technology matures, its use has expanded to include prehospital, military, medical evacuation, and expeditions. It is probable that the utility of portable ultrasound will continue to evolve in a rapid and dramatic manner, offering an excellent resource for improving care in austere environments.

References

1. Kirkpatrick AW, Sirois M, Laupland KB, et al. Prospective evaluation of hand-held focused abdominal sonography for trauma (FAST) in blunt abdominal trauma. *Can J Surg.* 2005;48:453–60.
2. Kirkpatrick AW, Simons RK, Brown DR, et al. Digital hand-held sonography utilised for the focused assessment with sonography for trauma: a pilot study. *Ann Acad Med Singapore.* 2001;30:577–81.
3. Kirkpatrick AW, Simons RK, et al. The hand-held FAST: experience with hand-held trauma sonography in a level-I urban trauma center. *Injury.* 2002 May;33(4):303–8.
4. Blaivas M, Lyon M, Duggal S. A prospective comparison of supine chest radiography and bedside ultrasound for the diagnosis of traumatic pneumothorax. *Acad Emerg Med.* 2005;12:844–9.
5. Kirkpatrick AW, Sirois M, Laupland KB, et al. Hand-held thoracic sonography for detecting post-traumatic pneumothoraces: the extended focused assessment with sonography for trauma (EFAST). *J Trauma.* 2004;57:288–95.
6. American College of Emergency Physicians. American college of emergency physicians. ACEP emergency ultrasound guidelines – 2001. *Ann Emerg Med.* 2001;38:470–81.
7. American College of Surgeons. *Advanced Trauma Life Support for Physicians.* 7th ed. Chicago: American College of Surgeons; 2005.
8. Lapostolle F, Petrovic T, Lenoir G, et al. Usefulness of hand-held ultrasound devices in out-of-hospital diagnosis performed by emergency physicians. *Am J Emerg Med.* 2006;24:237–42.
9. Melanson SW, McCarthy J, Stromski CJ, et al. Aeromedical trauma sonography by flight crews with a miniature ultrasound unit. *Prehosp Emerg Care.* 2001;5:399–402.
10. Roberts J, McManus J, Harrison B. Use of ultrasonography to avoid an unnecessary procedure in the

prehospital combat environment: a case report. *Prehosp Emerg Care.* 2006;10(4):502–6.

11. Heegaard W, Plummer, D, Dries D, et al. Ultrasound for the air medical clinician. *Air Med J.* 2004;23(2): 20–3.

12. Brooks AJ, Price V, Simms M. FAST on operational military deployment. *Emerg Med J.* 2005;22:263–5.

13. Blaivas M, Kuhn W, Reynolds B, et al. Change in differential diagnosis and patient management with the use of portable ultrasound in a remote setting. *Wilderness Environ Med.* 2005;16:38–41.

14. Kimura A, Otsuka T. Emergency center ultrasonography in the evaluation of hematoperitoneum: a prospective study. *J Trauma.* 1991;31:20–3.

15. Ma OJ, Mateer JR, Ogata M, et al. Prospective analysis of a rapid trauma ultrasound examination performed by emergency physicians. *J Trauma.* 1995;38:879–85.

16. McElveen TS, Collin GR. The role of ultrasonography in blunt abdominal trauma: a prospective study. *Am Surg.* 1997;63:181–8.

17. Bode PJ, Edwards MJ, Kruit MC, et al. Sonography in a clinical algorithm for early evaluation of 1671 patients with blunt abdominal trauma. *Am J Roentgenol.* 1999;172:905–11.

18. Melniker LA, Leibner E, McKenney MG, et al. Randomized controlled clinical trial of point-of-care, limited ultrasonography for trauma in the emergency department: the first sonography outcomes assessment program trial. *Ann Emerg Med.* 2006;48:227–35.

19. Blood CG, Puyana JC, Pitlyk PJ, et al. An assessment of the potential for reducing future combat deaths through medical technologies and training. *J Trauma.* 2002;53(6):1160–5.

20. Walcher F, Weinlich M, Conrad G, et al. Prehospital ultrasound imaging improves management of abdominal trauma. *Br J Surg.* 2006;93(2):238–42.

21. Sarkisian AE, Khondkarian RA, Amirbekian NM, et al. Sonographic screening of mass casualties for abdominal and renal injuries following the 1988 Armenian earthquake. *J Trauma.* 1991;31(2):247–50.

22. Sztajnkrycer MD, Baez AA, Luke A. FAST ultrasound as an adjunct to triage using the START mass casualty triage system: a preliminary descriptive study. *Prehosp Emerg Care.* 2006; 10(1):96–102.

23. Steffen H, Eifert B, Aschoff A, et al. The diagnostic value of optic disc evaluation in acute elevated intracranial pressure. *Ophthalmology.* 1996;103(8):1229–32.

24. Blaivas M, Theodoro D, Sierzenski PR. Elevated intracranial pressure detected by bedside emergency ultrasonography of the optic nerve sheath. *Acad Emerg Med.* 2003;10:376–81.

25. Tayal VS, Neulander M, Norton HJ, et al. Emergency department sonographic measurement of optic nerve sheath diameter to detect findings of increased intracranial pressure in adult head injury patients. *Ann Emerg Med.* 2007;49(4):508–14.

26. Bokhari F, Brakenridge S, Nagy K, et al. Prospective evaluation of the sensitivity of physical examination in chest trauma. *J Trauma.* 2002;53:1135–8.

27. Lichtenstein D, Meziere G, Biderman P, et al. The comet-tail artifact: an ultrasound sign ruling out pneumothorax. *Intensive Care Med.* 1999;25:383–8.

28. Kirkpatrick AW, Brown DR, Crickmer S, et al. Hand-held portable sonography for the on-mountain exclusion of a pneumothorax. *Wilderness Environ Med.* 2001;12: 270–2.

Disability

Assessment during the primary survey for trauma-related disability primarily focuses on evaluation of mental status. As described earlier, confusion, agitation, and lethargy may all be signs of traumatic brain injury. For the sake of consistency, the Glasgow Coma Scale (GCS) (Figure 34.4) is used most commonly to evaluate the severity of head injury. The most important component of this score in regards to outcome is the motor score. The simplest approach to assessing and calculating the GCS is to initially observe the patient and see if the eyes are open spontaneously. Subsequently, speak to the patient and ask him or her to verbally respond and follow a simple command. If the eyes are not open spontaneously, or do not open to verbal commands, or the patient does not follow simple commands, then a noxious stimulus such as a sternal rub is required. Response to this noxious stimulus should be observed. A GCS < 9 is consistent with severe traumatic brain injury and requires the airway to be secured. A GCS between 9 and 13 is consistent with moderate brain injury, and clinical judgment is required in regards to airway. A GCS of 14 or 15 suggests minimal or no brain injury. In a patient with traumatic brain injury, every attempt should be made to avoid hypoxia and hypotension[13] because these secondary insults significantly worsen outcomes. Hypoventilation should also be avoided. The victim's pupils should be assessed for reactivity. If pupils are unequal, or reactivity is sluggish, this is suggestive of increased intracranial pressure, and the administration of mannitol should be considered if available. Although steroids are used for high-altitude cerebral edema, there is no evidence that they have any benefit in traumatic brain injury and may actually cause harm.[27]

A brief assessment for spinal cord injury should be conducted during the primary survey by either observing or asking the patient to move his or her extremities. The presence of gross motor function will help preclude complete proximal spinal cord injury and preclude neurogenic shock as a possible etiology of hypotension. Complete spinal immobilization should be maintained throughout the primary survey until a complete evaluation is conducted during the secondary survey. In an unconscious patient who is unresponsive to painful stimuli below clavicles, a painful stimulus should be applied to the supraorbital area to detect reaction.

Glasgow Coma Scale

Eyes
4 - Patient opens eyes spontaneously
3 - Patient opens eyes to speech
2 - Patient opens eyes to pain
1 - Patient does not open eyes

Verbal
5 - Patient oriented and speaks with normal conversation
4 - Patient confused
3 - Patient uses inappropriate words
2 - Patient utters incomprehensible sounds
1 - Patient makes no sounds

Motor
6 - Patient obeys commands
5 - Patient localizes painful stimuli
4 - Patient withdraws from painful stimuli
3 - Patient flexes with painful stimuli (decorticate posturing)
2 - Patient extends with painful stimuli (decerebrate posturing)
1 - Patient makes no motor response

Figure 34.4. The Glasgow Coma Scale. The patient is given his best score for each category and the results are reported in a Glasgow Coma Score. A perfect score is 15. It should be noted that the minimum score a patient can receive is 3.

Exposure and Environment

The trauma victim ideally should be fully exposed to facilitate complete evaluation and minimize the risk of missing injuries. However, complete exposure also places the patient at risk for hypothermia, especially in extreme environments, so the recommendation for exposure in the field is local exposure for evaluation of injuries. Avoiding hypothermia is one of the most important underlying principles in caring for the injured patient. If hypothermia does exist, external measures such as warm blankets and internal measures such as warmed intravenous fluids should be instituted as soon as possible. Helmets should be removed using a two-person technique: one person maintaining cervical spine immobilization from below as another person carefully removes the helmet from above. Clothing and gear is expeditiously removed by cutting the garments, and wet clothing should be removed immediately.

SECONDARY SURVEY

Head

Examination of the head during the secondary survey is a complete examination of the scalp, face, eyes, ears, nose, and oropharynx. However, assessment should begin with a reevaluation of the GCS and the pupillary exam. One of the important underlying principles of managing traumatic brain injury is maintaining euvolemia. Thus, intravenous fluids should be administered as needed. Diuretics should be avoided. If mannitol is administered during the primary survey, one must be wary of an osmotic diuresis and potential hypovolemia. Ecchymoses or contusions around the eyes (Raccoon's eyes) or behind the ears (Battle's signs) may be signs of brain injury or skull fractures. Drainage of clear fluid from the ears or nose is also a sign of brain injury and/ or skull fracture. If head injury is suspected, and the patient is not in shock, then efforts should be made to elevate the patient's head. However, care must be taken to maintain spine precautions because patients with head injury have a higher incidence of associated spine injury. Although minimal interventions may be possible in the austere environment, documentation of baseline exam is useful in subsequent care of the patient. Every effort should be made to evacuate patients with potential brain injury as quickly as possible.

The scalp is very vascular, and bleeding can be significant. Initially, it should be controlled with direct pressure. If suture is available, a running closure with locking stitches can temporarily control hemorrhage. Palpation of the skull may demonstrate skull fractures; however, these should not be manipulated in the field. The eyes should be examined for the presence of any foreign bodies. If the patient is complaining of irritation, it may be a foreign body or corneal laceration or abrasion. The eyes may be irrigated with clean water, and then taped shut to prevent further injury. Profuse epistaxis may require packing of the nasal cavity.

Chest

The chest is a commonly injured area of the body after both blunt and penetrating trauma and one of the leading causes of death after trauma. It is often quite difficult upon initial examination to know the full extent of injuries and how much eventual therapy is needed. The majority of patients with thoracic trauma will need minimal therapeutic intervention. However, in the small percentage of patients that do need an intervention, these simple maneuvers can be life-saving.

Immediately life-threatening injuries to the chest include tension pneumothorax, open pneumothorax ("sucking chest wound"), flail chest, massive hemothorax, and cardiac tamponade. In patients with any of these injuries, physiologic derangements are readily apparent on the primary survey and rapid intervention is necessary. Other injuries such as simple pneumothorax, hemothorax, pulmonary contusion, tracheobronchial tree disruption, blunt cardiac injury, blunt aortic injury, and blunt esophageal rupture are often not quite as noticeable. Patients may have normal vital signs and not be in immediate distress. However, all these injuries can be life-threatening if the diagnosis is not considered and/or treatment is delayed.[7]

Patients with thoracic trauma can have many different types of pathophysiology leading to clinical deterioration. These injuries often result in hypoxia either from changes in intrathoracic pressure (such as tension or open pneumothorax) or low cardiac output states such as patients with tension pneumothorax, cardiac tamponade, or hemorrhagic shock. Patients with multiple rib fractures and significant chest wall pain may have underlying pulmonary contusions with direct lung injury or be hypoventilating due to pain and splinting or anatomic derangements due to a flail chest.

Physical examination of the patient should direct the first responder to the appropriate diagnostic and therapeutic maneuvers. Physical examination of the chest should only be undertaken after the airway has been deemed appropriate or secured with endotracheal intubation (if available). Only then can breathing be examined, which will be the next step. Dyspnea, cyanosis, or significant accessory muscle use are signs of impending respiratory failure and when these are noted, prompt intubation is necessary (if available).

Visualization of the chest wall should note symmetric rise and fall with respiration. Any major flail segments with paradoxical motion (it will move in while the rest of chest wall expands) should be noted because these will impede normal respiratory function. Breath sounds must be auscultated bilaterally. When breath sounds are absent or diminished, percussion of that side of the chest is invaluable, especially in patients in whom a chest X-ray is not immediately available. The main differential of pneumothorax (air in the pleural space) versus hemothorax (blood in the pleural space) can often be differentiated by physical exam alone. The hemothorax will be dull to percussion, whereas patents with pneumothorax will be hyper-resonant.

Further physical examination of the chest should be performed to palpate for any areas of significant tenderness or chest wall instability looking for associated rib fractures. The rescuer should also examine the clavicles, sternoclavicular joint, and the sternum itself for areas of significant tenderness as injuries to these bony structures can be a marker of significant internal damage. Subcutaneous emphysema is an abnormal collection of air within the subcutaneous tissues that, upon palpation, has a characteristic crunchy feel beneath the skin. Subcutaneous emphysema should be sought in the neck and over both sides of the chest, as this finding is always abnormal and is associated with pneumothorax, esophageal injury, and/or major tracheobronchial disruption.

The ideal treatment for any type of pneumothorax is decompression by tube thoracostomy that should be available in any hospital. However, in wilderness situations in which the ideal tools or equipment are not available, other techniques may be used to decompress air from the pleural space. In patients with a penetrating injury into the chest, a finger may simply be placed through the wound into the pleural space to let the accumulated air evacuate. The first-aid provider should always be careful of any sharp edges of broken ribs or retained foreign bodies if this technique is used. If needle decompression is available with a large-bore needle (or any other type of plastic tubing), it is important to have a one-way valve (i.e., Heimlich valve) attached to the pleural decompression tube. A one-way valve can be improvised by placing an IV catheter through the end of an examination glove to create a "flutter-valve." This will allow air to leave the pleural space but not reenter. If one is not available, it can be improvised using a simple latex examination glove or even a plastic bag. The needle can be placed through the finger of a glove and the collapsed glove will act as a one-way valve to let air escape from the pleural space, but not go back in. Other types of makeshift tubes (such as IV tubing or any other hollow tube) may be placed into the chest to drain a pneumothorax if a chest tube is not available.

Open pneumothorax (sucking chest wound) is defined as a large hole in the chest wall with communication from the outside world to the pleural space. When the patient attempts to inspire, the negative intrathoracic pressure drives more air into the pleural space through this abnormal communication instead of into the lung through the airways because this will be the path of least resistance for the air. The patient's lungs will be underventilated leading to severe hypoxia. The common treatment for this injury is to cover the large chest wall defect with an occlusive dressing taped on three sides, the theory being that this type of dressing will prevent air from entering the pleural space while allowing air to escape if it becomes trapped. (Current military recommendations advise the taping of all four sides of the dressing and using needle decompression if a tension pneumothorax develops.) Any type of airtight dressing such as a plastic bag or other occlusive material may be used.

Some chest injuries require significant surgical or major invasive procedures to treat and prevent death. The rare patient with blunt aortic injury, blunt cardiac injury, tracheobronchial disruption, cardiac tamponade, or esophageal injury will need rapid transfer to the highest level of medical care for any chance at survival.

Abdomen

Life-threatening hemorrhage can occur within the abdomen; however, interventions in the austere environment are limited. The abdomen should be examined for tenderness and muscular rigidity. The presence of these physical findings is suggestive of injury. If ultrasound is available, it may be used to detect the presence of fluid within the abdomen. Fluid in the abdomen following trauma is assumed to be blood until proven otherwise. If abdominal injury is suspected in blunt injury, it is potentially a surgical emergency and the victim should be evacuated to a definitive care facility as rapidly as possible.

Anatomical surface markers can be used to define the borders of the abdominal cavity. Anteriorly, these markers are the nipple/areola complex superiorly and the pubic symphysis inferiorly. Posteriorly, they are the inferior tips of the scapulae superiorly and the pelvis inferiorly. If penetrating injury occurs within these landmarks or the potential trajectory crosses them, abdominal injury should be suspected. All gunshot wounds to the abdomen require formal evaluation and should be evacuated immediately. Stab wounds to the anterior abdomen may be examined with local wound exploration. This may require basic knowledge and expertise to extend the initial wound to obtain adequate exposure. An attempt should be made to evaluate the depth of the wound – if the anterior fascia is violated, then the possibility of intraabdominal injury exists, and the patient should be evacuated. However, if the wound is superficial and the anterior fascia is intact, then the wound may simply be irrigated and dressed, and evacuation is not necessarily mandatory. If the abdomen is penetrated by a foreign object, the object should not be removed in the field. If intraabdominal contents are protruding externally, reducing them back into the abdominal cavity should not be attempted – they should be covered with a moist, clean dressing until a formal exploration can be performed at a health care facility. Broad-spectrum antibiotics should be administered for penetrating injury to the abdomen as soon as possible.

Pelvis

Patients with pelvic injury can be some of the most difficult and complex trauma patients to treat. Complex pelvic fracture causes significant long-term morbidity and mortality after trauma. It is also a significant marker for other associated injuries (i.e., head, thoracic, etc.).

Although not logically intuitive, one always must consider significant pelvic fracture with internal hemorrhage as a potential injury in the hypotensive blunt trauma patient. After all other potential areas of hemorrhage (chest, abdomen, retroperitoneum, thighs, and external blood loss) have been ruled out, the pelvis remains a significant anatomic location for ongoing hemorrhage.[14] Physical examination evaluating for pelvic stability is an important maneuver in the early evaluation of the hypotensive blunt trauma patient. Examination of the pelvis should first begin with lateral compression by placing one hand on each anterior superior iliac spine (ASIS) and pushing them together (medially). A normal pelvis should not move. If no motion is noted on compression, pelvic stability should be confirmed by pushing down on both anterior superior iliac spines. When pushing simultaneously,

there should be no give. In a normal pelvis, pushing down on one ASIS will make the other side come up. This physical exam finding is often reported as the pelvis being "stable to rock." In the patient in whom movement is felt on compression, there is an unstable pelvic fracture. If the pelvis does move with medial compression, the rocking portion of the physical exam should not be performed. Any excess manipulation can precipitate worse internal pelvic bleeding. Pubic symphysis diastasis can be noted on physical examination as a depression between the two halves of the pubic symphysis. Physical examination should also search for common associated injuries. Blood at the urethral meatus, a high-riding prostate and/or scrotal hematoma may indicate a disrupted urethra. When evaluating for penetrating trauma, it is important to perform a rectal and vaginal exam to rule out occult injuries in these locations.

In patients with an unstable or a large complex pelvic fracture, internal bleeding will be the norm, and some sort of pelvic stabilization must be performed as soon as possible to help minimize this internal bleeding. Classically, a sheet tied around the pelvis and tightened to help cinch down the pelvis back into its normal anatomically structure has been used.[15] Military Anti-Shock Trousers (MAST) have also been used in the past for a similar pelvic stabilization, although their use has more recently fallen out of favor. More recently, commercially available pelvic binders (i.e., PelvicBinder and Trauma Pelvic Orthotic Device, or TPOD) using pulley systems (somewhat like a corset) are used to help close down the pelvic volume.[16] Their placement should be directed by physical exam findings, especially in situations where X-ray may not be immediately available to confirm the diagnosis. Pelvic binders can do an excellent job at temporarily reducing the pelvis to its preinjury anatomic state. The beneficial effects of this may help stop cortical bone bleeding and venous bleeding as well as arterial hemorrhage that can be noted with pelvic fractures such as these.

Spine

Injuries to the spine should be suspected in all trauma victims, and spine immobilization should be maintained until a thorough examination can be performed. A trauma victim can have vertebral fractures with or without spinal cord injury. Symptoms of spinal cord injury include sensory deficits (e.g., numbness/tingling, loss of sensation, inability to differentiate between sharp and dull) and motor deficits (e.g., weakness or incontinence). A physical examination involves palpating the entire length of the spine and evaluating for abnormal step-offs or tenderness. If the patient's mental status is altered, then tenderness cannot be reliably ascertained, and spine precautions should be maintained. Spine

Box 34.2. Evaluation of potential cervical spine injuries in austere environments

Gregory H. Bledsoe, MD, MPH

Evaluation of the cervical spine (c-spine) for potential injuries can be difficult even in a fully equipped tertiary-care facility. In the austere environment – without the aid of radiologic investigation – cervical injuries must be evaluated clinically. Maintaining c-spine immobilization for patients with minor trauma can lead to prolonged and sometimes hazardous evacuations requiring much time and costly resource utilization. However, improperly "clearing" a patient with an occult injury could lead to a disastrous outcome. The expedition medical officer needs to be aware of the clinical protocols for the evaluation of cervical spine without the aid of radiologic investigation.

Two large studies have been published in the medical literature reviewing the clinical evaluation of potential cervical spine injuries. Both studies were designed to help reduce unnecessary radiologic investigation and have been used with success in many academic and community emergency departments. The first of these studies was the National Emergency X-Radiography Utilization Study (NEXUS) group that developed five clinical criteria to determine whether an X-ray series was necessary for a patient following cervical spine trauma. If the patient had these five criteria – absence of midline cervical tenderness, normal level of alertness, no evidence of intoxication, absence of focal neurologic deficit, and absence of painful distracting injury – then the patient could forgo cervical spine radiographs and be "cleared" clinically for significant c-spine injury.[1] The NEXUS guidelines demonstrated a sensitivity of 99% for detecting cervical spine injuries.[2]

The second protocol developed to clinically evaluate cervical spine injury was the "Canadian C-Spine Rule for Radiography" and is based upon asking three questions to clinically identify patients in need of further investigation.[3] The clinician asks the following:

1. Are there any high-risk factors that mandate radiography?
2. Are there any low-risk factors that would allow a safe assessment of range of motion?

3. Is the patient able to rotate the neck 45 degrees to the left and to the right?

High-risk factors include age over 65 years old, a fall from height greater than 1 meter, an axial loading injury to the head, a high-speed motor vehicle crash or a crash that includes a rollover or ejection, or the presence of neurologic deficits such as paresthesias in the extremities. Low-risk factors include patient ambulatory at the scene and able to sit up without difficulty, delayed neck pain, no midline cervical spine tenderness, or minor motor vehicle crash such as a simple rear-end collision. These Canadian c-spine rules have been shown to have a "100 percent sensitivity and 42.5 percent specificity for identifying patients with 'clinically important' cervical spine injuries".[2]

In the field, the expedition medical officer can use these guidelines to identify patients at risk for possible occult cervical spine injuries and to "clear" those who are clinically stable. Patients suspected of occult injury must have their cervical spine protection maintained and be evacuated with spinal precautions. Those clinically cleared can be escorted out without c-spine precautions in place.

References

1. Hoffman JR, Mower WR, Wolfson AB, Todd KH, Zucker MI. Validity of a set of clinical criteria to rule out injury to the cervical spine in patients with blunt trauma. National Emergency X-Radiography Utilization Study Group. *N Engl J Med.* 2000;343(2):94–9.
2. Baron BJ, Scalea TM. Spinal cord injuries. In: Tintinalli JE, Kelen GC, Stapczynski, eds. *Emergency Medicine: A Comprehensive Study Guide.* 6th ed. New York: McGraw-Hill; 2004.
3. Stiell IG, Wells GA, Vandemheen KL, Clement CM, Lesiuk H, De Maio VJ, et al. The Canadian c-spine rule for radiography in alert and stable trauma patients. *JAMA.* 2001;286(15):1841–8.

precautions include log-rolling the patient, and securing the patient to a stiff board for transport. If the patient is altered or intoxicated or has other injuries causing pain and thereby distracting the spine exam, tenderness cannot be reliably evaluated, and spine precautions should be maintained. However, if a patient is awake and alert without signs of head injury or altered mental status secondary to altitude or medications, and does not have distracting injuries, then a more reliable examination of the spine may be possible. The risk/benefit ratio between "clearing" the spine to allow ambulation and make evacuation easier and potentially missing an injury that could result in paralysis must be considered in every situation. (See Box 34.2.) If the patient does have signs of spinal cord injury, then an attempt should be made to

determine the level of injury. Sensory deficits should be correlated with dermatomes, and motor deficits should be correlated with myotomes.[7] Once again, although interventions for spinal injuries in the austere environment are minimal, documentation of a baseline exam will be useful in subsequent evaluation and care.

Extremities

Injuries to the extremities are some of the more common injuries dealt with in remote and extreme environments. In general, isolated extremity and musculoskeletal injuries are rarely life-threatening and only slightly more commonly limb-threatening. However, they can be debilitating and have significant long-tem impact on the patients who suffer them. In the multiply injured patient, injuries to the extremity fall relatively low on the priority list and should only be addressed after the ABCDE of the primary survey is complete. Only in the case of ongoing extensive extremity hemorrhage, as is found in major peripheral arterial injury, should these wounds be dealt with early in the resuscitation under the category C for circulation. When identified and appropriately treated early, lives may be saved.

Major extremity arterial hemorrhage is encountered from both blunt and penetrating trauma. This type of injury is more commonly seen in the military setting, especially in soldiers with protective body armor that preferentially protects the head and torso. First line treatment (after airway and breathing, if necessary) is attempted direct pressure control to areas of active arterial hemorrhage. If direct digital pressure is attempted and this does not control the hemorrhage, early consideration of the use of a tourniquet must be considered (Figure 34.5).[17] In the past, the use of tourniquets has been discouraged in both civilian and military setting; however, there has been resurgence in recent years with suggestions that tourniquet use may actually improve care and salvage patients more so than thought of before. Ideally, a commercially available tourniquet such as a Combat Application Tourniquet supplied to the military should be used. Alternatively, a blood pressure cuff, if available, can be inflated above systolic blood pressure to occlude arterial inflow above the wound. If these methods are not available, tourniquets are easily improvised with common household, camping, or expedition gear. A piece of rope or webbing is placed around the extremity above the site of arterial injury. A simple knot tied around a stick can be placed above the initial knot and twisted, tightening down the tourniquet and occluding arterial inflow. In patients whom a tourniquet must be left on to occlude arterial inflow for a prolonged period of time, there is the potential of limb loss due to ischemia to the extremity. A common error in tourniquet use is placement proximal to a major venous injury. In this case, placement of a tourniquet which does not prevent arterial inflow but prevents venous outflow may actually worsen bleeding as blood can still come to the injured limb, but cannot drain back toward the heart. Once a tourniquet has been applied, the patient must be rapidly evacuated for definitive treatment of the arterial injury. Other potential treatments of major hemorrhage include topical hemostatic agents. Some of these specialized bandages (i.e., QuikClot or Celox) are also being used in both the civilian and the military settings for external hemorrhage control.[18] They are small, lightweight, and easy to use – often ideal for an expedition medical kit.

Another potentially life-threatening type of musculoskeletal trauma is a crush injury of an extremity. The crushed and mangled extremity may have active arterial hemorrhage or the bleeding may be easily controlled. However, the massive tissue destruction can set up the patient for a significant inflammatory response and need for large-volume fluid resuscitation. This resuscitation is necessary to compensate for the large amount of fluid sequestration into the injured limb. The primary tissue injury and ischemia that has occurred has significant impact on outcome, but the secondary injury caused by reperfusion may be even more harmful. This reperfusion injury often leads to compartment syndrome and/or rhabdomyolysis. Rhabdomyolysis is caused by muscle cell necrosis and release of myoglobin and can lead to acute renal failure, electrolyte abnormalities, and arrhythmias, which put patients at risk for death. If the patient with a crushed limb will have a prolonged extrication time, the fluid administration should begin before the limb is released. Even at trauma centers with the combined expertise of trauma, orthopedic, and plastic surgeons and significant resources, amputation may be necessary. Injuries such as these may involve the

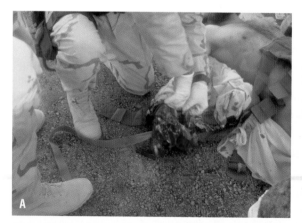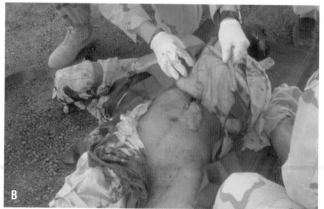

Figure 34.5. Tourniquet application in a patient with an extremity arterial bleed can be a life-saving measure. (A) Here a military medic assesses the upper extremity of a civilian patient who was injured after handling an unexploded ordnance. (B) Application of a tourniquet to the extremity controls the bleeding and allows the medic to assess for other injuries. Photos courtesy of Carol Noriega.

skin, soft tissue, bone, nerve, and blood vessels. Many scoring systems such as the Mangled Extremity Severity Score (MESS)[19] have been suggested to help predict which patients will eventually need amputation. If the amputation is performed early, then some of the systemic physiologic alterations can be avoided.[20] A large prospective observational study has actually shown that functional outcomes at 2 years after injury are similar in patients who received early amputation versus reconstruction.[21] It is better to have a live patient with an amputation than a dead patient whose limb was unsuccessfully salvaged despite utilization of significant resources and expense. In truly austere environments, primary amputation should be considered, if the appropriate surgical expertise is available.

After major injury has been ruled out and the airway, breathing, circulation has been confirmed, orthopedic or musculoskeletal injuries should then be evaluated. Clearly, physical exam plays the most important role in this type of injury.

Few other traumatic extremity injuries are life-threatening, although many others put the patient at risk for limb loss. These often look quite terrible and draw immediate attention. However, we should once again reiterate the importance of assessing the ABCDEs before these extremity injuries are addressed. Types of injuries that may lead to eventual limb loss include open fractures, open joint injuries, compartment syndromes, and neurologic and vascular injuries.

Open fractures or joint injuries are at high risk of infection even in the best of circumstances. The basic premise based on physical examination is that a wound near a fracture or joint is considered an open fracture (or joint) until proven otherwise. In the hospital, these wounds are interrogated with X-rays and prompt operative debridement and washout. Ideally, this is performed within 6 hours of injury;[22] however, this is not always possible in more remote locations. These patients should also receive tetanus prophylaxis and systemic antibiotics if available. Oral antibiotics can be substituted for intravenous if this is all that is available. In addition, gross contamination should be washed away, often with simple soap and water.

Patients with compartment syndrome have ongoing swelling within the muscle compartment enclosed by the tight fascia. This edema causes decreased muscle perfusion and increased cell death that leads to swelling and worsening perfusion into a rapid cycle of decline. If not treated promptly, limb loss will be the unfortunate result. Compartment syndromes are most commonly found in the lower leg, but they can be seen in any muscle group contained by a fascial compartment (i.e., thigh, buttock, forearm, hand). The diagnosis must always be considered in any type of extremity injury. The earliest sign and symptom is pain (often described as "pain out of proportion" to what is expected and worsened with passive range of motion). Neurologic findings (decreased sensation) will follow. Only in the late stages will motor function decline, the compartment become extremely tense, and the patient have the eventual loss of peripheral pulses. Surgical decompression by release of the fascia is necessary to preserve limb integrity.

Significant neurologic injury also leads to eventual limb loss from either sensory deficiencies or motor deficiencies. Distal neurologic exam should be performed (both a sensory and motor examination) before any manipulation of an obviously injured extremity is performed. After this quick neurovascular examination in a threatened limb, obvious fractures should be reduced and splinted, if possible. The old adage "splint it where it lies" is a reasonable approach in patients who will be rapidly transported to appropriate medical care. However, in expedition medicine or wilderness evacuation, it is not always a feasible option. In this case, fracture reduction and joint relocation are often preferable choices.

The benefits of reducing and splinting a fracture include decreased pain, tissue destruction, and bleeding. A femur should be pulled out to length to help with internal hemorrhage control. A shortened thigh with two ends of the femur overriding, has ongoing muscle bleeding and ongoing bone bleeding into the thigh compartment. After the extremity is distracted, the fascial compartment tightens, which helps tamponade and slow down further ongoing bleeding. If available, traction can be performed by using a commercially available hare traction splint. The splint is placed with multiple straps around the lower extremity and a pulley system that pulls on the ankle and helps to stop ongoing bleeding. If a system such as this is not available, other types of traction may be improvised. A simple method is to pull the limb out to length and to attach the injured extremity to the noninjured extremity to keep it at full tension. Dislocations of extremity joints should be reduced promptly. After these are reduced, pain will decrease significantly. This early relocation will also help long-term function because these dislocations are often associated with tension on nerves. The sciatic nerve is commonly stretched with posterior hip dislocations or the axillary nerve with shoulder dislocations.

The vascular system should be examined for hemorrhage and for signs and symptoms of distal ischemia such as weakened or diminished pulses. The opposite extremity is often an excellent reference point in patients with isolated extremity trauma. A young healthy person with a normal exam in the affected leg should, in general, have the same exam on the contra-lateral leg. If the injured leg is clearly ischemic (no palpable pulse, cold, pale, pain, and paresthesias), vascular compromise must be considered, and the problem should be addressed immediately. Peripheral vascular injuries in the extremities must be promptly treated to allow any chance of limb salvage. The hard signs of vascular injury include absent or diminished pulses, active hemorrhage, expanding hematoma, palpable thrill, audible bruit, or any signs of distal ischemia and require prompt surgical intervention or rapid evacuation and transfer for further management. Soft signs of vascular injuries include a stable hematoma, unexplained hypotension, proximity of an injury to a major vessel, or an associated neurologic deficit, all of which are potential markers of vascular injury.

As with any other injury, options for evacuation must be considered. Some extremity injuries are managed in the field in the same way that it would be managed in an acute care hospital setting. In a patient with a dislocated or fractured finger, it may be appropriate to simply buddy tape the injured digit to the adjacent digit and let it heal on its own. Similarly, other simple musculoskeletal injures such as sprains, strains, and even a dislocated shoulder may not require evacuation.

SUMMARY

Traumatic injury is an inevitable risk of traveling in remote or extreme environments. However, with proper education and experience, a medical officer can make a considerable difference and reduce potential morbidity and mortality even while working without typical hospital resources.

ACKNOWLEDGMENTS

Special thanks to Carol Noriega, RN, and Dennis Hutchins, RN, for their help with the airway photos.

REFERENCES

1. World Health Organization Mortality Database. Available at: *http://www.who.int/violence_injury_prevention/resources/ publications/en/injury_factsheet.pdf*. Accessed December 25, 2006.

2. MacKenzie EJ, Rivara FP, Jurkovich GJ, Nathens AB, Frey KP, Egleston BL, Salkever DS, Scharfstein DO. A national evaluation of the effect of trauma-center care on mortality. *N Engl J Med*. 2006;354(4):366–78.

3. Demetriades D, Martin M, Salim A, Rhee P, Brown C, Doucet J, Chan L. Relationship between American College of Surgeons trauma center designation and mortality in patients with severe trauma (injury severity score > 15). *J Am Coll Surg*. 2006;202(2):212–5; quiz A45.

4. Demetriades D, Martin M, Salim A, Rhee P, Brown C, Chan L. The effect of trauma center designation and trauma volume on outcome in specific severe injuries. *Ann Surg*. 2005;242(4):512–17; discussion 517–19.

5. Demetriades D, Berne TV, Belzberg H, Asensio J, Cornwell E, Dougherty W, Alo K, DeMeester TR. The impact of a dedicated trauma program on outcome in severely injured patients. *Arch Surg*. 1995;130(2):216–20.

6. Cornwell EE 3rd, Chang DC, Phillips J, Campbell KA. Enhanced trauma program commitment at a level I trauma center: effect on the process and outcome of care. *Arch Surg*. 2003;138(8):838–43.

7. American College of Surgeons Committee on Trauma. *Advanced Trauma Life Support (ATLS) Student Course Manual*. 7th ed. Chicago; 2004.

8. Lefrançois DP, Dufour DG. Use of the esophageal tracheal combitube by basic emergency medical technicians. *Resuscitation*. 2002;52(1):77–83.

9. Davidoff J, Fowler R, Gordon D, Klein G, Kovar J, Lozano M, Potkya J, Racht E, Saussy J, Swanson E, Yamada R, Miller L. Clinical evaluation of a novel intraosseous device for adults: prospective, 250-patient, multi-center trial. *JEMS*. 2005;30(10):Suppl 20–23.

10. LaRocco BG, Wang HE. Intraosseous infusion. *Prehosp Emerg Care*. 2003;7(2):280–5. Review.

11. Frascone RJ, Jensen JP, Kaye K, Salzman JG. Consecutive field trials using two different intraosseous devices. *Prehosp Emerg Care*. 2007;11(2):164–71.

12. Calkins MD, Fitzgerald G, Bentley TB, Burris D. Intraosseous infusion devices: a comparison for potential use in special operations. *J Trauma*. 2000;48(6):1068–74.

13. Brain Trauma Foundation and American Association of Neurological Surgeons, Joint Section on Neurotrauma and Critical Care. Management and Prognosis of Severe Traumatic Brain Injury. Available at: *http://www2.braintrauma. org/guidelines/*. Accessed July 6, 2007.

14. DiGiacomo JC, Bonadies JA, Cole FJ, Diebel L, Hoff WS, Holevar M, Malcynski J, Scalea T. Practice Management Guidelines for Hemorrhage in Pelvic Fracture. The Eastern Association for the Surgery of Trauma. Available at: *http://www.east.org/ tpg/pelvis.pdf*. Accessed July 6, 2007.

15. Simpson T, Krieg JC, Heuer F, Bottlang M. Stabilization of pelvic ring disruptions with a circumferential sheet, *J Trauma*. 2002;52:158–61.

16. Nunn T, Cosker T, Bose D, Pallister I. Immediate application of improvised pelvic binder as first step in extended resuscitation from life-threatening hypovolaemic shock in conscious patients with unstable pelvic injuries. *Injury*. 2007;38(1):125–8. Epub September 22, 2006.

17. Welling DR, Burris DG, Hutton JE, Minken SL, Rich NM. A balanced approach to tourniquet use: lessons learned and relearned. *J Am Coll Surg*. 2006;203(1):106–15.

18. Wedmore I, McManus JG, Pusateri AE, Holcomb JB. A special report on the chitosan-based hemostatic dressing: experience in current combat operations. *J Trauma*. 2006;60(3):655–8.

19. Johansen K, Daines M, Howey T, Helfet D, Hansen ST Jr. Objective criteria accurately predict amputation following lower extremity trauma. *J Trauma*. 1990;30(5):568–72; discussion 572–3.

20. American College of Surgeons Committee on Trauma. Management of Complex Extremity Trauma. Available at: *http:// www.facs.org/trauma/publications/mancomplextrauma.pdf*. Accessed July 6, 2007.

21. Bosse MJ, MacKenzie EJ, Kellam JF, Burgess AR, Webb LX, Swiontkowski MF, Sanders RW, Jones AL, McAndrew MP, Patterson BM, McCarthy ML, Travison TG, Castillo RC. An analysis of outcomes of reconstruction or amputation after leg-threatening injuries. *N Engl J Med*. 2002;347(24): 1924–31.

22. Bednar DA, Parikh J. Effect of time delay from injury to primary management on the incidence of deep infec-

tion after open fractures of the lower extremities caused by blunt trauma in adults. *J Orthop Trauma.* 1993;7(6): 532–5.

23 Bickell WH, Wall MJ Jr, Pepe PE, Martin RR, Ginger VF, Allen MK, Mattox KL. Immediate versus delayed fluid resuscitation for hypotensive patients with penetrating torso injuries. *N Engl J Med.* 1994;331(17):1105–9.

24 Dutton RP, Mackenzie CF, Scalea TM. Hypotensive resuscitation during active hemorrhage: impact on in-hospital mortality. *J Trauma.* 2002;52(6):1141–6.

25 Salomone JP, Ustin JS, McSwain NE Jr, Feliciano DV. Opinions of trauma practitioners regarding prehospital interventions for critically injured patients. *J Trauma.* 2005;58(3):509–15; discussion 515–7.

26 Krausz MM. Related Articles, Initial resuscitation of hemorrhagic shock. *World J Emerg Surg.* 2006;1:14.

27 Edwards P, Arango M, Balica L, et al. Final results of MRC CRASH, a randomised placebo- controlled trial of intravenous corticosteroid in adults with head injury – outcomes at 6 months. *Lancet.* 2005. Jun 4–10;365(9475):1957–9.

35 | Principles and Practice of Expedition Wound Management

James M. Marinucci

Author's Note: The topic of expedition wound management is, in itself, worthy of an entire publication. The inherent difficulty in writing this chapter is to determine which key elements of the subject are exclusive to expedition practice or merit further discussion and exclude those common in most quality wound management texts. The goal is not to burden the reader with a review of technical skills he or she should already possess or provide lists of wound care supplies that might be packed for the generic expedition. The rationale behind this chapter is to consider the overall approach to the wound care patient in the context of a remote setting.

All wounds can be more severe than a given first impression allows, even potentially life-threatening, therefore, "tunnel vision" must be avoided when assessing and treating the patient.

EXPEDITION VERSUS CONVENTIONAL WOUND MANAGEMENT

The treatment of acute traumatic wounds suffered during an expedition often demands a significant portion of the clinician's attention. The idea that the practice of wound management during an expedition might somehow be different than performed in a "brick and mortar" setting is, by no means, a revolutionary concept. It is easy to feel quite comfortable when closing a wound in a well-stocked, climate-controlled Procedure Room. It is another matter when your Procedure Room is a poorly lit tent, the galley of a ship, the bed of a pickup truck or, maybe, the floor of the closest four-walled structure. While the former environment is certainly preferable for most complicated cases, both settings are not without their advantages and disadvantages. A conventional treatment area can accommodate nearly all available options with regard to pre- and postprocedure imaging studies, anesthesia, methods of closure, dressings, splints, access to subspecialists, and so on. However, the clinician cannot often reliably predict the volume of patients that might arrive at any given time. He or she cannot anticipate the mechanism of their injuries or obtain an accurate picture of their past medical history if they are unable to communicate. The expedition medical provider, while limited in both the amount and diversity of supplies carried, can foresee many inherent threats in a given environment, access and review participants' medical histories prior to departure and construct a specific wound care arsenal based upon known variables. In spite of its obvious limitations, the practice of wound management in the expedition setting can certainly be looked upon as *a glass half full.*

Predeparture Preparation

Doing your homework prior to departure is essential for anyone serving as the expedition's medical provider. Given a proper amount of lead time, there is no excuse for the provider not to become familiar with readily available information concerning the expedition environment, attain any additional skills to effectively carry out their job, and assemble the necessary equipment to provide the highest level of wound care under the circumstances.

Anticipating the Expedition Environment

The expedition's setting will exert a great deal of influence on your approach to wound management. The geographic location itself will suggest many indigenous hazards that can easily affect a traumatic wound's cause, treatment modality, and aftercare instructions. The medical provider supporting an African safari would anticipate very different types of wounds than someone preparing for an Everest climb. Likewise, certain medications, dressings, and other wound care components are sensitive to extreme climates.

The number of personnel, their past medical histories, and the expedition's length will certainly affect the amount and allocation of supplies carried. A large-scale undertaking over a longer period of time will demand a judicious use of wound management resources. Only so much space can be dedicated to this category of provisions. Regardless of the team's size, increased length of an expedition will yield a higher number of injuries. The clinician must understand from the onset of a mission that compromise is often necessary when addressing traumatic wounds in the field. Do the most good with the supplies on hand.

Let's not forget, however, that certain injuries occur often enough regardless of any variation in an expedition's size, duration, or location. Simple lacerations, minor burns, abrasions, contusions can happen as often in your own home as they can while hiking the Inca Trail. Treatment of these common wounds should be expected.

The stated mission of the expedition will, understandably, play a significant role in anticipating injuries. Is your team's goal to photograph exotic birds in East Africa or provide humanitarian assistance to refugees constantly under threat in the Sudan?

When planning wound management (as well as general medical capabilities), the clinician must consider two extremely important, but often overlooked, aspects of the expedition environment: (1) What is the general assessment of the nearest health care facility or system? (2) Who will assess and treat *you* if needed? The location and capabilities of the nearest health care system can guide your decision as to the variety and amount of wound care supplies that must be packed, the scope of any potential evacuation in the event of a severe injury, and the level of training required preexpedition. More than a passing thought should be given to the fact that traumatic injury can strike the primary medical provider on even the most benign excursion. It may not be feasible for more than one person to have advanced wound management training. However, at least one additional team member should have basic first responder training and be familiar with the medical supplies chosen for the expedition.

Attain the Appropriate Level of Training

At this point, it must be clearly stated that good wound management is much more than apposing two sides of a laceration and neatly bandaging the patient. It takes very little training to actually *close* a wound. The skill lies in understanding the kinetics of an injury, its subsequent evaluation, and the long-term consequences based on many different treatment options. Recognizing which situations allow for a continued presence on the expedition and which require evacuation may not always be so obvious. The patient with a small finger laceration transecting a neurovascular bundle may require evacuation while another with a larger wound may be allowed to continue. When participants invest a significant amount of time and money, the decision to cut the expedition short may not come easily. The medical provider's job is to offer guidance, but he or she may often be required to make the tough call for them.

As previously stated, the medical provider can anticipate much about the nature of potential injuries based upon readily available data before departure. The medical provider then needs to take a long, hard look at his or her own skill level and decide which areas, if any, need improvement. Reference material in the form of texts, online resources, hands-on classes, or preexpedition consultation can prove invaluable.

Because of the inherent nature of an expedition and the fact that *normal* pathways to care may not be available, the primary medical provider needs to possess certain skills to compliment his or her wound management abilities. Basic first-aid and first responder training are a must. You and others on the team are the prehospital providers.

Construct the Proper Wound Management Kit

A number of companies produce high-quality wound management kits specifically for use under austere conditions. These kits come with a variety of supplies for practitioners of all levels. Unfortunately, the author has not yet seen one single pack that addresses the range of injuries that is typically planned for. However, most companies allow you to customize their products according to your specifications.

The amount and variety of supplies will vary according to the details of an expedition. Ask the following questions:

- What is the location and purpose of the expedition?
- What is the expected duration of the trip?
- What intrinsic hazards exist in the expedition environment?
- Can I anticipate the treatment area prior to departure?
- Will the treatment area be fixed or mobile?
- How many team members will I be responsible for treating?
- What is their past medical history with particular regard for any adverse drug reactions?
- Will I be responsible to treat anyone else who may not be part of the core group?
- If so, can I predict the potential number of patients?
- What was the injury trend in previous similar expeditions?
- What is my level of training with regard to wound management?
- Who else might be responsible for using the wound management provisions and what are their levels of training?

- What additional outside medical resources, if any, are available during the expedition?
- What additional medical and dental supplies will be taken?
- Have I established evacuation criteria and procedures prior to departure?
- What is the budget for wound management supplies?

After you have answered these questions satisfactorily, you can decide upon the scope and quantity of supplies.

MEDICAL DOCUMENTATION

The role of proper medical documentation in the pre-expedition phase is clear. Medical histories and recent exams are documented. Personal contact information is collected. In the course of the expedition, illness, injury, and any other medical changes – major or minor – must be noted. This record is especially important with regard to wound management. A documented baseline sensory/motor/vascular examination prior to any procedure is a tremendous tool when, and if, the patient requires additional follow-up. It can also serve as a legal safeguard for the medical provider should an undesired outcome or permanent disability result. After the expedition, data fields gathered from injury documentation should be examined and catalogued. This information can and should be used to do a risk analysis for future expeditions, determine the average scope and frequency of various wounds, and adjust the medical supplies accordingly.

SELECTING THE APPROPRIATE TREATMENT AREA

The lack of a fixed location during an expedition presents the medical provider with several difficulties when treating open wounds: issues of maintaining a hygienic treatment area, adequate space and lighting, patient privacy, and ease of access in the event an evacuation is required. In a more stable location, finding an appropriate treatment area may also be difficult, but the provider has certain advantages. A larger and broader selection of wound care supplies can be brought due to the fact that they would not have to be transported from location to location. Sanitary conditions are often easier to maintain. Evacuation protocols can more accurately be executed when a changing location is no longer a considerable variable.

CLASSIFICATION OF ACUTE WOUNDS

Before a discussion of the principles and practices in expedition wound management can begin, a brief description of the subject's building blocks should be established. One of the most elemental aspects of acute wound management is very often the one that tends

to be somewhat inconsistent in much of the literature: acute wound nomenclature. It is a mind-numbing experience to try to find a consistent definition regarding soft tissue wounds. Most definitions are either too simplistic or incomplete. For example, one source has the definition of "laceration" as "an injury to the skin and the soft tissue underneath it."[1] When documenting a patient's wound care, it's important to describe the injury without any ambiguity.

Characteristics of Common Soft Tissue Wounds

In adding my voice to the chorus of definitions, it's my preference that acute wounds be categorized either by *mechanism of injury* or by their *wound geometry*.

Laceration: A tissue separation that, regardless of its mechanism, tends to be longer than it is deep. Lacerations can occur as a result of something quite sharp, leaving either a *clean* or *jagged* edge. They can also result from a blunt impact, splitting the tissue, not necessarily in a straight line or even with a single edge. A blunt impact to the forehead can result in a stellate, or multiple pedicles, flap laceration. Lacerations can also be partial-thickness (superficial) or full-thickness (completely through the dermis).

Puncture wound: A wound that is deeper than it is long. Puncture wounds can be superficial or deep. They can be relatively clean or exceedingly dirty. They all tend to be problematic because they are difficult to clean and irrigate effectively.

Abrasion: A wound caused by a tangential force applied to the skin resulting in a wearing away of the epidermis and varying depth of the dermal layer. Abrasions are most often caused by friction and may be superficial, deep, irregularly shaped, or even somewhat linear. Underlying tissue may be crushed, and the edges may be devitalized. These wounds are often painful and heal over a longer period of time because the wound must granulate.

Avulsion: A wound resulting in a portion of soft tissue completely removed from the body. Avulsions can be full or partial thickness. They are measured in terms of area, not length. Their definitive treatment is dependent upon their size. Avulsions that exceed anything much larger than 1.0 cm^2 often require a skin graft. Smaller ones are usually dressed and allowed to granulate.

Amputation: A wound similar in mechanism to an avulsion but involving bone. Amputations need not only refer to whole extremities. They may also be complete or incomplete, transverse or oblique.

Burn: Damage to skin and other tissues as a result of temperature extremes, electricity, radiation, or caustic substances. "The depth of burn is related to the amount of energy delivered in the injury and to the relative thickness of the skin (the dermis is thinner in very young and very old people)."[2] Currently, burns are classified by the amount of tissue loss: superficial (epidermis), superficial dermal (through epidermis and into the upper layers of dermis), deep dermal and full thickness (through all layers of skin).

Bite: A wound caused by the "teeth of an animal or the mouthparts of an insect or similar organism." Bites can result in nearly every category of wound but they are treated separately because of their highly infectious nature.

Sting: A puncture, laceration, or abrasion caused by a sharp, pointed structure, or organ. Stings are commonly associated with retained foreign bodies, localized swelling, and, occasionally, anaphylactic reactions.

PRINCIPLES AND PRACTICE OF EXPEDITION WOUND MANAGEMENT

Now that the precursors to providing effective wound care in the field have been explored, we must now examine the process by which a patient suffering an acute wound is approached, evaluated, prepped, and treated. The following principles and practices serve as a general guide for this task. Many of these themes are commonplace in the conventional realm, but many others are unique to field practice.

... the first ten minutes

Initial Steps

1. **Body Substance Isolation (BSI).** As soon as the provider is alerted to a potential patient, he or she must take the first step in shielding him- or herself against the transmission of infectious disease. Similar to the Occupational Safety and Health Administration's (OSHA) *Universal Precautions*, the Centers for Disease Control (CDC) published guidelines setting a new standard. These guidelines include the use of Personal Protective Equipment (PPE), handwashing, and proper cleaning as well as disinfection and/or sterilization of equipment.[3]

   IMPORTANT! In a multiple casualty incident, the medical provider's gloves *do not* repeatedly become clean as they move from patient to patient. Don't forget to change your gloves.

2. **Basic first-aid/first responder duties.** In many cases, the patient may require immediate medical care to prevent permanent disability or even death. Remember that you will most likely be the principal responder to any and all medical or traumatic emergencies. As such, your primary responsibility is to the general well-being of the patient, not just their wound. These responsibilities may include, but not be limited to:

   Maintaining or establishing a patent airway

   Patient assessment

   Cardiopulmonary Resuscitation (CPR)

   Initial hemostasis

   Stabilization of injuries to the spine and/or extremities

   IMPORTANT! Place a tourniquet on an arm or leg *only* to save a life! Small digital tourniquets placed no longer than 30 minutes are acceptable for minor wound exploration and repair.[4,5]

3. **Patient comfort and safety.** Without a relative comfort level and a feeling that they are out of immediate danger, it will be extremely difficult to treat, let alone approach, the patient. Hemostasis will go a long way in accomplishing this task. Both provider and patient need to understand, however, that wound hemostasis does not necessarily mean that the bleeding will stop altogether. Venous or capillary bleeding may go on throughout the case even, to a degree, after the wound is closed. Inform the patient of each step you intend to take prior to treatment. Generally, the expedition party's level of anxiety is directly proportional to that of the conscious patient.

4. **Jewelry removal.** Whether the trauma sustained is a crush injury to the hand or a superficial burn to the shoulder, all upper extremity jewelry must be removed as soon as possible. Any offense to an extremity will cause varying degrees of edema. This will be exacerbated by bandaging. It is much easier to get a ring off of a finger at the onset of a case than after the digit is changing color.

5. **Establish the treatment area.** If the expedition is *on the move*, the criteria for establishing an appropriate treatment area can take into consideration the wound itself. The space needed to treat a simple abrasion would not necessarily be the same space desired for the treatment of a large, deep dermal burn.

6. **Delay in definitive care.** In the event that definitive wound care cannot be provided at the time of injury (if, for example, the patient with a possible cervical spine injury and large facial laceration with underlying fracture must be evacuated), careful thought should be given to the possibility that avascular structures may have been violated, requiring antibiotic prophylaxis. In wounds that cannot be readily closed due to lack of a suitable treatment area, special attention should be paid to the application of the proper dressing to minimize the risk of infection and desiccation. Patients requiring transportation to a desired treatment area might have to be splinted to reduce the risk of further injury and increased edema.

7. **Number of people in the treatment area.** Keep in mind that wound care is not a spectator sport! It is not necessary to have an audience while treating the patient. This is true not only to maintain the patient's privacy but also to avoid generating additional patients from onlookers who thought they were tougher than they actually were.

General Physical Examination

Before passing any anesthesia or giving any other medications, some basic information should be obtained.

1. **Basic vital signs.** These signs are always taken prior to dispensing medication or starting a procedure. They can often provide clues as to the cause of a patient's trauma.
   - Blood pressure
   - Respiration rate
   - Heart rate
   - Temperature and occasionally
   - Glucose level
   - Oxygen saturation
   - Glasgow Coma Scale
   - Subjective pain scale

2. **Past medical history.** The past medical history should be checked face to face with the patient and compared to what the patient said on his or her pretrip medical forms. When an injury occurs, details are sometimes forgotten.

   Allergies – not only "to what" but "what happens when you're exposed"

   Current medical problems – patients sometimes need to be reminded that chronic medical conditions count as current medical problems

   Current medications – not only "what are you taking" but also "what are you *supposed* to be taking"

   Prior injury to currently affected area – if there is a deficit, it will be important to know when it actually occurred

History of Present Injury

The history of the present injury is critical information that can be obtained very often without even unwrapping the injury and will allow the provider to tightly focus his or her examination:

1. **Mechanism of injury.** "What happened?" Blunt mechanism versus sharp mechanism: Injury to the dermis may look the same but the damage to the underlying structures and surrounding tissue might be vastly different. A volar finger laceration from a broken piece of glass might look identical to one

sustained from a closing door but the risk of an open fracture is much higher in the latter.

2. **Time from injury.** "When did the injury occur?" It can be difficult to tell the age of a wound solely by exam. The treatment options for a 16-hour-old lower leg laceration are far less than a 1-hour-old wound in the same location.

3. **Prior treatment rendered.** Ask not only "what was done *for* the wound" but also "what was done *to* the wound." Patients do not always clean and dress a wound properly before seeking treatment. A wound cleaned with soap and water, and then dressed with gauze will most likely do better than one that was spit on and packed with tobacco.

4. **Degree of contamination.** This consideration is a purely subjective method of gauging wound healing probability. The more *tidy* the wound, the better chance for a complication-free healing process. A tidy wound typically exhibits one or more of the following characteristics:

   - Generally short-time lapse from wounding
   - Usually secondary to sharp trauma
   - Clean, nonabraded wound edges
   - No surrounding contusion
   - Minor contamination

   An untidy wound typically exhibits one or more of the following characteristics:

   - Generally longer time lapse from wounding
   - Usually secondary to blunt trauma
   - Contused and abraded wound edges
   - Jagged and devitalized wound edges
   - Larger degree of contamination

   Ultimately, the provider will determine if the wound is tidy or untidy based on his or her overall impression. A simple, uncomplicated hand laceration from a clean piece of metal might be considered tidy, but the same wound presenting 20 hours later would be considered untidy and have a higher risk of a poor outcome.

5. **Wound size.** What are the wound's dimensions?

   Length in centimeters. If the wound is dressed, ask the patient how long the wound is. After the wound's mechanism is established, the provider can then have an idea of what structures may have been damaged.

   Depth by tissue layers, not centimeters. A wound 1.0 cm deep to the thigh would barely extend into the subcutaneous tissue, whereas a 1.0 cm deep wound to the eyelid could be devastating.

   Width doesn't necessarily say much about the wound.
   - Because of the tissue structure, a self-approximating elbow laceration may extend as far as

joint space, but a 2.0-cm-wide thigh laceration may only extend into subcutaneous tissue.

- This information can occasionally be helpful provided the clinician has a good understanding of the wound's underlying anatomy. A self-approximating palm laceration may only be partial thickness, but one that is 1.0 cm wide will probably extend into muscle. After the wound's width is visualized and prior to exploration, the provider can assume that the extremity will have a larger degree of edema, higher risk of infection, and longer recovery time, in addition to requiring splinting for the first 48 hours. All of this can be assumed just by seeing the width of the injury.

6. **Possible foreign bodies.** Although it may seem a bit unbelievable, the evidence tends to suggest that patients who claim to feel the presence of a foreign body are very often mistaken. However, when practicing in an unconventional setting in which the use of traditional imaging is more of a wish than a reality, the patient's complaint of a retained foreign body cannot be minimized. Consider the mechanism of injury, the anatomic location, and the patient's level of certainty. In my practice, I've observed far more often than not, with particular regard for injuries to the volar hand and plantar foot, that when a patient claims "something is still in there," it usually is. Remember, on the expedition, your clinical evaluation is extremely important. It's tough to get an X-ray or ultrasound on the shores of Lake Titicaca!

7. **Obvious sensory, motor, and/or vascular deficits.** When there's no doubt about it, prophylactic antibiotics are a must!

  Patients with vascular injuries require constant reevaluation.

  Many arterial transections have associated nerve injuries and vice versa.

  Consider immediate evacuation of patients with obvious deficits.

  These types of deficits do not have an infinite amount of time in which to be surgically repaired, generally 7–10 days.

  Consider a primary wound closure with understanding that further surgery may be required.

  ... the next ten minutes

Inorganic objects – lower risk of infection[6]
Organic objects – higher risk of infection[7]
Most glass is radio-opaque
Most wood is translucent

Simple removal versus extraction

- The extraction procedure usually requires an elective incision to remove the object.
- Consider a regional nerve block instead of local infiltration because there is less possibility of damage.
- Avoid exploring more than 30 minutes without a break. It's easy to become frustrated. Technical skills become less precise. If another qualified individual is present, ask them to assist with the exploration. Sometimes another set of eyes is all that's needed.
- Under certain circumstances retained foreign bodies can be left in place. This is the general rule if the object in question is relatively small, inert (usually inorganic in nature), and not particularly noticeable to the patient and, most importantly, poses no threat of damage to a nerve, vessel, organ, or joint space.
- The clinician must also consider the possible damage caused by an aggressive attempt at foreign body removal. The clinician must decide, "Is removal a necessity *now* or would conservative treatment be in the patient's best interest?" Consider the object and the risk it poses, access to available outside resources, necessity for evacuation, time remaining in the expedition, and the patient's comfort level.
- Antibiotics are not required for every patient with a foreign object. Consider the object and the patient's underlying medical condition.
- With the "splinter problem," a patient may present several days after sustaining a splinter to their finger. They may claim that it is still there. It may be but if the digit is infected, their sensation of a retained foreign body may only be the indurated tissue still present. If the object isn't found after an appropriate amount of exploration time, it may not be there regardless of what the patient says. Treat the digit (draining any abscess, if necessary) and observe closely.

Preparation for Definitive Care

Once the patient is secured and removed from any threat of additional injury, the bleeding controlled, the treatment area is established, and the history taken, the second phase of wound management can proceed.

IMPORTANT! All aspects of the history and wound exam are really just pieces of a puzzle. Do not rush to judgment about any wound based on only one or two parts of the exam.

1. **Thorough and specific wound area exam:** After the patient is in a position conducive to wound repair (most often supine) and the provider has "set up shop" in the best possible location, a comprehensive wound assessment can be done.

  General appearance: What is your *gut* reaction to the appearance of the wound and the involved anatomy? Is it what you'd expect given the history? Is the wound causing an asymmetry?

Sensory exam

- Regardless of which exam is used to check sensation, give the patient a recognizable baseline before proceeding.
- Examine each area distal to the wound that might be affected.
- Light Touch or Sharp/Dull are simple, quick, and generally reliable methods for checking sensation in most anatomic regions.
- Administer the two-point tactile discrimination (2pd) exam.
  - The 2pd exam is for use primarily with injuries on the volar aspect of the hand or digits.
  - Gently use the tips of a scissors, a paper clip, or any similar object.[8]
  - Place the instrument on the volar aspects of the digits, distal to the proximal interphalangeal joints (PIPJ) or interphalangeal joint on the thumb (IPJ).
  - Accuracy drops significantly for many individuals if the instrument is placed proximal to those points.
  - Place points along radial and ulnar aspects only.
  - Normal range is between 5 and 8 mm.[9]
  - Document the minimum distance at which both points are felt simultaneously on both the radial and ulnar aspects of the digit.
  - The 2pd exam may be widened or absent for reasons other than a nerve laceration (e.g., edema, constriction from a digital tourniquet, previous injury).

Motor exam

- A patient may have a significant muscle or tendon laceration and still have good strength.[10]
- Check movement against resistance.
- Extension is generally weaker than flexion.
- When in doubt, compare to the opposite extremity.
- Do not mistake the pain from the wound with pain from a possible muscle or tendon injury.
- Quantify muscle or tendon lacerations:
  - Orientation – longitudinal versus transverse in centimeters
  - Depth – approximate percentage

Vascular exam

- More than just Capillary Refill Time!
- Has there been, or is there currently, arterial or venous bleeding?
- Is the temperature of the extremities equal bilaterally?
- Is the color of the extremities equal bilaterally?
- Is there a larger than expected amount of edema and/ or ecchymosis present?

IMPORTANT! Be aware that an arterial laceration often goes hand-in-hand with a nerve transection.

2. **Effective local and regional anesthesia:** "How to remain friends with your patient." (See Tables 35.1, 35.2, and 35.3.)

   Why is it used?
- Patient comfort means reduced anxiety for both patient and clinician!
- More effective wound prep, exploration, and procedure completion
- Avoid possible medicolegal complications

   When is it used?
- Wound preparation, exploration, and repair
- Foreign body removal
- Orthopedic, dental, and other surgical procedures
- Incision and drainage

Table 35.1. Common agents

Agent	Route	How supplied	Onset	Duration	Maximum dose
Lidocaine	Injection	½, 1, 2%	Immediate	60–90 minutes	4.5 mg/kg up to 300 mg
Lidocaine w/epi	Injection	1:200,000 = ½% 1:100,000 = 1&2%	Immediate	1.5–2 hours	7 mg/kg up to 500 mg
Lidocaine	Topical	2% jelly	3–5 minutes	< 5 minutes	4.5 mg/kg
Lidocaine	Topical	4% liquid	30 seconds	< 5 minutes	4.5 mg/kg
Bupivacaine	Injection	¼, ½%	5–20 minutes	6–8 hours	175 mg
Bupivacaine w/epi	Injection	1:200,000	5–20 minutes	6–8 hours	225 mg
Mepivicaine	Injection	1 & 2%	Immediate	1.5–2 hours	400 mg
TAC	Topical	Liquid mix w/ methyl cellulose	20–40 minutes	30–45 minutes	5 cc
Cocaine	Topical	4% liquid	3–5 minutes	30–45 minutes	5 cc
Cetacaine	Topical	oral spray	Immediate	< 5 minutes	NA
Diphenhydramine HCl	Injection	50 mg syringe mixed w/3–5 cc sterile saline	Immediate	20–40 minutes	100 mg

U.S. National Library of Medicine, National Institutes of Health, Health & Human Services. Available at: *http://dailymed.nlm.nih.gov*. Accessed May 1, 2007.

Table 35.2. Common additives to local anesthesia

Anesthetic additive	Properties

Epinephrine	• Vasoconstriction delays absorption into bloodstream prolonging anesthesia
	• Increased hemostasis
	• Absolute contraindications: end arterial points
	• Relative contraindications:
	  • Tidy vs. untidy wounds
	  • Underlying pathology
	  • Anatomic location
	  • Severe head injuries, hypertensive crisis, beta-blockers (propranolol)

Methylparaben	• Preservative in multidose vials • Ester (metabolite PABA) • Frequently source of true allergic reaction • Should not be given in a spinal or epidural anesthetic because of concerns about neurotoxicity • Often not listed as ingredient
Sodium bicarbonate	• Buffer (raises pH) • Decreases "sting" of injection • Decreases shelf life (≤24 hour) • Increases amount of anesthesia in base form thereby shortening onset time

Roberts JR, Hedges J. *Clinical Procedures in Emergency Medicine.* 4th ed. Philadelphia: Saunders.
Xia Y, Chen E, Tibbits, DL, et al. Comparison of effects of lidocaine hydrochloride, buffered lidocaine, diphenhydramine, and normal saline after intradermal injection. *J Clin Anesth.* 2002;14:339–43.

- General pain relief
- Etc., etc., etc. . . .

IMPORTANT! When considering the maximum dosage of an agent, calculate the *equivalent volume* of the agent prior to starting the case. This will add perspective when treating the patient.

Methods of administration

- Anesthetic delivery – What is the basic equipment?
  - Recommended syringes: 1, 3, 10 cc
  - Recommended needles: 27 gauge 0.5 inch, 27 gauge 1.25 inch (28–30 gauge needles are equally acceptable)
- Connsiderations for approach – How to decide between topical/local/regional approaches.
  - Is there a continuous need for hemostasis?
  - What is the possibility that foreign bodies are present?
  - What are the general wound characteristics?
  - Are there multiple lacerations?
  - How much anesthetic has been used and what is the anticipated additional need?

- Are there any dosage variations for infants and children?
- Will the approach be affected by *difficult* patients (patients who may have an altered mental status, possibly uncooperative, or extremely anxious)?
- How will distortion of the anatomy be affected by the approach?

- Topical
  - It may be applied to skin, mucosa, and open wounds.
  - The surrounding anatomy is not distorted.
  - It should not be used on mucosa or areas with end-arteriolar circulation when combined with epinephrine.
  - Careful attention must be paid to the volume (dosage) used.
  - Reliability in coverage and duration varies.
- Local infiltration
  - Injection is made from within wound margins into the subcutaneous tissue.
    - Subdermal plexus injection is less painful than intradermal injection.[11]
    - Subcutaneous tissue is less dense than connective tissue of intact dermis; therefore, injection requires lower pressure.
  - Start at edge most proximal to the origin of the nerve(s) innervating the tissue to be anesthetized then infiltrate distally.
  - Consider the size of needle and syringe.
    - Use the smallest diameter needle suitable for the particular wound.
    - Increased pain from injection due to increased hydraulic pressure is a result of a large syringe + a small needle.
    - Increase the size of the needle, increase the size of the syringe.
  - Advantages of local infiltration
    - Ease of technique
    - Generally reliable
    - Good hemostasis from both the anesthetic's volume and any added epinephrine
  - Disadvantages of local infiltration
    - May require higher volumes of anesthetic agent
    - Distortion of anatomical landmarks occurs more easily than a regional nerve block would allow
    - Increased possibility of contaminants introduced into "good" tissue
    - Can be excessively painful in areas such as extremities, volar hand, plantar foot, infected or burned tissue
- Regional nerve and field blocks
  - Field blocks (Figure 35.1) are
    - Defined as the distribution of anesthesia across multiple nerve pathways without direct injection of wound margins.

Table 35.3. Common reactions to local anesthesia

Anesthetic reaction	Reason for occurrence	Signs and symptoms	Treatment	Prevention
Toxic	Plasma concentration exceeds maximum allowable dosage due to: Excessive bolus amount given Decreased rate of absorption Liver and/or renal failure	Disorientation metallic taste, circumoral tingling Tinnitus/auditory hallucinations Muscle spasms Seizures Coma Respiratory arrest Cardiac arrest	Treatment of adverse reactions is supportive Seizure prophylaxis Airway control and support Cardiovascular support Immediate evacuation	Pay strict attention to recommended dosage and amount of anesthetic given
Allergic	Patient receiving ester-linked local anesthetics Amide reactions are rare No cross-sensitivity between the ester and amide groups Allergic reactions more common to preservative methylparaben	Urticaria, generalized edema, anxiety Bronchospasm, laryngeal edema, and shock may rapidly follow The patient may be tachycardiac and hypotensive	Airway evaluation and support, IV access, O$_2$ Subcutaneous injections of 0.3 to 0.5 ml epinephrine 1:1,000 and intravenous diphenhydramine HCl (Benadryl), 50 to 100 mg, may be indicated Steroids may also be of some value Cardiopulmonary support or resuscitation may be required Immediate evacuation	Obtain a good history from the patient
Vasovagal	Hemodynamic instability when exposed to a specific psychologically stressful trigger (administration of anesthesia)	Cardioinhibitory response: Drop in heart rate Drop in blood pressure Vasodepressor response: Vasodilation Drop in blood pressure Minimal drop in heart rate Majority have a mixed response	Protect, reassure, and ease the patient into a supine position with legs elevated Continue to monitor	*Never* unveil, anesthetize, clean, explore, or repair a wound in a nonsupine patient!!

Rutten A, Nancarrow C, Mather L, et al. Hemodynamic and central nervous system effects of intravenous bolus doses of lidocaine, bupivacaine, and ropivacaine in sheep. *Anesth Analg*. 1989;69:291–9.
Tetzlaff JE. The pharmacology of local anesthetics. *Anesthesiol Clin North America*. 2000;18(2):217–33.
Strichartz G, Berde C, Miller RD, eds. *Miller's Anesthesia*. 6th ed. Philadelphia: Churchill Livingstone; 2005: 593–4.

- Utilized when region to be anesthetized has multiple nerve innervations and/or when local infiltration is contraindicated.
- Regional nerve blocks are
  - Defined as the blockade of peripheral sensory nerves proximal to wound
- Regional nerve and field blocks are more effective when a higher percentage solution is used (e.g., lidocaine 2% or bupivacaine 0.5%).
- Advantages of regional nerve and field blocks
  - Does not distort anatomy
  - Fewer contaminates introduced into wound
- Generally requires lower volume of anesthetic agent
- Fewer injections required relative to local infiltration
- Broader coverage for special cases
- Allows coverage of several nerves and branches
- Accommodates for individual variability in nerve pathways
- Disadvantages of regional nerve and field blocks
  - Limited locations
  - Not as reliable as local infiltration

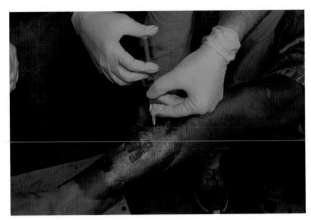

Figure 35.1. Field block of contaminated wound. Photo courtesy of James Marinucci.

- Hemostasis not as effective
- Too large an area may become anesthetized leading to unnecessary further injury

Alternative anesthetic strategies

- Use no anesthesia at all – *not* recommended! Even the toughest patients may move inadvertently when stuck with a needle. This can easily lead to an unnecessary exposure for the provider.
- Use multidose normal saline alone (actually, its preservative, benzyl alcohol). It has low toxicity but is very short acting.
- Place on and around the wound – can cause tissue damage.
- When an ester allergy is suspected, use single dose vials of amide anesthetic agent not containing the preservative methylparaben.
- If allergic to one class of anesthetic, use the other.
- Use diphenhydramine (Benadryl) – 50 mg (1 cc) in 4 cc of normal saline = 1% solution (100 mg maximum dosage).[12]

Recognizing and reducing anesthetic complications

- Complications most often seen:
  - Generally low reported incidence[13,14,15]
  - Inadvertent needle placement
  - Frank injection into vasculature
  - Neurotoxicity of local anesthetics
  - Infection at the site(s) of injection
  - Neuronal ischemia/compartment syndrome
  - Mechanical trauma
    - Needle trauma
    - Intraneuronal injection
- Minimizing complications
  - Practice aseptic technique!
  - Use needles of appropriate length.
  - Always aspirate prior to injection.
    - Smaller gauge needles may not provide adequate flash – aspirate slowly.
  - Avoid injection into foramen.

- Avoid injection under high pressure. Consider size of both needle and syringe. Large syringes with very small gauge needles (e.g., 30 ml syringe with 27 g needle) will create excessive pressure.
- Paresthesias during injections are normal, radiating pain is not!
- Choose your anesthetic agent wisely.
- Instruct patient on care of insensate extremity to prevent unnecessary additional injury.

3. **Wound preparation and debridement in the field.** "Wound prep" refers to the antisepsis of both the wound and surrounding tissue. Whether practiced in the field or in a more traditional acute care setting, this topic is understandably looked upon as the least glamorous facet of acute wound management. In reality, this is one of the most important elements in the process. A hastily done primary closure or wound dressing without due regard for preparation will increase the probability of enhanced scarring and decreased functionality. Reducing the risk of infection and other complications through adequate wound preparation and appropriate debridement must be the primary goal of the provider. This objective should always take precedence over the desire for an aesthetically pleasing repair.

   Aseptic technique: Employing the aseptic technique while practicing wound management in the field is no small task. Logistical complexities in establishing an appropriate treatment area, maintaining both the integrity of that area and the sterility of the supplies contribute to the burden placed upon the provider. Recent studies have suggested, perhaps counterintuitively, that in the emergency or outpatient setting, wound infection rates were not affected by the provider's use of a surgical cap, mask, irrigation with tap water instead of sterile saline, or even the use of sterile technique.[16,17,18] While these studies might give the prospective expedition medical provider some degree of comfort, the benefits of the use of aseptic technique – to the extent it is possible – far outweigh the risks.

   Hair removal: Certainly, the process of wound repair would be much simpler and faster if the removal of hair around the wound was a standard part of any procedure. This course of action is ill-advised. It is true that hair frequently tends to find its way into wounds. It's also true that hair can be prepped as easily as skin. Its penchant to get caught while suturing is not in question. However, removing trapped hair or minimizing the amount of hair finding its way into a wound is a straightforward task. In the field, it serves as an additional barrier against debris.

   Even the most experienced provider can become frustrated with a patient's long hair. In these cases, clipping is advised over shaving. Studies indicate that the shaving of hair actually increases the infection risk relative to clipping.[19,20] The reason is that disturbing the follicles introduces bacteria into the wound area. Another option is coating the hair with a sterile, topical antimicrobial ointment. This works well not because of its antimicrobial properties but, simply because it's *greasy*. This method also facilitates hair removal from the wound postclosure.

Still another reason not to shave hair is the fact that it often provides a good landmark for approximating anatomic borders. This is especially true in the eyebrow. Eyebrows frequently do not grow back in the same way, if at all, after being shaved. If they do, and the wound is not approximated well, the visibility of the resulting scar may actually be dwarfed by the step-off to the eyebrow.

Skin prep: Clinicians tend to use the terms "skin prep" and "wound prep" synonymously. They are not the same. "Skin prep" refers only to the cleaning of the skin around the wound. There are over 20 different brands of skin antisepsis agents on the market, but all belong to only two general groups: iodophor or chlorhexidine. The latter has been shown to be slightly more effective than the former.[21] They are both bactericidal as well as cytotoxic.[22] Therefore, care must be taken in preventing these agents from filling the wound trough or soaking the wound directly in the agent. These were meant to clean *intact* skin only. Cleaning the skin outward from the wound edges with a sponge or gauze is the preferable method for the task.

When preparing for the expedition, consideration should be given to the packaging of the skin prep product. Due to the frequency of minor and major traumatic wounds, a significant amount of prep agent should be part of any wound management kit. For anything more than a simple abrasion, the skin prep as well as the closure should be done using sterile technique. An agent that can be poured into a sterile basin or smaller amounts that are part of a prepackaged wound prep kit are ideal.

Wound irrigation: The most efficient method of removing contaminants from a wound is through irrigation (Figure 35.2). This is where the *actual* wound cleaning occurs. It is a mechanical, not chemical, process.[23] It is a function of three equally important components: irrigate solution + volume + pressure. Regardless of the solution tested, normal saline remains the irrigate of choice. It is an isosmotic or isotonic solution and, therefore, less harmful to exposed tissue. Other solutions used in wound irrigation but known to cause tissue damage or add nothing but cost over normal saline include various agents used for skin prep, hydrogen

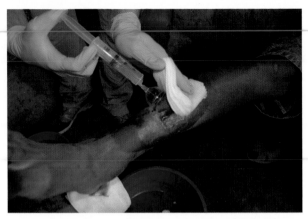

Figure 35.2. Irrigation. Photo courtesy of James Marinucci.

peroxide, alcohol, povidone-iodine, a solution of saline plus antibiotic.[24] The use of tap water has also been studied with rates of infection virtually equal to that of saline.[25,26] However, when one considers the many contaminants found in much of the world's tap water, the use of it as an irrigate should be avoided. It may be acceptable, on the other hand, if it is filtered, brought to a boil, and allowed to cool prior to use.

The volume range of irrigate is based more on tradition than documented evidence. The general practice is to use between 50 and 100 ml/cm wound length. The *dirtier* the wound, the higher the volume of irrigate used.[27]

Many studies have been done over the years examining optimal pressure for the irrigation of wounds: the pressure of irrigate exiting the syringe, the pressure of the irrigate hitting the wound, and the trough pressure within the wound. These studies have incorporated several variables: wound length, syringe size, needle gauge, and the use of commercially available splash shields. For expedition medicine, the bottom line is clear: Use the syringe that fits most comfortably in your hand (usually a 30- to 60-ml syringe) and a commercially available splash shield (with tapered lumen) to reduce the risk of exposure.[28] This equipment, coupled with normal saline will provide the most effective method of wound irrigation in or out of the hospital.

Wound debridement: The removal of devitalized and/or grossly contaminated tissue serves two purposes. First, it significantly decreases the risk of infection. Second, it increases the probability of less scarring resulting in better cosmesis and increased functionality.[29,30]

IMPORTANT! Conservative debridement in the field, as in the conventional acute care setting, should be a principal focus of the provider. Tissue cannot be replaced after it has been removed.

Foreign matter and tissue of questionable viability increases the likelihood of an inflammatory response from the body. This response can quickly lead to infection.[31] Nevertheless, before aggressively debriding a wound, the provider must consider the end result. Anytime tissue is removed, the ensuing tension on the wound edges increases. The increase can be minimized when debriding by making the edges as close to perpendicular as possible. The exception to this rule is that rare occasion when debridement within an eyebrow becomes necessary. Because eyebrow hair grows at an angle, debridement should also be done along that same angle.

Occasionally, trauma to wound margins is beyond simple debridement. Extensive devitalized tissue or gross contamination can lead the provider to the conclusion that the preferred management includes *excision*, a surgical removal of the entire wound periphery. This is done by placing a wider field of anesthesia or the utilization of a regional nerve block, scoring the wound elliptically with a #15 blade scalpel, debriding the tissue with the appropriate scissors, and undermining postdebridement. The result is a slightly longer, slightly wider wound that can then be closed.[32] In wounds with a significant risk of infection, a *delayed primary closure* may be more desirable. This closure option will be discussed in the following section.

Undermining: Separating the dermis from the underlying tissue manually[33] or with a surgical instrument is another effective method of reducing tension. The provider must be aware that undermining a wound will often generate increased bleeding from the disruption of small blood vessels. The subsequent hematoma can lead to an increase in the patient's discomfort and a wound environment slightly more at risk for infection. Hematoma is an optimal nidus for bacteria growth.

Providing Definitive Care in the Field

As with many dealings in expedition medicine, proper wound management in the field requires the provider to have both a knowledge base rooted in traditional, proven techniques and the ability to prioritize, compromise, and improvise. To that end, the treatment modality chosen in the field will depend, to a large degree, upon not only the wound but additional factors unique to the expedition environment. Factors include the types of supplies on hand, the amount of supplies remaining, the duration and mission of the expedition, and the *injury trend* during the expedition, as well as potential difficulties with the time and method of evacuation.

Types of Wound Healing

Taking into account all available information regarding the patient, the *specific* wound, and any other issues surrounding the expedition environment, the clinician must then decide which approach will be implemented when providing definitive care.

Primary closure: In this method, it is determined that the benefits of closure outweigh the risks. The wound edges are approximated at or near the time of injury. Most acute lacerations will require definitive management via sutures, adhesive tape, cyanoacrylate (tissue adhesive), staples, or a combination of closure methods.

The preference to opt for this type of closure is based upon a set of five criteria. They include time from injury, past medical history, anatomic location, degree of contamination, and desired cosmetic outcome.

1. **Time from injury.** Studies have been inconsistent with regard to the upper range of when a safe primary closure should be performed, but the basic conclusion is the same. The longer a wound remains open and untreated, the higher the risk of infection.[34,35,36] To the degree that the remaining criteria do not pose a significant threat to wound healing, we can formulate the primary closure timetable shown in Table 35.4.

   It is possible for the risk of infection to actually decrease after a wound remains open for several days. At that point, if no signs of infection are present, a delayed primary closure should be considered. This technique will be explored later.

2. **Past medical history.** Any medical condition or medication affecting wound healing will negatively influence the decision to perform a primary closure. Patients who are currently immunocompromised, diabetic, receiving radiation or chemotherapy, or taking steroids are at a higher risk of infection. [37]

3. **Anatomic location.** Wounds in areas of poor vascular supply are at greater risk. Distal extremities often present an increased likelihood of infection for two reasons. The area tends to have a decreased blood supply relative to the rest of the body, and the injuries sustained tend to be of higher contamination.[38,39]

4. **Degree of contamination.** The degree of contamination plays a large role in selecting a method

Table 35.4. Wound closure	
Anatomic location	**Hours**
Neck/face/scalp	12—24
Upper extremity	8—12
Lower extremity	6—10

of closure. Wounds with minimal contamination have a longer period of time in which to be closed. Grossly contaminated wounds are more problematic. If they are to be closed, they must be thoroughly cleaned and debrided. In many cases, however, a primary closure of grossly contaminated wounds is ill-advised. Open wound management for four days followed by delayed closure (delayed primary closure) is the preferred means of treatment.[40,41]

5. **Desired cosmetic outcome.** Cosmesis also plays a part in determining if and when a primary closure is to be attempted. The degree to which a cosmetic outcome is sought may lead the provider to choose among a primary, secondary, or tertiary closure.

   For example, an adult male might suffer a dog bite to the thigh. Because these wounds tend to be longer than deep, it may be advisable to clean, irrigate, debride, and close the wound loosely. This primary closure will decrease both the healing time and scarring as compared to letting it granulate and contract (secondary closure). The degree of scarring resulting from this wound might be of little consequence to the patient. The fact that the wound is closed acutely and, thus, easier to manage than leaving it open, is more important. However, if the same injury occurred to a young girl, the scar resulting from a primary or secondary closure may be unacceptable. In this case, a delayed primary closure would be considered.

Secondary closure: The wound is allowed to heal by contraction, epithelialization, and granulation. A variety of wounds would be allowed to heal secondarily. These would include wounds that may be grossly contaminated and unable to be excised later, wounds presenting beyond a safe time for primary closure or wounds that are simply unable to be closed (burns, abrasions, avulsions).

Tertiary closure (delayed primary closure): Wounds that would have an exceedingly high risk of infection if closed primarily or that can only be closed loosely might be considered for a delayed closure.[42] In this technique, the wound is cleaned, irrigated, debrided and packed with moist, saline-soaked gauze for 4 days.[43,44] Prophylactic antibiotics can be given if the situation necessitates, such as a mammalian bite or a wound on a patient with diabetes. The dressing is left in place and undisturbed but may be uncovered to examine for signs of infection. If, after 4 days, no signs of infection are present, the wound may be approximated as is or excised and closed.[45] Keep in mind that if the wound is to be excised, the closure must not alter symmetry or prevent a full range of motion to an extremity. In other words, make sure you have the excess tissue available when planning a delayed primary closure.

Methods of Wound Closure

In expedition wound management, there are a variety of wound closure methods, conventional and unconventional, available to the provider. Each has its own advantages and disadvantages. These methods, under certain circumstances, may be used in combination. (See Table 35.5.)

Postrepair Field Wound Management

While the actual treatment of the wound is primarily the domain of the clinician, postrepair field wound management is truly a joint venture. In the expedition environment, both clinician and patient share follow-up responsibilities. The patient's tasks are not unlike those required in the conventional setting. He or she needs to be diligent with regard to wound care instructions: elevation, keeping the wound clean and dry until directed otherwise, taking the prescribed regimen of medication, activity restrictions, and the like. Additionally, the expedition's provider does not have the luxury of jotting down a few instructions and perhaps scheduling one or more follow-up appointments. The clinician quickly realizes that the follow-up component to expedition wound management must often be more aggressive than when practiced in the conventional setting. Many field operations will necessitate the provider and patient remain in close proximity for some time. Because of this unique situation and the fact that many expeditions do not take place in the most hospitable environment for proper wound care, this gives the clinician an opportunity to monitor the patient's progress closely and intervene quickly, if needed.

1. **Wound dressings:** A key component to follow-up care is the initial and subsequent dressing and bandaging of the wound. During the first 24–48 hours, most wounds below the neck should have a nonadherent dressing with a topical antimicrobial agent to promote both rapid epithelialization and a lower risk of infection.[55,56,57] After that, the wound should be washed regularly with a mild surfactant and redressed appropriately according to the environment. There are many different types of dressings designed for a variety of environments.[58,59] Part of the clinician's initial preparation should be to evaluate which dressings and bandages are most suitable for the setting.

   Most sutured wounds above the neck are at a very low risk of infection and can be left open using only a topical antimicrobial ointment for coverage.[60] The exceptions would be the following:

   • There has been significant disruption of the vasculature secondary to penetration, tissue loss, or undermining. In these circumstances, a pressure dressing is applied for the first 48 hours followed by reevaluation.

Table 35.5. Suture and staple removal

Technique	Advantage	Disadvantage
Conventional methods		
Sutures	1. Most precise method of approximation 2. Lowest dehiscence rate over time 3. Retains the greatest tensile strength over time	1. Requires the greatest technical skill 2. Highest cost method of closure 3. Highest tissue reactivity 4. Removal is often required 5. Highest risk of provider exposure
Surgical adhesive tape	1. Good approximation when used properly 2. Lower cost 3. Rapid application 4. Low associated rate of infection[46] 5. Very low risk of provider exposure	1. Low tensile strength 2. Rapidly fall's off (increased rate if wet) 3. Use in areas of hair or moisture is not advisable 4. High rate of dehiscence[47]
Cyanoacrylate (tissue adhesive)	1. Good approximation when used properly 2. Water-resistant 3. Does not require removal 4. Better acceptance by patients 5. Relatively lower cost 6. Rapid application 7. Low associated rate of infection 8. Provides a degree of antimicrobial protection[48] 9. Very low risk of provider exposure	1. Clinicians have a tendency to become "lazy" and neglect good wound prep and exploration. Subsequently, infection rates rise. 2. Lower tensile strength relative to sutures[49] 3. Breakdown can vary between 5 and 10 days 4. Does not allow drainage, therefore, should not be used in the following areas: Jagged or stellate lacerations Bites, punctures, or crush wounds Grossly contaminated wounds Mucosal surfaces High-moisture areas High tension areas esp. hands, feet, and/or joints[50]
Surgical staples	1. Low cost 2. Rapid application 3. Low tissue reactivity[51] 4. Low risk of provider exposure[52]	1. May be difficult to approximate many acute traumatic wounds 2. Should not be used in the face, feet, hands, joints 3. May interfere with older generation imaging studies
Improvised methods		
Hair apposition technique (plus tissue adhesive)	1. Provides rapid and effective hemostasis if no significant bleeding[53,54] 2. Low risk of provider exposure 3. Rapid application 4. Low tissue reactivity 5. Low cost	1. Low tensile strength 2. May be difficult technique for the unskilled practitioner 3. May come undone rapidly 4. Practitioner may not perform adequate prep and exploration
Sutures through surgical tape	1. Reinforces tissue prior to suturing (great for friable skin esp. on older individuals or those taking steroids)	1. Requires sufficient technical skill 2. High tissue reactivity 3. Removal is often required 4. Highest risk of provider exposure
Commercial tape	1. Good temporary approximation when used properly 2. Rapid application 3. Very low risk of provider exposure 4. Provides rapid and effective hemostasis	1. High possible tissue reactivity 2. Unsterile packaging 3. Unpredictable retention 4. Low tensile strength 5. Use in areas of hair or moisture is not advisable 6. High risk of dehiscence
Commercial adhesive	1. Good approximation when used properly 2. Rapid application 3. Very low risk of provider exposure 4. Provides rapid and effective hemostasis	1. Higher risk of tissue reactivity or possibly thermal burn 2. Unsterile packaging 3. Unpredictable breakdown rate 4. Lower tensile strength 5. Use in areas of hair, moisture, or high tension is not advisable 6. Use in areas of high infection risk is not advisable 7. High risk of dehiscence

- The wound was closed with a tissue adhesive. The use of an ointment will increase the risk of dehiscence by breaking down the adhesive.
- The wound is infected and actively draining. Abscesses, lacerations, puncture wounds, bites, or any other wound that becomes infected should be covered with an absorbent dressing, but the use of an ointment should be avoided in most cases. These wounds heal by secondary intent and should be allowed to granulate and contract. Rapid epithelialization should be discouraged.
- The patient is in an environment that may cause the wound to become grossly contaminated. In such cases, a simple dressing will alleviate that risk.

2. **Splinting:** The use of a splint of any kind on any extremity should be given careful consideration prior to placement. Splints can be both beneficial and detrimental but rarely benign. The benefits of splinting a fracture are well known. Splints can also be used in areas of soft tissue trauma to minimize edema through restrictive movement and uniform compression. When a splint is used to minimize edema, it should remain in place for approximately 48 hours. Tendon or ligamentous injuries frequently benefit from splinting. It can also provide protection in an environment where the patient cannot always remain vigilant.[61]

   Again, the use of a splint can be advantageous to the healing process, but when it is used inappropriately, it can actually be injurious. Splinting is not often required simply because a wound is over a joint. Restricted movement can quickly lead to a contraction of tendons and ligaments as well as muscle atrophy. Even when the splint is suitably placed, these outcomes can occur. However, the clinician must decide when the benefit outweighs the risk.

3. **Indication and selection of antibiotics:** Antibiotic therapy in expedition wound management should be used judiciously. As previously stated, knowing the past medical histories of the expedition members, their allergies, and their current medications is invaluable. Careful consideration should be given to the expedition environment and the most likely encountered offending pathogens. Remember, the quantity of supplies will be limited and the formulary established prior to departure. The clinician can only use what he or she packed.

   Infected wounds should be treated appropriately, including, when necessary, incision and drainage, debridement, cleaning, and/or removal of contaminants. Antibiotic therapy should be initiated when the clinician's evaluation suggests a tangible benefit.[62]

   Studies suggest that decontamination is far more beneficial in routine laceration repair than is the use of prophylactic antibiotics.[63] Do not substitute good wound care with antibiotics. The use of prophylactic antibiotic therapy on the expedition should not exceed 3–5 days and should be used in the following cases:[64]

   - Confirmed or highly suspected open fractures
   - Confirmed or highly suspected open joints
   - Lacerated tendons, cartilage or ligaments
   - Grossly contaminated wounds
   - Through and through oral lacerations
   - Most bites
   - Puncture wounds to the plantar foot and volar hand
   - Suspected globe penetration
   - Patients who may be immunocompromised or at elevated risk for systemic complications
   - Patients with a current localized or systemic infection

4. **Postclosure follow-up:** Suture and staple removal can be done on the schedule shown in Table 35.6.

Postrepair Complications

Occasional complications in field wound care are an unfortunate, yet inevitable, aspect of numerous expeditions. Many of these can be prevented by thorough examination, diligent wound prep, meticulous treatment, and attentive follow-up. Others, however, occur despite our best efforts.

Common Wound Complications

The variations of poor outcomes that can arise due to clinician error, patient neglect, or a host of unknown reasons are, quite frankly, too numerous to count. Nonetheless, there are several complications that are seen more frequently than others.

- Missed fracture or retained foreign body
  Causes:

  Failure to obtain accurate history or ascertain exact mechanism of injury

  Lack of available imaging studies to assist with diagnosis
  Inability to locate with direct visualization

- Missed neurological, motor, or vascular damage
  Causes:

Table 35.6. Wound closure	
Anatomic location	**Days**
Scalp	7—10
Face/neck	3—5
Anterior/posterior trunk	8—14
Upper/lower extremities	8—14
Hand/fingers	7—10
Foot	10—14

Inadequate exam performed due to:

Uncertainty with regard to underlying anatomy

Patient's altered mental status

Patient's physical location while treatment is initiated

Extreme environmental conditions

- Excessive edema and/or ecchymosis
  Causes:

Lack of postoperative elevation

Required splint not placed or removed too soon

Initial unnoticed vascular damage

Improper bandaging and/or poor patient aftercare

- Poorly healing or nonhealing wound
  Causes:

Extensive tissue damage

Excessive maceration of surrounding tissue

Past medical history indicates predisposition toward poor healing

Inadequate wound prep and/or repair

Improper follow-up instructions and/or poor patient aftercare

- Wound dehiscence
  Causes:

Wound is under excessive tension

Method of closure is removed too soon

Inadequate repair technique (inversion or over-eversion of wound edges)

Excessive maceration of surrounding tissue

Improper follow-up instructions and/or poor patient aftercare

- Wound infection
  Causes:

Inadequate wound prep

Aseptic technique was not maintained

Retained foreign body

Avascular structures exposed to environment

Prophylactic antibiotics not given when required

Improper follow-up instructions and/or poor patient aftercare

- Poor cosmesis
  Causes:

Poor repair technique

Extensive tissue damage

Past medical history indicates predisposition toward poor healing

Improper follow-up instructions and/or poor patient aftercare

Reasons for Elevated Concern and/or Evacuation

At some point, the expedition's provider may come to the conclusion that the medical needs of a patient exceed the resources available. Even with the most meticulous predeparture planning, this might be unavoidable. Participating in an expedition is a costly venture, as is evacuation. Neither decision should be made lightly. A medical evacuation can potentially put more people at risk than just the patient. Transportation in and out of remote areas is often hazardous under the best of circumstances. Contingency plans need to be in place prior to departure, and participants need to be briefed. All parties must understand prior to departure that unavoidable contraindications to immediate evacuation, such as poor weather conditions, security concerns, or medical instability, might adversely affect the long-term outcome. These situations are unfortunate but also an intrinsic risk in expedition travel.

From the wound management perspective, possible evacuation should be considered for any number of reasons:

- Uncertainty with the extent of the injury
- Tissue defects with avascular structures unable to be covered
- Penetration of avascular structures:

Tendon

Ligament

Joint

Bone

Cartilage

- Deep penetration of certain anatomic regions:

Eyes

Neck

Chest

Abdomen

Groin

- Compression and injection injuries
- Suspected arthropod or venomous bites
- Significant burns and electrical injuries
- Severely impaired mobility
- Wounds in patients with serious underlying systemic disorders

SUMMARY

In conclusion, it must be remembered that expedition wound management is as much an art as it is a science. Relative to the conventional arena, there is less emphasis on rigid algorithm and greater focus on how the patient might be affected by the entire expedition environment. The ever-changing number of variables influencing even the simplest wounds forces the provider to exercise a certain amount of clinical agility when practicing in the field. Remember . . . *prioritize, customize,* and *improvise*!

ACKNOWLEDGMENT

Research assistance was provided by Amy Keim, PA-C, MPAS.

REFERENCES

[1] *http://www.healthtouch.com/bin/EContent_HT/cnote-ShowLfts.asp?fname=00730&title=LACERATION+&cid=HTH LTH.*

[2] *http://www.bmj.com/cgi/content/full/329/7457/101.*

[3] *http://www.cdc.gov, http://www.osha.gov.*

[4] Lubahn JD, Keoneman J, Koser K. The digital tourniquet: how safe is it? *J Hand Surg.* 1985;10A:664.

[5] Shaw JA, Demuth WN, Gillespy AW. Guidelines for the use of digital tourniquets based on physiological pressure measurements. *J. Bone Joint Surg.* 1985;67A:1086.

[6] Lamers RL, Magill T. Detection and management of foreign bodies in soft tissue. *Emerg Med Clin N Am.* 1992;10:767–81.

[7] Capellan O, Hollander JE. Management of lacerations in the emergency department. *Emerg Med Clin N Am.* 2003;21:205–31.

[8] Finnell JT, Knopp R, Johnson P, et al. A calibrated paper clip is a reliable measure of two-point discrimination. *Acad Emerg Med.* 2004;11(6):710–14.

[9] Sloan EP. Nerve injuries in the hand. *Emerg Med Clin North Am.* 1993;11(3):651–70.

[10] Canale ST, Beaty JH. *Campbell's Operative Orthopedics.* 10th ed. New York: Elsevier; 2003.

[11] Bartfield JM, Sokaris SJ, Raccio-Robak N. Local anesthesia for lacerations: pain of infiltration inside vs. outside the wound. *Acad Emerg Med.* 1998;5(2):100–4.

[12] Xia Y, Chen E, Tibbits DL, et al. Comparison of effects of lidocaine hydrochloride buffered lidocaine, diphenhydramine, and normal saline after intradermal injection. *J Clin Anesth.* 2002;14:339–43.

[13] Faccenda KA. Complications of regional anesthesia incidence and prevention. *Drug Saf.* 2001;24(6):413–42.

[14] DeJong RH. Toxic effects of local anesthetics. *JAMA.* 1978; 239:1166.

[15] Gall H, Kaufamann R, Kalveram CM. Adverse reactions to local anesthetics: analysis of 197 cases. *J All Clin Immun.* 1996;97(4): 993–1038.

[16] Ruthman JC, Hendrickson D, Miller RF, et al. Effect of cap and mask on infection rates. *Ill Med J.* 1984;165:397–9.

[17] Whorrall GJ. Repairing skin lacerations: does sterile technique matter? *Can Fam Phys.* 1987;33:1185–7.

[18] Perelman VS, Francis GJ, Rutledge T, et al. Sterile versus nonsterile gloves for repair of uncomplicated lacerations in the emergency department. *Ann Emerg Med.* 2004;43:362–70.

[19] Seropian R, Reynolds BM. Wound infections after pre-operative depilation vs. razor preparation. *Am J Surg.* 1975;129:251–4.

[20] Alexander JW, Fischer JE, Boyajian M. The influence of hair removal methods on wound infections. *Arch Surg.* 1983; 244:1353.

[21] Brown, CD, Zitelli JA. A review of topical agents for wounds and methods of wounding. *J Dermatol Surg Oncol.* 1993;19:732–7.

[22] Wilson JR, Mills JG, Prather ID, et al. A toxicity index of skin and wound cleansers used on in vitro fibroblasts and keratinocytes. *Adv Skin Wound Care.* 2005;18:373–8.

[23] Stevenson TR, Thacker JG, Rodeheaver GT, et al. Cleansing the traumatic wound by high pressure syringe irrigation. *JACEP.* 1976;5:17–21.

[24] Dire DJ, Welsh AP. A comparison of wound irrigation solutions used in the emergency department. *Ann Emerg Med.* 1990;19:704–8.

[25] Bansal BC, Wiebe RA, Perkins SD, et al. Tap water for irrigation of lacerations. *Am J Emerg Med.* 2002;20(5):469–72.

[26] Fernandez R, Giffiths R, Ussia C. Water for wound cleansing. *Cochrane Database Sys Rev.* 2002;(4):CD003861.

[27] Fesmire FM, Dalsey WD, Howell JM, et al. American College of Emergency Physicians: clinical policy for the initial approach to patients presenting with penetrating extremity trauma. *Ann Emerg Med.* 1999; 33(5):612–36.

[28] Singer AJ, Hollander JE. Wound preparation. In: Singer AJ, Hollander JE, eds. *Lacerations and Acute Wounds: An Evidence-Based Guide.* Philadelphia: F. A. Davis; 2003: 13–22.

[29] Haury B, Rodeheaver G, Vensko J, et al. Debridement: an essential component of traumatic wound care. *Am J Surg.* 1978;135:238.

[30] Singer AJ, Quinn JV, Thode HC, et al. Determinants of poor outcome after laceration and surgical incision repair. *Plast Recon. Surg.* 2002;110(2):429–37.

[31] Dubay DA, Franz MG. Acute wound healing: the biology of acute wound failure. *Surg Clin N Am.* 2003;83:463–81.

[32] Roberts JR, Hedges J. *Clinical Procedures in Emergency Medicine.* 4th ed. Philadelphia: Saunders.

[33] Edlich RF, Rhodeheaver GT, Thacker JG, et al. Management of soft tissue injury. *Clin Plast Surg.* 1977;4:191.

[34] Lammers RL, Hudson DL, Seaman ME. Prediction of traumatic wound infection with a neural network–derived decision model. *Am J Emerg Med.* 2003;21(1).

[35] Berk WA, Osboure DD, Taylor DD. Evaluation of the "golden period" for wound repair: 204 cases from a third world emergency department. *Ann Emer Med.* 1988;17(5):496–500.

[36] Fesmire FM, Dalsey WD, Howell JM, et al. American College of Emergency Physicians: clinical policy for the initial approach to patients presenting with penetrating extremity trauma. *Ann Emerg Med.* 1999;33(5):612–36.

[37] Hollander JE, Singer AJ, Valentine SM, Shofer FS. Risk factors for infection in patients with traumatic lacerations. *Acad Emerg Med.* 2001;8(7):716–20.

[38] Stamou SC, Maltezou HC, Psaltopoulou T, et al. Wound infections after minor limb lacerations: risk factors and the role of anti-microbial agents. *J Trauma.* 1999;44(6):1078–81.

[39] Singer AJ, Quinn JV, Thode HC, et al. Determinants of poor outcome after laceration and surgical incision repair. *Plastic Recon Surg.* 2002;110(2):429–37.

[40] Tobin GR. Closure of contaminated wounds. *Surg Clinics North Am.* 1984;64(4):639–52.

[41] Fesmire FM, Dalsey WD, Howell JM, et al. American College of Emergency Physicians: clinical policy for the initial approach to patients presenting with penetrating extremity trauma. *Ann Emerg Med.* 1999;33(5):612–36.

[42] Tobin GR. Closure of contaminated wounds. *Surg Clin North Am.* 1984;64(4):639–52.

[43] Fesmire FM, Dalsey WD, Howell JM, et al. American College of Emergency Physicians: clinical policy for the initial

approach to patients presenting with penetrating extremity trauma. *Ann Emerg Med.* 1999; 33(5):612–36.

44 Edlich RF, Rogers W, Kasper G, et al. Studies in the management of the contaminated wound: I: optimal time for closure of contaminated open wounds; II: comparison of resistance to infection of open and closed wounds during healing. *Am J Surg.* 1969;117:323–9.

45 Roberts JR, Hedges J. *Clinical Procedures in Emergency Medicine.* 4th ed. Philadelphia: Saunders.

46 Hirshman HP, Schurman DJ, Kajiyama G. Penetration of *Staphylococus aureus* into sutured wounds. *J Orthop Res.* 1984;2:269–71.

47 Hollander JE, Singer AJ. Laceration management. *Ann Emerg Med.* 1999;34:356–67.

48 Howell JM, Bresnahan KA, Stir TO, et al. Comparison of effects of suture and cyanoacrylate tissue adhesive on bacterial counts in contaminated lacerations. *Antimicrob Agents Chemother.* 1995;39:559–60.

49 Farion K, Osmond MH, Hartling L, et al. Tissue adhesives for traumatic lacerations in children and adults. *Cochrane Database Syst Rev.* 2002;3:CD003326.

50 Shapiro AJ. Tensile strength of wound closure with cyanoacrylate glue. *Am Surg.* 2001;67(11):1113–15.

51 Brickman KR, Lambert RW. Evaluation of skin stapling for wound closure in the emergency department. *Ann Emerg Med.* 1989;18:1122–5.

52 Ritchie AJ, Rocke LG. Staples versus sutures in the closure of scalp wounds: a prospective, double blind, randomized trial. *Injury.* 1989; 20(4): 217–8.

53 Singer AJ. Hair apposition for scalp lacerations. *Ann Emerg Med.* 2002;40:27–9.

54 Ong MEH, Ooi BS, Saw SM, et al. A randomized control trial comparing the hair apposition technique with tissue glue to standard suturing in scalp lacerations. *Ann Emerg Med.* 2002;40:19–26.

55 Watcher M, Wheeland R. The role of topical antibiotics in the healing of full thickness wounds. *J Dermatol Surg Oncl.* 1989; 15:1188.

56 Dire DJ, Coppola M, Dwyer DA, et al. A prospective evaluation of topical antibiotics for preventing infections in uncomplicated soft-tissue wounds repaired in the ED. *Acad Emerg Med.* 1995;2:4–10.

57 Geronemus RG, Mertxz PM, Eaglstein WH. Wound healing: The effects of topical antimicrobial agents. *Arch Dermatol.* 1979;115:1311–14.

58 Brown CD, Zitelli JA. Choice of wound dressings and ointments. *Otolaryngol Clin North Am.* 1995;28:1081–91.

59 Vermeulen H, Ubbink D, Goossens A, et al. Dressings and topical agents for surgical wounds healing by secondary intention. *Cochrane Database Syst Rev.* 2004;2:CD003554.

60 Goldberg HM, Rosenthal SAE, Nemetz JC. Effect of washing closed head and neck wound on wound healing and infection. *Am J Surg.* 1981;141:358–9.

61 Edlich RF, Thacker JG, Buchanan L, et al. Modern concepts of treatment of traumatic wounds. *Adv Surg.* 1979;13: 169–97.

62 Cummings P, Del Baccaro MA. Antibiotics to prevent infection of simple wounds: a meta-analysis of randomized studies. *Am J Emerg Med.* 1995;13(4).

63 Cummings P, Del Baccaro MA. Antibiotics to prevent infection of simple wounds: a meta-analysis of randomized studies. *Am J Emerg Med.* 1995;13:396–400.

64 Moran GJ, House HR. Antibiotics in wound management. In: Singer AJ, Hollander JE, eds. *Lacerations and Acute Wounds: An Evidence-Based Guide.* Philadelphia: F. A. Davis; 2003: 194–204.

Stanley L. Spielman, MD

INTRODUCTION

The prevention and treatment of expedition-related eye problems are an important part of the overall medical plan. Exposure to ocular disorders is often increased by the extreme conditions and circumstances of expeditions. Unfortunately, loss of vision and ocular pain can be incapacitating, rapidly placing the victim in a precarious and dangerous situation.

The eye is a complex organ, and for practical purposes, this chapter is not a substitute for more comprehensive ophthalmic texts that address numerous eye conditions not commonly related to expeditions. However, it recognizes that a random ocular problem may arise or a preexisting eye condition may recur during an expedition. Certain of these problems and their symptoms could be confused with an expedition-related injury or condition; therefore, an accurate history is essential under these circumstances. Some of these conditions are briefly discussed.

Attention is focused on the identification and therapy of common expedition-related eye conditions that can be reasonably managed within the expedition environment. Certain disorders that require evacuation are identified and described – although they are important, they are rare. When a serious disorder is evident, difficult evacuation decisions must be made; evaluation and therapy may be required by an experienced ophthalmologist using office equipment and tests not available on expeditions; hospital care and surgery may also be necessary. Guidelines for such circumstances are addressed.

EXPEDITION EYE SUPPLIES

Individuals with chronic or recurring eye conditions (i.e., glaucoma and allergic conjunctivitis) are advised to carry their own supply of personal tried and tested eye medications on expeditions. Expedition medical supplies are limited and not intended to replace those available in the neighborhood drug store.

If possible, it is wise to carry extra topical antibiotics and antiinflammatory medications; amounts supplied in one eyedropper bottle for example, may not last several weeks or be sufficient to treat more than one individual – extra eye medications require little additional personal space.

Eye supplies discussed here do not include various systemic medications utilized to treat medical conditions that may have occasional ocular symptoms. It is also expected that the expedition's general medical kit will include certain medications (i.e., antihistamines for treating allergies, and narcotics for pain).

Special care is required in cold climates and at high altitudes to prevent freezing of eyedrops and ointments.

Certain expeditions do not require strict constraints upon the weight and space (e.g., research vessels, remote hospitals and medical clinics); working in these circumstances allows additional elective items to be included with the expedition's eye supplies.

It is advised to consult the current *Physicians' Desk Reference* and the *Physicians' Desk Reference for Ophthalmology* for any questions regarding side effects, complications, and alternatives of medications suggested in this chapter.

Topical Medications

Topical medications are summarized in Table 36.1.

Topical anesthetic drops (tetracaine 0.5% solution) are helpful when it is difficult to examine the eyes because of severe pain and blepharospasm secondary to surface injuries and foreign bodies. The drops must not be applied excessively because they tend to delay wound healing; however tempting, it is necessary to withhold continued applications in patients enduring the pain of corneal abrasions, keratitis, and corneal ulcers. Topical anesthetics are not effective in relieving pain in iritis, acute glaucoma, or other nonsurface painful inflammations; if no significant relief is experienced after instillation of tetracaine, it is assumed the condition is not

Table 36.1. Topical medications[a]

Tetracaine drops 0.5% solution
Neosynepherine 2½% solution
Bacitracin/polymyxin B ophthalmic ointment 500 units/g
Ofloxacin 0.3% solution
Prednisolone 1% solution
Diclofenac 0.1% solution
Pilocarpine 2% solution
Scopolamine 0.25%solution
Artificial tears
Hypertonic sodium chloride 5% solution (high altitudes)
Hypertonic sodium chloride 5% ointment (high altitudes)
Irrigating saline solution (elective)

[a] Solutions = eyedrops

surface related (corneal foreign body or, etc.) but internal (iritis, hyphema, etc.). This fact can be used to assist in diagnosis.

Diclofenac 0.1% solution is a nonsteroidal antiinflammatory agent that has been used for the control of postoperative inflammation and is useful in moderating pain associated with corneal surface defects.[1]

Neosynepherine 2½% solution is advised when it is important to dilate the pupils in order to examine the fundus. The 2½% dilution is a relatively mild dilating agent and can usually be counteracted with pilocarpine 2% solution (drops that dilate the pupils present the occasional possibility of precipitating an attack of acute angle closure glaucoma – the treatment is emergency laser therapy or surgery). Pilocarpine usually counteracts dilating drops by constricting the pupils. Therefore, instill several drops of pilocarpine 2% immediately after examining the fundus and repeat every 30 minutes for several hours or until the pupil is no longer dilated. If the pupil does not respond but remains dilated after several hours, acute glaucoma may be suspected; treat as described in the "Glaucoma, Acute Angle Closure" section.

Bacitracin/polymyxin B 500 units/g ophthalmic ointment is used to treat conjunctivitis, blepharitis, and defects in the corneal epithelium – abrasions, erosions, and ulcers. It is unusual to see toxicity or allergy to either polymyxin or bacitracin. Blepharitis is commonly caused by *Staphylococcus* species of bacteria and herpes and *Moraxella* viruses. Conjunctivitis is principally caused by *Staphylococcus aureus*, *Streptococcus* species, *Hemophyllis influenzae*, *Moraxella* species, *Neisseria gonorrhoeae*, and *Chalmydia trachmatomatis* bacteria. It is also caused by the herpes simplex virus and adenoviruses (extremely contagious).[2] Ocular ointments are used whenever sustained effect is desired (during the night, under patches and when compliance to a regular schedule is uncertain) for their ability to cling to eyelashes and eyelid margins, and for their lubricating properties. A side effect of ointments is blurring of vision

secondary to the prolonged corneal film the ointment creates. Therefore, it is common practice to apply antibiotic ointments at bedtime and drops throughout the day. The blurring effect may persist after awaking in the morning if excessive amounts of ointment are applied at bedtime the night before. Ofloxacin 0.3% solution is an effective antibiotic drop for the therapy of conjunctivitis; it is instilled four times a day, or more frequently, for empirical therapy of bacterial infections; eye drops do not create a blurring corneal film.[3,4]

Prednisolone 1% solution is used to treat moderate to severe ocular inflammations. Unless administered by an ophthalmologist, prednisolone drops should usually be restricted to about 3–4 days to guard against delayed wound healing, the spread of infection, and glaucoma and cataracts. Topical prednisolone is primarily useful in treating allergic inflammations, acid and alkali burns, and anterior uveitis (iritis). Because it delays healing, it should be avoided in the therapy of corneal abrasions.

Scopolamine 0.25% solution is used to relax ciliary and iris spasm that accompany anterior uveitis; it moderates pain of corneal abrasions, ulcers, and foreign bodies; and it is used for penetrating injuries and blunt trauma. A prominent symptom of uveitis is deep pain over the eye in the vicinity of the eyebrow. It is accompanied by miosis (constricted pupil).

Artificial tears are used when a lubricant is needed. They are helpful for treating dry eyes, tight contact lenses, and keratitis.

Hypertonic (hyperosmolar) sodium chloride 5% solution and ointment are dehydrating agents that temporarily reduce corneal edema. They relieve corneal edema that blurs vision at high altitudes; therapy allows the patient to see well enough to descend without assistance. Treatment also assists in healing certain recurrent corneal erosions.

When instilling eyedrops, the lower eyelid is retracted downward; drops are instilled directly on the eye or within the pouch formed between the lower eyelid and the globe; the eyelid is released after several seconds. One to two drops usually provide an adequate therapeutic dose; additional solution often overflows and is wasted. In cases of acid and alkali burns, avoid substituting prednisolone 1% drops for an irrigating agent – the limited supply must last for extended therapy; instill the drops after irrigation is completed. If a more lasting effect of eyedrops is desired, after the eyelids are closed press a finger firmly and broadly against the side of the nose where it meets the inner corner (canthus) of the eye; this is continued for several minutes. Finger pressure blocks tear outflow from the eye through the lacrimal ducts (canaliculi) that connect to the tear (lacrimal) drainage system, thereby allowing prolonged contact of the medication with the surface of the eye. When using several different medications, several minutes should elapse between each application to ameliorate dilution and overflow; if ointments are added, they should be applied last to allow adequate dispersion and absorption of eyedrops before coating the eye with an ointment film.

Ointments are applied across the inner surface of the lower eyelid in the pouch formed at the eyelid's junction with the globe. In cold environments, before application the tube should be held within the closed warm hand for several minutes to achieve softening. Ointments are preferred at bedtime because they have a longer duration of effect than drops.

Systemic Medications

Systemic medications are summarized in Table 36.2.

It is preferred that prednisolone tablets are dispensed by a physician because of possible harmful side effects; the professional has a better chance of establishing the correct diagnosis and rationale for therapy. Development of glaucoma and cataracts, delayed wound healing, and spreading of infections are examples of possible complications. The use of corticosteroids is primarily for the therapy of inflammations, when necessary, rather than infections. After administration of prednisolone tablets for several days, the dose must be tapered off for another several days, rather than abruptly stopped. The primary ocular inflammatory conditions treated with oral corticosteroids are anterior uveitis and posterior optic neuropathies that cause visual deterioration; several periocular inflammations are also treated.

Acetazolamide (250 mg) is used to reduce elevated intraocular pressure of acute glaucoma and also to treat high-altitude (mountain) sickness. It is taken two to four times daily. Acetazolamide increases the urinary excretion of potassium creating low blood potassium levels (hypokalemia); potassium may be replaced by eating foods with high potassium content: prunes, apricots, raisins, bananas, oranges, figs, carrots, tomatoes, and fish. Acetazolamide often causes a tingling sensation in the finger tips and toes that may be confused with symptoms of altitude mountain sickness (AMS). It also gives a metallic taste to carbonated beverages including beer. Acetazolamide should not be taken by patients allergic to sulfonamides (sulfa drugs).

Levofloxacin (500 mg tablets) is a fluoroquinolone with excellent ocular penetration and effective against a broad spectrum of Gram-positive and Gram-negative organisms; it is not as effective against anaerobic bacteria.[3,5] The usual dosage is 500 mg every 24 hours,

Table 36.2. Systemic medications
Prednisolone 20 mg tablets
Acetazolamide 250 mg tablets
Levofloxacin 500 mg tablets
Ciprofloxacin 500 mg tablets (alternative to levofloxacin)

Table 36.3. Miscellaneous items
Near vision card
Amsler grid
Pinhole occluder
Penlight with cobalt blue filter
Fluorescein strips
Cotton-tipped applicators – sterile
50 cc hypodermic syringe
Eye patches – sterile
2 × 2 inch gauze pads – sterile
Metal shield
Tape (1 inch nylon and 1 inch paper)
Wound closure strips (1/4 inch)
Magnifying lens
Binocular loupe (elective)
Portable tonometer (elective)
Ophthalmoscope (elective)

although 750 mg is given in critical situations. . An alternative is ciprofloxacin 500 mg tablets every 12 hours.

Miscellaneous Items

Most of the items listed in Table 36.3 require little space and are of little weight, a primary consideration on expeditions. The Amsler grid is an important asset when evaluating status of central vision and is critical in decision making regarding evacuation in cases of ocular trauma and high-altitude retinal hemorrhage. This is especially important when no ophthalmoscope is available. (See Figure 36.1.) Even though a battery-powered ophthalmoscope is desirable, the batteries are relatively heavy, so an ophthalmoscope may have to be excluded. It is

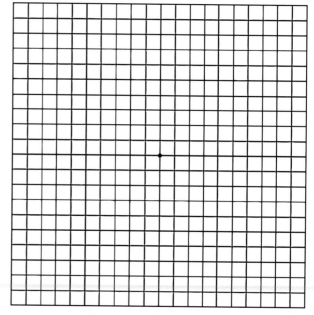

Figure 36.1. Amsler grid. Graphic services provided by Vishnu Hoff, Coordinator of Ophthalmic Imaging, Macular Foundation, Manhattan Eye, Ear, & Throat Hospital.

noted, however, that (C) batteries are carried on many expeditions and, therefore are available to power a portable ophthalmoscope. Binocular loupes are pricey; however, they are a great asset, especially when substituting for the slit lamp microscope.

The author always carries a 6× binocular loupe fastened to a pair of prescription eyeglasses. Before the advent of operating microscopes, all eye surgery was accomplished using binocular loupes; microscopes remain unavailable in certain remote hospitals and clinics – using a loupe the author successfully repaired a globe perforated by a 3-inch-long glass shard from an exploding soda bottle, and also operated upon cataracts in a small mountain hospital in Western Papua, New Guinea. On expeditions, a binocular loupe can be utilized for suturing lacerations of the eyelids or wherever fine sutures are required; it is also useful for removing splinters and thorns embedded in the skin.

Personal Items

Table 36.4 lists personal items that all expeditioners should consider carrying.

Sunglasses

Ultraviolet (UV) blocking, polarized, polycarbonate, impact-resistant lenses provide protection against high levels of harmful ultraviolet B (UVB) radiation found in many extreme environments – ranging from the subtropics and tropics to high mountain altitudes and deserts. Ultraviolet radiation is especially enhanced by reflection from water, snow, and sand. When the sun is no longer directly overhead, it is often incorrectly assumed that, because it is lower in the sky, it is too weak to become a significant hazard. While hats with long peaks or wide brims and overhead tops on boats are useful in preventing excessive direct overhead UV radiation, they are of less value protecting against exposure to both direct and reflected rays found later in the day. This becomes an important factor near the equatorial regions of the earth, on the sea, and also in the thin air and snow found at high altitudes. At high altitudes, specialized glacier glasses and goggles have side panels or are wrap-around styles that provide protection against harmful incident UVB rays from reaching the eyes. (See the following discussions in the "Keratitis" and the "Snow Blindness [Solar Keratitis]" sections.)

Polycarbonate lenses are lightweight and impact-resistant; they act like protective work goggles to help

Table 36.4. Personal items

Sunglasses
Contact lenses and related supplies
Medications (see preceding discussion)

guard against direct physical damage to the eyes from rigid and often sharply pointed foreign objects such as palm fronds, thorns, and broken branches. They also protect against wind-driven foreign bodies and blunt injuries from various sources. The lenses should be large enough to provide an adequate physical barrier to eye injury, and the frames should fit tightly enough to avoid displacement of the glasses by glancing blows or slipping due to excess perspiration, rain, ocean spray, and the like. Clear polycarbonate safety glasses or goggles provide eye protection when night treks are planned in heavy shrub and forested areas. The designation of CR-39 specifies plastic lenses other than polycarbonate; they are not impact-resistant and are therefore not advised for expeditions.[6]

The color of tinted lenses is usually an individual preference and provides no actual medical benefit; tints can enhance contrast under certain circumstances. Color tints do not block ultraviolet light but plastic does. Specialized lenses designated as UVB-blocking or polarized lenses are advised. However, according to cataract studies at the Wilmer Institute at Johns Hopkins Medical Institutions, "Even inexpensive, plastic sunglasses are good absorbers of UV-B . . . and how dark the glasses are isn't an issue . . . dark glasses are needed to block the visible light from the sun." Dark tints provide comfort from bright and glaring light.[7]

Polarized lenses reduce glare of reflected light and are particularly useful on water and snow. They are available in either neutral gray (often referred to as gray-green) or brown-amber tints. In my neighborhood of the Florida Keys and the Bahama Islands, neutral gray is often chosen by open-water boatmen, whereas brown-amber is usually desired by flats fishermen and divers to best visualize and locate shallow coral reefs, fish, and underwater obstructions; darker tints can be added if desired, for additional comfort from glaring sunlight. Mirror reflective coatings give additional protection and are commonly used in glacier glasses at high altitudes.

In hot humid conditions (i.e., tropical rainforests), a narrow space may be left between the frames and the face to allow adequate air exchange for the amelioration of lens fogging. Vented goggles are also available.

In addition to proper sunglasses, artificial tears (tear substitutes) may also be used to keep the corneal surface wet and lubricated in dry environments of deserts and high altitudes. Instillation of one to two drops of artificial tears, four or more times daily is usually adequate. Lubricating ointments have a longer duration of action than drops but are best applied in small amounts before sleep – they impart a greasy film to the cornea that tends to fog vision when awake. In individuals with chronic dry eyes it is advised to instill artificial tears prophylactically to prevent exposure keratitis.

Contact Lenses

Extreme conditions of expeditions can provide a harsh environment for contact lenses. Deserts and high altitudes cause impaired lubrication and dry eyes; blowing dirt and sand enter the tear film and lodge between the cornea and the contact lens, abrading the corneal epithelium; divers develop superficial punctuate keratitis from salt water and mask-clearing solutions; contact lenses dislodge in leaking masks and become lost. The most serious problem of contact lens wear is infection.

Contact lenses are a predisposing factor for microbial and parasitic infections of the cornea and sclera; extended wear and continuous overnight wear increase the chance of microbial keratitis (corneal ulcers) by approximately 15 times.[8] In tropical and subtropical environments, this figure may be higher, with a greater opportunity to acquire dangerous fungus and protozoan infections; these infections are difficult to treat and can be extremely devastating to the eye.

Infection from unsanitary conditions is usually caused by manipulating contact lenses, cases, and solutions with unclean hands. It is often not possible to adequately cleanse the hands when clean water is not available; infection can result. Infections are enhanced by dry eyes, prolonged lens wear, and corneal abrasions associated with improper handling and fit. It is often inconvenient to take adequate time for the proper care required with contact lenses when occupied with other pressing expedition tasks – setting up camp in approaching darkness or in early morning preparations for the day's adventure. When clean water and towels are not available, it is better to cleanse hands thoroughly with one of the sanitizing gels that contain 60–62% alcohol before handling lenses; the gels are available in 2 fl oz (59 ml) travel containers and larger sizes as desired; antiseptic hand tissues can also be used, although they are bulkier to carry. The gels dry in several minutes without the necessity of using contaminated towels. When clean water is available, use antibacterial soap routinely when cleansing the hands. It is also better not to bathe than to utilize water that is likely contaminated; if absolutely necessary to bathe, avoid flushing the eyes, nose, and mouth with the water.

Contact lens wear should be eliminated if there are signs of eye or eyelid infection (blepharitis), or if there is an epidemic of conjunctivitis among expedition members.

Caution is advised with overnight wear of extended wear contacts; the maximum duration is one week with fresh new lenses inserted after a night's sleep. At the first sign of infection (red or pink eye), excess tearing or discharge, photophobia and foreign body sensation – lenses should be discarded and topical antibiotics initiated four times a day. Eyeglasses should replace the contacts until 3 days after all symptoms have terminated. Eyeglasses

---

Table 36.5. Expedition contact lens guidelines (includes military guidelines)

1. Do not use an expedition as an opportunity to wear contact lenses unless experienced in their use.
2. Always have backup glasses and extra contact lenses.
3. Carry your own private supply of topical fluoroquinolone antibiotics, rewetting solutions, and artificial tears.
4. Use sanitizing hand cleansers (60–62% alcohol gels or antiseptic/antibacterial tissues) before handling contact lenses, whenever sanitation and hygiene are questionable.
5. Wear polycarbonate sunglasses over contact lenses for physical protection and to avoid symptoms of increased sensitivity to sunlight and other elements.
6. Disposable extended wear contact lenses must be removed and discarded after one week; insert new lenses the following morning.

Butler FK. The eye at altitude. *Int Ophthalmol Clin.* 1999;39(59).

---

have an additional advantage over contact lenses by physically protecting the eyes from injury; however, eyeglass lenses can fog. If keratitis remains after antibiotic therapy, fungus or protozoan infection is likely and is reason for evacuation – corneal ulceration may result.[9]

Contact lens problems associated with underwater diving and at high altitudes are addressed later in the "Special Locations" section.

Guidelines for contact lens wear and care are outline in Table 36.5.

EYE EXAMINATION

Anatomical

The customary comprehensive ocular examination is not usually possible in the field due to a lack of cumbersome office equipment and the professional expertise required in its use (e.g., slit lamps, automated visual field testing equipment, and indirect ophthalmoscopes). On expeditions, a practical examination, more consistent with available resources and experience, is therefore desirable. A history is first taken to establish details of the antecedent injury or ocular disorder and related symptoms (i.e., pain, blurred vision, areas of visual field defects, opaque spots [scotopsia], light flashes [photopsia], double vision [diplopia], photophobia, itching, and pink or red eye).

Eyelids

The condition of the eyelids and ocular surface is noted regarding swelling, exudates, hemorrhages, hematomas, inflammation, injury, or other pathology. If swollen, the eyelids are palpated for tenderness and pain. Soft puffy swelling without pain usually indicates an allergy or noninfected insect bite or sting; cold compresses are helpful to reduce symptoms. If pain is experienced, it is a

Anatomy of the Eye

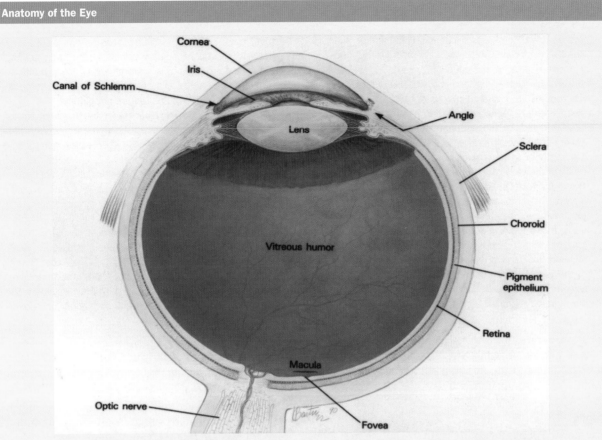

Figure 36.2. Anatomy of the eye. Courtesy of National Eye Institute, National Institutes of Health, Department of Health and Human Services.

The diagram in Figure 36.2 illustrates the anatomy of the eye.

- *Conjunctiva.* Thin clear membrane that coats the exposed surface of the sclera and inner surfaces of the eyelids.
- *Cornea,* Clear circular dome-shaped window of the eye, centrally located and directly anterior to the iris. Contact lenses fit upon the cornea. The cornea, together with the lens focuses light upon the retina.
- *Sclera.* White tissue comprising the major portion of the rigid wall that gives the eye its globular shape. It is limited by the cornea anteriorly and pierced by the optic nerve posteriorly. The sclera provides attachment for six extraocular muscles in each eye.
- *Corneal epithelium.* Thin, extremely sensitive, outer surface tissue of the cornea, directly exposed to the environment, frequently the location of foreign bodies and injuries (e.g., corneal abrasions and lacerations). The epithelium is bathed in tears; it is dependent upon an adequate flow of tears for its integrity.
- *Anterior chamber.* Space between the cornea and iris, occupied by clear aqueous fluid.
- *Posterior chamber.* Shallow space between the iris and the lens and its zonules. It is also occupied by aqueous fluid with which it is continuous into the anterior chamber through the pupil's aperture.

- *Anterior segment.* The forward portion of the eye extending from the front surface of the cornea to the back surface of the lens.
- *Posterior segment.* Extends from the back surface of the lens to the posterior surface of the globe. It includes the choroid, vitreous cavity, and retina.
- *Iris.* Colored tissue that lies within the eye directly behind the cornea. The pupillary opening is located in its center. When healthy, the pupil is round and will constrict upon exposure to a light source and upon movement of an object from far to near (accommodation). The pupils of both eyes normally respond equally to these stimuli. An irregular pupil or a dilated pupil that does not react briskly to light and accommodation can be a sign of ocular injury.
- *Lens.* The crystalline lens is a biconvex transparent body lying between the aqueous and vitreous chambers. The lens focuses light rays to form sharp images upon the retina. If the lens becomes cloudy or opaque (cataract) it interferes with transmission of these rays to the retina causing blurred vision. Cataracts occur as a natural process of aging, trauma, excess ultraviolet radiation, excess heat and electrical exposure, and certain chemicals and drugs (i.e., corticosteroids).
- *Choroid.* Vascular layer sandwiched between the sclera and retina. It joins the ciliary body anteriorly. An inner

(Continued)

layer of fine blood vessels (choriocapillaris) is adjacent to Bruch's membrane, which separates the choroid from the pigmentary layer of the retina.

- *Ciliary body*. The lens attaches to the ciliary body through the zonules. The ciliary body secretes the aqueous fluid that fills the anterior and posterior chambers of the eye; it also joins with the peripheral iris, which it serves to anchor in its circumference.
- *Retina*. Inner sensory layer, lining the posterior (vitreous) cavity of the globe and equivalent to the film in a camera. The retina receives light energy through its visual sensory organs (the rods and cones); this energy is converted into electrical impulses that are transmitted through the optic nerve to the brain where images are perceived.
- *Macula*. Small central area of the retina where light is focused; located on the visual axis at the posterior pole of the eye. As seen through the ophthalmoscope, it lies temporal to the optic disc and appears darker than the surrounding retina. The center of the macula (fovea cen-

tralis) contains the greatest concentration of cones (no rods); it is critical for sharp central vision (e.g., reading, and color vision in daylight illumination). Rods dominate the peripheral retina and detect lower levels of colorless light (scotopic vision); images are not distinct.

- *Optic disc*. The optic disc is located in the posterior portion of the globe and is observed as a pale pink round area with fairly distinct margins; it is seen at the point where the optic nerve pierces the sclera, it lies nasal to the macula. Nerve fiber continuations of retinal ganglion cells form the optic nerve, which connects through synapses with the brain. The terminal portions of the central artery and vein, branch out across the retina from the optic disc. Complete occlusion of either results in blindness; blockage of their branches gives segmental vision impairment.
- *Vitreous*. Consists of a transparent gel mass that fills the large cavity of the eyeball between the lens and retina. The gel tends to liquefy with aging. Opaque objects within this tissue are perceived as spots or floaters (scotopsia).

sign of infection or cellulitis. A systemic antibiotic, levofloxacin 500 mg is administered bid (twice a day); warm compresses are applied.

Pupils

Examine the pupils for symmetry in size and shape. They are tested with a penlight in a dark location for normal response to light and accommodation. Normal pupils are round and equal in size. Shining a light in the eye normally causes prompt constriction, producing a miotic or small pupil. The pupils should normally constrict consensually when the light is shined into either eye (the opposite pupil constricts in the same manner as the stimulated pupil). Accommodation is tested by moving a finger toward the patient's eye; normal pupils constrict with this maneuver. The common written designation of normal pupils, PERLA, indicates the pupils are equal, round and react normally to light and accommodation. Anisocoria refers to pupils of unequal diameter.

The inability of one pupil to constrict promptly, or a pupil that remains dilated or irregular after acute injury, may be a sign of iris tear or sphincter damage, clouding of the optical system, or damage to the sensory system – optic nerve or retina. Although not usually incapacitating, it may signal other associated injuries of the eye.

When clarity of the optical system is obstructed, insufficient light reaches the retina to initiate the normal pupillary constriction (afferent pupillary defect) (e.g., hyphema with blood obstructing the pupil or vitreous hemorrhage); it is also possible the retina and/or the optic nerve may be significantly damaged, interfering with the direct light reflex. These sensory impairments can be tested by swinging a light between the pupils; if

there is impairment of one pupil's direct reflex to light, it will constrict promptly to a light stimulus directed into the opposite normal eye (consensual reflex) but not as rapidly when shining the light directly into the affected eye (it remains dilated) – the sensory component of the reflex is impaired (Marcus Gunn pupil).

A dilated pupil following head trauma associated with decreased consciousness is usually caused by brain injury with oculomotor (third cranial nerve) dysfunction. Surgical intervention is often necessary and accelerated evacuation is required. Oculomotor nerve damage may also be associated with fractures of the orbital apex.

Anterior Segment

The cornea, iris, and lens are examined with a penlight. The cornea and anterior chamber are checked for clarity. The cornea is searched for evidence of wounds or foreign bodies. The anterior chamber is examined for blood (see following discussion in the "Hyphema" section). The lens may be cloudy (cataract) or displaced causing an irregular pupil and/or deeper than normal anterior chamber (posteriorly displaced lens and iris) when compared to the uninjured eye. Another sign of a displaced lens is a tremulous iris – the iris will appear to quiver upon movements of the eye or head. An iris defect or tear (coloboma) and irregular pupil may indicate blunt or penetrating injury.

Posterior Segment

Examination of the posterior segment (fundus exam) is performed by a health care professional experienced with using the direct ophthalmoscope. While slowly approaching the eye and searching for the familiar anatomy and the orange color of the fundus, the diopter power is reduced from + 9 toward zero and if necessary, to minus until focus is attained; this is done by dialing the ophthalmoscope click stops counterclockwise. If clear focus is not possible, the ocular media may be cloudy secondary to the following conditions: cornea abraded or edematous, the lens displaced or opaque (cataract), or hemorrhage in the anterior chamber (hyphema) or vitreous body. These disorders can be recognized by adjusting ophthalmoscope click stops, while focusing upon each structure of the eye from cornea to retina.

When the posterior pole of the fundus is in focus, the macula and optic disc are examined; particular notice is taken of any disturbance in the usual anatomy. Hemorrhages or macular edema should be noted. While hemorrhages can be identified rather easily as dark red, usually well-defined features, macular edema can be more difficult to discern with the direct ophthalmoscope; the macula may appear pale gray and elevated when compared to the uninvolved eye. In either case, the diagnosis can be verified if there is evidence of central vision impairment; test central vision with the reading card and with the Amsler's grid (the pinhole test and confrontation visual fields can further confirm central vision function).

Definitive examination of the peripheral retina and choroid of the eye is limited to experienced physicians using office instruments. The 110-volt slit lamp microscope and indirect ophthalmoscope, so vital to office examinations, are not practical to carry into the field; these instruments have the benefit of providing magnified stereoscopic views. The indirect ophthalmoscope also gives a clear wide angle view of the most peripheral structures in the posterior segment; it is especially useful in identifying peripheral retinal tears, detachments, and hemorrhages (the pupils must be widely dilated). Physicians, who are experienced in the use of a direct ophthalmoscope, may carry a battery-operated model on expeditions. Although limited in observing the periphery of the fundus, examination with the direct ophthalmoscope may assist in identifying many serious injuries and disorders. By searching the periphery, a traumatic retinal detachment may be observed; if it is large, it may be easily recognized near the central vitreous cavity. Many other important disorders can also be observed (e.g., retinal and vitreous hemorrhages, macular damage – edema, holes and hemorrhages). (See discussion in the "Retinal Detachment" section.)

Vision Testing

Vision testing is of great importance in the field because of the limited availability of specialized ophthalmic diagnostic instruments, as previously described. Therefore, many injuries to internal eye structures cannot be directly recognized. In this situation, visual testing, as well as symptoms and signs of ocular injuries, can provide important clues to diagnosis. Do not instill eye drops or shine a light into the eyes before conducting vision tests because testing may be altered.

With eyeglasses in place (if normally used), test visual acuity with a near reading card. If acuity does not approach 20/40 or better, injury should be suspected. When vision is lost or persistently blurred after an accident, the patient must be evacuated to an ophthalmologist to ensure proper diagnosis and optimum therapy.

Confrontation visual fields and the Amsler grid test are performed to identify peripheral and central vision impairment. The Amsler grid test can either eliminate or suggest significant macular pathology; critical central vision (reading and color discrimination) can be permanently lost (central scotoma) if disorders are not recognized.

When evaluating vision testing, all examinations must be taken into consideration before arriving at a diagnosis; because of the subjective nature of the tests, all may not agree.

Visual Acuity

It is not practical to test visual acuity as routinely tested in an office, with a standardized and properly illuminated Snellen vision chart at a measured distance of 20 feet from the patient's eye; the near vision card (small and convenient to carry on expeditions) is a practical alternative. Holding the card at approximately 14 inches from the eye in adequate illumination, the near vision in each eye is recorded while the patient wears prescription eyeglasses. Poor visual acuity is an indication of an ocular disorder but it does not always correspond with the severity of a problem; the loss of central vision, however, does suggest a serious disorder. See the Amsler grid in Figure 36.1. In cases of complete vision loss (amaurosis), the designation of no light perception (NLP) is used – the patient cannot perceive a bright light shining directly into the eye; a blind painful eye is a major reason for enucleation.

Pinhole Vision

If prescription glasses are usually worn but are damaged or lost, the vision is tested with the patient looking through a pinhole occluder positioned in front of the eye. As with early cameras, the pinhole takes the place of a lens. The patient adjusts and centers the pinhole himself. If a pinhole occluder is not available, punch a small hole through the center of a paper card with a pointed object. Occlude the opposite eye; a hand can be used. The pinhole reveals the best possible vision (when the ocular media are clear); it detects central vision defects caused by macular pathology. However, clouding of some portion of the eye's optical system (e.g., hemorrhage or cataract) will also reduce pinhole visual acuity and can be confused with macular dysfunction. If the patient can read better without utilizing the pinhole, media clouding may be suspected (numerous peripheral light rays entering the pupil are able to be gathered and focused through the cloud by the cornea and lens; total light intensity is greater than with the pinhole). The pinhole functions by eliminating all but the central axis of direct light rays that enter the eye and continue directly to the macula (focusing is not necessary to give a clear image); however, any obstruction along that narrow line greatly diminishes vision as detected through the small aperture of the pinhole. When the optical media are clear, poor pinhole vision suggests macular pathology is present.

Depending upon degree of visual loss, it must be decided if evacuation is necessary. Although normal visual acuity is an encouraging sign that the macula is not injured, it is no guarantee that a serious problem does not exist elsewhere; when central vision is normal but the patient complains of blurring, it is possible that peripheral vision is reduced by a retinal and/or choroidal detachment or hemorrhage, vascular occlusion, or some other problem in the fundus of the eye (or central nervous system). If it is not possible to examine these areas, confrontation visual field examination may demonstrate evidence of such a problem.

Amsler Grid Examination

The Amsler grid is a small handheld chart composed of numerous uniform squares and a central fixation dot. The test is used to detect abnormalities within the central 20° of the visual field and is especially useful in evaluating macular function. By comparison, the total monocular visual field measures approximately 120°. Patients with macular degeneration routinely use the grid to monitor the status of their own disease; they accomplish this at home with no physician present. In the field, the Amsler grid is a valuable tool of self-examination; because of the high frequency of retinal hemorrhages at high altitudes, a grid should be carried by every mountain climber to monitor central vision daily. It is especially useful when no ophthalmoscope is available to evaluate the retina.

The subject should wear reading glasses if needed, and the contralateral eye must be occluded. While holding the chart at the usual reading distance, the patient adjusts it inward and outward until the central fixation dot and surrounding lines are in best focus. It is always advisable to test the uninjured eye first; this helps introduce the person to the test and establishes a normal baseline to compare with the injured eye. When the test suggests questionable or minimal findings, always repeat, and monitor daily; for comparison purposes, diagram the area of vision impairment.

When abnormalities are revealed in the grid, an ophthalmoscope is used to search the macula and peripheral retina for evidence of the responsible pathology. It is important to note that pathology (i.e., retinal

---

Amsler grid questions

Following trauma, the patient is asked the following questions while focusing upon the central fixation dot; they may also be a used for self-testing:

1. Can you recognize the center dot?
   If the patient cannot recognize the fixation dot he may have a central visual field defect (central scotoma) suggesting macular pathology.
2. Can you recognize the four sides of the grid? Are the lines straight and clear?
   If while focusing upon the center dot, the patient cannot recognize all four sides – and those sides are not clear, complete, and straight – a retinal detachment or hemorrhage may be encroaching into the macula or adjacent area. Chronic glaucoma, brain and optic pathway impairment (optic nerves, tracts, and radiations) and droopy upper eyelids (blepheroptosis) can also cause this finding.
3. Are all lines indistinct or evenly blurred? Uniform blurring indicates a disorder causing reduced clarity or focusing of the optical system (i.e., corneal defects [abrasions, keratitis, edema], hyphema, lens dislocation, traumatic cataract, or vitreous hemorrhage).
4. Are there any blurred, distorted, double, or curved lines within the entire grid? If a particular segment is involved outside the center portion of the grid, a paracentral scotoma is present, and a retinal detachment or hemorrhage may be encroaching upon the edges of the macular area. It may also indicate a branch vascular occlusion.

---

detachment) will involve the opposite side of the eye from the direction of the visual field defect. Macular or retinal pathology associated with injury and vision loss requires evacuation. The eye may remain white, and pain may be negligible or nonexistent. It is not necessary for the eye to have an obvious wound; retinal detachments can occur after blunt ocular trauma, jarring head trauma as experienced in auto accidents, head punches, and falls. Highly myopic people especially, are prone to retinal detachments with no apparent proximate cause.

Confrontation Visual Field Examination

This is a rapid screening test that depends on the patient's subjective response to a stimulus. No specialized equipment is required. As with the Amsler grid, the uninjured eye is tested first to familiarize the patient with the test and establish a normal baseline for comparison. The examiner sits face-to-face with the patient, and compares his or her own peripheral vision to that of the patient. Their faces are positioned approximately 1 meter apart. The examiner's fingers are used as targets while extending one arm in the extreme periphery midway between himself and the patient. With corresponding eyes occluded, the patient and the examiner concentrate, without deviation, upon the pupil of the other's eye on the corresponding side (patient's left eye to examiner's right eye). The examiner occludes the opposite eye, as does the patient (it is best to occlude the patient's eye with a patch or hand; it should remain open); if the eyelids are voluntarily closed it can cause the eyelids in the tested eye to partially close, resulting in an erroneous reduced visual field.

The fingers, invisible in the extreme periphery, are slowly moved toward the center until detected by both examiner and patient. The patient is requested to count the number of fingers presented. Assuming the examiner has normal visual fields, if he or she can detect the moving finger targets significantly before the patient, it is indication that the patient has a field defect in that particular position. The patient's eye is constantly observed to ensure it does not drift from focusing upon the examiner's pupil. This test is repeated from four different quadrants of the visual field. It may be further refined by testing in eight meridians. If the patient has difficulty in detecting the fingers in a particular peripheral position, it is assumed that there is corresponding visual impairment in the contralateral (opposite) portion of the posterior segment of the eye; examination with an ophthalmoscope can then be concentrated in that area. The optic nerve and retinal blood vessels are also examined; vascular occlusions and optic nerve damage may cause visual field defects. Brain injury can also be responsible for these findings. A generalized constriction of the visual field in all positions indicates impaired clarity of the optical system as previously described.

In addition to testing for peripheral visual field defects, the central field is evaluated as well; this can assist in detecting macular pathology. Central field loss is demonstrated as the fingers disappear approaching the center, testing from each quadrant as with peripheral field testing. When associated with reading difficulty, these defects suggest retinal pathology in the macular region (retinal detachment, hemorrhage, hematoma, and edema – central serous retinopathy). Macular edema often occurs as the result of direct blunt trauma when abrupt force is transmitted through the globe to the macula region. Central vision may also be impaired or lost secondary to a retinal hemorrhage or detachment that progresses to involve the macular region. Confrontation visual fields help confirm Amsler grid findings in establishing central vision impairment. An abnormal test of the injured eye is always compared with the opposite eye. Color vision, although not tested on expeditions, is also impaired when central vision is lost.

If an ophthalmoscope is not available, these tests along with other evidence of injury should be sufficient to arrive at reasonable evacuation decisions. It is always possible, however, that the injured person is unreliable or is insufficiently cooperative to give accurate results. In questionable cases, the tests are repeated and compared with one another – they require little time.

PERIORBITAL INFLAMMATIONS

- Blepharitis, chalazion and hordeolum. Blepharitis is an inflammation of the eyelids. Although it may lead to a red eye (blepharoconjunctivitis), it is typically a chronic process; it is therefore included here rather than in the classification of acute red eye.
- Orbital cellulitis, preseptal and postseptal
- Dacriocystitis
- Orbital pseudotumor
- Giant cell arteritis

Blepharitis

Anterior blepharitis is a chronic inflammation along the eyelid margins at the base of the lashes usually accompanied by crusting. (See Figure 36.3.) It is frequently associated with seborrhea, acne rosacea, and bacterial infection of the glands of Zeiss and Moll. When an abscess forms, it is commonly known as a stye (hordeolum).[11] It is treated with warm, moist compresses applied to the eyelids for 5 minutes several times a day. Bacitracin/polymyxin B ointment 500 units/g is applied along the eyelid margins at bedtime (after warm compresses) for at least 4 weeks. The problem often recurs. If associated with chronic seborrheic dermatitis of the scalp (white flakes, "dandruff" on the scalp and eyelid margins) it will not completely resolve until the scalp is adequately treated with a medicated shampoo. Posterior blepharitis involves the Meibomian glands, located more deeply within the eyelids. The glands have ducts located within the cartilaginous tarsus; the ducts are oriented vertically – perpendicular to the eyelid margins where they exit.

Chalazion

A swelling (chalazion) forms when gland secretions plug the Meibomian ducts. It presents as a soft inflamed

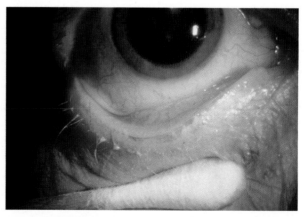

Figure 36.3. Blepharitis. Courtesy of Professor Richard K. Forster, MD, Bascom Palmer Eye Institute, Miller School of Medicine, University of Miami, Miami, Florida.

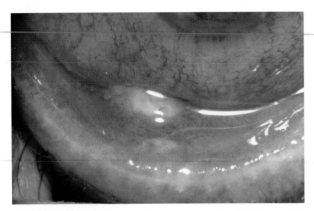

Figure 36.4. Chalazion. Courtesy of Professor Richard K. Forster, MD, Bascom Palmer Eye Institute, Miller School of Medicine, University of Miami, Miami, Florida.

swelling on the inner surface of the eyelid that becomes firmer over several weeks. If allowed to progress, the inspissated matter within the ducts can form pale hard concretions[12] or may become infected. (See Figure 36.4.) Therapy consists of warm compresses and oral tetracycline for 1–2 months; this tends to decrease and soften the matter plugging the ducts. If secondary infection is suspected, apply warm compresses followed by Bacitracin/polymyxin B ointment 500 units/g to the inner eyelid surfaces at bedtime. Warm compresses soften the inspissated material and often assist in causing the lump to rupture and drain at its apex on the tarsal or skin surface. Finger massage through closed eyelids can expedite the rupture. Surgical evacuation from the everted inner (tarsal) eyelid surface is a common treatment when the mass persists. The procedure can be deferred until return from the expedition. If exudates collect on the eyelid margins, they often dry, becoming crusty and irritating to the eyes; scrubs across the eyelid margins are advised using moistened cotton-tipped applicators; small amounts of baby shampoo applied to the cotton expedite the process.

If necessary a large soft chalazion can be drained from the underside of the eyelid (tarsal surface) using a #11 BP blade and quickly stabbing horizontally across the involved duct(s), parallel to the eyelid margin and through the apex of the pointing mass. Incision should be approximately 2–3 mm in length. It is important that

The definitions and anatomical locations of hordeola and chalazia are frequently interchanged and/or confused. See, for example, "Internal hordeola occasionally evolve into chalazia ..." American Academy of Ophthalmology, External Disease and Cornea, Basic and Clinical Science Course, Section 8 (2006–7):168. The same reference describes both inflammatory disorders as involving either meibomian or Zeis glands (pp. 87, 168).

the eyelid is everted away from the globe (a special metal chalazion clamp is routinely used to protect the eye when this procedure is performed in the office); prior to incision, tetracaine is applied to the area for several minutes with a saturated cotton applicator. Additional tetracaine is applied after drainage. Applicators can be used to massage and assist in drainage and evacuation of the exudate. Bacitracin/polymyxin B ointment 500 units/g is applied directly from the tube into the remaining cavity. Warm compresses should be continued every morning and night for several days to assist drainage; bacitracin/polymyxin B ointment 500 units/g is applied afterward.

Preseptal Orbital Cellulitis

The orbit is divided into two compartments by the orbital septum. The septum is a sheet of connective tissue that connects the orbital rim to the upper and lower tarsal plates of the eyelids. Preseptal cellulitis involves the anterior or forward compartment and presents with markedly swollen, tender, and reddened eyelids. The upper eyelid may droop (ptosis). The most common etiology on expeditions is usually due to envenomation from an insect bite or puncture by a contaminated sharp object (i.e., thorn or fishhook). Levofloxacin 500 mg should be administered every 12 hours (bid); ampicillin is an alternative, 250 mg four times a day (QID). If symptoms worsen or do not subside, emergency evacuation is required. The patient should be given a travel supply of the medication to continue daily until professional help is attained. Intravenous antibiotics are frequently necessary, and tetanus prophylactic therapy is given if required.

Postseptal Orbital Cellulitis

This most serious infection is usually secondary to chronic sinusitis, but during an expedition, it can be caused by an injury that penetrates deeply into the posterior compartment of the orbit. The infection occurs within the fat and connective tissue and involves the posterior compartment, behind the orbital septum. In addition to swollen erythematous eyelids as in preseptal disease, most symptoms are due to proximity of infection to important structures within the posterior compartment. History and symptoms of preexisting sinus disease (sinus pain and rhinitis) are clues to diagnosis of the usual form of the disease; however, during an expedition, proximate trauma is the most likely cause. Symptoms include fever, unilateral headache, orbital pain, protruding eye (proptosis), and blurred vision. Multiple cranial nerves may become involved and cause double vision (diplopia). Treat as with preseptal disease, however evacuate immediately. The condition can lead to septic cavernous sinus thrombosis, meningitis, and encephalitis; it can be life-threatening.[13] Accelerate evacuation; airlift to a hospital if possible; intensive care usually includes culture, sensitivity, and intravenous antibiotics.

Giant Cell Arteritis (Temporal Arteritis)

Giant cell arteritis is a systemic inflammation of arteries that originates from the aortic arch. The disorder is not related to expeditions but could be confused with other causes of vision loss. It causes vascular occlusion with inflammation and ischemia of the optic nerve; ischemic optic neuropathy can lead to optic atrophy and blindness. Temporal arteritis usually occurs in people older than 55–60 years of age. Patients often experience transient visual blurring and double vision (diplopia) several days before more complete vision loss. This may be accompanied by headache, fever, and tenderness to firm palpation over the inflamed temporal artery (located between the eye and upper ear). One or both eyes may be affected. Diagnosis is confirmed with an elevated Westagren sedimentation rate (ESR) and temporal artery biopsy. Suspicion of this condition dictates evacuation. Oral corticosteroids in high doses (prednisolone 80–100 mg daily) is occasionally administered in desperate cases of rapidly deteriorating vision; however, this practice is not desirable before diagnostic studies are completed because corticosteroids alter results of diagnostic tests; confirmation of the diagnosis is always preferred before lengthy corticosteroid therapy is undertaken. Clinical improvement following this therapy is suggestive of giant cell arteritis. Orbital pseudotumor is in the differential diagnosis.[14]

Dacriocystitis

An infection of the nasolacrimal sac, located just below and nasal to the inner corner (canthus) of the eye, the disorder is not expedition related. The sac normally drains tears from the eye into the nose via the nasolacrimal duct. Infections of the lacrimal sac are usually the consequence of an obstruction of the duct, although infection may spread from the sinuses, nose, or conjunctiva. Swelling, erythema, pain, and tenderness are common symptoms of the infection. The most common causative organisms are *Staphylococcus aureus*, *Staphylococcus epidermidis*, and *Streptococcus pneumoniae*.[15] Treatment consists of warm moist compresses applied over the swelling twice daily, followed by massage and ofloxacin 0.3% drops instilled in the eye. Levofloxacin 500 mg is administered daily. If improvement is not noticed within the first few days, evacuation is required.

Orbital Pseudotumor

An orbital pseudotumor is a nonspecific inflammation of the soft tissue in the posterior compartment of the orbit. A characteristic symptom is painful proptosis (prominence) of the globe (one or both orbits may be involved) due to inflammation and tissue pressure from within the confines of the posterior orbit. Symptoms include periorbital pain, swelling and erythema of the eyelids, conjunctival injection, ophthalmoplegia, and restricted movements of the globe with diplopia. The etiology of the inflammation is unknown. The diagnosis may be confused with orbital cellulitis and Graves' thyroid ophthalmopathy. Initiate levofloxacin therapy and evacuate. Systemic prednisolone is added 80 mg daily if no improvement is noted within 1–2 days. The response to corticosteroids is dramatic.[16]

ACUTE RED EYE

A red eye is a prominent symptom common to many acute ocular disorders experienced on expeditions. It indicates an inflammatory or infectious process that requires attention; this is especially true when there is an antecedent injury. The category also applies to pink eyes; in common usage pink eye often connotes infectious conjunctivitis. An acute red eye is usually accompanied by symptoms, and signs other than red discoloration, that assist in diagnosis. However, an injured or diseased eye may not always be red, and a red eye may not always be injured (e.g., inflammatory and infectious disorders of the anterior segment are red, whereas most disorders of the posterior segment are associated with a white eye unless associated with anterior segment injury). See Table 36.6.

In a preponderance of surface eye problems, the connective tissue membrane covering the white sclera (bulbar conjunctiva) becomes pink or reddened with inflammation; the conjunctiva lining the inner surfaces of the eyelids (palpebral conjunctiva) may also become

Table 36.6. Differential diagnosis of acute red eye
• Burns
• Conjunctivitis – allergic, bacterial, viral, foreign substance, and chemical
• Contact lens complications
• Corneal abrasion
• Corneal and conjunctival (surface) foreign bodies
• Corneal erosion
• Corneal ulcer – infectious keratitis
• Dry eye
• Endophthalmitis
• Episcleritis
• Glaucoma, acute
• Herpes simplex
• Hyphema
• Iritis, traumatic
• Keratitis
• Pterygium
• Subconjunctival hemorrhage
• Trauma – blunt, penetrating, perforating, and ruptured globe

similarly inflamed. If the inflammation is not generalized but concentrated in a localized segment, it may point to a foreign body or reveal the area involved with an irritant or injury (e.g., conjunctival inflammations adjacent to the cornea may indicate a nearby corneal abrasion or foreign body). Therefore, if a foreign body is suspected but not detected, it is prudent to search the cornea adjacent to the localized conjunctival injection. Opaque or darkly colored foreign bodies are more obvious when located over the white sclera rather than the cornea. Use a penlight with a concentrated halogen beam for identifying ocular surface injuries and foreign bodies. Direct the light across the ocular surface from various directions to avoid glare and better accentuate a tiny foreign body. A magnifying lens is desired when searching for tiny particles such as sand or metallic fragments; a binocular magnifying loupe is ideal for this purpose and allows better evaluation of the depth embedded foreign bodies penetrate into the cornea.

Conjunctivitis (commonly referred to as pink eye) is one of the most common nontraumatic eye conditions treated in emergency rooms and is one of the most common eye conditions to be expected on expeditions. It may be contagious and frequently extends to involve the cornea causing keratitis–keratoconjunctivitis (see discussion later in the chapter). The conjunctiva is exposed to airborne and waterborne irritants and a variety of pathologic organisms. For practical reasons, exact identification of most infectious microorganisms is not possible during expeditions; treatments advised are therefore empirical. However, a new method of identification of adenoconjunctivitis has now become available. (See following discussion in the "Viral Conjunctivitis" section.)

Burns

Burns may be either chemical or thermal. Chemical burns are treated as outlined in the "Conjunctivitis caused by Foreign Substances and Chemicals" section. They create corneal defects that can be large in the case of acids and alkalis. In severe cases, the entire epithelium may be eroded away. Alkalis tend to be more damaging than acids because they continue to erode long after initial contact. Powders (i.e., lime) that burn into the corneal surface are especially difficult to irrigate free from the eye.

Thermal burns of the eye and eyelids are unusual and usually accompany related facial burns of a wider scale or small areas struck by sparks from campfire embers, grinding wheels, and other power tools; they may also result from splashing boiling water. Eyelid burns are treated as other skin burns with antiseptics and antibiotics, avoiding eye contact. If the cornea is involved, remove any foreign substance from the eye and treat as a corneal abrasion. (See following discussion in

"Conjunctivitis caused by Foreign Substances and Chemicals" section.)

Allergic Conjunctivitis

Allergic conjunctivitis presents with pink, itchy, and watery eyes. It may be associated with rhinitis, sinusitis, and sneezing. Allergic inflammations of the conjunctiva are often a recurring problem of seasonal pollen allergies or contact with specific allergens from many sources; through experience, these are often known to the patient. During travel, however, exposure is often related to high levels of local pollens or other airborne irritants (e.g., smog in Katmandu, Nepal, and Mexico City). Topical eye medications and contact lens solutions (especially their preservatives) can also cause allergies. If there is a history of allergies, the individual should carry his or her own supply of antihistamine drugs and corticosteroid nasal spray; they may not be available in the expedition's general medical kit. In cases of allergic conjunctivitis, diclofenac 0.1% drops and cold compresses are applied four times a day. Various corticosteroid nasal sprays are effective in controlling allergies to airborne allergens when prolonged exposure is expected. Only in instances of acute severe allergic conjunctivitis should prednisolone drops be instilled in the eyes.

Bacterial Conjunctivitis

In the absence of trauma, an irritated red eye, with or without obvious discharge, may indicate viral or bacterial conjunctivitis (surface infection). The viral variety is the most common and most contagious. On expeditions, conjunctivitis is often caused by bathing in contaminated water, sharing face towels, general unsanitary conditions, contact lenses, and touching one's face with unclean hands.

Very few natural sources of water can be considered uncontaminated by pathogenic microorganisms; Giardia cysts have been found in alpine mountain headwaters freshly supplied by rainwater. It is always dangerous to bathe downriver from other humans or animals that carry and excrete a multitude of enteric pathogens. Immersing the face in a stream or river is not advised.[17,18]

The dangers of contaminated water are emphasized by the case of a 54-year-old patient of the author, Miguel Arellano; he went into a coma, and then died 5 days after washing his face in river water on a farm in Venezuela; his daughter relates he had aspirated the water into his nose as was his custom "to clear his sinuses." Amoebae from the water most probably entered his nose – many were detected in spinal fluid. The invading organisms apparently had traveled the short distance to his central nervous system via the facial venous and/or lymphatic systems.

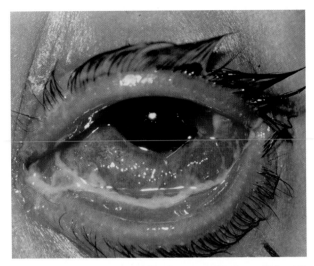

Figure 36.5. Bacterial conjunctivitis. Courtesy of Professor Richard K. Forster, MD, Bascom Palmer Eye Institute, Miller School of Medicine, University of Miami, Miami, Florida.

Symptoms of bacterial conjunctivitis include itching, burning, and a dry or gritty sensation. The eyelids may be stuck together with exudates and crusting upon waking. (See Figure 36.5.) When the cornea is involved, keratoconjunctivitis (see keratitis), it is generally a more incapacitating condition – symptoms are more pronounced and vision may be reduced. In conjunctivitis without corneal involvement, unless a significant discharge is present, vision is usually not significantly reduced. Treat with ofloxacin 0.3% eye drops four times daily and bacitracin/polymyxin B ointment 500 units/g at bedtime; apply a bead along the deep inner surface of the retracted lower eyelid. Tobramycin 0.3% solution is an alternative therapy. The condition is usually self-limiting over a period of several weeks.

Conjunctivitis Caused by Foreign Substances and Chemicals

Eye wash preparations (irrigating solutions) are available in handy plastic bottles that are usually too bulky to carry on many expeditions. They contain buffered saline solutions that are well tolerated by the eye. If not available, intravenous (IV) saline or properly disinfected drinking water may be irrigated from a 50 cc hypodermic syringe without needle; this method can be used to flush eyes clear of foreign substances (i.e., sand, chemicals, or irritating toxic substances – cactus sap, dive mask antifogging solutions, and sun block). The cornea, sclera, and inner surfaces and recesses of the eyelids should be irrigated using measured force. During this procedure, tetracaine drops can be instilled as a topical anesthetic. Copious irrigation is usually necessary if a toxic substance is tenacious. Exudates containing foreign matter often collect in the fornices (recesses) under the eyelids,

and at the inner corners of the eyes. After flushing these locations they may be cleaned of residual matter with cotton-tipped applicators. After a foreign substance has been irrigated free, a foreign body sensation may persist due to fine corneal abrasions, keratitis, and/or conjunctival inflammation. This will usually pass after several hours or one night's sleep; if persistent, stain the cornea with fluorescein dye and search for corneal defects and foreign bodies.

If acid or alkali is being flushed, the procedure should begin immediately at the site of injury with almost any available nontoxic solution. Within limits, if it is safe to drink (alcohol, citric juices, and spicy liquids are excluded), it should be suitable. Retract the eyelids and pour into the eye if no syringe is available; immediate treatment is critical to minimize damage, seconds are important! Continue irrigation for at least 30 minutes to ensure adequate dilution of residual amounts. It is customary to instill topical prednisolone 1% drops every hour to reduce intense ongoing inflammation and scarring. Although it is possible that complications may result from the application of topical corticosteroids, in these cases the benefits far outweigh the risks – continue application every hour for several days if significant inflammation persists; reduce the dosage schedule as the inflammation subsides. Instill scopolamine 0.25% four times a day to ameliorate painful ciliary spasm. Also apply ofloxacin 0.3% four times a day to prevent bacterial infection

Severe acid and alkali burns of the cornea can lead to permanent blindness due to neovascularization and opaque scarring. Persistent conjunctival inflammation can cause scarring with adhesions between the globe and eyelids. Iritis often accompanies severe inflammations. In chemical burns of a lesser degree, topical prednisolone 1% may be avoided. The nonsteroidal antiinflammatory drops diclofenac 0.1% can be instilled four times a day to reduce inflammation and pain. (See the following discussion in the "Viral Conjunctivitis" section.) After initial irrigation, do not apply topical anesthetics because they delay healing.

While acid and alkali burns can be treated with corticosteroids in the emergency situation, they are ideally treated by an ophthalmologist knowledgeable about possible complications. If significant corneal epithelium is damaged or healing is prolonged, evacuate after initial treatment. The patient should continue topical prednisolone 1% during evacuation travel. Dispense oral narcotics or other suitable pain medications.

Corneal irritants may cause *superficial punctuate keratitis*. If an office slit lamp examination were performed with fluorescein dye stain, disseminated fine punctuate corneal defects would be observed. In more serious cases, the stain would reveal larger defects of the corneal epithelium. On expeditions, larger fluorescein stained defects can also be observed using a magnifying lens with a cobalt blue penlight and even the naked eye in many instances. This should be done in a dark place with the light directed obliquely. The cornea may also appear cloudy from edema secondary to marked keratitis.

Viral Conjunctivitis

Viral conjunctivitis is the most common variety of conjunctivitis and is frequently highly contagious. Some varieties are associated with corneal inflammation (keratoconjunctivitis). Viral conjunctivitis should be suspected if topical antibiotics do not resolve symptoms of red (pink eye), itching, and photophobic eyes; symptoms spread from one eye to the other. The most common viral infections are adenovirus – adenoconjunctivitis (pharyngeal conjunctival fever and epidemic keratoconjunctivitis, or EKC); and herpes simplex keratitis. Pharyngeal conjunctival fever presents with an upper respiratory infection. Viral conjunctivitis spreads rapidly because of close human contact and poor sanitary conditions during expeditions; it is prevalent in certain areas where expeditions are common. EKC has spread through eye offices and clinics, settings that attract and concentrate patients and where the disorder can be spread by patients and examiners alike; extreme precautions and sanitizing measures must be taken. Preauricular lymph nodes are enlarged and tender and assist in the diagnosis of adenoconjunctivitis including EKC. (See Figures 36.6 and 36.7.) In the subacute stage of EKC, characteristic opaque white subepithelial corneal infiltrates form. If present in large numbers, they may blur vision and are frequently treated with topical prednisolone. There is no effective therapy for most cases of viral keratoconjunctivitis; they usually run their course in several weeks. Consideration should be given for evacuation because the disorders are so contagious and disabling. When more than one or two people related to the expedition develop symptoms in rapid succession, the diagnosis should be suspected. Warm compresses, cycloplegics, artificial tears, and diclofenac drops may give a degree of symptomatic relief.

In acute herpes simplex keratoconjunctivitis, typical dendritic (branching) corneal ulcers are diagnostic. The

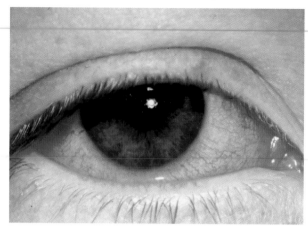

Figure 36.6. Adenoconjunctivitis (pharyngeal conjunctival fever). Courtesy of Professor Richard K. Forster, MD, Bascom Palmer Eye Institute, Miller School of Medicine, University of Miami, Miami, Florida.

branching configuration that identifies these ulcers can be readily observed using fluorescein dye. (See following discussion in the "Herpes Simplex Keratitis" section.) Prednisolone 1% therapy is contraindicated.

A rapid (10 minute) immuno-diagnostic (chromatographic) point of care test for adenoviruses is now available; the kit weighs 15 grams. Clinical trials are in progress for diagnosing allergic conjunctivitis and herpes simplex keratoconjunctivitis. Eye fluid for testing is taken from the conjunctiva of the lower cul de sac. The test is 88% sensitive and 91% specific when compared with standard testing methods (*As of this writing, the author plans to become a shareholder in the company that is developing these tests*).[19]

Contact Lens Complications

Acute red eyes associated with contact lenses are due to poor fit or damaged lenses, traumatic corneal epithelial defects caused during insertion or removal, allergy to solutions, foreign substances or irritants, displaced lenses, dry eyes, and hypoxia due to low levels of available oxygen (high altitudes). Corneal infection leading to ulcerative keratitis is the most serious complication of contact lens wear and was discussed previously in the "Expedition Eye Supplies, Personal Items" section.

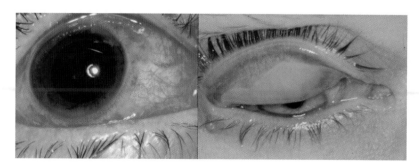

Figure 36.7. Adenoconjunctivitis (epidemic keratoconjunctivitis). Courtesy of Professor Richard K. Forster, MD, Bascom Palmer Eye Institute, Miller School of Medicine, University of Miami, Miami, Florida)

Corneal Abrasions

These defects in the corneal epithelium are caused by physical damage from foreign objects, including contact lens manipulation. They take the configuration of scrapes, scratches and patches of denuded epithelium.

Symptoms of corneal abrasions include pain associated with foreign body sensation, photophobia, blepharospasm, and a pink or red eye. Similar symptoms and signs also occur with corneal ulcers, corneal foreign bodies, open wounds, and serious internal ocular conditions – iritis (anterior uveitis) and acute glaucoma. Topical tetracaine does not relieve pain symptoms when used to treat internal ocular conditions however, and can therefore assist in differentiating these problems from surface conditions. Also the pain of internal ocular conditions is characteristically deep and in the vicinity of the eyebrow. This is helpful for suggesting diagnoses when a slit lamp is not available.

Defects in the corneal epithelium can be identified by staining with fluorescein dye and illuminating with a cobalt blue light (penlight with a blue filter attached) in a dark environment. Fluorescein dye may also be applied to the eye to assist in identifying other corneal disruptions – superficial punctuate keratitis (slit lamp required), ulcers and lacerations. Moisten a fluorescein paper strip slightly with a trace of antibiotic solution touched lightly to the edge of the strip and apply to the inner corner of the eye. Excess dye interferes with recognition of the stained defect and requires considerable tearing to dissipate. Blinking spreads the dye across the surface of the eye; when exposed to UV light in a dark environment, it renders a green tint to defects in the corneal surface epithelium. A compact binocular magnifying loupe or magnifying lens is helpful in identifying small abrasians and removing corneal foreign bodies.

To prevent most infections of the disrupted corneal surface, antibiotic drops such as ofloxacin 0.3% solution should be applied four times during the day and Bacitracin/polymyxin B ointment 500 units/g applied at bedtime. If infection occurs, the drops should be instilled every one to two hours while awake and the ointment applied at bedtime. To reduce pain associated with iritis, scopolamine 0.25% is applied twice daily; this cycloplegic medication relaxes ciliary and iris spasm and dilates the pupil. Non-steroidal diclofenac 0.1% is also helpful.

If the environment is clean and organic materials have not come in contact with the eye, a pressure patch may be applied; it has been determined that small corneal abrasions less than 10 square millimeters, heal faster and with less discomfort when treated without a pressure patch.[20] A pressure patch keeps the eyelids closed and prevents blinking; this moderates pain and enhances healing. Every day the patch is changed, the eye is examined, and medications repeated. On expeditions it is understood that the patient may not be able to tolerate wearing a patch because of important visual requirements.

If injury is caused by a soil or vegetation related item, or occurs in a likely contaminated environment (e.g., tropical rainforest), the pressure patch is avoided altogether in preference to frequent instillations of topical antibiotics. Pressure patches are conducive to fungal infections because of trapped body temperature and moisture, and limiting exposure of the eye to atmospheric oxygen.

Prior to applying a pressure patch scopolamine 0.25% drops, diclofenac 0.1% drops, and Bacitracin/polymyxin B ointment 500 units/g are applied to the eye. The pressure patch is composed of sterile eye pads and/or 2 × 2 inch gauze pads, if eye pads are not available. The first pad is placed against closed eyelids and the second pad is folded to fit within the eye socket over the first. Additional pads are then stacked exceeding the depth of the eye socket, to form an elevated dressing that can transfer reasonable pressure against the deeper pads and cornea. The skin, excluding eyebrows, is shaven prior to application; it should be clean and dry. If available, tincture of benzoin solution (avoid the eyelids and eyes) may be applied to the skin for better adhesion of the tape. About eight strips of one-inch wide times six to seven inches long tape usually applied obliquely, from the side of the cheekbone to the center area of the forehead; after anchoring over the cheekbone the tape is pulled toward the forehead, stretching the skin and applying indirect pressure to the underlying pads before attaching firmly to the skin. Complete recovery can usually be anticipated and the patient should be reassured.

The patch is removed daily for inspection and instillation of antibiotic and cycloplegic agents. It is then reapplied with fresh tape. Although improvement will usually be noticed in one to two days, the patch may have to remain in place longer to ensure more complete healing. Often, closing the fellow eye is required to assist in restricting eye and eyelid movements. If the abrasion and pain persist and the eye remains red, it should be examined for signs of infection and the pressure patch avoided.

Corneal and Conjunctival Foreign Bodies

When searching for ocular foreign bodies that are not readily evident on the exposed surfaces, the eyelids must be retracted away from the eye to allow examination of the complete surface of the cornea and sclera, as well as under the eyelids. A topical anesthetic drop, tetracaine, is useful to ameliorate blepharospasm – avoid excessive use.

Cotton-tipped applicators may be used to retract the eyelids (apply on the skin surface only). Clean fingers may be used for retraction if no applicators are available. The conjunctiva covering the exposed sclera of the eye (bulbar conjunctiva) often becomes inflamed in the vicinity of an irritating surface foreign body, offering a clue to its location.

In addition, the undersurface of the upper eyelid and the pocket (fornix) may be exposed by everting the eyelid upon itself. Carefully place the wooden end of a cotton applicator horizontally across the outer surface of the eyelid (toward the nose bridge) in the skin crease under the orbital rim (at the upper border of the tarsal plate) and maintain pressure gently inward and downward. With the other hand grasp the eyelashes at the eyelid margin and fold it upward over the applicator while pulling slightly outward; the stick firmly anchors the upper portion of the eyelid in place acting like a hinge while the semi-rigid tarsal plate is everted over it; the maneuver usually takes some practice.

A handheld light is used and foreign bodies are best detected by illuminating from different directions across the ocular and inner eyelid surfaces. Magnification may be required. Removal can often be accomplished by using irrigation. Conjunctival foreign bodies that are not readily irrigate free may be removed with a cotton-tipped applicator. Corneal foreign bodies that remain after irrigation may be embedded. Use of a moistened cotton-tipped applicator in an attempt to remove them usually results in an extensive corneal abrasion. It should only be attempted with great care. A magnifying lens is used to determine if the foreign body is loose or embedded (not always easy to determine). Remove excess cotton from the applicator and create a pointed brush-like flexible shape to the cotton, dampen the cotton with antibiotic solution, irrigate the cornea and gently brush off the foreign body. A moistened applicator is not as abrasive to the ocular surface as a dry one. If the foreign body does not readily respond it may be embedded.

Although extremely tiny particles are not always visible (i.e., glass, fiberglass, and sand) they may be removed by gently brushing a moistened cotton-tipped applicator across conjunctival surfaces, and especially the undersurface of the eyelid adjacent to the margin; take care not to touch the cornea. An occasional contact lens lost in the deep pocket (fornix) under the upper eyelid, can be identified and removed with an applicator utilizing this technique.

If a corneal foreign body is not easily removed, it is probably embedded in the superficial cornea. This usually requires the skilled steady hands of an ophthalmologist using a sharp instrument (foreign body spud, specialized small curette, or hypodermic needle) and stereoscopic magnification (loupe or slit lamp). The object is then scooped out. The procedure is not advised for a nonprofessional. In the field, the surgeon uses the point of a 19- to 22-gauge hypodermic needle attached to a 1 cc tuberculin syringe or short pencil to serve as a

stabilizing handle. This should only be attempted in a desperate situation. The process is easier after several days have passed and the immediately adjacent cornea has softened. With deeply embedded corneal foreign objects, especially in those instances where penetration into the anterior chamber is suspected, it is advisable to remove in a hospital. When ferrous metallic objects containing iron or its derivatives are removed they usually leave ring shaped rust deposits (rust rings); if small and not too painful they can be removed later by an ophthalmologist using a slit lamp microscope and a small curette or burr. Metallic foreign bodies often originate as sparks from a grind wheel and are therefore sterilized by heat before striking the eye. Foreign bodies are most painful when they protrude from the corneal surface and scratch against the upper eyelid. Ofloxacin 0.3% solution is instilled four times a day when foreign bodies remain. It is also applied four times a day for several days, after foreign objects have been removed. Bacitracin/polymyxin B ointment 500 units/g is applied inside the lower eyelid at bedtime.

Recurrent Corneal Erosion

Occasionally the corneal epithelium doesn't heal completely following a corneal abrasion and symptoms may recur many months or even years after the corneal defect was considered healed. The symptoms of these erosions are usually experienced upon waking from sleep. It is thought that during sleep there is adhesion between the inner surface of the eyelids and the damaged corneal epithelial cells; when the eyelids open upon waking, they pull these cells loose from the corneal epithelium. This causes the appearance of a fresh epithelial defect or abrasion and may exhibit the same symptoms as the original – red eye, foreign body sensation, increased tearing and photophobia. It is often a recurring problem regardless of therapies attempted. The clear cornea may appear normal unless examined with a slit lamp microscope and fluorescein dye during an actual episode. Hypertonic sodium chloride ointment or antibiotic ointments are applied at bedtime as a physical barrier to prevent adhesion of the eyelid to the corneal epithelium. It is thought that hypertonic ointment may benefit healing by reducing edema. Pressure patches and debridement are sometimes useful therapies in chronic cases.

Corneal Ulcers – Infectious Keratitis

Ulcers are defects in the corneal surface caused by invasion of microorganisms. Bacteria that normally reside without harm in the surface flora of the eye are considered pathogens when they invade through damaged corneal epithelium. Defects in this corneal barrier provide an opening to invading microorganisms; trauma and contact lens wear are a common source of such infection. *Staphylococcus aureus, Staphylococcus epidermidis*, corynebacteria, and streptococci, along with a variety of Gram-negative and anaerobic organisms are frequently found in the flora. In the expedition environment, in addition to bacteria, fungus and protozoa are frequent invaders difficult to identify and eradicate.

Corneal ulcers cause pain, photophobia, foreign body sensation, lacrimation, and blepharospasm. They can be recognized by the same techniques as used to identify corneal abrasions. The associated corneal inflammatory condition is keratitis, and secondary iritis is common; the surrounding cornea may become hazy with edema; large numbers of inflammatory cells, leukocytes, respond by chemical attraction to the cornea and form a visible white infiltrate. Ulcers can extend through the epithelium and Bowman's membrane into the corneal stroma where they become necrotic. (See Figure 36.8.) As a consequence of stromal involvement, permanent white scars, leucomas, result; vision is significantly impaired when the central cornea (optical axis) is involved. Ulcers can progress more deeply and penetrate into the anterior chamber by eroding through the final barriers of the cornea (Descemet's membrane and endothelium). Penetration can result in aqueous leakage, herniation of uveal tissue, and devastating endophthalmitis. In addition to bacteria, fungi and protozoa have this capability and are difficult to eradicate; if not rapidly controlled, the eye will be lost. Treat bacterial ulcers with ofloxacin 0.3% every 1–2 hours while awake and antibiotic ointment at bedtime. While topical and systemic antimicrobial therapy is instituted under field conditions, a progressing ulcer requires evacuation to properly identify and intensively treat the invading organism; special fortified antibiotic preparations are utilized.[5]

There is a higher than normal incidence of ocular fungus infections in the subtropics and tropics due to their increased prevalence and enhanced incubation secondary to elevated temperatures and humidity. Diagnosis may be confused with bacterial infections. Corneal infiltrates of *Aspergillus* and *Fusarium* usually have filamentous margins characteristic of many fungus infections. Unlike bacterial infections, fungus and protozoan infections are refractory to usual antibiotic and antiviral therapy; therefore, any serious ocular infection, if not improving within the first few days of antibiotic treatment, requires evacuation to the care of an ophthalmologist. Proper therapy of fungal and amoebic corneal ulcers requires identification through stained scrapings and cultures. Natamycin 5% solution instilled every 1–2 hours is recommended for the initial treatment of fungus corneal ulcers.[21]

Protozoa such as acanthamoeba are common inhabitants of fresh water and soil and therefore present a serious threat of ocular infection. It is important to be aware of the dangers associated with bathing in fresh water where contamination is possible. Appearance of the ulcers can be confused with herpetic keratitis because of irregular dendritic-like forms; acanthamoeba ulcers may be distinguished by subepithelial infiltrates and multiple noncontiguous patterns. Therapeutic agents are often unsuccessful, and penetrating keratoplasty is frequently necessary. Cysts in particular are difficult to eradicate. Recently, it has been recommended to treat these ulcers with chlorhexidine 0.02% or in combination with polyhexamethaline biguanide (PHMB) 0.02%.[22,23]

Dry Eye

For more on dry eye, see the following discussion in the "Acute Keratitis" section.

Endophthalmitis

Endophthalmitis is an infection within the eye; dominant symptoms are red eye, pain, increased lacrimation, blepharospasm, and progressive vision loss occurring shortly after an open wound injury. The protective walls of the eye, the cornea and sclera, normally resist internal infection from an exogenous source. Endophthalmitis usually results when a microorganism gains entry through an open wound; it may be introduced or inoculated into the eye by a foreign object or by an eroding surface infection such as a corneal ulcer. Foreign objects are prone to contamination by a variety of virulent pathogens frequently present in an organic environment. Endophthalmitis is one of the most serious and disastrous disorders of the eye; the eye's interior provides an excellent culture medium at a temperature conducive to infection. In addition, access to the entire vitreous cavity by antibiotics is limited because of the lack of the generous blood supply common to other organs. The

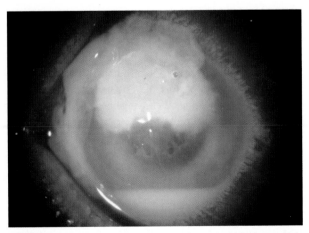

Figure 36.8. Corneal ulcer with hypopyon. Courtesy of Professor Richard K. Forster, MD, Bascom Palmer Eye Institute, Miller School of Medicine, University of Miami, Miami, Florida.

danger of endophthalmitis is a primary reason to expedite evacuation of any expedition member who has suffered an open wound of the eye. The infection is capable of rapidly destroying the eye (e.g., if evacuation of an open wound case is delayed, by the time endophthalmitis is recognized it is usually too late to salvage the eye). Initiate levofloxacin 500 mg tablets every 24 hours and continue during evacuation.

Adequate management and treatment of endophthalmitis is impossible during an expedition. Usual procedures for management include B-scan ultrasound, cultures, and sensitivities – aqueous and vitreous samples are tested, vitrectomy is performed, antimicrobial agents are injected directly into the vitreous and also administered intravenously and topically. Vancomycin and ceftazidime are drugs of choice in bacterial disease and amphotericin-B is commonly administered in fungal infections. Additional therapy consists of systemic corticosteroids, topical cycloplegic agents, and systemic medications to relieve pain.[24,25]

Surgically induced endophthalmitis and those cases caused by endogenous sources of infection are not considered relevant to expeditions. The endogenous form is most prevalent in debilitated patients, patients with septicemia, and drug users.

Episcleritis

Episcleritis is a relatively harmless inflammation limited to the surface and superficial layers of the sclera; it may be confined to only one segment; cases may demonstrate nodules. The symptoms are usually similar to corneal surface inflammations but are milder. Vision is usually not affected; photophobia is usually absent and, if present, suggests another diagnosis; episodes often recur. The condition is self-limited to several weeks and seldom requires therapy. The more severe condition of scleritis is chronic and rare; it is not addressed.

Acute Angle Closure Glaucoma

Acute angle closure glaucoma is not usually associated with special conditions of expeditions, but it may occur when the pupil dilates (secondary to blunt trauma or dilating drops) or along with hyphema. In certain predisposed individuals, dilating the pupil with eye drops causes iris tissue to jam into the peripheral angle of the anterior chamber, damming up the aqueous outflow channels (trabecular meshwork). Acute angle closure glaucoma can result in permanent damage to the optic nerve and retina resulting in blindness. In acute glaucoma, pain and blurred vision suddenly occur, the eye becomes red, and the affected pupil enlarges reacting poorly to light and accommodation. If a portable tonometer is available, the intraocular pressure can be

measured and will usually be elevated into a range of 30 to 60 mmHg. If a tonometer is not available, test the intraocular pressure by gently pressing the tips of your forefingers upon the corneas through closed eyelids and compare both eyes; the affected eye may feel relatively firm. In severe cases, the cornea may cloud over, and the pain will become intense; deep pain is usually perceived in the region of the eyebrow. Medical therapy may succeed in controlling the problem, but acute glaucoma usually represents an acute surgical emergency. Laser therapy or surgery is used to create an opening near the iris root, allowing trapped aqueous fluid to circumvent the obstruction and permit aqueous outflow. Although angle closure glaucoma is not common, pupils should not be dilated with drops during expeditions unless necessary.

Acute glaucoma therapy involves the following:

1. Pilocarpine 2% eye drops are instilled every 15–30 minutes for several hours in an attempt to constrict the pupil, lower the intraocular pressure, and possibly avoid evacuation.
2. Acetazolamide (Diamox) 500 mg should be given orally and 250 mg continued two to four times a day for several days if required. This therapy can compliment the effect of pilocarpine. (See precautions offered in the "Systemic Medications" section).
3. After approximately 1–2 hours, gentle pressure may be applied to the eye through closed eyelids (limit to several minutes); as the pressure is gradually increased, the globe may be noted to soften. Avoid if hyphema is present. Experience is advised.

All these measures are taken in an attempt to break the glaucoma attack and soften the globe. If no significant response is noted within 3–4 hours, accelerate evacuation; continue therapy during evacuation. If the intraocular pressure is successfully reduced, the drops should be continued four times daily to ensure pressure control during the expedition; Diamox therapy may be tapered off over several days.

Acetazolamide is a diuretic and depletes potassium; supplement with high-potassium foods (i.e., apricots, prunes, bananas, figs, dates, fish, orange juice, and tomato juice). Acetazolamide also causes a tingling sensation in the fingertips and toes and gives a metallic taste to carbonated beverages including beer. At high altitudes paresthesias can cause confusion with the diagnosis of acute mountain sickness.

Herpes Simplex Keratitis

This disease, a viral infection of the cornea, is a common cause of blindness. The virus remains dormant within neurons of the trigeminal (fifth cranial nerve) ganglion until it manifests itself with acute corneal ulceration.

In addition to supplying the face, these sensory nerves also supply the cornea. The condition has a tendency to recur and can be difficult to resolve. Corneal ulcers have a characteristic branching (dendritic) configuration visible with the slit lamp and fluorescein dye; the ulcers can also be recognized by using a magnifying lens and, in some cases, the unaided eye. Treat with vidarabine 3% ointment five times a day or acyclovir 3% ointment five times a day for 10 days.[26] These specialized medications are not included in routine medical supplies. Cycloplegics are used to relieve the discomfort of ciliary spasm; diclofenac 0.1% solution is instilled to relieve inflammation. Topical corticosteroids are contraindicated in treating acute herpes simplex keratitis.

Traumatic Hyphema

Traumatic hyphema is defined as blood in the anterior chamber of the eye secondary to injury. It often accompanies blunt trauma. Hyphema represents a serious emergency with possible disastrous consequences. The pupil is often dilated and does not constrict, as does the fellow pupil, upon exposure to light – traumatic mydriasis. This usually indicates that the force of trauma was sufficient to damage the pupillary sphincter muscle. Sometimes irreparable damage occurs, and the pupil remains permanently dilated. The patient remains sensitive to bright light, and vision is usually impaired. Dark blood is visible within the anterior chamber, either obscuring the colored iris entirely or in its lower portions; resolution depends upon absorption of the blood until it is no longer evident within the anterior chamber. Blood cells can be seen with the slit lamp when not visible to the naked eye. (See Figure 36.9.) The head should be upright during examination to allow blood to gravitate into the lower portion of the anterior chamber and expose the pupil. When the blood sinks to the bottom of the

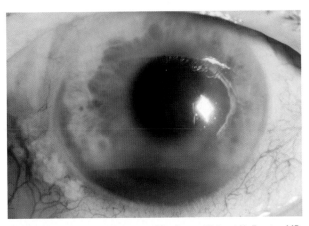

Figure 36.9. Hyphema. Courtesy of Professor Richard K. Forster, MD, Bascom Palmer Eye Institute, Miller School of Medicine, University of Miami, Miami, Florida.

anterior chamber, it creates a flattened surface (meniscus) across the top. It may be impossible to examine the vitreous cavity and retina because of blood cells obstructing the pupil. The same disorders that may be overlooked with orbital fractures – vitreous hemorrhages and retinal detachments frequently coexist with hyphema; monitor visual acuity and central vision. The degree of impaired vision should be consistent with the amount of clouding of the anterior chamber; if there is no additional damage to the eye, vision should improve as the blood absorbs; if not, further investigation is required. Caution is advised if dilating the pupil because it can cause rebleeding and also contribute to glaucoma. All cases should be evacuated. Chances of rebleeding are greatest during the first 10 days following onset.

Hyphema is frequently associated with elevated intraocular pressure (traumatic glaucoma), a dislocated or partially dislocated lens (subluxed), a posteriorly displaced iris, and additional internal ocular injuries. Glaucoma occurs when blood cells mechanically obstruct the outflow channels (trabecular meshwork) in the angle of the anterior chamber. Traumatic glaucoma may cause extreme pain and permanent damage to the optic nerve and retina if allowed to persist. Intraocular pressure should be evaluated with a tonometer and if over 22–25 mmHg, glaucoma should be suspected. High pressures can cause the cornea to cloud with edema. When glaucoma is suspected, measure intraocular pressure with a tonometer; treat as previously but avoid massage. If hyphema is associated with deep ocular pain, circumcorneal injection, a dilated pupil, and a cloudy cornea it is highly suggestive of acute glaucoma. This is a serious emergency. Treat as described in the "Acute Glaucoma" section and evacuate. Treatment must be continued during evacuation.

During evacuation, head and eyes should be moved as little as possible to prevent rebleeding common during the first 10 days. If possible, the head should be elevated at approximately 30° to 45° during bed rest and transport. If walking is necessary, every attempt should be made to avoid a bouncing gait or bending forward (e.g., food should be lifted to the mouth when eating and feet are raised to tie shoe laces); eyes should be moved as little as possible (they may be lightly patched if necessary), and reading should be avoided.

Iritis (Anterior Uveitis)

Iritis is an inflammation of the iris and usually includes the connecting ciliary body (iridocyclitis, anterior uveitis); the terms are commonly used interchangeably. Iritis occurs secondary to blunt trauma, open wounds, and other ocular inflammations and infections. The ciliary body connects with the choroid posteriorly. The choroid is the vascular tissue in the posterior segment of the eye sandwiched between the sclera and retina; when inflamed, the condition is defined as posterior uveitis and can damage the contiguous retina. All three tissues, iris, ciliary body, and choroid, are interconnected comprising the uveal tract. Clinically it is often difficult to delineate exactly where the inflammation process begins and ends. Iritis and cyclitis (anterior uveitis, iridocyclitis) is usually associated with brow pain, photophobia, and a miotic (constricted) pupil that reacts poorly to light and accommodation. A pink or red corona (ciliary injection or flush) surrounding the corneal limbus (junction of cornea and sclera) is usually evident. Miosis and ciliary injection indicate significant inflammation and warrant therapy. The classical office slit lamp sign of inflammatory cells dispersed in the aqueous humor is not helpful in diagnosis under field conditions. In severe cases of iridocyclitis, so many inflammatory cells may be present that they gravitate and layer out as a white mass in the bottom of the anterior chamber (hypopyon); this can be grossly visible without benefit of magnification. (See Figure 36.8.) Dilating the pupil and relaxing spasm of iris and ciliary muscles with mydriatic/cycloplegic drops, scopolamine 0.25% two times a day, moderates pain. It also assists in preventing inflammatory adhesions between the iris and lens (posterior synechiae) that can distort the pupil and ultimately inhibit pupillary mobility. Topical corticosteroid drops, prednisolone 1%, are instilled four times a day or more frequently depending upon severity of symptoms; they reduce inflammation and also assist in preventing posterior synechiae. If anterior uveitis is secondary to infection (e.g., corneal ulcer), it is problematic to treat with prednisolone (it can enhance the spread of infection); this decision is based upon the degree of inflammation and requires professional judgment.

Unless iridocyclitis is mild, evacuation is necessary; it is certainly necessary whenever hypopyon is recognized. During expeditions, iridocyclitis usually accompanies trauma to the eye or infection; it subsides after the primary problem is controlled.

Acute Keratitis

Acute keratitis denotes a sudden inflammation of the cornea. It is often secondary to other corneal problems such as corneal abrasions, dry eyes – inadequate tears (keratitis sicca), infections (ulcerative keratitis), irritants, and foreign bodies (including contact lenses). Chemical irritants, such as dive mask antifogging solutions, and exposure to high levels of solar ultraviolet radiation (snow blindness) is especially related to expeditions. (See following discussion in "High Altitudes" section). Under the slit lamp microscope, superficial punctuate keratitis (SPK) is evident as multiple scattered pinpoint epithelial defects; when caused by excessive UVB exposure, it is termed solar keratitis. Symptoms are similar to

those of corneal abrasions: red eye, blurred vision, pain, photophobia, foreign body sensation, compensatory reflex lacrimation, and blepharospasm. When severe, it may be accompanied by iritis with deep eyebrow pain, a miotic (constricted) pupil, and circumcorneal flush (injection). Causative agents must be avoided. Artificial tears, a cycloplegic such as scopolamine 0.25%, and a nonsteroidal antiinflammatory such as diclofenac 0.1% can be administered. Topical anesthetics like tetracaine are avoided because they delay healing. A pressure patch may be applied when infection is not suspected; if bacterial infection is suspected, topical antibiotics are applied. (See previous discussion in "Corneal Ulcer – Infectious Keratitis" section). Herpes simplex keratitis, a viral infection, requires special topical agents. (See preceding discussion in the "Herpes Simplex Keratitis" section.)

Pterygium

A pterygium is a fibrovascular growth on the cornea that originates from the adjacent conjunctiva at the corneal limbus. It usually has a triangular shape and may progress across the cornea until it encroaches upon the optical (pupillary) axis and interferes with vision. The progression takes many months to years. Pterygia involve only the exposed areas of the ocular surface between the open eyelids and usually occur on the nasal side of the cornea. They may remain quiet without significant inflammation or become acutely inflamed and red when exposed to ultraviolet radiation, wind, and wind-borne irritants (i.e., smoke). As with keratitis, artificial tears and diclofenac drops are used to reduce acute inflammation. In addition, proper sunglasses protect against excessive corneal drying as well as ultraviolet light exposure. Surgical excision is necessary when the optical axis is threatened; when inflammation becomes chronic, severe, and painful; or for cosmetic considerations. Recurrence is a problem in people predisposed to keloids, in dark-skinned people, and in chronically inflamed eyes.

The etiology of pterygiums and related measures of prevention are topics of interest. During an Amazon expedition in 2005, the author examined the eyes of numerous Indians of different tribes located on various upper tributaries of the Amazon River. No pterygia or red eyes were observed in the Matis Indians of Brazil (also called the Jaguar or Cat People); however, in Colombia, about 500 miles distant and living in a similar lifestyle, climate, and habitat, numerous Ticuna Indians displayed red eyes with markedly inflamed and advanced pterygia, many impinging upon the pupillary axis of the cornea; the two groups also displayed major differences in anatomical facial features. Although this is anecdotal evidence, it strongly suggests a genetic predisposition to the condition.

In New Guinea, indigenous people cook and sleep in huts with fires burning to avoid night chill and to repel insects (i.e., malaria mosquitoes). Chronic exposure to irritating smoke undoubtedly contributes to the numerous cases of pterygia observed, as well as prevalent chronic obstructive pulmonary disease.

Subconjunctival Hemorrhage

Occasionally small splinter and flame hemorrhages occur on the surface of the sclera. Although the hemorrhages are not dangerous they are of concern to many patients. They can enlarge by dissecting between the conjunctiva and sclera to form elevated hematomas (more prevalent in people taking aspirin or anticoagulants). Following injury, a large hematoma may mask a more serious underlying injury to the globe (e.g., a ruptured or lacerated globe may be concealed by the hemorrhage). Subconjunctival hemorrhages can result mechanically from incidental rubbing the eyes or accidental abrasions that break capillaries and also by physical straining, retching or coughing – probably caused by Valsalva-precipitated pressure surges within capillaries. The hemorrhages may be associated with the prolonged retching sometimes present in severe motion sickness and can occur when a diver pulls his dive mask from his face attempting to relieve a mask squeeze (barotrauma). No specific therapy is required for the hemorrhages.

Ocular Injury

Injuries to the eyes present a great challenge on expeditions. Diagnosis is often difficult, and therapy is limited. Most serious eye injuries require sophisticated ocular surgery with specialized operating microscopes, lasers, and microsurgical instrumentation. Most remote hospitals do not have these items or the eye surgeons required for their use. As previously described, sophisticated instruments are also necessary for exact diagnosis. Surgery is usually performed on an emergency or urgent basis; most significant trauma requires accelerated evacuation if vision is to be preserved. See Table 36.7.

Closed Globe Injuries

Blunt Trauma (Contusion and Concussion)

Contusion eye injury is caused by acute and forceful compression and traction distortions of the globe; it is possible there is no outwardly visible wound. Concussive injuries are the result of sudden jarring of the head with force transmitted through the eye causing damage to various internal tissues (e.g., whiplash and boxing injuries). See Tables 36.8 and 36.9 for classification of anterior and posterior segment injuries.

In the United States, blunt trauma causes the majority of eye injuries. In sports, most blunt trauma to the eye results directly from finger poking (basketball and

---

Table 36.7. Ocular injuries

Closed globe; blunt trauma (contusion, no wound entrance on the globe)
- Lamellar laceration (partial thickness wound)
- Superficial foreign body

Open globe
- Penetrating (entrance wound only), includes puncture wounds
- Laceration (sharp object is usually involved)
- Perforating (entrance and exit wounds caused by same object)
- Intraocular foreign body
- Ruptured globe (blunt trauma, full thickness opening)

Kuhn F, Morris R, Witherspoon CD, et al. A standardized classification of ocular trauma. *Ophthalmol.* 1996;103:240–3.

Table 36.8. Blunt trauma injuries, anterior segment[a]

- Corneal abrasion
- Corneal edema
- Iris tears
- Mydriasis (dilated pupil)
- Iritis (iridocyclytis)
- Dislocated or subluxed (partially displaced) lens
- Glaucoma, acute
- Hyphema

[a] See discussion in the "Acute Red Eye" section.

Table 36.9. Blunt trauma injuries, posterior segment

- Vitreous hemorrhage
- Choroidal rupture
- Retinal detachment, hemorrhage
- Maculopathy
- Ruptured globe
- Orbital fracture

---

football) and balls small enough to fit past the protective bony rim of the orbit – hand balls, racquet balls, and tennis balls. Larger objects can fracture the bony rim and gain access to the eye: fists, hockey sticks, hockey pucks, baseballs, and softballs. Any blunt object that strikes the eye with sufficient force during expeditions can cause serious contusion injuries to the globe.[28,29]

Eye injury caused by blunt trauma may result from the same trauma that causes orbital fractures and may be masked, or overlooked, by the more dominant symptoms of fractures (orbital pain, marked periorbital swelling, ecchymosis, hematomas, and bone displacement). Therefore, the eye must be carefully examined in all cases of suspected orbital fracture; ocular pain, blurred and/or double vision, and/or red eye, together with a history of trauma require careful evaluation. Emergency treatment of serious ocular injuries has a priority over fractures in making decisions for treatment and evacuation; however, it is frequently difficult to examine the eye due to poor exposure secondary to marked swelling of surrounding tissues.

Vitreous Hemorrhage

Traumatic vitreous hemorrhage is the presence of blood in the vitreous cavity caused by blunt or open eye injury. It causes cloudy vision that may fluctuate; blood clots are perceived as floaters (scotomata), shadows, and cobwebs. Bleeding usually originates from penetrating and lacerating wounds through the sclera and choroid, tears in retinal vessels, and globe ruptures. Recognition of retinal detachments and macular damage is often obscured. Recovery can take many months as blood slowly absorbs; rebleeding, hemosiderosis, permanent opacities, and fibrovascular proliferation with eventual retinal detachment can result. Diagnostic B-scan ultrasonography, CT scans, and MRI are not available in the field, and little treatment can be provided. Excessive head movement should be avoided. If visual acuity is low and blood obstructs a satisfactory view of the fundus, confrontation visual fields using a penlight (rather than fingers as targets) can be helpful in detecting a poorly responsive segment of the visual field, suggesting a retinal detachment, choroidal rupture, or macular pathology. Although useful, the test is not accurate because it is not possible to properly fixate and hold a steady gaze due to poor vision. However, light is a strong stimulus that can be seen through many vitreous hemorrhages. Evacuation is usually indicated – it is not possible to accurately diagnose the cause of bleeding or the extent of injury. However, improving vision over several days is a sign that the hemorrhage is clearing and may allow more accurate evaluation using the Amsler grid, confrontation field testing, and the ophthalmoscope.

Choroidal Rupture and Detachment

Bruch's membrane is a connective tissue layer that is fused between the retinal pigment epithelium and the choriocapillaris (vascular layer) of the choroid. Rupture occurs following blunt trauma when Bruch's membrane cannot stretch and distort sufficiently to contain the compression forces that develop within the globe; when it ruptures, the damage extends through the choroid and retina. This produces a white scar with pigmented margins that is usually oriented concentrically to the optic disc. Approximately 5–10% of people who have had blunt trauma injury to the eye develop choroidal rupture; the macula is damaged in 66% of the cases, and 80% are located temporal to the disc.[30] Blunt trauma damage to a choroidal vessel can produce choroidal hemorrhage; subretinal and vitreous hemorrhage often obscure a clear view of the problem. Most choroidal injuries can be monitored, and the decision to evacuate can be made according to visual status and field testing (as with vitreous hemorrhage). Management is similar to that of vitreous hemorrhage.

Retinal Detachment

Retinal detachments result from blunt or penetrating trauma to the eyes; they are more frequent in highly myopic eyes. In blunt trauma, retinal tears are often caused by sudden forceful traction placed upon the retina through vitreous attachments at foci along the vitreous base; retinal tears often lead to retinal detachments and may cause retinal hemorrhages if the tear involves retinal blood vessels. Retinal detachments can be suspected following trauma whenever the patient complains of a shadow, curtain, or blurred vision in a particular segment of the visual field; symptoms of photopsia (light flashes) and scotopsia (opaque spots) can precede or accompany retinal detachments. Sudden jarring of the vitreous during trauma produces traction at foci of attachment on the retina causing photopsia.

The area of involvement of retinal detachment can be identified by performing a confrontation visual field examination. Retinal detachments may be recognized by focusing within the peripheral vitreous cavity and varying direct ophthalmoscope lens positions to adjust levels of focus.

If dilating drops are not available, the retina may be searched in a dark environment using the ophthalmoscope with the light adjusted to a low illumination setting and a small circle of light; the technique requires experimentation and patience to find the most opportune combination of settings and usually requires some experience. It allows the pupil to dilate a sufficient amount to detect elevated retinal detachments. The detached retina will appear as a gray billowing or ballooning thin tissue mass, contrasting sharply with the characteristic orange color of adjacent attached retina. The elevated (balloonous) retina often jiggles upon movements of the head or eyes.

In February 2006, the author utilized this method to diagnose and evacuate a patient from a ship in the Pacific Ocean near Indonesia, to Hong Kong, China, for successful retinal surgery. However, low retinal detachments, especially those occurring in the far periphery, are difficult to recognize with the handheld direct ophthalmoscope. The diagnosis or strong suspicion of retinal detachment requires immobility with the patient remaining on his or her back and urgent evacuation. Bending forward is avoided. Excess movements of the head and eyes often result in the retinal detachment enlarging and detaching the macula. The macula is considered threatened when the nearby retina is detached; it represents a surgical emergency – evacuation is advised.

As long as the macula remains attached, central vision is preserved; the patient is able to read. Once detached, the macula rapidly loses its capability to function and vital central vision is lost (central scotoma). It is therefore especially important to avoid excess motion, including reading. Once the macula detaches, it should be reattached within 5–7 days in order to preserve critical central vision.[31] The macula can be threatened by a nearby enlarging retinal hematoma that can dissect into the area: Hemorrhages may also involve the macula directly, as a result of contusion injury.

Photopsia unrelated to trauma may occur as random light flashes associated with vitreous degenerative changes and traction. They may also appear as jagged arcs of flickering lights, usually originating centrally and expanding into the temporal visual field (scintillating scotoma) – symptoms of ocular migraine. Ocular migraine can be associated with temporary loss of central vision. The disorder can be followed by headache. Migraine is thought to be caused by vascular spasm followed by dilatation on the surface of the brain. On expeditions, symptoms can sometimes be caused by electrolyte imbalance associated with dehydration, exertion, and high altitudes. Certain foods – red wines, sharp cheeses, and chocolate – are thought to precipitate ocular migraine episodes. Typical ocular migraine episodes are self-limited to approximately 15–20 minutes and are not usually dangerous; episodes tend to recur. No therapy is required. Migraine symptoms originate in the brain, not in the retina.

Traumatic Maculopathy

Various forms of macular pathology can result from blunt trauma to the eye (e.g., hemorrhage, edema [central serous retinopathy], choroidal rupture, localized retinal detachment, and retinal holes); all demonstrate impaired central vision. (See previous discussion in the "Eye Examination" section.) Treatment may not be effective in changing the outcome of these conditions. The possibilities of threatened macular involvement (see earlier discussion) must be considered in making evacuation judgments. It is a more urgent problem to prevent macular involvement than to deal with it once it has occurred.

Orbital Fracture

Fractures of the orbital bones are usually determined by a history of forceful trauma to the orbital region plus swelling and ecchymosis (purple-blue discoloration secondary to bleeding into skin) of the eyelids and adjacent periorbital areas. In fractures of the orbital rim, palpation of the bones may elicit point tenderness and bone irregularity or displacement. Fractures may involve the rigid orbital rim directly or the more delicate bones that comprise the walls of the orbital sinuses indirectly (blowout fracture). When fracture is diagnosed, evacuation is usually required. This is especially true when the fracture is complex, bone fragments are displaced, or there is associated ocular injury.

Blowout Fracture

In a blowout fracture, the orbital rim is preserved but the orbital floor is fractured secondary to trauma directly upon the globe itself; thin bones of the orbital floor fracture and displace downward into the maxillary sinus through pressure instantly transmitted by compression of the globe and orbital contents within the confined space of the orbit. The eye may be sunken (enophthalmos) and motility limited; vision may be impaired due to eye injury, and double vision (diplopia) may be present – an indication that ocular muscles are injured or trapped in a blowout fracture. Diplopia and hypesthesia occur when the infraorbital nerve is damaged secondary to fracture of the orbital floor. Along with orbital fat and connective tissue, ocular muscles may herniate into the maxillary sinus and become trapped by displaced bone fragments; diplopia results.[32] Forced duction testing may be conducted: Tetracaine is applied to the inferior conjunctiva with a soaked cotton applicator; the tissue near the insertion of the inferior rectus muscle on the globe is broadly grasped at the six o'clock position with forceps and attempt is made to rotate the eye upward; when muscles are trapped, rotation is impaired. Diplopia may also result from hematomas within the ocular muscles secondary to orbital trauma in the absence of fracture; they resolve without treatment; without X-ray studies, they are difficult to differentiate from entrapped muscles.

Although orbital fractures usually present the dominant symptoms of orbital injury, always examine the eye for associated injuries. Near reading vision with glasses gives a rapid indication of possible ocular injuries. Eye injuries must have priority over fractures in evacuation decision making, although evacuation judgment must take all factors into account.

Open globe injuries (Table 36.10) are full-thickness wounds; usually identified by evaluating the proximate causative factors and examining the eye. All wounds in this category are serious emergencies that require immediate evacuation to professional care. The smallest wounds present a conduit for infectious organisms to invade the ocular interior; the invasion of these organisms can cause overwhelming internal infection (endophthalmitis) with rapid loss of the eye. In larger

Table 36.10. Open globe injuries, standard classification

- Penetrating
- Lacerating
- Perforating
- Foreign body
- Ruptured globe

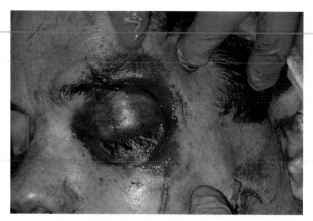

Figure 36.10. Ruptured globe caused by a golf ball. Edematous and ecchymotic eyelids. Courtesy of Adrian Lavina, MD, treating physician; Anita Agarwal, MD, Associate Professor of Ophthalmology, Vanderbilt Eye Institute, Nashville, Tennessee.

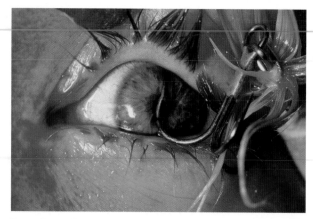

Figure 36.12. Fishing hook penetration, left cornea. It is taped to the forehead and a shield applied for transport to the ophthalmologist. Courtesy of Adrian Lavina, M.D., treating physician; Anita Agarwal, MD, Associate Professor of Ophthalmology, Vanderbilt Eye Institute, Nashville, Tennessee.

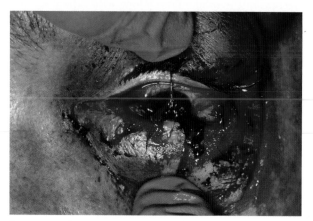

Figure 36.11. Ruptured globe caused by a golf ball. Eyelid and corneascleral laceration; uvea prolapsed on the eyelid. Courtesy of Adrian Lavina, M.D., treating physician; Anita Agarwal, M.D., Associate Professor of Ophthalmology, Vanderbilt Eye Institute, Nashville, Tennessee.

open globe injuries, the contents of the eye (fluid aqueous and/or gel vitreous and darker uveal eye tissues, even retina) may herniate from the wound; they can be observed externally extruding from the wound and lying upon the ocular surface (see Figures 36.10 and 36.11). The eye may lose its internal pressure and deflate or collapse, losing its characteristic globular shape (phthisis bulbi). Projectile injuries can be especially damaging causing both an open globe wound, as well as contusion injury from instantaneous pressure shock waves.

Penetrating Injuries

Penetrating injuries have a single entrance wound. (See Figure 36.12). The injuries are not always clearly evident under field conditions (e.g., a subconjunctival hematoma may obscure an open globe wound and certain sharply pointed objects can puncture/penetrate without leaving an obvious entrance opening). This is true of small puncture wounds (e.g., those caused by the end of a rigid

wire, sharply pointed thorns, fish hooks, or other similar items). Tiny puncture wounds may not leak and require no repair; however, they can cause internal hemorrhage and directly damage ocular structures (e.g., iris and lens). After injury into the anterior segment by a sharp object, a distorted or peaked pupil indicates iris damage or adhesion to the cornea at the point of injury; the iris may be trapped within the wound or prolapsed onto the ocular surface; the anterior chamber often collapses.

Most open globe injuries cannot be repaired without the assistance of an experienced eye surgeon and proper operating conditions. During expeditions, these injuries are true ocular emergencies. Proper care must be rapidly obtained; chance of salvage is dependent upon reaching proper professional care as rapidly as possible. Treat with levofloxacin 500 mg twice a day and give the patient a supply to continue therapy during evacuation. Apply bacitracin/polymyxin B ointment 500 units/g to the eye and eyelids. Lightly patch the eye. If available, narcotics may be administered (question the patient regarding previous sensitivity to narcotics with vomiting; retching can increase hemorrhage and cause additional extrusion of ocular contents).

Lacerating Injuries

Lacerating wounds can be either partial thickness (closed globe wounds) or full thickness penetrating wounds. Lacerating wounds are linear or jagged and usually caused by sharp objects. Ocular contents can herniate outward through the wounds; vitreous loss usually accompanies deep wounds – the globe may collapse.

Perforating Injuries

In perforating injuries, an object enters the globe at one position and exits at another, producing two wounds; the exit wound is usually in a posterior obscured location; ocular contents can extrude posteriorly; in addition to creating open wounds, the foreign object directly damages ocular tissues. Fortunately, this is a rare occurrence, and many ophthalmologists have never had occasion to treat such a case. If the object remains lodged in the eye, it must be removed by an eye surgeon. If this is not immediately possible, a long object is shortened, if possible, before evacuation to minimize additional damage to the eye. Stabilize close to the globe with a forceps, surgical clamp, hemostat, or vice-grip pliers, and break off (thin branch) or cut off as closely as possible. In order to avoid additional damage, an alternative with short objects is to tape the exposed portion firmly to the face; it must not be moved but supported if not lying directly upon the face.

Foreign Body, Intraocular

This category usually refers to a foreign object that remains contained within the globe (intraocular foreign body). When acquired on an expedition, it presents a serious danger of endophthalmitis (infection within the globe). Retained intraocular foreign bodies are removed surgically. Accelerated evacuation is vital.

Ruptured Globe

A sudden blunt impact compresses and distorts the globe creating elevated hydraulic pressures that exceed the elasticity of the scleral wall to expand. The globe cannot contain these extreme forces and bursts; contents extrude and the globe collapses. This is a major ocular disaster that is seldom salvageable. The emotional reaction can be extreme; if available, narcotics may be administered. Accelerated evacuation is required.

SPECIAL LOCATIONS

Underwater (SCUBA Diving)

Contact Lenses and Diving

Contact lenses may easily become displaced from the eye and lost in the underwater environment. A common problem is clearing the dive mask when flooded. (See following discussion in "Mask Squeeze" section.) Salt water is an irritant when it comes in contact with the surface of the eye; therefore, when it enters the mask, it causes stinging and tearing. A similar problem (with more intense pain) occurs when residual lens antifogging solutions (usually detergents) come in contact with the ocular surface; contact lenses may become displaced and lost. Pain and blepharospasm (forceful closing of the eyelids, a reflex to intense eye pain) may occur. During blepharospasm, reflex production of extra tears serves to dilute the irritant and lubricate the cornea, reducing the pain and discomfort; while the eyelids are temporarily closed, blepharospasm can prevent the contact lenses from drifting off the corneas. During this time, the mask may be cleared of water with the usual mask-clearing procedure.

After resurfacing, the diver should apply lens rewetting solution or artificial tears if necessary. Punctate corneal defects (superficial punctate keratitis) may remain causing pain and photophobia; this usually resolves by the next morning. Dry eyes are especially prone to marked symptoms from this exposure.

Disposable soft contact lenses are preferable to the extended wear variety because they are less susceptible to infections caused by marine microorganisms. Bubbles may collect under contact lenses, causing corneal dry spots with keratitis and corneal edema. This has been noted even with rigid gas permeable contact lenses. Hard lenses reduce the amount of oxygen supplied to the cornea causing corneal edema; they also trap bubbles. A 0.4-mm hole (fenestration) can be drilled through the apex to reduce this problem.[33]

Decompression Sickness

Decompression sickness (DCS), or arterial embolism, is characterized by nitrogen bubbles forming emboli within blood vessels at depth. In addition to many systemic complications, the emboli can cause various ocular problems depending upon which blood vessels are affected: retinal and subconjunctival hemorrhages, transient and permanent blindness, double vision (diplopia) secondary to extraocular muscle palsies, pain in the eye muscles, swelling and hemorrhages (ecchymosis) of the eyelids. There may be loss of a portion or one half of the visual field (hemianopsia). Nitrogen bubbles in cerebral vessels as well as ocular vessels can result in visual field loss, diplopia, and blindness. In addition, the bubbles may cause dizziness, paralysis, staggering, and convulsions. If emboli involve the spinal cord, loss of feeling and paralysis can occur. When emboli form in bones, joints, or muscles, pain may be experienced in these areas. In order to avoid DCS, adhere to diving guidelines for depth/time limits and ascent/decompression standards. Therapy is emergency oxygen breathing and recompression. It is wise to know the location of the nearest recompression facility beforehand and to have a plan for emergency evacuation.[34,35,36]

To avoid DCS, the diver should avoid flying over 8,000 feet in a nonpressurized aircraft for 12 hours after no-decompression dives and should wait 24 hours after decompression diving before flying in pressurized aircraft.[37]

Keratitis

Keratitis, or superficial punctate keratitis (SPK), is corneal inflammation secondary to the surface corneal defects discussed earlier. In diving it is usually the result of excessive residual amounts of antifogging solutions incompletely flushed from dive masks. These solutions are detergents (surfactants) that rapidly erode the corneal epithelium causing painful fine defects similar to those seen in snow blindness. Toothpaste is as an effective antifogging agent and not quite as irritating as commercial antifogging solutions; using a clean finger, it is vigorously smeared (it helps clean the faceplate) across the inner surface of the faceplate; it is then thoroughly flushed from the mask, leaving a thin film on the glass; excess gel may be removed by agitating with a clean finger with water and flushing. It is also comfortable and helpful for corneal protection to wear ultraviolet blocking sun glasses whenever on the surface. The combination of corneal contact with seawater and antifogging agents, plus exposure to ultraviolet radiation all contribute to painful keratitis.

Mask Squeeze, SCUBA Diving, and Barotraumas

Mask squeeze is not a common diving disorder but an understanding of the hydrodynamics and principles involved help in preventing and responding to problems associated with the unique underwater environment. The condition can usually be avoided when proper precautions are taken. It is associated chiefly with goggle-type masks that cover the nose but not the mouth. If the mask style includes the mouth in the mask space, the glottis would have to close to create the conditions required for mask squeeze.

The dive pressure regulator normally equalizes external water pressure with the air pressure within the respiratory system and the mask as the diver descends – the diver is able to blow through his nose into his mask to accomplish this equalization. Mask squeeze is associated with any condition that prevents this process by interrupting adequate air continuity between the upper respiratory passages and the dive mask. It results from obstruction of the nasal airways caused by any of several factors: a tight mask that pinches the nose closed, internal swelling of nasal tissues, and mucus plugging of nasal airways. The obstruction is precipitated by any of the following or combinations: poor mask fit, narrow nasal airways, upper respiratory infection, and seawater and allergic irritation/inflammation of nasal mucosa.

At sea level the total weight of a column of air one 1 by 1 inch is one atmosphere (ATM); it exerts a pressure of 14.7 pounds per square inch (14.7 PSI). As the diver descends, the mounting column of seawater adds this same weight, 14.7 PSI for every 33 feet of descent, increasing the ambient pressure upon the diver. Therefore at 33 feet, two atmospheres of pressure (the air column at 14.7 PSI plus the water column, 14.7 PSI = 29.4 PSI) surrounds the diver. The pressure within the dive mask is equalized with this ambient pressure by blowing through the nose.

In SCUBA diving, air pressure from the dive tank is distributed to the respiratory system through the pressure regulator and transmits air into the mask space at a pressure equal to the ambient water pressure – equalization. The air at sea level remains confined within the mask at 1 ATM (14.7 PSI); with descent the pressure increases above 1 ATM (through equalization) until a nasal obstruction occurs. The air confined within the mask space is then blocked from connecting with the respiratory system and therefore can no longer equalize with the external (ambient) water pressure; as a result, upon further descent, a relative difference in pressures between the mask space and surrounding water develops. The confined air within the mask space shrinks in volume and its pressure slightly increases as the mask compresses more tightly against the face – according to Boyle's laws of gas physics (this slightly counteracts but does not significantly negate the negative pressure differential).

Without proper equalization, the rubber mask flange continues to press against the face; the glass face plate presses inwardly with an added 14.7 PSI for every 33 feet of additional descent. This causes discomfort and pain. As long as the mask remains sealed against the face, the degree of compression (squeeze) is limited by the rigidity of the rubber flange against the face, and the mask against the nose. This is mask squeeze; a positive pressure of at least 1 ATM remains within the mask. Although a pressure differential exists, no true vacuum is created, as often described; however, a relative vacuum-like condition does exist. These mechanisms and conditions are commonly confused and distinctions should be properly understood to address associated problems.

During mask squeeze, it is possible that several factors affecting hydrodynamic pressure differentials act independently or together to cause facial barotraumas (subconjunctival hemorrhage, eyelid edema, chemosis, and ecchymosis) within the dive mask:

1. Hydrodynamic pressure differentials exist between the mask space and the water pressing upon the remainder of the body's surface; these differentials redistribute blood and tissue fluid from the body into blood vessels and lymphatic channels (engorgement, hemorrhages, and ecchymoses) and soft tissues (edema) within the mask. Body tissues are commonly considered to act as solids relative to air (gases) in response to underwater pressure differentials; however, these significant fluid shifts within the body are usually overlooked. (Fighter pilots use pressure suits that utilize this principle to counteract loss of consciousness from excessive (G) forces).
2. A Valsalva reflex can result from increasing intrathoracic pressure caused by straining to force expiration against blocked nasal airways.[38] Pressure surges within blood vessels may then cause barotrauma.

3. If the diver suddenly attempts to pull the compressed mask away from his or her face, against the opposing hydraulic pressure of the squeeze, the relative pressure differential is elevated; this may suddenly increase venous and capillary engorgement within the mask and lead to barotraumas. The diver should ascend to relieve the pressure of the dive mask pressing against the face, rather than attempt to pull off the mask at depth or strain excessively to force the nasal airway open.

Table 36.11. Medications that assist in the prevention of mask and ear squeeze

- Decongestant, topical: nasal spray, oxymetazoline HCl 0.5% – two sprays in each nostril every 12 hours
- Decongestant, systemic: Pseudophedrine HCl 60–120 mg every 4–6 hours
- Decongestant/antihistamine combination, systemic: Fexofenadine HCL 60 mg and pseudoephedrine HCL 120 mg extended-release tablets
- Nonsteroidal antiinflammatory drugs (NSAIDs)

Mask Leak

Mounting water pressure upon descent may force air to leak from the rubber mask seal as the rubber mask walls distort and collapse inwardly; seawater floods into the mask as it replaces the air. If the nose remains blocked, clearing the mask of seawater will not be possible; water remains in the mask and impairs vision. The diver must ascend and equalize.

Mask Squeeze Compared with Ear Squeeze

The same general mechanisms of relative unequal pressures that cause mask squeeze can cause ear squeeze. This occurs when blocked eustachian tubes (comparable to the blocked nasal passageways that cause mask squeeze) trap air within the inner ear cavities at 1 ATM (comparable to the space within the dive mask); therefore, equalization of pressure between air trapped within the inner ear cavities and the chest cavity is not possible. As ambient water pressure increases above 1 ATM with descent, the tympanic membrane (comparable to the glass plate and rubber wall of the face mask) squeezes inwardly and becomes traumatized (barotrauma); hemorrhage can occur behind the tympanic membrane (eardrum), and if the pressure differential becomes too great, the membrane can rupture. If cold water forces through the rupture, it can affect the ear's vestibular apparatus causing vertigo.

Mask Squeeze and Leak Prevention

To ensure a good mask seal and prevent leaks, it is best to store dive masks alone in small rigid containers; rubber dive mask flanges can become deformed and leak if not handled with gentle love and care. This occurs when rubber mask walls and flanges are compressed and folded in crammed dive bags for extended periods under the usual assortment of dive gear, including lead weights.

Various medications (Table 36.11) prevent the swelling of mucosal tissues and the accumulation of mucus that obstruct vital respiratory airways; these medications assist equalization of pressures within dive masks and also the clearing of ears and sinuses. If diving is prolonged, it is important to retake the medications before their effects fully dissipate or rebound congestion may occur. One particular medication may be preferred over another on the basis of an individual's experience. It is advised to check with one's personal physician before taking decongestants that may increase heart rate and elevate blood pressure and anti-inflammatory medications that can enhance bleeding.

Preexisting Eye Problems

Postoperative eye surgery with residual air or gas (e.g., certain retinal detachment procedures) is a contraindication to diving as long as the gas remains. Recent eye surgery should be completely healed before diving, and this is best judged by the surgeon; wounds that are not completely healed are subject to wound failure and to invasion by marine microorganisms. It is generally advised to delay diving several months after glaucoma filtering surgery.

Refractive Surgery

Radial keratopathy is no longer a preferred procedure for refractive surgery; the procedure involves almost full thickness radial corneal incisions – therefore, the corneal integrity is weakened and always presents a risk of late wound failure – especially if exposed to contusion injury. This is also true of penetrating keratoplasty, in which a full thickness corneal graft is sutured in place. However, to the author's knowledge, there are no reported cases of diving complications attributed to LASIK (laser in situ keratomileusis); it is recommended to wait 1 month after the procedure is performed before diving.

High Altitudes

Acute Mountain Sickness

The symptoms of acute mountain sickness (AMS) include various combinations of headache, fatigue, anorexia, nausea, vomiting, and dizziness. Symptoms are usually worse during the night. The onset of symptoms occurs upon ascent to high altitudes when low available oxygen (hypoxia) combines with low barometric pressure (hypobaria) to cause oxygen deprivation. High-altitude cerebral edema (HACE) with increased intracranial pressure can result. Oxygen, dexamethasone, and hyperbaric therapy are advised; descent is the treatment of choice.[39,40,41,42] High-altitude pulmonary edema (HAPE) also occurs, with shortness of breathe (dyspnea) at rest, pulmonary congestion (wheezing and rales), cough, weakness, elevated heart and respiration rates, and cyanosis. Noncardiogenic HAPE is the most common cause of high-altitude death. For emergency hyperbaric oxygen therapy, portable hyperbaric bags, Gamow or Chamberlite, are used; immediate descent is advised.[39,40,43,44]

Corneal Edema

The cornea is a clear tissue devoid of blood vessels; consequently, most of its oxygen supply is derived via diffusion from the air and adjacent scleral blood vessels. Anoxia, therefore, affects the cornea's contact lens tolerance at high altitudes. Vision may blur due to corneal swelling (edema) secondary to oxygen deprivation. Hyperosmolar agents (sodium chloride 5% solution and sodium chloride 5% ointment) may be used to assist in dehydrating and clearing edematous corneas; although they are of temporary value, the medications can restore vision long enough to allow descent. The edema will usually be temporary with full recovery of vision expected after return to lower altitudes and adequate oxygen. As a general rule, drops are instilled throughout the day, and longer-acting ointments are applied at bedtime to avoid daytime blurring.

High-Altitude Retinal Hemorrhage (HARH)

High-altitude retinal hemorrhage (HARH) is a common eye problem, although most individuals do not manifest visual symptoms. On Mt. Everest, McFadden et al. reported that 56% of climbers had retinal hemorrhages at an altitude of 5,630 m (13,917 feet).[45] They may be associated with high-altitude mountain sickness. Cortical blindness has also been reported and must be considered when vision is lost; treatment with hyperbaric recompression and oxygen is recommended.[46] Remaining at the same altitude does not seem to cause progression of hemorrhages, although additional ascent may increase hemorrhages and be dangerous to vision.[47,40,48]

Retinal changes noted at high altitudes are primarily related to blood flow compensation mechanisms in response to low levels of available oxygen. The fundus displays increased vascular engorgement and tortuosity, and the usually pale optic disc becomes hyperemic; the blood may thicken (vessels can obstruct from clots) due to increased numbers of red blood cells (polycythemia) and dehydration – for these reasons it is advised to maintain good hydration.[40,49,50] Factors such as altitude acclimatization, cardiovascular conditioning (exercise tolerance), lung capacity, the blood's oxygen-carrying capacity (red blood cells and hemoglobin), ambient temperatures, hydration, and amount of physical effort expended, may all influence oxygen availability to the retina.

Retinal splinter and blot-shaped hemorrhages and possible cotton-wool spots (infarcts) observed with the ophthalmoscope indicate occlusions in vascular branches affected by oxygen deprivation. Most individuals are not aware of acute visual loss secondary to these hemorrhages until they encroach upon the macula and involve central or paracentral vision (central or paracentral scotomata); in some cases, it is possible that glacier glasses with side shields interfere with the perception and awareness of peripheral visual field loss.

Although visual loss is not usually permanent, when central vision is involved or threatened it is wise to descend; it is possible that macular hemorrhage can enlarge and cause permanent damage to central or paracentral vision – permanent visual impairment has been reported.[51,52] When attempting to make judgments regarding evacuation or descent to a lower altitude, it is best to monitor the progression of retinal bleeding with the ophthalmoscope and/or special vision examinations, rather than relying entirely on the patient's subjective opinion regarding symptoms; adventurers with so much invested and with so much zeal to achieve mountain-climbing accomplishments, may not be completely objective about symptoms of visual impairment; awareness may also be compromised under conditions of oxygen deprivation. The Amsler grid test, confrontation visual field examination, pinhole test, and near visual acuity test described earlier (see the "Eye Examination" section) can be superb aids for rapidly judging central vision impairment. Confrontation visual fields may also help delineate extent of the impairment and whether the macula is threatened by a nearby hemorrhage. If patient cooperation is adequate, an examiner should take no longer than 10 minutes to complete the tests; the examinations can provide a valuable asset for critical decision making. Without assistance and in about one minute, the Amsler grid test and reading of small print can be accomplished daily by each climber to monitor status of critical central vision; these are the most practical visual examinations that can be done at high altitudes. When there is evidence that central vision is threatened or impaired, immediate descent is advised.

Snow Blindness (Solar Keratitis)

Special eye problems encountered at altitudes above 4,573 meters (15,000 feet) are associated with low oxygen levels, low ambient oxygen pressure, dry air, and increased exposure to ultraviolet radiation. Ultraviolet radiation increases 4% for every 300 meters increase in altitude.[53] The Sun is our natural source of ultraviolet radiation; the shortest wavelengths of solar radiation that reach the eye are the most damaging. (See Table 36.12.)

Table 36.12. Four wavelengths of UV radiation, from the shortest to the longest[54]

1. UVC (220–290 nm) is absorbed by the ozone layer of the atmosphere and therefore doesn't reach the eyes in any significant amount.
2. UVB (290–320 nm) can damage the cornea causing solar keratitis (snow blindness). UVB is required by our body for synthesis of vitamin D, but it also causes photochemical damage to cellular DNA; UVB radiation causes skin cancer and cataracts.
3. UVA (320–400 nm) is absorbed by the lens of the eye and as with UVB is thought to cause cataracts. It is also helpful in vitamin D synthesis.
4. Visible light (400–760 nm) is perceived as color and is responsible for the sensations of brightness and glare.

Solar keratitis is a common problem in high dry altitudes, in glaring snow of mountains (snow blindness), in deserts, at sea, and in any other environment where the eyes are exposed to high levels of UVB radiation. Damage to surface corneal epithelium may be due to direct and reflected UV radiation from the Sun. Reflected UV rays cause more damage than often recognized because they access the eyes underneath protective hat peaks and brims. Keratitis is usually identified as multiple dispersed pinpoint epithelial defects (SPK) when examined under the magnification of the slit lamp microscope and fluorescein dye; the defects appear in those areas of the cornea exposed between open eyelids. Dry air and wind enhance the epithelial damage. Corneal damage and symptoms are the same as the flash burns encountered by welders. In severe cases, secondary swelling (edema) of the cornea further reduces vision. The condition causes blurred vision; extreme pain usually manifests itself 8 to 10 hours after exposure. Patients should be reassured that the disorder is reversible and vision will return. Lubricating tear substitutes, cycloplegics–scopolamine 0.25% drops, topical antibiotics, and overnight pressure patching assist in relieving discomfort and promoting healing. Bacitracin/polymyxin B ointment 500 units/g is applied before patching as a precaution against infection and to guard against recurrent corneal erosions; infection is always possible whenever the protective corneal epithelium has been compromised.

Hats with brims or peaks and specialized glacier sunglasses, as discussed earlier, should be worn whenever possible as a barrier to excessive UV radiation exposure at high altitudes. The same precautions should be taken on cloudy days as are taken on bright sunny days because a significant amount of UVB radiation can penetrate clouds. Although UVA radiation is greatly blocked, cloudy conditions give a false perception that all the Sun's harmful UVB rays are also blocked. UVB radiation is harmful to the eyes because it damages DNA.[54,55] People with chronic dry eyes are predisposed to keratitis and should instill prophylactic artificial tears several times a day in addition to wearing appropriate sunglasses; goggles and glasses that fit close to the face retain moisture and reduce evaporation from the ocular surface. However, if not vented, they have a predisposition to fog over and must be occasionally pulled a short distance away from the face to allow adequate air exchange. As with dive masks, lens antifogging agents may be helpful. Polarized polycarbonate glasses with side panels or wraparound styles, are advised to give maximum protection against UV radiation. (See the preceding discussion of sunglasses.)

Tropical Environment

The unsanitary, septic conditions that commonly prevail in the tropics are due to high temperatures and humidity, combined with an abundance of pathogenic infectious organisms, including fungi and protozoa; contact lenses and wounds are frequently contaminated and diseases are readily transmitted in this environment. When hands cannot be safely washed with disinfectant soap and uncontaminated water, the transmission of infections can be reduced by cleaning the hands with one of the easily carried, 60–62% alcohol-based gel preparations or antiseptic/antibacterial paper wipes (containing 0.3% benzethonium chloride). Aside from the subject of eye care, this precaution should also be considered by anyone on expeditions in the tropics and mandatory with those involved in food preparation.

Parasitic ocular disorders are common to tropical habitats and may present with chronic systemic disorders that must be addressed after return from expeditions; acute parasitic ocular disorders can result directly from contamination of contact lenses (keratitis) or eye injury (See the previous discussions in the "Corneal Ulcer" and "Contact Lens Complications" sections). The diseases are endemic to certain geographical regions where they are acquired by the local people. They are transmitted by insect bites and contaminated soil, food, and drink. Diagnosis requires specialized laboratory testing and frequently includes biopsy. River blindness (ocnhocerchiasis), amebiasis, loiasis, Kala-azar (leishmaniasis), trichinosis, Chagas' disease (trypanosomiasis), and traucoma are examples of such diseases. Traucoma (chlamydia), are small bacteria that multiply within host cells.[17]

EVACUATION

- Philosophy
- Symptoms and signs that require evacuation
- Diagnoses that require evacuation

Philosophy

There are limitations in diagnosing and treating many ocular disorders; therefore, one of the most important and difficult decisions to be made on expeditions is whether or not to evacuate the injured individual and how to best manage the evacuation. When symptoms and signs indicate a serious problem, it is prudent to evacuate to the care of an ophthalmologist with access to customary diagnostic and treating assets. Inability to reach adequate medical care in a timely manner is one of the greatest risks associated with many expeditions; it is often not fully appreciated by those who accept the challenge and frequently presents a greater hazard than more publicized dramatic aspects of expeditions.

In hindsight it is understood that decisions to evacuate will not always be correct – it will be determined that the individual could have continued without significant harm. It is unrealistic to believe that under expedition conditions, one can sort through a complex differential diagnosis and make correct evacuation decisions 100% of the time. This is especially true without the benefit of medical office and hospital-based assets; even under the best of circumstances, certain eye conditions are difficult to diagnose and are considered interesting cases when presented at hospital grand rounds. The objectives and benefits of an expedition must be weighed against the risk of permanent visual impairment or sacrifice of an eye. In addition, when binocular vision or the visual field is compromised in a hazardous or unfamiliar environment, the explorer is at heightened risk for other injuries (i.e., trauma to the uninjured eye, bumping the head, tripping and falling).

Whenever there is reason for evacuation, required medications should be carried to sustain therapy throughout the evacuation process. In many cases, the evacuated individual must travel with a responsible team member.

Tables 36.13 and 36.14 provide outlines to expedite evacuation decision making following trauma to the eye and periorbital area; they do not anticipate every possible condition or situation. The outlines in general compliment one another.

Table 36.14. Diagnoses requiring evacuation

1. Open eye wound
2. Orbital cellulitis
3. Acute glaucoma
4. Corneal ulcer (infectious keratitis)
5. Iritis, significant
6. Subluxed and dislocated lens
7. Hyphema
8. Orbital fracture, complex or displaced
9. Vitreous hemorrhage
10. Retinal detachment
11. Maculopathy
12. Central artery or vein occlusion
13. Diplopia
14. Endophthalmitis
15. Amaurosis

LOCAL PEOPLE AND EYE CARE

In remote locations, the ophthalmologist is frequently called upon to provide eye care to tribal or indigenous people; many of these people have had no dental or medical care whatsoever; eye surgery, antibiotics, and eyeglasses are widely needed. The greatest problem in these situations is lack of adequate follow-up care and compliance in continuation of therapy (e.g., with people who have never kept time, it is doubtful that eyedrops will be applied four times a day on a regular schedule as instructed). Antibiotic ointments, used only once or twice daily, are therefore preferred over eyedrops for treating bacterial infections under these circumstances.

In addition to eye disease, respiratory infections are common and can be treated with systemic antibiotics. Unfortunately, it is difficult to remedy parasitic and fungus disease without eliminating poor hygiene and predisposing environmental conditions.

CONCLUSION

This discussion has been an attempt to assist with the prevention and care of certain common eye disorders encountered during expeditions. Guidelines have been discussed for expedient, first-aid eye care in remote areas and should not be understood as a substitute for professional or definitive care provided by a qualified ophthalmologist under controlled conditions. Injuries and circumstances vary widely; therefore suggestions herein must be tempered with good judgment and common sense.

Table 36.13. Symptoms and signs requiring evacuation

1. Vision is significantly impaired with or without apparent injury.
2. Vision impairment is protracted and/or progressive.
3. Vision impairment is associated with poorly controlled periocular or ocular pain.
4. Central vision is threatened, impaired, or lost.
5. Peripheral vision is significantly impaired.
6. An open wound is apparent.
7. Red eye is associated with persistent vision loss.
8. There is acute diplopia.
9. Pupil is irregular.
10. Pupil is dilated after head trauma; consciousness is diminished.

REFERENCES

1 Jayamanne DG, et al. The effectiveness of topical diclofenac in relieving discomfort following traumatic corneal abrasions. *Eye.* 1997;11:79.

2 Sutphin JE, et al. Amer Acad of Ophthalmol, External Disease and Cornea, Basic and Clinical Science Course, Section 8 (2006–7): 119.

3 Gerhard WC, et al. Foundation of Amer Acad of Ophthalmol, Fundamentals and Principals of Ophthalmology, Basic and Clinical Science Course, Section 2 (2001–2): 439.

4 O'Brien TP, Maguire MG, Fink NE, Alfonso E, McDonnell P. Efficacy of ofloxacin vs cefazolin and tobramycin in the therapy for bacterial keratitis. *Arch Ophthamol.* 1995;113(10): 1257–65.

5 Sutphin JE, et al. Amer Acad of Ophthalmol, External Disease and Cornea, Basic and Clinical Science Course, Section 8, (2006–7):181–3.

6 West S, et al. Sunlight poses universal risk of cataracts. *JAMA.* 1998;27(42); *http://www.jhu.edu/~gazette/julsep98/sep0898/ 08eyes.html.*

7 Lambert G. Glossary of optical terms St. Paul: Sunray Optical; 2006; *http://www.heavyglare.com/glossary.php.*

8 Sutphin JE, et al. Amer Acad of Ophthalmol, External Disease and Cornea, Basic and Clinical Science Course, Section 8 (2006–7): 179.

9 Alfonso E, et al. Ulcerative keratitis associated with contact lens wear. *Am J Ophthalmol.* 1986;101(4):429–33.

10 Butler FK. The eye at altitude. *Int Ophthalmol Clin.* 1999;39(59).

11 Sutphin JE, et al. Amer Acad Ophthalmol, External Disease and Cornea, Basic and Clinical Science Course, Section 8 (2006–7): 87, 168.

12 Sutphin JE, et al. Amer Acad of Ophthalmol, External Disease and the Cornea, Basic and Clinical Science Course, Section 8 (2006–7): 168.

13 Glasser JS. *Neuro-ophthalmol.* 2nd ed. Philadelphia: J. B. Lippincott Company; 1990: 450.

14 Glasser JS. *Neuro-ophthalmol.* 2nd ed. Philadelphia: J. B. Lippincott Company; 1990: 138–40.

15 MacCumber MW. *Management of Ocular Injuries and Emergencies.* Philadelphia: Lippincott–Raven; 1998; 121–3.

16 Glasser JS. *Neuro-ophthalmol.* 2nd ed. Philadelphia: J. B. Lippincott Company; 1990: 384.

17 Mahmoud AF. *Tropical and Geographical Medicine.* 2nd ed. New York: McGraw-Hill; 1993:42–60.

18 Meyer K. *How to S— in the Woods.* Berkley, Calif: Ten Speed Press; 1989: 20.

19 Samburskry R, et al. The RPD adeno detector for diagnosing adenoviral conjunctivitis. *Ophthalmol.* 2006;10: 1758–64.

20 Kaiser PK, the Corneal Abrasion Patching Study Group. A comparison of pressure patching versus no patching for corneal abrasions due to trauma or foreign body removal. *Ophthalmol.* 1995;102:1936.

21 Naradzay JFX. Corneal ulceration and ulcerative keratitis. *eMedicine.* 2006. *http://www.emedicine.com/emerg/topic115. htm.*

22 MacCumber MW. *Management of Ocular Injuries and Emergencies.* Philadelphia: Lippincott–Raven; 1998: 203.

23 Sutphin JE, et al. Amer Acad of Ophthalmol, External Disease and the Cornea, Basic and Clinical Science Course, Section 8 (2006–7): 187–9.

24 Brinton GS, Topping TM, Hyndiuk RA, Aaberg TM, Reeser FH, Abrams GW. Posttraumatic endophthalmitis. *Arch Ophthalmol.* 1984;102:547.

25 MacCumber MW. *Management of Ocular Injuries and Emergencies.* Philadelphia: Lippincott–Raven; 1998: 279–81.

26 Sutphin JE, et al. Amer Acad of Ophthalmol, External Disease and the Cornea, Basic and Clinical Science Course, Section 8 (2006–7): 141–2. Standardized classification of ocular injury.

27 Kuhn F, Morris R, Witherspoon CD, et al. A standardized classification of ocular trauma. *Ophthalmol.* 1996;103:240–3.

28 Rodreguez JO, Lavina AM, Agarval A. Prevention and treatment of common eye injuries in sports. *Am Fam Physician.* 2003;(67):1481–8, 1494–6.

29 Vinger PF. The eye and sports medicine. In: Tasman WJ, ed. *Duane's Clinical Ophthalmology.* Philadelphia: Lippincott–Raven Publishers; 1994.

30 Lihteh W. Choroidal rupture. *eMedicine.* 2005. *http://www. emedicine.com/oph/topics533.htm.*

31 MacCumber MW. *Management of Ocular Injuries and Emergencies.* Philadelphia: Lippincott–Raven; 1998: 87.

32 MacCumber MW. *Management of Ocular Injuries and Emergencies.* Philadelphia: Lippincott–Raven; 1998: 110.

33 Brown MS, Siegel IM. Cornea-contact lens interaction in the aquatic environment. *CLAO J.* 1997;23(4) 237–42.

34 Butler FK. Diving and hyperbaric ophthalmology. *Surg Ophthalmol.* 1995;(39):347–66.

35 Jeppesen S, ed. *Open Water Sport Diving Manual.* 4th ed. Englewood, Colo: Jeppesen Saunderson; 1984: part 2, 34, 41–8.

36 Rutkowski D. *Diving Accident Manual.* 3rd ed. Miami: Dick Rutkowski; 1985: 2–15.

37 Jeppesen S, ed. *Open Water Sport Diving Manual.* 4th ed. Englewood: Jeppesen Saunderson; 1984: part 2, 48.

38 MacCumber MW. *Management of Ocular Injuries and Emergencies.* Philadelphia: Lippincott–Raven; 1998: 321.

39 Dietz T. The Lake Louise consensus on the definition of altitude illness. Himalayan Rescue Association, Nepal. Available at: *http//www.gorge.net/hra/us/AMS-Lake Louise.html.* Accessed November 11, 1997.

40 Harris MD, Terrio MC, Miser MD, Yetter III MC. High-altitude medicine. *Amer Fam Physician.* 1998;57(8); *http://www. aafp.org?afp/980415ap/harris.html.*

41 Roach RC, Loeppky JA, Icenogle MV. Acute mountain sickness: increased severity during simulated altitude compared with normobaric hypoxia. *J Appl Physiol.* 1996;15:191.

42 Tom PA, Garmel GB, Auerbach PS. Environment-dependant sports emergencies. *Med Clin North Am.* 1994;78:305–25.

43 Hultgren HN. High-altitude pulmonary edema: current concepts. *Annu Rev Med.* 1996;47:267–84.

44 Shimada H, Morita T, Saito S. Immediate application of hyperbaric oxygen therapy using a newly devised transportable chamber. *Am J Emerg Med.* 1996;14:412–15.

45 McFadden DM, et al. High altitude retinopathy. *JAMA.* 1981;245:581.

46 Hackett H. Cortical blindness in high altitude climbers and trekkers: a report on six cases (abstract). In: Sutton JR, Houston CS, Coates G, eds. *Hypoxia and Cold.* New York: Praeger; 1987.

47 Butler FK. The eye at altitude. *Int Ophthalmol Clin.* 1999; 39:50.

48 Lang GE, Kuba GB. High altitude retinopathy. *Am J Ophthalmol.* 1997; 123:418–20.

49 Rennie D, Morrissey J. Retinal changes in Himalayan climbers. *Arch Ophthalmol.* 1975;93(6); *http//archopht.*

ama-assn.org/cgi/content/abstract/93/6/395 http://www.aafp. org?afp/980415ap/harris.html.

50 Wielochowski A. Medical aspects of high altitude moun- taineering, Andrew Wielochowski, The Kilimanjaro Map and Guide, 13/04/02. *http//www.ewpnet.com/OEDEMAS. HTM.*

51 Shults WT, Swan KC. High altitude retinopathy in mountain climbers. *Arch Ophthalmol.* 1997;93(6).

52 Weidman M. High altitude retinal hemorrhages: a classifica- tion. In: Henkind P, ed. *Acta XXIV International Congress of Ophthalmology.* Philadelphia: J. B. Lippincott; 1990.

53 Zafren K, Honigman B. High-altitude medicine. *Emerg Med Clin North Am.* 1997;15:191–222.

54 Zeman G. Ultraviolet radiation. Health Physics Soci- ety. 2006. *http://www.hps.org/hpspublications/articles/uv. html.*

55 Sutherland BM. Ultraviolet radiation hazards to humans. In: Hardy K, Meltz M, Glickman R, eds. *Nonionizing Radiation: An Overview of the Physics and Biology.* Madison: Medical Physics Publishing; 1997.

INTRODUCTION

Common oral and dental emergencies encountered on field research expeditions and explorations in remote areas will be discussed in this section. Examples include fractured or broken teeth and jaws; tooth, jaw, and mouth trauma; loose, broken, or missing fillings; dislodged or fractured crowns or bridges; cracked or broken partial or full dentures; dislodged orthodontic brackets and wires; gum abscesses; tooth nerve inflammation; and other acute dental and oral swellings. The reader will learn how to recognize certain dental and oral conditions and treat them temporarily. A list of instruments and medications will be included as guides for the expedition dental emergency kit. Options for the kit are included and are based on risk in the field and treatment capability. Duration of the expedition, number of team members, and weight of supplies will also determine the size and weight of the dental kit.

PREPARATION

How do expedition team members prepare for the dental emergency? Roald Amundsen's notes from the Norwegian Antarctic Expedition of 1910–12 give some insight into the training that helped prepare that expedition for such an event. [1]

Lieutenant Gjertsen, who had a pronounced aptitude both for drawing teeth and amputating legs, went through a "lightning course" at the hospital and the dental hospital. He clearly showed that much may be learnt in a short time by giving one's mind to it. With surprising rapidity and apparent confidence, Lieutenant Gjertsen disposed of the most complicated cases – whether invariably to the patient's advantage is another question, which I shall leave undecided. He drew teeth with a dexterity that strongly reminded one of the conjurer's art; one moment he showed an empty pair of forceps, the next there was a big molar in their grip. The yells one heard while the operation was in progress seemed to indicate that it was not entirely painless.

Still, even with preparation, the unexpected situation can arise. Physician, Everest climber, and extreme medicine pioneer, Dr. Kenneth Kamler describes this incident:

Sometimes there are lines of people who wait for my treatment in Nepal. One lady had waited in line for over two hours and came to me with a sore tooth. She held her jaw in desperation and I gave her some anesthetic and told her to wait for awhile while the anesthetic set in and I could start some other treatments. When I saw her again and was ready to extract her infected tooth, she told me it was "cured." I told her, "No, it will come back after the medicine wears off." She went off convinced that I had cured her and would never let me remove the tooth.

The single most important factor in avoiding dental emergencies on expedition is the preventive care planned before departure to the field site. Each member of the expedition team should have a complete and recent dental examination including dental radiographs at least 3 months in advance of the departure date. Expeditions lasting more than 3 months should allow participants a 6-month period for any necessary treatment that may be recommended. This allows sufficient time for any needed treatment to be completed before departure. The recommended form shown in the following section should be completed, signed and submitted to the expedition leader or appointed medical resource team member.

All of the training and treatments that follow are secondary to the preparation that should be completed prior to the departure date. Even with preventive measures taken, programs like NASA document their astronauts on the Apollo missions as having 1 in 9,000 man-days lost because of a disabling dental emergency and 1 in 1,500 man-days lost from significant discomfort. [2] Thus, it may be difficult to monitor preventive care in some instances. Risk factors are hard to measure for every situation, but they are certainly multiplied when given members of the team have not been screened before departure.

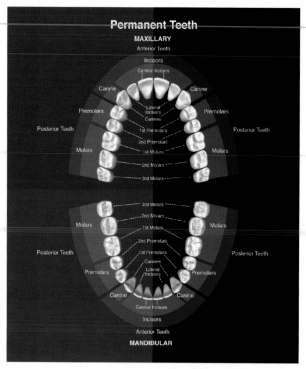

Figure 37.1. Tooth nomenclature and position.

Even with the best preventative care for expedition participants, other dental emergencies may arise with members of the team who join closer to the departure site (e.g., sherpas, guides, and indigenous peoples living in remote regions). Customs such as betel nut chewing practiced by people in India, Southeast Asia, and some parts of Africa may affect some treatment outcomes. Often, individuals with medical and dental backgrounds want or try to assist those in need who may live in the area of the expedition. Additional equipment can be brought for this purpose as often these resources may be the only way for some indigenous peoples to get medical care. Their gratitude may be a priceless reminder of the value of such actions.

DESIGNATING A MEDICAL AND DENTAL RESOURCE PERSON

Someone should be designated to collect and organize medical and dental history background before departing on the expedition. That person should also be responsible for treatment of possible injuries and follow-up care

Anatomy of a Tooth

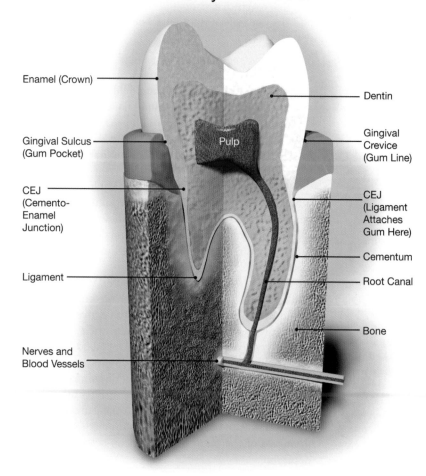

Figure 37.2. Anatomy of a tooth.

that may be needed. In the absence of a person with medical or dental background, the designated person should at least be familiar with basic emergency care covered here.

KNOW YOUR TEAM MEMBERS

Part of the preparation includes documenting health history background that may influence emergency treatment. Do any members have antibiotic allergies? How about reactions to local anesthetics? Are there any medical conditions like prosthetic joints or valves, heart disease, diabetes, hypertension, or other conditions that may influence the risks of treatment? This can be coordinated with a general medical history, but it should include the questions that follow.

DENTAL HISTORY FORM

Date: _____

Name: _____

      Last   First   Middle

Home: (   ) _____ - _____

Business/Cell Phone: (   ) _____ - _____

Address: _____

City: _____ State _____

ZIP: _____

Emergency Contact: _____

Relationship: _____

Phone: (   ) _____ - _____

Dental Information: *For the following questions, please circle your responses.*

Do your gums bleed when you brush or floss?   Yes   No   DNK

Are your teeth sensitive to cold, hot, sweets, or pressure?   Yes   No   DNK

Does food or floss catch between your teeth?   Yes   No   DNK

Do your upper front teeth protrude abnormally?   Yes   No   DNK

Is your mouth dry?   Yes   No   DNK

Have you had any periodontal (gum) treatments?   Yes   No   DNK

Have you ever had orthodontic (braces) treatment?   Yes   No   DNK

Have you had any problems associated with previous dental treatment?   Yes   No   DNK

Are you currently experiencing dental pain or discomfort?   Yes   No   DNK

Do you have earaches or neck pains?   Yes   No   DNK

Do you have any clicking, popping or discomfort in the jaw?   Yes   No   DNK

Do you clench or grind your teeth?   Yes   No   DNK

Do you have sores or ulcers in your mouth?   Yes   No   DNK

Do you wear dentures or partials?   Yes   No   DNK

If yes, has any section broken within the last year? Specify. _____

_____

Have you ever had a serious injury to your head or mouth?   Yes   No   DNK

Do your lips touch, or nearly touch when your mouth is closed?   Yes   No   DNK

Do you use your teeth as functional tools opening wrappers or cutting thin line or thread?   Yes   No   DNK

Date of last dental X-rays?

_____

Date of your last dental exam?

_____

What was done at that time?

_____

Allergies: *Are you allergic to or have you had a reaction to:*

To all **yes** responses, specify type of reaction.

Local anesthetics   Yes   No   DNK

_____

Penicillin or other antibiotics   Yes   No   DNK

_____

Barbiturates, sedatives, or sleeping pills   Yes   No   DNK

_____

Sulfa drugs   Yes   No   DNK

_____

Codeine or other narcotics   Yes   No   DNK

_____

Metals   Yes   No   DNK

_____

Latex   Yes   No   DNK

_____

Iodine   Yes   No   DNK

_____

Hay fever/seasonal   Yes   No   DNK

_____

Animals	Yes	No	DNK
Food	Yes	No	DNK
Other	Yes	No	DNK

Has a physician or previous dentist recommended that you take antibiotics prior to your dental treatment?

Yes   No   DNK

Name of physician or dentist making recommendation

_____

Phone: (   ) _____ - _____

Do you have any disease, condition, or problem not listed above that you think I should know about?

Yes   No   DNK

Please explain. _____

_____

_____

Have a dentist sign a statement 3–6 months before expedition departure that reads as follows:

As of _____ (date), I certify that _____

_____ (name) is in good oral health. There is currently no active treatment required or needed and minimal risk associated with this patient for dental problems that might occur in a remote area.

_____

_____ (treating dentist)

Depending on the length of field work, possible problems or risks include: _____

_____

_____

PREVENTION ON THE EXPEDITION

Avoid placing yourself at risk for tooth problems by staying away from hard, chewy foods including indigenous delicacies that may challenge the strength of your teeth. Likewise try to avoid using your teeth as instruments for opening packages, untying knots in rope, cutting fishing line, or holding hard objects. The more you ask your teeth to do, the more risk they take.

There are also predisposing factors that place certain individuals at risk. Questions included in the dental health history will identify such people. "Do your front teeth protrude abnormally?" "Do your lips have trouble meeting when your jaw is closed?" Yes to these questions identifies people who are more likely to have dental injuries.[3–10] Prevention on expedition is especially important for these people.

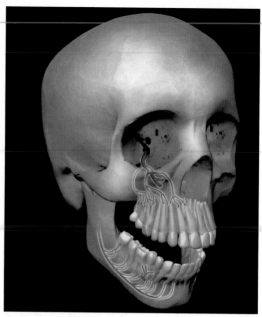

Figure 37.3. General anatomy of nerves in the head, anterior view. In the upper jaw is pictured the maxillary nerve branching into the posterior, middle, and anterior superior alveolar nerves, innervating the molar, bicuspid, and anterior teeth. In the lower jaw is pictured the inferior alveolar nerve with the mental foramen and associated nerves that innervate the lower teeth.

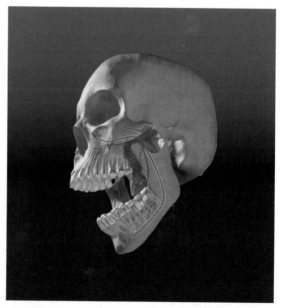

Figure 37.4. General anatomy of the nerves in the head, lateral view. Located in the upper jaw and in the most posterior region is the trigeminal ganglion, a connecting point for nerve pathways of the trigeminal or fifth cranial nerve, including the ophthalmic branch to the eye, maxillary division to the upper teeth, mandibular division to the lower teeth, and long buccal nerve located above the mandibular nerve which innervates the surrounding gums of the lower teeth.

TRAUMATIC INJURIES TO TEETH AND THE ORAL REGION

Oral Mucosa and the Skin

Lip and oral region lacerations often involve the impact of a foreign object to the mouth or a blunt force that forces the teeth into the lips and surrounding oral tissue. Because this is a highly vascularized region[1] seldom does one need to worry about serious tissue reactions. However, one needs to be thorough about cleaning such areas.[11,12] For lacerations extending to the vermilion border, one should suture the area by the skin border first and then use interrupted sutures for the remaining closure.

If there is blunt trauma to the mouth with no noticeable breaks or fractures in the teeth, one should check to see if the area affected has loose or painful teeth. These areas can be diagnosed by lightly tapping on the affected teeth with the blunt end of a dental mirror. Areas of external tissue damage or trauma should be treated with ice, if available, for the first 24 hours, altering 20 minutes on and 20 minutes off.[13] A soft diet and plenty of liquids will keep any pressure off these affected tissue areas until healing takes place.

If lip or cheek laceration is associated with tooth fractures, one must be sure to clean out the laceration, removing any foreign debris and tooth fragments that may have become lodged in the tissue. Such injury can often occur when a hard object strikes the mouth forcing the tooth into the lip region. Clean the affected area with an antiseptic-soaked gauze and irrigate with purified water. Tooth fragments can become embedded in the tissue and are often difficult to detect by palpation.[14,15] Such fragments can eventually cause fibrosis,[18] so an X-ray should be taken at the first opportunity. Oral tissue lacerations are almost always associated with some contamination and foreign body penetration. Thus, individuals affected, should be given 1.2 g penicillin at once followed by 1.2 grams twice a day for 2 days.[19–21] If the lesion is on the gum tissue, tongue, or lips and is extensive or deep, one should place sutures to close the wound after a complete cleansing of the area. Only use external sutures and none that are buried. As a general rule on expedition, use a 7-day resorptive suture material. For experienced doctors on expedition, silk suture material will be ideal as there is less tissue reaction associated with this material.[16,17]

Ideally, in an office setting, traumatic lesions associated with fractured and loose teeth are treated by splinting the teeth together and repairing exposed fractured areas. Because this is not possible in field conditions, one must be sure to keep pressure off these areas by limitations in diet. Extreme temperatures should also be avoided, especially to exposed areas of fractured teeth. Lukewarm liquids and pureed or soft solids are most easily tolerated in such conditions.

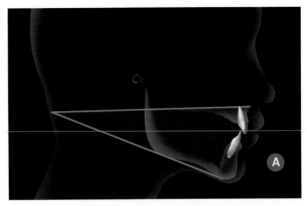

Figure 37.5. Normal bite relationship.

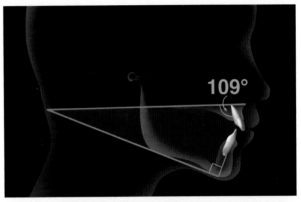

Figure 37.6. Protrusive overbite relationship.

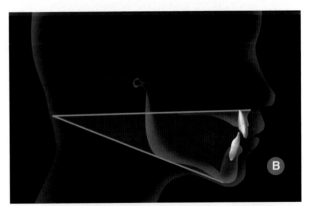

Figure 37.7. Overbite relationship.

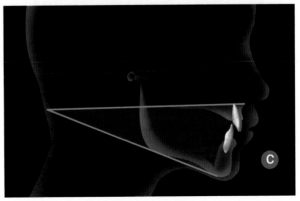

Figure 37.8. Deep overbite with some overjet relationship.

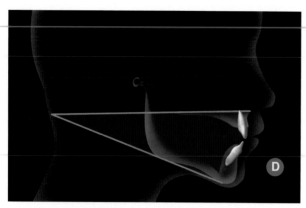

Figure 37.9. Anterior open bite relationship.

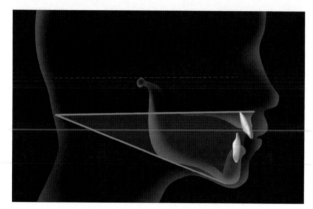

Figure 37.10. Deep overjet and overbite relationship.

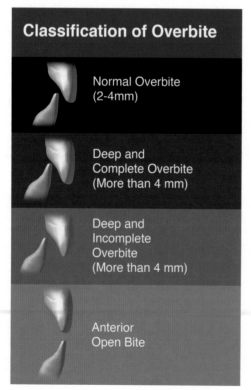

Classification of Overbite

Normal Overbite
(2-4mm)

Deep and
Complete Overbite
(More than 4 mm)

Deep and
Incomplete
Overbite
(More than 4 mm)

Anterior
Open Bite

Figure 37.11. Variability in bite relationships.

FIELD EXAMINATION AFTER A TRAUMATIC INJURY

What to Do

1. Note when and how the injury took place.
2. Was the trauma associated with loss of consciousness, vomiting, or headache?
3. Are the associated teeth sensitive? Does temperature change, either ice or heat, stimulate pain? Are the teeth painful without any stimulus?
4. Do the affected teeth hurt when chewing or applying light pressure? Do they hurt with finger pressure either around the neck of the tooth or below where the root extends?
5. Has the bite changed and have any of the teeth moved? Often lacerations are associated with tooth movement. If the gum tissue immediately surrounding the neck of the erupted tooth bleeds easily, even though it is not directly associated with the laceration, then trauma and some movement to the tooth has occurred.
6. Are any teeth broken and is there any coloration change, particularly dark red to blue, to the surrounding tissue, which may be evidence of a subdermal hematoma resulting from underlying bone trauma?

FRACTURING OR BREAKING A PORTION OF TOOTH

Dental injuries are dependent on three variables; the degree of impact, the direction of impact, and the ability of the surrounding tooth structures to withstand the impact.

Most tooth fractures involve the upper anterior teeth, specifically the front two teeth or maxillary central incisors.

Tooth fractures may occur with biting or chewing trauma, direct impact with an object, or indirect impact with a blow or fall to an area of the mouth. Breaks can also occur with seemingly no traumatic event. Such incidents happen because a stress fracture already exists from a prior traumatic event (Figures 37.12 through 37.14). Once the piece is dislodged, there may be some sensitivity to temperature or air and sweet foods. The edge of the remaining tooth's also may be sharp or bothersome to the tongue or cheek depending upon the area where the break occurred. Usually the piece is small, one-quarter to one-third of the tooth's total area. In these cases, a temporary filling can be placed directly on the missing or fractured area or it can be left alone if there is no discomfort.

There are three broad categories of crown (portion of tooth above the gumline) fractures.

1. Those involving small chips of just the enamel or outer tooth layer (Figure 37.15)[16]
2. Those involving fractures of enamel and dentin combined (Figure 37.16)[17,19]
3. Those involving enamel and dentin and pulp exposure (Figure 37.17)[18,20]

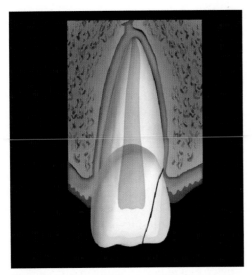

Figure 37.12. Stress fracture in dentin with retained piece.

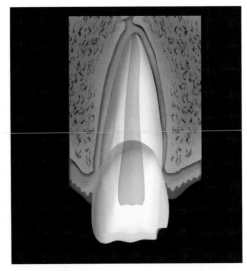

Figure 37.15. Small chips of enamel.

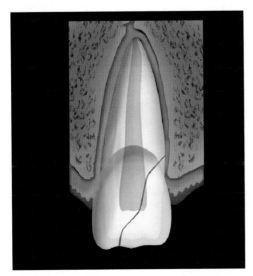

Figure 37.13. Stress fracture with pulp involvement.

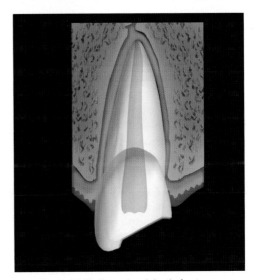

Figure 37.16. Enamel and dentin fractures.

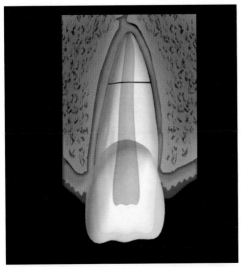

Figure 37.14. Stress fracture with root involvement.

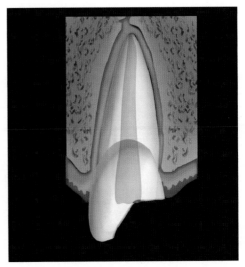

Figure 37.17. Fractures involving pulp exposure.

In the first case, if there is little or no sensitivity, no treatment is recommended. In the first and second cases, if the exposed area is sensitive to air or cold then a temporary covering is recommended. For fractures involving pulp exposure, the area exposed should be dried first and then a pulp covering and temporary cement should be applied. If the exposed pulp area is painful to touch, the prior application of a benzocaine topical anesthetic for 30 seconds is recommended before drying with a cotton pellet and applying the pulp covering.

For fractures involving the crown and roots of teeth, the same steps should be followed for crown fractures with pulp exposure. If there is a moveable section of tooth involving the root below the gumline, it is usually best to remove that section and then place a temporary filling.

Fractures may occur with the fractured piece still attached to the tooth. These can be uncomfortable because the fractured piece, often movable during biting or chewing, aggravates the gum tissue. In these cases, the removal of the fractured piece may be required.

TOOTH TRAUMA DIAGNOSIS

How an injury to the teeth and jaw occurred can tell you about the resulting effect to the traumatized area. For example in direct trauma, there is a blow that directly impacts the teeth. Such trauma usually affects the front teeth and results in fractured crown sections of the teeth following the impact. Though fractured teeth are the most obvious sign of such trauma, one must be aware of nonvisible effects to surrounding teeth as these may have root fractures or displacement caused from the traumatic event.[1–4] In indirect trauma, there is usually a blow to an area of the jaw or chin that impacts the teeth. Posterior premolar and molar teeth are usually affected by such trauma, and the resulting damage can be fractures in the crowns or combined crown and root fractures.[22]

The degree of traumatic impact can also be useful in the dental trauma record. High-velocity impact usually results in fractured pieces. Low-velocity impact often results in the greatest damage to tooth supporting structures. Root and bone fractures, for example, are more likely evident in such injuries.[21]

Often after tooth or jaw trauma, it can be difficult to assess damage to the affected teeth. Though fractures and chips broken off are obvious, there can be fractures to the underlying roots of a tooth or bone supporting a tooth or multiple teeth. Because you do not have the diagnostic tool of radiographs in field conditions, it can be difficult to assess the full extent of damage. What you cannot see may be the worst of the trauma. For example, there are situations where multiple teeth receive an external blow that results in fracture of one or more teeth. In such instances, the fractures to the crown or erupted portion of the teeth may suggest the possibility of underlying root or bone fracture in surrounding teeth, even though appearing unaffected.[6–9]

The best way to diagnose nonvisible or underlying tooth and bone fracture is by signs you can detect and symptoms of the affected person. Such fractures are often sensitive to palpation around the roots and to light percussion on the erupted crown position of the tooth. Ideally, in an office setting, such teeth would be splinted together for stability. Because this is often not an option in the field, measures should be taken to cover a fractured tooth area and have the person on a soft diet. Food and liquid should be ideally temperate with no extreme variations in cold or hot as this can exacerbate pain. A soft diet will prevent any undue stress on the affected area. If the food is tough or cannot be pureed, then smaller sections can be cut for more localized chewing in the unaffected areas.

Bone fractures can be detected by observing blood clots in the gum tissue around the affected area of the jaw bone. Without proper training, it is not advisable to reposition bone sections.

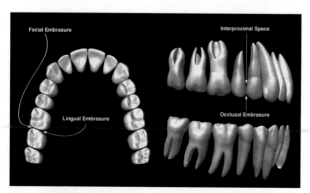

Figure 37.18. Left image erupted crown anatomy of the upper jaw. Right image overall general tooth morphology of teeth in upper and lower jaws.

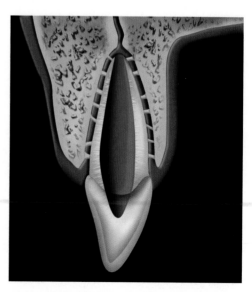

Figure 37.19. Normal tooth position.

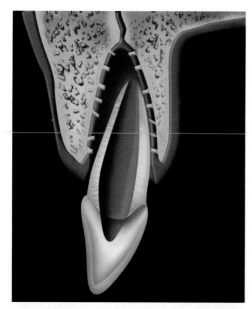

Figure 37.20. Direct trauma causing displacement of the root.

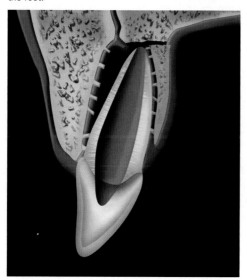

Figure 37.21. Direct trauma associated with displacement of the root.

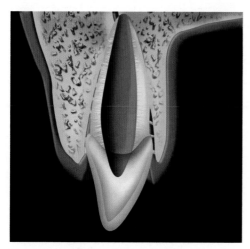

Figure 37.22. Intrusion of tooth from direct vertical impact.

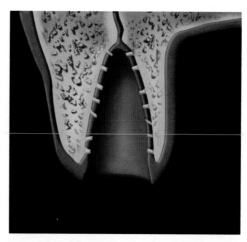

Figure 37.23. Complete luxation of tooth and root from either direct or blunt trauma.

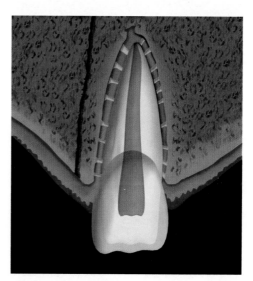

Figure 37.24. Vertical bone fracture associated with blunt trauma.

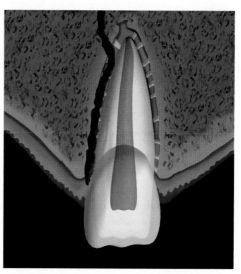

Figure 37.25. Alveolar or tooth socket trauma from blunt injury.

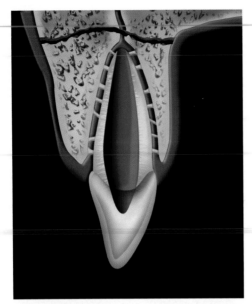

Figure 37.26. Horizontal bone fracture in association with blunt traumatic injury.

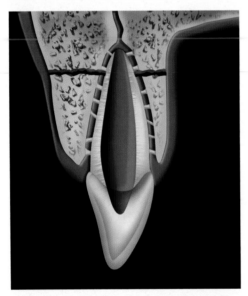

Figure 37.27. Horizontal bone fracture involving the base of the tooth's root and caused from blunt trauma.

PREPARING THE PATIENT AFTER TOOTH FRACTURE

For lower teeth, place two cotton rolls on either side of the affected area, one in between the tongue and tooth and one between the tooth and cheek. Upper teeth only require one cotton roll between the teeth and the cheek. Use the spoon excavator to clean any soft material still attached to the decayed or fractured area of tooth. Then dry the area as best you can with cotton pellets. The dryer the area, the better the temporary material will cling to the tooth.

TREATMENT OF TOOTH FRACTURES

For small fractures, cover the damaged area with a thick paste of temporary cement (IRM, or intermediate restorative material). The consistency should be thick enough that you can mold it with your fingers. The paste is too thin if it sticks to your fingers and is not moldable, and too thick if portions break off when you try to mold it. Roll the cement into a tube-like shape (diameter no larger than 1/8 inch and length approximately 1 inch) with your finger using light pressure against a small mixing pad. Using the metal plastic instrument, take a small portion from the tube onto the instrument and place in the fractured area. After wiping the instrument clean, use it to mold the cement covering the area and finishing it smoothly. Keep the repaired area of temporary cement smaller than the piece dislodged. This will help avoid any biting interferences when you are done.

TOOTH LUXATION

With severe trauma, a tooth may completely come out.[5] The area should be closed with sutures and/or bite firmly on cotton gauze for one hour. If the incident occurs within 20 minutes, repositioning can be attempted after cleaning the tooth with saline or whole milk if available. In most situations, it is best not to reinsert the tooth especially after a blood clot has formed. Do not attempt repositioning a tooth without additional training. With training, one can find the proper orientation and fit in the socket if inserted promptly within the first 20 minutes. However, if additional care is much more than a day away, adequate stabilization can be difficult and problematic.[23] For any area sutured, the diet should consist of soft food for at least 3 days. If soft food is unavailable, drinking additional liquids and cutting foods into small pieces is recommended.

Should a traumatic injury occur on expedition, a simple notation record should document the incident to assist any follow-up care.

DENTAL TRAUMA RECORD

Name _____

When did the injury occur?

_____

Where did the injury occur?

_____

How did the injury occur?

_____

Was a headache associated with the injury?	Yes	No
Was nausea associated with the injury?	Yes	No
Was vomiting associated with the injury?	Yes	No
Was there bleeding from the nose?	Yes	No
Were there any palpable signs of jaw fracture?	Yes	No
Was there any loss of consciousness during the injury?	Yes	No

Were abrasions, lacerations or contusions associated with the trauma and resulting injury? Yes No

LOST FILLINGS, CROWNS, OR BRIDGES

Once the restoration is recovered, clean the interior or underlying surface of the filling or crown. Next remove any debris or food that may still be visible around the affected area. Then place the restoration back onto the area. Slowly have the person bite together and make sure they can close normally. Clean any soft material on the tooth where the restoration came off using the spoon excavator. Dry the tooth with cotton pellets and place cotton rolls on either side of the area. Mix the temporary cement (IRM) into a paste with the consistency of toothpaste. Once mixed, you will have about 3 minutes of working time. Fill the crown or bridge half full with cement or cover the underlying surface of the filling. Place the restoration back onto the tooth and have the patient again slowly close together. Make sure that the bite is okay. Let the cement dry until it is hard. Using the explorer and floss, remove any excess cement. Be sure when flossing that once you floss downward, you thread the piece out instead of coming back up. One should note the following on mixing temporary cement: Keep in mind that cements are temperature-sensitive. Expect longer setting times in cold arctic-like climates and shorter ones for sea level hot equator-like climates.

BROKEN PARTIAL OR FULL DENTURES

If a piece of acrylic breaks off of a denture, file down the remaining sharp edge. The same should be done for a broken clasp or metal component.

TREATING INFECTIONS

Whether you are treating an infected tooth or jaw area at Massachusetts General Hospital or atop Annapurna 2, standard protocol should be followed. Four considerations need to be made. First, find and remove the source of the infection; second, drain the infection; and third, irrigate the infected area. Finally, give a standard 10-day course of antibiotics for infection.

GUM ABSCESS OR SWELLING

If you notice an unusual swelling in the gum or around a tooth, take a cotton pellet and lightly cover the area with some benzocaine gel. Some local anesthetic may also be needed. After a minute, take a sterile needle and probe no deeper than 1/8 inch into the affected part. If there is a yellowish white fluid draining, there is likely a bacterial infection present. In such instances, you may cut a small slit into the area and gently press against the swollen area to milk the fluid from the surrounding area. Be sure to have some cotton ready to absorb the fluid. If the swelling is larger than 1/8 inch in diameter, take dry gauze and place it at or below the affected area to absorb the bacterial fluid. The patient should take a standard 500-mg course of penicillin every 6 hours for 10 days.

For swellings whose cause cannot be determined, do not attempt any further treatment. A regimen of antibiotics should be initiated. If the swelling persists after 2 days or gets larger and is accompanied by elevated body temperature, then you should arrange to have the person removed from the expedition so that he or she can get prompt care. In certain instances, large swellings of oral origin that involve swelling of the neck can indicate a cellulitis and can become serious if left untreated for more than a couple of days.

PULPITIS AND PULPAL ABSCESS

Pulpitis occurs when the inner blood and nerve supply of the tooth has been traumatized or partially exposed. The inner pulpal tissue may be exposed during a tooth fracture or recurrent decay underneath an old restoration. Usually a pulpitis is reversible and most sensitive to cold. If there is any sign of pulp exposure during the placement of a temporary filling or before recementing a filling or crown, place a light covering of benzocaine paste on the area, then dry the area with a cotton pellet and use IRM paste for repairing the affected area or recementing a crown or bridgework.

A pulpal abscess occurs when the tooth aches when any pressure is applied or when finger pressure around the tooth elicits a pain that continues when the pressure is discontinued. The tooth may also have a dull continuous ache. In such cases, the standard antibiotic regimen for 10 days with penicillin should be initiated. Pain medication may be helpful as well. If pain persists, the affected individual may need to leave the expedition.

Note for anesthetic use: In situations where treatment is not possible and/or when severe pain will not subside, give an injection of marcaine, which numbs the area for about 8–10 hours, giving relief.

MOUTH SORES

Among mouth ulcers that may present on expedition are those associated with herpes labialis, primary herpetic gingivostomatitis, and recurrent aphthous stomatitis. Differentiation of the ulcers is not critical as treatment for both is to let the infection run its course for approximately 10 days. Primary herpetic gingivostomatitis may present with multiple painful sores, headache, and an elevated temperature. Avoiding recurrent aphthous ulcers is best achieved by maintaining a proper diet since they are associated with iron, vitamin B-12 and folate deficiencies. Taking a multivitamin on expeditions should be recommended for these individuals with a prior history of such ulcers. Herpes labialis is associated with sunlight, stress, and other unknown factors. For these individuals, frequent use of a lip balm with a high SPF is recommended.

PERICORNITIS

This gum swelling created by a flap of tissue partially covering the back portion of the biting surface of the wisdom teeth can be painful and should be treated with an antibiotic for 10 days and with use of warm salt rinses to keep the swelling down. Apply benzocaine topical a couple of minutes prior to eating to relieve that pain when chewing food. A diet free of hard-crusted breads, chips, or other foods that can potentially lodge in such swollen areas of gum tissue is recommended. Under conditions where such foods cannot be avoided, as previously discussed, cut foods into smaller pieces so that chewing can be done on unaffected areas.

TOOTH REMOVAL

When minor repairs to fractured teeth are not effective and associated pain is extreme, there may be a need for tooth extraction or removal. Though every measure should be explored and attempted before making such a decision, tooth extraction can be accomplished on expedition. Usually weight concerns on expedition do not merit bringing surgical forceps. However, if one forcep is brought, the pediatric 150A is the forcep of choice.

After adequately anesthetizing the area, separation of the gumline immediately attached to the root surface should be established. Forcep jaws should be held tightly against the root at the gumline, and a slow rocking figure-eight action should be initiated to separate the tooth from the attached bone. Tooth and root fractures

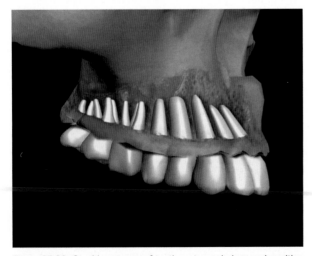

Figure 37.28. Graphic cutaway of tooth root morphology and position as a guide for upper tooth extraction.

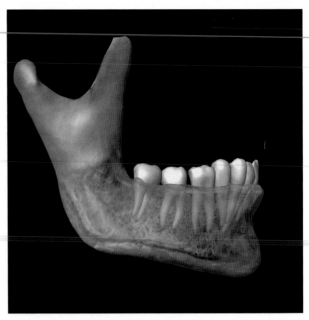

Figure 37.29. Tooth morphology and position as a guide for lower tooth extraction.

occur most often when undue force or rapid removal is attempted. Because you will not have the benefit of radiographs on expedition, there is no confirmed way to know the angle or orientation of roots in a tooth.[10,23] As a general rule, if the tooth feels solid with little or no give or movement after initial attempts of extraction, leave it alone. Even seemingly simple extractions can pose an unexpected challenge.

BARODONTALGIA

Trapped air pockets in the interior of a tooth can cause severe pain for those who undergo pressure changes in either high-altitude climbing or deep undersea dives. It is imperative for these explorers to alert their dentists about their travels. Extra precaution needs to be taken for any filling material applied to their teeth. A tiny air bubble trapped in the cement while attaching a crown, for example, can later have a dramatic effect when the body undergoes pressure changes. The air in the pocket or cement remains the same while the pressure around it changes. The force of such air pressure has been documented to crack and shatter filling material and tooth. Should any cement or filling material be used during an emergency treatment for high-altitude climbers or undersea divers, a smooth consistency must be maintained.

If one is undergoing root canal treatment or has other temporary restorations, then some attention must be paid to potential air pockets. Though not customary for most explorers, areas undergoing such treatment should have such voids temporarily filled with a cement that alleviates these air pockets.

ANESTHETICS

Two anesthetics[11,12] should be brought on expedition. Carbocaine or lidocaine would be a good choice for a single local anesthetic. There are several formulas to choose from and Cook-Waite Carbocaine 2% with Neo-Cobefrin is one that should be considered. This gives approximately 1 hour of anesthetic to the teeth and approximately 2 hours of soft tissue anesthetic. Marcaine, also referred to as sensorcaine or bupivacaine hydrochloride, is a good choice for longer-acting anesthesia to an affected area. In severe cases of trauma, marcaine may be an effective pain reliever until assistance or help arrives. Marcaine provides 6 hours of anesthesia to the teeth and 7 hours to the soft tissue.

On larger expeditions, there may be anesthetic overlap with the medical emergency kit. Lidocaine or Xylocaine are commonly selected anesthetics in both medicine and dental medicine. If you have already selected one of these, then you can opt for bringing more Carbocaine.

INJECTIONS

You should be familiar with two types of injections in the mouth. The first is infiltration, which is direct application of the anesthetic to the problem tooth. The needle should be inserted into the gum vestibule directly around the outside of the tooth.[28] A 32-gauge short needle should be inserted into the tissue about halfway, and the anesthetic should be deposited. Approximately half of a carpule is normally required. The injections are useful for all anterior teeth, and some posterior teeth. They are less effective for back molar teeth. (See Figures 37.30 through 37.33.)

The second type of injection is a nerve block. Such injections numb the trunk of a nerve that eventually reaches multiple teeth. Useful block injections for the

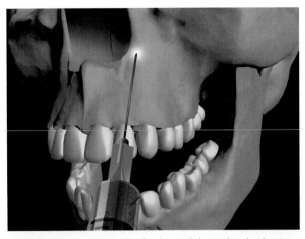

Figure 37.31. Injection location for the medial superior alveolar nerve block and/or infiltration area to attain numbness for the premolar or bicuspid teeth.

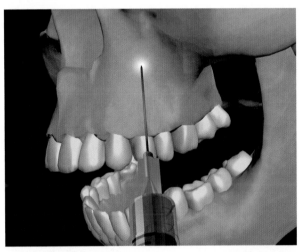

Figure 37.32. Injection location for the anterior superior alveolar nerve block and/or infiltration area to attain for the anterior teeth.

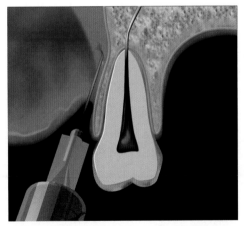

Figure 37.33. Needle location for infiltration injections.

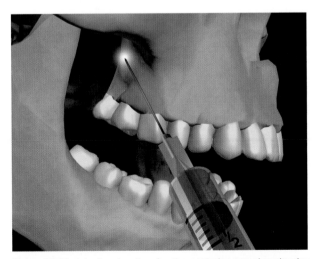

Figure 37.30. Injection location for the posterior superior alveolar nerve block and/or infiltration area to attain numbness for the posterior molar teeth.

upper jaw include the posterior and middle sections of the main nerve supplying the upper teeth, the superior alveolar nerve. For the lower jaw, the mandibular block is the only injection needed. This nerve lies within bone and must be injected at its trunk before entering the lower

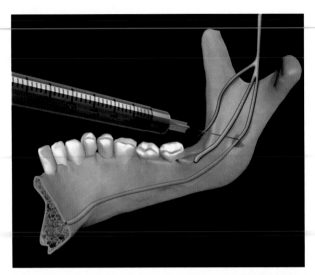

Figure 37.34. General anatomy and nerve location for the inferior alveolar nerve.

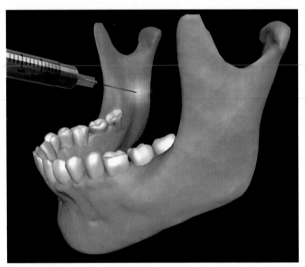

Figure 37.35. Needle location for delivery of anesthetic.

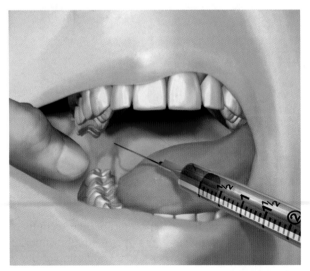

Figure 37.36. Appearance of tissue in relative position for needle placement.

jaw.[13–15] As with all injections, aspiration is imperative to avoid injecting into a blood vessel. (See Figure 37.34 through 37.36.)

ANTIBIOTICS

Penicillin is still considered to be the drug of choice in oral and dental infections. Most conditions requiring antibiotic therapy should proceed with a 10-day course of 500 mg penicillin V every 6 hours. It is most effective taken on an empty stomach. Clindamycin 300 mg is the antibiotic of choice for those individuals allergic to penicillin. One 300-mg tablet is taken every 6 hours for 10 days. A broad-spectrum antibiotic should be taken for resistant infections. Augmentin for patients who can tolerate penicillin, or Biaxin for patients with penicillin allergy, is recommended. The dosage for both antibiotics is 500 mg every 8 hours for a 10-day period.

PAIN MEDICATIONS

Advil, Motrin, ibuprofen, and Tylenol are effective pain medications for tooth and gum discomfort. At 200-mg doses, these can be taken three at a time per single dose, though constant use over several days can result in stomach discomfort. In certain instances, carrying prescription pain medications can be considered illegal for international travel, and if they are brought, especially in any large quantity, they can be confiscated. You may want to avoid this potential problem. A formal document from a doctor should always be carried when bringing any narcotic pain reliever on such trips. Prescription pain medications may also impair judgment and depth perception and have many more side effects that may not be conducive to remote field expedition work.

THE DENTAL EMERGENCY KIT

The Basics
  Mouth mirror #5, front surface
  Explorer #6DE
  Spoon excavator Hu Friedy 19W
  Cotton rolls #2
  Cotton gauze 2 × 2s
  Cotton pellets #4
  Cotton pliers
  Floss, Glide waxed

Materials
  Zinc and Eugenol temporary cement (IRM recommended)
  Orthodontic wax
  Calcium hydroxide paste
  Benzocaine topical anesthetic (Hurricaine brand)

Instruments
  30 G Short, 27 L needles
  Mixing pad, small, roughly 2 in. × 2 in
  Mixing spatula, Hu Friedy CS24
  Metal plastic instrument for temporary material application
  Hemostat and surgical scissors
  Absorbable suture material, C-6, 3/8ths circle, reverse cutting needle
  Dental syringe, self-aspirating

Anesthetic
  Carbocaine
  Marcaine long acting, 8–10 hours

Additional Items for Expeditions or Research for Periods of 6 Months and Longer
  Surgical curette #10
  Straight elevator #1
  Pediatric 150A forcep
  Tooth chart showing the roots underlying bone (Guide to understanding the usual shape you will be removing)

When Time and Storage Space Are Critical

Orthodontic wax is useful when time and supply space is critical. With little effort, a piece of wax can be easily placed on a defect or broken area and provide temporary relief.

OBTAINING DENTAL EMERGENCY KITS

Assistance with assembling dental emergency kits, and additional training for those interested, can be obtained by contacting your family dentist or the author, E-mail at mnweeia@gmail.com, or writing to 6 New Street, P.O. Box 35, Sharon, CT 06069.

Glossary

Abscess: Collection of pus collected in a cavity formed by the tissue on the basis of an infectious process or other foreign materials.

Abrasion: Superficial damage to the skin, usually within the epidermis layer.

Antiseptic: A substance that retards, destroys, or inhibits the growth of microorganisms.

Anesthetic: A substance that blocks the sensation of pain.

Aspiration: To draw in using suction.

Carpule: A 1.8 cc glass container for the delivery of anesthetic

Cellulitis: An acute, edematous, diffuse, suppurative inflammation of the connective tissues that can be associated with a dental abscess and lead to systemic infection if left untreated.

Contusion: A bruising that is caused by a blunt trauma and has no break in the skin.

Explorer: A dental instrument with a straight or curved needle-like point used to detect decay in dentistry.

Fibrosis: Formation of fibrous or scar tissue around an area.

Forceps: A tong-like or pinching instrument used to remove or luxate teeth.

Laceration: A tear, cut, or opening in the skin that may involve multiple layers of tissue.

Lesion: An altered or damaged area of tissue.

Luxation: Displacement or dislocation of an anatomic structure, referring to tooth.

Metal plastic instrument: A dental instrument with narrow short flat ends at differing angles to the handle used in placement of paste-like materials.

Mucosa: The moist soft tissue lining the mouth. In reference to the gingival, that portion covered by keratinized epithelium.

Orthodontics: Involving the movement of teeth, from *ortho* ("move") and *dontics* ("referring to teeth").

Pericornitis: The inflammation of the flap of tissue sometimes partially covering an erupted wisdom tooth.

Spoon excavator: A dental instrument with small curved spoon-like ends at varying angles from the handle used primarily for the removal of decayed or foreign material from a tooth.

Subdermal hematoma: A blood clot formed beneath the dermis layer of skin.

Vermilion border: The line formed around the lips between where the outer moist red tissue meets the skin.

Vestibule: Small tissue-lined areas of the oral cavity formed by different anatomic locations (e.g., the inner lining of the cheek and the gum tissue lining below the level of the teeth).

Treatments and advice given in this text are no supplement for training in dental medicine and the author claims no legal responsibility for the actions of those practicing dentistry without proper license credentials, and resulting in any permanent damages either to the teeth, oral cavity, or general health of the person being treated. Instruments and materials for the dental emergency kit were selected for their ease of use and not for any contract, agreement, or affiliation with any company or product line. Options for any and all instruments may also be suggested by your family dentist or the author. All illustrations courtesy of Kevin Hand.

SUGGESTED READINGS

Andreasen JO, Andreasen FM. *Textbook and Color Atlas of Traumatic Injuries to the Teeth.* 3rd ed. Copenhagen: Mosby; 1994.

REFERENCES

[1] Amundsen R. Plans and preparations. *The South Pole: An Account of the Norwegian Antarctic Expedition in the Fram, 1910–1912.* Northampton, Mass: Interlink Publishing Group; 2003.

[2] Hawkins MD, Royce W, Ziglschmid J. Clinical aspects of crew health. *Biomedical Results of Apollo.*

[3] Hardwick GL, Newmann PA. Some observations on the incidence and emergency treatment of fractured permanent anterior teeth of children. *J Dent Res.* 1954;33:730.

[4] Lewis TE. Incidence of fractured anterior teeth as related to their protrusion. *Angle Orthod.* 1959;29:128–31.

[5] Hallet GEM. Problems of common interest to the paedodontist and orthodontist with special reference to traumatised incisor cases. *Eur Orthod Soc Trans.* 1953;29:266–77.

6 Eichenbaum IW. A correlation of traumatized anterior teeth to occlusion. *ASDC J Dent Child*. 1963;30:229–36.

7 McEwen JD, McHugh WD, Hitchin AD. Fractured maxillary central incisors and incisal relationships. *J Dent Res*. 1967;46:1290.

8 Omullane DM. Some factors predisposing to injuries of permanent incisors in schoolchildren. *Br Dent J*. 1973;134: 328–32.

9 Wojciak L, Ziolkiewics T, Anholcer H, Frankowska-Lenartowska M, Haber-Milewska T, Zynda B. Trauma to the anterior teeth in school-children in the city of Poznan with reference to masticatory anomalies. *Czas Stomatol*. 1974;27:1355–61.

10 Jarvinen S. Incisal overjet and traumatic injuries to upper permanent incisors: a retrospective study. *Acta Odontol Scand*. 1978;36:359–62.

11 Ghose LJ, Baghdady VS, Enke H. Relation of traumatized permanent anterior teeth to occlusion and lip condition. *Community Dent Oral Epidemiol*. 1980;8:381–4.

12 Hughes NC. Basic techniques of excision and wound closure. In: *Operative Surgery: Plastic Surgery*. 4th ed. London: Butterworths; 1986.

13 Hunt TK, ed. *Wound Healing and Wound Infection. Theory and Surgical Practice*. New York: Appleton-Century-Crofts;1980.

14 Hughes NC. Basic techniques of excision and wound closure. In: *Operative Surgery: Plastic Surgery*. 4th ed. London: Butterworths; 1986.

15 Schultz TC. *Facial Injuries*. 3rd ed. Chicago: Year Book Medical Publishers; 1988.

16 Bergenholz A, Isaksson B. Tissue reactions in the oral mucosa to catgut, silk and merilene sutures. *Odontologisk Revy*. 1967;18:237–50.

17 Lilly GE, Armstrong JH, Salem JE, Cutcher JL. Reaction of oral tissues to suture materials. Part II. *Oral Surg Oral Med Oral Pathol*. 1968;26:592–9.

18 Edlich RF, Rodeheaver G, Thacker JG, Edgerton MT. Technical factors in wound management. In: Hunt TK, Dunphy JE, eds. *Fundamentals of Wound Management*. New York: Appleton-Century-Crofts; 1979: 364–454.

19 Zallen RD, Black SL. Antibiotic therapy in oral and maxillofacial surgery. *J Oral Surg*. 1976;34:349–51.

20 Paterson JA, Cardo VA, Stratigos GT. An examination of antibiotic prophylaxis in oral and maxillofacial surgery. *J Oral Surg*. 1970;28:753–9.

21 Yrastorza JA. Indications for antibiotics in orthognathic surgery. *J Oral Surg*. 1976;34:514–6.

22 Ingle JI, Frank AL, Natkin E, Nutting EE. Diagnosis and treatment of traumatic injuries and their sequelae. In: Ingle JI, Beveridge EE, eds. *Endodontics*. 2nd ed. Philadelphia: Lea & Febiger; 1976: 685–711.

23 Andreasen JO. Luxation of permanent teeth due to trauma. *Scand F Dent Res*. 1970;78:273–86.

38 | Foot Injuries

John VonHof, EMT-P, OT, and Zak H. Weis, DPM, MS

ANKLE SPRAINS AND STRAINS

A sprain is a stretching or tearing injury to the ligaments that stabilize bones together at a joint. Sprains are usually associated with traumas such as falling or twisting, and ankles are frequently the sprained or strained joint. If the patient cannot walk after a few minutes of rest or if they heard the infamous "pop," you can be fairly certain they have a sprain. After a sprain occurs, the fibrous joint capsule swells and becomes inflamed, discolored, and painful. A strain is the overstretching of a muscle or tendon – but without the significant tearing common to a sprain. There may be bleeding into the muscle area that can cause swelling, pain, stiffness, and muscle spasm followed by a bruise. Strains can come from overuse, repetitive movements, excessive muscle contractions, or prolonged positions.

The most common ankle injury sprain is an inversion sprain and strain. The injured area is the anterior tailofibular and calcaneal fibular ligament just at the ankle joint on the outside of the foot. An eversion sprain, where the medial deltoid ligaments are injured, is less common. In some very serious trauma sprains, both the lateral and medial ligaments can be injured. An anterior drawer test, application of a tuning fork on the bony prominences, pain on palpation, palpation of a dell, or decrease in muscle strength can all be indications that there is a more serious condition and immediate transfer to an emergency room is indicated. An X-ray, CT, and/or MRI will reveal whether there is a bone fractured or a tendon has been torn, and this may require immobilization of the joint.

There are three degrees of an ankle sprain. A grade 1 sprain has some soft tissue tearing with intact structures and minimal swelling, and the athlete can still put weight on the leg with the twisted ankle. The ankle's ligaments have been stretched, and some are partially torn. A grade 2 sprain has moderate swelling and moderate pain when weight is put on the injured ankle. There is a more significant tear of the ligament and increased swelling. A grade 3 sprain has a large amount of swelling; a clinical exam of 0/4 muscle strength, and weight placed on the ankle cannot be tolerated. Great care needs to be taken when examining the muscle strength in that the muscle in question is isolated and tested along with palpation of the muscle and tendon. Many muscles have cross-contributory motions and can give a false positive exam. Grades 1 and 2 will heal in about 4–6 weeks with full recovery in 10–12 weeks. A grade 3 sprain requires medical attention. With a severe sprain, there is the possibility of a related fracture or avulsions so attention should be focused not only on the joint or tendon in question but also on at least one joint proximal and one joint distal to the site. If there is a great deal of pain and swelling, and the patient is unable to bear weight on the foot, an emergency room visit and an X-ray are in order, and the clinician should not hesitate to refer to a center of greater care.

Treating a Strain or Sprain

The treatment goal is to return the ankle to normal motion and to be weight bearing as soon as possible. The initial treatment for a strain or sprain includes the classic RICE treatment: rest, ice, compression, and elevation. Ice the injury within 30 minutes if possible. Have them apply ice for 20 minutes at a time at least four times daily. In the field, a cold stream river or lake can be used. Early treatment within the first 24 hours decreases swelling and lessens the risk of additional injury. Initial rest of the foot is also important. A lightly applied Ace wrap or Coban will provide compression to help keep swelling down while providing support. Apply the compression dressing from the forefoot (distal) toward the ankle (proximal). Warn the patient not to wear the Ace wrap at night and that it may need to be reapplied as it will loosen when the edema starts to resolve.

Elevate the injured area above the level of the heart as much as possible during the first 48 hours. This keeps blood away from the injured area and reduces pain and swelling. When resting and sleeping, the ankle should be elevated.

Heat causes a hyperemic response that will increases blood flow to an injured area, which makes swelling worse. For this reason, the use of heat is not recommended for at least a week after an injury. Moist heat can be applied by using a moist heating pad, a warm towel, or a warm bath. Dry heat can be applied by using a heating pad for 20 minutes at a time.

NSAIDs are used to control pain and swelling after an injury. Urge care if continuing in the event because the NSAIDs block pain signals that would warn of further injury. The use of NSAIDs and the hydration state of the athlete must be taken into consideration prior to prescribing.

There are two schools of thought on how soon to start bearing weight on an injured ankle. One says to get out on it as soon as possible and let pain be your guide. Advise the athlete that if the ankle is stiff and sore when starting out, keep going and see if it loosens up. If the pain increases, the patient should get off the ankle and use the RICE treatment. If it doesn't get worse or feels better, they are probably OK. The other says to work through the healing process at the ankle's speed. The patient must make an informed choice.

Proprioception is key to nonsurgical rehabilitation, but many fail to strengthen the peroneal muscles on the lateral side of the leg (the ankle everters). If the lateral ligaments are stretched out, then the muscles must be very strong to help stabilize against recurrent sprains. The other thing that is very important is protecting the ankle from reinjury. Wearing a brace will not make the ankle weak; not doing the strengthening and proprioception exercises leaves the ankle weak. The brace may prevent a severe injury and should be prescribed during a race if a grade 1 or 2 sprain or strain is identified.

Two tips will help athletes more quickly and completely recover following an ankle sprain. First, the use of crutches for even a few days can dramatically improve recovery time. Encourage walking using the crutches to reduce weight on the ankle instead of keeping the foot off of the ground. Second, a compression wrap with the addition of a horseshoe-shaped felt pad, greatly reduces the effects of swelling.[1]

Wrapping an Ankle

To wrap an ankle sprain, cut ¼-inch thick felt into a horseshoe shape and place it so that the "U" cradles the malleolus. Then use an elastic wrap to firmly compress the entire horseshoe against the ankle. The horseshoe and wrap should be used until the swelling is nearly gone. Then wrap the ankle in the following manner to provide compression and support:

1. Elastic wrap that is 2-in wide works best, and the tension should be firm but still allow normal circulation.

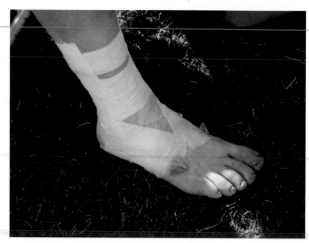

Figure 38.1. Ankle taped with white athletic tape. Credit: John Vonhof.

2. Start the wrap 3–4 inches above the outer side of the ankle. Pull the wrap straight down under the heel and around to the arch.
3. From the arch proceed around to the front of the ankle and then around to the back of the heel/Achilles.
4. From the Achilles, continue diagonally along the inner side of the heel, then wrap under the arch to the outer side of the ankle and up to the front of the foot.
5. Proceed around the inside of the ankle and pull the wrap behind the heel/Achilles. Continue around the outer ankle diagonally coming under the foot again and around to the front of the ankle. This pattern can be repeated for additional support and compression.
6. With any additional wrap spiral up the lower leg.[1]

An ankle can be taped with white athletic tape, although other tapes can be used. Figure 38.1 shows a taped ankle. The yellow prewrap is visible under the tape and should always be used. The three tape wraps around the lower leg serve as anchors for the strips of tape applied as a stirrup. Finally, several strips are applied around the back of the heel to lock the ankle.

If an ankle is wrapped or taped, it is imperative that the patient carefully bunches up his or her socks and rolls them over the wrap or tape. This should be done when putting socks on and taking them off.

BLISTERS AND HOT SPOTS

In an article in the *Journal of Emergency Medicine*, "Event Medicine: Injury and Illness During an Expedition-Length Adventure Race," the authors reported: "blisters on the feet represent the single most common injury at 32.8 percent of all reported and treated cases."[2] The article confirms what many medical teams know. The majority of their time is spent on blister control. The authors [of this chapter] patched feet in a 7-day stage race in Costa Rica. Every night, three medical staff patched an orderly queue of runners. A more in-depth presentation on blister prevention and management can be found in the book, *Fixing Your Feet: Prevention and Treatments for Athletes.*[3]

Blisters start out as hot spots, which can be caused by friction, moisture, heat, poor-fitting footwear, bunched-up socks, and debris in the shoe. If caught in time and treated, hot spots can be controlled. Left to their own, they will develop into an irritating blister that can stop athletes in their tracks, end their event, and sideline them for weeks.

Blisters can be painful, changing an athlete's gait to avoid putting pressure on the spot, thereby changing stride, which can lead to injuries. Hot spots are simple to prevent and treat. Blisters are different. This section will consider many different ways to manage blisters. Some are simple and quick. Others are complex and take more time – because they are meant to last during a multiday event.

It is important for medical staffs of large events to make sure participants are educated in foot care, blister repair, and taping. Participants should carry a basic foot care kit.

Hot Spots

Most athletes experience hot spots in the areas where they are susceptible to blisters forming. The area will become sore and red – thus, the name "hot spot." They may also experience a stinging or burning sensation. Around the reddened area will be a paler area that enlarges inward to where the skin is being rubbed.[4] The epidermis becomes elevated because it fills with fluid. The hot spot has then become a blister. Untreated hot spots usually turn into blisters, which are harder to treat.

Treating Hot Spots

Use your choice of one of the tapes or blister care products to protect the area. Clean the affected area with an alcohol wipe before applying tape, adhesive felt, or moleskin. Have athletes smooth wrinkles in socks and check inside their shoes for rough seams and debris. One of the commonly used lubricants can also be applied over the hot spot.

Blisters

Blisters are an injury and come in a variety of sizes. They start small, from a hot spot, and can continue to grow until they are treated. Athletes may describe a sudden stinging or burning sensation as the blister forms.[5] Multiply the pain of one well-placed blister times three or four, and you can imagine how severe a seemingly minor problem can become.

The time and conditions required for blisters to develop will vary from individual to individual. Runners and hikers tend to get either "downhill" blisters on the toes and forefoot caused by friction while going downhill, or "uphill" blisters on the heel and over the Achilles tendon caused by friction while going uphill. Blisters on the heel can also mean the heel cup is too wide. Blisters on the top or front of the toes or the outsides of the outer toes can indicate friction in the toebox.

Because patching blisters can be time-intensive, it is wise to train participants to care for their own feet. It is not unusual to spend an hour or more on one person's feet. Unless the medical team is large and foot care can be delegated to specialists, much of your time can be spent each day patching everyone's feet. Expecting athletes to carry a foot care kit and know how to use it can help the whole medical team. At the end of this chapter is a section on participant's foot care kits and an expedition kit for medical teams.

Blisters 101

A basic understanding of how blisters are formed is necessary to successfully treat them. Heat, friction, and moisture contribute to the formation of blisters. Studies have shown that the foot inside a shoe or boot is exposed to friction at many sites as it experiences motion from side to side, front to back, and up and down. These friction sites also change during the activity as the exercise intensity, movement of the sock, and flexibility of the shoe or boot changes.[6]

The outer epidermis layer of skin receives friction that causes it to rub against the inner dermis layer. This friction between the layers causes a blister to develop. As the outer layer of the epidermis is loosened from the deeper layers, the sac in between becomes filled with serous fluid. A blister has then developed. Figure 38.2 shows a blister that started small and grew from the base of the fifth toe, to the middle of the foot, and up to the other side of the foot. This type of blister requires special care in patching. The large surface area of loose skin is easily ruptured resulting in painful raw skin.

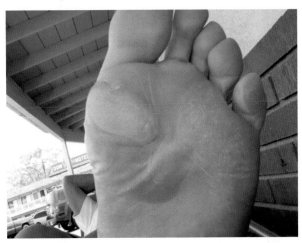

Figure 38.2. Full bottom of foot blister. Credit: John Vonhof.

If blisters are deep or traumatically stressed by continued running or hiking, the lymph fluid may contain blood. When the lymph fluid lifts the outer layer of epidermis, oxygen and nutrition to this layer is cut off and it becomes dead skin. This outer layer is easily drained. The fluid then drains and the skin loses its natural protective barrier. The underlying dermal layer is raw and sensitive. At this point, the blister is most susceptible to infection.

The friction against whatever is touching the skin causes the friction between the layers of skin. As identified earlier, the majority of foot problems can be traced back to socks, powders, and lubricants – or the lack of them. In order to prevent blisters, friction must be reduced. Friction can be reduced in three main ways: wearing double-layer socks or one inner and one outer sock, keeping the feet dry by using powders, or using a lubricant to reduce chafing. It has been found that rubbing moist skin tends to produce higher friction than does rubbing skin that is either very dry or very wet.[7] Eliminating pressure points caused by poor-fitting insoles and/or ill-fitting shoes can also reduce friction.

Because footwear can cause blisters, and irritate existing blisters, the healing process truly begins when these are removed. Encourage athletes to remove shoes and socks when stopping to rest or sleep. Wearing sandals without socks exposes the blister to the air, which aids in healing by helping dry the lesions.

Electrolytes and Blisters

Dehydration and the loss of important electrolytes can have a negative effect on the skin of athlete's feet. Toes often swell as they retain fluid because of hyponatremia. The foot's soft, waterlogged tissues become vulnerable to rubbing and pounding. Using a sodium replacement product in prolonged physical activity can help in the prevention of blisters.

Athletes who maintain proper electrolyte levels will reduce swelling of hands and feet even after many hours of exercise and reduce hot spots and blisters on the feet. In heat and humidity, the sweat rate is high resulting in significant amounts of sodium being lost. The sodium comes from the blood stream, and when the plasma gets too low, the body reacts to maintain the minimal tolerable level by pushing water from the blood into extracellular spaces. As the tissue on the feet swells, the feet become soft and more susceptible to blisters and damaged toenails. Feet swell inside the running shoes, putting extra pressure on the tissues, and those tissues can be rubbed to the point of physical damage. Blisters form as layers of skin separate, and toenails move more, damaging the weakened tissues that normally anchor them. Figure 38.3 shows a severely macerated foot.

Proactive Blister Prevention – Lubricants

The use of a lubricant on feet can help prevent blisters. BodyGlide, Blistershield Roll-On, and SportsSlick are

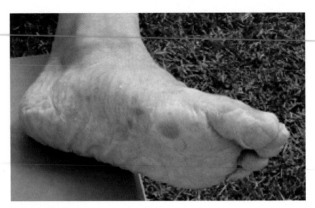

Figure 38.3. Maceration makes blister patching difficult. Credit: John Vonhof.

petroleum-free, waterproof, nonsticky, and hypoallergenic. Some athletes use Bag Balm. Athletes in conditions where their feet are exposed to extended periods of moisture often prefer Hydropel, an advanced skin protectant with silicone that is water-repelling and sweat-resistant. It is an excellent tool to control moisture and maceration. Avoid Vaseline as it is greasy, can cake up on socks, and tends to attract grit particles that can become an irritant and themselves cause blisters.

Studies have shown that lubricants may initially reduce friction, but over long periods of time they may actually increase it. After 1 hour the friction levels returned to their baseline factor, and after 3 hours the friction levels were 35% above the baseline. As the lubricants are absorbed into the skin and into the socks, friction returns and increases.[8] Based on this study, lubricants should be reapplied at frequent intervals.

The important thing to remember about lubricants is to clean off the old coating before applying the new one. Wipe off the old stuff with a cleansing towelette or an alcohol wipe.

General Blister Care

The goal of blister treatments is to make the foot comfortable since often travel by foot must continue. Blister management has four therapeutic goals:[9]

1. Avoiding infection
2. Minimizing pain and discomfort
3. Stopping further blister enlargement
4. Maximizing recovery

The best method of repairing a blister is to apply a blister patch with tape over the top, or tape alone. When using any product over a blister, apply it as smoothly as possible. Use finger pressure to smooth it evenly across the blister, and then repeat the smoothing process several more times after the initial application. Remember to cut the tape large enough to extend well beyond the edges of the blister and the patch underneath. The most common failure in using tape is not allowing enough

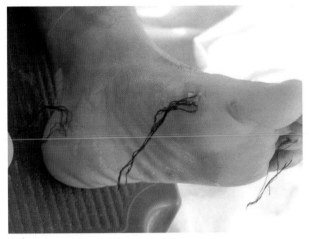

Figure 38.4. Blisters with side-to-side thread to promote draining. Credit: Rob Conenello.

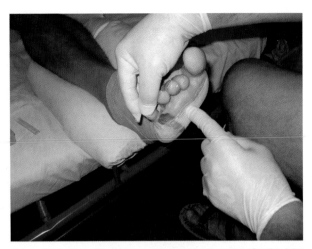

Figure 38.5. Blood-filled blister spreading under tape. Credit: John Vonhof.

necessary for good adherence. The larger the blister, the more the tape should extend past its edges.

Optimally, repair blisters before they enlarge and rupture. The recommendation is to drain the blister prior to applying a dressing when it is in a weight-bearing area and larger than ⅕ inch in diameter.[10] In a multiday event, however, any size blister is drained and patched. There are several ways to drain a blister, with a needle and syringe, a needle alone, a lancet, or a pointed scissors.

Another method helps blisters drain better when further walking or running is required. After draining the blister, add another step: Sterilize a needle and a few inches of thread with alcohol. Then thread the needle and run it and the thread through one side of the blister and out the other, leaving the thread in place with at least a 1-inch tail hanging out either end as shown in Figure 38.4. The thread acts as a wick to further drain any moisture in the blister while one is running or sleeping. This method has been successfully used in multiday stage races. Alternatives for a more effective drain are Nugauze or Iodoform.

Blood-Filled and Infected Blisters

Extra care is required for blood-filled blisters and infected blisters. When a blister is blood-filled, there is risk of infection as bacteria are easily introduced into the dermis layer of skin and into the blood system. Normal blister fluid is clear and if the fluid inside appears to be either cloudy or hazy, the change indicates that an infection has set in. In either case, drain the fluid, and apply an antibiotic ointment and a protective covering. Recheck the blister daily. Each time you check, apply a new coating of antibiotic ointment and change the dressing. Figure 38.5 shows a blood-filled blister likely caused by the tape being not close enough to the toes.

Ruptured Blisters

If the blister has ruptured, the degree of repair depends on the condition of the blister's outer covering. Figure 38.6

shows a ruptured blister on a foot in the Sahara Race. Clean around the blister and apply one of the blister products based on the condition of the blister.

If the outer layer of skin is torn off or only a flap of skin is left, carefully cut off the loose skin, clean the area, and cover the new skin with one of the blister patches described at the end of this section. The use of a light coating of zinc oxide or Desitin Ointment under a blister patch or tape can help to dry out the skin and repel moisture.

If the blister's roof is completely torn off, or the blister cavity is large and/or deep, consider using use one of the wound care products, like PolyMem or AmeriGel's Wound Dressings, mentioned at the end of this section. A sterile AmeriGel premoistened Wound Dressing was used on the heel wound in Figure 38.7. Also recommended are Ferris' PolyMem Wound Care Dressings.[11]

After debridement of the blister's roof with iris scissors, cleanse the area with normal saline. Cut the patch to fit the shape of the blister and cover with tape. This packs the blister and can greatly reduce the pain.[12]

Patching Blisters

Practice on good feet so you will know how to make the patch or tape stick when feet go bad. Learn how to patch intact blisters, drained blisters, and blisters with the skin torn off. The more you practice taping and patching blisters, the better you will become.

For years, the main product for patching blisters has been the familiar blue squares of Spenco 2nd Skin. 2nd Skin has two downsides though. It requires a tape or dressing to hold it in place, and over long periods of time, the gel softens the skin – leading to maceration requiring a drying agent.

Most blister care products described at the end of this section are applied to the skin. They can be used over intact or torn blisters. The exception is the Engo Blister Prevention Patches that are applied to footwear or on the sock.

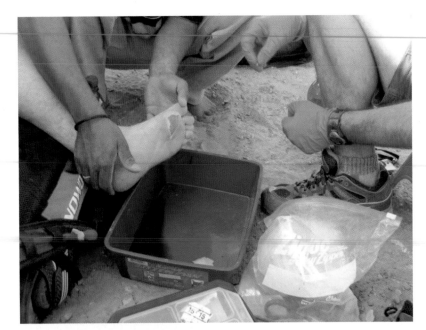

Figure 38.6. A ruptured ball of the foot blister. Credit: Rob Conenello.

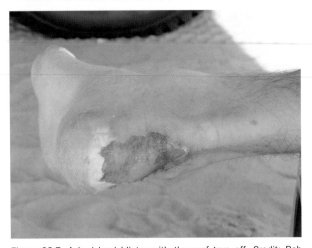

Figure 38.7. A bad heel blister with the roof torn off. Credit: Rob Conenello.

Tincture of benzoin applied to the area around a hot spot or blister will help blister products or tapes stick to the skin more effectively. Avoid getting tincture into a ruptured blister or other broken skin – it momentarily burns. After the tincture has dried, apply one of the blister care products or tape. Be sure to apply a light coating of powder or lubricant to counteract the still exposed tincture of benzoin to prevent socks or contaminants from sticking to the skin. Be aware that some individuals may contact dermatitis from the tincture.

After cleaning the skin, draining the blister if necessary, and applying benzoin, decide whether you will cover the blister with a blister patch or tape. Place a dab of zinc oxide or an antibiotic ointment on the blister and apply the covering. Commonly used blister patches are Spenco 2nd Skin, QuikStik Pads, and Sports Blister Pads; Blist-O-Ban; and Engo Blister Prevention Patches. The

Taping for Blisters section describes how to tape any part of the foot.

After patching, be sure to apply a dab of lubricant or powder to the bandage and surrounding skin, and then carefully roll socks on. Instruct athletes to roll socks on and off in the same way to preserve the patch or tape job. This keeps the patch from catching on the socks and pulling off or bunching up. The use of a shoehorn will save patches applied to heels.

Blister, Maceration, and Moisture

Patching blisters on macerated feet is difficult and the feet must be dry before patching. The use of Betadine or a drying agent, like Lazerformalyde Solution (Pedinol Pharmacal) can be beneficial in managing maceration prior to patching. In order for blister patches to stick, a tape adherent like tincture of benzoin must be used. The use of waterproof tape, like Kinesio-Tex, or a very sticky tape, like duct tape, is recommended. The section on Extreme Conditions covers maceration and moisture.

Treating Infected Blisters

If infected, blisters can become serious health issues. For open blisters, using soap and water, and an antibiotic ointment, Betadine, or hydrogen peroxide is important for avoiding infection. A broad-spectrum antibiotic ointment like Neosporin or Polysporin provides protection against both Gram-positive and Gram-negative pathogens. If ascending cellulitis is noted, a broad-spectrum oral antibiotic is indicated and possibly an oral antifungal too. Levoquine 750 mg QD is an excellent choice due to its Gram-positive and -negative coverage. Lamisil 250 mg QD × 14 days can be used if a fungal component is suspected. With Lamisil, a thorough history of liver problems and/or intolerances to medications should be obtained. With a 2-week course, tests for liver functions are not needed. It is advisable to make an outline of the cellulitis with a permanent marker so that the progression can be monitored.

Recheck blisters daily for signs of infection: redness, swelling, red streaks up the limb, pain, fever, and pus. Treat the blisters as wounds. Clean them frequently and apply an antibiotic ointment. Frequent warm water or Epsom salt soaks can also help the healing process. Although difficult in the field, encourage the athlete to stay off the foot as much as possible and elevate it above their heart.

If the blister is infected with pus, remove the roof of the blister and flush the blister cavity with betadine or normal saline, and apply a thin layer of antibiotic ointment. Cut a piece of wound dressing or Spenco 2nd Skin in the shape and size of the open blister. Place it inside the blister cavity. This soothes the wound, fills the empty space inside the blister, and helps with pain control. Tape over the patched blister with cover-roll or other sterile bandage. Early treatment can keep the infection from becoming more serious (see Figure 38.8).

Gluing Blisters

There are several techniques to "glue" the blister's roof to the skin underneath. These methods have helped many adventure racers finish their events. The methods should not be used if the blister is infected. These methods of gluing blisters should be used at your discretion. Although there is a chance of infection from the

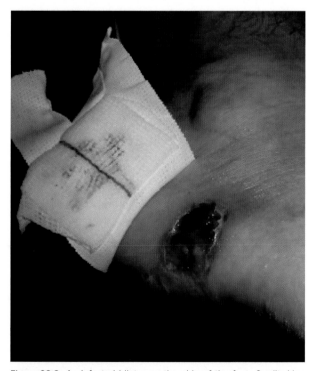

Figure 38.8. An infected blister on the side of the foot. Credit: Lisa de Speville.

nonsterile products, gluing the blister is a common technique used by many athletes – particularly where racing must continue.

After the blister has been drained thoroughly, and the skin is dry, use one of the following methods to seal down the blister roof:

- Use a syringe, without a needle, to inject tincture of benzoin directly into the blister. Immediately apply pressure across the top of the blister to evenly seal down the blister's outer layer to the underlying skin. This also pushes out any extra benzoin. Be forewarned that injecting the benzoin is momentarily painful. It has been rated as an eight on a one to ten pain scale.
- Use New-Skin Liquid Bandage, instead of benzoin, injected into the blister. This does not seal the blister as well as benzoin, but it is less painful.
- Krazy Glue and Orajel (Orajel Maximum Strength Toothache Pain Relief Gel) can also be used. Krazy Glue has better sticking power but Orajel has the added benefit of 20% benzocaine that helps soothe the burning. With either of these, just squirt a drop in the hole you've cut to drain and press down firmly. The application of a dressing or tape over the top is still recommended.

Deep Blisters

Deep blisters on the heels and the balls of the feet are usually under calluses. The only way to treat deep blisters is to use a syringe and needle to drain the fluid. The blister is so deep that nothing else can get in that deep. The athlete knows there is a blister there, but it is almost impossible to drain. Pressing on the callus to try to expel the fluid by hand is too painful. Lidocaine can be injected to numb the area but this technique will open up another portal for possible infection and should only be used in severe cases.

Blister Care Products

- Adhesive Felt is extra thick, and compared to moleskin, provides extra cushioning and a stronger adhesive base.
- Band-Aid Blister Relief, Blister Block, and Advanced Healing Blister Cushions are blister patches made with an elastic polyurethane film over a hydrocolloid layer or gel (*http://www.bandaid.com*).
- Blist-O-Ban patches are two layers of breathable plastic film bonded together, except for a collapsed dome type air bubble in the center. The bubble provides a gliding surface, reducing friction and shear forces (*http://www.blistoban.com*).
- Coban is a self-adherent wrap that can be used around feet, ankles, and heels to hold blister products in place (available at most drugstores).
- Dr. Scholl's Blister Treatment sterile pads (available at most drugstores).

- Engo Blister Prevention Patches are ultra-thin, slippery patches applied to footwear and socks – not to skin – significantly reducing friction (*http://www.GoEngo.com*).
- Moleskin is a soft, cotton padding that protects skin surfaces against friction and has a medium grade adhesive backing that adheres to the skin.
- Mueller's More Skin pads have the feel and consistency of human skin and remove friction between two moving surfaces (*http://www.muellersportsmed.com*).
- New-Skin comes in two forms: a Liquid Bandage useful as a skin protectant or toughener, and a Wound & Blister Dressing (available at most drugstores).
- Spenco 2nd Skin Blister Pads are a hydrocolloid pad bordered with a thin adhesive film (*http://www.spenco.com*).
- Spenco 2nd Skin Dressings are unique skin-like hydrogel pads that can be applied directly over closed or open blisters. They can also be used over abrasions, cuts, or similar wounds. Use one or more pads to cover the blister area. The pads do not stick to the skin and require tape to hold them onto the skin.
- Spenco QuikStik Pads and Sports Blister Pads contain a soft hydrocolloid pad covered by an ultra-thin film dressing to promote faster healing (*http://www.spenco.com*).
- Spyroflex is a thin two-layered polyurethane membrane with a moisture-vapor–permeable and microporous outer layer (*http://www.outdoorrx.com*).
- Gel toe caps will protect the whole toe if athletes have toe hot spots or blisters. The caps are either solid gel or a fabric with gel inside. Bunga Toe Caps (*http://www.bungapads.com*), Bunhead's Jelly Toes (*http://www.bunheads.com*), Hapad's PediFix Visco-Gel Toe Caps (*http://www.hapad.com*), and Pro-Tec's Toe Caps (*http://www.pro-tecathletics.com*) are examples of these caps. With care, these caps can be washed and reused.

Sterile Wound-Dressing Products

Sterile dressings are useful to manage extreme blisters and cases where the skin has separated from the foot. Apply these products over open blisters or raw skin. The dressings require a tape covering or self-adhering wrap to hold them in place. These dressings are typically available only through medical supply stores but may also be found through an Internet search:

- AmeriGel's Wound Dressings and Hydrogel Saturated Gauze Dressings
- Cramer Products' Nova Derm Wound Dressings
- Ferris' PolyMem Wound Care Dressings
- Mueller Sports Medicine's Dermal Pads
- Spenco 2nd Skin Moist Burn Pads
- Spyroflex Wound Care Blister Dressing Pads
- Xeroform

Taping for Blisters

The benefits of taping are well proven. Tape can be applied before an event as a proactive preventive measure or in a reactive mode after hot spots or blisters develop; to socks over where hot spots or blisters typically develop; and inside their shoes or boots to cover irritating footwear seams. The friction points on the feet will also have what amounts to an additional layer of skin.

Types of Tape

The following tapes are well suited for taping feet:

- Duct tape is a 2-inch-wide, very sticky silver tape with a fabric core that has excellent adhesive qualities. It does not breathe but is very strong and tough and can withstand almost unlimited friction. Use only a single thickness because additional layers become too hard and unyielding. Buy high-quality duct tape, which is available at any hardware store.
- EnduraFix is a 2-inch-wide breathable tape, with a removable backing, that provides extra comfort and protection especially to sensitive skin. It works well on toes, over hot spots, on heels, and for anchoring tape between the toes. It is similar to HypaFix (*http://www.optp.com*).
- EnduraSports tape is breathable and has a specially formulated zinc-oxide heat-sensitive adhesive that is triggered to ensure secure adhesion – even with perspiration, water, or cold weather. This 1-inch-wide tape is strong and similar to Leukotape, working well on the balls of the feet and heels (*http://www.optp.com*).
- HypaFix is a 2-inch-wide woven, breathable tape with a removable backing. It works well on toes and between toes and around the heels.
- Kinesio Tex tape is a ribbed tape that stretches longitudinally. Designed for muscle taping, it comes in 2-, 3-, and 4-inch widths. This tape has a removable paper backing and is very smooth and breathable. After applying, rubbing the tape briskly generates heat, which bonds it to the skin. Be sure to use the water-resistant type (*http://www.KinesioTex-tape.com*).
- Leukotape P is a nonbreathable 1½-inch tape made by BSM Medical. It is strong and very sticky – a good choice as an alternative to duct tape. It works well on the bottom of the feet and heels.
- Micropore is a paper tape made by 3M that comes in ½- and 1-inch widths. It's an excellent tape for toes. The ½-inch width is sometimes used to anchor the edges of tape as is described in the next section.
- Athletic white tape is not well suited for taping feet.

Taping Tips

Preparation of the skin is important. Before taping, clean the feet of their natural oils, dust, and dirt. This is vital to getting a good stick with the tape. Wipe the feet with a towel to remove any lubricants and grit. Then use rubbing alcohol to clean the feet. Next, apply tincture of benzoin as a taping base to hold the tape to the skin and let it dry. Then apply the tape based on the athlete's specific needs or problems.

When the tape is applied, that part of the foot should be flexed to its maximum extension. Cut the ends of the tape so they are rounded. A thin layer of a lubricant under the tape at problem areas like the ball of the foot or the heel can help with the removal of the tape. When applying the tape, keep it as smooth as possible. Ridges in the tape may cut into the skin and lead to irritation that may cause blisters. If the tape must be overlapped, be sure the overlapping edge of the tape is in the same direction as the force of motion. The less overlap the better. Generally speaking, do not tape all the way around toes or the foot because of possible circulation problems. If after applying tape, the skin or portion of the foot farthest from the body becomes discolored, cool, or numb, loosen the tape.

Place a single layer of toilet paper or tissue, or a dab of zinc oxide or Desitin, over any existing blisters where the outer skin has pulled loose from the inner skin. This keeps the adhesive from attacking the sensitive area and protects the blistered skin when the tape is removed. Do not to use gauze because it is too abrasive.

After the foot is taped, choose from one of the finishing touches. Apply a sprinkling of powder to the sticky areas that are not taped to counteract any adhesive left uncovered. Or run a thin layer of a lubricant over the tape and around the edges. This allows the taped surface to slip easily across friction points without snagging. Figure 38.9 shows an example of preventive taping with a coating of powder to cut any exposed adhesive.

As important as taping the feet is, all those benefits can be lost if the athlete is not careful in putting on or taking off his or her socks. The socks should be rolled on and off. All the time and value of a good tape job can be ruined when changing socks too fast. The use of a

shoehorn is recommended to keep additional friction off the heel as it is lowered into the shoe.

When removing tape, work slowly and carefully. You do not want to pull off a layer of skin or a toenail with the tape. Work from the sides to the center, using the fingers of one hand to hold the skin while pulling the tape with the other hand. The use of baby oil and gentle massage to roll off the tape and excessive adhesive can help. Use fingernail polish remover to get rid of any leftover adhesive on skin or toenails.

In events where there are nightly rest periods, patients can benefit from removing the tape, cleaning their feet and allowing them to dry as much as possible. The downside of this is they will then need new taping or patching before starting the next day.

Taping the Ball of the Foot

The easiest method of taping the ball of the foot is to apply a strip of tape at a right angle, with the trouble spot dead center on the tape. Then pull the ends of the tape up, cutting them an inch up on either side of the foot. Cut the tape at the forward edge of the ball of the foot so it does not contact or cut into the crease at the base of the toes or the toes themselves. Figure 38.10 shows Kinesio-Tex tape on the ball of the foot. Kinesio-Tex tape is especially good because it stretches lengthwise and can be stretched to the shape of the foot.

Taping the Heel

Many times, feet blister at the area where the insole meets the inside of the shoe. After prepping the skin, the side of the heel can be taped by either running a piece

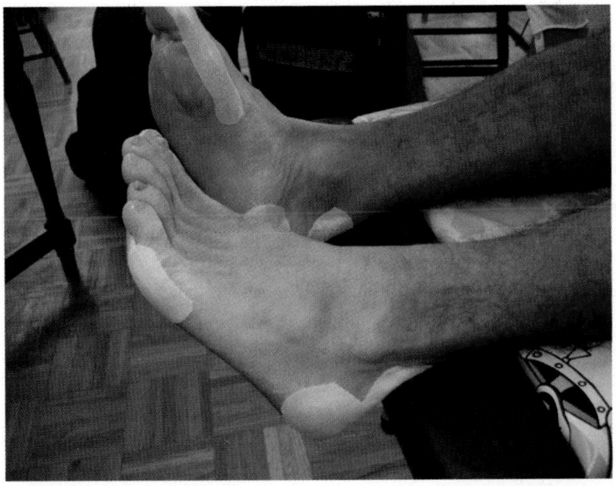

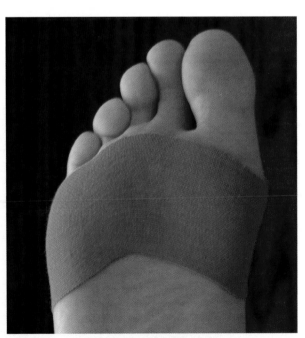

Figure 38.9. Preventive tape on the Achilles, heels, and sides of the forefoot. Credit: John Vonhof.

Figure 38.10. Ball of the foot tape, applied to follow the curve of the foot at the base of the toes. Credit: Denise Jones.

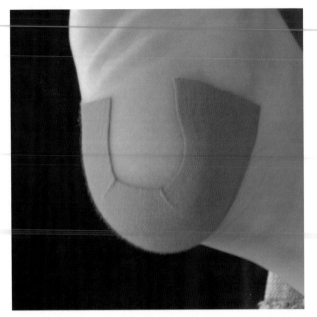

Figure 38.11. The first strip to tape a heel. Credit: Denise Jones.

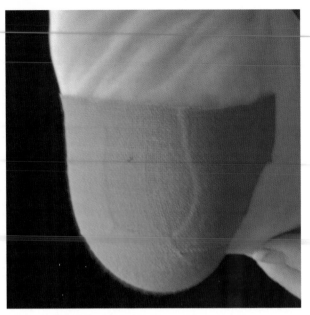

Figure 38.12. The second strip side to side over the first strip. Credit: Denise Jones.

of tape around the back of the heel or under the heel from side to side. With either method, cut the tape into a V as necessary to avoid folds in the tape. Try to avoid taping over the two anklebones. Figure 38.11 shows Kinesio-Tex tape around the back and sides of the heel. Note the V cuts to avoid folds. Then Figure 38.12 shows a strip of tape under the heel from side to side. The heel is now completely protected with tape. In Figure 38.13, note the Micropore tape applied to help anchor the edges of Kinesio-Tex tape. This is optional when taping large areas. An alternative is to have the patients wear socks over the tape to hold it in place and maintain its integrity.

Taping the Bottom of the Foot
Apply tape to the ball of the foot as described previously; then tape the heel as is described next. Add one or more strips between the ball of the foot and the heel. Figure 38.14 shows how five strips of tape have completely taped the bottom of the foot. Benzoin should be applied to all areas being taped.

Taping the Toes
Following skin prepping, the first piece of tape goes from underneath the toe, just before the crease, over the tip and finishes on top of the toe (Figure 38.15). Fold the excess over at the tips of the toes, pinching the top and bottom together. Cut off any wrinkles or V corners of the tape with sharp scissors, so it conforms to the toe perfectly (note the trimmed V in Figure 38.16). The second piece starts inside the toe, goes around the tip of the toe to the other side (Figure 38. 17). When the toes are finished, bend them back and forth to make sure they feel good and are not restricted. Make sure that all areas of

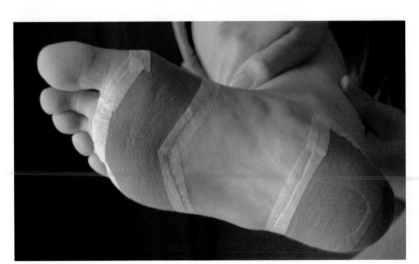

Figure 38.13. Ball of the foot and heel taped with Kinesio-Tex and anchored with Micropore tape. Credit: Denise Jones.

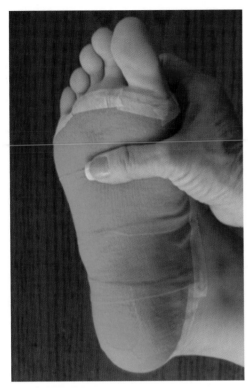

Figure **38.14.** A complete bottom of the foot taping. Credit: Denise Jones.

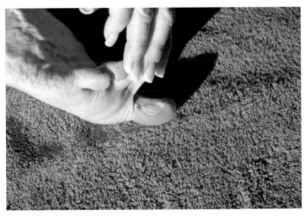

Figure **38.15.** Kinesio-Tex tape bottom to top, medial view. Credit: Denise Jones.

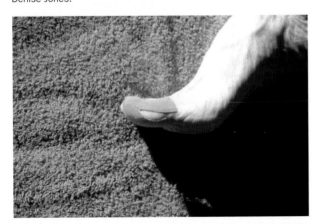

Figure **38.16.** Kinesio-Tex tape bottom to top, lateral view. Credit: Denise Jones.

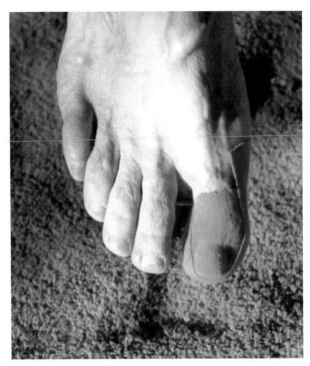

Figure **38.17.** Kinesio-Tex tape around the toe, side to side. Credit: Denise Jones.

the toe are secure with no gaps and no ridges. After taping, use foot powder to keep feet dry within the socks.

Toes can also be taped as needed without covering the whole toe. Figures 38.18 and 38.19 show Hypafix applied to sides of toes. Both Micropore and Hypafix tapes hold well and are smooth.

Taping between the Toe and Foot

This important method comes in handy for those hard-to-tape areas at the base of toes or between the toes. If there is a blister at the base of the toes or between the toes, apply a patch of your choice. Then apply a piece of tape on the ball of the foot as described previously. Now cut a short strip of Hypafix or EnduraFix tape in a figure-eight, spread the toes, and apply the tape first to the tape on the ball of the foot, pulling it fairly tight between the toes and adhere it to the top of the foot. Now you have a patch on the blister protected by tape, and the whole thing is held firmly in place by the figure-eight tape anchoring the edge of the tape at the base of the toes. In Figure 38.18, you can see Leukotape tape on the ball of the foot and the bottom of the figure-eight piece of tape. Figure 38.19 shows the top of the foot with the figure-eight piece of tape anchored on the top of the foot.

Tape Alternatives

There are several good products to use in addition to or instead of taping. Engo Performance Patches are low-friction patches uniquely applied to blister-prone areas of footwear, insoles, socks, and athletic equipment – not

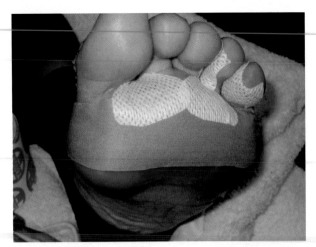

Figure 38.18. Two pieces of Hypafix figure-eight cut tape between the toes. Credit: John Vonhof.

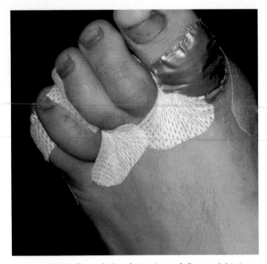

Figure 38.19. Top of the foot view of figure-eight tape between toes. Credit: John Vonhof.

skin (*http://www.GoEngo.com*). Bunhead Gel Jelly Toes (*http://www.bunheads.com*), Hapad PediFix Visco-Gel Toe Caps (*http://www.hapad.com*), and Pro-Tec's Toe Caps (*http://www.pro-tecathletics.com*) are made of polymers to cushion and protect toes from friction trauma.

BUNIONS

A bunion or hallux abductor valgus (HAV) is an exostosis located at the dorsal and medial aspect of the first metatarsal phalangeal joint. A displacement of the first metatarsal bone medial and a simultaneous displacement of the hallux lateral cause this bump to appear. Over time, the hallux can come to rest plantar, or occasionally dorsal to the second digit. The bony bump is most often a form of degenerative arthritis. A similar bump at the outer head of the fifth metatarsal is called a bunionette or Taylor's bunion. These are formed when the fifth metatarsal moves laterally and the fifth digit then starts to move toward the midline.

The deformity widens the forefoot and can exaggerate the pronatory forces, thus resulting in a decreased medial arch. The motion of the joint and shoe pressure can cause pain. There may be corns on the adjacent sides of the digits. A callus may develop over the bunion, and bursitis can form.

Treating Bunion Pain

* Footwear needs to be wide and deep enough in the forefoot and toebox.
* Encourage the use of wider shoes, pads between the big and first toes, arch supports, and warm soaks.
* The use of antiinflammatory medication may be warranted.
* Elevate the foot and apply ice.
* Lace the first few loops of the shoelace loosely, tie a knot, and then lace the rest of the way up the shoe.
* Cutting an aperture in the shoe can prove some relief.

DISLOCATIONS

A dislocation is a complete displacement of bone from its normal position at a joint's surface, which disrupts the articulation of two or three bones at that junction and alters alignment. The dislocation may be complete, where the joint surfaces are completely separated, or incomplete (subluxation), where the joint is only slightly displaced. The dislocation may be caused by a direct blow or injury, or by a ligament's tearing.

In the foot, the most common dislocations are the toes. Any of the toes can be dislocated, but the most typical are the big toe or the small toe. The ankle can be dislocated by any combination of fractures of the tibia or fibula, resulting in a displaced talus. Ankle dislocations can be a major lower leg injury with severe consequences if the circulation to the foot is compromised. When viewing a gross deformity, it should be assumed that a fracture or avulsion fracture is present, and the patient once stabilized should be transferred to an emergency room for an X-ray.

Treating Dislocations

Dislocated toes are fairly simple to treat. First, access the neurovascular status. Does the patient have palpable dorsalis pedis (DP) and posterior tibial (PT) arteries along with capillary fill time (CFT) to the digit? Can the patient feel the difference between sharp and dull with the end of a Q-tip? Second, prepare for reduction. Several types of anesthesia can be used. Local injection of 3–6 cc of 1 or 2% lidocaine plain or 0.25 or 0.5% marcaine plain. Valium 5 or 10 mg PO can easily be used for severe muscle spasms. The injection for a digital block can be

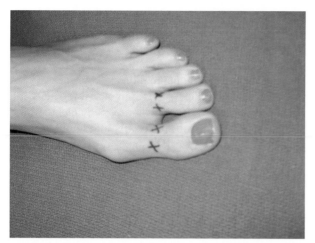

Figure 38.20. Marked injection sites at the intermetatarsal space. Credit: Zak H. Weis.

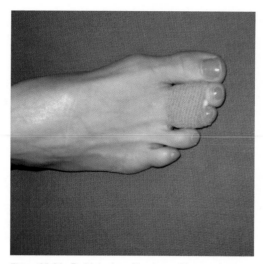

Figure 38.21. Buddy-taping of two toes with gauze between toes. Credit: Zak H. Weis.

done in the intermetatarsal space on the adjacent sides of the digit (Figure 38.20). Anesthetic can be placed in all four quadrants by starting your injection from the dorsal aspect proceeding plantar. The plantar digital nerves supply the distal tuft and nail bed. Avoiding a pure digital block is recommended so the clinician will not be fighting the hydraulic effects upon reduction.

To effect the reduction, with one hand, stabilize the metatarsal heads and midfoot, with your thumb plantarly and your fingers dorsal to the injured toe. With the other hand, increase the deformity, exert traction to the toe while pulling slowly and steadily on the displaced section of toe, and then reduce the deformity. Pull firmly enough that it clears the previous section of toe. The connecting ligament will then pull the toe back into place almost automatically. Examining the CFT and neurological status is of utmost importance at this stage. If the neurovascular state has been compromised, then attempting the reduction over again can be of great benefit and may release impingement of the neurovascular bundle.

The toe then needs to be buddy-taped to the toe or toes next to it for stabilization. The less stable digit should be splinted to a more stable digit. For example, the dislocated fifth digit should be taped to the fourth, and the dislocated fourth should be taped to the third. If the second is dislocated it should be taped to the third digit due to the instability of the first ray and the often-large gap in the first interspace. If the hallux is dislocated, it should be splinted to the second digit. This will aid in the inherent stability. As shown in Figure 38.21, a small piece of gauze, cotton, or tissue between the taped toes will prevent skin breakdown if the tape or Coban is on for any great length of time. After this has been completed, a reassessment of the neurovascular status should be accessed for any changes.

A firm-soled shoe like a surgical shoe will prevent toe off and help keep the toe in line and prevent motion at

the metatarsal phalangeal joint. Frequent icing and elevation in the next 48 hours is recommended.

Ankle dislocations should be approached in a stepwise fashion. The assessment of the neurovascular status should be accessed (sharp/dull, CFT, DP & PT). Anesthesia should be used. A local injection 10–15 cc of 1 or 2% lidocaine plain or 0.25 or 0.5% marcaine plain in an ankle block should be performed (tibial, sural, cutaneous saphenous, intermediate dorsal cutaneous, superficial and deep peroneal – Figures 38.22, 38.23, and 38.24). Valium 5 or 10 mg PO can easily be used for severe muscle spasms to ease the reduction. The injection can be done in the following steps:

1. **Ankle block sural** (Figure 38.22) – posterior and inferior to the lateral malleolus. This site may be used to incorporate the intermediate dorsal cutaneous nerve that communicates dorsally.
2. **Ankle block peroneal** (Figure 38.23) – the deep and superficial peroneal. This site may also be used to

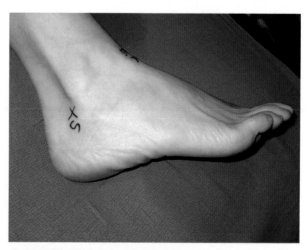

Figure 38.22. Marked site for ankle block sural. Credit: Zak H. Weis.

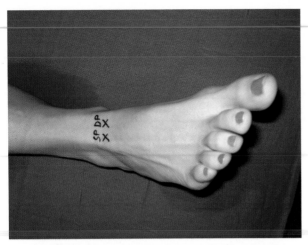

Figure 38.23. Marked site for ankle block peroneal. Credit: Zak H. Weis.

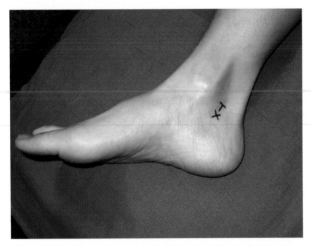

Figure 38.24. Marked site for ankle block tibial. Credit: Zak H. Weis.

incorporate the cutaneous branches of the saphenous nerve medially.

3. **Ankle block tibial** (Figure 38.24) – posterior to the medial malleolus. This site may also be used to incorporate the cutaneous branches of the saphenous nerve medially.

Temporary correction and stabilization of an ankle dislocation and related fracture can be accomplished by

stabilizing the lower leg, increasing the deformity, distracting the deformity, and then reducing the deformity to its natural neutral position. Palpating the subtailor joint with the thumb and forefinger in the medial and lateral gutters can help guide the ankle into place. After this has been completed, it is imperative to check the DP and PT with CFT. If these are not palpable, than the reduction technique must be reattempted until the vascular status has been reestablished.

The foot, ankle, and lower leg then need to be stabilized with a splint. Use any available materials to keep the extremity stable. Check the toes frequently for normal skin color and warmth, which indicates good circulation during the splinting. Two different splinting techniques are common – the sugar tong and the posterior splint. In the opinion of the authors, a posterior splint for this particular set of fractures is more stable. The posterior splint allows for swelling and prevents dorsal, plantar, medial, and lateral motion around the ankle and subtailor joints. Careful attention needs to be addressed so as not to compress the common peroneal nerve that is by the head of the fibula. A dislocated ankle needs to be treated by an emergency room as soon as possible. Below are step-by-step instructions and photos of how to apply a posterior splint (Figures 38.25 through 38.28):

1. Place one or two rolls of web roll or cast padding round the foot, ankle, and leg. Do not cover the digits or compress the common peroneal nerve (Figure 38.25). In a pinch, pre-tape-wrap can be used.
2. Wrap a 3-inch Ace wrap around the foot, ankle, and leg – no more proximal than the cast padding (Figure 38.26).
3. Conform the cast to the back of the leg, ankle, and foot. See the next paragraph for information on the angle of the foot to the leg. Extend the cast beyond the digits to act as a protective shield. It is helpful to have an assistant hold the leg and bend the knee to reduce the effects of the gastrocnemius. In the absence of casting materials, a Sam Splint works well (Figure 38.27).
4. Wrap a 6-inch Ace wrap around the foot, ankle, and leg, and check the common peroneal and CFT of the digits (Figure 38.28).

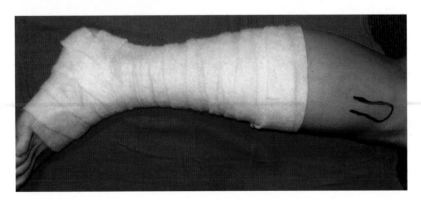

Figure 38.25. Posterior splint – step 1, web roll wrapped. Credit: Zak H. Weis.

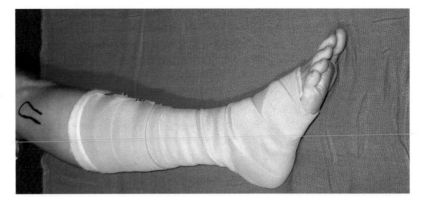

Figure 38.26. Posterior splint – step 2, application of Ace wrap. Credit: Zak H. Weis.

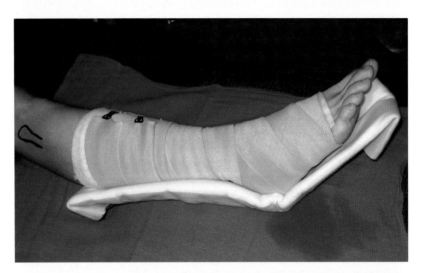

Figure 38.27. Posterior splint – step 3, application of casting material. Credit: Zak H. Weis.

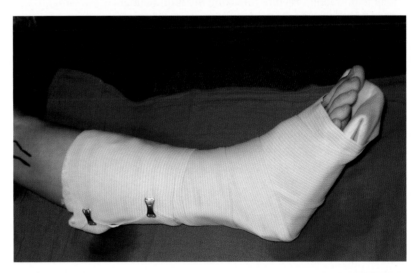

Figure 38.28. Posterior splint – step 4, final Ace wrap applied. Credit: Zak H. Weis.

When a posterior splint is applied, the angle of the foot, relative to the leg, depends on the condition being treated:

- Neutral or 90° is standard for most soft tissue and fractures.
- Plantarflexed for Achilles tendon injury.
- Do not move it for fractures that you are concerned about neurovascular compromise with motion.

- Dorsiflexed and later deviation for peroneal tendon tears.
- Move the ankle and foot joints in a triplanar manner to take the pressure off the tendon or structure in question.

If either a toe or ankle dislocation is an "open" dislocation, where the bone has come through the skin, extra care must be taken. This open, or complex, dislocation is usually associated with a fracture, and the bone may still be outside of the skin or may have pulled back inside. First, clean the wound with a lavage of normal saline or sterile water. A 20-cc syringe should provide enough hydraulic pressure to void the area of most particulate matter. Avoid closing the wound at this time due to the nonsterile environment. Packing the wound with betadine-soaked gauze can be helpful to keep the flora count to a minimum. Then proceed with the reduction and apply a splint to the extremity. Check the end(s) of the extremity farthest from the body to be sure there is adequate circulation, adjusting the extremity as necessary. Starting the patient on oral antibiotic can be very helpful especially if your location is remote. Use a broad-spectrum antibiotic such as Levaquin 750 mg QD or a combination of Clindamycin 300 mg QID/Ciprofloxacin 500 mg BID. When the open dislocation is stabilized, seek out immediate medical attention.

FRACTURES

Any bone in the foot can fracture; however, some are more prone to injury than others. The terms "break" and "fracture" are synonymous – both describe a structural break in the continuity of the bone. A fracture may occur from a fall, the twisting motion of a turned ankle, a blow from hitting a foot on a rock or tree root, or simply from a bad foot plant. The toes are the most likely bones to fracture in the foot – usually the first (big toe) and the fifth (small toe). A Jones fracture (breaking the fifth metatarsal base on the outside of the foot) is common. This type of fracture is common with a fall or loss of balance where a sudden and undue amount of pressure is put on the outside of the foot to force an inversion injury. But there are many types of fractures:

- *Avulsion* – the tearing away of a part of the bone attached to a ligament or tendon.
- *Butterfly* – a bone fragment shaped like a butterfly and part of a comminuted fracture.
- *Comminuted* – more than two fragments; may be splintered.
- *Complete* – the bone is completely broken through.
- *Displaced* – bone fragments are moved away from each other.
- *Impacted* – fragments are compressed by force into each other or adjacent bone.
- *Incomplete* – the continuity of the bone is destroyed on only one side.
- *Nondisplaced* – the bone pieces are still together in the correct locations/angles.
- *Segmental* – several large fractures in the same bone.
- *Spiral* – the fracture line is spiral in shape.

Fractures usually manifest themselves with a great deal of pain and tenderness directly above the fracture site. When a soft tissue injury has occurred, there will also be discoloration of the skin proximal and distal to the fracture. Fractures that are ignored can result in a malunion or nonunion of the pieces of bone as they heal. This could require surgery to correctly align the bone ends.

Emergency room physicians and sports specialists often use tuning forks and the Ottawa ankle rules[13] to determine the likelihood of an ankle fracture before an X-ray is taken (and to avoid unnecessary X-rays). The tuning fork is only 50% predictive of a fracture; however, it can provide a diagnostic aid when no further equipment is available. This technique is best used when the tuning fork is struck and the base is placed on the bony prominence close to the fracture. The patient will elicit a painful response to the slight vibration of the fragment; however, too much edema and improper technique can mislead the clinician. The Ottawa study takes two approaches:

- Pain in the malleolar (ankle bones) zone and either an inability to bear weight immediately and in the emergency room, or bone tenderness at the posterior (back) edge of either malleolus
- Pain in the midfoot zone and either an inability to bear weight immediately and in the emergency room, or bone tenderness at the navicular (the bone at the top front of the foot at the curve up the ankle) or fifth metatarsal (the midfoot bone on the outside of the foot)

Treating Fractures

When treating digital fractures that are grossly displaced, first assess the neurovascular status. Does the patient have palpable DP and PT arteries along with CFT to the digit? Can the patient feel the difference between sharp and dull with the end of a Q-tip? Second, prepare for reduction. Several types of anesthesia can be used. Local injection of 3–6 cc of 1 or 2% lidocaine plain or 0.25 or 0.5% marcaine plain. Valium 5 or 10 mg PO can easily be used for severe muscle contractures. The injection for a digital block can be done in the intermetatarsal space on the adjacent sides of the digit (see Figure 38.20). Avoiding a pure digital block is recommended so the clinician will not be fighting the hydraulic effects upon reduction. With one hand, stabilize the metatarsal heads and midfoot, with your thumb plantarly and your fingers dorsal to the injured toe. With the other hand increase the deformity, exert traction to the toe while pulling slowly and steadily on the displaced section of toe, then reduce the deformity. Pull firmly enough that it clears the previous section of toe. The connecting ligament will then pull the toe back into place almost automatically.

Examining the CFT and neurological status is of utmost importance at this stage. If the neurovascular state has been compromised, attempting the reduction over again can be of great benefit and may release impingement of the neurovascular bundle. The toe then needs to be buddy-taped to the toe or toes next to it for stabilization (see Figure 38.21). The less stable digit should be splinted to a more stable digit. For example the dislocated fifth digit should be taped to the fourth and the dislocated fourth should be taped to the third. If the second is dislocated it should be taped to the third digit due to the instability of the first ray and the often large gap in the first interspace. If the hallux is dislocated it should be splinted to the second digit. This will aid in the inherent stability. A small piece of gauze, cotton, or tissue between the taped toes will prevent skin breakdown if the tape or Coban is on for any great length of time. Once this has been completed, a reassessment of the neurovascular status should be assessed for any changes. A firm-soled shoe, like a surgical shoe, will prevent toe off, and help keep the toe in line and prevent motion at the metatarsal phalangeal joint. Frequent icing and elevation in the next 48 hours is recommended.

Ankle, midtarsal and metatarsal fractures should be approached in a stepwise manner. The assessment of the neurovascular status should be accessed (sharp/dull, CFT, DP, and PT). The use of an anesthesia is recommended. Local injection 10–15 cc of 1 or 2% lidocaine plain or 0.25 or 0.5% marcaine plain in an ankle block should be performed (tibial, sural, cutaneous saphenous, intermediate dorsal cutaneous, superficial, and deep peroneal, see Figures 38.22 through 38.24). Valium 5 or 10 mg PO can easily be used for severe muscle spasms to ease the reduction.

To temporarily correct and stabilize an ankle dislocation and related fracture, stabilize the lower leg, increase the deformity, distracting the deformity, and reduce the deformity to its natural neutral position. Palpating the subtailor joint with the thumb and forefinger in the medial and lateral gutters can help guide the ankle into place. After this has been completed, it is imperative to check the DP and PT with CFT. If these are not palpable, the reduction technique must be reattempted until the vascular status has been reestablished. The foot, ankle, and lower leg then need to be stabilized with a splint. Use any available materials to keep the extremity stable. Check the toes frequently for normal skin color and warmth, which indicates good circulation during the splinting. Two different splinting techniques are common – the sugar tong and the posterior splint. In the opinion of the authors, the posterior splint for this particular set of fractures if more stable. The posterior splint allows for swelling and prevents dorsal, plantar, medial, and lateral motion around the ankle and subtailor joints. Refer to the instruction and photos on applying a posterior splint (Figures 38.25 through 38.28). Careful attention needs to be addressed to not compress the common peroneal nerve by the head of the fibula. A dislocated ankle needs to be treated in emergency room as soon as possible.

Standard practice with fractures is to immobilize the joint proximal and the joint distal to the fracture. Sam Splints are a good addition to the medical kit to use when splinting is necessary.

Stress Fractures

Stress fractures are a common sports injury. Sudden or repetitive stress, usually from overuse without proper conditioning, results in a small crack in the outer cortex of the affected bone. Over time, if not treated, this crack will develop into a through and through fracture of the bone. Often the patient will have no recollection of having injured the foot and will disregard its severity.

The most common foot bones to stress fracture are the second and third metatarsal bones in the forefoot. These are referred to as "march fractures." Some doctors will use an X-ray to make the diagnosis, but often a stress fracture does not show on an initial X-ray because the bone's callus formation has not yet taken place at the fracture site. A bone scan or MRI is useful for a questionable diagnosis and will usually confirm whether it is a stress fracture.

Other possible causes of stress fractures include wearing worn-out or poor-fitting shoes, or ill-fitting insoles; abnormal foot structure or mechanics (pathologic supination and or pronation problems or leg-length discrepancies); or tightness and inflexibility as seen in muscular imbalance. You may recommend additional supplements or prescription medication in the patient's diet and/or a DEXA scan bone-density test. Female athletes who have infrequent periods are most at risk for stress fractures.

At the point of the stress fracture, there is typically pain to the touch, often first felt as a dull ache or soreness. The pain usually becomes worse as the fracture progresses and more soft tissues and periosteum become compromised. Swelling is common. Stress fractures are most common from overuse, overtraining, or a change in running surfaces – from a softer to a harder surface.

Treating Stress Fractures

Stress fractures should be treated just like a fracture in the triage phase. The importance of identifying the fracture is imperative to the treatment. This can only be done in the hospital setting.

An Ace wrap or compression sock will help control swelling. An orthopedic or wooden shoe may be used to splint the foot. Antiinflammatories are helpful. Elevation of the foot above the level of the heart will help reduce pain and swelling. Ice the area 20 minutes at a time three to four times a day. Difficult cases may require splinting, casting, or surgery.

HAGLUND'S DEFORMITY

Haglund's deformity, or retrocalcaneal bursitis, is a bump in the form of an enlargement of the posterior lateral aspect of the calcaneus at or near the area of the insertion of the Achilles tendon. Sometimes it has the appearance of a square, shelf-like bump. When the wearing of shoes irritates the bump, it becomes red, swollen, and painful. The tissues over the bone bump may thicken forming a callus, which can grow quite thick and become inflamed. The enlarged bone may also irritate the Achilles tendon, resulting in pain with motion of the ankle joint and foot. It may be present in conjunction with Achilles tendonitis, but it is a separate diagnosis. Shoes with a rigid heel counter tend to rub up and down on the calcaneus. There is a bursa sac between the Achilles tendon and the calcaneus that becomes irritated and over time bursitis may develop.

Treating Haglund's Deformity

* The focus of treatment should start with reducing the painful pressure on the bump.
* Changing to shoes with a lower or softer heel counter or a heel counter that is notched for the Achilles tendon can help.
* A heel pad can lift the heel up above the part of the heel counter that is rubbing on the bump.
* Cut a donut out of molefoam to pad the bump and distribute the pressure.
* NSAIDs can be taken to reduce the pain.
* If this condition becomes unbearable during an event, cutting a notch or slice into the heel counter can relieve some of the pressure off the bump.
* Application of an Engo Blister Prevention Patch at the point of friction on the shoe can provide some relief, but it should be applied when the shoe is dry.
* Avoid steroid injections due to its proximity to the Achilles tendon and the contraindications of increased risk of rupture.

METATARSALGIA/CAPSULITIS

Metatarsalgia/capsulitis is pain underneath the metatarsal heads of the foot. It typically occurs when one of the metatarsal is plantarflexed (i.e., points downward). Typically the second metatarsal head is affected, but it can also be any of the metatarsal heads. The patient may complain of a small stone in their shoe, or feeling pain, a burning sensation, or swelling at the ball of the foot. By dorsiflexing the digit and then slightly pressing dorsally on the affected metatarsal head, you can usually identify the painful area. Typically the metatarsal head that is lower then the others is causing the pain and pressure. There will often be a callus at the pressure point. Metatarsalgia/capsulitis is often associated with Morton's foot.

Shoes that are too narrow in the forefoot or laced too tight over the forefoot area, or an insert that has been crushed down over time and miles can aggravate this problem. To see how the pressure in a narrow shoe affects the metatarsals, try this simple test. Grasp the foot around the base of the toes and squeeze gently. See how it forces the metatarsals downward (on the bottom of the foot) and results in increased impact to the area with each step. For proper prevention, athletes should wear shoes that fit correctly, use lacing techniques that do not put pressure on the forefoot, and have accommodations made to the insole to off-weight the affected area of tenderness.

Treating Metatarsalgia

A cushioned metatarsal pad made of ¼- or ⅛-inch plastizote or felt can provide relief from metatarsalgia. These pads can be fashioned in a "cookie" style or in a "horseshoe" shape, to float the metatarsal head (see Figure 38.29 for an example). If a pad does not help, try cutting a small hole in the insole under the painful metatarsal head. This is done to off-weight the callused area and/or tender metatarsal phalangeal joint. With the plantarflexed metatarsal, the cookie will raise the metatarsal base and shaft, thus raising the head and off-weighting the lesion. To find the right position for a pad, first make a mark at the sore area with marking pen or lipstick. Then have the patient stand on the insert that you have taken out of the shoe. Stick felt or plastizote pad to the insole (the patient may want to have the pad on the bottom of the insert) with the opening toward the toes. Wearing shoes with a wide forefoot and high and wide toebox is also recommended. A custom orthotic may be necessary and can more easily incorporate these concepts. The adjunctive therapy of NSAIDs can be added (ibuprofen 800 mg TID). This will act as an analgesic and an antiinflammatory.

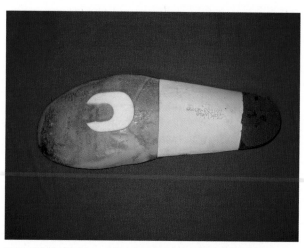

Figure 38.29. Metatarsal float pad cut in a horseshoe shape, applied on the underside of the insole. Credit: Zak H. Weis.

Treatment of this condition should be first attempted with biomechanical changes and by NSAIDs as noted previously. If these options fail, the clinician can attempt a medrol Dose Pak or the use of injectable steroids can also be used. Mix 1 cc of injectable steroid (such as Kenalog 40, methylpredinsolone 20 mg, or dexamethasone sodium phos.) with 1 cc of 0.5 or 0.25% marcaine or 1 or 2% lidocaine. Placement of the injection should be made from the dorsal aspect of the metatarsal phalangeal joint. Avoid a plantar injection; it is very painful and unnecessary. It is very important to clean the area thoroughly prior to use. It is normally in the best interest of the patient to avoid an injection for this condition in the field. Extremely unclean environments are normally present and opening up a possible pathway for infection in a chronically contaminated environment should be used with extreme caution.

MORTON'S NEUROMA

Morton's neuroma is pain associated with a nerve inflammation usually affecting the third and fourth toes. It will sometimes be felt between the other digits. The common digital nerves running between the metatarsal heads and the toes have become inflamed and irritated as they are squeezed and stretched at the base of the toes. The painful, swollen nerve is the neuroma. There is typically tingling, burning, or a pins-and-needles sensation that radiates to the medial side of one digit and the lateral side of the adjacent digits. Some people describe the sensation as walking on a pebble. If you press with your thumb at the base of the fourth toe and the patient indicates pain, it could be a neuroma. Often if the clinician pinches down on the space between the metatarsal shafts, the same discomfort can be elicited. Another way to diagnose this is to squeeze all the metatarsal heads together, and often an audible click or pain will be elicited. If untreated, scar tissue forms around the nerve, and it becomes more painful.

This condition can be caused by a shoe's tight toebox that compresses the forefoot or by the nerves being pressured by the metatarsal heads and the bases of the toes. This condition can also be caused by metatarsals that are congenitally close together and, when squeezed, irritate the nerve. Sports that place a significant amount of pressure on the forefoot area can cause inflammation of the nerves. When walking or running, the motion of coming up onto one's toes can cause the ligaments supporting the metatarsal bones to compress the nerve between the toes.

Treating Morton's Neuroma

Treatments include applying ice to the pain area, wearing wider shoes, and employing a more lax forefoot lacing technique, using a more cushioned insole, and inserting

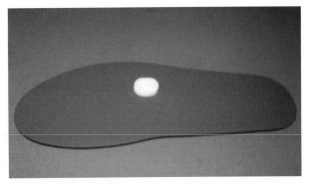

Figure 38.30. A neuroma pad applied to the top of an insole. Credit: Zak H. Weis.

in shoes metatarsal splay pads that take pressure off the metatarsal heads and nerve. The pad reduces forefoot pressure and spreads the toes and metatarsals, which can relieve the pain. To find the right position for a pad, first make a mark at the metatarsal heads of the digits that are causing the discomfort with a marking pen or lipstick. Then take the insert out of the shoe and transfer the mark onto the insole by having the patient stand on the insole. Stick the pad to the top of the insole with the small cookie at the base of the metatarsals. Care needs to be taken to make sure that the pad is placed proximal to the neuroma and not under it. Figure 38.30 shows a neuroma pad, ¼-inch felt applied to insert in the proximal half of metatarsal shaft region

Massaging the foot usually helps to relieve the pain. Use ice to help reduce pain and inflammation. Relief may also be gained by inserting a piece of lamb's wool between the toes.

A course of oral antiinflammatory medication may be suggested (ibuprofen 800 mg TID). Treatment of this condition should be first attempted with biomechanical changes and by NSAIDs as noted previously. If these options fail, the clinician can attempt a medrol Dose Pak, or injectable steroids can also be used. Mix 1 cc of injectable steroid (such as Kenalog 40, methylpredinsolone 20 mg, or dexamethasone sodium phos.) with 1 cc of 0.5 or 0.25% marcaine or 1 or 2% lidocaine. Placement of the injection should be made from the dorsal aspect in the distal third of the metatarsal shaft as shown in Figure 38.31. Splaying the metatarsal heads with your other thumb can be helpful. The clinician will need to make sure he or she is injecting plantar to the transmetatarsal ligament. A common mistake is to inject too far distal to the split of the common digital nerve into its associated digital branches. Avoid a plantar injection if at all possible; it is very painful and unnecessary. It is very important to clean the area thoroughly prior to use. It is normally in the best interest of the patient to avoid an injection for this condition in the field. Extremely unclean environments are normally present and opening up a possible pathway for infection in a chronically contaminated environment should be used with extreme caution.

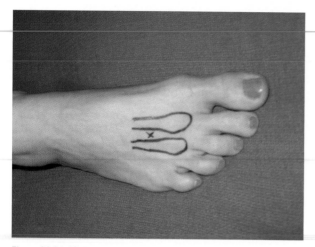

Figure 38.31. Marked site for a neuroma injection. Credit: Zak H. Weis.

NAIL AND DIGITAL PATHOLOGY

Black Toenails

A black toenail, or subungual hematoma, describes a blood-filled swelling under the nail. This common occurrence is caused by the trauma of the toe or toes repetitively bumping against the front of the shoe. Blood pools in the space between the nail plate and nail bed as they separate or compress from repeated trauma. Individuals with Morton's toe are most susceptible to experiencing black toenails. The nail becomes discolored and usually has associated pain. Most often the nail bed turns dark, almost black or blue because of the blood.

Black toenails are often a result of insufficient electrolyte management. Too little sodium makes hands and feet swell. As the tissues swell, the mechanical strength of the nail footing goes down. Then any movement will do tissue damage.

Prevention for those prone to black toenails can be done by properly trimming and filing toenails short (see Toenail Trimming, p. 633), cutting slits in the shoe's toe box, or applying Spenco 2nd Skin under tape wrapped bottom to top around the tip of the toe. Be sure the tape does not irritate adjoining toes.

Treating Black Toenails

If there is no pain from the black toenail, no action may be necessary. If the pain and pressure increases, the pressure must be relieved. To relieve pressure from a black toenail, use one of the following methods, depending on the look of the toenail. The treatment may have to be repeated several times on the same nail or after a period of time. Although the two methods below might sound painful, they are usually not. The blood has separated the nail from the nail bed and is a barrier between the nail and the live skin underneath.

If the discoloration does not extend to the end of the toenail, swab the nail with an alcohol wipe, and use a small nail drill or hypodermic needle (18 gauge) to gently drill a hole in the nail with light pressure and rolling the needle/bit back and forth between your thumb and fingers. The blood will ooze through the hole. Keep slight pressure on the nail bed to help expel the built-up blood. Stopping too soon will cause the blood to clot in the hole and the problem will reoccur. A syringe can be used to extract the fluid (Figure 38.32). An alternative method is to use a match to heat a paper clip and gently penetrate the nail with the heated point. The heat in this method can cauterize the blood and stop the flow of blood out from under the nail. Press on the nail to expel the blood. If the discoloration extends to the end of the toenail, lance the blister under the nail and release the pressure. Holding slight pressure on the nail bed will help expel the blood.

Care must be taken to prevent a secondary bacterial infection through the hole in the nail or at the end of the nail by using an antibiotic ointment and covering the site with a Band-Aid or cover-roll. If the hole seals up, use the drill, needle, or paper clip to open it up again. Loss of the nail usually follows in the months ahead. If the nail is loose, use tape or a Band-Aid to keep the nail from tearing off. When taping the nail apply skin prep, and then apply one piece of tape from the dorsal proximal aspect of the nail, going distal applying pressure to the nail to the nail bed, then proximal around to the plantar aspect of the nail. The second piece of tape may want to be applied starting from the dorsal aspect of the digit then going medial or lateral to anchor the edges of the first piece of tape. Care should be taken not to have a tape edge between the digits.

Typically, reliving pressure under the nail will immediately ease the pain. If the toe is still painful, either pad

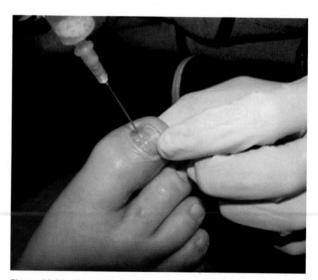

Figure 38.32. Extracting fluid from under a toenail. Credit: Lisa de Speville.

the toe with Spenco 2nd Skin or cut away part of the shoe over the toe. A metatarsal pad can be used to push up the ball of the foot and drop the toes down to a more rectus position, taking pressure off the toenails.

Hammertoes, Claw Toes, and Mallet Toes

Hammertoes are dorsiflexed at the metatarsal phalangeal joint (MPJ), plantarflexed at the proximal interphalangeal joint (PIPJ), and then dorsiflexed at the distal interphalangeal joint (DIPJ). Claw toes are rectus at the MPJ, plantarflexed at the PIPJ, and plantarflexed again at the DIPJ. Mallet toes are rectus at the MPJ and PIPJ and plantarflexed at the DIPJ.

The ligaments and tendons have tightened and are forcing the toes to curl. This can lead to severe pressure and pain. Blisters or corns may form on the dorsal aspect of the joints and calluses at the ends of the toes. Many times when these digits contract, they produce a plantarflexion force on the associated metatarsal head, thus causing a callus on the plantar aspect of this metatarsal head.

Treating Hammertoes, Claw Toes, and Mallet Toes

First step is to address the etiology of the associated digit pathology. Many times if the digits are flexible, an arch support can be applied. This will help reduce the plantarflexion of the metatarsals and also help decrease the bowstringing effect of the flexor and extensor tendons. Another possible treatment is to apply ⅛-inch felt cut out to the plantar aspect of the insert in the shoe. This is done to off-weight the area in pain. If these methods are not successful or if the digits are rigidly contracted, cutting away part of the shoe's toebox over the affected toes will relieve pressure on the toes. This usually allows the other toes additional room so there is less friction against the individual toes. Taping the individual toes can protect them from friction.

Ingrown Toenails

Ingrown toenails or onychocryptosis or paronychia, most common to the big toe, may cause infection and require medical attention. One or both of the medial or lateral nail borders grow into the flesh of the associated labial borders of the toe. The result is erythema, edema, calor, pus, and possible ascending cellulitis proximal to the interphalangeal joint or distal interphalangeal joint. It is sensitive to any degree of pressure. The most common cause of an ingrown toenail is improper nail trimming. Trauma from a stubbed toe or someone stepping on a toe can cause the nail to be jammed into the skin. Repeated trauma, such as the pounding to which athletes typically subject their feet, also can lead to ingrown toenails.

Treating Ingrown Toenails

For nails that are not infected and just painful, an easy way to repair an ingrown toenail requires only a metal nail file and cuticle trimmers. File the entire top surface of the nail from near the cuticle to the tip until you get it as thin as possible. This weakens the nail. Then soak the foot in warm water for about 30 minutes to soften and further weaken the nail or apply hydrogen peroxide–soaked gauze to the nail for 10 minutes.

Then use the cuticle trimmer to free the ingrown portion. A slant back procedure is recommended. Using a standard medical-grade nail nipper or tissue nipper is much more effective than your typical pair of clippers. Start from the distal edge and work proximal, using force to lift the affected border toward the median aspect. If the athlete cannot tolerate the discomfort, do not hesitate to inject with 3 cc of lidocaine (1–2% plain) or marcaine (0.25–0.5% plain) into the middle portion of the proximal phalanx.

Remember the dorsal and plantar digital nerves are on their respective medial and lateral borders. The plantar digital nerve supplies the terminal tuft area and often reaches to the dorsal and distal tip of the digit. Once anesthesia has been tested with a sharp dull test, the athlete may experience pressure but should not experience pain. If pain is elicited 20 minutes after injection, the clinician may want to inject another 3 cc of anesthetic. Diphenhydramine may be used as an injectable local anesthetic when the athlete is allergic to amines. After anesthesia has been obtained, the digit should be cleaned with Betadine.

A finger of a surgical glove can be used as a tourniquet at the level of the proximal phalanx. The nail should be freed with the use of a freer elevator, or the serrated edge of a hemostat can be used (serrated portion always touches the nail and not the tissue). Then, the border can be cut with an English anvil or a medical-grade nail nipper and removed with a hemostat. Care must be taken when cutting the nail portion plantar to the epinychium (within the cuticle or nail fold) to avoid lacerating this tissue if possible. When the offending border has been removed, use the serrated edge of a hemostat or a curette to check for any loose spicules or fragments. Clean the wound with Betadine, apply antibiotic ointment, 2 × 2 gauze, remove the tourniquet and check for capillary fill time, and apply a few layers of Coban to the digit.

The athlete now has several open wounds from the injection and the removed nail. The use of Levaquin 750 mg QD × 10 days or Keflex 500 mg QID × 10 may be needed. Have the athlete check with you every day and change the bandage once to twice a day with antibiotic ointment and a dressing of Band-Aid or cover-roll, or 2 × 2 and Coban. The clinician should keep a close eye on ascending cellulitis, pus, or odor. Soaking the affected foot in warm water with Epsom salts with dressing changes may reduce the infection. Soaking of the foot is not always necessary and is the judgment of the clinician if needed or appropriate based on conditions.

Morton's Foot

Morton's foot, often called Morton's toe, is a common problem in which the second toe, next to the big toe, is longer than the big toe. The first metatarsal is shorter than normal, and this makes the second toe appear longer than it actually is. The constant pressure placed on the longer second toe while walking or standing can lead to callus formation under the second metatarsal head due to this excessive pressure. Because of the excessive pressure on the second metatarsal head in the forefoot, Morton's foot is often associated with metatarsalgia.

Treating Morton's Foot
A metatarsal pad under the metatarsal heads with a cut-out to float the second metatarsal head can relieve some pressure. The use of a nonslippery insole will keep the foot from sliding forward. Consider applying tape to the insole to hold the foot in place. Other options include cutting a slit over or on either side of the insole around the toe to relieve pressure or cut out a small piece of the toebox over the toe. Make sure the toenails are trimmed smooth to keep socks from catching on the nail and putting backward pressure on the toe's nail.

Tape over the top of the toe will protect it from blistering and help pad a corn. If the athlete has pain at the base of the toe, cut a U-shaped pad and position the cutout area at the site of the pain on the underside of the insert. To find the correct position, first make a mark at the sore area with marking pen. Then slide the foot inside the shoe or on the insole that you have removed and have them step down to transfer the ink onto the insole. Stick the pad to the underside of the insole with the opening toward the toes. Make sure the insole is clean and dry or the pads will not stick.

Overlapping Toes

Overlapping toes can lead to hot spots and blisters. This can occur with any toes and cause extreme irritation. Overlapping toes typically involve one toe lying on top of an adjacent toe. The fifth toe is the most affected digit.

Treating Overlapping Toes
Shoes with a high and wide toebox can give toes the space they need. Cutting into the shoe's upper over the affected toes can reduce pressure. Another option is removing the shoe's insole and cutting out a portion of the insole under the affected toes, making a depression for the toes to fit into. Taping the toes with cover-roll is an option to reduce friction of skin against skin. Check the toes for callus and file smooth to reduce irritation on

neighboring toes. Silicone toe spacers can also be used, but they may come loose or move over time.

Stubbed Toes

Stubbed toes can result in a hematoma, a bruise, or even a fracture. They are more common in running shoes than in hiking boots. Check the toe for discoloration that can indicate a deep bruise or a fracture. There may be a laceration into the nail bed or into the toe itself.

Treating Stubbed Toes
Treatment includes buddy-taping, icing the toe, elevating the foot, and wearing a firm-soled shoe or boot. Buddy-taping provides support and a limited degree of immobilization to the toe. Lightly tape the injured toe to the toe next to it after placing a piece of gauze between toes. Do not tape skin to skin. When a stubbed toe does not respond to treatment, an X-ray may be necessary.

If the patient's toenail on the stubbed toe is injured, it's important to prevent the toenail from catching on a sock and tearing off. Wrap either a Band-Aid or tape around the toe to hold the toenail in place. Trimming off any loose parts of the nail can help prevent the nail from lifting off further. When taping the nail, apply skin prep and apply one piece of tape from the dorsal proximal aspect of the nail, distally to the nail and nail bed, and then proximal around to the plantar aspect of the nail. The second piece of tape should be applied, starting from the dorsal aspect of the digit and then going medial or lateral to anchor the edges of the first piece of tape. Take care not to have a tape edge between the digits.

Toenail Fungus

Nail fungus, also known as onychomycosis, is a persistent fungal infection of the nails that occurs when fungi called dermatophytes, invade the nail. Toenails infected with a fungus usually become thick, friable, and deformed. The infection may cause the nail to have a brown, white, or yellowish discoloration. The nail may become brittle and give the appearance of debris under the nail. As the fungus progresses, the nail thickens, which can cause pressure inside footwear. It is important to know that there are many other reasons that cause a nail to be long, yellow, thick, and friable, such as trauma, age, and a veritable array of medical conditions.

Treating Toenail Fungus
Because the fungus gets into the nail bed and spreads, it is important to stop the progression when symptoms of infection are first seen. It is not in the best interest of the athlete to start treatment in this setting. To properly diagnose a fungus, a culture must be taken. Topical and oral treatments are options and should only be considered when the athlete's home clinician can be consulted.

For best results in the field for a painful thick nail, file the top of the nail down. If the thickened nail is painful from pressure from a tight toebox, slits can be cut into the shoe's toebox, part of the toebox can be removed, or partial or complete removal of the nail can be performed (see previous section on ingrown nails).

Toenail Trimming

Improperly trimmed toenails can lead to socks catching on nails that are too long or that have rough edges. This puts pressure on the hyponychium, nail bed, and epinychium, leading to blisters under the toenails, at the tips of the toes, or painful toenails as they are pushed back into the cuticle. Nails that are too long are also prone to pressure from a shoe or boot toebox that is too short or too low.

Toenails, especially on the big toe, should be trimmed regularly, straight across the nail – never rounded at the corners. Leave an extra bit of nail on the outside corner of the big toe to avoid an ingrown toenail. After trimming toenails, use a nail file to smooth the top of the nail down toward the front of the toe and remove any rough edges. If you draw your finger from the skin in front of the toe up across the nail and can feel a rough edge, the nail can be filed smoother or trimmed a bit shorter. Shoes that are too tight in the forefoot or too short can cause the nail to press into the sides of the toe. Use a metal nail file and large clippers.

Turf Toe

Turf toe commonly occurs at the first metatarsal phalangeal joint. The cause is typically either hyperextending the toe, jamming the toe, or pushing off repeatedly when running or jumping. There may also be an associated stiffness and swelling. The injury is actually a tear of the capsule and ligament that surround the joint and are within the metatarsal sesamoid complex. Tearing this joint capsule and ligament can be extremely painful and can lead to instability and even dislocation of the joint at the base of the toe. Stress fractures of the sesamoids are very possible and should be ruled out if pain swelling continues after attempted treatment fails.

Treating Turf Toe

The common treatment consists of resting the sore toe, icing the area, and elevating the foot. Using a pad (e.g., ⅛- or ¼-inch felt) under metatarsal heads 2 through 5 to off-weight the first MPJ with a cutout may relieve the pain. An antiinflammatory medication may be prescribed. Injectable steroids can be used, but it is not advised in the field due to the possibility of opening another portal for infection and the possible delayed healing if a stress fracture is suspected. The use of conservative padding is the treatment of choice. If the athlete does not respond, it is advised that an X-ray be obtained. Like many injuries, the condition can recur, and the rate of rehabilitation can slow with each occurrence.

NEUROPATHY/NUMB TOES AND FEET

Transient Paresthesia

Transient paresthesia is a temporary nerve-compression that can be caused by a gradual buildup of fluids in feet and legs during extended on-your-feet activity. As the extremity swells and blood flow decreases, ligaments and the retinaculum of many tendons and nerves become compressed. During the compression, the nerves do not receive the oxygen-rich blood they need and have mechanical constriction, resulting in numbness and/or tingling. Tight shoes and/or tightly laced shoes contribute to the problem. Shoes with poor cushioning, coupled with a heavy, pounding gait with strong pronatory forces can also be a contributing factor. The nerves most commonly affected are the common peroneal, tibial, and superficial peroneal. These will show a positive tennell and velox with a diminished sharp/dull test and possibly a positive straight leg test.

If the problem continues after the activity has stopped, suggest changing to more cushioned shoes and changing insoles and arch supports. There may be some lymph system breakdown in the foot caused by microtrauma.

Peripheral Neuropathy

Peripheral neuropathy is a nerve condition that can manifest itself as a burning, tingling, numbness, pain, itching sensations in the feet but that sometimes will appear as a cold sensation. It may start as a mild tingling in the toes and progress to searing pain. It can spread upward in the body, even to the thighs. Other symptoms might include prickling, or the sensation of having an "invisible sock" on your feet; a sharp jabbing or electric-type pain; extreme sensitivity to touch; muscle weakness; and a loss of balance or coordination. The pain results from damage to peripheral nerves that can come from a myriad of causes. A partial list of causes includes poor blood flow to the feet caused by diabetes, kidney or liver disease; an underactive thyroid, viral and bacterial infections, vitamin deficiencies, and pressure on a single nerve, although often no cause is identified.

Treating Peripheral Neuropathy

Treatment often depends on the cause and symptoms of the neuropathy and should be addressed from this perspective:

- Oral treatments can include over-the-counter or prescribed pain relievers for mild symptoms and tricyclic and SSRI antidepressants for burning pain. Antiseizure medications are also utilized, but these are not normally given in the field and are not indicated in acute cases.

- Self-care treatments include proper care of the feet with loose socks and padded shoes, cold water soaks and skin moisturizers, massage to improve circulation and stimulate nerves.
- Local injections of steroids can be given in a 1 cc of Kenalog 40 mixed with 2 cc of 0.5% marcaine plain in and around the specific nerve. These injections should be avoided if at all possible due to the possible point of infection.

Raynaud's Syndrome

Raynaud's syndrome affects 5–10% of the population. The discomfort is caused by a decreased blood supply to the fingers and toes. Attacks are precipitated by exposure to cold and stress. Although the severity, duration, and frequency of attacks vary both among individuals and over time, the primary symptoms of Raynaud's syndrome are changes in skin color. The affected areas turn white from the lack of circulation, then blue and cold, and finally become numb. When the attack subsides, the affected parts may turn red and may throb, tingle, or swell.

Treating Raynaud's Syndrome

- Keep the whole body warm.
- Wear wind- and water-resistant socks.
- Wear wool or wool-blend socks that retain warmth.
- Wear shoes that block wind and moisture, and tape over mesh in the shoe's upper.
- The patient must be careful not to injure the skin in affected areas, and to treat injuries without delay. Even minor cuts and scrapes take longer to heal and may be more susceptible to infection when circulation is impaired.
- Oral medication such as aspirin and niacin can be used.

PODIATRIC DERMATOLOGY

Athlete's Foot

Athlete's foot, tinea pedis, is a skin disease caused by a fungus. The combination of a dark, warm, and humid environment in the shoes or boots, excessive foot perspiration, and changes in the condition of the skin combine to create a setting for the fungi of athlete's foot to begin growing. The fungal infection usually occurs between the toes or under the plantar arch of the foot (moccasin tinea pedis). Typical signs and symptoms of athlete's foot include itching, dry and cracking skin, inflammation with a burning sensation, and pain. Bulla and vesicles with swelling may develop if left untreated. When these bullae are opened, small, red areas of raw tissue are exposed with some serous fluid. As the infection spreads, the burning and itching will increase and a subsequent secondary bacterial infection can occur from the open lesions. The most common pathogen of tinea pedis is *Trichophyton rubrum*, most often associated with the plantar and side of the foot distribution. Another common pathogen is *Trichophyton mentagrophytes*, which is responsible for inflamed vesicles or bullae.

Treating Athlete's Foot

Treatment includes keeping the feet clean and dry, changing socks frequently, and using antifungal medications and foot powders. An antiperspirant may also help those with excessive foot moisture.

In the field, use an antifungal cream with active ingredients of clotrimazole, econazole, ketoconazole, miconazole – all very effective. Other topical emollients such as Betadine and gentian violet are also efficacious against dermatophytes, *Canidida*, and Gram-positive and -negative organisms. Most topical medications are applied BID to TID until symptoms resolve. Vicks Vapo-Rub and homeopathic remedies such as tea tree oil are touted to kill the fungi and help relieve the associated itching. Apply a few drops to the affected areas two to three times daily with a cotton ball held in place with tape. Test a drop or two on the athlete's skin to be sure they are not allergic to the oil.

Calluses

A callus is an abnormal amount of dead, thickened skin caused by recurring pressure and friction, called hyperkeratosis, usually on the plantar aspect of the foot, most often on the heels and plantar metatarsal heads, or on the digits. Figure 38.33 shows a ball of the foot callus. Calluses may be yellowish in color, layered, or even scaly due to excessive dryness. They can form over any bony prominence. Common callus are called heloma molle, an interdigital callus often in the fourth interspace. A

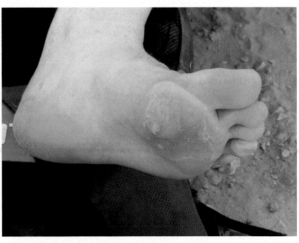

Figure 38.33. Large ball of the foot callus. Credit: Rob Conenello.

heloma dura is a hard callus that is usually found on the lateral side of the fifth digit, and the dorsum sides of the second, third, and fourth digits. Heloma dura can often be found on deformities such as hammertoes, mallet toes, and claw toes. Intractable plantar keratosis is a localized callus buildup at or near the metatarsal heads on the ball of the foot.

Some calluses may have a deep-seated core, called nucleation or porokeratosis that can be painful to pressure. Many athletes will state that they feel a grain of sand within the callus. When debrided, however, it is noted to be a papule that is very tender to pressure, not compression. This is hypertrophy of the stratum corneum over and around a sweat gland. Close attention should be made to differentiate this from a wart or a callus. If the athlete complains of point tenderness, cut a donut or horseshoe out of moleskin to relieve pressure.

Blisters under calluses are common and are difficult to treat. Refer to the blister section of this chapter for information on how to manage these blisters.

Treating Calluses

Use a callus file or surgical blade (#15, 62, and 64 are often helpful) to remove dead skin and any rough edges of skin. These edges can catch on socks and lead to the start of a blister. They can also open up into a fissure, a crack in the skin. Debriding too deeply into a corn or callus can cause an open lesion. A pumice stone will work as well as a file and is often something that the athletes can use on their own feet. Do not encourage the athletes to debride their own lesions.

A cushioned insole with a good arch support can help equalize the weight load of the foot, while pads around or near the callus can relieve pressure. To relieve heel discomfort from calluses, a heel cup or heel pad will distribute body weight evenly across the heel.

Hydrostat, Keralac ointment, or urea cream can be used on calluses. Encourage athletes, at night or before sleep breaks, to apply cream or lotion to callused areas. File the callus prior to the next bout of activity. Hydrostat and Keralac are also good treatments for daily skin care.

Corns

A corn is a hard, thickened area of skin, generally on the dorsal aspect of the digit or between the toes, usually caused by friction and pressure. A corn is usually like a kernel of corn, round and yellowish in color. Corns on the outer surface of the toes are usually hard, whereas those between the toes are usually soft and macerated. The larger the corn and the more it rubs against the shoe, the more painful it becomes. Typically the corn is an inverted cone shape with a point that can press on a nerve or bony prominence below, causing pain.

Tight-fitting socks and footwear or the foot sliding around the shoe can cause corns. Heloma molles are soft corns, caused by prominent, irregularly shaped bones and exostosis that occur between the toes.

Treating Corns

Warm water and Epsom salt soaks or the application of hydrogen peroxide may help soften corns prior to mechanical debridement with a surgical blade (#15 is very commonly used). After debridement, gently buff off any dead tissue with a callus file or pumice stone. You can also pad around the corn with corn pads, felt, small pieces of tape, or Spenco 2nd Skin. Lamb's wool can be wrapped around the toe for cushioning. To control corns, the pressure and friction must be eliminated, usually from improper fitting shoes.

Fissures

Fissures often develop in the thickened, callused skin on our heels, but they also occur on callused skin on the plantar metatarsal heads. They can become infected, bleed, and split open into the deeper exposed underlying granular tissues. Like many foot conditions, fissures, if left untreated, can lead to secondary bacterial or fungal infection.

Treating Fissures

Keep the fissure clean, covered, with an antibiotic ointment applied. Watch for signs of infection. Use a callus file and moisturizing cream on callused feet to help prevent fissures. When possible, before rest breaks or sleep, the athlete should apply lots of moisturizing cream or Vaseline, slip a plastic bag over the feet, and then elevate the feet and sleep. In the morning, the athlete's heels will be moist and flexible. Treating these fissures is very difficult and there are not many very successful treatment options.

Plantar Warts

Plantar warts are found on the plantar aspect of the foot (the plantar surface) and can cause severe foot pain. Already painful from the pressure of standing and walking, plantar warts can become more painful due to sports activities. They are typically small, hard, granulated lumps on the skin that can be flesh-colored, white, pink, brown, or gray. The spongy appearance, punctuate bleeding, and pressure with compression are hallmarks and can aid in clinical diagnosis. They can also feel thick, and scaly. Plantar warts are often irregular in shape and have noted skin lines that go around the lesion. The athlete may complain of a small stone in his or her shoe when a wart appears.

Plantar warts are contagious benign tumors caused by common viral infections, usually the human papillomavirus. Moist, cracked skin and open or healing blisters leave one susceptible to the virus. While usually small on the skin's surface, they penetrate deep into the foot, where they can cause deep pain.

Treating Plantar Warts

Plantar warts thrive in the warm, moist environment found in sports shoes, so encourage athletes to air their feet when able and change into fresh shoes and socks as often as possible. Most warts disappear without treatment in 4–5 months. Sometimes though, when the wart is bothersome or has not gone away on its own, treatment is necessary. Treating plantar warts in the field with over-the-counter plantar-wart removal compounds is unrealistic. Use moleskin with a hole cut out or other pressure-relieving treatments to relieve painful pressure on the wart. If a salicylic acid compound is available, apply the product then tape over the wart each time the treatment is applied. Advise the athlete to seek medical attention after he or she has returned home. Debriding the lesion down to the pinpoint bleeding in the field only makes the athlete more susceptible to a secondary infection.

Rashes

Capillaritis or topical dermatitis is a common rash that affects the legs of athletes. It is a harmless skin condition in which reddish-brown patches are caused by leaky capillaries, often after exercise. Many times the rash will appear under the socks and gaiters. The rash may be caused by a topical reaction to detergents, or to clothing products such as Lycra, sock fabrics, or other fabrics that irritate skin. It could also be a heat rash from the combination of trapped sweat and hot temperatures. In extreme cases it will present with serous-filled blisters. It can reoccur and even persist for years.

Heat rash is caused by a blockage of sweat glands in areas of heavy sweating, usually beneath clothing. This rash appears as red, itchy, inflamed bumps. Figure 38.34 shows a common rash.

Treating Rashes

Capillaritis will disappear on its own over a few weeks. The use of a topical hydrocortisone 1% cream or Benadryl will help control the rash and any related itching. Heat rash usually lasts for a few days and then disappears on its own, although it may last longer if hot and humid conditions continue. Other treatments can be made by mixing ingredients such as triple antibiotic ointment, Benadryl, and hydrocortisone. Holistic treatments can also be used such as Bag Balm and either tea tree oil or Manuka oil. Another solution to those affected by rashes is to try different socks, apply powder under their socks, or wear thin sock liners made from silk. Oral Benadryl with its sedative side effects during an athletic activity is not advised, but it may be helpful after the event has been completed.

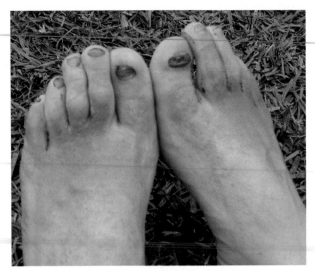

Figure 38.34. Common heat rash. Credit: John Vonhof.

SESAMOIDITIS

Sesamoiditis is an inflammation of the soft tissue and the sesamoid bone, most commonly on the plantar aspect of the first metatarsal head but, it can be at almost any joint in the foot. These two sesamoid bones can become bruised and inflamed, resulting in either sharp, constant pain or pain that occurs with range of motion of the hallux and or compression of the sesamoids against the head of the first metatarsal. The bones can also fracture, resulting in sudden, intense pain and the inability to bear weight on the foot. Repetitive and excessive pressure on the forefoot area and shoes with poor cushioning that offer inadequate protection against rocks can cause trauma to the sesamoid bones.

Treating Sesamoiditis

- Avoid using soft pads under the sesamoid bones because this will take up room in the shoe and press the sesamoids against the first metatarsal.
- Cut a small hole in the insole under the sesamoid bones or pad around the sesamoids to off-weight or "float" the area of discomfort.
- Loosen shoelaces over the forefoot to relieve pressure.
- Use ice.
- Buddy-tape the big toe to the second toe for stabilization.
- Wear a firm-soled shoe to help keep the toe in line and the foot–toe joint stable and reduce the amount of motion in the first MPJ.
- Surgical shoe with crutches and a trip to the emergency room may be necessary if no other conservative treatment option are successful and a fracture is suspected.

TENDON AND LIGAMENT INJURIES

The primary function of tendons is to transmit muscle force to the moving joints with limited elongation. Tendons attach muscles to bones. Ligaments are similar structures that attach bones to other bones. When muscles and bones move, they exert stresses on the tendons and ligaments that are attached to them. With 26 bones, 33 joints, 107 ligaments, 19 muscles, and tendons to hold the structure together and allow it to move in a variety of ways, the foot offers all kinds of opportunities for tendon and ligament injuries. Soft tissue injuries often result from overtraining and or a sudden traumatic event like an ankle sprain or strain.

The terms "tendinitis," "tendinosis," and "tendinopathy" all refer to tendon injuries. These terms are commonly confused and misused. Tendinitis is inflammation, irritation, and swelling of a tendon. Tendinosis, sometimes called chronic tendinitis, chronic tendinopathy, is damage to a tendon at a cellular level. Tendinopathy is used to describe tendinitis (inflammation) and tendinosis (microtears) collectively.

When muscles and tendons move in new ways or do more work than they can easily handle, they can sustain damage. If the increase in demand is made gradually, muscle and tendon tissues will usually heal, build in strength, and adapt to new loads.

Many athletes, however, participate in activities that injure a tendon or ligament on a microscopic scale and then do more injury before the tendon heals. Continuing the injurious activity can gradually accumulate these microinjuries. When enough injury accumulates, pain is felt. This kind of injury comes on slowly with time and persists as a chronic injury; acute tendon injuries are sudden tears that cause immediate pain and obvious symptoms. Tendon injuries often require patience and careful rehabilitation because tendons heal more slowly than muscles primarily due to their limited blood flow.

There are three grades of classification and treatment of tendon and ligament injuries:[14]

* *Grade 1* – A mild sprain or strain of the ligament or tendon with mild to moderate pain and inflammation. Responds rapidly to rest, ice, compression, and elevation. Supportive taping decreases the chance of reinjury as the athlete returns to competition.
* *Grade 2* – A moderate sprain or strain of the ligament or tendon with hematoma formation. Excessive pain and swelling with activity. Treatment is supportive therapy of the inflammation with use of crutches until weight-bearing is comfortable; then physical therapy and rehabilitation. Bracing and/or taping should be used with competition for approximately 2 months.
* *Grade 3* – A severe sprain or strain with total disruption of the ligament or tendon with palpable void or

rift and positive anterior drawer test (calcaneus pulled forward and tibia pushed posterior). Treatment is a posterior cast, non-weight-bearing on crutches and immediate emergency room evaluation.

Tendons are critical for converting the movement of muscle contraction to movement of the foot and/or ankle. The most common tendon injury is to the Achilles tendon, which connects the muscles of the posterior calf (gastrocnemius, soleus, and plantaris) to the middle one-third of the calcaneus bone and mediates plantar flexion function across the ankle and subtalor joints. Injuries to other tendons that cross the ankle are usually the result of lacerations or direct trauma.

A common tendon problem affects the ankle flexors. These tendons are caught under the pressure of the shoe's tongue and laces across the front top of the foot. Walking or running steep hills can also cause this problem. Another common tendon injury is posterior tibial tendinitis. This affects plantarflexion and inversion of the ankle and the foot. The peroneus longus and brevis tendons are also common tendons that are injured. The peroneus brevis tendon directly opposes the posterior tibial tendon in that it abducts, dorsiflexes, and everts the foot.

How Tendons and Ligaments Heal

Tendons have limited blood supply, and nutrition is often supported via synovial fluid within the presence of a tendon sheath. In other words, tendons and ligaments are designed to transmit tensile loads, have limited elastic properties, and heal slowly compared to other more oxygenated tissue. This is important to know as one begins to understand the basis of optimal healing after injury and repair. It is very important to understand if prevention and performance is in mind.

Optimal healing consists of three major phases, namely, inflammation, repair, and remodeling. Within the first week after acute tendon or ligament injury, there is inflammation. During this time there is an influx of neutrophils, macrophages, and a proliferation of granulation tissue angiogenesis. At this time, the soft tissues are most sensitive to mechanical load. Relative rest is indicated. Interestingly, after about 3 weeks, inflammatory cells are not present, and medications may lose the desired effect.

Repair of damaged tissue lasts from about the end of week one for the next 4–6 weeks and consists of the deposition of new fibroblast (mitogenesis) and collagen (fibrogenesis) by capillary infiltration.[15] Early mobilization is a key factor for strengthening the repairing tendon and begins the process of organizing the new collagen along the lines of functional stress. Collagen deposition will follow the lines of tissue stress. Prolonged rest may not provide the controlled loading stimulus necessary for maturation of the healing tissue and may actually set up a degenerative process – a condition referred to as tendinosis. This early graded controlled mobilization is only indicated in grade one and two injuries. Grade three ruptures should be immediately immobilized and the athlete should be taken to the nearest emergency room for proper imaging and treatment due to the high probability of adjacent soft tissue and osseous injury.

Remodeling is the process of reorganizing collagen fibers. This is the process of macrophages that remove debris, vascular granulation, fibroblast proliferation, and collagen deposition. This process ends in a dense collagen scar fibrocytes (fibroblast become inactive) and vascularity reduction.[16] Effective remodeling requires a graded return to normal weight-bearing and activity to prevent contractures and to promote strength and flexibility. This process may take anywhere from a few months to a year. Rehabilitation should include all three cardinal planes of functional motion and is best done under the supervision of a physical therapist.

Achilles Tendinitis

The Achilles tendon connects the gastrocnemius and the soleus, the two major muscles of the calf, to the posterior middle one-third of the calcaneus. It stabilizes the heel every time we take a step. The tendon makes it possible for us to rise up on our toes, run, and jump. Achilles tendinitis occurs when the sheath surrounding this cord becomes inflamed. There may be small tears in the tendon, or sudden and repeated stretching of the tendon may cause an inflammation that is painful behind the heel, ankle, and lower calf while walking and running. The pain may be felt during the early part of a run or hike, and then subside, only to worsen after stopping. This pain is the first warning, followed by swelling of the Achilles tendon, and pain to touch at the base of the heel.

A mild first-degree injury makes it difficult to rise up on our toes or walk on our heels. With proper treatment, athletes should be able to walk with little pain after about 48 hours. They should not resume normal athletic activity for several weeks. A second-degree injury is when there is partial tearing of the tendon. This injury will take from 6 to 8 weeks to heal, with an additional 2–4 weeks of stretching exercises before normal athletic activity can be resumed. In a third-degree injury, an extreme case, the Achilles tendon ruptures. This requires immediate medical intervention, usually surgery, and a long healing and strengthening process. There is sudden calf pain and usually an audible snap if the tendon ruptures. The tendon will ball up in the calf with a related defect in the lower tendon. A positive Thompson's sign may be present. This is when the athlete is in the prone position and the calf muscle is squeezed. When the foot does not plantarflex like the contralateral side, a rupture is

suspect. If the tendon is swollen, or you suspect a tear, usually a second- or third-degree injury, the athlete should not risk running on it. It can further damage or rupture the tendon. If the pain is mild and goes away in 5 minutes with a warm-up, it is typically a first-degree injury.

A sudden increase in activity, increasing mileage too fast, or running steep hills can lead to an inflamed Achilles tendon. To prevent Achilles tendon problems, suggest increasing activity, mileage, and hill training gradually, no more than 10% a week. Proper lower leg muscle stretching can also help prevent problems. Overpronators, whose arch collapses when walking or running, are more prone than others to Achilles problems.

Enthesopathies of the Achilles tendon is when calcium deposits form in and on the tendon. These deposits provide a considerable amount of irritation with the range of motion and may be permanently debilitating or require surgery. If you grasp the tendon between your thumb and forefinger, move the foot up and down, and feel a grating or crepitus, this is a sign of serious tendinitis. Crepitus can represent severe inflammation. If not treated appropriately, it can lead to calcific tendinitis. You must slow the athlete's exercise regimen as much as possible. Some authorities recommend casting until this goes away. Ice and antiinflammatories in the form of NSAIDs and oral steroids may be helpful. The use of local steroid injected into the Achilles tendon insertion should never be performed and is highly contraindicated.

Ignoring the signs of Achilles tendinitis and not seeking treatment can lead to a chronic inflammation or even tendon rupture. The pain may occur when warming up and then ease up. The athlete continues to train, and the pain returns after the session has ended. Over time, the periods of pain-free training become shorter and shorter. Eventually, training may become impossible and treatment mandatory. This can lead to formation of a cyst in the tendon. As the cyst expands, the tendon thins out and becomes more susceptible to rupture if overstressed.

Treating Achilles Tendinitis

The major causes of Achilles tendon problems are a lack of strength and flexibility in the calf muscles, a weakness in the tendon, or a weak ankle joint. Treatment may include any or all of the following: icing as described later, doing stretching and flexibility exercises, wearing flexible shoes or boots with a well-padded heel counter, and avoiding the ups and downs of hills.

If Achilles tendinitis is suspected, the athlete should stop running – running through the pain is not advised. Ignoring the symptoms may cause the tendon to rupture, which usually requires surgery. The patient may be put in either a flexible or immobilizing cast to reduce movement and weight-bearing. Once the cast is removed, stretching exercises to strengthen the tendon before resuming normal athletic activity will be necessary.

The treatment for Achilles tendinitis is the same RICE treatment used for ankle sprains and strains: rest, ice, compression, and elevation. The first 24 hours are the most critical for beginning treatment. Early treatment decreases swelling and lessens the risk of additional injury. Initial rest of the foot is also important. A lightly wound Ace wrap will provide compression to help keep swelling down while providing support. Apply the Ace wrap from the forefoot upward toward the calf. The Ace wrap should not be worn at night. Apply ice for 20 minutes at a time three to four times daily. Ice can be very helpful in the healing process.

The injured area should be elevated above the level of the heart as much as possible during the first 48 hours. This keeps blood away from the injured area and reduces pain and swelling. The use of antiinflammatory medications is usually warranted. Ibuprofen 800 mg TID or the use of a Medrol dose pack can be utilized.

A small heel lift will help alleviate the stresses on the tendon. This heel lift can be made of ⅛- to ⅜-inch felt or plastazote (PPT). Some people prefer cork or other accommodative material. Hard materials are usually not recommended for heel lifts. For some individuals, wearing low-heeled shoes will take some of the pressure off of the Achilles tendon. An Achilles notch in shoes or mid- and low-top boots will accommodate the Achilles tendon by relieving the friction force of the tendon on the shoe. Use a scissors or scalpel to cut a notch in the shoe's heel counter. The use of an Engo Blister Prevention Patch in the heel counter will also aid in the gliding motion of the tendon over the shoe.

A lightweight plastic or fabric night splint worn to bed can help to stretch the foot, limit contraction of soft tissues at night, and avoid morning stiffness. Night splints help keep the foot in a dorsiflexed position and avoid accompanying muscle tightening. Night splints are proven as a treatment method for preventing the plantar fascia and Achilles tendon from contracting during the night.

Bursitis

Bursae are small fluid-filled sacs found between areas of high friction such as where muscles or tendons glide over bone. The bursa acts as a shock absorber, allowing movement between neighboring structures, usually in opposite directions. Bursitis is the formation of an inflamed fluid-filled sac from trauma or overuse. On the feet, bursitis may develop beneath a callus or a bunion; under the metatarsal heads; at the insertion of the anterior and posterior tibial tendons, or the insertion of the peroneal brevis and tertius; along the contour of the peroneal longus tendon primarily through the notch in the cuboid; at the heel around the Achilles tendon; or along the course of the flexor hallucis longus through the posterior aspect of the talus.

Typical causes of bursitis in the feet can be repetitive motions or an injury or sustained pressure to a joint or motions that are outside the normal course of the tendon. As the usually slippery bursa sac becomes inflamed, it loses its gliding capabilities and becomes gritty and rough. Inflamed bursas are painful and irritating.

Treating Bursitis

The first action is to stop or reduce the motion or action that is causing the bursitis. The use of NSAIDs or a Medrol dose pack will temporarily help reduce the inflammation. Care should be taken to avoid injection of the inflamed bursitis in the expedition races if at all possible due to the possibility of introducing an extra portal for infection. Focusing attention on the biomechanics pathology can be much more successful. Treating a forefoot or rearfoot varus, valgus, or equines can often provide much more relief for the athlete than the temporary treatment with steroids. Many of the accommodations can be made with felt, PPT, foam, or cork. These can be taped or glued to the athlete's insole or shoe. Ice and cold will reduce the inflammation and should be used when possible. Care should be used to properly warm up the affected area prior to activity.

In severe cases, fluid may need to be drawn from the sac to relieve pressure. A proximal nerve block should be performed prior to this procedure and the injection of steroid into the exsanguinated sac may be therapeutic. It is not advised to inject more than 1 cc of steroid into the area. This steroid is most often mixed with marcaine or lidocaine to aid in the comfort of the athlete.

Plantar Fasciitis

The plantar fascia is a band of connective fibrous tissue that runs from the medial tubercle of the calcaneus along the medial aspect of the median band of the plantar fascia that fans to attach to the metatarsal heads of the foot, forming the foot's arch. The band helps in support and stabilization of the foot during gait. Pronation of the arch occurs when standing and during midstance in the gait cycle, as the arch of the foot is flattened in order to accommodate changes in the terrain. As toe off begins, the heel lifts up, and the foot begins to supinate as the plantar fascia tightens to form the curve of the arch. This provides a strong lever for push off with the toes. An inflammation of the fascia, called plantar fasciitis, occurs most often with overuse. The inflammation is caused by the stretching and tearing of some of the fibers in the plantar fascia and intrinsic muscles of the foot as it inserts into the calcaneus and along its course. The plantar fascia is strained, mainly at the heel, in athletes with flat feet, high arches, or overpronation. The stresses of impact sports, running, and hiking may flatten, lengthen, and eventually cause small tears in the plantar fascia. Tears near the calcaneus often result in calcaneal spurring and enthesopathies.

Athletes who are predisposed to plantar fasciitis injuries typically have increased their mileage too fast, have increased the frequency and intensity of their workouts, have increased the amount of hill work, and/or lack flexibility and strength in their ankle and foot. Other factors that may contribute to plantar fasciitis are an increase in weight, such as carrying a pack or the breakdown of shoes due to age or wear. Some athletes may also have a foot imbalance such as flat feet or high arches. Many pathologic conditions such as forefoot and rearfoot varus, valgus, and equinus also contribute to plantar fasciitis.

Plantar fascia pain is commonly felt with activity after prolonged periods of rest, such as in the morning or after long periods of sitting. This condition is referred to as post static dyskinesia. The first steps at these times cause a sudden strain to the band of tissue that has started to heal itself during the night. The pain and stiffness is usually centered at the plantar aspect of the heel, but symptoms may radiate into the mid portion or distal aspect of the arch. Although the pain may decrease somewhat with initial activity, as the day progresses, it may return and be quite painful.

Treating Plantar Fasciitis

Generally prescribed treatments for plantar fasciitis include rest, stretching in the morning and/or before activity, icing massage after activity, using heel cups, changing insoles or adding an arch support, and taping the foot or using an arch brace, orthotics, foot exercises, and shoe modifications. Usually you need either to provide more support to the arch or lessen the amount of overpronation. An arch support or arch pad can provide pain relief.

Addressing the pathologic biomechanical etiology is the best way to alleviate the discomfort long term; however, adjunctive therapy may be needed. Oral NSAIDs and steroids can be very helpful. In extreme cases, cortisone injections can be administered with 1 cc injectable steroid (such as Kenalog 40, methylprednisolone 20 mg, or dexamethasone sodium phos.) mixed with 2 cc of marcaine or lidocaine. The injection should be administered from the medial aspect of the foot and placed superior and inferior to the plantar fascia and at the medial tubercle of the calcaneus. The clinician should avoid injection of the plantar fascia in the expedition races if at all possible due to the possibility of introducing an extra portal for infection. Focusing attention on the biomechanics pathology can be much more successful.

Regaining flexibility and elasticity of the soleus muscle/sheath helps to prevent the condition from reoccurring. Stretching is the way to do that, but the patient has to start out slow and easy, that is, a calf stretch and circular stretching motions with the foot, for example, writing the alphabet with their foot. It is known that some fibers of the Achilles tendon extend down to and around the calcaneus into the plantar fascia. Stretching out the Achilles tendon can help stretch out the plantar fascia and also alleviate the pathologic equinus.

Studies have shown that stretching and off-the-shelf shoe inserts were just as effective as stretching and the more costly orthotics.[17] If the athlete chooses to wear heel pads, they must be worn in all the athlete's shoes.

Orthotics will often help relieve plantar fascia pain. It is recommended that the athlete try an inexpensive orthotic shoe insert before having expensive orthotics made. No matter if it is custom or over-the-counter, it should have some flexibility. The orthotic fitted for an athlete is going to be different than those given to people standing on their feet. A gradual break-in period should be used prior to full exercise. The patient should wear the inserts for no more than one hour the first day and gradually increasing the time by one hour a day until they can ambulate without discomfort. A gradual increase in exercise regimen should also be followed until the athlete is slowly brought up to a full exercise bout.

It is possible to tape the plantar fascia area under the foot for support, though doing so can be hard to manage. The longitudinal arch (low die) technique is commonly used. The tape, however, loses strength as it moves with the skin – 40% of its strength can be lost within 20 minutes. It is preferable to wear an arch brace wrapping around the arch to provide support and decrease the pull of the plantar fascia on the calcaneus.

Lightweight plastic and fabric night splints are proven as a treatment for preventing the plantar fascia and Achilles tendon from contracting during the night. The splint helps stretch the foot, limit contraction of soft tissues at night, and avoid morning stiffness by relieving the pathologic equinus. These devices can be worn during a multiday event during rest periods and at night.

Plantar Fasciitis Stretches

Before getting up in the morning or after resting, these stretches can be helpful in making the patient's first steps less painful:

- Lie on your stomach, put your toes and forefoot against the mattress/ground, and straighten your leg so your heel stretches your calf muscle.
- Slowly stretch the toes upward toward the head at least three times per day, holding the stretch for at least 15 seconds.
- Stretch the Achilles tendon by bending the knee with the ankle flexed back toward you and gently pulling your toes back toward your knee. Hold this pull to a count of 10 and repeat six to ten times a day.

Ruptured Tendon

The seriousness of a rupture of a tendon requires specialized care, and the athlete should be taken to an emergency room as soon as possible. An Achilles tendon rupture can be diagnosed with evidence of severe ecchymosis, palpable dell or void, a positive Thompson sign, calcaneal gate, and/or the inability to raise up on toes. If a rupture is suspected, a posterior splint should be applied in a plantarflexed position. The patient should be made non-weight-bearing with the aid of crutches or wheelchair or the aid of other personnel if no supplies are available. If the rupture is fresh, within hours of the injury, surgical repair of the tendon is usually done. Older injuries may also be treated surgically, though many patients will improve by casting the leg. Diminished strength and rerupture is more frequently seen in patients who are casted without surgery, so preference is to surgically repair the rupture.

EXTREME CONDITIONS

Aching Feet

Athletes often complain of foot pain, an aching pain that many people get on the bottoms of their feet from overuse. It can feel like someone has repeatedly taken a hammer to the bottom of one's feet. The aching pain can be caused by undue pressure on the bones, tendons, ligaments, and muscles of the feet from a number of causes:

- Day after day stresses to one's feet
- Trying to do too many miles too fast
- A lack of proper conditioning
- Pushing too hard in an event or race that one is not fully trained for
- Encountering conditions one is not prepared for
- Worn-out footwear (shoes, insoles, and socks)
- Preexisting foot conditions (like flat feet or plantar fasciitis)

Treating Aching Feet

- Change to a more supportive and/or cushioned footwear.
- Take off shoes and socks and elevate feet and legs – this can provide immediate relief.
- Elevate feet and legs while sleeping.
- Massage feet.
- Soak feet in ice or ice water.
- Reduce pack weight.
- Take a rest day, an often overlooked remedy.

Frostbite/Chilblains

Frostbite, sometimes called chilblains, occurs when tissue actually freezes. Toes are particularly susceptible to this serious condition. Factors that contribute to frostbite include exposure to wind, wet skin (even from sweat), and tight socks and shoes that constrict blood flow.

First degree or early signs of frostbite include numbness, a waxy or pale discoloration of the skin, tissue that has become firm to the touch, and pain in the area, but no blistering. Second degree will see clear blistering with superficial freezing. Third-degree frostbite includes hemorrhagic bulla and subcutaneous deep-freezing of the skin. As the frostbite progresses, the skin gets paler, and the pain ceases. When the full thickness of freezing results in loss of the body part, dry gangrene sets in; this is the fourth degree. Often frostbite will thaw on its own as the person keeps moving or gets into a warm environment and out of the wind, wet, and cold. As the tissue warms, there can be redness, itching, and swelling.

Tips for Managing Frostbite/Chilblains

- Do not rub toes to warm them – that causes even more tissue damage.
- Unless absolutely necessary, don't allow the person to walk on frostbitten feet or toes.
- Get the person into a warm environment as soon as possible.
- Immerse the affected area in lukewarm (104–106°F) water for approximately 30 minutes or warm the affected area with the body heat from another person. Do not use hot water.
- Do not use a heating pad, heat lamp, or the heat of a stove, fireplace, or radiator for warming.
- Do not rewarm or thaw a person's frostbite unless you are sure you can keep them warm.
- It is important to remember that thawing the tissue and then allowing it to refreeze can be devastating.
- Dehydration will make the athlete more susceptible to frostbite.
- Local injection of marcaine plain proximal to the area can be very therapeutic in two ways. It will relieve some discomfort and it will cause some hyperemic response.
- Use of aspirin, Pletal, and niacin are also helpful.
- It is imperative to start the athlete on PO antibiotics if any open lesions are identified.
- Dressing open lesions with Betadine and a dry sterile dressing can help keep the area clean of infection until transfer to a higher-care facility can be arranged.

Heat

- Pretape any potential hot spot or blister problem areas. In the desert, a breathable tape is essential.
- Wear moisture-wicking socks.
- Orthotics or extra insoles can provide extra insulation from the heated pavement.

- Encourage larger-sized shoes to accommodate swelling feet.
- Be watchful of water poured over athlete's heads to cool off running down their legs and into their shoes. This can lead to moisture and maceration problems.

Jungle Rot/Tinea Vesicularis

Jungle rot is a skin disorder induced by a tropical climate. In long adventure races or ultra-marathons, particularly in foreign countries, feet are often exposed to all sorts of organisms. Many of these parasites enter the skin through open blisters, cracks between the toes, fissures on the skin, and scratches. Some may lead to a hemorrhagic appearance under the skin. They may ooze fluid, often yellow with pus, from infection. The feet may be painful and itch unrelentingly. In some cases, oral antibiotics and oral antifungals need to be prescribed. With a 2-week course of Lamisil, liver function tests do not need to be run and the choice of a broad-spectrum antibiotic such as Levaquin is indicated to combat the host of Gram-positive and -negative bacteria often found. Some of these organisms will take weeks or months to be eliminated. Many times the race organizations will be aware of the potential for this type of exposure and have medical recommendations for its control.

Tips for Controlling Jungle Rot

- Keep feet as dry as possible.
- Air feet whenever possible, exposing them to sunlight when resting.
- Use a water-repelling ointment mentioned in the maceration section that follows to control moisture.
- Change into dry clean socks as often as possible.
- When changing socks and shoes, check feet for open skin and treat those areas with Betadine and an antiseptic ointment.

Maceration

Maceration of the skin can cause a great deal of pain and interfere with walking and running. Figure 38.35 shows how painful skin folds can occur. Steps can be taken prior to exposure for the best effect:

- Use Betadine or a drying agent like Gordon Lab's Forma-Ray or Formalyde-10 Spray or Lazerformalyde Solution (Pedinol Pharmical) to dry the skin.
- Apply Hydropel Sports Ointment, which is used by many adventure racers because of its moisture-repelling capabilities, or a beeswax and lanolin preparation such as Atsko's Pro-Tech-Skin or Kiwi's Camp Dry.
- Coat feet with Desitin or zinc oxide.

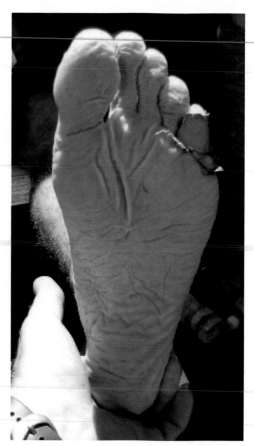

Figure 38.35. Severe maceration with skin folds. Credit: John Vonhof.

- Reapply the skin protectant at frequent intervals or when changing socks, even during the middle of a race, always cleaning off the old coating.
- When resting or sleeping, remove footwear, dry feet, and allow them to air but keep them warm.

Moisture and Cold

Consider the following pointers when helping at any event in which moisture and cold will be an issue:

- For high-intensity, fast-paced sports, lightweight and fast-drying and -draining shoes are the best bet.
- Moisture-wicking socks should always be worn.
- Encourage wearing thicker socks for better insulation and more water absorption (which keeps the feet drier at the skin surface).
- If shoes have a breathable upper, a layer of duct tape over the upper can keep the wind and moisture out.
- Wearing shoes that do not have adequate draining capabilities will subject feet to extended periods of moisture. Use a heated nail or a drill to make a few small holes where the upper attaches to the lower part of the shoe or boot. Make one at the heel and one on each side of the forefoot.

- In humid conditions, make a "cuff" out of a highly absorbent, microfiber towel. A 3-inch-wide cuff around the top of socks will catch much of the moisture running down legs.
- Foot powders that absorb moisture can help keep feet dry.
- When resting or sleeping, athletes should take off wet shoes and socks to allow feet to dry and breathe.
- A foot massage can restore capillary flow to the skin.

Sand

Because sand can be an extreme irritant, the goal is to keep it out of shoes and socks:

- Avoid double-layer socks that trap sand between layers.
- Avoid shoes that are made with mesh uppers.
- Wear gaiters.
- If athletes use a lubricant, watch for sand buildup on toes and feet.
- Wipe off any old lubricant before applying a new coat.
- Keep feet as clean as possible.
- Stop and check feet regularly.

Trench Foot

Trench foot is a serious nonfreezing cold injury that develops when the skin of the feet is exposed to a combination of moisture and cold for extended periods. Tissue death can occur in feet exposed to moisture and cold in boots or shoes that constrict the feet for periods of 12 hours or longer. It can occur in temperatures as high as 60°F if the feet are constantly wet – in other words, it does not have to be winter conditions.

Trench foot is caused by factors common to athletes participating in extreme sports: dehydration, wet shoes and socks, poor nutrition, inadequate footwear that is too tight, and cold. Many of the multiday ultramarathons and adventure races can create conditions right for trench foot. Under the right conditions, even a one-day event could jeopardize feet. Figure 38.36 shows a case of trench foot on a participant in a stage race in Chile.

Due to the cold, wet, and constricting environment inside the shoe, vasoconstriction and arterioconstriction reduce circulation to preserve heat loss. With the resulting lack of oxygen and nutrients in the blood, toxins build up and skin tissue begins to die. The skin reddens and becomes numb with a waxy and possibly mottled appearance. Pitting edema follows with associated itching and tingling pain. When the skin rewarms, blisters form, and when they are deroofed, an ulcer is present, exposing open granular tissue with serosanguineous drainage. If trench foot is left untreated, amputation may

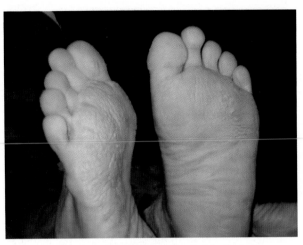

Figure 38.36. Trench foot. Credit: John Vonhof.

be required. It can take 24–48 hours before the severity of the damage is fully apparent.

Tips for Managing Trench Foot

Trench foot is caused by factors common to athletes participating in extreme sports: dehydration, wet shoes and socks, poor nutrition, inadequate and too tight footwear, and cold. There are specific ways to reduce chances of getting trench foot:

- Wash and dry feet.
- Do not sleep in wet socks.
- Avoid socks and shoes that are too tight.
- Do not add socks if it causes constriction inside shoes. Move up to a larger shoe.
- Rewarm gently; do not use a strong heat source.
- Do not rub the skin; instead, use passive skin-to-skin contact.
- Elevate the feet above the level of the heart.
- Do not pop blisters, apply lotions or creams, or walk on injured feet.
- Start an antiinflammatory drug program.
- Start PO antibiotics if open lesions are present.
- Dress lesions with antibacterial ointment and a dry sterile dressing.

MULTIDAY EVENTS

Daily foot care should be emphasized. This includes cleaning, inspecting, and repairing blisters; sandpapering any dry, rough, or cracked areas; trimming and smoothing nails; and applying a favorite conditioner, such as a lotion, salve, alcohol, or powder. Shoes should also be inspected. Take out the insoles so dirt can be removed and an inspection can be made for nasty little sharp burrs and stickers that like to work their way through the fabric, padding, and linings. Encourage participants to take the following steps to be proactive in foot care:

- If toe swelling is an issue or there are toenail injuries, cut the toebox out of shoes (if the location and terrain allow). A piece of Lycra or other stretch material can be sewn or glued over the hole to keep out junk.
- Frequently immerse feet in cold water during breaks and then thoroughly dry them off prior to putting on fresh socks and shoes.
- Elevate feet above the heart when resting.
- Rotate socks to keep feet as dry as possible, multiple times during the day if needed.
- Have extra shoes a size or two larger than normal, with interchangeable insoles.
- If participants cannot change into larger shoes, start with shoes larger than normal and add a flat insole to help them fit from the start. Remove the insole as their feet swell.
- Use different thicknesses of socks.
- Use antiinflammatory medications.
- Use Betadine or an antibiotic ointment to keep feet as healthy as possible.

MODIFYING FOOTWEAR

Footwear can be modified with an EMT scissors, utility shears, or a surgical blade. Be careful when modifying shoe gear as it is very easy to injure oneself. The toebox can be removed to allow for swelling in the toes or to accommodate bandaged or splinted toes. The shoe's upper can be cut vertically or horizontally to allow for swollen feet or bandages. Here are a few tips for removing the toe box:

- Cut from just below the bottom pair of eyelets or the trim piece of fabric that the eyelets go through.
- Cut down to where the upper joins the sole, from one side around to the other side.
- Trim as much as necessary to clear the toes.
- If trimming the heels, keep the top part of the heel counter. Trim under this down to where the upper joins the sole.
- Use duct tape to cover any rough edges.

POSTEVENT TREATMENTS

The most common foot care injury requiring postevent treatment is blisters. If the blister is still intact, but in an area where pressure may cause it to rupture, drain it and apply a dressing. Instead of tape, use a self-adhering wrap to cover the blister such as cover-roll and/or Coban. Spenco 2nd Skin can be used to protect the blister and make it more comfortable. Blood blisters, unless they are large and prone to rupture, should be left intact. The use of Desitin or zinc oxide can speed up the drying process of a ruptured blister. Soaking one's feet in warm or hot water with Epson salts several times a day will help dry blisters.

COLD AND HEAT THERAPY

Several foot injuries can be helped through the use of cold and heat therapy. Each has its place in the rehabilitation phase of an injury as they help healing by reducing swelling, reducing pain, and promoting circulation. Cold and heat therapy can be used for sprains and strains, contusions and bruises, muscle pulls, and postexercise soreness. Those with Raynaud's syndrome or former frostbite sufferers should not use ice on affected body parts.

The rule of thumb is to start with cold and switch to heat or a cold/heat combination later. Do not use cold or heat therapy on an area where the skin is broken. First treat the wound. Individuals with known or suspected circulatory problems or cold hypersensitivity, paralysis, areas of impaired sensation, or rheumatoid conditions should consult a physician before using cold compression therapy.

Cold Therapy

Cold therapy, often called cryotherapy, is an essential part of rehabilitation after an injury, as well as a preventive measure to avoid problems. Icing is usually done in combination with all the other RICE components: rest, compression, and elevation. Remember that all four are important and should be used together for faster recovery from an injury.

Icing progresses through four stages – cold, burning, aching, and finally numbness, usually taking about 20 minutes in all. The numbness stage should be reached in order to receive the full benefits of icing; when the area goes numb, stop applying ice. The duration of icing depends on the type and depth of the injury. Body areas with less fat and tissue should be iced for less time than fatty or dense areas. After an injury, soft-tissue damage can cause uncontrolled swelling. This swelling can increase the damage of the initial injury and increase the healing time. The immediate use of ice will reduce the amount of swelling, tissue damage, muscle spasms, inflammation, and pain.

Cold therapy works by decreasing the tissue's temperature and constricting the blood vessels in the injured area. This decreases blood flow, venous/lymphatic drainage, and cell metabolism, reducing the chance of hemorrhage and cell death in an acute injury. Once the fourth stage of icing, numbness, is reached, light range-of-motion can be started. Avoid strenuous exercise during cold therapy.

Homemade ice packs can be made with three parts water and one part rubbing alcohol. Mix in a zip-top bag. The result is a hard slush. If the mix is too hard, let it melt and add a little more alcohol. If it is too liquid, add a little more water. The right consistency will allow the bag to be formed around the patient's foot, ankle, or other body part. Use a towel between the ice bag and the skin. Because the alcohol can make them colder then over-the-counter ice packs, care must be taken not to get an ice burn from these packs.

Do not place ice directly on the skin. Always use a thin towel, washcloth, or T-shirt between the ice bag and skin. If you have an Ace wrap on the injured part, apply the ice directly over the wrap. Ice cubes in a plastic bag will work, but crushed ice conforms better to the body. Use an Ace wrap or other type of compression wrap to hold the ice against the injured area. Apply ice three to four times daily to the injured area for 15–20 minutes at a time.

Heat Therapy

Heat therapy is used less often than cold therapy. It is recommended only after swelling and inflammation have subsided (usually at 48–72 hours postinjury). The heat increases blood flow to the injured area, allowing the blood's nutrients to help in the healing process, aid in the removal of waste products from the injured site, and promote healing. Heat can help reduce muscle spasms and pain. Stiffness decreases as tissue elasticity increases. Heat should not be applied for longer than 15–20 minutes at a time and should not be applied to areas of broken skin.

Combination Cold and Heat Therapy

A combination of cold and heat therapy can be used 48–72 hours after an injury. This can be easily accomplished by alternating the use of cold and heat packs, 10–15 minutes at a time. An alternative is a contrast bath. Fill two buckets or basins, one with cold water and some ice and the other with tolerable hot water. Alternate soaking in each for 2 minutes. With combination therapy, the cold keeps the swelling down while the heat keeps the blood and its nutrients circulating through the injured area.

FOOT CARE KITS

It is important to have a high-quality foot care kit. The expedition kit described here is a good example that can be modified for your trips. Additionally, the medical team can encourage or require event participants to have an adequate participant's kit and know how to patch their own feet. If participants spend time preparing their feet before the trip and learning patching techniques, they reduce the chances of needing many of the supplies in the expedition kit. Pretrip preparation includes three steps: reducing calluses with a callus file or creams; getting the skin on their feet in the best possible condition; and trimming toenails correctly.

Participant Kits

It is imperative that those who are involved in extreme team sports or who often cover long distances without crew support carry a small foot care kit. The following items are recommended as a minimum:

- Tincture of benzoin swab sticks or squeeze vials
- Alcohol wipe packets
- A pin and matches for blister puncturing
- A small container of lubricant and/or foot powder
- Selection of tapes wrapped around a pencil
- A plastic bag with their choice of blister patching materials and several pieces of toilet paper or tissues
- A small pocketknife with a built-in scissors

Depending on team or personal needs, they could add a lightweight ankle support and pads for metatarsal, arch, or heel pain.

Expedition Kits

An expedition foot care kit can be customized according to the type of event, the length, and the number of participants. If the medical team will be supplying aid station or transitions areas, additional supplies are warranted. The following materials form the core of the kit. Add or eliminate materials based on personal preferences and experience. Look in the tool section of your local hardware stores for a plastic toolbox with trays in which to store the materials.

Instruments
- Sharp-pointed small scissors
- Sterile needles (18 and 25 gauge)
- Sterile scalpels (#15 and 11)
- Syringes (3 and 5 cc)
- EMT or utility scissors for cutting tape and shoes
- Nail drill
- Toenail clippers
- Nail or pedicure files
- Callus file
- Tweezers for pulling blister skin to cut a hole in it
- Shoehorn

Blister-patching materials
- Lubricant of choice
- Powder of choice
- Blister patches of choice in various sizes (e.g., Spenco 2nd Skin, QuikStik Pads, and Sport Blister Pads)
- Engo Blister Prevention Patches
- Tapes of choice in a variety of sizes (e.g., Leukotape, Kinesio-Tex, and boxes of cover-roll)
- Tincture of benzoin or other tape adherent
- Swabs for applying benzoin
- Alcohol pads
- Tubes of zinc oxide

- Tubes of 2% Xylocaine jelly
- ~~Gauze pads (2 × 2 and 4 × 4) for draining blisters~~

Miscellaneous

- Betadine for cleaning dirty wounds/blisters
- Antiseptic ointment
- Hydrogen peroxide
- Coban – 1 and 2 inch
- Ace wrap – 4 inch
- Sam Splint
- Ankle support
- Pads for metatarsal, arch, or heel pain
- Latex gloves
- Antibacterial hand wipes
- Small basin for soaking feet
- Sponge for cleaning feet
- Hand towel for drying feet
- Plastic bags for garbage
- Injectable steroid (Kenalog 40, Depo-Medrol, methylprednisolone 20 mg, or dexamethasone sodium phos.)
- 2% lidocaine with and without epinephrine
- 0.5% marcaine with and without epinephrine
- 1% hydrocortisone cream
- Injectable Benadryl
- Levaquin 750 mg
- Augmentin 875 mg
- Kerlix bandages
- Roll of ¼-inch adhesive felt
- Veritable array of pads for the metatarsals and arch
- Athletic tape for ankle taping

REFERENCES

1. Bryan Whitesides, MPT, OCS, is a board certified orthopedic clinical specialist and founder of The Injured Runner, *http://www.injuredrunner.com*.
2. Townes DA, Talbot TS, Wetmore IS, Billingsly R. Event medicine: injury and illness during an expedition-length adventure race. *J Emerg Med.* 2004;27(2):161–5.
3. Vonhof J. *Fixing Your Feet: Prevention and Treatments for Athletes*. 4th ed. Berkeley, Calif: Wilderness Press; 2006.
4. Knapik JJ, Reynolds KL, Duplantis KL, Jones BH. Friction blisters: pathophysiology, prevention and treatment. *Sports Med.* 1995;20(3):138.
5. Ibid., p. 138.
6. Ibid., p. 140.
7. Ibid., p. 139.
8. Ibid., p. 139.
9. Bergeron B. A guide to blister management. *Physician Sportsmed.* 1995(February):40.
10. Ibid., p. 43.
11. Rob Conenello, DPM.
12. Hamilton DL. Foot care at Nijmegen 2000. *J Special Operations Med.* 2002;2(3).
13. Auleley GR, et al. Validation of the Ottawa ankle rules. *Ann Emerg Med.* 1998;32(1):14–18.
14. Subotnick S. *Sports Medicine of the Lower Extremity*, vol. 13. 2nd ed. New York: Churchill Livingstone; 1999: 201–4.
15. Lippincott. *Pathophysiol.* 1998;45:1081.
16. Lowe J. *Pathology.* 1995;5:71.
17. The Conservative Treatment of Plantar Fasciitis: A Prospective Randomized, Multicenter Outcome Study. American Orthopaedic Foot and Ankle Society; October 1996.

39 | Expedition Orthopedics

Alan Gianotti, MD, and Swaminatha V. Mahadevan, MD, FACEP, FAAEM

INTRODUCTION – INITIAL APPROACH TO TRAUMA IN THE FIELD

Traumatic events in the wilderness are dramatic. It is easy to become emotional. The victim may be a friend. The scene is often witnessed. A calm, rational approach is essential for proper assessment, stabilization, and treatment of the victim – saving lives and salvaging limbs. This chapter will focus on orthopedic diagnostic and stabilization techniques without the aid of radiography and without the burden of documentation.

INITIAL EVALUATION

In cases of wilderness trauma, always ensure the scene is safe before proceeding toward the victim. Never assume that the scene of any injury is safe. Do not magnify the problem by becoming a statistic yourself. An unstable debris field in an avalanche zone or a hidden crevasse field on a warm, sunny day may also prove hazardous to potential rescuers.

As you arrive at the victim's side, begin with the ABCs (airway, breathing, circulation). This is often difficult because the victim's orthopedic injuries may be very dramatic, and human nature draws our focus to them. Begin by assessing his or her airway and breathing. Call out to the patient to see if they can talk with you. Under most circumstances, hearing the victim speak with a normal voice suggests that the airway and breathing are adequate for the moment. If the victim does not respond to you, assess the airway and breathing by using the look, listen, and feel approach. Look for the symmetric, smooth rise and fall of the chest associated with normal breathing. Listen for air flow from the nose or mouth. Feel for air exchange at the patient's mouth and nose.

Next, evaluate the victim for the presence of shock and/or active bleeding. Begin by feeling for the victim's pulse. The pulse may be assessed at his or her wrist (the radial artery), groin (femoral artery), or neck (carotid artery). Check for the presence, rate, and strength of the radial pulse. A rapid, weak, or absent radial pulse suggests shock. A patient who lacks a palpable carotid or femoral pulse is in cardiopulmonary arrest. Then, assess the color, temperature, and moisture of the extremities. Pale, cool, or clammy skin is worrisome for shock. Next, briefly apply pressure to the patient's nail bed and release. A delay (> 2 seconds) in the return of blood to the nail bed is also of concern for shock.

The initial rapid neurologic evaluation includes assessment of the patient's level of consciousness, gross motor and sensory function, and pupillary reactivity. The AVPU approach assesses if the patient is Alert, responds to Voice or Painful stimulus, or is Unresponsive. Assessment of movement and sensation in all extremities is a gross evaluation of spinal cord function. A detailed neurologic exam is impractical during the initial evaluation and may be delayed until the patient is stabilized.

Any significant mechanism of injury necessitates a rapid yet thorough patient assessment (including vital signs) and vigilant attention to the ABCs. It is imperative to continually reassess patients while en route to definitive medical care.

ORTHOPEDIC EVALUATION

Once the patient is deemed stable, determine the extent of the patient's orthopedic injuries. (See Table 39.1.) The primary areas of focus include the spine, pelvis, and extremities. The cervical spine is evaluated for point tenderness, swelling, or step-off. The pelvis may be gently compressed once (down and in, concurrently) to assess for pain, crepitus, and stability. While maintaining spinal alignment, the back is inspected for point tenderness and any signs of trauma. Finally, the exposed extremities should be assessed for deformity, crepitus, tenderness, swelling, and open wounds. Every joint should be evaluated for range of motion.

Evaluation of the extremities requires assessment of circulatory, nerve, skeletal, and joint function. Determining the extent of the injury, including soft tissue damage, fractures, dislocations, and neurovascular compromise, is imperative. In the field, inspection is often difficult. Layers of clothing and harsh environments are

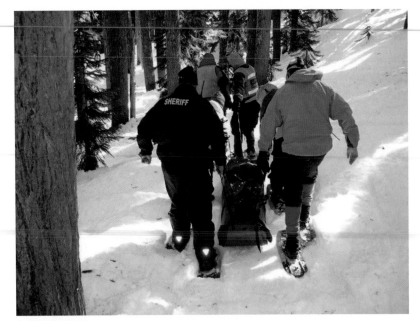

Figure 39.1. Long board evacuation. Courtesy of Deschutes County Search and Rescue.

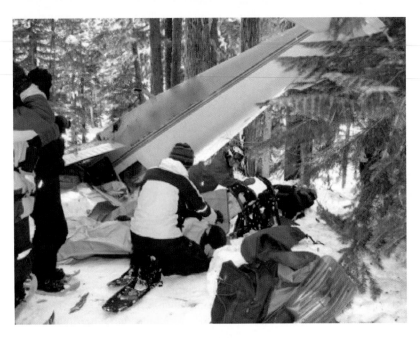

Figure 39.2. Backcountry plane crash in Deschutes County, Oregon. Courtesy of Deschutes County Search and Rescue.

two common obstacles involved in "total" exposure of the patient and the injury. Palpation provides further information: swelling, tenderness, joint involvement, and so on. Only then can a complete assessment be made. Is the injury open or closed? If open, is it reparable in the given environment or is an extensive transport required? Is there joint involvement? Is there ligamentous involvement? Is there neurovascular compromise? Is compartment syndrome a consideration? Has the bleeding been controlled? Is this injury stable or unstable? How will it be splinted and then transported?

Palpable extremity pulses and normal skin color distal to an extremity injury suggest adequate peripheral perfusion. Normal motor and sensory function distal to an extremity injury suggest normal peripheral nerve function (Table 39.2). Specific extremity injuries are associated with specific nerve deficits (Table 39.3).

In the absence of an intact neurovascular exam, gentle traction and repositioning of a fracture, even in a limb that is relatively aligned, will offer the best chance of neurovascular recovery in the field.[1,2] Splinting the injury (post-reduction) while maintaining alignment and traction will provide the best chance of stabilizing the limb. Limb stabilization is essential to limit mobility, reduce pain, slow bleeding, and "contain" the injury.

Table 39.1. Rapid orthopedic assessment

Vascular
  Assess the color and warmth of the extremity distal to the injury.
Nerve
  Assess for light touch and pinprick sensation and motor function.
  For suspected spinal injuries, check the dermatomal distribution.
Skeletal
  A visible deformity may be present with a fracture or dislocation.

In the case of a dislocated joint, attempts at reduction (realignment to a normal anatomic position) should be considered if (1) you are sure it is a dislocation (and not a fracture), (2) there is neurovascular compromise, or (3) transport to definitive health care is delayed (1–6 hours depending on the joint).[3,17] Reductions begin with proper analgesia and proceed with traction of the affected limb, slowly separating the bone surfaces and allowing them to return to their natural anatomic position. Reduction should always

Table 39.2. Peripheral nerves: sensory and motor function [11]

Nerve	Sensory	Motor
Axillary (C5,6)	Lateral aspect of deltoid	Shoulder abduction
Median (C6–8)	Lateral palmar aspect of hand (including lateral palmar half of ring finger)	Abduction of thumb
Radial (C6–8)	Lateral dorsum of hand	Thumb/wrist extension
Ulnar (C8,T1)	Medial palmar aspect of hand (including medial palmar half of ring finger)	Finger abduction
Femoral (L2–4)	Anterior aspect of thigh	Knee extension
Saphenous (L2–4)	Medial aspect of leg and foot	
Sciatic (L4–S3)	Posterior aspect of thigh	Knee flexion
Tibial (L4–S3)	Sole of foot	Plantar fexion (posterior compartment)
Common peroneal (L4–S2)	Posterior aspect of lower leg	
Superficial peroneal (L4–S2)	Lateral aspect of lower leg Dorsum of foot	Foot eversion (lateral compartment)
Deep peroneal (L4–S2)	First toe web space	Dorsiflexion (anterior compartment)

Table 39.3. Extremity injuries and associated nerve deficits [11]

Injury	Possible nerve deficit
Anterior shoulder dislocation/fracture	Axillary nerve Musculocutaneous nerve
Humeral shaft fracture	Radial nerve
Fracture of distal third of radius	Radial nerve
Supracondylar fracture of humerus	Median nerve Radial nerve Ulnar nerve
Posterior elbow dislocation	Median nerve Ulnar nerve
Wrist fracture/dislocations	Median nerve
Posterior hip dislocation	Sciatic nerve
Anterior hip dislocation	Femoral nerve
Knee fracture/dislocation	Peroneal nerve Tibial nerve
Proximal fibula fracture	Peroneal nerve

be followed by reevaluation of perfusion, sensation, and motor function. The realigned joint should then be splinted for stabilization and transport.

EVACUATION

Evacuation is the key to survival with most catastrophes in the wilderness. Preparation is paramount. An evacuation plan includes communication capabilities, transportation techniques, evacuation routes, and a definitive medical destination. Preplanning for any wilderness expedition is essential.

Patient movement techniques vary based on the geography, injury, and number of rescuers involved. Rescuer safety is of primary importance. As noted previously, evaluate the scene and determine its level of safety.[3] Care must then be taken to protect the victim's spine and airway. Bleeding should be controlled, and fractures should be splinted (and typically reduced) in the case of prolonged evacuations. If there is an immediate life-saving reason to move a victim, a variety of transport techniques can be utilized.

"Dragging" a patient (along his or her "long axis") is a common one-rescuer technique when the patient is unresponsive and there is a significant size disadvantage for the rescuer.[2] Shoulder drags, foot drags, blanket drags, and clothes drags are commonly utilized. These are considered "emergency" move techniques and involve keeping the spine forces in line, and the head position low at all times.

One-rescuer carrying styles commonly include piggyback, cradle, pack strap, and firefighter positions.[2] (See Figure 39.6.) These usually require at least partial assistance from the victim. These techniques are contraindicated when there is concern for cervical spine injury. Two- and three-rescuer lifts include direct ground and extremity lifts.[2] The former involves three rescuers assigned to the head, midsection (straddling the buttocks), and legs. Lifting directions are given from the rescuer at the "head." The extremity lift requires a rescuer from behind the victim, lifting under the arms and holding the wrists of the victim. The second rescuer is in front of the patient, turned forward, grasping the legs from behind the knees.

The recovery position is an important positioning technique for the unconscious patient without suspected spine injury.[2] This position helps maintain a patent airway and prevent aspiration. Kneeling on the patient's left, the victim's left arm is placed straight out above the head, and the right arm is stretched across the chest with the right knee completely flexed. The victim is pulled onto his or her left side, resting the victim's head on their left arm.

The log roll technique is important for the unconscious patient who is face down (prone).[2] One rescuer kneels at the head and stabilizes the cervical spine in a neutral, in-line position. The second rescuer kneels at the patient's side, positioning the arms along the side. At the signal from the "head" rescuer, the second rescuer gently pulls at the shoulders and hips while maintaining the spine in a neutral, in-line position until supine.

Many types of specialized equipment are utilized in the evacuation of victims depending on the wilderness location. While baskets are the preferred transport mechanism on the trails of Nepal and Pakistan, scoop (orthopedic) baskets, stair chairs, wheeled litters, long boards, flexible stretchers, and a variety of rescue sleds are available in many of the North American National Parks. (See Figures 39.1, 39.3, 39.4, and 39.5.)

COMMON ORTHOPEDIC CONDITIONS

Definitions

Extremity soft tissue injuries may occur alone, or in association with fractures and dislocations. Sprains,

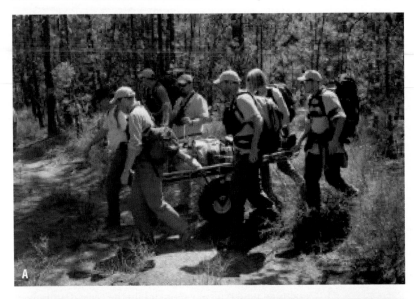

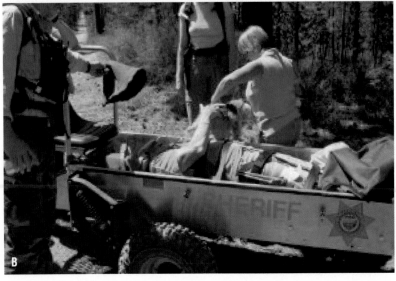

Figure 39.3. Wheeled litters. Courtesy of Deschutes County Search and Rescue.

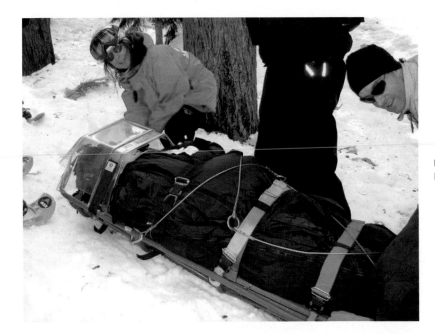

Figure 39.4. Rescue sled. Courtesy of Deschutes County Search and Rescue.

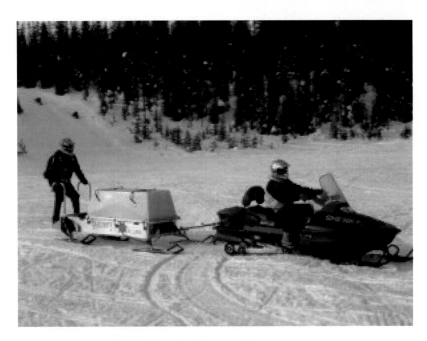

Figure 39.5. Rescue sled. Courtesy of Deschutes County Search and Rescue.

strains, abrasions, avulsions, bruises, lacerations, puncture wounds, and contusions all denote soft tissue injuries that are usually diagnosed and managed in the field. Soft tissue injuries that require immediate evacuation include compartment syndromes and amputations.

A *strain* involves the tearing or stretching of a muscle and its associated tendon. A *sprain* involves the tearing or stretching of ligaments as they attach to bone. These injuries may be further classified by the degree of injury. First-degree injuries have limited fiber involvement; second-degree injuries represent incomplete disruption of the tissue. A third-degree injury designates a complete tear with marked swelling, tenderness, joint laxity,

and functional loss.[4] A person suffering a third-degree ankle sprain in the wilderness would be unable to weight bear and would require ambulatory assistance, such as a crutch, for evacuation.

Tendons are capable of inflammation as well as tearing. Inflammation of a tendon is called *tendonitis.* This condition is a result of overuse. The tendons at high risk for inflammation include the rotator cuff muscles of the shoulder (shoulder impingement), the forearm extensors of the wrist (lateral epicondylitis), the patellar tendon of the knee (jumper's knee), and the posterior tendon of the leg (shin splints). Chronic tendonitis can lead to weakening of the tendon and subsequent rupture.

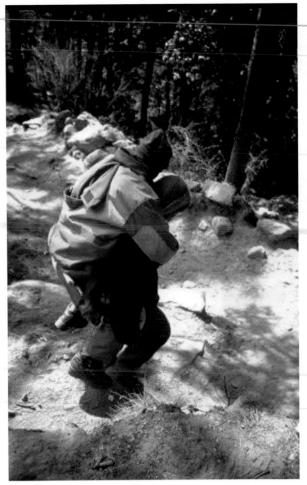

Figure 39.6. Piggyback evacuation in Khumbu, Nepal. Photo courtesy of Alan Gianotti.

Middle-aged adults are most susceptible to tendonitis, but this condition can occur at any age. Antiinflammatory medication, activity modification, and splinting of the affected joint are typically indicated.

An inflamed bursa or *bursitis* usually results from overuse, repetitive movement, or prolonged and significant pressure. Any movement of the joint in question will exacerbate this condition. Stabilization with splinting or drainage may be indicated.

Arthritis encompasses numerous etiologies leading to joint inflammation. In this discussion, we will limit our focus to osteoarthritis, or degenerative joint disease: the destruction of a joint from bone on bone friction following the deterioration of the cartilaginous "cushion" between the bones. Acute inflammation of an arthritic joint may be managed with activity modification and antiinflammatory medication.

Injuries to the soft tissues of the extremities may lead to bleeding. Arterial bleeding is bright red, pulsating, and profuse. Venous bleeding is often "oozing" and dark maroon in color. Significant blood loss can lead to shock.

The four steps to stop bleeding include: direct pressure, elevation, pressure placed at proximal artery points, and, as a last resort, a proximal tourniquet (only if prior steps have failed).[2] Shock management is discussed further in other chapters.

A *fracture* is any break in the continuity of the bone. Fractures may be closed or open (associated with a break in the skin). Fractures of the long bones (e.g., femur fracture) may result in loss of up to 2 L of blood.[3] Fractures typically present with pain, swelling, deformity, and crepitus (the palpable movement of a bone).

Dislocations are the traumatic displacement of a bone out of a joint. Dislocations are frequently associated with ligamentous injury and may be associated with fractures (*fracture dislocation*). Dislocations are commonly diagnosed in the field, and knowledge of reduction techniques is useful for the expedition physician. The common dislocations involve digits, elbows, shoulders, hips, and ankles. Hip and knee dislocations are generally considered medical emergencies that require emergent transfer if the dislocation cannot be reduced in the field. Field reductions are recommended for all dislocations with prolonged transfer times (greater than 1–6 hours depending on the joint) or distal neurovascular compromise.[1,11,17]

GENERAL TREATMENT PRINCIPLES

Pain Management

All expeditions should anticipate the need for analgesic medications. Orthopedic injuries may cause unimaginable pain. Medical kits should include a combination of opioid and non-opioid analgesic agents. Nonsteroidal antiinflammatories (NSAIDs) are effective for mild pain and swelling. NSAIDs should be used cautiously in those at risk for gastrointestinal bleeding, dehydration, and renal impairment.[5] Narcotics (opioid analgesics) such as morphine are extremely effective in reducing severe pain and often anxiety. In general, morphine at 0.1mg/kg IV/IM is a standard initial dose for the treatment of severe pain.[6] The onset of action for an intramuscular shot of morphine is 15 minutes, while the duration can be as long as 5 hours.[6] Opioid analgesics have no antiinflammatory function. Nausea, vomiting, and constipation are common side effects among all narcotics. Respiratory depression and an altered sensorium can be seen at high doses.

RICE

RICE is a mnemonic for Rest, Ice, Compression, and Elevation. It is a time-honored initial treatment for extremity soft tissue injuries. Rest and protect the injured area. Apply ice or a cold pack to reduce pain and

Table 39.4. Backcountry pain management: opioid and nonopioid analgesia [11]

Generic (proprietary)	Dose	Pediatric dose	Toxic dose	Maximum dose
Acetaminophen (APAP)	650–1000 mg PO q4–6h 1 g PR q6h 1–2 g PR q12h	10–20 mg/kg PO 20–40 mg/kg PR q4h	Not an NSAID. Exact mechanism unknown. Liver toxicity possible when above 150 mg/kg is taken in 24 hours	100 mg/kg/day.
Aspirin (ASA)	650–975 mg PO q4h	10–15 mg/kg PO	Reye's syndrome in children who subsequently get flu or chickenpox. Tinnitus Toxic dose 150 mg/kg	60 mg/kg/day
Ibuprofen	600 mg q6–8h	10 mg/kg q6–8h	GI irritation Platelet dysfunction Renal dysfunction Bronchospasm	40 mg/kg/day

Generic (proprietary)	Oral equipotent dose	Parenteral	Duration (in hours)	Comments	Precautions
Morphine	30–60 mg (0.5 mg/kg)	10 mg (0.1 mg/kg)	3–5	Standard for comparison	Respiratory depression Hypotension Sedation Histamine release
Hydrocodone (Vicodin, Lortab)	5–10 mg	N/A	3–4	Good cough suppressant Fewer side effects than codeine and greater potency	Greater abuse potential
Oxycodone (Percocet, Tylox)	5–10 mg	N/A	3	Parenteral form not available in the US. Very effective analgesic	Euphoria, abuse potential

MAOI: monoamine oxidase inhibitor; IV:intravenous

swelling. Ice should never be applied directly to exposed skin; rather, place a towel or cloth under the ice to prevent skin injury. Gentle compression with an elastic bandage will help decrease swelling and augment venous and lymphatic drainage. Signs of overcompression include numbness, tingling, increased pain, reduced circulation, or worsening swelling below the bandage, and necessitate loosening the compressive bandage. Elevate the injured extremity above the level of the heart (if possible) to reduce swelling.

Irrigation

Cleaning open wounds greatly reduces the risk of infection. High-pressure irrigation is the most important aspect of wound cleaning. By applying at least 7–8 psi (e.g., 30-ml syringe and 18-gauge angiocatheter), the irrigation fluid can wash out foreign bodies, contaminants, and bacteria. Tap water is as efficacious as sterile water in most studies.[7,8] Soap and water is effective for out-of-hospital settings. A common practice is to irrigate with about 100 mL for every 1 cm of wound length. Avoid applying peroxide, Beta-iodine, or chlorhexidine directly into the wound because these agents can damage the tissues and impair wound defenses.[9,10]

Antibiotics

The literature suggests a handful of indications for prophylactic antibiotics to prevent wound infections.[10] Complicated wounds such as intraoral lacerations, human or dog bites, cat bites, foot puncture wounds, open fractures, and clearly contaminated wounds should receive antibiotic prophylaxis. In the case of an "open fracture" or an "open joint," the wound is considered contaminated and is at high risk for posttraumatic infection (osteomyelitis).

The time frame for initiating antibiotics is controversial and depends in part on the transport duration to a medical facility. In general, for short transport times, the wound can be bandaged, the extremity splinted, and the patient transported. If the expected duration is greater than 6–8 hours, the wound should be irrigated, debrided and bandaged, the extremity reduced (if indicated) and splinted, and antibiotics initiated.[11] Broad-spectrum antibiotics are indicated for the bacteria commonly implicated in these wounds (oral ciprofloxacin 750 BID and cephalexin 500 QID).[17]

Empiric use of fluoroquinolones (e.g., ciprofloxacin) is controversial for the nail-through-the-tennis-shoe foot puncture wound.[12] The risk of infection (osteomyelitis)

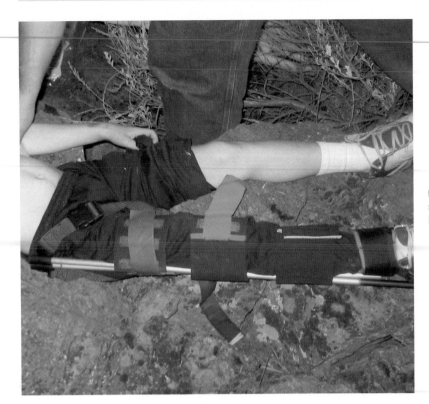

Figure 39.7. Improvised long leg splint with tent stakes and Velcro straps. Photo courtesy of Deschutes County Search and Rescue.

from this mechanism of injury is 1.5%.[13,14] Frequent wound checks and follow-up exams are an alternative to prophylactic antibiotics.

Tetanus

There are approximately 60 cases of tetanus in the United States annually.[10] International rates are even higher. Deep, dirty, and devitalized wounds are tetanus-prone. The unimmunized patient (i.e., < 3 lifetime doses) requires active and passive immunization for the tetanus-prone wound. If the patient is poorly immunized (> 3 doses but last dose given > 5 years prior), give active immunization only. Active immunization is tetanus diphtheria (Td) or tetanus toxin (TT) (0.5 ml IM). Children less than 8 years require diphtheria, pertussis, and tetanus (DPT). Passive immunization is tetanus immune globulin (TIG) 500 units deep IM.[10]

Splinting

Knowledge of splinting techniques is essential in the wilderness. All fractures, dislocations, sprains, strains, and inflammatory conditions may benefit from splinting. In the case of fractures, splinting immobilizes bone ends and protects them from further trauma and bleeding. Splinting, especially in the case of a reduced fracture, minimizes swelling and bleeding and protects against further injury by relieving pressure on compressed nerves and vessels. Splinting allows for the transfer of

a victim out of the wilderness while minimizing movement, injury, and pain.

Splinting guidelines are universal. Expose the fracture site. Control the bleeding. Dress all open wounds. Check circulation. Apply manual traction by gently pulling on the injured limb. Immobilize the fracture as well as the joints above and below the injury. Secure the splint. Elevate the extremity. Maintain body temperature. Reassess the injury and transport.

Virtually any device with structural integrity can be used to splint an injury. Wood, metal, cardboard, rolled newspapers, and even a folded blanket can be used to restrict movement of an injured body part. Soft splints such as pillows, towels, and blankets have a role in support and limiting pain and swelling. Soft splints for the upper extremities are secured with a sling and swathe, such as a triangular bandage, for added support. Rigid splints are more common for the forearm and lower extremities. Rigid splints are commercially available or may be improvised in the field. (See Figures 39.7, 39.8, 39.11, 39.13, 39.20, and 39.22.)

CERVICAL SPINE

An unstable cervical spine is prone to additional injury from manipulation. Spinal immobilization can limit unwanted motion. Proper and secure spinal immobilization is accomplished with a long backboard, a rigid cervical collar, lateral support devices such as tape blocks or towel rolls, and tape or straps to secure the patient to the backboard. Padding may improve positioning and comfort. A rigid cervical collar and tape should be included in all orthopedic first-aid kits. Immobilization of the cervical spine can be improvised in the field. Two rolled sleeping pads placed on either side of the head, taped across the forehead and chin and secured to the supporting stretcher is common in the backcountry.

UPPER EXTREMITY SPLINTING

The hand should always be maintained in the neutral position, also known as the "position of function." This is the position a hand would be in while, say, holding a beer can. A distal neurovascular assessment should always follow placement of any splint. The splint should be removed or repositioned if there are any signs or symptoms of neurovascular compromise.

Rigid splints are not appropriate for shoulder injuries. Shoulder and upper arm (humerus) injuries are secured with a sling and swathe, elevating the wrist above the elbow. Padding may be placed between the chest and arm for additional comfort. A rigid splint is preferred for elbow injuries, although the specific technique (straight or bent position) depends on the initial presentation. Commonly, the elbow is immobilized in the position it is found unless there is distal vascular compromise. Elbow splinting techniques also include immobilization of the shoulder and wrist. Forearm injuries require a rigid splint that should extend from the elbow to beyond the fingertips. Vacuum and air splints are popular for

forearm fractures but require vigilant monitoring of distal perfusion.

Wrist injuries should also be splinted in the position in which they are found unless there is distal neurovascular compromise. Wrist, hand, and finger splints typically include joints proximal and distal to the injury. Buddy-taping an injured finger to its adjacent healthy finger is a common way of immobilizing a finger fracture.

LOWER EXTREMITY SPLINTING

Pelvis fractures are suggested by pelvic, hip, or groin pain, which is exacerbated by palpation or gentle compression. Pain with hip movement is worrisome for a hip fracture. High force pelvic girdle injuries can cause major venous blood loss (in excess of 2 liters).[1] A variety of antishock compression garments are now available to limit pelvic hemorrhage and provide pelvic support. Tied sheets and blankets have also been used in the field for such purposes.[15] (See Figure 39.13.) Transport is usually in the form of long boards or scoop stretchers to further stabilize the fracture.

Posterior hip dislocations present with a medially (inward) rotated leg and bent knee. An anterior dislocation presents with lateral (outward) leg rotation and a bent knee. Supporting the leg in its "found" position with soft splinting is helpful until definitive reduction can take place.

Traction splints and long rigid splints are indicated for thigh (femur) fractures.[1] These rigid splints extend from the groin to beyond the foot. Cravats (straps) are

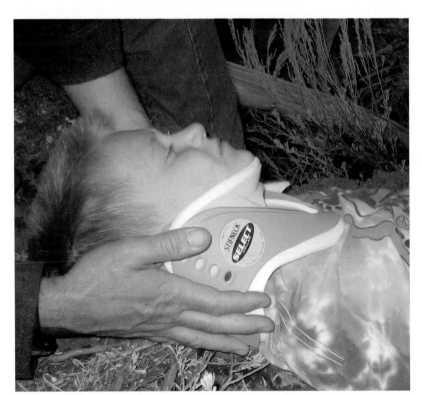

Figure 39.8. Rigid cervical collar. Courtesy of Deschutes County Search and Rescue.

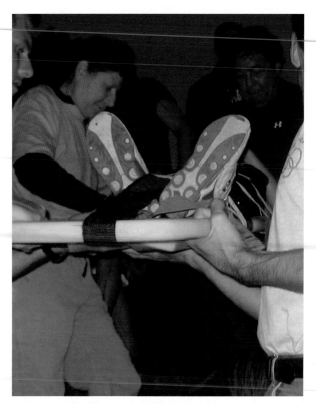

Figure **39.9**. Improvised leg traction. Photo courtesy of Deschutes County Search and Rescue.

used to secure the splint. Traction splints utilizing an ankle hitch involve a frame braced against the trunk and apply a pull to the affected limb. (See Figures 39.7, 39.9, 39.10, and 39.20.) This traction counteracts thigh muscle spasm and allows for bone reduction, pain control, and hemorrhage control.

Rigid splints are most effective for immobilizing an injured knee. These can be placed posterior in the case of an extended knee, or anterior across the thigh and leg (in the case of a flexed knee). Soft or rigid splints are used with lower leg injuries. Pillow splints are common for the

ankle and foot, applying gentle and uniform pressure to immobilize the extremity.

SPINAL INJURY

Spinal Injuries

The spine is susceptible to trauma in the backcountry. Any injury (e.g., diving, falls) that transmits force to the head, neck, or back can result in spinal injury. These injuries may take the form of bony vertebral injury, spinal ligamentous injury, spinal cord injury (SCI), or a combination of these. Spinal injuries should be suspected in any trauma patient with significant mechanism of injury, altered mental status or intoxication, midline spinal tenderness, neurologic symptoms (e.g., numbness, tingling, weakness), or distracting injury (another painful injury that diverts the patient's attention from their spinal injury).

Primary spinal cord injury can vary from microvascular neural tract injuries to complete spinal cord transection.[16] Symptoms can range from pain and paresthesias to complete flaccidity and death. With complete spinal cord transection, symptoms include paralysis with a loss of both sensation and deep-tendon reflexes (below the level of the injury). Prognosis is poor without improvement after 24–48 hours.[16] Cervical spinal cord injury (especially above C4) is usually catastrophic and may require respiratory and circulatory support in the backcountry. Secondary spinal cord injury is further progression of primary SCI and can be minimized through restriction of spinal motion, and maintenance of oxygenation and perfusion.

The mainstay of suspected spinal injury management includes immobilization and evacuation. Immobilization begins with the cervical collar (see Figure 39.8). Many wilderness medical kits do not routinely include immobilization collars. However, most do include materials that are flexible yet rigid, such as Ensolite sleeping pads, rolled bath towels, or empty water bottles. When

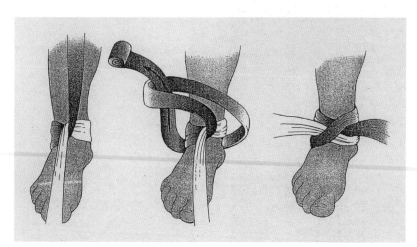

Figure **39.10**. Traction ankle hitch. Redrawn from Auerbach PS, *Wilderness Medicine*, 5th ed, St. Louis: Mosby; 1997: 577.

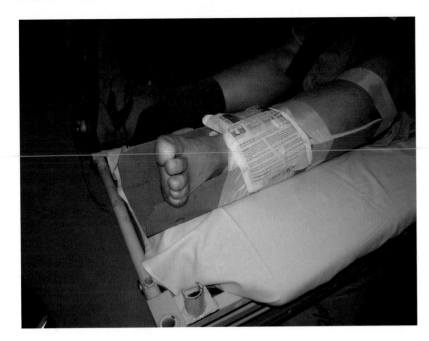

Figure 39.11. Cardboard shortleg splint. Photo courtesy of S.V. Mahadevan.

improvising an immobilization collar, care must be taken to make the collar comfortable and secure (typically with duct tape), and provide access to check anterior carotid pulses. Long spinal boards help reduce spinal motion but require significant manpower and are not always feasible in the backcountry. (See Figure 39.1.) High-dose IV steroids, begun within 8 hours of the injury, may be of benefit with spinal cord injuries but this is controversial.[16]

PELVIC INJURIES

Low-energy pelvic fractures typically result from falls from standing and are stable fractures (do not deform the pelvic ring with normal pressure or weight-bearing). Examples include athletic overuse and avulsion fractures, iliac wing fractures, and low sacral and coccyx fractures. High-energy forces (e.g., falls from height, crush injury) are required to fracture the ischial and pelvic rings. While pubic rami and single pelvic rim fractures are typically stable, open-book and double ring pelvic fractures are not. Gentle palpation may identify crepitus or focal tenderness suggestive of a pelvic fracture. Manual compression along the iliac crests can provide a tactile assessment of pelvic stability. Impaired active leg flexion is predictive of a pelvic fracture (90% sensitivity/95% specificity).[15] Severe pelvic pain and abnormal vital signs (hypotension, tachycardia) may reflect significant blood loss. Venous hemorrhage from an unstable pelvic fracture can be in excess of 2 liters. Unstable pelvic fractures are life-threatening emergencies and early mortality may be as high as 50%.[15]

The stable pelvic fracture can be managed with analgesia, weight-bearing or crutches as tolerated, and activity modification. However, initial field management for unstable fractures includes external compression to control blood loss and IV fluids for circulatory support. Not all expeditions will carry sterile IV fluids, but this is one indication for aggressive fluid administration. IV fluids should be given to maintain a blood pressure of 90 mmHg – external pulses may be used as a rough guide to systolic pressure. A variety of commercial devices are available to provide external pelvic compression including medical antishock trousers and SAM slings. Tied bed sheets or blankets can substitute if these compression devices are not available.[15] (See Figure 39.13.) Transport is usually in the form of long boards or scoop stretchers to further stabilize the fracture.

High-energy pelvic fractures are commonly associated with other significant traumatic injuries, especially abdominal and genitourinary injuries. Therefore, besides death secondary to exsanguination, expected complications include injuries to the abdominal organs, bladder, urethra, anus, rectum, prostate, uterus, as well the lumbar and sacral nerve roots. Emergent transport is essential.

UPPER EXTREMITY INJURIES

Shoulder

The shoulder is composed of three bones (scapula, proximal humerus, and clavicle) and three joints (glenohumeral, acromioclavicular [AC], and sternoclavicular). The rotator cuff, a series of four muscles, surrounds and supports the glenohumeral joint. The deltoid muscle lies just inferior to the rotator cuff. Because the

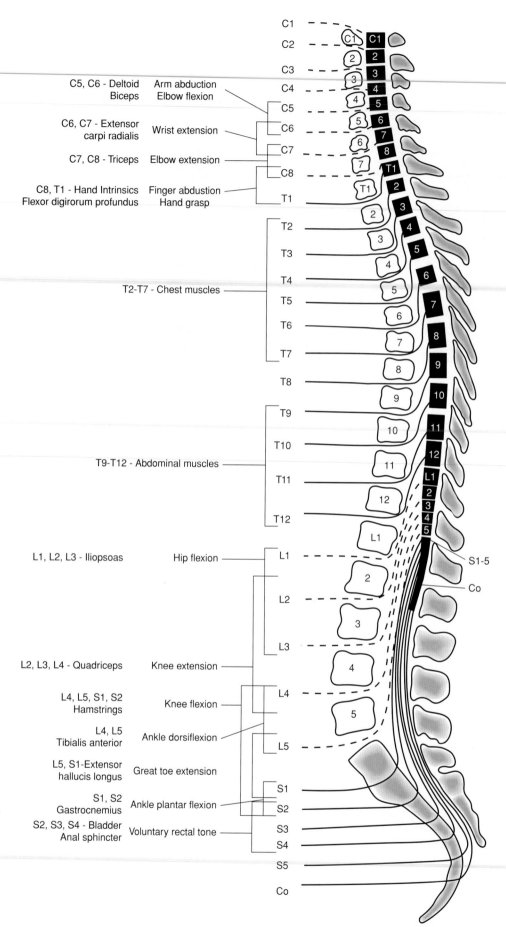

C5, C6 - Deltoid | Arm abduction
Biceps | Elbow flexion

C6, C7 - Extensor carpi radialis | Wrist extension

C7, C8 - Triceps | Elbow extension

C8, T1 - Hand Intrinsics
Flexor digirorum profundus | Finger abdustion
Hand grasp

T2-T7 - Chest muscles

T9-T12 - Abdominal muscles

L1, L2, L3 - Iliopsoas | Hip flexion

L2, L3, L4 - Quadriceps | Knee extension

L4, L5, S1, S2
Hamstrings | Knee flexion

L4, L5
Tibialis anterior | Ankle dorsiflexion

L5, S1-Extensor hallucis longus | Great toe extension

S1, S2
Gastrocnemius | Ankle plantar flexion

S2, S3, S4 - Bladder
Anal sphincter | Voluntary rectal tone

S1-5

Co

Figure 39.12. Spinal cord levels and corresponding motor functions. From Tintinalli JE, Ruiz E, Krome RL, eds., *Emergency Medicine – A Comprehensive Study Guide.* 5th ed. New York: McGraw-Hill; 1996: Figure 256–6.

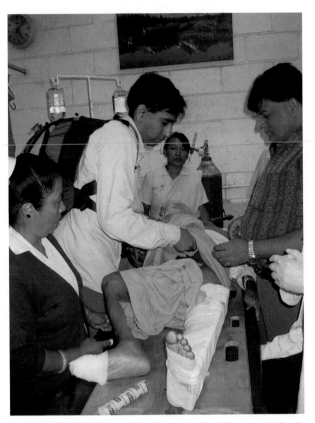

Figure 39.13. Author improvising "bed sheet" pelvic compression in Kathmandu, Nepal. Long leg splint is also seen. Photo courtesy of Alan Gianotti.

shoulder is often the first point of contact in most gravity "mediated" injuries, it is commonly injured. Shoulder injuries include fractures of the clavicle, proximal humerus, and scapula; dislocations of the glenohumeral joint; and injuries to the AC joint and rotator cuff.

Fractures

Shoulder injuries account for 11% of all alpine ski injuries.[3] and clavicle fractures are the most common childhood fracture.[4] Shoulder fractures typically present with localized tenderness and swelling, decreased range of motion, and ecchymoses. All shoulder fractures are initially managed alike, utilizing a sling and swathe. Clavicle and scapula fractures may be associated with serious injuries including cardiac, pulmonary, vertebral, brachial plexus, and great vessel injury. Complications of proximal humerus fractures include impingement syndromes, axillary nerve injury, avascular necrosis, and adhesive capsulitis.[16]

Dislocations

The most common shoulder dislocation (anterior dislocation) occurs when the arm is raised and forced posteriorly (abduction with external rotation).[4] The clinical appearance is a "squared off" shoulder, with loss of the rounded deltoid contour compared to the unaffected side. (See Figure 39.15.) The patient typically holds their arm in slight abduction and external rotation and resists abduction and internal rotation. The humeral head is palpable anteriorly in the subcoracoid region, beneath the clavicle. The axillary nerve may be injured with anterior shoulder dislocations so sensation over the deltoid should be tested.

Numerous techniques have been described for reducing anterior shoulder dislocations. For the traction-countertraction technique, the patient is supine with the arm abducted and flexed 90 degrees at the elbow. The primary care provider applies traction to the arm while a colleague applies steady countertraction with a sheet tied around the patient's torso until the shoulder

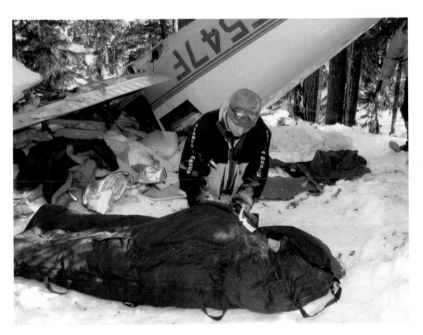

Figure 39.14. Warming blanket. Courtesy of Deschutes County Search and Rescue.

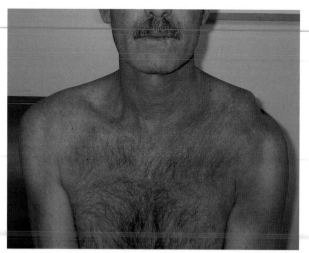

Figure 39.15. Anterior shoulder dislocation. Photo courtesy of S.V. Mahadevan.

is reduced. Narcotic analgesics and benzodiazepines are quite helpful, allowing the patient to relax and limiting resistance.[4]

Scapular manipulation (or rotation) is another reduction technique that enjoys a high success rate (See Figure 39.16.) With the patient sitting upright, traction is applied to the affected arm by pulling on the wrist with one hand and bracing the chest with the other. A second provider then manipulates the scapula, simultaneously rotating the inferior scapula medially (towards the spine) and the superior scapula laterally (away from the spine). Repetitive dislocations can often be reduced quickly without analgesia.[4] Following reduction, the shoulder should be immobilized with a sling and swathe.

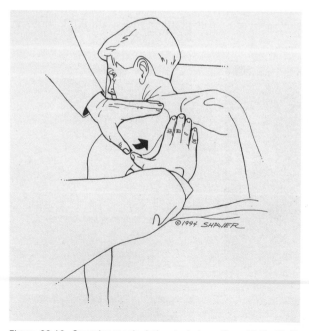

Figure 39.16. Scapular manipulation technique. From Tintinalli JE, Ruiz E, Krome RL, eds. *Emergency Medicine – A Comprehensive Study Guide.* 5th ed. New York: McGraw-Hill; 1996.

AC Joint Separation

A direct blow to an adducted shoulder is the common mechanism of an acromioclavicular (AC) joint separation. Picture the rock climber pendulating into the cliff – shoulder first. Findings include acute shoulder pain, point tenderness over the AC joint, and prominence of the distal clavicle (due to the downward pull of the shoulder). Severity ranges from ligamentous sprains (first-degree separation) to complete ligamentous tears (second-degree) to superior clavicle dislocation (third-degree). Initial management includes ice, sling and swathe, and antiinflammatories. Early range of motion is encouraged, and long-term complications include degenerative joint disease.

Shoulder Impingement

The rotator cuff consists of four muscles and their musculotendinous attachments that abduct and rotate the shoulder. Rotator cuff injuries and other conditions that narrow the space between the acromion and the humeral head can cause impingement. Repetitive overhead arm movements are often to blame and are the primary cause of shoulder impingement pain in adults over 35.[16] Other common causes of shoulder impingement are bursitis, arthritis (AC joint), and tendonitis.

Symptoms of impingement vary from shoulder pain after activity, to a dull, nocturnal discomfort that can evolve into widespread shoulder pain with paresthesias. Painful abduction to 90° with internal rotation against resistance is considered a positive impingement sign. Weak resisted abduction (70–120°) with external rotation is considered a positive goal post test and may represent an advanced injury or tear.[16]

Management of a shoulder impingement involves modifying overhead activity, ice therapy after activity, and NSAIDs. Lidocaine and steroid injections into the subacromial bursa are indicated when conservative measures fail.[16] Surgery is indicated in the athletic patient with a complete tear.

Arm

In layman's terms, and for the sake of this discussion, the proximal humerus will be considered part of the shoulder; the distal humerus part of the elbow; and the arm will represent the shaft of the humerus.

Arm fractures result from either direct blows or falls onto outstretched hands. The clinical exam reveals tenderness, swelling, and deformity, and the patient will usually resist motion secondary to pain. Fractures of the proximal humerus may be difficult to differentiate from a shoulder dislocation.

Proximal humerus fractures may be splinted with a sling and swathe. Midshaft humerus fractures may be treated with a coaptation (sugar tong) splint. Proximal and midshaft humeral fractures are not treated with mechanical traction as this approach can compress the axilla (and axillary artery) and compromise circulation.

Worrisome complications of humeral shaft fractures include brachial artery damage, and injury to the radial, ulnar, and median nerves.[4] Displaced humeral fractures may require reduction in the field to restore neurovascular function.

Elbow

The elbow is an inherently stable joint formed by the articulations of the distal humerus, proximal radius, and proximal ulna. The elbow is traversed by the brachial artery and the radial, ulnar, and median nerves. The superficial olecranon bursa overlies the olecranon process. Elbow injuries include fractures of the distal humerus (e.g., suprcondylar), proximal ulna (e.g., olecranon), and proximal radius (e.g., radial head). The elbow may also suffer from dislocation, overuse syndrome (e.g., tennis elbow), and bursitis.

Fractures

Fractures involving the elbow most commonly result from a fall on an outstretched hand, direct trauma, or an avulsion of bone. On examination, these patients may have bony tenderness, crepitus, swelling, and reduced range of motion. Joint effusions are best palpated between the lateral epicondyle, olecranon, and radial head. Patients with tenderness of the radial head or pain with pronation/supination may have a radial head fracture. A careful neurovascular exam is important with elbow injuries because ulnar nerve injury is common with olecranon fractures, and the median nerve and brachial artery may be injured with supracondylar (distal humeral) fractures.[4] Acute vascular injury should always be suspected with supracondylar fractures, and absence of radial pulse is a worrisome finding mandating immediate reduction. Fracture reduction involves longitudinal traction and elbow flexion to 90° with pulse monitoring for vascular restoration. The arm should be splinted in the position where vascular supply is restored.

The management of suspected elbow fractures (not requiring emergent reduction) involves a long-arm posterior splint (from axilla to palm) with the elbow at 90° of flexion and the forearm in neutral (thumb-up) position. Alternatively, a double-sugar tong splint may be used to prevent pronation and supination of the elbow. Some patients with elbow fractures and significant effusions may benefit from joint aspiration to relieve pain. Aspiration should be performed between the radial head, lateral epicondyle, and olecranon process (20-cc syringe, 18 gauge needle, and aspiration of 4 cc blood).[4] Radial head fractures can alternatively be treated with a sling and early range of motion exercises.

Children with supracondylar fractures are at risk for complications such as compartment syndrome and Volkmann's ischemic contractures.[4] Complications of radial head fractures include restricted range of motion and chronic pain.

Posterior Elbow Dislocation

Posterior and posterolateral dislocations account for 90% of all elbow dislocations. Posterior elbow dislocations result from a fall onto an extended, abducted arm. The clinical exam reveals the elbow held in flexion (45°), with an obvious deformity and a prominent olecranon posteriorly.[4] (See Figure 39.17.) Posterior, medial, and lateral dislocations are reduced with gradual traction along the long axis of the forearm and while an assistant provides countertraction of the upper arm. This is followed by flexion of the elbow; a palpable "clunk" confirms successful reduction. Downward pressure on the forearm may assist with dislodging the coronoid process from the olecranon fossa. Following reduction, immobilize with a long-arm posterior splint and the elbow flexed to 90°. Fractures are common following elbow dislocations. Neuropraxias can occur but are usually transient (ulnar nerve most commonly).[4] The patient should also be assessed for brachial artery injury.

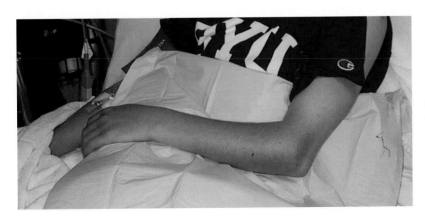

Figure 39.17. Posterior elbow dislocation. Photo courtesy of S.V. Mahadevan.

Radial Head Subluxation (Nursemaid's Elbow)

Subluxation of the radial head most commonly occurs in children, usually younger than 3 years of age. The mechanism of injury is a sudden jerking or lifting of the forearm resulting in some fibers of the annular ligament lodging between the radial head and capitellum. The affected child will usually avoid moving his or her arm and hold the elbow in slight flexion with pronation of the forearm. Treatment consists of application of thumb pressure to the child's radial head and then flexing and supinating in one continuous motion. With a successful reduction, the child will begin using the affected arm within minutes. No other treatment is necessary.

Lateral Epicondylitis (Tennis Elbow)

The elbow is sensitive to overuse. A lateral epicondylitis (tennis elbow) results from repetitive rotary motion of the forearm. Dorsiflexion of the wrist and supination of the forearm against resistance will reproduce the discomfort. Tennis elbow is treated with moist heat, antiinflammatories, and avoidance of the inciting activity. A posterior splint may be applied with the elbow flexed at 90°, the forearm supinated, and the wrist slightly extended. Local injection (at the point of maximum tenderness) of 1–2 ml of a corticosteroid-anesthetic mixture may be helpful in the wilderness setting.

Olecranon Bursitis

Olecranon bursitis may result from trauma, overuse, or infection. The classic exam reveals focal swelling and tenderness to palpation over the posterior elbow. Elbow range of motion is usually normal. If there is a high suspicion for an infected (septic) bursitis, needle aspiration and oral antibiotics are indicated in the field. Noninfectious bursitis may be managed with sterile aspiration, compression (Ace wrap), immobilization (sling), and nonsteroidal antiinflammatory medications.

Forearm

The forearm is made up of two long bones (radius and ulna) that may fracture as a result of direct blows (nightstick fracture) or falls. (See Figure 39.18.) Though forearm shaft fractures are uncommon in adults, three are worth mentioning: ulnar shaft fractures, Monteggia fractures, and Galeazzi fractures.

The Monteggia fracture is a proximal ulnar shaft fracture with radial head dislocation. The Galeazzi fracture is a distal radial shaft fracture with dislocation of the distal radioulnar joint. The joint injuries associated with these fractures may be easily missed so it is important to assess the elbow and distal radius and ulna for tenderness and swelling. Management of forearm fractures includes long-arm posterior splinting with 90° elbow flexion and the wrist in the neutral position. Most forearm fractures require emergent surgical correction.

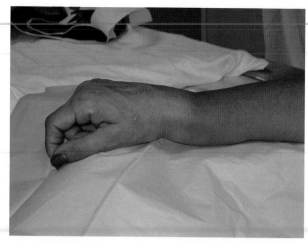

Figure 39.18. Distal radial fracture with dorsal angulation. Photo courtesy of S.V. Mahadevan.

Complications of forearm shaft fractures include malunion, recurrent joint subluxations, and radial nerve contusions (impaired finger and wrist extension) with Monteggia fractures. Ulnar nerve injuries are rare. Compartment syndromes can be seen with any high-energy injury.[4]

Wrist

The wrist is formed by the distal ulna and the distal radius, which independently articulates with the carpal bones, a group of eight bones joined by a complex set of ligaments.

Fractures

The common mechanism of wrist fracture is a fall onto an outstretched hand (FOOSH injury). This fall may result in a Colles' fracture (extension fracture of the distal radius) which presents with dorsal wrist swelling and deformity. (See Figure 39.18.) Rarely, the distal radius may flex "south," resulting in a Smith's fracture (reverse Colles') because of the volar angulation. This fracture occurs when the wrist is flexed or the fall is backward onto a supinated forearm. In the field, the indication for emergent reduction of a wrist fracture is neurovascular compromise (dusky or numb hand) or prolonged time to evacuation.[17]

Emergent reduction in the field can be accomplished by injecting 5–10 cc of 1% lidocaine (or 0.5% bupivacaine) into the fracture site (hematoma block). Aspirating blood with the syringe will ensure proper needle placement. Reduction of a Colles' fracture involves hyperextending and then applying pressure to the distal fragment with both thumbs until it can be "hooked over" the proximal fragment. Having an assistant provide countertraction above the elbow may facilitate reduction. Special attention needs to be paid to the median nerve compression (palmar pain and paresthesias). Splinting involves a short-arm or double sugar tong splint with the forearm neutral and the wrist in slight flexion with ulnar deviation. Smith's fractures are splinted similarly, but with the forearm in supination with slight wrist extension.

The second most frequently fractured wrist bone is the scaphoid. The mechanism is a hyperextension injury or a direct blow. The exam displays point tenderness over the anatomical "snuff box" on the dorsal wrist (ulnar border: extensor pollicis longus; radial border: extensor pollicis brevis and abductor pollicis longus).[4] Any tenderness in this area with the aforementioned mechanism should be considered a fracture in the field. Splinting consists of a radial gutter (thumb spica) splint. Common complications with scaphoid fractures include malunions and avascular necrosis.

Carpal Tunnel Syndrome

The median nerve runs through a carpal tunnel at the wrist, overlaid by the transverse carpal ligament. Overuse syndromes and systemic illness can cause inflammation of this narrow pathway causing compression of this nerve. This syndrome presents with paresthesias, numbness, and pain at the palmar surface of digits 1–3 (and the radial half of digit 4), worsened by repetitive gripping or prolonged flexion of the wrist (e.g., holding a book). It is often worse at night. Atrophy and weakness are late findings. Initial treatment is conservative with antiinflammatories, continuous wrist splinting, and activity modification. Surgical release is reserved for refractory cases.[15]

Hand

Hand injuries are very common (accounting for up to 20% of ED visits) and can be quite complicated.[15] The hand consists of 19 separate bones: the five metatarsals forming the infrastructure of the palm and 14 phalanges forming the digits (three for each finger and two for the thumb). The muscles that control hand function are divided into the extrinsic muscles (originating from the forearm) and the intrinsic muscles (originating from the hand). Two major arteries supply blood to the hand (radial and ulnar arteries), and share extensive collateral blood flow. Three nerves (median, ulnar, and radial) supply sensory innervation and motor function to the extrinsic and intrinsic muscles of the hand.

Fractures

Hand injuries to the digits or metacarpals are primarily caused by axial loads or direct trauma, and are as likely in the wilderness as they are in your local bar. The clenched fist axial load is the most likely cause of a fifth metacarpal neck fracture, aptly named the Boxer's fracture. Wilderness management of these injuries is difficult because the location, angulation, and rotation determine fracture management, and radiographs are not available in the field. Rotational deformities are suspected when digits 2–5 of a closed fist do not point to the tubercle of the scaphoid. Metacarpal reduction is indicated if angulation is greater than 15–40° in metacarpals 4 and 5, or if greater than 10° in metacarpals 2 and 3. Displaced phalanx fractures may be reduced by applying traction to correct the deformity. Though fractures of the first metacarpal are rare, they may be complicated by the MCP joint involvement (Bennett fracture). In the field, all metacarpal and phalanx fractures should be splinted. Ulnar gutter splints are utilized for metacarpals 4 and 5, while radial gutter splints are utilized for metacarpals 1, 2, and 3. The splint should extend from the distal elbow to the proximal interphalangeal (PIP) joints. The wrist joint should be splinted in 20° of extension and the metacarpophalangeal (MCP) joint in 60° of flexion.[4] For splinting isolated digit injuries, buddy taping (to an adjacent digit) or a foam padded aluminum splint may be employed.

The major complication with metacarpal fractures is the high incidence of open fractures. Unfortunately, these are commonly infected with organisms from the human mouth – the common end point of an axial load. These wounds need to be extensively irrigated. Dead and devitalized tissue should be debrided. Most contaminated wounds should be initially left open. The preferred drug for prophylaxis and treatment is amoxicillin-clavulanate (875/125 mg BID for 5 days).[14]

Dislocation

Disolocations at the proximal interphalangeal (PIP) joint occur commonly while distal interphalangeal (DIP) joint dislocations are much less common. The mechanism associated with PIP dislocations is forced hyperextension with axial loading (e.g., outstretched finger is struck by a thrown object). The distal phalanx displaces dorsally over the head of the more proximal phalanx. PIP dislocations typically include at least one collateral ligament injury and rupture of the volar plate.[4]

Management is reduction. A digital block (4 cc of 1% lidocaine without epinephrine) is utilized as a regional anesthetic. Reduction is performed with gentle hyperextension followed by axial (longitudinal) traction. Postreduction, the joint is splinted at 15-30° of flexion for 3–5 weeks to allow healing of the volar plate.[4] Long-term complications of a closed injury may include residual periarticular swelling.

Ulnar Collateral Ligament (Gamekeeper's Thumb)

A fall onto an outstretched thumb causing hyperabduction at the MCP joint is capable of tearing the ulnar collateral ligament. This injury, known as gamekeeper's thumb, is now more likely to be seen with falls on the ski slope with the ski pole in hand. Clinically, patients have difficulty touching their thumb to their little finger (pinch and/or grasp). Holding a beer can is an appropriate test in this case. The examination may reveal tenderness and swelling over the ulnar aspect of the first MCP joint. The severity of the injury is based on the degree of laxity with passive abduction. Surgical repair within one week of injury is indicated for greater than 20 degrees of ulnar ligament instability when compared to the unaffected side.[4] Lesser injuries can be treated with extended (3 weeks) immobilization (thumb-spica splint). Long-term complications include chronic weakness, pain, and instability.

Subungual Hematoma

Crush injuries to the distal digit may lead to subungual hematoma (bleeding in the space between the nail bed and fingernail). Dark discoloration under the nail and associated point tenderness confirm the diagnosis. Subungual hematomas are managed with nail trephination (e.g., electrocautery, heated paper clip). Previously, larger hematomas (< 50%) were commonly managed with nail removal to allow evaluation of the underlying nail bed. Currently, nail removal is only recommended with associated nail avulsion or surrounding nail fold disruption.[5] Nail removal and the repair of nail bed lacerations require a digital block for anesthesia and repair with absorbable, 6–0 Vicryl sutures.

Felon

Infection of the distal digit pulp-space is termed felon. These infections result from minor trauma to the finger pad. Patients present throbbing pain, pressure, and a red, swollen finger pad. *Staphylococcus aureus* is the most common bacterial culprit. Management is surgical with a digital block for anesthesia. A simple midline incision of the pad is made with a sterile #11 blade at the point of maximum tenderness, directly over the abscess. A small clamp or blunt instrument can be used to break up septa and ensure complete drainage. With larger incisions, insertion of a wick allows for continued drainage. Warm soaks, elevation, splinting, and oral antistaphylococcal antibiotics should be routinely initiated. Complications include spread of the infection to the flexor tendon sheath, osteomyelitis, chronic pain, and loss of sensation.[5]

Paronychia

A paronychia is a soft-tissue infection at the lateral nail fold. Conservative therapy involves antistaphylococcal antibiotics and warm soaks 3–4 times per day. A small abscess may be drained by lifting the nail fold off the nail with a blunt instrument. A larger abscess requires a digital block for anesthesia and incision with a #11 blade. Paronychia with pus extension beneath the nail require partial or complete nail removal.

De Quervain's Tenosynovitis

Repetitive thumb activity can cause inflammation of the thumb tendons (abductor pollicis longus and extensor pollicis brevis) where they cross the radial styloid, also known as De Quervain's tenosynovitis. An overuse history, tenderness over the radial styloid, and a painful Finklestein's test (pain with the thumb tucked closed fist and ulnar deviation of the wrist) are diagnostic. Management is usually conservative with immobilization (a thumb-spica splint) and antiinflammatories. Injection of the tendon sheath with a steroid and local anesthetic may provide relief if conservative therapy fails.

Extensor Tendon Injuries

Boutonniere Deformity

A boutonniere deformity is typically a delayed complication following injury to the PIP joint, specifically the central slip of the extensor mechanism. The patient presents joint tenderness associated with flexion of the PIP joint and hyperextension of the DIP joint. Treatment consists of a volar or safety-pin splint for 6 weeks to maintain the PIP joint in extension and referral to an orthopedic surgeon. Complications include contractures and permanent loss of motion.

Mallet Finger

A jamming injury causing forced flexion of an extended DIP joint can lead to an avulsion of the extensor tendon and subsequent mallet or swan neck deformity. With this injury, the distal phalanx appears slightly flexed and the patient is unable to actively extend at the DIP joint. Management is strict, uninterrupted splinting of the DIP joint in extension (6-8 weeks) to allow complete healing.

LOWER EXTREMITY INJURIES

Hip

The hip is a protected ball and socket joint formed by the head of the femur and the acetabulum of the pelvis. The joint is supported by a strong fibrous capsule, which then forms three separate ligaments by capsular thickening. There are three sources blood to the femoral head: the retinacular arteries, the nutrient artery (superior branch), and the artery of the ligamentous teres. The muscles surrounding the hip joint are massive and, in turn, powerful.

Hip Fracture

A hip fracture implies a fracture to the femur proximal to the subtrochanteric region. The mechanism of hip fractures differs depending on the age of the patient. A low-energy fall is sufficient to fracture an elderly (osteoporotic) or cancerous hip, while overuse can cause a stress fracture in an endurance athlete. In the wilderness, most hip fractures result from high-impact trauma in young healthy victims. The diagnosis can often be made clinically on the grounds of a shortened, externally rotated leg in a patient unable to bear weight. Pain is typically localized to the anterior thigh or groin. Effective splinting is maintained by a long spine board (or similar object) while supporting the leg as found with pillows and blankets for comfort. Aseptic necrosis of the femoral head (from the disruption of blood flow) is a significant long-term complication of this fracture and may be reduced by early orthopedic management.

Posterior Hip Dislocation

Hip dislocations are generally a high-force, high-velocity injury. This injury can occur in major traumas and falls, such as on a ski slope or into a crevasse. Trivial injuries may lead to hip dislocations in two specific groups – young children and individuals with "prosthetic" artificial hips.

Clinical findings include hip and buttock pain, and limited range of motion. In the field, visual deformity may help distinguish between hip fracture and dislocation.[11] The characteristic posture of the more common posterior dislocation is a shortened leg, slightly flexed knee and hip with the leg internally rotated and adducted, and the foot turned inward. Anterior dislocations are less common and may appear similar to hip fractures with the leg shortened, abducted, and externally rotated (foot turned outward), except that the head of the femur protrudes in the inguinal area and not posteriorly.

In the case of traumatic hip dislocations, immediate transfer to an orthopedic facility is desirable because of the high incidence of concurrent hip fracture and risk of avascular necrosis of the femoral head. In the field, if the diagnosis is assured and transfer is delayed (>6 hours), attempts to reduce the posterior hip dislocation are recommended.[11,22] In the case of neurovascular compromise (decreased distal circulation, sensation or motor function), attempts at reduction should be considered immediately.[1]

Reduction of a posterior hip dislocation is facilitated by having the patient lie supine on the ground or a firm surface. Pre-procedure narcotic analgesia is essential. An assistant should hold the pelvis firmly by placing downward pressure on the iliac crests. Then, the primary care provider should apply slowly increasing traction along the axis of the femur to a flexed (90°) hip and knee. Gentle internal and external rotation may help. The muscles may take some time to relax but the provider will feel the hip pop back into position following successful reduction. The leg should be splinted supine, in full extension. If the reduction is unsuccessful, the leg should be splinted in its "found" position on a long spine board utilizing pillows for support/comfort.[1]

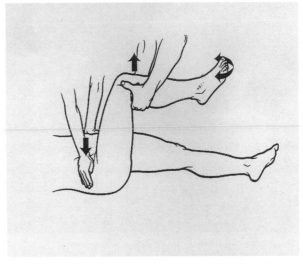

Figure 39.19. Allis method for posterior hip reduction. From Marx JA, et al., ed., *Rosen's Emergency Medicine*. 5th ed. St. Louis: Mosby; 2002: 64.

Complications of hip dislocations include ligamentous injury, acetabular fractures, concurrent knee injury (up to 50%), and sciatic nerve injury (8–13%). Delayed reduction increases the risk of aseptic necrosis of the femoral head.[16]

Thigh

The thigh represents one bone – the femur. This bone is surrounded on three sides by the large quadriceps muscles (vastus lateralis, intermedius, medialis, and rectus femoris). The gluteus maximus and hamstring muscles support the femur from posterior aspect. The femoral artery and vein become the popliteal artery and vein posterior to the knee. The femoral nerve runs through the anterior thigh while the sciatic nerve courses the posterior thigh.

Femur Fracture

A femur fracture (shaft fracture) results from a violent force, and may be associated with other serious injuries including hip dislocations, pelvic fractures, and internal bleeding. These fractures are painful and blood loss from an isolated femur fracture may exceed 1 liter. The diagnosis of a femur fracture can be made clinically in the field by visualization of deformity or swelling, and palpation tenderness on examination. These fractures warrant narcotic analgesia, splinting, and rapid transport. Traction splints help reduce blood loss and alleviate pain by reducing femur fractures to near anatomic alignment. (See Figures 39.20 and 39.21.) Traction splints are contraindicated if the lower extremity or pelvis is fractured in addition to the femur.[1] Pneumatic (air) splints may have a role in controlling blood loss by direct pressure.

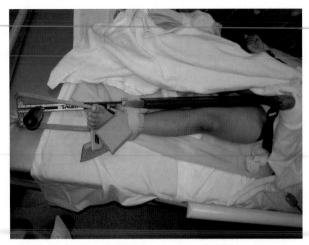

Figure 39.20. Sager traction splint. Femur fracture. Photo courtesy of S.V. Mahadevan.

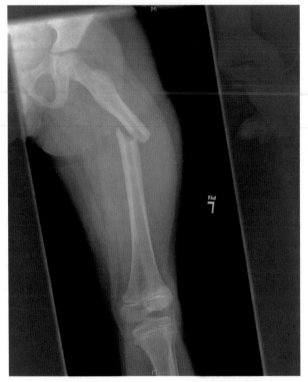

Figure 39.21. Femur fracture. Photo courtesy of S.V. Mahadevan.

Knee

The knee is a complex hinge joint, formed by articulations of the distal femur, proximal tibia, and proximal fibula, as well as the patella and its patellofemoral joint. Intrinsic ligaments and external tendons from the quadriceps and hamstring muscles support the knee joint. The fibrous iliotibial tract also supports the knee joint laterally. Internally, the anterior and posterior cruciate ligaments stabilize the knee. Blood is supplied from the popliteal artery. It has a posterior tether and is susceptible to injury by traction forces, such as dislocations

and fractures. Collateral circulation is poor, and so the viability of the distal limb is at risk with popliteal injury. The sciatic nerve separates prior to the knee. The tibial branch courses posterior with the popliteal artery and is susceptible to the same forces as the popliteal artery. The peroneal branch courses superficially around the lateral aspect of the knee to the proximal fibula and is susceptible to superficial external compression forces (i.e., high ski boots).

Fractures

Knee fractures occur commonly. Patella, distal femur, and tibial plateau fractures result from direct blow or axial compression injuries. The clinical examination in patients with knee fractures commonly reveals a large joint effusion, focal bony tenderness, and the inability to bear weight. Patients with patella fractures may be capable of bearing weight. Field treatment of knee fractures includes immobilization and non-weight-bearing transport. Complications include popliteal artery injury as well as common peroneal and tibial nerve injury. Tibial plateau fractures with concurrent knee dislocation are at especially high risk for a popliteal artery injury that could jeopardize the viability of the leg.

Knee Dislocation

Knee dislocations are another high-force, high-velocity injury. These injuries are typically manifested by a gross knee deformity associated with swelling and immobility. Some dislocations may reduce spontaneously making the diagnosis challenging. Clinical exam may reveal joint laxity to varus and valgus stress, and to anterior and posterior stress, though excessive swelling makes these exams difficult.

Emergent reduction is essential in all cases of distal neurovascular compromise or when transport time will exceed 2 hours.[1] If reduction is not performed, the knee should be splinted in the position found. Both anterior and posterior knee dislocations are reduced by applying longitudinal traction to the lower leg.[15] Having an assistant apply downward pressure on the distal femur may be helpful in reducing posterior dislocations.[1] The liberal use of analgesia is essential and the knee should be immobilized following successful reduction.

Knee dislocations have associated vascular injuries in 40–50% of cases.[11] Emergent evaluation for a popliteal artery injury is indicated in all cases. Presence of a normal distal pulse does not preclude occult popliteal artery injury.[5] Knee amputation rates are reported at 86% for those vascular injuries not repaired within 8 hours of dislocation.

Patellar Dislocation

Patellar dislocations are more common than knee dislocations and result from a twisting injury or direct patellar trauma with the knee in slight flexion. The injury occurs primarily in adolescents (85%), is more common in girls, and may be recurrent.[16] The patient usually presents with the knee flexed and the patella displaced laterally. Patella reduction is accomplished by simple extension of the lower leg (straightening at the knee) with gentle pressure on the patella, pushing it back into its femoral articular groove. Successful reduction commonly relieves the pain and should be followed by bracing/splinting the knee in full extension.

Soft Tissue Injuries

Patella and quadriceps tendon injuries historically occur with direct knee trauma, but they also may result from an indirect distracting force (quadriceps contraction with knee flexion). These injuries can be identified by a mobile or high-riding patella, knee tenderness and swelling, and inability to extend the knee. A gentle evaluation is essential as forceful extension may complete a partial tear.

Ligamentous knee injuries are typically associated with falls or forced twisting injuries. Anterior cruciate ligament injury may be accompanied by an audible "pop." Patients with ligamentous knee injuries complain of knee pain and may describe a feeling of joint instability. The clinical examination of ligamentous knee injuries may include focal tenderness, knee effusion, and joint laxity. Fractures should be suspected with any history of direct trauma and inability to bear weight. Ligamentous knee injuries may benefit from immobilization to prevent further injury. Secondary treatments target pain and swelling and include ice, elevation, crutches, and antiinflammatories.

Leg

The tibia and fibula run parallel in the lower leg and are tightly bound by ligamentous connections. The tibial and peroneal nerves and anterior/posterior tibial arteries supply this area and are at risk of injury with associated shaft fractures.

The two forces responsible for leg fractures are direct trauma and twisting or rotary injuries, such as skiing accidents (i.e., "boot top" fractures). The bones may fracture independently or together. Since the tibia is a weight-bearing bone and the fibula is not, you cannot walk on a broken tibia. Tibial fractures are often open and are the most common open fracture in the wilderness setting.[17] Management of leg fractures includes alignment of the injured limb, assessment of neurovascular status, and immobilization with a long leg rigid splint.

Peroneal nerve injuries (impaired plantarflexion) complicate fibula fractures, while anterior tibial nerve injuries (impaired dorsiflexion) complicate tibial fractures. The most devastating complication for any leg shaft fracture (and unfortunately common in tibial shaft fractures) is a compartment syndrome. They are usually present within the first 24–48 hours,[4] and limb salvage is unlikely if ischemia exceeds 6 hours.[16]

Ankle

The ankle is a weight-bearing saddle joint. The ankle joint allows plantar- and dorsiflexion while inversion and eversion take place within the subtalar joint. The ankle joint is formed by the distal tibia, fibula, and talus. Strong ligamentous support allows the ankle to function under significant weight. Lateral support is from the anterior/posterior talofibular ligament, and the calcaneofibular ligament. Medial support is from the deltoid ligament, a combination of three separate tibial ligaments. The tibiofibular ligaments that serve to strengthen the ankle mortise also join the tibia and fibula distally.

Ankle Fracture

Ankle fractures should be suspected in patients with ankle or foot trauma (e.g., twisting, rolling, axial load) who are unable to bear weight. Fractures may be difficult to distinguish from severe ankle sprains. Patients with ankle fractures may have swelling, bruising, and focal tenderness of the malleoli, proximal fifth metatarsal or talus. An obvious ankle deformity suggests a fracture, dislocation or combination of the two. Ankle fractures may involve the medial and lateral malleoli (distal tibia and fibula, respectively), the intrarticular tibia (trimalleolar fracture), and the talus. Ankle fractures should be gently realigned and splinted with either a posterior lower leg splint or a long rigid splint on either side of the limb. Apply ice, elevate the extremity (if possible), and keep the patient non-weight-bearing.

Ankle Dislocation

One of the more disabling, and surprisingly common injuries in the wilderness is the ankle fracture/dislocation (tibiotalar dislocation). (See Figures 39.22 and 39.23.) The injuring force is often torsional and significant. Ankle dislocations (commonly accompanied by fractures) are defined by ligamentous disruption, involving the deltoid ligaments medially and the talofibular ligaments laterally, and may include the central tibiofibular ligaments.

Gross deformity, pain, swelling, and ecchymosis are common with tibiotalar dislocations. Neurovascular compromise is possible. Management in the wilderness typically involves pain management and immediate reduction to maintain neurovascular integrity. Narcotic analgesia is imperative. To perform the reduction, the patient's knee should be flexed and the caregiver should grasp the patient's heel with one hand and the metatarsal arch with the other. Longitudinal traction should be applied until the bone ends have disengaged and the joint is allowed to fall into

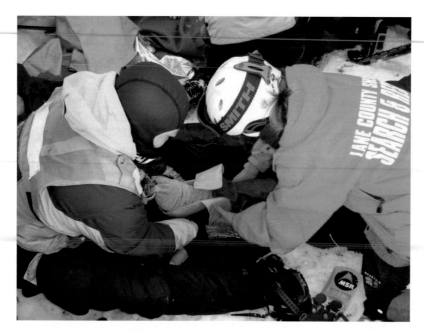

Figure 39.22. Ankle fracture with SAM splint. Courtesy of Deschutes County Search and Rescue.

its normal anatomical alignment. Lateral dislocations (most common) may require medial rotation for proper alignment.[6]

Immobilization with a posterior splint after reduction is essential for stabilization. SAM splints are commercial splints, reportedly advantageous for use in the wilderness.[11] (See Figure 39.22.) Definitive management

of ankle fracture/dislocations includes open reduction and internal fixation to realign the ankle mortise and limit future instability, arthritis, stiffness, and pain. Open injuries are common orthopedic emergencies. Initial field management of open injuries includes sterile irrigation, a wound dressing, empiric antibiotics, and splinting. Emergent reduction is indicated with open fractures complicated by neurovascular deficits or in the face of transport delays.

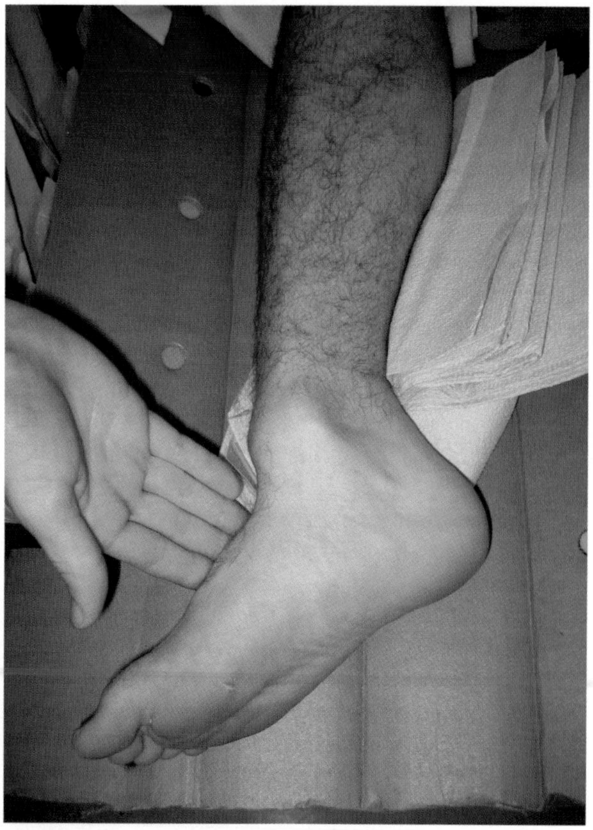

Ankle Sprains

Ankle sprains are the most common soft tissue injury in the expedition setting.[11] (See Figure 39.24.) A lateral ankle sprain involves forced inversion of the talofibular ligament and encompasses 85% of these injuries.[16] Forced eversion injuries are less common and are the cause of medial ankle sprains (deltoid ligament). A deltoid

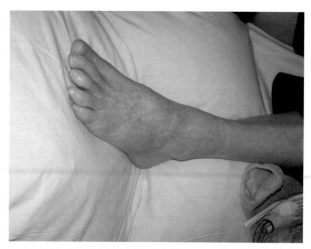

Figure 39.23. Ankle fracture dislocation. Photo courtesy of S.V. Mahadevan.

Figure 39.24. Fifth metatarsal base fracture after an ankle sprain. Photo courtesy of S.V. Mahadevan.

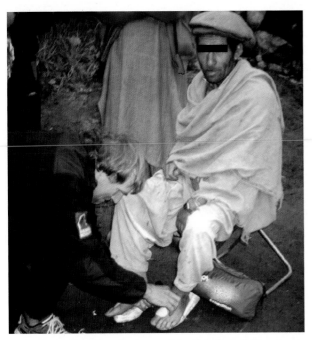

Figure 39.25. Phalange fracture and buddy-taping. Balti porter in Karakorum, Pakistan. Photo courtesy of Alan Gianotti.

ligament injury is commonly associated with fractures of the medial (tibia), posterior (tibia), and lateral (fibula) malleoli.

The patient with an ankle sprain may report a "pop" sensation, and physical examination findings include tenderness, swelling, and inability to bear weight. Joint laxity is present with severely sprained ankles. Joint immobilization is indicated in all patients. Stabilization of the joint reduces pain and swelling and limits further damage to the ligaments. Splint the ankle at 90° of flexion. Secondary treatments target pain and swelling, and include ice, compression, elevation, antiinflammatories, and crutches. Taping may be indicated in the backcountry for support. The ability to bear weight suggests a sprain and is a nice stress test for excluding serious fractures in the field.

High ankle sprains involve the anterior inferior tibiofibular ligament and occur in 10% of ankle sprains. Pain is localized to the distal syndesmosis high above the ankle joint and the initial management is similar to that of an ankle fracture. Complete ligamentous tears and associated fractures will eventually require orthopedic evaluation.

Foot

The foot is a relatively simple structure made up of three bony parts: the hindfoot (calcaneus and talus), the midfoot (navicular, cuboid, and cuneiforms), and forefoot (metatarsals and phalanges). Blood is supplied from two main sources: the dorsalis pedis artery off the anterior tibial artery and the posterior tibial artery. The deep peroneal and tibial nerves course with these arteries, respectively.

Foot fractures vary depending on mechanism. Calcaneus fractures result from heavy axial loading (landing on your feet) after falls from significant height in the wilderness setting. Metatarsal fractures result from direct blows, rotational forces, axial loading while plantarflexing (Lisfranc fracture dislocation) or repetitive stress injuries (marathoners and "march" fractures). The fifth metatarsal base is commonly fractured with jumping injuries such as in ballet and basketball. (See Figure 39.24.) Phalanx fractures are usually from axial (stubbed toe) or crushing forces. (See Figure 39.25.) These fractures can be distinguished by point tenderness and deformity. Foot and ankle fractures are immobilized similarly (rigid or soft splints) and are non-weight-bearing injuries. Toe fractures can be buddy-taped, securing them to their adjacent unaffected toes.

Calcaneal fractures may be associated with concurrent thoracolumbar vertebral fractures. Displaced metatarsal fractures may result in malunion. Vascular foot injuries are uncommon. Osteomyelitis rates for foot puncture wounds are low (1–2%).[13,14] Pseudomonal infections (93%) have been implicated in tennis shoe puncture wounds, but most soft tissue infections are from *Streptococcus* and *Staphylococcus*.[15]

Plantar Fasciitis

Plantar fasciitis causes pain on the plantar surface of the foot in a physically active adult. This inflammation of the plantar aponeurosis is thought to be secondary to overuse and poor arch support. It is worse with activity including stair climbing (dorsiflexion of the toes). Examination reveals tenderness over the plantar fascia (anterior medial aspect of the calcaneus). Treatment is conservative with activity modification, antiinflammatories, ice, rest, arch support, and dorsiflexion night splints. Steroid injections are not indicated secondary to risk of plantar fascia rupture.[5]

SPECIAL INJURIES

Amputation

An amputation consists of a traumatic avulsion of a body part, commonly a digit. (See Figure 39.26.) Immediate consideration should be given to hemorrhage control via direct pressure and elevation. If this approach fails to control bleeding, application of manual pressure to distinct pressure points (locations where an artery courses just below the skin and directly over the bone) is indicated. The primary pressure points are the brachial artery, for bleeding from the forearm; the axillary artery, for upper extremity bleeding; the popliteal artery, for bleeding from the lower leg; and the femoral artery, for proximal lower-extremity hemorrhage. Tourniquets are recommended only as a last resort in the control of

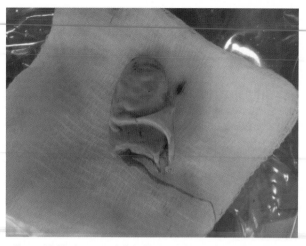

Figure 39.26. Amputated digit. Photo courtesy of S.V. Mahadevan.

hemorrhage.[1] Circumferential pressure (as opposed to point pressure) can damage distal tissue and must be used with caution. Anticoagulation medications, alcohol, nonsteroidal antiinflammatories, and hypertension will all aggravate bleeding.

The amputated "part" should be cleaned with water, wrapped in moistened gauze, and transported in a plastic bag on (not in) ice, snow, or cold water. Successful reimplantation mandates transportation to an appropriate facility within 6 hours. An amputated limb can survive 6 hours of warm ischemia and 12 hours of cold ischemia.[15] Digits can survive even longer.

Open Fracture

A compound or open fracture indicates broken skin (an open wound) overlying a fracture. (See Figure 39.27.) All open fractures are considered contaminated and high risk for posttraumatic infection (osteomyelitis). Initial management depends on the estimated transport duration to an orthopedic facility. In general, if the expected time is less than 4–6 hours, the injured extremity can be bandaged and splinted, and the patient transported. If the anticipated transport duration is greater than 6–8 hours, the wound should be irrigated with available clean water; the fracture reduced or realigned (if displaced) and splinted; and antibiotic therapy should be initiated (typically first-generation cephalosporin plus fluorquinolones).[11,17] Analgesics are indicated in both scenarios.

Compartment Syndrome

Fractures, severe contusions, and crush wounds are at high risk for developing considerable swelling. Swelling in a confined fascial compartment may restrict blood flow to the distal extremity. The resultant condition is called a compartment syndrome (see Figure 39.28). Obstructed venous outflow from the affected compartment only amplifies the injury. Diagnosis is based on a high clinical suspicion. Compartment pressures above 30–40 mm Hg are capable of causing injury, but having access to a pressure monitor in the field is unlikely. Late symptoms include severe pain (out of proportion to the injury itself), weak pulses, paresthesias, and sensory loss. Resultant injuries are tissue ischemia, necrosis, and limb death. Treatment in the field should focus on elevation of the extremity to level of the heart (not above), application of ice, removal of any constricting clothing or splinting material, and urgent evacuation for surgical compartmental release (fasciotomy) within 6–8 hours. Limb salvage is unlikely if ischemia exceeds 6 hours.[16]

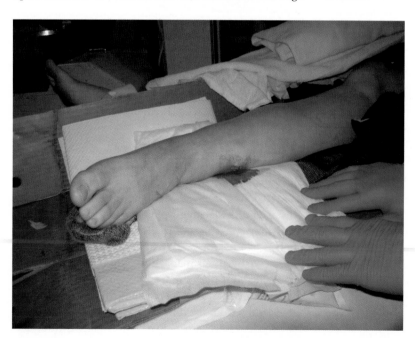

Figure 39.27. Open fracture Photo courtesy of S.V. Mahadevan.

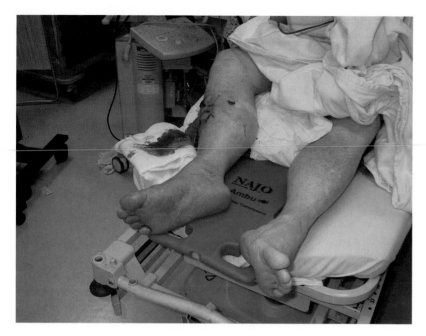

Figure 39.28. Clinical evidence of compartment syndrome in a patient with lower extremity injury. Photo courtesy of S.V. Mahadevan.

The 5P mnemonic characterizes the classic symptoms of the syndrome: Pain, Pallor, Paralysis, Pulselessness, and Paresthesia. Unfortunately, by the time all these symptoms are present, limb ischemia has caused irreversible tissue damage. The key to early diagnosis is a high index of suspicion.[6] Non-orthopedic causes of compartment syndromes include circumferential swelling from snakebites and burns.

Crush Injury

A torso crushed from a fall or extremities pinned by falling debris are examples of crush injury. Crush injuries result from blunt or compressive trauma. Internal organ rupture and fractures are immediate life- and limb-threatening consequences, respectively. Prolonged muscle compression (> 4–6 hours) can lead to muscle cellular death. Sudden release of an entrapped, compressed limb could lead to systemic absorption of the by-products of muscle cell breakdown, primarily potassium, lactic acid, and myoglobin. Field treatment of crush injury aims to prevent and treat complications from this sudden toxin release, namely hyerkalemia and renal failure. Intravenous NS or D5NS is recommended to maintain a urine output of 2 cc/kg/hr.[5] Additionally, sodium bicarbonate (44 mEq in 1 L 0.5 NS, or 88 mEq in 1 L D5W run at 100 cc/hr) is recommended to keep the urine pH at around 6.5 and prevent acute renal failure.[5] Intravenous calcium can be used to treat hyperkalemia-induced cardiotoxicity.

Mammalian Bites

The most common animal bites are dog bites (80%). The majority of animal bites usually involve the hand or forearm. While few dog bites (5%) will become infected, most cat bites will (60–80%).[5] Infections are usually polymicrobial, including anaerobes, *Staphylococcus* and *Streptococcus* species, and *Pasteurella multocida* (especially with cat bites).

The management of an animal bite wound includes high-pressure irrigation and wound debridement. Wound closure is recommended in large dog bites less than 6 hours old. Immobilization and antibiotics are advisable in high-risk patients (elderly, diabetics, alcoholics, and the immunosuppressed) as well as with cat and human bites (amoxicillin and clavulanate, 875/125 mg BID × 7 days).[5]

Tetanus prophylaxis varies based on history of immunizations and quality of the wound (see preceding discussion). Rabies prophylaxis must be considered for bites from unvaccinated, unobserved animals.

EXPEDITION MEDICAL KIT

Be prepared. When planning for an expedition, get to know your supplies – the only thing more important than the medical gear you carry is the knowledge to use it. Be familiar with your kit, and be comfortable with what it can (and cannot) accomplish. Every medical kit should be customized for each individual adventure taking into account environmental extremes, endemic disease, pre-existing illnesses, the number of people your kit will support, the trip duration, and, most importantly, the goal or purpose of the adventure. However, it is difficult to imagine preparing for any "adventure" scenario without packing basic orthopedic supplies.

A basic orthopedic medical kit should include splints, wraps, bandage supplies, and analgesics. In a pinch, just about anything of substance can improvise as a splint. If you carry nothing else, Duct tape, a SAM splint, and an Ace wrap are essential orthopedic tools in the backcountry. The most important orthopedic rescue device, however, continues to be the satellite or cellular telephone (with a spare battery).

Basic Orthopedic Medical Kit

    Sat/cell phone

    SAM splint

    Ace wrap

    Cervical collar

    Warming blanket/sleeping bag

    Duct tape/adhesive tape

    Bandage scissors/shears

    Analgesics

    Masks/gloves

    Triangular bandages

    Elastic roller-type bandages

    Gauze dressings (4 × 4)

    Nonadherent sterile dressings

    Strip and knuckle adhesive bandages

    Occlusive (airtight) dressings

    Molefoam/moleskin (blister material)

    Eye protector

    Blanket/pillow/Ensolite pad (soft splint material)

    Rigid splint sets (upper and lower extremity)

    Cotton-tipped applicators

    Lidocaine scrub brush

Advanced Orthopedic Medical Kit

    Wound management/suture, staple, and glue kits

    Lidocaine and steroid injectables

    Needles and syringes

    Chemical ice packs

    IV starter kit and IV fluids

    IV sodium bicarbonate

    Antibiotics (oral and parenteral)

    Stethoscope

    Chest tubes

    Airway supplies (oral and nasal airways, endotracheal supplies)

    CPR microshield

    Extreme temperature thermometer (85–107°F)

REFERENCES

1. Bledsoe BE, Cherry RA, Porter RS, eds. *Intermediate Emergency Care: Principles and Practice.* Upper Saddle River, NJ: Pearson Education; 2004.

2. Bergeron JD, Bizjak G, Krause GW, LeBaudour C. *First Responder.* 7th ed. Upper Saddle River, NJ: Pearson Prentice Hall; 2005.

3. Johe DH, Bowman WD. *Outdoor Emergency Care: Comprehensive Prehospital Care for Nonurban Settings.* 4th ed. Sudbury, Mass: Jones & Bartlett; 2003.

4. Simon RR, Koenigsknecht SJ. *Emergency Orthopedics the Extremities.* 4th ed. New York: McGraw-Hill; 2001.

5. Tintinalli JE, Kelen GD, Stapczynski JS. *Emergency Medicine – A Comprehensive Study Guide.* 6th ed. New York: McGraw-Hill; 2004.

6. Mahadevan SV, Garmel GM. *An Introduction to Clinical Emergency Medicine – Guide for Practitioners in the Emergency Department.* New York: Cambridge University Press, 2005.

7. Valente JH, Forti RJ, Freundlich LF, Zandieh SO, Crain EF. Wound irrigation – tap water or saline? *Acad Emerg Med.* 2001; 8(5):539.

8. Moscati RM, Reardon RF, Lerner EB, Mayrose J. Wound irrigation with tap water. *Acad Emerg Med.* 1998:5:1076–80.

9. Edlich RF, Rodeheaver GT, Morgan RF, et al. Principles of emergency wound management. *Ann Emerg Med.* 1988;17(12):1284–302.

10. Li J, Hiller KM, Brainard D. Antibiotics: a review of ED use. In: Keim SM, Talavera F, Weiss EL, Halamka J, Adler J, eds. eMedicine Specialties. Available at: *http://www.emedicine.com.*

11. Farrar EL. Fractures and dislocations in the wilderness. Presented at: Wilderness and Travel Medicine 2000. Big Sky, Mont; February 12–17, 2000.

12. Pennycook A, Makower R, O'Donnell AM. Puncture wounds of the foot: can infective complications be avoided? *J R Soc Med.* 1994;87(10):581–3.

13. Fitzgerald RH, Cowan JDE. Puncture wounds of the foot. *Orthopedic Clinic North Am.* 1975;6:965–72.

14. Gilbert DN, Moellering RC, Sande MA. *The Sanford Guide to Antimicrobial Therapy.* 33rd ed. Sperryville, Va: Antimicrobial Therapy; 2003.

15. Wolfson AB, et al., eds. *Clinical Practice of Emergency Medicine.* 4th ed. Philadelphia: Lippincott Williams & Wilkins; 2005.

16. Green WM. *Manual of Emergency Orthopedics for Emergency Physicians.* Davis, Calif: Division of Emergency Medicine, University of California, 1990.

17. Auerbach PS. *Wilderness Medicine.* 5th ed. St. Louis: Mosby; 1997.

40 | Expedition Self-Rescue and Evacuation

Ken Zafren, MD, and Urs Wiget, MD

INTRODUCTION

Few expeditions in modern times are prepared to go to the lengths of an earlier era when it comes to self-rescue. With satellite phones, GPS positioning, and modern air transport, it is unlikely that any major expedition to any area on earth, no matter how remote, will ever again be as isolated as famous expeditions of the past. The epic survival stories, such as that of Ernest Shackleton and his stranded *Endurance* crew in Antarctica, are largely the stuff of history. However, even today, ships still sink with all hands on board, and climbers still are lost and their bodies never recovered.

Expeditions have limited resources for treating threats to life and limb. Prevention of injury and illness is therefore extremely important on expeditions. For example, it is better to ascend slowly to high altitudes than to rush up a mountain and be forced to treat expedition members with high-altitude illness. If proper prevention measures fail, however, then the expedition physician must be prepared to deal with untoward events.

It is in the spirit of preparation for untoward events that this chapter on expedition self-rescue is written. Some of the measures taken in advance will complement self-rescue planning. These include provision of communications gear, such as satellite phones and external rescue plans. Other measures, such as including expedition members with search and rescue experience, self-rescue experience, and medical skills and bringing along rescue and medical equipment may enhance the ability of an expedition to perform a self-rescue and evacuation of ill or injured patients.

PREVENTIVE DECISION MAKING

Expeditions cannot bring along unlimited equipment. Smaller expeditions, especially those in which the members must transport the gear using small boats, sleds, or backpacks, may be quite limited in this regard. In small expeditions, also, there may be no member with medical or rescue training. The expedition should carefully consider the likely hazards, how to prevent them, and how to provide for their successful resolution if prevention measures fail.

In many remote areas, the consequences of loss of equipment or injury might be so severe that evacuation might be impossible or nearly so. Expeditions operating in such environments might take stringent precautions against such eventualities or might make a conscious decision that the risks are acceptable to the members. Military expeditions in particular must accept a level of risk that is considered unreasonable in civilian endeavors. The transition of mountaineering expeditions in the Himalayas from "expedition style," with fixed camps and a supply chain, to "alpine style," with climbers moving quickly and with limited food and equipment up a mountain, has carried with it an increase in risk for those at the "thin end" of the rope.

Decisions that an expedition must make prior to departure include whether to bring backup equipment in case of failure of necessary equipment, specialized rescue equipment, and medical supplies and whether to bring members with rescue or medical skills either as full members of the expedition or as resource members. Some of these extra personnel may have support roles and not participate in the expedition. Examples include those who stay in base camp on a mountaineering expedition and those who stay on the surface in a diving expedition. There may also be support personnel who do not even go on the expedition, but who can do such tasks as coordinating the sending of extra supplies during the expedition or the launching of a rescue, if needed.

Some of the most important decisions an expedition must make have to do with standard operating procedures, especially standard safety protocols. Often, these decisions are not made consciously. When the consequences of failure are high, the consequences of an inadequate safety culture can be grave. Routine activities that clearly exemplify these principles are the operation of commercial airplanes and the provision of anesthesia for surgical operations. Both of these activities have become extremely safe in recent years because of their safety cultures. The rates of human error and equipment failure have been reduced through the use of checklists, standard procedures, and redundancy. Vertical rescue is another example of an inherently dangerous activity that has been made safer by these principles.

When applied to expeditions, adequate safety culture has the potential to decrease the rate of equipment failure, illness, and injury. Adequate training is essential. Even with training, fail-safe measures are needed to decrease human error. Basic measures such as ensuring that all members wash their hands after defecating and before meals and requiring the use of sun protection in high-exposure areas can prevent serious problems. Ensuring safe practices, including use of appropriate safety equipment in such hazardous activities such as boating, diving, mountaineering, canyoning (known as canyoneering in the United States), and caving also can dramatically reduce the chances and consequences of "accidents."

RECOGNITION OF A PROBLEM

During an expedition, when something goes wrong that threatens the health or survival of one or more members, the leader or other members must first recognize this fact and then decide on a course of action. Even though this may seem obvious, it is human nature to ignore problems until they are clearly threatening. For instance, there is a natural tendency to ignore fire alarms in large buildings and to carry on with work as usual.

Recognition of a problem is an important first step. Proper communication with the entire expedition team is necessary as soon as a problem is identified. In some situations, communication may be nonexistent or may be interrupted. The famous self-rescue of Joe Simpson (*Touching the Void*) was a result of his partner being sure he had died in a fall. Many expeditions have had a tragedy occur to one group while base camp or other groups are completely unaware.

DECISION MAKING IN SELF-RESCUE

After the problem has been defined, the leader and other members of the expedition must attempt to solve it. The ultimate success of the expedition may depend on the solution. In many cases, an ill or injured member may be unable to move under his or her own power, or as in cases such as high-altitude pulmonary edema (HAPE), allowing a patient to move under his or her own power may worsen the prognosis. Patients with frostbite of the feet can often self-evacuate, for example, but frostbite of the hands may make it impossible to do necessary tasks, such as descending technical terrain using fixed lines.

If a member is ill or injured enough to require evacuation, the expedition must devote sufficient resources to the task. Before proceeding with the rescue, the team should spend adequate time discussing the plan. Every member should be given a defined role and the techniques to be used should be determined. A few minutes spent in planning will prevent many mistakes and delays later on.

SEARCH AND RESCUE

In this chapter on expedition self-rescue the emphasis is on improvised techniques. On larger expeditions with multiple teams in the field and possibly a support group in base camp, expedition rescue may sometimes take on certain aspects of organized search and rescue. Search and rescue skills are best acquired through formal training and participation in rescue missions in an organized rescue group. These skills can be adapted to the expedition setting. Written resources include several useful books (Table 40.1).

In the expedition setting, search is usually limited or unnecessary, either because the location of the party or parties needing rescue is known to the rest of the expedition or is inaccessible to them. If the expedition is broken into teams, an injury or equipment malfunction may break the chain of communications and the only knowledge that one team may have is that another team failed to arrive at a destination or failed to communicate as scheduled. When this occurs, the rest of the expedition will initiate a search for the missing party.

Search is an emergency. The common wisdom is that the person or group that is overdue is very capable is often the opposite of the correct interpretation, which is that this very capable party may be in real trouble because they missed a rendezvous or radio call. Like a pilot using flight tracking, expeditions can increase safety by frequent radio contact with moving parties. With the increasing availability of passive global positioning systems, expeditions can potentially keep track of the location of every member and every equipment cache in real time. However, this technology is not yet used on most expeditions.

There are many ways to conceptualize the search phase of search and rescue. A common schema breaks search into subphases of "first notice," planning or strategy, and tactics. First notice on an expedition may consist of a radio call from a team that is in trouble and at an unknown location or may be inferred from the failure

---

Table 40.1. Useful books – search and rescue

William G. May's *Mountain Search and Rescue Techniques* – written as a training manual for an active mountain rescue group; out of print but basic techniques have not changed

Slim Ray and Les Bechdel's *River Rescue: A Manual for Whitewater Safety*, 3rd ed.

John C. Hempel and Annette Fregeau-Conover's *On Call: A Complete Reference for Cave Rescue*

Tim J. Setnicka's *Wilderness Search and Rescue* – general text that covers related areas such as whitewater and cave rescue; out of print but basic techniques have not changed

of a team to arrive at a location or to communicate as planned. The expedition leader or a designated member then determines the search strategy.

Search strategy should be mostly preplanned. For example, a series of steps would be initiated if a team fails to arrive at a rendezvous as planned. These steps could include extra radio calls and the use of alternate means of communication, including whistles, or flares, followed by sending out a search party toward the expected location of the missing team.

In organized search and rescue, subjects are often found with the aid of a strategy that includes determining their last known location ("point last seen"), and confining the search area by defining the perimeter beyond which the missing subject is unlikely to be found. The next step is to determine likely routes of travel and then perform a "hasty" search with small fast teams or airborne searching along these likely routes. A large search often culminates in saturation searching with large numbers of searchers looking for clues. At this phase, there are often very formal estimates of the likelihood of finding a lost subject in each part of the search area based on the likelihood of the subject being in the given part and the probability of detection using different search methods.

For an isolated expedition, search tactics will likely start with survey methods, including contacting other teams that might be in contact with the missing team and the use of noise and flares, to be answered in kind. The next step, for expeditions without motorized or airborne resources, will likely employ old-fashioned methods such as sending a team or teams to the likely location(s) of the lost team and along likely routes of travel (a "scratch" or hasty search). Scratch teams will carry a radio and a minimum amount of survival, rescue, and medical gear. If the expedition has motorized resources such as wheeled

vehicles, snow machines, or boats, these can be used in this phase and may be able to carry more gear than self-powered teams.

Depending on the nature of the expedition and the terrain, there may be no role for saturation search. In vegetated areas or avalanche debris, there may be a role for specialized line searches. These are beyond the scope of this book.

METHODS FOR CARRYING AN ILL OR INJURED PATIENT

There are many stretchers available for organized rescue groups. These stretchers are often used for formal rescues and usually will not be available on most expeditions. In rescue work, these stretchers are usually referred to as litters and include basket litters, flat litters, and soft litters. (See Figure 40.1.)

While it might conceivably be worthwhile under unusual circumstances to have a litter available at a base camp, most expeditions will have little use for heavy, bulky equipment. If long overland evacuation with a litter from base camp is a real possibility, an expedition should also consider having a wheeled litter available because it makes it much easier for a small number of rescuers to move a patient in a litter over long distances.

One item, which might prove useful under some circumstances and could be brought on an expedition, would be a vacuum mattress (also referred to as a full-body vacuum splint). These devices are the best means of immobilizing a patient for long transports. They are far superior to backboards for stabilizing spinal injuries because they are far more comfortable and much less likely to lead to decubitus ulcers from pressure points. Vacuum mattresses are essentially a mattress-shaped

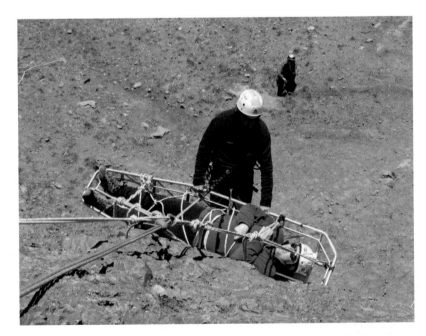

Figure 40.1. Vertical evacuation with a Stokes litter using the one-rope technique with one litter bearer and improvised rigging. A second line, next to the lowering line, is the belay line. For safety reasons, the rescuer and patient are both tied into the lowering line and the belay line, rather than the litter. Photo courtesy Ken Zafren.

bean bag with a valve so that air can be evacuated. Once the air is removed, atmospheric pressure outside the mattress causes it to assume a rigid shape that conforms to the patient. Vacuum mattresses can be used alone as a stretcher in nontechnical terrain, but they more commonly are placed in a litter for ease of transport. In a large expedition, a vacuum mattress could be kept at a base camp.

Improvised techniques, while not as satisfactory as using commercial equipment, have the advantage that they can be used immediately where needed. On most expeditions, the initial stages of transport, if not the entire rescue will utilize improvised techniques. The basic improvised litter is the rucksack stretcher, the production of which will be described later in this chapter.

PATIENT PACKAGING

No matter what type of litter is used, whether commercial or improvised, patients must be protected from further injury. All injured parts must be stabilized using dressings and splints, including traction splints and cervical collars as appropriate. The patient must be kept warm, even though immobile, while still allowing for reassessment of injuries during transport, with the least possible interruption of the actual transport. The patient must be protected from hazards of transport, including falling objects or other potentially threatening structures such as tree branches. The patient must be secured to the litter (except for some forms of water transport) and in technical terrain must be belayed independent of the litter.

Most commercial litters come with tie-in straps of some sort. If a vacuum mattress is being used, the mattress is easily secured to most litters. For the rucksack stretcher, the hip belts serve as the tie-in straps. The patient's head can usually be secured by placing the hip belt of the last pack around the forehead. The last pack is the one in which the hip belt is not part of the assembly. Care must be taken not to secure the hip belt of the next pack too tightly around the patient's chest, which would restrict breathing. Depending on the specific injuries, some adjustments will be necessary to avoid placing pressure in certain areas. Slings, short lengths of rope, and tape can all be used to improvise systems to immobilize patients and specific injured parts so that they don't slide around in the litter and sustain further injury.

Rucksack stretchers, with clothes in the backs of the rucksacks, provide some padding for patient comfort. If backboards or commercial litters are used, the patient should be placed in (or on) a sleeping bag, preferably with sleeping pads underneath the sleeping bag for padding. The vacuum mattress is the only really ideal solution to prevent pressure sores, however.

If there is risk of the patient vomiting, the patient should be transported on one side in the "recovery position" in order to protect against aspiration after vomiting. However, no good method to secure the patient in that position has been developed. It is also usually not feasible to elevate injured parts, as advocated by some authors, although one should try to protect injured parts from excessive pressure. As a practical matter, most patients are transported supine. They must be secured in the litter and monitored, so that in the case of vomiting, the whole unit of litter and patient can be turned to one side and the airway protected. If pelvic or leg injuries do not prevent it, padding placed under the knees will greatly increase patient comfort in the supine position.

The patient will usually be placed in a sleeping bag for warmth. In any case, the patient's body should be covered for protection against falling or wind-blown objects, especially if there is any chance that a helicopter will be used for evacuation. The patient's face and head should be covered for the same reason, although the use of goggles is recommended to reduce claustrophobia. In steep terrain, the patient should wear a climbing helmet. The patient's arms should be restrained in the litter for ease of packaging and to avoid injury.

If there is any chance that the litter will be upended, the patient should be protected against sliding downward. Because they conform to the patient, vacuum mattresses do not have the problem of the patient shifting, either lengthwise or from side to side. Commercial litters sometimes have leg dividers, which help, as does padding under the knees. Leg straps, tied around the foot and secured to the side of the litter are sometimes used, but they don't work if the knees are bent or if there is a lower extremity injury. In mountainous or glaciated terrain, the patient will wear a climbing harness. This will be used to secure the patient to any lowering or belay ropes as well as to prevent sliding lengthwise in the litter.

HIGH-ANGLE TERRAIN

In high-angle terrain (also referred to as technical terrain), the expedition will already have ropes and anchors. An ill or injured patient who can assist the rescuer can be lowered on vertical terrain using a tragsitz (German for "carry seat"). The original tragsitz was made of canvas, but there are now other commercial fabric tragsitz products. The rescuer splits a long coil of rope into two joined coils and puts the coils over the shoulders. The patient then puts the legs through the coils, which can also be joined in front of the rescuer. The rescuer and the patient are then lowered down a cliff or very steep slope. This technique is easiest in truly vertical terrain. Both the patient and the rescuer must be tied into the lowering line. Another technique, which accomplishes the same purpose, is the single rucksack technique. It is also possible for a single rescuer to lower him- or herself and the patient down a fixed line with the tragsitz technique as a rappel. In this case, the brakes are located well above both the rescuer and the patient, both of whom are secured to the braking system.

Rescuing an unconscious or severely injured patient in vertical terrain using improvised gear is somewhat desperate. Many rope and fabric stretchers have been described elsewhere, but none of these provide significant back support. Some of them can be stiffened with skis or ski poles, but these are not often available in the vertical environment. In a pinch, the patient could be lowered in a sleeping bag, especially if there is a bivouac sack and sleeping pad and preferably some other means to stiffen the system for back support. Suspension of some rope litters would be straightforward using loops as tie-in points, but fabric methods, sleeping bags, and bivouac sacks typically lack tie-in points, so a harness for the litter would still need to be constructed. As with all rescue systems on technical terrain, the patient and rescuers must be secured to the lowering line or to a separate belay line, either directly or indirectly via the suspension system and not just to the stretcher (Figures 40.1 and 40.2). Lowering systems for litters, using one rope with a belay line or two load-bearing ropes, are beyond the scope of this chapter.

There seems to be no compelling reason why the rucksack stretcher cannot be used. Rucksacks are certainly not designed to hold this sort of load, but they are generally quite strong, and this system provides substantial back support. Properly suspended horizontally from a harness, which is often referred to as spiders,

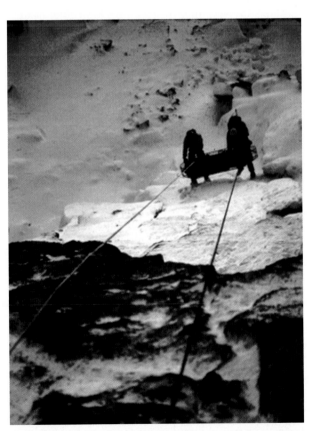

Figure 40.2. Vertical evacuation using the two-rope technique with two litter bearers in a high-mountain environment (organized rescue with a Stokes litter). Photo courtesy of Charley Shimanski.

the rucksack stretcher would function like a litter on a vertical or near-vertical evacuation. As with all evacuations in technical terrain, the rescuers and patient must both be belayed, with both wearing climbing harnesses. This is usually done by having both the patient and the rescuer tied in to the spider system, but never directly into the litter. If the litter system fails, the result is not a catastrophic fall of the rescuer or patient. Although many rescue groups use a single rescuer to guide the litter, it is easier in all but vertical or overhanging terrain to use two rescuers. These litter bearers ideally will wear their own packs. In the case of rockfall or other falling objects, the litter bearers attempt to lean over the patient for protection, while their own packs protect their backs.

The spiders can also be improvised. One easy method of improvising spiders is to use a double bowline on a bight, with the end loop of the rope tied as long as the other two loops, forming a knot with three loops that can then be attached to two sides and an end of the litter. A single 15-meter length of climbing rope would suffice to make two spiders (with six points of suspension) using this method. This would be tied into a long loop with the spiders suspended from the lowering rope at the top and a shorter connection along the long axis of the litter between the two spiders, which could be formed into a patient tie-in.

When using a rucksack stretcher, it would probably be preferable to make the loops longer and run them completely under the rucksacks, so that the rucksacks are supported by the rope rather than by the straps of the rucksacks. In less-than-vertical terrain, the potential for abrading the rope supporting the side of the litter that faces the cliff is always present. Tape can be used to pad the rope in areas likely to rub on the rock.

INTERMEDIATE TERRAIN

On steep terrain, the litter is usually oriented parallel to the slope angle, rather than horizontally as on vertical terrain. The litter is lowered on a rope from above. On very steep terrain, two litter bearers are sufficient because much of the weight of the litter is taken by the rope. The litter bearers are positioned on either side of the litter. As the terrain becomes less steep, it becomes very difficult for two litter bearers to carry the litter because less weight can be borne by the rope. Four litter bearers are better than two in lower-angled terrain. The rucksack stretcher can be used for this purpose, but it will require some ingenuity in creating an appropriate tie-in system for the litter. As in all technical rescue systems, the patient must wear a climbing harness and be secured directly to the lowering rope in case of litter failure.

On snow slopes, it is often possible to lower a patient in a sleeping bag (well padded below using a sleeping pad) in a bivouac sack. This is a better technique for ill rather than injured patients. On steeper slopes, the bivouac sack usually slides nicely and can be lowered from a fixed anchor. The patient wears a climbing harness and is tied into the lowering line. On gentler slopes, the bivouac sack can slide with assistance from rescuers, usually with a rescuer using a rope from above to belay the patient in case the bivouac sack slides out of control of the other rescuers. This rescuer may move with the litter on very gentle slopes and safeguard the patient with a short line tied to the rescuer's harness. This is safe only if the rescuer can reliably self-arrest or even just lie down in order to stop the litter from sliding downhill, generally only on soft snow.

FLAT TERRAIN AND GENTLE SLOPES

On gentle terrain, where there is no chance of the patient and litter falling or sliding down a slope, the rucksack stretcher is superior to most of the other commonly advocated techniques, although there is still a limited role for short drags or carries.

Dragging or carrying an unconscious patient is indicated only in the most hazardous or dire conditions. The patient can be dragged without use of any special device, especially if wearing smooth synthetic expedition outerwear, but preferably on a sleeping pad, in a bivouac sack, or on any fabric, such as a tent. For very short carries of patients who are able to assist to some extent, a simple piggyback carry is a useful method. Even a heavy patient can be carried uphill by a single rescuer, but only for very short distances. It is easier if there are two other rescuers to help support the weight from the sides.

For longer, but still short, carries, a four-handed technique may be useful. The patient sits between two walking rescuers, supported on the joined right arm of the rescuer on his or her right and the left arm of the rescuer on his or her left. The rescuers' other arms support the back and the patient's arms are wrapped around the necks of the rescuers. The patient can also be supported in a similar fashion between two rescuers on a coil of rope suspended over the rescuers' shoulders. This has the advantages of leaving the rescuers' outer arms free and having the patient's weight supported by the rescuers shoulders rather than the forearms. The disadvantage is the need to reposition the rope every time the rescuers change off. Two rescuers cannot carry an adult patient very far using either method.

For longer carries, the rucksack stretcher is the most useful technique under most circumstances. Fabric techniques, using tarps, tents, or blankets without poles, provide very little support for the patient's back and rapidly become uncomfortable. Rope techniques are usually quite elaborate and take a long time and a lot of practice to assemble. They also provide very little back support. Both fabric and rope litters can be made more rigid by use of poles (ski poles, skis, or tree branches), but they

still are more difficult to construct and offer less support than the rucksack stretcher. Rucksacks are almost invariably present on expeditions, while the other methods require special equipment and do not solve the problem of what to do with the patient's rucksack.

Some pole litters are designed to be carried by two rescuers from the ends. This is only practical for very short distances unless the patient is very light. However, it is sometimes necessary to carry a patient in a litter in this manner for short stretches on narrow sections of trails or across bridges.

Travois stretchers and improvised "sledges" have also been described. These are theoretically useful on quite smooth ground, especially on snow, but they are difficult to construct. Polar expeditions and mountaineering expeditions in other glaciated areas are likely to have sleds available. These can be commercially available, heavy-duty sleds or children's plastic sleds with some additional rigging. Either of these types is quite adaptable for transporting patients with suitable padding, even though few of them are long enough to be ideal. The patient, like any important load, must be tied into the main rope in crevassed areas.

CARRYING THE LITTER ON NONTECHNICAL TERRAIN

The optimum number of litter bearers on nontechnical terrain is six, with three on each side. More litter bearers just get crowded and get in each other's way. Fewer carry too much weight and risk dropping the litter if one person stumbles. On level and uphill terrain, the patient is carried head end first, but on downhill terrain, the litter is turned around to keep the patient's head higher than the feet. If there is some variation in the heights of the litter bearers, the pairs should be matched for height across the litter, except on sidehills, where the taller litter bearers should be on the downhill side.

Sometimes a seventh rescuer will act as litter captain. The captain stays in front on level terrain, sometimes supporting the heavier head end, but may also steady the litter from behind on downhill stretches. The captain or the litter bearers in front call out obstacles to those behind because those behind will have a hard time seeing ahead. If there are enough people, the person who is providing medical care will walk behind the litter and monitor the patient.

Even with six litter bearers, carrying a litter with an adult patient for any significant distance is quite strenuous. If the expedition is large, there may be enough members to carry the litter in rotation. Some members will go ahead and scout the route stopping in pairs at intervals of 50–100 meters. They then station themselves on either side of the trail and as the litter passes they replace the pair of litter bearers at the back of the litter. This back pair moves forward to become the middle pair, while the middle pair moves forward and the front pair walk ahead of the litter. All of this is done simultaneously. It may help to have a leader who stations the next pairs. The pairs also can switch sides of the litter each time, so that they use different muscles in consecutive carries. In complex terrain, such as woods or very rocky terrain, this technique can be modified by having the next pairs in front of the litter and a hand-off done to them from the front pair, who then moves to the middle, while the middle pair moves to the back and the back pair drops off (Figure 40.3). In either of these sequences, the litter keeps moving continuously, with only occasional interruptions in complex terrain.

If there are not enough litter bearers to rotate, the litter bearers can use slings to help carry the litter. A 3-meter length of sling can be fixed to the litter or clipped with a carabiner and passed over the bearer's shoulders to the outside hand. If commercial litters are used, this method transfers some of the weight of the litter to the shoulders of the bearers, which makes it much less strenuous to carry the litter. The slings can also be used to adjust the height of the litter to compensate for variations in terrain. The litter bearers should not be tied to the litter.

WATER RESCUES

On flat water, such as lakes and protected harbors, a boat or raft may be valuable for avoiding a long difficult way around by land. A six-person raft is adequate, but is best for a single rescuer to row along with the patient. Not only does an eight-person raft allow two rowers and an additional one or two rescuers, but it is also more stable. All rescuers should wear personal flotation devices, and the patient should not be strapped into the litter.

AIRPLANES AND HELICOPTERS

In many parts of the world, rescue has been revolutionized by the use of aircraft, which enable long transports that were almost unimaginable in the pre–aircraft era. For expeditions operating in suitable terrain, fixed-wing aircraft (airplanes) have many uses for rescue. Many expeditions in remote areas will arrive and leave by airplane. These can be adapted for take-off and landing in areas not suitable for wheels with the use of skis for snow and floats for water. Airplanes can also be used to airdrop supplies in areas in which they are unable to land, either because of terrain or weather. Rotorcraft (helicopters)

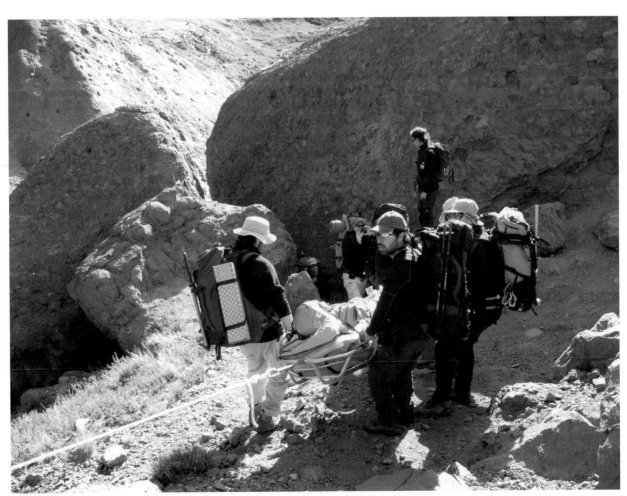

Figure 40.3. Passing the litter. Preparing to pass a litter in complex terrain. Photo courtesy of Ken Zafren.

have additional capabilities in mountainous, canyoned, or forested terrain, which make them useful for expedition transport or rescue.

A detailed discussion of the use of aircraft for expedition logistics and expedition rescue is beyond the scope of this book; however, a general knowledge of aircraft operations can be crucial for the success of expedition rescue. The aeromedical chapter covers medical aspects of flight and the use of aircraft for evacuation of ill or injured patients. One important principle for using aircraft in remote areas cannot be overemphasized: *Nobody should ever be separated from personal survival gear.* An expedition member should never board an aircraft, take off in an aircraft, or leave an aircraft without his or her own pack, even if two aircraft are flying the same route at the same time or if the aircraft is expected to return immediately for gear. Aircraft can be diverted by weather, mechanical problems, or, most unfortunately, by crashing.

To use aircraft successfully for expedition rescue, the expedition should have a plan for activating air rescue, be able to communicate successfully with the pilot of an aircraft used for rescue, define or construct a safe landing zone, and assist the pilot with the landing. Every member of the expedition should be familiar with safety in aircraft operations.

Preplanning will include a plan for activating air rescue if the expedition does not have its own aircraft. In many countries, including most developing countries, arranging air rescue will require either prepayment or a guarantee of payment. Expeditions from many developed countries can count on their embassies in the host country to guarantee payment. The expedition should contact their embassy in the host country to ascertain their policy. In the past, an alternative to guaranteed payment was to make funds available in case of emergency in the form of a cash deposit or bond with the embassy of the expedition's home country. Nowadays, credit card authorization to the aircraft operator is usually sufficient.

The expedition should know the requirements for landing zones for any aircraft likely to be used in a rescue or evacuation. Airplanes will need a runway for wheeled aircraft, a large area of snow if on skis, or a large body of water – usually a lake – if on floats. The pilot will want to know the altitude, slope, and nature of the surface, especially if it is uneven or if there is soft snow into which a ski could stick in addition to whether there are any obstacles on the approach or take-off route. Helicopters can land and take off vertically, but it is safer to have a route for gradual descent and take-off. Although this is usually described as two routes – one for ingress and another for egress – helicopters can often turn 90° while still near the ground and take advantage of the same path for landing and take-off. The larger the landing zone, the safer it will be. There should be no objects, such as shrubs or tree stumps sticking up, and all loose objects must be secured so that they do not become a hazard in the "rotor wash." The helicopter pilot will also want to know if the surface has loose snow, gravel, or dust that will limit visibility on take-off or landing when blown up by rotor wash.

Airplane and helicopter pilots will want to know the weather conditions at the landing zone, including visibility, temperature, and wind speed and direction. Ideally at least one radio should be available for ground-to-air communications. Ground-to-air signaling can be used. A visible indicator of the wind speed and direction is often very helpful. This can be a wind sock or any flagging (e.g., a short length of brightly colored surveyor's tape); a flare or smoke grenade is also a useful option. It may be helpful to mark the landing zone, especially on snow. Dark-colored garbage bags filled with snow or rocks give the pilot a visual reference, which would otherwise be lacking. Some pilots will throw these out of the airplane onto snow on a first pass before landing. Any object used to mark the landing zone or give wind direction should be well secured or should be heavy enough not to blow in propeller wash or rotor downwash.

All personnel and equipment should be out of the landing zone, except in some helicopter operations in which the terrain requires that the helicopter land right next to a rescue team. In this case, the team crouches down and doesn't move while the helicopter lands. There should be no loose equipment or clothing in the landing zone. If the landing zone has gravel, dust, or loose snow, anyone near the landing zone should wear eye protection and face away from the helicopter during landing and take-off. In an emergency, putting a hand in front of the eyes and squinting will help somewhat. A windbreaker with a hood is also helpful.

Hot loading and unloading (with the engine running and rotors turning) is more hazardous than cold loading and unloading, but it is often necessary. During hot loading, the tail rotor may be nearly invisible.

Passengers should approach or leave helicopters only from the front and sides (except in the case of rear-loading Chinook helicopters) and only after a signal or radioed permission from the pilot or a crew member. They should stay in the pilot's line of sight during the entire process. If the helicopter is sitting on a slope, passengers should approach and leave from the downhill side of the helicopter. This helps to maintain a safe distance below the rotor blades. Sometimes it will be necessary to circle partway around the helicopter. This should always be done around the front rather than the rear of the helicopter. Passengers should crouch down while approaching or leaving the helicopter and should carry any objects horizontally below waist level. On some types of helicopters, the ends of the rotor blades may be as little as 1.5 meters (5 feet) above level ground. Some helicopters have rear doors. Crew members will generally assist directly with approaching and leaving these helicopters because of the proximity to the tail rotor.

Other safety rules for approaching or leaving a helicopter include removing hats, holding on to loose objects and never reaching up or running after a loose object that is blown away. If blinded by dust, crouch lower or, if possible, sit down and await help.

Passengers boarding a helicopter should generally place their gear inside first and then board, moving over if other passengers are going to board. The pilot or a crew member will give them instructions about where to put gear, where to sit, and how to put on seat belts and shoulder harnesses. Any changes in location of passengers or gear may affect the helicopter's center of gravity and must be cleared with the pilot or other crew member in advance.

On occasion it will be necessary to board or exit a helicopter while it is hovering just above the ground or on one skid. Because the pilot must compensate for any weight shifts or changes, all movements in and on the helicopter must be done slowly and as gently as possible. Passengers boarding a hovering helicopter should gently place packs and other equipment on board before boarding, and when leaving a hovering helicopter, should gently put (or occasionally drop) the pack and any other baggage on the ground. Sometimes a short jump to the ground will be necessary, and communication with the pilot is important in this case. Rappelling out of a helicopter is potentially very dangerous and must only be done by those with special training and only when no other method of reaching the ground is feasible.

If there is an injured patient on a litter, the method of loading will vary depending on the type of helicopter. In small helicopters, the litter may fit only longitudinally next to the pilot or in another specified configuration.

When a load is not put into the helicopter, it is referred to as an external load. Some helicopters have external baskets; loads must be secured in these by the crew. In rescue work, ropes or cables may be used to carry a load below the helicopter or to hoist a load into or out of a helicopter. People or gear can be attached to a line underneath the helicopter and flown from one location to another in that position, to be deposited (gently) on the ground at the destination. This is referred to as long-line or, confusingly, short-haul operation. In the case of gear, often placed in a net, it is usually termed sling loading. Long-line operations differ from winch or hoist operations in which the external load is lowered from the helicopter or raised into the helicopter by means of a winch (Figure 40.4). Members of expeditions who are not specially trained for long-line or hoist operations should await instruction from a helicopter or ground crew member. Never touch a load hanging from a helicopter until it has touched the ground and discharged the often considerable static electricity built up in flight. Also beware of loads hanging from helicopters because they can pendulum or spin unexpectedly and injure those on the ground. Some helicopters with suitably trained crew may be able to pick patients or stranded climbers off cliffs or other technical terrain. Generally, a rescuer

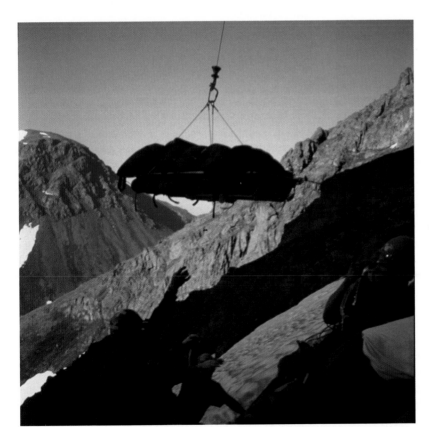

Figure 40.4. Raising a victim into a helicopter using a winch. A tag line is being used to prevent the litter from spinning. Photo courtesy of Ken Zafren.

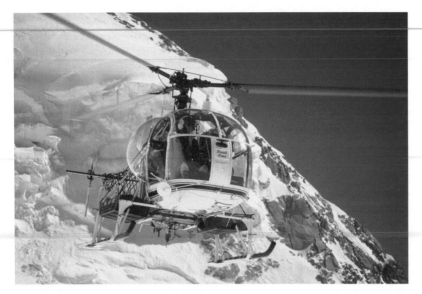

Figure 40.5. The Aerospatial Lama is an example of a helicopter that is ideal for high-altitude rescue by virtue of its high performance, but with very limited aeromedical capability. A standard rescue litter fits in the *Lama* only with the head somewhat elevated. The *Denali Lama* used in Denali National Park, Alaska, is outfitted for short-haul operations. Photo courtesy of Ken Zafren.

will descend first and secure the external load for this delicate and potentially hazardous operation.

Airplanes are usually safer to approach than helicopters, but precautions must be taken around the propellers. The pilot or another crew member will give signals or instructions. In general, hot loading and unloading is avoided. Sometimes one engine will be left running on the side of the aircraft opposite the main cabin door. Most of the other safety principles are the same as for helicopters. Movement of people and gear in light aircraft can change the center of gravity just as in a helicopter and must be avoided without approval of the pilot or crew.

There are many types of helicopters, not all of which are suitable for rescue. Most aeromedical helicopters are not well suited for rescue and vice versa (Figure 40.5). In certain mountainous areas, such as the Alps, rescue helicopters typically have significant aeromedical capabilities. In other areas, there are major dangers to helicopter crews and those who would be rescued associated with the use of aeromedical and other helicopters in technical terrain. Any helicopter used for rescue should meet specific qualifications for performance and crew training.

Wilderness rescue is the art of the possible. It is usually better to transport an ill or injured patient in a suitable helicopter initially and then transfer to an aeromedical helicopter unless the aeromedical helicopter has adequate performance and the crew are specially trained for operations in mountain terrain. For high-altitude and mountain operations, most helicopters, including helicopters not routinely used for rescue (such as news helicopters, sightseeing helicopters, and air taxis) are frankly dangerous to the rescuers and should be used only for the most limited tasks, such as ferrying gear or equipment to optimal landing zones that are well within the performance capability of the helicopter and crew. The same principles apply to airplanes.

IMPROVISED RESCUE TECHNIQUES

There are many improvised techniques that can be useful for expedition self-rescue. The following are a few very useful techniques. In some cases, such as the rucksack stretcher, these techniques are not generally found in printed reference materials and have advantages over those found elsewhere. The selected techniques are basic, but most require practice. They are best learned prior to the expedition and ideally practiced during it from time to time.

TRANSPORTATION TECHNIQUES

Split Coil Rope Technique

Transportation techniques should be easy to perform, even in cold, windy conditions, and should require only material that is already carried by the group.

If a climbing rope is available, one may use it as an improvised device for a conscious patient without severe injuries. The rope is rolled up as a ring with its diameter chosen according to the rescuer's height. The knot must be located at the back of the patient on a level with the rescuer's belt. One disadvantage of the rope technique is that the patient's leg can hang down very near the ground, especially if the rescuer is going downhill and is shorter than the patient. Another disadvantage is the fact that the patient and the rescuer can carry only one rucksack including essential survival gear.

To use this technique the rescuer divides a standard coil of rope into two rings (Figure 40.6). The patient steps through the rope and the rescuer slides his arms through the coils (Figure 40.7). The knot in the coils should be located on the patient's back and near the rescuer's belt (Figure 40.8).

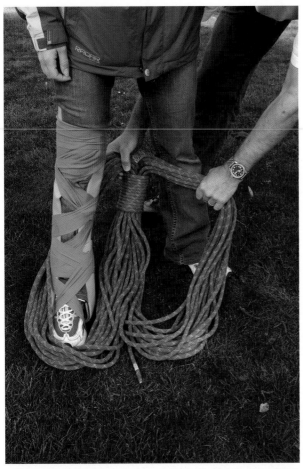

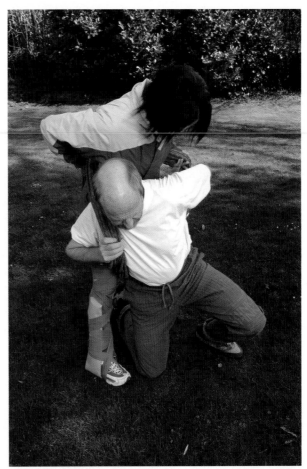

Figure 40.6. Photo credit: Reavita AG, Franco Bottini, Zürich (Switzerland) and Urs Wiget.

Figure 40.7. Photo credit: Reavita AG, Franco Bottini, Zürich (Switzerland) and Urs Wiget.

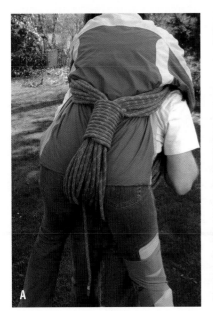

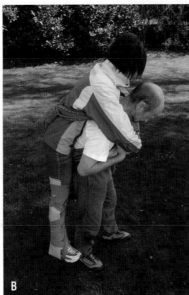

Figure 40.8. Photo credit: Reavita AG, Franco Bottini, Zürich (Switzerland) and Urs Wiget.

Rucksack Techniques

On expeditions, rucksacks are generally available. Techniques for carrying patients using rucksacks can be improvised very quickly. There is another advantage using these techniques: The group will be able to carry the most important survival gear (sleeping bag, stove, food) with them.

Single-Rescuer Technique

This technique is excellent for patients with a lower limb injury or who are ill but conscious and able to sit and to hold themselves on the back of a rescuer. Both rescuer and patient carry a rucksack with their most important personal gear (Figure 40.9).

Procedure

- Choose the rucksack with the longest straps.
- Prepare some spare gloves or other clothing to pad the rescuer's shoulder.
- Help the patient (while sitting or standing) to sit in both straps so that the rucksack is partially under the bottom and against the back of the patient.
- The patient should pull the rucksack as high on his or her back as possible.
- Make sure that the waist belt of the rucksack is located between the thighs of the patient.
- The rescuer slips between the legs of the patient and places the straps on his or her own shoulders.
- Pad the rescuer's shoulders before he or she stands up.
- Inform the patient that he or she will bend high over the head of the rescuer and should hold him- or herself around the shoulders of the rescuer.

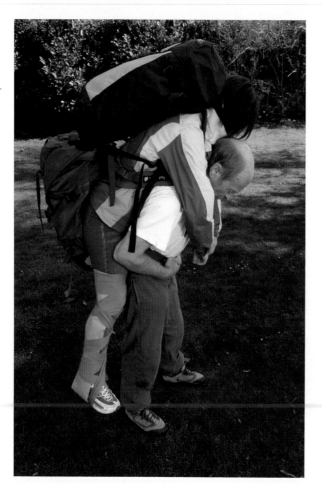

Figure 40.9. Photo credit: Reavita AG, Franco Bottini, Zürich (Switzerland), and Urs Wiget.

- The rescuer should then stand up, if possible with the help of another person, and adjust the load.
- The patient is given his or her own rucksack by a helper (if the patient and the rescuer are alone, the patient may put on his or her rucksack before the rescuer stands up).
- While traveling, the rescuer may search for stones/ice blocks on the way in order to rest letting the patient sit on the block without slipping out of the rucksack straps.

Rucksack Stretcher

Patients who should be carried in a lying position are unconscious patients and patients with femur/pelvis/spine lesions. If the rucksack stretcher is made using fairly full rucksacks (survival gear) and carried by at least three or four rescuers on each side, the patient will be well stabilized. While restrained with the hip belts of the rucksacks, the patient will not fall off the stretcher if one of the rescuers slips. This stretcher can literally be made in one minute and gives good support to the patient, while improvised rope stretchers described in many texts take a long time to construct and provide very poor support.

Procedure

- Choose three or four rucksacks (depending on the height of the patient) and put them on fairly flat ground top to bottom in line with each other (carrying sides up) (Figure 40.10).
- Undo the shoulder straps of the middle or middle two rucksacks; this may require cutting the security seams at the ends of the straps).
- Run the shoulder straps of each rucksack except the top one through the shoulder straps of the one above it.
- Reattach the shoulder straps of each rucksack.
- Do not tighten the straps before putting the patient on the stretcher, and make sure that the hip belts of the rucksacks lie flat and wide open.
- Put the patient flat on the stretcher (Figure 40.11). It may be easiest to lift the patient by his or her clothing. The patient's head can be placed between the upper ends of the straps of the first rucksack or can be stabilized by the hip belt of the "bottom" rucksack. If the patient is unconscious, first stabilize the neck with a SAM splint.
- Restrain the patient firmly with the hip belts; then tighten the straps under the patient (Figure 40.12).
- Before lifting the stretcher, make sure that one of the rescuers will give the commands.
- Lift and carry the patient (Figure 40.13).
- One of the rescuers at the head end should continuously observe the breathing of the patient.
- When the group stops to rest, make sure that the rucksacks do not roll over with the patient on them.

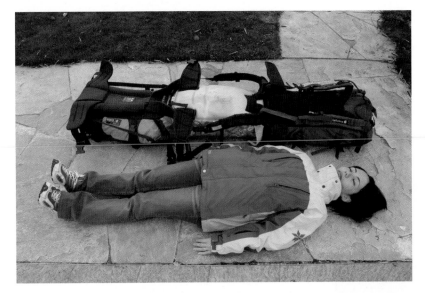

Figure 40.10. Photo credit: Reavita AG, Franco Bottini, Zürich (Switzerland), and Urs Wiget.

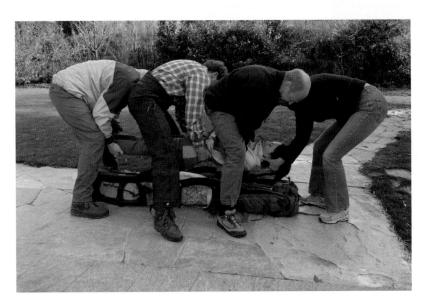

Figure 40.11. Photo credit: Reavita AG, Franco Bottini, Zürich (Switzerland), and Urs Wiget.

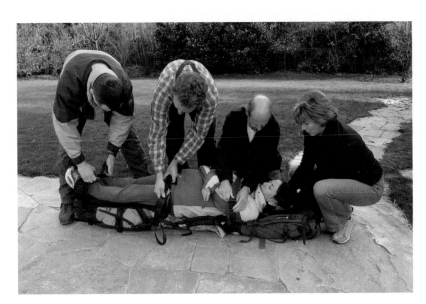

Figure 40.12. Photo credit: Reavita AG, Franco Bottini, Zürich (Switzerland), and Urs Wiget.

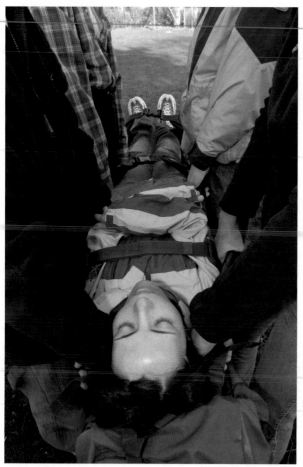

Figure 40.13. Photo credit: Reavita AG, Franco Bottini, Zürich (Switzerland), and Urs Wiget.

There are many improvements possible. Ski poles may be inserted in the straps in order to clip in a shoulder-carry sling with a carabiner. Without a sling and a carabiner, it is easier to carry the rucksacks and patient directly by the straps. Ski poles are too small to be held for a long time. The patient may be placed in a sleeping bag.

If the unconscious patient vomits, turn the packs with the patient on command by pulling up one side and putting down the other side of the stretcher: the patient will be held by the hip belts and the forearms of the rescuers.

IMPROVISED IMMOBILIZATION TECHNIQUES

SAM splints (SAM Medical) allow improvised immobilization of nearly all parts of the body. We advise lay rescuers use SAM splints instead of circumferential wraps in order to avoid complications by compression. Many techniques exist, some of which are quite complicated. Here is one of the simplest:

Improvised Neck Collar

Always stabilize the neck of an unconscious patient during transportation. A SAM splint may be applied quickly even if the patient is lying in deep snow.

Procedure

- One helper stabilizes the head and neck of the patient with both hands.
- The SAM splint is rolled around the neck like a bandage and may be tightened a bit (Figure 40.14).
- Be sure that the chin has not rolled into the SAM splint (Figure 40.15) – the head should be stabilized in a slightly extended position (Figure 40.16).
- Adjust the rim by folding it if it forms pressure points.
- The end of the SAM splint may be closed by using tape or a short bandage.

Simple and Rapid Immobilization of Shoulder–Arm–Hand

The following immobilization techniques can be used for a patient with a lesion of the upper extremity (from the clavicle to the fingers) who is still able to walk.

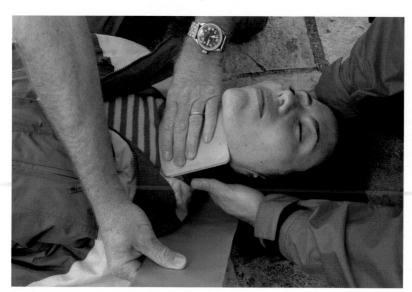

Figure 40.14. Photo credit: Reavita AG, Franco Bottini, Zürich (Switzerland), and Urs Wiget.

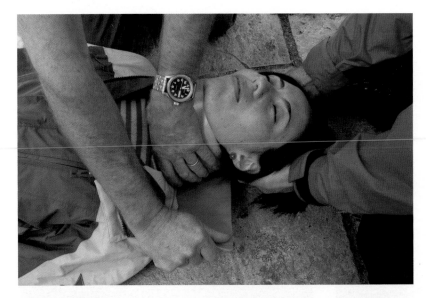

Figure 40.15. Photo credit: Reavita AG, Franco Bottini, Zürich (Switzerland), and Urs Wiget.

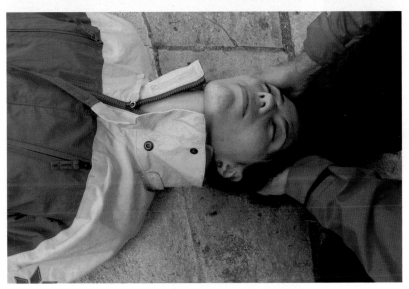

Figure 40.16. Photo credit: Reavita AG, Franco Bottini, Zürich (Switzerland), and Urs Wiget.

Using a T-shirt

Procedure

- Hold the injured arm.
- Flex the elbow over the abdomen.
- Roll the bottom of the T-shirt up over the forearm and the upper arm as high as possible so that the lower edge of the T-shirt reaches the shoulder (Figure 40.17).
- Secure the bottom of the T-shirt using a small stone (or a pocket knife or other convenient item) inside the T-shirt and a shoelace or other string or thread (Figure 40.18).

Using an Anorak or Jacket

Procedure

- Turn the sleeve of the anorak on the patient's injured side inside out.
- Put the uninjured arm in its sleeve and put the anorak over the shoulders and the flexed injured arm.
- Close the anorak over the injured arm, which is located over the abdomen.
- Put a string or a belt over the anorak around the abdomen so that the injured arm cannot fall down (Figure 40.19).

The anorak technique is ideal in cold weather. The injured part of the body will not move even while walking over uneven ground.

IMPROVISED WOUND CARE – SOME PRACTICAL TIPS FOR WOUND CARE IN THE FIELD

Nonstick Dressings of Superficial Wounds in the Field

Abrasions and superficial wounds cannot be left open because clothes and sleeping bags may rub and cause further damage. Most dressings will stick to the wet wound surface and cause pain and injury when removed.

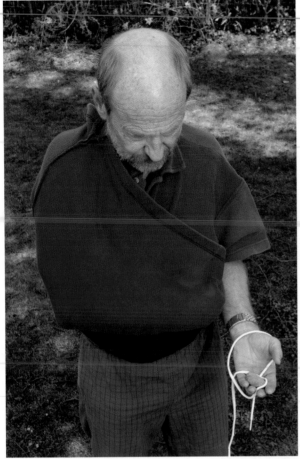

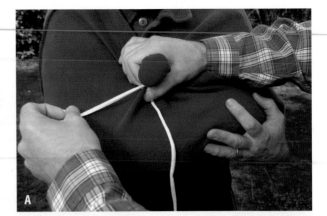

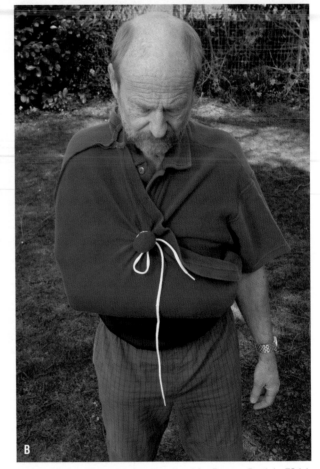

Figure 40.17. Photo credit: Reavita AG, Franco Bottini, Zürich (Switzerland), and Urs Wiget.

Procedure

- Clean the wound.
- Cut a piece of a plastic bag a bit larger than the surface of the wound.
- Put the nonprinted side of the plastic directly on the wound and apply a bandage.
- Remove the dressing every 12–24 hours, recleaning the wound as necessary.
- Continue to dress the wound in this way until the wound surface is dry.

This idea comes from Dave Allan, a surgeon in Bangor, UK. He points out that the plastic remains more or less sterile even when carried in a rucksack because the material is not a tissue but a "frozen liquid" without pores.

The wound may be covered with a yellow "jelly" and smell like fresh meat when the dressing is removed. After cleaning, it is unlikely that one would see a wound infection but rather neat granulation tissue.

Closure of Skin Cracks

In dry or wet cold conditions, skin cracks are common on fingers and hands. Barefoot porters in the Himalayas

Figure 40.18. Photo credit: Reavita AG, Franco Bottini, Zürich (Switzerland), and Urs Wiget.

and elsewhere often suffer from deep and painful skin cracks of the soles of the feet. Skin cracks may not heal because of a humid and dirty local milieu.

Procedure

- Carefully apply a drop of skin glue in the crack and wait until the glue dries.
- Be careful not to splash drops of the glue in the eyes and not to touch the glue as long as it is moist because it will stick to whatever touches it.

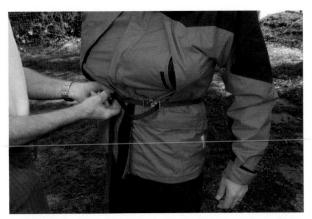

Figure 40.19. Photo credit: Reavita AG, Franco Bottini, Zürich (Switzerland), and Urs Wiget.

The crack will heal from the inside and the glue will progressively appear at the surface of the skin where it will wear off. Sometimes it may be necessary to repeat the application.

DISLOCATIONS

Finger Dislocations

A dislocated finger should be reduced immediately in order to avoid injuries of cartilage and/or soft tissues. The reduction is easy, but one should be careful not to pull straight along the axis of the finger. This may cause a fracture of the articular surface. The dislocation should be reduced by "milking out" the dislocated finger by pushing the proximal end of the dislocated phalanx, with the finger in the position of function.

Reduction of Shoulder Dislocations in the Field

Untrained rescuers should not reduce a shoulder dislocation in the field if professional help will be available in less than one hour. If immediate transportation is not possible, try to reduce a shoulder dislocation as soon as possible. Many shoulder dislocations can be reduced without the use of analgesics or muscle relaxants, especially if done very early.

Before trying to reduce a shoulder dislocation, one must be sure that it is really a dislocation and not a subcapital fracture of the humeral head. A dislocated shoulder joint is locked and cannot completely be adducted to the body. The palpation of the empty glenoid fossa may also be an indication, but it is not as convincing as the lack of the ability to abduct. A patient with a dislocated shoulder should not be able to touch the thorax with the elbow.

There are many techniques. The technique described by Rudi Campell, an orthopedic surgeon from Pontresina, Switzerland, in 1929 is quite popular in Europe and has been extensively used by one of the authors (UW). This technique provides a measure of safety in the field. If the patient who has not received pain medication feels more pain the more one pulls on his arm, the rescuer will stop the procedure before nerves or tendons in the dislocated joint are damaged further.

Procedure

- Explain the procedure to the patient.
- Grasp the injured arm at the elbow and apply traction along the axis of the upper arm. With the other hand, hold the neck of the patient firmly to help him or her lie down with minimal motion of the injured arm (Figure 40.20).
- Grasp the patient's hand as if shaking hands and apply progressive traction on the arm.
- With the hand that held the neck of the patient before, grasp the wrist of the injured arm and with both hands apply continuous traction, without interruption (Figure 40.21).
- Elevate the injured arm under traction slowly so that you are able to pull directly over the injured shoulder (Figure 40.22).

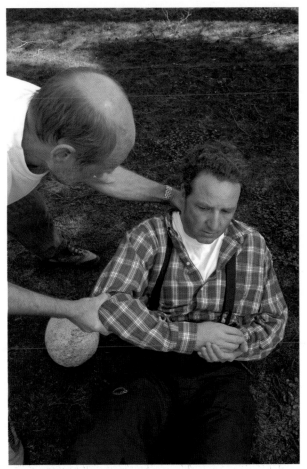

Figure 40.20. Photo credit: Reavita AG, Franco Bottini, Zürich (Switzerland), and Urs Wiget.

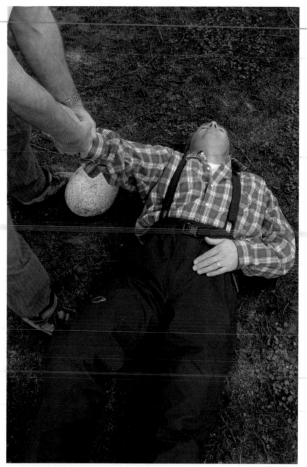

Figure 40.21. Photo credit: Reavita AG, Franco Bottini, Zürich (Switzerland), and Urs Wiget.

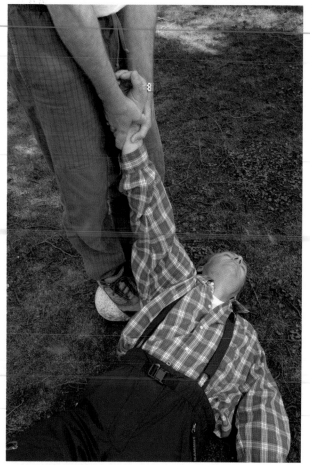

Figure 40.22. Photo credit: Reavita AG, Franco Bottini, Zürich (Switzerland), and Urs Wiget.

- In most cases, it will be necessary to lift the shoulder and a part of the thorax of the patient from the ground.
- Try to relax the patient by saying, for example, "try to push your fist very fast toward the sky." In many cases, the patient will relax the chest and shoulder muscles.
- Sometimes the rescuer will feel a pop when the head of the humerus slips into the glenoid fossa.
- It is often necessary to pull for several minutes. The rescuer will stop when unable to pull any longer.
- Whether successful or not, immobilize the arm in an anorak and try to get care as soon as possible.

While the rescuer is pulling, the patient should feel real pain only at the wrist and the hand of the injured arm. If the shoulder joint becomes progressively more painful, stop and immobilize the arm.

It may be helpful to put a towel or handkerchief around the wrist of the patient in order to prevent slipping.

Even a reduced shoulder dislocation may become more painful, especially at night. Pain medication may be indicated.

An alternative technique, which also is quite safe, involves having the patient continue to sit up. With the elbow bent, use the proximal forearm as a handle to apply progressively increasing traction to distract along the axis of the arm to distract the femoral head. After some movement is felt in the shoulder joint (often after a minute or more), externally rotate the humerus, again using the forearm as a handle. This technique is often so atraumatic that one does not feel any pop. Immobilize the arm after reduction as in the Campell technique. One of the authors (KZ) has used this technique frequently without the need for any medication.

RING REMOVAL (IN CASE OF HAND INJURIES)

With any hand injury, rings should be removed immediately to prevent circulatory problems of the fingers. With the thread technique, it will be often possible to remove rings even from a mildly swollen finger. The technique works well with fine fishing line or dental floss. If these materials are not available, extract a fine nylon thread from a small climbing rope. The more slippery the thread, the easier it will be to remove the ring.

Procedure

- Prepare a piece of thread of 50–70 cm length.
- Insert one end carefully under the ring (perhaps with a knife blade) in order to have the long end hanging in the direction of the fingertip (Figure 40.23).

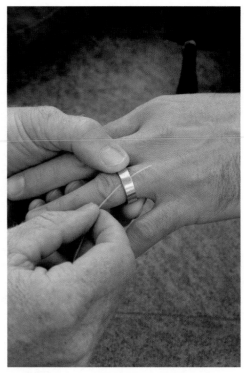

Figure 40.23. Photo credit: Reavita AG, Franco Bottini, Zürich (Switzerland), and Urs Wiget.

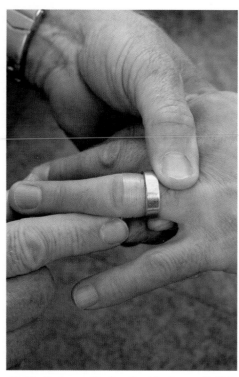

Figure 40.25. Photo credit: Reavita AG, Franco Bottini, Zürich (Switzerland), and Urs Wiget.

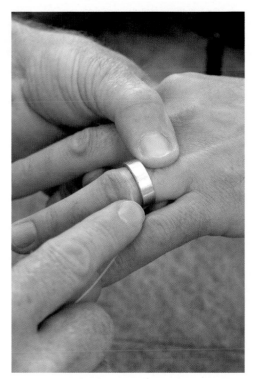

Figure 40.24. Photo credit: Reavita AG, Franco Bottini, Zürich (Switzerland), and Urs Wiget.

- Push or pull the ring downward toward the knuckle as much as you can, then start to roll the thread around the finger including the knuckle (Figure 40.24). Do not hurry. Wrap the thread very carefully with each layer touching the next one. This procedure may hurt a bit, and the finger may become blue.

- When the thread is completely wrapped (Figure 40.25), start to pull the upper end of the thread slowly, firmly holding the bottom end of the thread (Figure 40.26). By unrolling the thread, the ring will slip over the knuckle (Figure 40.27).
- If the ring is not freed, repeat the procedure. Pull the bottom end of the thread carefully under the ring (don't cut the skin by pulling too fast) and roll the thread around the finger again.

OTHER IMPROVISED TECHNIQUES

There are many additional improvised techniques, which may be useful on expeditions. Table 40.2 summarizes a list of texts that include further information on rescue techniques.

CONCLUSION

Expeditions are inherently risky enterprises. Risk can be minimized by taking preventive measures and by being prepared to manage untoward events. Preparing for the possibilities of injury or illness during an expedition is important to ensure the best outcome. There are many useful improvised techniques for self-rescue, a few of which are presented in this chapter. Expeditions should be prepared to take at least the initial steps to rescue ill or injured members.

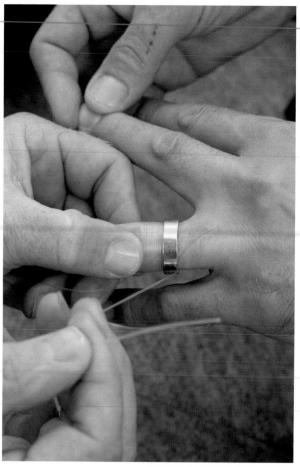

Figure **40.26**. Photo credit: Reavita AG, Franco Bottini, Zürich (Switzerland), and Urs Wiget.

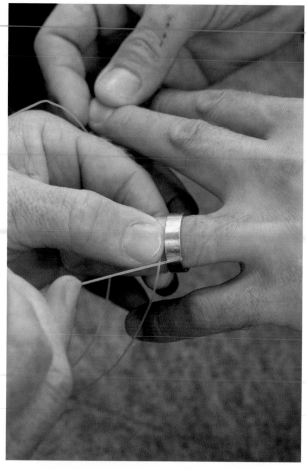

Figure **40.27**. Photo credit: Reavita AG, Franco Bottini, Zürich (Switzerland), and Urs Wiget.

Table 40.2. Useful books – rescue techniques

David J. Fasulo's *Self-rescue* – geared to self-rescue in rock climbing and contains many useful strategies for self-rescue in a vertical environment

Bill March's *Improvised Techniques in Mountain Rescue* – a classic text, but now almost impossible to find; first published as a spiral bound guide for mountaineering students and later included in his *Modern Rope Techniques in Mountaineering Incorporating Improvised Techniques in Mountain Rescue*

Andy Selter's *Glacier Travel and Crevasse Rescue*, 2nd ed. – a clearly written guide to glacier safety and rescue with information about self-rescue

Andy Tyson and Molly Loomis's *Climbing Self Rescue: Improvising Solutions for Serious Situations*

Eric A Weiss and Howard J Donner's chapter on wilderness improvisation in *Wilderness Medicine*, 5th ed. (P. S. Auerbach, editor) – contains many improvised techniques, which may be useful on expeditions, including many techniques for using SAM splints; Weiss coined the phrase "101 uses for a safety pin" and 22 of these are listed here

SUGGESTED READINGS

Auerbach PS, ed. *Wilderness Medicine*. 5th ed. St. Louis: Mosby; 2007.

Fasulo DJ. *Self-rescue*. Evergreen, Colo: Chockstone Press; 1996.

Hempel JC, Fregeau-Conover A. *On Call: A Complete Reference for Cave Rescue*. Huntsville, Ala: National Speleological Society; 2001.

March B. *Improvised Techniques in Mountain Rescue*. Self-published.

March B. *Modern Rope Techniques in Mountaineering Incorporating Improvised Techniques in Mountain Rescue*. New York: Hippocrene Books; 1984.

May WG. *Mountain Search and Rescue Techniques*. Boulder, Colo: Rocky Mountain Rescue Group; 1973.

Ray S, Bechdel L. *River Rescue: A Manual for Whitewater Safety*. 3rd ed. Boston: Appalachian Mountain Club; 1997.

Selters A. *Glacier Travel and Crevasse Rescue*. 2nd ed. Seattle: The Mountaineers; 2006.

Setnicka TJ. *Wilderness Search and Rescue*. Boston: Appalachian Mountain Club; 1980.

Tyson A, Loomis M. *Climbing Self Rescue: Improvising Solutions for Serious Situations*. Seattle: The Mountaineers; 2006.

41 | Aeromedical Evacuations

Eugene F. Delaune III, MD

INTRODUCTION

Moving patients by air is in some ways very similar to moving patient by ground transport and in some ways very different. A patient must be stabilized as much as possible prior to moving, and problems that could arise during transfer must be anticipated. Plans must be made to addresses any potential complications that may occur en route and the stresses to the patient inherent to the chosen mode of transport must be considered in the planning process. During any flight, outside assistance is at least 30 minutes away. Extremes of temperature, pressure, noise, and relative hypoxia may be encountered. Awareness of these unique stresses and accounting for them will ensure that all aeromedical evacuations are conducted as safely and efficiently as local conditions and the patients' disease processes allow.

REPATRIATION VERSUS EVACUATION

Although grouped together as *aeromedical evacuations* for the purpose of this chapter as well is in common usage, medical evacuation and repatriation are actually two distinct activities. "Evacuation" usually implies that a patient cannot receive the appropriate care locally and is being moved to the closest suitable facility. "Repatriation," on the other hand, involves taking the patient home. In some situations, patients cannot receive appropriate care locally, and it makes sense to return them home for definitive care. More often, repatriation involves a patient who has been stabilized at a facility away from home, and will then require on-going care or rehabilitation. Repatriation patients tend to be more stable, and there is less urgency in moving them.

MODES OF AEROMEDICAL EVACUATION

The most common and flexible means of aeromedical evacuation over long distances are the fixed-wing air ambulance (Figures 41.1 and 41.2) and rotary wing aircraft (helicopters). In general, a helicopter is useful for the patient requiring urgent evacuation when the distance to travel is 150 miles or less, and/or either patient condition, local environment, or patient location make ground transport impractical. There are many different types of fixed-wing aircraft, from the small propeller planes, which barely have enough space for the patient and two attendants, to the large jet aircraft with space enough for a full medical team, the patient's family, and room to spare. An additional means of aeromedical transport that is often overlooked is the commercial aircraft (Figures 41.3 and 41.4). When patient movement can be planned around scheduled commercial flights, commercial airlines often provide an efficient, safe, and cost-effective alternative to moving patients, especially when moving patients over long distances. Each of these modes of transportation will be discussed later in this chapter.

AEROSPACE PHYSICS

To accurately plan for evacuating patient by air, a basic understanding of aerospace physics is essential. The laws of science describing the relations of volume and pressure, as well as the effects of these variables on the human body should be clear. Simply stated, increasing altitude corresponds to decreasing ambient temperature and decreasing ambient pressure. It is useful to look at decreasing ambient temperature and decreasing ambient pressure separately because they may each have an impact on patient care and condition in different ways during aeromedical transports.

REDUCTION IN TEMPERATURE

After the ambient temperature drops below freezing, the humidity (i.e., water content of the ambient air) quickly falls, and any significant moisture that is present freezes and precipitates. Even in pressurized aircraft, the cabin air is mixed with outside air, which is bled into the aircraft from outside. The cabin is then pressurized to a set equivalent barometric pressure. As a result, the humidity

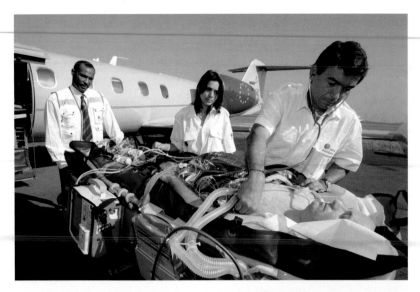

Figure 41.1. Fixed-wing air ambulance. Photo courtesy of The Europ Assistance Group.

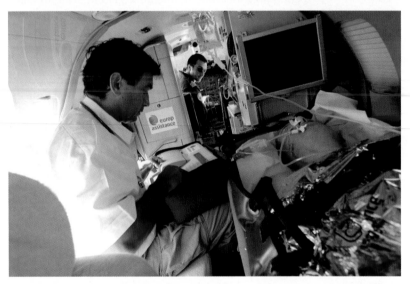

Figure 41.2. Limited space on an air ambulance. Photo courtesy of The Europ Assistance Group.

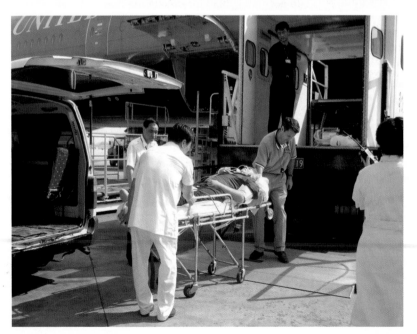

Figure 41.3. Elevator truck for boarding patient. Photo courtesy of Eugene F. Delaune, III.

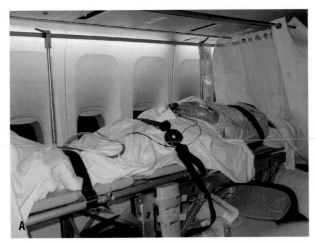 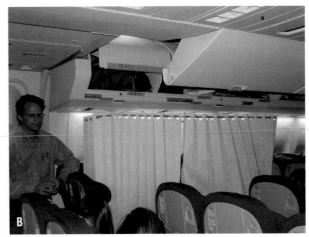

Figure 41.4. Stretcher on commercial aircraft. Photo courtesy of Eugene F. Delaune, III.

of the partially recirculating air inside any aircraft flying at cruising altitude is less than 25%.[1]

REDUCTION IN PRESSURE

All elements, including gases, have mass and weight. The gases that make up the earth's atmosphere extend several miles up from the ground. At sea level, there are several miles of gas molecules pressing down on any given point on the earth, thus exerting pressure. As one moves away from the ground, more and more of the atmosphere's gas molecules are below, rather than above, any given point; therefore, they are no longer exerting pressure – this explains why atmospheric pressure decreases as altitude increases. In aviation, the most common means of expressing ambient pressure is in terms of pressure altitude (i.e., equivalent feet above sea level). Even in pressurized aircraft, as the aircraft ascends, the equivalent pressure altitude in the cabin decreases, albeit at a slower rate than outside the pressurized cabin. In an unpressurized aircraft, the cabin pressure corresponds to the outside pressure. Generally, unpressurized aircraft fly no higher than 10,000 feet, as the decreased partial pressure of oxygen above this altitude (discussed later is this chapter) makes supplemental oxygen during extended flight for all occupants of the aircraft essential.[2] An aircraft capable of being pressurized is usually recognizable by its rounded doors and windows as well as the seals on the doors. The cabins in these aircraft can be pressurized relative to the outside pressure. As the plane ascends, the difference between the cabin pressure and the outside pressure gradually increases. The type of aircraft being used determines the maximum differential that can be achieved. As a result, even in a pressurized aircraft, the pressure inside the cabin may be as low as the equivalent of 6,000–8,000 feet above sea level (8,000 feet is the maximum allowed by the FAA for general aviation, i.e., private aircraft).[3] Because of the structural limits of the aircraft, if sea level pressure must

be maintained in the cabin, the maximum altitude of flight must be reduced to maintain an acceptable and safe inside – outside pressure differential. The exact maximum altitude that can be flown while still maintaining sea level pressure in the cabin is a function of the aircraft design and therefore specific to each particular type of aircraft. Limiting the aircraft altitude will also limit the aircraft speed, increase fuel consumption, and may necessitate additional refueling stops, significantly increasing the duration of the transport.

As stated in Boyle's Law, pressure and volume are inversely proportional.[4]

$$PV = k$$

or, stated differently,

$$P_1/V_1 = P_2/V_2$$

Stated differently and as shown in Table 41.1, as pressure goes down, volume goes up. Because, even in a pressurized aircraft, pressure decreases as the aircraft ascends and the volume of all confined (nonvented) gases expands. This is a linear relationship, meaning that a halving of the pressure altitude results in a doubling of volume of all gases in enclosed spaces. This phenomenon is easily demonstrated with a bag of chips or bottle of shampoo, which is sealed at sea level and then examined during a commercial flight or after ascending into the mountains. The bag of chips will appear inflated, and may even burst from the increased pressure in the bag. Similarly, a bottle of shampoo sealed at sea level may open spontaneously at altitude with a resultant venting of the accumulated pressure. Conversely, if a sealed container is closed at altitude, it will appear to be under a vacuum when observed back at sea level.

As stated in Dalton's law of partial pressures, the total pressure exerted by a gaseous mixture is equal to the sum of the partial pressures of each individual component in a gas mixture.[5]

$$P_{total} = P_1 + P_2 + P_3 + \ldots$$

Table 41.1. Increasing altitude with corresponding increases in volume of gases

| Altitude | | Atmospheric | | Volume of 1 liter | Percentage increase |
Feet	Meters	pressure (mmHg)	Bars	of gas	in volume
0	0	760	1	1	0
1,000	305	734	0.97	1.03	3
2,000	610	710	0.94	1.06	6
3,000	915	686	0.91	1.1	10
4,000	1,219	662	0.88	1.14	14
5,000	1,524	639	0.85	1.17	17
6,000	1,829	617	0.82	1.22	22
7,000	2,134	595	0.79	1.27	27
8,000	2,439	574	0.76	1.32	32
9,000	2,743	554	0.73	1.37	37
10,000	3,048	534	0.71	1.41	41

The air in our environment is roughly composed of a relatively constant mixture of 80% nitrogen and 20% oxygen.[6] Even at 40,000 feet, the higher end of the range where commercial aircraft fly, the proportion of this mixture remains relatively constant. Because the overall atmospheric pressure decreases with altitude, the pressure exerted by the individual gases decreases as well. Physiologically, this means that the approximate 20% oxygen that is present at a higher altitude is exerting less pressure and therefore has less of a pressure gradient to drive oxygen molecules across the alveolar membranes in the lungs to oxygenate the blood. This leads to a falling PaO_2 as altitude increases. Notice in Table 41.2 that although the atmospheric pressure and the ambient pressure of oxygen both fall with altitude, the partial pressure of the oxygen remains constant at just above 20%. Also demonstrated is the partial pressure of the oxygen in the alveoli, where the oxygen must travel down a pressure gradient in order to be taken up by the hemoglobin molecules in the blood.

As the amount of oxygen that is able to transverse the alveolar membranes decreases with increasing altitude, the oxygen content of the blood decreases; thus, the oxygen saturation of the blood begins to fall. This phenomenon is demonstrated in Table 41.3. Note that in normally functioning lungs, the hemoglobin oxygen saturation falls to 90% at 8,000 feet, the highest allowable altitude in general aviation without the use of supplemental oxygen.

AEROSPACE PHYSIOLOGY

Physiological Effects of Decreased Pressure

Conditions That May Be Aggravated by Decreases in Relative Pressure

The most relevant effects of decreased pressure on the body in-flight are the expansion of gases and the reduction of the blood's oxygen content. As explained earlier, the volume of enclosed gases increases linearly with altitude. (See Table 41.1.) If the gases that are trapped in an enclosed space are not allowed to vent, the pressure within this space will increase and/or the volume in which they are enclosed will increase. With air trapped in the intestines, for example, the expansion of the gases leads to intestinal and corresponding abdominal bloating. If the gas is near the mouth or anus, it will be vented in the form of belching or flatus. Because the walls of the intestine are elastic, they allow for some expansion, and there is the possibility of venting some of the increased volume. Therefore the expansion of normal intestinal gas at altitude during gradual ascent to normal commercial cabin pressure altitude is a relatively harmless event, usually only minimally uncomfortable.

In situations where there are abnormal collections of gas in the body, the effects of gas expansion can have significantly more noticeable and potentially harmful effects. It is therefore worth discussing, in more detail, some of the medical conditions in which gas expansion at altitude must be considered when planning an aeromedical evacuation.

Table 41.2. Actual measured alveolar oxygen and carbon dioxide concentrations at different pressure altitudes

Pressure Altitude (feet)	Atmospheric Pressure (mmHg)	Ambient O_2 (mmHg)	Alveolar O_2 (mmHg)	Alveolar CO_2 (mmHg)
0	760	159	103	40
5,000	632	133	81	37
10,000	523	110	61	35
12,000	483	101	54	34
13,000	465	97	51	33
14,000	447	94	48	33
15,000	429	90	45	32
20,000	350	73	34	29
25,000	282	59	30	27

http://www.dr-amy.com/rich/oxygen/.

Table 41-3. Oxygen content of human blood by pressure altitude

Pressure altitude (feet)	Alveolar partial pressure of O_2 (mmHg)	Dissolved O_2 (ml O_2/100 ml blood)	Hemoglobin saturation (%)	O_2 carried by hemoglobin (ml O_2/100 ml blood)	Total O_2 in blood (ml O_2/100 ml blood)
0	103	0.32	97	20.22	20.54
5,000	81	0.25	94	19.60	19.85
10,000	61	0.19	90	18.77	18.96
12,000	54	0.17	87	18.14	18.31
13,000	51	0.16	84	17.51	17.67
14,000	48	0.15	82	17.10	17.25
15,000	45	0.14	80	16.68	16.82
20,000	34	0.11	67	13.97	14.08
30,000	30	0.09	57	11.88	11.97

Assumes that alveolar O_2 = arterial O_2, pH 7.40, T = 37°C, 1.39 ml O_2 per gram of saturated hemoglobin (actual physiologic probably approximates 1.31).
http://www.dr-amy.com/rich/oxygen/.

Recent Brain Surgery or Head Injury

The cranial vault is a relatively stiff and confined space. Under normal circumstances it contains no air and therefore should be unaffected by decreases in ambient pressure. Any condition that introduces air into the cranial vault changes this situation. Air can be introduced into the cranium by any injury that leads to penetration through the skull or by any procedure that may be performed upon an injured brain. The insertion of ventricular drains and intracranial pressure monitors are common procedures in head-injured patients in which some air may remain in the brain for several days, even after the device is removed. As long as the drain is still in place, with one end of the drain communicating with the trapped air, pressure will not accumulate in the skull as there exists a route for the air and cerebrospinal fluid to be vented to the outside. If there is no drain in place, however, and air has entered the skull, either through a procedure or from the original injury, the trapped air can become problematic at altitude. Because the skull is a closed, noncompliant structure, even small increases in the size of a retained pocket of air can exert significant pressure on the entire brain. This increased pressure can be manifested by symptoms as innocuous as a headache and nausea or as extreme as seizures, reduced brainstem function, or, ultimately, herniation and death.

Eye Injuries or Recent Eye Surgery

Like the cranial vault, a normal eye contains no air and has no means of venting air. If air has been introduced into the globe, either by injury or as part of surgical therapy, expansion of this gas at altitude will cause problems. As the pressure from the expanding air inside the globe increases, blood flow to the retina decreases, eventually leading to permanent visual loss. Baroreceptors in the eye respond to increased pressure by causing severe pain and changes in nonrelated functions, such as a potentially dramatic decrease in heart rate. Because there is no means of venting trapped air in the eye, patients with this condition must be maintained at their present equivalent altitude until all air has been resorbed. In the past, there has been some reluctance to fly patients with detached retinas or some other ocular pathologies; however, experience in the U.S. military aerovac community shows that, as long as no air has been introduced into the globe, flying these patients poses no unique risk.

The Middle Ear

The middle ear contains three small bones that articulate to transmit sound from the outer ear, through the eardrum to the inner ear where the brain is able to process the sound. These three bones of the middle ear are contained in a small, air-filled cavity. This cavity is vented to the nasal pharynx via the narrow, collapsible eustachian tube. Under normal conditions, as the air in the middle ear expands with altitude, it passively inflates the eustachian tube and easily vents the expanded air to the nasal pharynx. As altitude decreases during descent of an aircraft (or diving underwater) the eustachian tube usually requires active opening, sometimes by yawning, chewing gum, or performing a Valsalva maneuver (attempting to force air through a closed mouth and occluded nose). In small children, or in conditions that cause inflammation in the back of the nose, the eustachian tube can become so narrowed that it is impossible to push air back into the middle ear because a vacuum develops during descent as the air in the middle ear contracts with decreasing altitude. This can be an extremely painful condition and can lead to tympanic membrane rupture. Once the tympanic membrane ruptures, most of the pain is resolved as the pressure is now equalized through the outer ear. The ear drum usually heals with no intervention over the ensuing months although in some cases it may require surgical repair.

Sinuses

Similar to the middle ear, the maxillary and frontal sinuses drain through small openings into the nasopharynx. When these openings become occluded, usually due to inflammation or viscous secretions, there is no opportunity for pressure in the sinuses to vent; therefore, pain can be experienced either during ascent or descent.

Teeth

Because teeth are very rigid structures, they provide no space for air to expand. Therefore, even small decreases in ambient pressure can cause an extreme elevation of the pressure exerted by trapped air in teeth and cause debilitating pain. Patients with caries or who have had procedures that involved drilling the teeth in the prior week or two are prone to this problem. Short of drilling a hole in the tooth and chemical pain control, little can be done to provide relief to a patient who experiences altitude-induced dental pain.

Chest/Lungs

Under normal spontaneous negative pressure ventilation, the lungs are inflated by the downward movement of the diaphragm and the outward expansion of the chest wall musculature. This creates in the chest a relative vacuum that pulls the lungs open, forcing them to expand and fill with air, which enters through the nose and mouth. If there is a leak from the lung into the chest cavity, air from the lung will migrate into the pleural space when the diaphragm moves down, thus hampering the development of appropriate negative pressure and the resultant inflation of the lung. This condition is referred to as a pneumothorax or a collapsed lung. In significant cases, the pneumothorax must be decompressed. This is usually accomplished by placement of a chest tube to remove accumulated air from the pleural space to reexpand the lung, until the leak resolves.

Patients with pneumothoraces have to be managed very carefully when they are evacuated by aircraft. Any air in their chest cavity should be expected to expand anywhere from 25 to 50% at the normal 8,000-feet relative cabin altitude. If there would be a sudden decompression of the aircraft, the expansion of air within the chest cavity would be significantly greater. As long as there is a vented chest tube in place connected to a chest tube, suction device, water seal, or Heimlich valve that is draining the accumulated air, expansion of the pneumothorax will quickly be reversed as the increased volume of air is vented out through the chest tube. If the chest tube has been removed, or occluded, there is danger that there could be some degree of collapse of the affected lung at altitude. Various recommendations

exist as to when a patient can fly after the removal of a chest tube. Although the U.S. military will fly patients within 24–48 hours after a chest tube is removed from a resolved pneumothorax, other professional organization recommend waiting 1–4 weeks.[12]

Another lung condition which can be impacted by decreases in pressure is the presence of lung blebs. Blebs are noncommunicating pockets of air, usually on the surface of the lung. As the volume of the air in these blebs increases with increasing altitude, they can rupture, possibly resulting in a spontaneous pneumothorax.

Patients who require mechanical ventilation, either as a result of lung pathology or another medical condition, need special attention in-flight. Most endotracheal tubes used to maintain the airway in a ventilated patient have an air-filled cuff at their distal ends. As the air in this cuff expands, it can exert damaging pressure in the trachea, or it can burst. In these patients, it therefore becomes necessary to either replace all the air in the cuff with a sterile fluid or to carefully monitor the cuff pressure both during ascent and descent.

Gastrointestinal Tract

As mentioned previously, gastrointestinal gas expands with altitude. In a normal gastrointestinal tract, the intestines are able to expand and eventually vent in response to the increased volume occupied by the expanded gases. There are, however, several pathological conditions where this expanding gas can become problematic. With some types of surgery on the intestines, a segment of the intestines is cut and then reanastomosed with staples or sutures. At the points where this reanastomosis of the intestines takes place, there is a resultant weak spot in the intestinal wall. If expanding gas in that region puts pressure on the newly closed defect, there is a real danger that the closure could fail, leaking bowel contents into the abdomen. This would rapidly make the patient very ill and guarantee that if the patient survived, the recovery period would be long and complicated. In addition to intraintestinal air, there is also residual atmospheric air left within the abdominal cavity following both open and laparoscopic abdominal surgery. Depending on the volume of this air, the patient can experience significant discomfort as the air expands at altitude. There are also nonsurgical conditions that can be reason for concern when the patient is exposed to an increase in altitude. Any condition that leads to an increase in luminal gas in the intestine can cause varying degrees of discomfort to a patient in flight. As this gas expands, it can exert pressure on the intestinal wall and the neighboring organs and can cause an increased heart rate due to the pain this causes.

Bone Fractures

Emergent care of any fracture, even prior to considering evacuation involves stabilizing the fracture and ensuring that the affected body part is positioned in such a way as to maximize the circulating blood and nerve function distal to the fracture. Both of these actions usually require the application of some type of splinting device. When flying a patient with a splint or a full cast, care must be taken to ensure that no small pockets of air are trapped by the splint or cast. If trapped air is not provided with some means of escaping as it expands, it will exert pressure on the adjacent skin and will likely damage this skin in an already compromised limb. This is especially important when transporting an unconscious or otherwise impaired patient who may be unable to communicate discomfort. If a circumferential cast has been recently applied and still fits snugly, it must be bivalved prior to flying the patient. This involves cutting the cast through its long axis, and then wrapping the cast with either an elastic bandage or some material that allows the cast to maintain its structural integrity while allowing it to vent or expand to accommodate trapped air. When moving these patients, frequent rechecks of distal pulses and sensation must be performed to ensure that repositioning or swelling have not compromised pulses and nerve function – failure to recognize this phenomenon could lead to permanent limb damage or loss. When air-filled splints are used, either the air must be vented in flight or the splint partially deflated prior to flying to ensure that the splint does not become too tight during the flight.

Diving-Related Illnesses

Divers can develop several conditions where pathological air bubbles develop in different parts of the body. In decompression sickness (DCS), nitrogen comes out of solution in the blood forming bubbles; these can occlude small capillaries. DCS is commonly divided into two categories: Type I, which only involves the musculoskeletal system (commonly called the bends), lymphatic vessels, and skin, and Type II, which involves any other organ – especially the nervous system. Type II DCS can be manifested by neurological dysfunction such as numbness, paresthesias, and changes in behavior. Type II DCS involving the inner ear presents similarly to vertigo and is sometimes called the staggers. When DCS involves the formation of air bubbles in the pulmonary parenchyma, it is sometimes referred to as the chokes.[13] Another phenomenon sometimes seen in divers is the formation of arterial gas emboli. In this case, increased air pressure in the alveoli during ascent forces air across the capillary membranes into the pulmonary venous circulation. These bubbles then travel through the left heart into the systemic arterial circulation. Another cause of arterial gas emboli could be the formation of air bubbles in the venous circulation in patients with a patent foramen ovale, allowing the free flow of the bubbles from the right to left heart without the lungs having the opportunity to filter them out. When these bubbles find their way into the coronary and cerebral circulations, myocardial infarction and stroke, respectively, can result.

Symptomatic patients are treated in hyperbaric chambers where ambient pressure is *increased* in an attempt to force the nitrogen air bubbles back into solution. As might be expected, the *decreased* ambient pressure usually associated with flight has the opposite effect on these bubbles, and therefore flying in a cabin which does not maintain sea level pressure is not advised until a hyperbaric physician has cleared the patient to fly. Even in divers who have not experienced symptoms following a dive, the general recommendation is for all divers to refrain from flying for anywhere from 12–72 hours after their last dive, depending on the duration and depth of their dives.[13] If a patient must fly to reach appropriate hyperbaric treatment, the plane should maintain a cabin pressure of 1,000 feet or less.[13]

Physiological Effects of Decreased Oxygen Concentration

Conditions That May Be Aggravated by Hypoxia

The most relevant indirect effect of decreased pressure on the body in flight is the reduced availability of oxygen at the cellular level. As previously described, with an increase in altitude, the pressure of the oxygen in the air decreases linearly with the decrease in atmospheric pressure. As the pressure gradient decreases, there is less oxygen transfer across the alveolar membranes in the lungs and into the red blood cells where it is then transported to the tissues of the body. As a result, the oxygen saturation of the blood falls, and less oxygen is delivered and made available for use to the cells of the body. (See Table 41.3.) In the typical aircraft, which is pressurized to the equivalent of 6,000–8,000 feet of altitude, this relative deprivation of oxygen has little effect on an otherwise healthy person with healthy organs. Certain disease states and medical conditions, however, make some individuals especially sensitive to this state of relative hypoxia.

Atmospheric oxygen can be considered to be 20%. For patients receiving supplemental oxygen via nasal cannula, the oxygen concentration (FiO_2) can be estimated by adding 4% for each liter of O_2 delivered per minute.[7] So a patient at sea level receiving oxygen at 4 liters per minute via nasal cannula is breathing 36% oxygen or has an FiO_2 of .36 (20 + [4 × 4]). In patients requiring supplemental oxygen, a useful equation helps to predict the amount of supplemental oxygen that will be needed in flight and at the final destination:[7]

(Pressure altitude at originating facility × Required FiO_2)/New Pressure Altitude = Required FiO_2 at a new pressure altitude

For example, a patient is transported from sea level (760 mmHg) to an altitude of 4000 feet (662 mmHg) (Table 41.1). The patient is on a mechanical ventilator with FiO_2 of 40% at the originating facility. The following would be used to determine the required FiO_2 at 4,000 feet to achieve the same level of hemoglobin saturation with oxygen;

$$(0.40 \times 760)/662 = 0.46 \text{ or } 46\%$$

In another example, if a patient is requiring 2 liters per minute via nasal cannula (an FiO_2 of approximately 28%) of supplemental oxygen at a referring facility at sea level and is to be transported on a commercial aircraft where the pressure altitude can be up to 8,000 feet (574 mmHg), the following would be the calculation to determine how much supplemental oxygen this patient will require in flight:

$$(0.28 \times 760)/574 = 0.37 \text{ or } 37\%$$

The patient would therefore require 4 L/m flow of 100% oxygen via nasal cannula to maintain the same degree of hemoglobin oxygen saturation in flight as at the originating facility.

Cardiac Diseases

The heart is a solid muscle with very high metabolic requirements. A normal heart has its metabolic requirements (including it oxygen delivery) satisfied by the coronary arteries, which run within the walls of the heart. In patients with coronary artery disease, these vessels become either partially or completely occluded, leading to angina or myocardial infarction. In these patients with reduced blood flow to the heart, it is vital that the reduced flow that is ultimately able to get through or around a stenosed vessel be completely saturated with oxygen to satisfy the metabolic needs of the heart muscle. Such a patient may compensate well at sea level, where the blood is close to 100% saturated with oxygen breathing only room air. When they get to altitude, however, with blood that is only saturated in the low 90%s, the heart's metabolic requirements may no longer be sufficiently satisfied and various degrees of ischemia can result. This negative effect of altitude on the heart will be magnified in patients with underlying lung disease, which further impairs the blood's ability to absorb oxygen in the lungs, and in anemic patients who have less oxygen-carrying capacity in their blood.

Lung Diseases

As blood circulates through the lungs, it absorbs oxygen and unloads carbon dioxide, a waste product produced by the body's cells. There are many lung diseases and conditions that impair the lungs' ability to perform this vital function. As a result, these patients tend to have more difficulty at altitude, where the availability of oxygen is even further reduced. To a certain point, most people can compensate for a drop in their oxygen saturation relatively well. Once the degree of hypoxia at which they can compensate is exceeded, a person

will rapidly decompensate with resultant organ dysfunction (e.g., mental status changes). Special care must therefore be taken when flying patients with lung diseases to ensure that they will be able to adequately oxygenate at altitude.

Neurological Diseases

Like the heart, the brain has a very high metabolic requirement, and it has little reserve capacity. When blood flow is limited to part of the brain (usually through blockage of blood vessels, as in an ischemic stroke, or because of brain swelling from any one of a number of insults to the brain), cell function is jeopardized. If the reduced volume of blood flowing to the compromised part of the brain is suboptimally oxygenated as a result of altitude-induced hypoxia, exacerbation of the detrimental effects of this hypoxia should be expected.

Patients prone to seizures could be more likely to experience a seizure during flight because many of the factors that can induce seizures in susceptible patients are found during air travel: hypoxia, fatigue, and overall physiological and psychological stress. When flying a patient with seizures, efforts should be made to minimize these factors, and medical attendants must be prepared to treat seizures should they occur.

Ophthalmological Disease

Because the cornea is an avascular structure, it is largely dependent upon diffusion of oxygen from the ambient air to meet its oxygenation requirements. Therefore, even patients who have adequate oxygen saturation of their hemoglobin can have a hypoxic cornea if there is relative hypoxia in the ambient air.[14] Patients with corneal disease are particularly sensitive to a decreased availability of oxygen in the ambient air. As a result, the decision to fly these patients must be carefully considered.

Pregnancy

Commercial air travel poses no special risks to a healthy pregnant woman or her fetus. However, certain conditions in pregnancy – such as severe anemia, sickle cell disease, clotting disorders and placental insufficiency – can increase the risk of problems.[8] Because the pregnancy does not generate any new air-filled organs, the pregnancy is not directly affected by changes in cabin pressure. At cruising altitude, both mother and baby will both have slightly lower hemoglobin oxygen saturations than at sea level; however, a healthy woman and fetus can easily compensate.[8]

According to the American College of Obstetricians and Gynecologists, the safest time for a pregnant woman to travel is during the second trimester (18–24 weeks). This is when a pregnant woman has the lowest risk of miscarriage or premature labor. Many doctors recommend that women avoid flying after 36 weeks of pregnancy or at any time if they are at risk of preterm delivery to avoid any potential onset of labor in flight.[8]

Other Conditions Affected by Flying

There has been much interest recently in the link between the development of deep vein thrombosis (DVT) and flying.[9] While the clot itself may cause some localized swelling and discomfort, the more serious medical concern is that one of these clots could break free and travel to the lung (or brain if the patient has an underlying heart defect resulting in the right to left shunt), causing serious impairment or even death. This effect would likely be potentiated by the relative hypoxia that would already exist at altitude if this event happened in flight. Many of the commercial airlines now actively educate their passengers on how to reduce the risk of developing this condition where a clot forms in the deep veins of the legs and pelvis. Conventional thinking is that the prolonged inactivity, combined with the maintenance of the leg in a bent position, kinking the leg veins, thereby reducing blood flow, lead to stasis and possible endothelium damage in the legs and therefore clotting of the blood contained in these veins. Because veins contain fluid blood and no air, the effects of changes in cabin pressure should have no effect on the blood, and therefore play no role in the increased incidence of clot formation in people who fly.[9] Any patient with a recent injury, especially a vascular or orthopedic injury, has had multiple chemical cytokines and other biochemical communicators released from the cells of their body, which makes their blood especially prone to developing clots. Smokers, patients using oral contraceptives, patients who are inactive, patients with a history of clotting disorders, pregnant women, patients with cancer, and obese patients are also at increased risk.

Some actions can be taken to reduce the risk of DVT from flying. Air travelers, especially those prone to developing clots, should avoid bending and crossing legs for an extended period. Frequent walks or at least isometric leg contractions are also recommended. Patients may also be advised to take aspirin prior to flying, or may even benefit from the administration of fractionated heparin, assuming no contraindications to either. Patients can also wear compression hose to reduce blood pooling in the legs.[10]

The effects of reduced cabin pressure on casted patients with orthopedic injuries were discussed earlier. Even in noncasted patients with orthopedic injuries, some special considerations are necessary during aeromedical transport. Injured limbs are prone to swelling. This swelling can be due to decreased muscle tone, reduced use, prolonged time in a dependent position, inflammation, and even damage to the venous or lymphatic drainage system. If an injured limb is allowed to remain in a dependent position for a long time during a flight, the increased swelling can lead to discomfort, skin damage, or even the formation of a deep vein thrombus.

For this reason, every effort must be made to elevate dependent limbs during air evacuation.

MODES OF AEROMEDICAL EVACUATION

Several modes of transportation can be used when evacuating an ill or injured patient. The most appropriate and safest means of patient movement will change according to the patient's pathology, local terrain, weather, distance to be traveled, time constraints, and availability of aircraft.

Types of Aircraft

Helicopters

Helicopters are frequently the first means of transportation that come to mind when considering the evacuation of a patient. Helicopters have the flexibility of being able to land any place there is a small flat surface, and even the ability to hoist patients out of locations where they cannot land. Helicopters can carry a limited medical staff and may have sufficient room for the medical attendants to perform emergency procedures on a patient. Despite these many advantages, helicopters do have limitations. The range of a helicopter is limited by the amount of fuel it can carry. As a general rule of thumb, an aeromedical evacuation helicopter can fly approximately 150 miles on a full tank of fuel.[11] When it is necessary to transport a patient over a greater distance, it is useful to consider fixed-wing aircraft, which are faster and have a much longer range. Because most helicopters fly by visual navigation using ground-based landmarks (VFR = visual flight rules), they may only fly in weather that allows for visualization of ground at all times during flight. Wind, rain, and freezing can all make it impossible to safely fly a helicopter at certain times. The altitude at which most aeromedical evacuation helicopters can fly is limited to around 15,000 feet, so some rescues at higher altitudes become impossible. Most helicopters are unable to achieve a significant pressure differential from inside to outside the cabin; therefore, when transporting patients with conditions that may be aggravated by the direct and/ or indirect effects of reduced relative pressure, the flight altitude may need to be severely restricted. This inability of helicopters to pressurize their cabins also limits their usefulness at high altitudes (e.g., high on mountains) as well as for transporting patients from one location to another when flying over a high mountain range is required. Because helicopters fly low, there is a danger of striking objects such as power lines, which are difficult to see, especially if they are not marked. The noise level, vibrations, and cramped space inside of most aeromedical helicopters make good patient care difficult. In summary, helicopters are a good choice for patients urgently requiring evacuation for a short distance, from a location that may have restricted landing possibilities, and where limited care is required in flight.

Fixed-Wing Air Ambulances

The traditional air ambulance actually comes in many varieties, from the most basic propeller-powered, non-pressurized airplane to the pressurized jet aircraft. These aircraft are typically small aircraft that would normally be chartered or owned by individuals and companies with a need for private aircraft. The cabin of the aircraft is retrofitted from a passenger-carrying configuration to an aeromedical configuration. Some aircraft remain in this configuration, while others may be changed from a passenger to aeromedical configuration on a flight-by-flight basis. The smaller, propeller-powered aircraft, which sometimes do not have the ability to pressurize, tend to be less expensive to operate, are able to land on shorter runways, but are noisier and have a more limited range. The larger, jet-powered aircraft are often better suited for longer distances as well as situations where more space and a pressurized cabin environment are required. Through the use of inverters, the aircraft power can be adapted for the use of most medical equipment.

If required, a sea level equivalent altitude that allows for pressurization can be maintained, although this limits the altitude, speed, and fuel efficiency of the aircraft. The exact altitude to which an aircraft is limited depends on the particular airframe. If a patient's condition would be aggravated by an increase in altitude, but absolute sea level altitude is not required, providing the pilot with a higher absolute altitude restriction can greatly increases speed and fuel efficiency of the aircraft and alleviate the need for extra fuel stops.

Certification of Rotary and Fixed-Wing Air Ambulances

There are no universally accepted regulations or certifications governing aeromedical evacuation aircraft. There are internationally accepted and enforced rules that dictate who can pilot aircraft. The type of training a pilot receives, medical fitness, drug testing, and flying experience are all monitored, and standards are enforced. Similarly periodic inspections, safety equipment, navigation, and communication capabilities of the aircraft are all carefully monitored by government agencies around the world to ensure that aircraft are safe. There are no such accepted standards for personnel or for equipment used in patient care during aeromedical evacuations.

The Federal Aviation Administration (FAA) in the United States and its equivalent international organizations are not in the business of certifying medical equipment or providers. As long as flight safety is not affected, the FAA is not concerned with the quality or type of care delivered in the back of the aircraft. In the United States and in some other countries, there have been attempts at regulating aeromedical crew, but enforcement is difficult and there are no universally accepted standards. The interstate and international movement of these aircraft makes the establishment of universally accepted aeromedical standard practically impossible. Within the United States, each state provides its own licensure of health care workers. This applies to all types of health care providers, including medical doctors, registered nurses, paramedics, respiratory therapists, psychologists, and any other provider who may be used during an aeromedical evacuation. The individual state in which a provider is licensed will dictate the type of prior and ongoing training required for certification, monitor complaints against the providers, and dictate the scope of practice allowed by a particular provider. For example, there is a wide range of procedures and types of intervention approved for paramedics, even between counties within a single state. Although most non-U.S. countries have similar types of certification processes for their health care providers, standards and scopes of practice vary from location to location. Individual certification and licensure is limited to the jurisdiction of the certifying body.

As a result of the regionally specific nature of medical certification, there is no universally accepted standard of certification by which to evaluate or control aeromedical crew. Similarly, the equipment and medications used in flight are determined by the aeromedical evacuation company, and there is no government-enforced quality control process.

Due to consumer demand, some countries and states have begun to establish their own standards and certifications for aeromedical evacuations. There are also private organizations, such as Commission on Accreditation of Medical Transport Systems (CAMTS) in the United States that, for a fee, offer independent evaluation and, if industry standards are met, certification of aeromedical evacuation companies. Similar to Joint Commission on Accreditation of Healthcare Organization (JACHO) in the United States hospital industry, these private certification authorities give some assurance to consumers that minimum standards of quality and competence are being met.[15]

Commercial Aircraft

For many patients, commercial airlines provide the ideal means for aeromedical evacuation. Each airline has its own policy on which types of patients it will transport. Some airlines will provide stretcher space and AC power for medical equipment and oxygen. It may also be possible to board nonambulatory patients using a lift. There are several advantages as well as disadvantages to using commercial airlines when transporting patients.

Commercial aircraft generally fly higher, faster, and longer legs than smaller fixed-wing air ambulances. There is significantly more space for medical equipment and medical crew, as well as patient's family members.

The spacious airline cabin offers more room to maneuver for the medical crew and generally a more comfortable flight for the patient and crew alike.

There are, however, some major disadvantages to using commercial aircraft for the aeromedical patient. The commercial airlines fly set schedules; therefore, patient movement must be coordinated around the airline schedules and seat availability. Commercial aircraft will not adjust cabin pressure or temperature for a particular patient and generally limit the flow of the oxygen provided to 4 liters per minute. There may be limited ability to provide the patient with privacy on commercial aircraft, and other passengers may be subjected to the odors and sounds associated with the patient's condition and the care required; thus, these types of patients may not be optimally suited for this environment. Clearance from the airline must be obtained prior to bringing any patient with a significant illness onboard the aircraft. The clearance process varies from airline to airline and can be very subjective, depending upon the airline personnel issuing the clearance. In addition to the safety of the patient, the airlines are concerned with the comfort (both physical and emotional) of their other paying passengers as well as adherence to scheduled flight times. Airlines are therefore reluctant to approve passengers who may require the timely installation of special equipment or boarding procedures. Airlines are reluctant to accept any patient who has any chance of becoming unstable during flight, as an emergency diversion to an unintended destination is extremely costly and logistically challenging. Many airlines limit the number of passengers who can use supplemental oxygen on a flight, the class of service in which oxygen can be used, and the type of medical equipment allowed onboard. For these reasons, among others, transporting patients onboard commercial airlines can take days to arrange and can be an unsuitable means of travel for many patients.

Disposition of Patients

As is done during interhospital transfers using ground transportation, a receiving facility and provider should be arranged prior to initiating an aeromedical evacuation. Many times, the reason for the evacuation is the need for a level of care that is not available at the patient's current location. If a patient cannot be transported to a facility or a provider equipped to take care of his or her needs, the risk and expense involved with moving the patient are hard to justify. Once a receiving facility is identified, as much information about the patient as possible should be provided to the accepting physician to ensure that proper arrangements are in place prior to the arrival of the patient. Any information, studies, tissue samples, or other items that may be useful in the future treatment of the patient should be transported with the patient to provide the receiving physician with all the information necessary to treat the patient.

Mass Casualty Evacuations

When several patients require medical transport, especially in a mass casualty setting, local resources may be insufficient to provide the necessary medical care and logistical support. In these situations, a patient, who under normal circumstances may have been treatable locally, will require movement to a facility outside of the region affected by the disaster.

There are two different scenarios to consider when discussing mass casualties. One occurs when there are multiple local casualties and possibly some damage to the local infrastructure. In these cases, patients are evacuated for medical care, which under normal circumstance would have been available from the local resources, now overburdened by the catastrophic event. The other scenario is one in which several patients from a single group or event require transport from an area with absent or limited medical resources to the closest appropriate facility.

Some classic recent examples of mass casualty situations where local medical resources were quickly overwhelmed, requiring aeromedical evacuation of large numbers of casualties, are the October 2002 bombing of a nightclub in Bali and the December 2004 tsunami, which affected several countries along the Indian Ocean. In both of these instances, the affected towns were relatively isolated, in less-developed parts of the world, which even under normal circumstances have limited medical resources. As is usually the case in such scenarios, the required aeromedical evacuation resources required in the initial response far exceeded the in-place civilian capabilities. Therefore, the local as well as foreign military became involved in evacuating patients out of the immediate disaster area to regional medical centers capable of initial stabilization and treatment of emergent conditions. At the same time, the military was conducting its initial evacuation, the civilian, governmental, and private agencies were initiating their own protocols for eventually transporting these patients home to their final destinations. In addition to the people directly affected by injuries or illnesses related to the disaster, other travelers found themselves stranded. With previously available transportation and logistical resources overwhelmed, these other travelers also required evacuation, albeit on a less emergent basis.

In the early stages of a disaster response, tracking patients is usually not the primary focus. Patients tend to be placed on the most immediately available means of transportation and end up at the destination where that means of transportation is headed. This means that there is no record of where patients were taken, and patients from a single group or even family may end up distributed over several hospitals or even several countries.

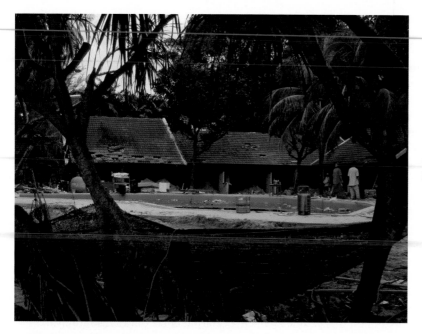

Figure 41.5. Beach front hotel damage in Phuket. Photo courtesy of Eugene F. Delaune, III.

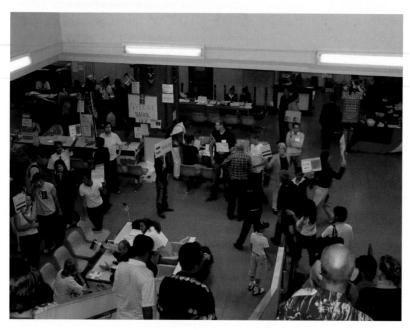

Figure 41.6. Coordinating relief in Bangkok Airport. Photo courtesy of Eugene F. Delaune, III.

Thus, an early challenge in these situations becomes locating survivors and assessing their further transportation needs. It may take days or weeks to locate patients who are unable to communicate or have perished.

After the majority of patients and other affected travelers are located following a mass casualty situation, the number and condition of patients to be evacuated will dictate the most appropriate means of transportation. When other travelers have also been affected, the usual aeromedical evacuation services (air ambulance companies) are in high demand and may not be an option. It is therefore necessary in these situations to consider bringing in aircraft from farther away, possibly with a larger load capacity, to take the patients to another part of the world where the smaller air ambulance and medical services are not stretched. Coordinating such an effort, possibly from thousands of miles away, thus becomes the most practical means of transporting the patients and other affected travelers in a timely manner. It is in these situations where the size and experience of the established travel assistance companies are a real advantage; it may be beneficial to enlist their services.

In some mass casualty situations, only a specific group of travelers are affected. A tour bus accident or a group of stranded hikers are some examples of such scenarios. In these situations, the goal becomes evacuation of the affected patients to the closest facility with the capability to provide the type of medical attention required. If the patients are in a remote location, the evacuation sometimes becomes a two-step process, first moving the patients to an area where aircraft can land and then flying them to a destination where the required medical attention can be obtained. When patients are in very remote locations, the extended time that this process may take sometimes makes it important to start some of the initial medical care prior to the patient's reaching the final destination. Anticipating the immediate needs of the patients is important, as these needs should be communicated to the evacuation providers so they can bring the required supplies and equipment.

ASSISTANCE COMPANIES

There are many forms of commercially available emergency assistance services that should be considered by individuals and groups making travel plans. These services can be purchased in many ways. Assistance services are sometimes attached to an insurance policy that subscribers already have purchased. Medical insurance, life insurance, or corporate benefit plans will often have travel assistance services as part of their benefits package. Other travelers may find that they have automatically acquired some emergency assistance coverage if they purchased their trip using a particular credit card, joined an association (e.g., a SCUBA or automobile club), or purchased trip cancellation insurance. Prior to traveling, subscribers should familiarize themselves with the services offered by their policy – the exclusions (e.g., some policies will have exclusions for travel to certain parts of the world or injuries relating to listed dangerous activities), the limits/deductibles, the periods of coverage, and the means of accessing the services should they become required. If an individual finds that he or she does not have coverage through any of these means, a number of companies will sell emergency travel assistance policies to groups or individuals.

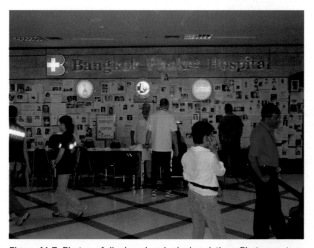

Figure 41.7. Photos of displaced and missing victims. Photo courtesy of Eugene F. Delaune, III.

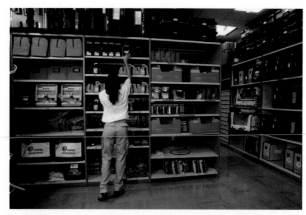

Figure 41.8. Assistance company medical warehouse. Photo courtesy of The Europ Assistance Group.

Whether already covered or seeking to obtain emergency assistance coverage, travelers need to consider several aspects of the types of services that are available. Emergency assistance policies may not cover medical expenses. A patient's regular medical insurance may not cover expenses incurred outside of a defined geographical area. Expenses related to injuries or illnesses obtained in the course of engaging in certain activities may be excluded. When evaluating emergency assistance coverage for adequacy, it is therefore necessary to first determine which services are included in the traveler's regular medical coverage and what the exclusions to this coverage are. Many non-U.S. medical insurers, for example, will exclude expenses incurred in the United States. Others may exclude coverage of expenses that an expatriate incurs when he or she is traveling in his or her home country. After the limitations of a subscriber's regular medical insurance are defined, the type of emergency assistance coverage to be purchased should be chosen to include the coverage that is lacking through the subscriber's other insurance policies. Some of the features to be considered include coverage for a family member to visit if the patient requires hospitalization away from home; the loss of the use of travel arrangements purchased prior to the medical event; and coverage for traveling companions who may have their intended travel plans interrupted as a result of the subscriber's illness or injury. The maximum coverage required is somewhat dependent on the planned activities. Excluding medical expenses, transportation via an air ambulance between any two parts of the world rarely exceeds $250,000. Air ambulance transport within a continent will generally be no more than $100,000. It is rare for an aeromedical transport to cost less than $20,000. Travel agencies and professional societies are good sources of information about which travel assistance companies are good options for any given trip.

Government Assistance

There are situations when local or even home government resources can be called upon for emergency aeromedical

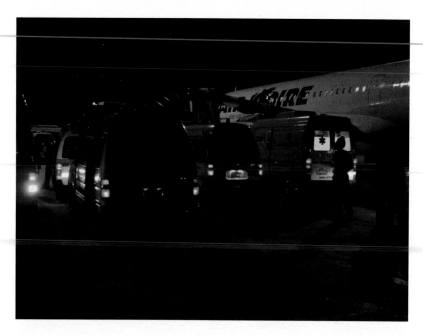

Figure 41.9. Loading tsunami patients in Bangkok. Photo courtesy of Eugene F. Delaune, III.

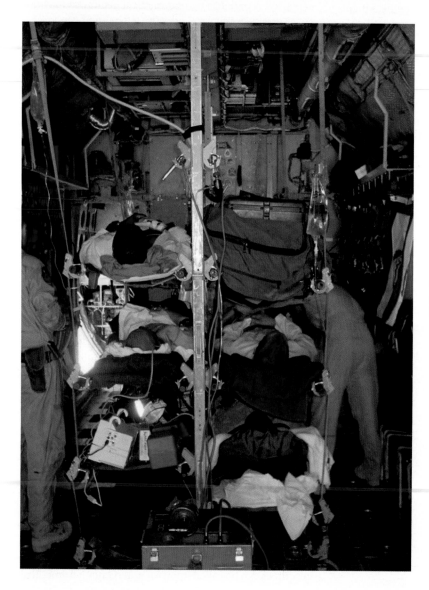

Figure 41.10. Patient evacuation on military aircraft. Photo courtesy of Eugene F. Delaune, III.

evacuations. In any significant mass casualty situation, military resources, which are well rehearsed and equipped for wartime operations, will usually be activated by the local governments where the event occurs as well as in the countries from which the affected patients originate. When patients are traveling in very remote areas or in areas that are unsafe for civilian aeromedical providers (e.g., in war zones and in environmental extremes, such as on the poles), a military organization may be the only one with the resources required to move a patient. Prior to planning a trip to areas where government-sponsored patient movement may be the only option, contact information for both host country resources as well as home country consulates should be obtained and readily available to all members of the traveling party. It is difficult in most situations to get a commitment from a government agent to be available for a theoretical aeromedical evacuation, so this option is usually reserved as a last resort option. If government-sponsored services are used, the charges will vary, but can be significantly less than alternative civilian options.

Repatriation of Remains

The logistics of repatriating the remains of travelers who perish while away from home will vary greatly depending on where the patient dies and the destination of the remains. Because the procedures for moving the remains will be specific to each country, good starting points in arranging such a transport are the deceased's home-country consulate as well as a funeral home in the country where the traveler perished. Some countries require that the body be embalmed prior to departing, or entering, the country. This would imply that, if an autopsy is required or requested, it would need to be performed prior to moving the body. Some countries require that caskets be permanently sealed prior to entering the country. If this is the case, caskets with small windows may be used so that when the remains are received in the home country, they can be visually identified without opening the casket. Cremating the remains prior to transport generally makes the entire process simpler and more expeditious. Although the expense of a repatriation of remains is significantly less than that of an aeromedical evacuation, the logistical maze that must be negotiated still makes the services of a travel assistance company useful. Many travel assistance insurance policies do include coverage for repatriation of remains.

SUMMARY

Moving patients by air is in many ways the same as transferring patients by ground. Once the patient is as stabilized as local capabilities allow, the most appropriate

destination and means of transport must be arranged. The destination should be chosen based on the patient's immediate as well as long-term medical needs. The mode of transportation should be chosen from available resources, considering how the stresses unique to each available option will affect the patient's condition. The equipment and personnel appropriate for the patient's condition should be available at all points during the patient movement. Whenever a group or individual is traveling, especially outside of an area with extensive local medical resources, it is important that a plan be in place, both for a situation requiring the evacuation of large numbers of patients or just one patient. Knowing what options for aeromedical evacuation exist, which ones are covered through insurance and how to access these resources will make the execution of an unplanned patient movement as smooth as possible. When one or several patients require aeromedical evacuation, it is usually the result of a very stressful and unplanned event. Having a preformed plan and knowledge of how to access evacuation resources will remove some of the stress and help expedite an eventual safe movement of the affected individuals.

REFERENCES

1. Lindgren T. Perception of cabin air quality in airline crew related to air humidification on intercontinental flights. *Indoor Air.* 2007;17(3):204–10.
2. Code of Federal Regulations, Aerunautics and Space (Chapter 14), Part 135.
3. Code of Federal Regulations, Aerunautics and Space (Chapter 14), Part 25.841(a).
4. Rodenberg H. *Rosen's Emergency Medicine: Concepts and Clinical Practice.* 3rd ed. St. Louis: Mosby; 1992: 235.
5. *Dorland's Illustrated Medical Dictionary.* 26th ed. Philadelphia: Saunders; 1985: 716.
6. *CRC Handbook of Chemistry and Physics.* 77th ed. Cleveland: CRC Press.
7. *http://www.healthsystem.virginia.edu/Internet/Anesthesiology-Elective/airway/supplementaloxygen.cfm.*
8. *http://mayoclinic.com/health/air-travel-during-pregnancy/AN00398.*
9. Deep-vein thrombosis is a serious risk in long-distance plane travel. *Time.* May 29, 2006: 73.
10. Eklof B, Maksimovic D, Caprini JA, Glase. Air travel-related venous thromboembolism. *Disease-A-Month.* 2005;51 (2–3):200–7.
11. Auerbach PS. *Wilderness Medicine.* 5th ed. St. Louis: Mosby; 2007. Chapter 35. Aeromedical Transport.
12. Delaune EF III. In-flight medical events and aircraft diversions: one airline's experience. *Aviat Space Eviron Med.* 2003;74(1):62–8.
13. Marx JA. *Rosen's Emergency Medicine: Concepts and Clinical Practice.* 6th ed. St. Louis: Mosby; 2006: 2288.
14. Auerbach PS. *Wilderness Medicine.* 4th ed. St. Louis: Mosby; 2007. Chapter 25. The Eye in the Wilderness.
15. *http://www.air-ambulance.net/industry_analysis.htm.*
16. *http://www.dr-amy.com/rich/oxygen/.*

The Expedition Medical Kit

William W. Forgey, MD

As discussed in Chapter 3, packaging the medical kit into modules, or functional units, aids the management and control of medical supplies. The items to be chosen and the quantities to be packed vary by the factors discussed in the referenced chapter. The basic modules listed below are divided into four functional groups: Topical Bandaging Module, Nonprescription (Non-Rx) Oral Medication Module, Prescription (Rx) Oral/Topical Medication Module, and a Prescription Injectable Medication Module. The functional utility of the items in the modules is described here. Various chapters in this book describe specific high-risk situations.

BASIC EXPEDITION MEDICAL KIT MODULES

This basic expedition kit consists of four modules: These kits and the use of each component have been described in detail in the referenced books (Forgey, 2002; 2007). The modules are capable of sustaining a group of six persons operating for 2 months in a very remote area, assuming a higher risk than was reported in the Boy Scout Adirondack study (Welch, 1997) or the NOLS data (Leemon and Schimelpfenig, 2003) and assuming the need for providing long-term and definitive care for expedition members. Because loss or consumption of kits can lead to shortages of items, a wilderness traveler must be adept at improvisation. Improvised alternatives to the kit components have been suggested.

As a minimum, the Topical Bandaging Module and Non-Rx Oral Medication Module will generally fulfill the vast majority of emergency treatment requirements. In that all components are nonprescription items, they can be readily obtained by any group requiring a basic expedition medical kit. The prescription modules are designed for long term and more advanced patient care. All items listed in the kit modules can be obtained without a prescription, except in the modules clearly marked "Rx." None of the basic modules contain schedule II (restricted) medications, which greatly aids in procuring and transporting these items across international boundaries.

Additional modules for the treatment of specific conditions will be detailed in the remaining chapters of this book. Therefore, components for modules for eye treatment, high-altitude illness prevention and treatment, and the like, are discussed in specific topic chapters.

All nonprescription medications have packaging that describes the official dosages and appropriate warnings or precautions concerning their use. Prescription medications have elaborate package inserts with this same information. When obtaining a prescription drug for your medical kit, request the package insert from your physician or copy the information for your use from the *Physicians' Desk Reference* (PDR), which is available at libraries and bookstores everywhere.

Topical Bandaging Module

Quantity	Item
10 pkg	Spyroflex 2 × 2 wound dressings (or carry two for each person)
4 pkg	Thick surgical gauze pads 5 × 7
15 pkg	Nu-Gauze, high absorbent, sterile, 2 ply, 3 × 3 pkg/2
25	Coverlet bandage strips 1 × 3
1	Tape, waterproof 1 × 5 yd
1	SAM splint, 36 inch
1	Elastic bandage, 3 inch
2	Elastic bandage, 4 inch
1	Elastic bandage, 6 inch
1	Maximum strength triple antibiotic ointment with pramoxine, 1 oz tube
1	Hibiclens® surgical scrub, 4 oz bottle
1	Tetrahydrozoline ophthalmic drops, 0.05%, 15 ml bottle
1	Carbimide peroxide otic drops, 6.5%, 15 ml bottle
1	Hydrocortisone cream 1%, 1 oz tube
1	Clotrimazole cream 2%, ½ oz tube
2 pair	Examination gloves
1	Irrigation syringe
1	Overpack container for above

- **Spyroflex® 2 × 2 wound dressings.** This multiuse bandaging system by PolyMedica Industries replaced wound closure strips *and* coverings. It accelerates blood clotting, hold's lacerations closed, is a barrier dressing to protect the wound from the outside, treats abraded skin as well as leaking and dry wounds, and is an excellent cover for first- and second-degree burns. Most importantly, it establishes a local environment that speeds up wound healing. The dressing is a "smart" dressing that absorbs and evaporates the correct amount of vapor to produce the proper healing condition. This dressing can be left in place for up to 10 days, thus decreasing the need for large quantities of bulky dressings.

Alternative Improvisation. Cellophane and duct tape: Cellophane, plastic food wrappers, or plastic sheeting of any kind makes an excellent wound covering. Held down with tape of any type, this dressing in nonadherent, seepage leaks from the unsealed edges, the wound can be observed, and the increased and appropriate moisture level of the dressing increases the rate of wound healing.

- **Thick surgical gauze pads 5 × 7.** These "battlefield" dressings provide absorption for large wounds and help provide hemostasis with pressure.

  Alternative Improvisation. Cotton clothing that is clean or that has been sterilized by boiling and then drying. Most synthetic garment pieces will also work as bulky dressings. These dressings can be washed, boiled, air dried, and used again if a survival situation so warrants.

- **Nu-Gauze pads.** J&J Company has developed a gauze that is 2-ply yet absorbs nearly 50% more fluid than conventional 12-ply gauze pads. This may not seem important until a rapidly bleeding wound needs care. For years J&J has made a "Nu-Gauze" strip packing dressing; the Nu-Gauze pads are a completely different material. They are a wonderful advance in gauze design.

  Alternative Improvisation. Cotton T-shirts or other clothing, bandanas.

- **Coverlet bandage strips.** A Beiersdorf product, these are common 1 × 3 bandage strips, but they are the best made. They stick even when wet, will last through days of hard usage, and stretch for compression on a wound and conform for better application.

  Alternative Improvisation. Duct tape, climbing tape.

- **Waterproof tape.** A tough tape that can be used for splinting or bandage application. There are no brand advantages that I can determine. A 1 × 5 yd roll on a metal spool is a usable size.

  Alternative Improvisation. Duct tape, climbing tape.

- **SAM Splint®.** A padded malleable splint that provides enough comfort to be used as a neck collar. It is adequately rigid to splint any extremity and universal so that only one of these need be carried for all splinting needs. It replaces the necessity for such items as ladder splints. I have never recommended the inclusion of splints in wilderness medical kits until this product was developed. It weighs less than 5 ounces.

  Alternative Improvisation. Malleable splints can frequently be made from stays found in internal backpack frames. Other stiff materials can be used such as strips of Ensolite foam pads or inflatable pads, held in place with tape or wraps of torn cloth.

- **Elastic Bandage, 3 inch, 4 inch, 6 inch.** Obtain good quality bandages that stretch without narrowing and that provide firm, consistent support. Self-adhering are best.

  Alternative Improvisation. Elastic bandages can be replaced with almost any cloth that is firmly wrapped in place. The most stretchy form of cloth usually available is from cotton T-shirts.

- **Maximum strength triple antibiotic ointment with pramoxine.** Each gram of this ointment contains bacitracin 500 units, neomycin sulfate 3.5 mg, polymyxin B sulfate 10,000 units, and an anesthetic pramoxine hydrochloride 10 mg for use as a topical antibiotic in the prevention and treatment of minor infections of abrasions and burns. This formulation is also an anesthetic that numbs the skin. A light coat should be applied twice daily. Neomycin can cause skin rash and itch in some people. If this develops, discontinue use and apply the hydrocortisone cream to counter this effect.

  Alternative Improvisation. Honey or granulated sugar placed on wounds is painless and kills germs by dehydrating them. A strong sugar solution draws the fluid from the bacteria, but human cells are able to actively avoid the dehydration process and are not injured with this technique.

- **Hibiclens® surgical scrub.** This Stuart product [chlorhexidine gluconate 4%] far surpasses hexachlorophene and povidone-iodine scrub in its antiseptic action. Its onset and duration of action is much more impressive than either of those two products.

  Alternative Improvisation. Many surgical scrubs are available without prescription and are ideal for wilderness use, but they can all be replaced with potable (drinkable) water irrigation.

- **Tetrahydrozoline ophthalmic drops 0.05%.** These eyedrops are used for allergy relief and to remove red color and discomfort due to smoke, eye strain, and so on. It will not cure infection or disguise the existence of a foreign body. Place 1 or 2 drops in each eye every 6 hours.

  Alternative Improvisation. Rinse eyes with clean water. A wet, cold compress relieves eye itch and pain.

- **Carbimide peroxide 6.5% otic drops.** This formulation is sold over the counter to treat ear wax. However, this solution is germicidal and fungicidal. A preparation may not be sold over-the-counter with an advertising claiming that it can cure ear infections, only for the purpose of softening wax and preventing infections. Use 3 drops 4 times a day, with a cotton plug.

  Alternative Improvisation. Warmed cooking oil is a soothing ear drop that relieves itching and pain. More than 90% of all external otitis (outer ear infection, swimmer's ear) can be treated with acetic acid (vinegar) in a vehicle such as glycerine or olive oil. However, an infected ear should be treated with prescription antibiotics.

- **Hydrocortisone cream 1%.** This nonprescription steroid cream treats allergic skin rashes, such as those from poison ivy. A cream is ideal for treating weeping lesions, as opposed to dry scaly ones, but it will work on either. To potentiate this medication, apply an occlusive dressing (plastic cover) overnight.

  Alternative Improvisation. Blistery rashes can be soothed and the leaking fluid dried by applying cloth made wet with concentrated salt solution.

- **Clotrimazole cream 2%.** This is one of the most effective antifungal preparations available for foot, groin, or body fungal infections. Brand names are Lotrimin® or Mycelex® (vaginal cream). The vaginal cream in a 2 ounce tube is less expensive per ounce and works well on the skin surface, as well as vaginally.

  Alternative Improvisation. Dry, itchy lesions of any type respond to a soothing coating of cooking oil.

- **Examination gloves.** Due to concerns with hepatitis B and C and AIDS, it is prudent to carry protective gloves for first-aid use. These can be nonsterile. Vinyl gloves will last much longer in a kit than latex gloves, but the best to obtain are the nitro or new barrier gloves. As mentioned in Chapter 3, the chance of catching HIV-1 infection from a healthy wilderness expedition participant is unlikely, but at times your group may be called upon to treat indigenous peoples or other persons in the area.

  Alternative Improvisation. Use an empty food bag or waterproof stuff sack as a glove, or wrap your hand in the most waterproof material available.

- **Irrigation syringe.** Required for forceful irrigation of wounds.

  Alternative Improvisation. The solution to pollution is dilution. Forceful irrigation is the best method to clean a wound and dilute the germ count to the point that the body's immune system can kill the remaining germs. Without a syringe, augment the volume of water that you are pouring on the wound with a brisk scrubbing action using a soft, clean cloth.

Non-Rx Oral Medical Module

Quantity	Item
24	Percogesic® tablets (pain, fever, muscle spasm, sleep aid, anxiety, congestion)
24	Ibuprofen 200 mg tablets (pain, fever, bursitis, tendonitis, menstrual cramps)
24	Diphenhydramine 25 mg capsules (antihistamine, antianxiety, cough, muscle cramps, nausea and motion sickness prevention)
10	Bisacodyl 5 mg tablets (constipation)
12	Loperamide 2 mg tablets (diarrhea)
24	Cimetidine 200 mg tablets (heartburn, certain allergic reactions)
1	Overpack container for above

Alternative Improvisation. Each of these medications has multifunctional uses as well as cross-therapeutic versatility. (See Table 3.7.) This means that each item can be used for more than one problem, and problems have more than one drug that can be used for treatment. This allows a minimal number of medications to be included in the medical kit, while providing depth of coverage.

- **Percogesic® tablets.** Relieves pain, fever, and muscle spasm. Each tablet contains 325 mg of acetaminophen and 30 mg of phenyltoloxamine citrate. It is ideal for injuries of joints and muscles, as well as aches from infections. Phenyltoloxamine is also a decongestant. It also induces drowsiness and can be used as a sleeping aid and to calm a hysterical person. Dosage is generally 2 tablets every 4 hours as needed. One of the most useful nonprescription drugs obtainable.

- **Ibuprofen tablets.** Brand names are Advil®, Nuprin®, among others. Relieves pain, fever, menstrual cramps, and inflammation. Overuse syndromes such as bursitis and tendonitis are common in wilderness-related activities, and this is an ideal treatment. The nonprescription dosage is 2 tablets, 4 times a day. It should be taken with food to prevent stomach irritation or heart-burn. The Rx dosage is 4 tablets taken 4 times daily, and this dose may be necessary for severe inflammation.

- **Diphenhydramine capsules.** The brand name is Benadryl®, but many variations of this medication, which contains ingredients other than just the diphenhydramine, are sold under this brand name. For antihistamine action, these capsules can be taken 1 or 2 every 6 hours. To use as a powerful cough suppressant, the dose is 1 capsule every 6 hours. For muscle spasm relief, 1 or 2 capsules at bedtime alone or in combination with 2 ibuprofen 200 mg tables. For nausea or motion sickness, 1 capsule every 6 hours as needed.

- **Bisacodyl.** This laxative works on the large bowel to form a soft stool within 6–10 hours. Use 1 tablet as needed.

- **Loperamide.** An anti-diarrheal with the brand name of Imodium®. Dosage for persons 12 or older is 2 tablets after the first loose bowel movement followed by 1 tablet after each subsequent loose bowel movement, but no more than 4 tablets a day for no more than 2 days. The prescription use of this medication is usually 2 tablets immediately and 2 with each loose stool up to a maximum of 8 per day. Follow the package instructions for children's dosages.

- **Cimetidine.** Brand name is Tagamet®. This medication suppresses acid formation. It may be used to treat certain allergic reactions. The nonprescription dosage is 2 tablets 4 times daily. Prescription use goes as high as 4 tablets 4 times daily for acid suppression.

Rx Oral/Topical Medication Module

Quantity	Item
20	Doxycycline 100 mg tablets (antibiotic)
12	Zithromax® 250 mg tablets (antibiotic)
16	Levaquin® 500 mg tablets (antibiotic)
2	Diflucan® 150 mg tablets (antifungal) (for a female trip participant and 1 additional pill for each additional female on trip)
24	Lorcet® 10/650 tablets (pain, cough)
24	Atarax® 25 mg tablets (nausea, anxiety, antihistamine, pain medication augmentation)
1	Topicort®.25% ointment, ½ oz tube (skin allergy)
1	Tobradex® ophthalmic drops, 2.5 ml (eye, ear antibiotic and antiinflammatory)
1	Tetracaine ophthalmic solution 0.5%, ⅛ oz tube (eye, ear anesthetic)
1	Denavir® (penciclovir) cream 1%, 5 g tube (antiviral, lip and mouth sores)
1	Stadol® nasal spray (severe pain)
*	Decadron® 4 mg tablets (10 per trip for allergy) (16 per climber at high risk for acute mountain sickness)

Brand Name

Brand names have been used to simplify spelling and product recognition or to minimize potential confusion between similar sounding and variations in generic names between U.S., Canadian, and British sources.

- **Doxycycline.** The generic name of an antibiotic that is useful in treating many travel-related diseases. The various sections of the text dealing with infections will indicate the proper dosage, normally 1 tablet twice daily. Not to be used in children 8 years or younger or during pregnancy. May cause skin sensitivity on exposure to sunlight, thus causing an exaggerated sunburn. This does not usually happen, but be cautious during your first sun exposure when using this product. Many people traveling in the tropics have used this antibiotic safely. Very useful in malaria prevention at a dose of 1 tablet daily. Common brand names are Vibramycin®, Vibra-tabs®, and Monodox®.

- **Zithromax®.** This is the brand name of azithromycin, a broad-spectrum antibiotic used to treat certain types of pneumonia, infected throats, skin infections, and venereal diseases due to *Chlamydia trachomatis* or *Neisseria gonorrhoeae* and genital ulcer disease in men due to *Haemophilus ducreyi* (chancroid). It is very effective in treating most forms of traveler's diarrhea caused by bacterial infections.

- **Levaquin®.** A broad-spectrum antibiotic of a group known as fluoroquinolones. This medication is useful in treating diarrhea and even organisms resistant to doxycycline and Zithromax. It is useful in treating sinus infections, bronchitis, pneumonia, skin infections and skin ulcers, and complicated urinary tract and kidney infections. Avoid excessive sun exposure while taking this medication. Avoid in persons under the age of 18 and during nursing and pregnancy. Drink extra water when on this medication. Do not take with antacid, vitamins containing minerals, and ibuprofen; otherwise, it may be taken at meal times. Some people are made dizzy by this medication. There is a possibility that it might cause tendonitis and should be stopped if muscle pain or tendon inflammation results. Even though it is used to treat diarrhea, it may cause diarrhea and may result in vaginal monilia infection.

- **Lorcet®.** The brand name of the combination of 650 mg of acetaminophen and 10 mg of hydrocodone, the principle use of the drug is in the relief of pain. Hydrocodone is a powerful cough suppressant and also useful in treating abdominal cramping and diarrhea. The dosage of 1 tablet every 6 hours will normally control a severe toothache. Maximum dosage is 6 tablets per day. It may be augmented with Atarax.

- **Atarax®.** A brand name of hydroxyzine hydrochloride (note also the listing under Vistaril in the Rx Injectable Medication Module section). These tablets have multiple uses. They are a very powerful antinausea agent, muscle relaxant, antihistamine, antianxiety agent, sleeping pill, and will potentiate a pain medication (make it work better). For sleep, 50 mg at bed-time; for nausea, 25 mg every 4–6 hours; to potentiate pain medication, take a 25 mg tablet with each dose of the pain medication. This medication treats rashes of all types and has a drying effect on congestion. The injectable version, Vistaril®, has identical actions.

- **Topicort® (desoximetasone) ointment 0.25%.** This prescription steroid ointment treats severe allergic skin rashes. Dosage is a thin coat twice daily. Occlusive dressing is not required when using this product. It should be used with caution over large body surface areas or in children. Use should be limited to 10 days or less.

- **Tobradex® ophthalmic drops.** This is a combination of a powerful antibiotic (tobramycin 0.3%) and steroid (dexamthasone 0.1%). It can be used to treat infections or allergies in the eye (for which it was designed) or the ear. It can be instilled in either location two or three times daily. This medication can cause complications in case of viral infections of the eye (which are rare compared to bacterial infections and allergy conditions). (See Chapter 36.)
- **Tetracaine ophthalmic solution (drops).** Sterile solution for use in eye or ear to numb pain. Do not reapply to eye if pain returns without examining for foreign body very carefully. Try not to use repeatedly in the eye as overuse delays healing. Continued pain may also mean you have missed a foreign body. Do not use in ears if considerable drainage is present for an ear drum may have ruptured. If this medication gets into the middle ear through a hole in the ear drum, it will cause profound vertigo (dizziness). (See Chapter 36.)
- **Denavir® (penciclovir) cream 1%.** An antiviral treatment that is a useful treatment for cold sores on the face and on the lips. Even though this product is not approved for use inside the mouth, it actually works well there and is not harmful if swallowed. This may be used at high altitude to prevent the cold sores caused by intense ultraviolet light. Apply every 2 hours during waking hours for a period of 4 days.
- **Stadol® nasal spray.** This is a powerful pain medication (generic name butorphanol) formulated to be absorbed by the lining of the nose. It is five times stronger than morphine on a milligram to milligram basis. Use only one spray up a nostril and wait, the instructions say 60 to 90 minutes before using a second spray in the other nostril. This process may be repeated in 3 to 4 hours. It should be working effectively within 20 minutes, however, after the first spray. Overspraying or allowing the medication to drain down the throat will waste it because it is inactivated by gastric fluids.
- **Decadron® (dexamethasone).** For allergy, take ½ tablet twice daily after meals for 5 days. For treatment of acute mountain sickness, take 4 mg every 6 hours until well below altitude at which symptoms appeared. (See Chapter 19.)
- **Nubain® (nalbuphine).** This strong, synthetic narcotic analgesic is available only by prescription, but it is not a controlled narcotic with the increased legal problems associated with those substances. It is equal in analgesic strength to morphine. The normal adult dose is 10 mg (½ ml) given intramuscularly every 3–6 hours. The maximum dose is 20 mg (1 ml) every 3 hours. It can be mixed with 25–50 mg of Vistaril® in the same syringe for increased analgesia in severe pain problems. It comes in 10 ml multiuse vials.

Rx Injectable Medication Module

Quantity	Item
1	Nubain® 20 mg/ml, 10 ml multiuse vial (pain)
1	Lidocaine 1%, 10 ml multiuse vial (local anesthetic)
12	3½ ml syringes with 25 gauge, ⅝ inch needles
1+	Decadron® 4 mg/ml, 5 ml multiuse vial (steroid) 1 per trip for allergy; 3 vials per climber at risk for acute mountain sickness
6–12	Rocephin®, 500 g vials (antibiotic)
1	Vistaril® 50 mg/ml, 10 ml multiuse vial (many uses)
2	Twinject® or EpiPen® (bee stings, anaphylactic shock, asthma)

- **Lidocaine 1%.** Injection for numbing wounds. Maximum amount to be used in a wound in an adult should be 15 ml. This fluid is also used to mix the Rocephin®. See the package insert that comes with the Rocephin®.
- **Syringes.** Many types of syringes are available, but for wilderness use I find the 3 ½ ml with the attached 25 gauge, ⅝ inch needle to be the most universal. An 18 gauge needle provides the best wound irrigation system, but it needs to be fitted to a larger syringe barrel to be the most efficient.
- **Decadron® (dexamethasone).** For use in allergic reactions, give 4 mg daily for 5 days IM. For acute mountain sickness give 4 mg (1 ml) every 6 hours until well below the altitude where symptoms started. (See Chapter 19.)
- **Rocephin® (ceftriaxone).** This broad-spectrum injectable antibiotic of the cephalosporin class has a wide range of bactericidal activities including pneumonia and bronchitis, skin infections, urinary tract and kidney infections, gonorrhea, pelvic infection, bone and joint infections, and many intraabdominal infections and some types of meningitis. Each vial will require 0.9 ml of lidocaine 1% to mix the contents. The reconstituted medication is stable at room temperatures for 3 days.
- **Vistaril®.** A brand name of hydroxyzine hydrochloride (note also the listing under Atarax® in the Rx Oral Medication Module section). Uses and dosages are the same as indicated in that listing. Obviously in the treatment of profound vomiting, injections of medication will work better than oral administration. This solution can be mixed in the same syringe as the Nubain® for administration as one injection.
- **EpiPen® or Twinject®.** Epinephrine injections of 0.3 ml of 1:10,000 solution for treating anaphylaxis or status asthmaticus. A commercial kit consisting of an automatic injection syringe of epinephrine. The Twinject has a second dose per unit, which can be activated manually. Multiple injection vials or single use ampoules of epinephrine with a syringe and needle can be substituted.

ADVANCED EXPEDITION MEDICAL KIT

Specialized Treatment Augmentation Modules

Expeditions expected to encounter specific high risks should augment their medical training and expedition medical kit so that these challenges can be adequately managed. Parts 2 and 3 have expanded treatment discussions on significant medical risks that expeditions might encounter.

Taking into account the possibility that one of these medical issues might be at high risk for the expedition, and the other factors of medical kit design discussed in Chapter 3, the diagnostic and therapeutic materials described in these clinical chapters should be added to either a basic medical kit module or carried as specialized treatment modules.

SUGGESTED READINGS

Forgey W. *Wilderness Medicine.* Guilford, Conn: Globe Pequot Press; 2002.

Forgey W. *Basic Essential of Wilderness First Aid.* Butte, Mont: Falcon Books; 2007.

Leemon D, Schimelpfenig T. Wilderness injury and evacuation: National Outdoor Leadership School's incident profile, 1999–2000. *Wilderness Environ Med.* 2003;14: 174–82.

Welch TP. Data-based selection of medical supplies for wilderness travel. *Wilderness Environ Med.* 1997;8(3):148–51.

Index